TUMORS OF THE CRANIAL BASE:
Diagnosis and Treatment

edited by

Laligam N. Sekhar, M.D.
Assistant Professor
Department of Neurological Surgery
Co-Director
Center for Cranial Base Surgery
University of Pittsburgh
School of Medicine
Pittsburgh, Pennsylvania

and

Victor L. Schramm, Jr., M.D.
Director
Center for Craniofacial and Skull Base Surgery
Colorado Ear-Head and Neck Clinic
Denver, Colorado

(formerly, Associate Professor
Department of Otolaryngology
University of Pittsburgh
School of Medicine
Pittsburgh, Pennsylvania)

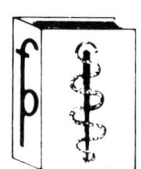

Futura Publishing Company, Inc.
Mount Kisco, New York
© 1987

Library of Congress Cataloging-in-Publication Data
Tumors of the cranial base.
  Includes bibliographies and index.
   1. Basicranium—Tumors. 2. Basicranium—Tumors—
Surgery. I. Sekhar, Laligam N. II. Schramm, Victor L.
[DNLM: 1. Brain Neoplasms—diagnosis. 2. Brain
Neoplasms—therapy. 3. Skull Neoplasms—diagnosis.
4. Skull Neoplasms—therapy. WE 707 T925]
RC280.H4T86 1987   616.99'281   87-149
ISBN 0-87993-302-X

Copyright 1987
Futura Publishing Company, Inc.
Published by:
  Futura Publishing Company, Inc.
  295 Main Street, PO Box 330
  Mount Kisco, New York 10549
LC#: 87-149
ISBN#: 0-87993-302-X
All rights reserved.
No part of this book may be translated or reproduced in any form without the written permission of the publisher.

*This book is dedicated to
   our patients,
      our teachers,
         and our families.*

Contributors

Dennis I. Bojrab, M.D.
Lakeshore Ear, Nose and Throat Center, P.C., Division of Otology and Skull Base Surgery, St. Clair Shores, Michigan

Joel-Pierre Bonnal, M.D.
Professor, Clinique Neurochirurgicale, Hospital Université de Baviere, Liège, Belgium

Jacques Brotchi, M.D.
Professor Agrege, Bruxelles, Belgium

Jacques Born, M.D.
Liege, Belgium

K. Ter Brugge, M.D.
Assistant Professor of Radiology, Toronto Western Hospital, Toronto, Canada

M. Chiu M.D.
Assistant Professor of Radiology, Toronto Western Hospital, Toronto, Canada

Hugh D. Curtin, M.D.
Associate Professor, University of Pittsburgh, Director of Radiology, Eye and Ear Hospital, Pittsburgh, Pennsylvania

Patrick J. Derome, M.D.
Chairman, Department of Neurosurgery, Hôpital Foch, Suresnes, France

Melvin Deutsch, M.D.
Professor of Radiology, University Health Center of Pittsburgh, Pittsburgh, Pennsylvania

Karen B. Domino, M.D.
Assistant Professor of Anesthesiology/CCM, University of Pittsburgh, School of Medicine, Director, Neurosurgical Anesthesia, Presbyterian-University Hospital, Pittsburgh, Pennsylvania

Benjamin H. Eidelman, M.D., Ph.D.
Associate Professor of Neurology, University of Pittsburgh, School of Medicine, Pittsburgh, Pennsylvania

Michael E. Glasscock, III, M.D.
Clinical Professor of Otolaryngology, Otology Group P.C., Nashville, Tennessee

Barry E. Hirsch, M.D.
Assistant Professor, Department of Otolaryngology, University of Pittsburgh, School of Medicine, Pittsburgh, Pennsylvania

L. Lopez Ibor, M.D.
Assistant de Neuroradiology, Hôpital Bicetre, Paris, France

Gary Jacobson, M.D.
Adjunct Assistant Professor, Department of Neurology, University of Cincinnati Medical Center, Chief, Auditory and Speech Pathology Section, Neurology Service, Veteran's Administration Medical Center, Cincinnati, Ohio

Peter J. Jannetta, M.D.
Professor and Chairman, Department of Neurological Surgery, University of Pittsburgh, School of Medicine, Pittsburgh, Pennsylvania

Neil Ford Jones, M.D.
Assistant Professor of Plastic and Reconstructive Surgery University of Pittsburgh, School of Medicine, Pittsburgh, Pennsylvania

Donald B. Kamerer, M.D.
Associate Professor, Department of Otolaryngology, University of Pittsburgh, School of Medicine, Chief, Division of Otology, Eye and Ear Hospital, Pittsburgh, Pennsylvania

Johannes Lang, M.D., Ph. D.
Professor of Anatomy, Anatomisches Institut, Koellikerstrasse, West Germany

Pierre Lasjaunias, M.D., Ph. D.
Praticien Hospitalier, Chef de travaux en anatomie, Service de Radiologie, Hopital Bicetre Universite Paris, Kremlin Bicetre, France

Richard E. Latchaw, M.D.
Professor of Radiology and Neurological Surgery, Chief, Division of Neuroradiology, University of Pittsburgh, School of Medicine, Pittsburgh, Pennsylvania

Edward R. Laws, M.D.
Professor of Neurological Surgery, Mayo Clinic, Mayo Medical School, Rochester, Minnesota

L. Dade Lunsford, M.D.
Associate Professor of Neurological Surgery and Radiology, University of Pittsburgh, School of Medicine Pittsburgh, Pennsylvania

J.L. Maestro, M.D.
Department of Otorhinolaryngology, Hopital Foch, Suresnes, France

Augusto Julio Martinez, M.D.
Professor of Pathology (Neuropathology), University of Pittsburgh, School of Medicine, Pittsburgh, Pennsylvania

David G. Mayernik, M.D.
Clinical Instructor of Medicine, University of Pittsburgh, School of Medicine, Pittsburgh, Pennsylvania

Aage R. Møller, Ph.D.
Research Professor of Neurological Surgery and Physiology, University of Pittsburgh, School of Medicine, Pittsburgh, Pennsylvania

Margareta B. Møller, M.D., Ph.D.
Associate Professor of Neurological Surgery and Otolaryngology, University of Pittsburgh, School of Medicine, Pittsburgh, Pennsylvania

J.P. Monteil, M.D.
Department of Otorhinolaryngology, Hopital Foch, Suresnes, France

Paul B. Nelson, M.D.
Associate Professor of Neurological Surgery, University of Pittsburgh, School of Medicine, Pittsburgh, Pennsylvania

Robert G. Ojemann, M.D.
Professor of Surgery, Harvard Medical School, Visiting Neurosurgeon, Massachusetts General Hospital, Boston, Massachusetts

Myles L. Pensak, M.D.
Assistant Professor, Department of Otolaryngology, University of Cincinnati Medical Center, Cincinnati, Ohio

Peter S. Roland, M.D.
Assistant Professor, Department of Otorhinolaryngology, University of Texas Health Science Center at Dallas, Dallas, Texas

Mark L. Rosenblum, M.D.
Associate Professor Department of Neurological Surgery, University of California, School of Medicine, San Francisco, California

James T. Rutka, M.D.
Fellow, Department of Neurological Surgery, Brain Tumor Research, University of California, School of Medicine, San Francisco, California

Victor L. Schramm, Jr., M.D.
Director, Colorado Ear, Head and Neck Clinic, Denver, Colorado *Formerly* Associate Professor, Department of Otolaryingology, University of Pittsburgh, School of Medicine, Pittsburgh, Pennsylvania

Charles H. Srodes, M.D.
Clinical Associate Professor of Medicine, University of Pittsburgh, School of Medicine, Pittsburgh, Pennsylvania

Laligam N. Sekhar, M.D.
Assistant Professor, Department of Neurological Surgery; Co-Director, Center for Cranial Base Surgery, University of Pittsburgh, School of Medicine, Pittsburgh, Pennsylvania

Karl W. Swann, M.D.
Chief Resident in Neurological Surgery, Massachusetts General Hospital, Boston, Massachusetts

John M. Tew, Jr., M.D.
Professor and Chairman, Department of Neurological Surgery, University of Cincinnati Medical Center, Mayfield Neurological Institute, Cincinnati, Ohio

William D. Tobler, M.D.
Assistant Professor, Department of Neurosurgery, University of Cincinnati Medical Center, Mayfield Neurological Institute, Cincinnati, Ohio

Andre Visot, M.D.
Department of Neurosurgery, Hôpital Foch, Suresnes, France

Foreword

The current era, beginning about 20 years ago, will be remembered among neurosurgeons, otolaryngologists, and plastic surgeons who deal with tumors othe skull base as an era of yeasty collaboration and exciting developments. These collaborations have superseded a time of competitiveness and lack of cooperation, a time when these specialty groups worked alone, often in isolated environments, vigorously trying to improve the lot of their patients afflicted with these lesions. Technology was not equal to the demands of surgery in the area of the skull base. Quality of patient survival was frequently dismal, despite the best efforts of many capable surgeons. The bony plates and buttresses, the dura mater, and the venous sinuses were walls separating the disciplines. Thinking was limited by the background and training of the surgeons and even by the tissues, bony, fibrous or vascular, which formed barriers to thinking, and to performance. The sigmoid sinus was a war zone; the temporal floor, a no man's land.

A number of developments altered the status quo. The first was technological. The application of the binocular dissecting microscope and of specific microscopic techniques to this area, as every reader knows, was a monumental advance in the area. The development and application of electrophysiologic monitoring techniques including, among others, brain stem auditory evoked responses, direct auditory nerve compound action potentials, and intraoperative electromyography of various cranial nerves have enabled even better precision in surgery, more complete removal of lesions, and better preservation of adjacent neural and vascular structures, even those directly involved by lesions. New radiologic diagnostic and interventional methods generated a better appreciation of the extent of lesions and the involvement of adjacent, often vital tissues, as well as a new way of treating some lesions primarily and of decreasing operative risk by decreasing the vascularity of many lesions. The utilization of safer anesthetic techniques and agents and better postoperative care contributed mightily to improvement in operative results.

Equally important, however, and perhaps more important was an attitudinal change. A generation of experts grew up in the various disciplines who were unhindered by the biases (often personal rather than scientific) of their predecessors and who were perhaps dissatisfied with what they saw in the management of patients with skull base lesions. They were more expert in the use of the newer techniques (because they had grown up with them rather than had them thrust upon them later in their set careers), and who were able to relate to their colleagues in other disciplines with a spirit of willing cooperation rather than the intellectual isolation of previous generations.

When people with different backgrounds and perspectives focus together on a scientific problem, wonderful things sometimes happen. Such has been the case in the evaluation and treatment of skull base lesions. A generation of experts have discarded or have never assumed the old biases and priorities. They have worked together fruitfully to set new standards for surgery in this area. The anatomical and professional barriers at the base of the skull have not only disappeared but become bridges which experts now cross together in the quest for excellence.

This volume brings together a distinguished group of such experts. They are from diverse disciplines. They work closely together in advancing an area of surgery. They have now synthesized their experience in a unified, well-organized, and well-written treatise. The authors are at the leading edge of the field. The reader will find, as I have, that thinking, action, and operative results will improve with the assimilation and application of the concepts in this volume.

PETER J. JANNETTA, M.D.

Preface

Cranial base tumors have evoked a great deal of interest in recent years among neurosurgeons, otolaryngologists, plastic surgeons, and other specialists. Many advances have taken place in this area within the past decade but many problems remain to be solved.

We have attempted to provide a comprehensive "state of the art" work in this multiauthored text. Contributions include experts from the United States and Europe brought together in the hope that this will provide a balanced viewpoint of the most recent material. A great deal of emphasis has been placed on skull base anatomy to overcome the limitations of specialty orientation and because knowledge of this anatomy is key to the understanding of the evolution of the disease and of the surgical treatment of these tumors. Emphasis has been placed on both the conventional and the innovative methods of treating skull base tumors. For example, the conventional view regarding the management of intracavernous tumors is emphasized in Chapter 22, whereas innovative methods of treatment are emphasized in Chapter 23. Discussions of techniques for diagnosis and treatment of skull base tumors which have become available only within the last five years are found in this book. These include the application of high resolution computed tomography and magnetic resonance imaging for diagnosis, the use of the balloon occlusion test of the internal carotid artery (ICA) in association with measurement of cerebral blood flow to predict the risk of ICA occlusion. New operative approaches to the cavernous sinus and the petroclival area, improved methods of managing petrous and upper cervical ICA and the cranial nerves, the use of neurophysiological monitoring to avoid intraoperative injury, and improved reconstruction of the skull base using vascularized flaps are further examples. However, wisdom gained from experience in the traditional treatment of patients over several years has also been emphasized.

The authors hope that the reader will not only benefit from the knowledge gained from reading this book, but would also be stimulated to contribute to progress in this field.

LALIGAM N. SEKHAR, M.D.
VICTOR L. SCHRAMM, JR., M.D.

Introduction

Tumors of the cranial base are defined here as those neoplasms which arise at the base of the brain, above the bones comprising the cranium (intradurally or extradurally), in the cranium itself, or below the cranium, often involving the paranasal sinuses, the infratemporal fossa, or the parapharyngeal space. Although the term "cranial base tumors" groups together a variety of neoplasms, they share certain common features and problems. In this book, we have attempted to bring together many different experts, to address many of these problem areas, and to illustrate the state of the art in the management of many of these lesions.

Diagnosis of cranial base tumors is often not made until they are of a large size. This is primarily because these tumors do not often manifest obvious symptoms until a late stage in their evolution. However, recognition of the significance of minor symptoms and their proper diagnostic evaluation may enable earlier diagnosis. Internists, neurologists, ophthalmologists, otolaryngologists, maxillo-facial surgeons, radiologists, radiation therapists, oncologists, and neurosurgeons may all be involved in the case of these patients at one stage or another. They all need to be aware of the special problems of these tumors and communicate freely with one another during a patient's management.

The biology of these tumors differs according to the type of the neoplasm. However, many of the malignant lesions remain locally confined for a long time, and metastasize relatively late in their course. Therefore, a radical or a near-total operative excision remains the best hope for achieving a cure of many of these lesions at present. Various forms of radiation therapy also play an important role in the control or cure of many of these tumors. Chemotherapy (including antineoplastic drugs and immunotherapeutic agents) for cranial base neoplasms remains in its infancy.

The surgical problems of cranial base neoplasms are similar. Because of their deep location at the base of the brain, different and innovative operative approaches are often required for adequate exposure. Brain tissue may have to be retracted during operations, potentially leading to postoperative problems. Injury to cranial nerves and blood vessels may occur during the operation or a preexisting problem may be worsened. This can lead to serious neurological and psychological disability. Repair of the cranial base is often a challenge, but needs to be adequately accomplished in order to prevent serious infection and death.

Several advances have occurred in the management of cranial base neoplasms in the past decade. The first is the recognition of the special problems of this group of lesions. The second is the increasing degree of collaboration between different disciplines, with consequent improvements of care. The third is improved radiological diagnosis, due to the advent of techniques such as computed tomography and magnetic resonance imaging, the improved knowledge of radiological anatomy, and the close collaboration between radiologists and surgeons. The fourth is through the advances of interventional radiology, making possible the balloon occlusion test and tumor embolization. The fifth is advanced neuroanesthetic technique, and the facility for intraoperative neurophysiological monitoring. The sixth is the application of microsurgical technique to the resection of these tumors, the availability of adjuvants such as the laser for tumor resection, and the progressive development of techniques for cranial nerve, vascular, and cranial base reconstruction.

In the next decade, there will be a need to study the problems of these tumors further in an organized fashion. Patients with these difficult lesions should preferably be concentrated at centers with established clinical and scientific programs for their management. Multi-institutional cooperative studies may be better able to optimize the numbers of patients with uncommon neoplasms and allow existing and new therapeutic modalities to be tested. Further human, cadaver, and animal scientific studies are definitely needed to resolve many of the current problems. Finally, the formation of support groups for the education, and psychological and financial support of patients' families is also very essential.

LALIGAM N. SEKHAR, M.D.
VICTOR L. SCHRAMM, JR., M.D.

Contents

I. Pathology and Biology of Cranial Base Tumors

1. Pathology of Cranial Base Tumors
   A. J. Martinez 3
2. The Biology of Skull Base Tumors
   J. T. Rutka, M. L. Rosenblum 25

II. Radiological Diagnosis and Embolization Techniques

3. Imaging of Tumors at the Base of the Skull: The Sphenoid Bone
   R. E. Latchaw 39
4. Radiology of Skull Base Lesions
   H.D. Curtin 65
5. Embolization and Balloon Occlusion Techniques
   in the Management of Cranial Base Tumors
   P. Lasjaunias, K.T. Brugge, M. Chiu, L.L. Ibor 95

III. Anesthetic and Monitoring Techniques

6. Anesthesia for Cranial Base Tumor Operations
   K. B. Domino 107
7. Electrophysiological Monitoring of Cranial Nerves in Operations
   in the Skull Base
   A. R. Møller 123

IV. Specialized Treatment Modalities

8. Use of the Laser for Resection of Cranial Base Tumors
   J. M. Tew, W. D. Tobler, M. L. Pensak, G. Jacobson 135
9. Stereotactic Methods for Diagnosis and Treatment of
   Skull Base Lesions
   L. D. Lunsford 151
10. Radiation Therapy in the Treatment of Tumors of the Cranial Base
    M. Deutsch 163
11. The Role of Chemotherapy in Management of Tumors of the Cranial Base
    C.H. Srodes, D.G. Mayernik 191

V. Reconstruction After Cranial Base Tumor Resection

12. The Exposure, Preservation, and Reconstruction of Cerebral Arteries
    and Veins During the Resection of Cranial Base Tumors
    L.N. Sekhar 213
13. Preservation and Reconstruction of Cranial Nerves
    During the Removal of Cranial Base Neoplasms
    L.N. Sekhar 227

14. Methods of Cranial Base Reconstruction
    N.F. Jones 233

VI. Anterior Cranial Base

15. Anterior Cranial Base Anatomy
    J. Lang 247
16. Anterior Craniofacial Resection
    V.L. Schramm, Jr. 265
17. Meningiomas of the Anterior Cranial Base
    R.G. Ojemann, K.W. Swann 279
18. Bony Lesions of the Anterior and Middle Cranial Fossa
    P.J. Derome, A. Visot 295

VII. Middle Cranial Base

19. Middle Cranial Base Anatomy
    J. Lang 313
20. Large Tumors of the Pituitary Gland
    P.B. Nelson 335
21. Craniopharyngiomas: Diagnosis and Treatment
    E.R. Laws, Jr. 347
22. Meningiomas of the Sphenoid wings
    J. Bonnal, J. Brotchi, J. Born 373
23. Operative Management of Tumors Involving the Cavernous Sinus
    L.N. Sekhar 393
24. Infratemporal Fossa Surgery
    V.L. Schramm, Jr. 421

VIII. Posterior Cranial Base

25. Posterior Cranial Base Anatomy
    J. Lang 441
26. Inferior Cranial Base Anatomy
    J. Lang 461
27. Clinical Syndromes of the Posterior Fossa
    B.H. Eidelman 535
28. Otoneurological Evaulation of Patients with Posterior Fossa Tumors
    M.B. Møller 553
29. Acoustic Neurinomas: Neurosurgical Approaches and Results
    P.J. Jannetta 563
30. Acoustic Neurinomas: Otologic Approaches and Results
    P.S. Roland, M.E. Glasscock, III, D.I. Bojrab 587
31. Management of Cranial Chordomas
    P.J. Derome, A. Viscot, J.P. Monteil, J.L. Maestro 607
32. Petroclival and Medial tenorial Meningiomas
    L.N. Sekhar, P.J. Jannetta 623
33. Paragangliomas ("Glomus Tumors") of the Temporal Bone
    D.B. Kamerer, B.E. Hirsch 641

34. Operative Management of Large Neoplasms
    of the Lateral and Posterior Cranial Base
        L.N. Sekhar, V.L. Schramm, Jr., N.F. Jones 655
35. Temporal bone Resection
        V.L. Schramm, Jr. 683

Pathology and Biology of Cranial Base Tumors

Pathology of Cranial Base Tumors

Augusto Julio Martinez, M.D.

Introduction

Various types of neoplastic lesions, including metastatic carcinomas, and non-neoplastic lesions (vascular lesions or inflammatory processes), may involve the base of the skull, the sellar, parasellar, and suprasellar region, producing similar clinical, endocrine, and ophthalmic signs and symptoms and generally identical radiological views.[8] There are no clear, typical clinical and radiological characteristics for a definite diagnosis. Therefore, the differential diagnosis of these lesions includes a long list of possibilities. They require biopsy for the demonstration of the histopathological pattern of the lesion, for the differential and for a conclusive diagnosis. Only microscopic examination, occasionally electron microscopy, immunocytochemistry, or other pathological or microbiological procedures can disclose their true character and the final diagnosis.

This chapter will review some of the clinical and epidemiological features and comments about the natural history of these lesions. The most important macroscopic appearances and histopathologic characteristics of these lesions will be described and some of them will be illustrated.

Classification of Lesions of the Base of the Skull

The word "tumor" means a space-occupying lesion (Tumere = to swell). Tumors occurring in the base of the skull can be divided into neoplasms and non-neoplastic lesions. The histological diagnosis of the tumors affecting the cranial base is of paramount importance because the proper surgical approach and adequate management depend on the type of lesion and its pathological diagnosis. The lesions affecting the base of the skull, the sellar, suprasellar, and parasellar regions may be classified according to the site of involvement, their radiological appearances, and their clinical signs and symptoms. In this review they will be classified mainly according to their histopathological features and embryonic tissue of origin into the following groups and entities:

A. *Neuroepithelial Neoplasms*
   1. Optic pathway or hypothalamic glioma
      a. Astrocytoma
      b. Glioblastoma multiforme
      c. Oligodendroglioma
      d. Ependymoma

From: Sekhar LN, Schramm VL Jr, eds: *Tumors of the Cranial Base: Diagnosis and Treatment.* Mount Kisco, New York, Futura Publishing Co, Inc, © 1987.

2. Olfactory neuroblastoma or esthesioneuroblastoma
3. Neurilemmoma or Schwannoma
B. *Mesodermal Neoplasms*
   1. Meningioma
   2. Fibroma
   3. Sarcoma
   4. Osteoma
   5. Chondroma
   6. Lipoma; Liposarcoma
   7. Chondrosarcoma (mesenchymal)
   8. Angioma; Hemangioma; Angiosarcoma
   9. Glomus tumor (paraganglioma)
C. *Ectodermal Tumors*
   1. Craniopharyngioma
   2. Pituitary adenoma
   3. Myoblastoma or granular cell tumor
D. *Congenital, Embryonic, and Malformative Tumors*
   1. Epidermoid cyst (Pearly tumor; Cholesteatoma)
   2. Dermoid cyst
   3. Arachnoid cyst
   4. Teratoma
   5. Chordoma
   6. Colloid cyst
   7. Aneurysm
   8. Mucocele of the sphenoid sinus
   9. Ectopic "pinealoma" or germinoma
   10. Hamartoma (Infundibuloma)
   11. Rathke's cleft cyst
E. *Inflammatory Lesions*
   1. Granulomas
      a. Tuberculoma
      b. Sarcoidosis
      c. Gumma
      d. Pituitary abscess
      e. Hypophysitis or lymphoid hypophysitis
   2. Parasitic
      a. Cysticercosis
      b. Ecchinococcal cyst
   3. Fungal
      a. Cryptococcosis (Torulosis)
F. *Metastatic Tumors*
   1. Carcinomas
   2. Lymphomas
   3. Sarcomas
   4. Melanomas
G. *Empty Sella Syndrome*

Local extensions from regional tumors: Among the neoplasms that may extend locally into the cranial cavity are glomus jugulare tumor (chemodectoma or paraganglioma), chordoma, chondroma and chondrosarcoma, olfactory neuroblastoma, and adenoid cystic carcinoma or cylindroma. In addition to these neoplasms, other tumors, such as the nasopharyngeal carcinoma and lymphomas, may involve and infiltrate the base of the brain.

Benign and malignant neoplasms of the tissues surrounding the central nervous system (CNS) may penetrate the base of the skull or they may grow through openings in the skull or foraminas (orbital tumors may penetrate the optic canal, while acoustic tumors may expand and penetrate through the porus acusticus), into the intracranial space, parasellar region, or the anterior, middle, or posterior fossas.

Benign tumors (osteoma, chondroma, osteochondroma) may arise extradurally and grow by expansion. They can lead to more or less severe compression of the underlying meninges and neural tissue displacing the cerebral cortex.

Malignant neoplasms (osteosarcoma, melanoma, lymphoma, carcinomas) may extend into the cranial cavity and compress or invade the meninges and the neural tissue.

Tumors from the soft palate or the sphenoid and maxillary sinuses can invade the base of the cranial cavity and the cerebral cortex. The epidural space is usually involved in the neoplastic process. Infiltration and compression of cranial nerves by the tumor may produce cranial nerve palsies.

Carcinomas and other primary tumors of the ethmoid area and of the mucosa of the nasal and paranasal cavities can penetrate into the cranial cavity and infiltrate the frontal, frontobasal, and temporal regions of the dura mater, leptomeninges, and cerebral cortex. Inflammatory lesions (granulomas, sarcoid, cysticercosis, and ecchinococcal cyst) may also act as space-occupying masses mimicking malignant tumors. All of these lesions should be included in the differential diagnosis of neoplastic and non-neoplastic lesions of the cranial base.

Nasopharyngeal carcinomas may be classified as squamous cell carcinoma, anaplastic carcinoma, spindle cell carcinoma, clear cell carcinoma, or lymphoepithelioma. These are malignant epithelial neoplasms arising in the nasal portion of the pharynx that may infiltrate and gain access to the base of the cranial cavity. These tumors may present with several histomorphological types depending on the predominant tissue involved. The mean age at time of diagnosis is about 50 years of age. Because of their anatomic location, they are difficult to remove completely.

Squamous cell carcinomas originating in the nasal cavity, maxillary sinuses, the external auditory canal, the middle ear, or in the mastoid may invade the cranial base.

Adenoid cystic carcinomas are also called cylindromas. These are malignant tumors that arise from the minor or major salivary glands. Occasionally, they may originate from the lacrimal glands. The ones that may infiltrate the base of the skull usually arise from the parotid gland, from the hard palate, nose, paranasal sinuses, or the maxillary sinuses. They are slow-growing tumors that recur locally and have a predilection to invade perineurial spaces. They also may involve bone without producing destruction or erosion of the bone.

Nasopharyngeal angiofibroma is a rare mesenchymal and vascular nonencapsulated, locally aggressive, and histologically benign tumor of the nasopharynx that occurs almost exclusively in adolescent males. This neoplasm may spread into the base of the skull, particularly the infratemporal fossa, middle cranial fossa, the orbit, the ethmoid sinus, the sphenoid sinus, and the cavernous sinus.

Neuroepithelial Neoplasms

Optic and Hypothalamic Gliomas

Optic and hypothalamic gliomas are rare tumors.[47,50] They comprise astrocytomas, oligodendrogliomas, ependymomas, glioblastoma multiforme, and mixed gliomas with the combination of two or more glial elements. They constitute about 4.0% of all intracranial tumors in children (the great majority occur in less than 10-year-old children). The optic chiasm and one or both optic nerves and adjacent brain are usually involved.

The clinical manifestations of optic nerve glioma depend on whether the tumor arises within or behind the orbit. In general, the intraorbital lesions present with proptosis, ipsilateral loss of vision, strabismus, and papilledema. Retroorbital lesions lead to loss of vision in both eyes and may be associated with symptoms of obstructive hydrocephalus or hypothalamic dysfunction. The areas involved (optic nerves, tracts, or optic chiasm) are grossly enlarged by a firm, pale gray tissue.[43]

Histologically, the majority of these tumors are astrocytomas, a few are oligodendrogliomas, others are glioblastoma multiforme and ependymomas. Orbital and intracanalicular optic nerve gliomas can extend into the suprasellar area. Lesions arising from the intracranial portion of the optic nerve and optic chiasm are primarily in the suprasellar region. The gliomas involving the optic tracts and hypothalamus are often difficult to differentiate from one another because of the frequent infiltration of the contiguous structures and the aggressive behavior of the lesions. The majority of optic nerve gliomas occurring in children are well differentiated low-grade astrocytomas. In adults they are aggressive, with areas of pseudopalisading, necrosis, hemorrhages, numerous abnormal mitotic figures and bizarre cells (Figs. 1A & B).

Hypothalamic gliomas occur primarily in young patients. They are also known as juvenile astrocytomas of the

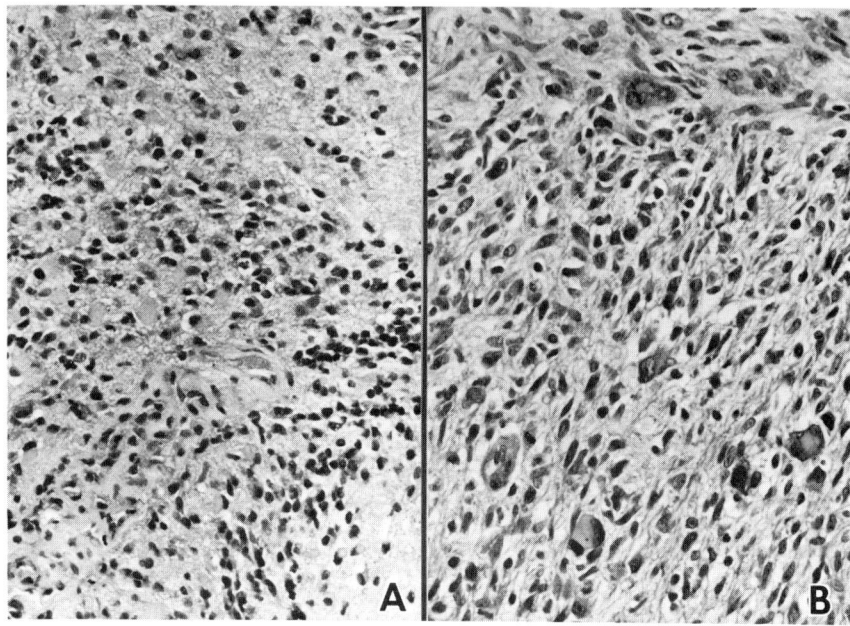

Figure 1: A: Optic nerve astrocytoma. There is replacement of the normal myelinated axons by neoplastic astrocytes with pleomorphic and hyperchromatic nucleus and abundant cytoplasm. (H&E, original magnification X315.) **B:** Glioblastoma multiforme arising in the optic chiasm. The neoplasm is composed of bizarre astrocytes, some of them very large with multiple pleomorphic nuclei. There is loss of polarity of the neoplastic astrocytes and vascular endothelial hyperplasia. (H&E, original magnification X315.)

hypothalamus or as diencephalic gliomas. These neoplasms usually arise from the floor or from the walls of the third ventricle and may infiltrate the optic chiasm, the thalamus, and the interventricular foramen.[2] They are slow-growing tumors which may appear circumscribed to the naked eye and may be cystic or solid.

Juvenile astrocytomas of the hypothalamus may cause hypothalamic dysfunction. Patients with this type of lesion suffer from emaciation, diabetes insipidus, or may complain of visual difficulties. In infants, hypothalamic glioma should also be considered as one of the possible causes of the diencephalic syndrome. Diencephalic gliomas comprise astrocytomas of different cellularities and pleomorphic characteristics, also including anaplastic features and mixed gliomas.[2]

Olfactory Neuroblastoma or Esthesioneuroblastoma

This neoplasm usually arises in the superior aspect of the nasal cavity of young adults and adolescents. These are tumors composed of neurosensory receptor cells of the olfactory mucosa. Grossly they are soft, friable tumors. Microscopically, they contain tightly packed undifferentiated neuroblasts, forming cords around blood vessels. Axons may be seen with silver impregnation. Rosettes and pseudorosettes may be seen.

Neurilemmoma, Schwannoma, or Nerve Sheath Tumor

The terms neurilemmoma (with 2 m's), neurilemoma (with 1 m), Schwann cell tumor, Schwannoma, lemmocytoma, neurinoma, neuroma, neurofibroma, and perineural fibroblastoma have been used synonymously. Here, for consistency, only the term *neurilemmoma* will be used. Neurofibromas and plexiform neurofibromas can be classified as developmental anomalies, rather than true neoplasms. They are usually seen in neurofibromatosis. The typical acoustic neurilemmoma may present with hearing loss, tinnitus, vertigo, and facial weakness.

Neurilemmomas may arise from any nerve of the parasellar region. The cell of origin is the Schwann cell. They are benign and slow growing. Fibroblasts may also be present particularly in cases of neurofibromatosis.[31] These nerve sheath tumors may occur at any age, usually as a solitary tumor. The vestibular portion of the acoustic nerve is the usual origin in tumors arising from this nerve. This is the most common intracranial site, near the cerebellopontine angle. In neurofibromatosis they may be multiple, located in different nerves, and associated with meningiomas (collision tumors) or even with gliomas (astrocytomas and ependymomas).[1] In neurofibromatosis peripheral plexiform neurofibromas may be found in the subcutaneous tissue or in other internal organs associated with other stigmata, such as café-au-lait spots, which give a clue in the differential diagnosis.

Neurilemmomas are usually well circumscribed, encapsulated, and frequently attached to a nerve. The cut surface is white, sometimes yellow, usually firm and solid, but often possesses a mucinous or gelatinous texture with cavitations.

Microscopically, neurilemmomas are composed of spindle-shaped cells, arranged in a palisading fashion (Antoni A pattern) with fibroblasts and a variable amount of intercellular collagenous tissue, and other elements from the endoneurium, perineurium, or epineurium. Verocay bodies are the parallel arrangement of neoplastic cells in a regular manner with acellular areas. In some neoplasms the palisading arrangement of nuclei is absent and numerous cavities with macrophages may appear with a loose meshwork of reticulum fibrils (Antoni B pattern), representing degenerative or retrogressive changes. Malignant nerve sheath tumors (malignant Schwannoma or neurilemmoma) are seen in the neurofibromatosis. Histologically, the malignant tumors consist of fusiform cells with nuclear pleomorphism, hyperchromatism, and marked mitotic activity. Necrosis is present and there may be infiltration of the adjacent tissues. Ultrastructurally, the neoplastic cells are surrounded by a well-defined basal lamina. Long-spacing collagen (Luse bodies) are frequently seen.

Mesodermal Neoplasms

Meningiomas

The term *meningioma* was introduced by Cushing in 1922, to describe a benign intracranial neoplasm which had been given different and often confusing names including epithelioma, sarcoma, fibroblastoma, mesothelioma, endothelioma, and psammoma. The word meningioma simply indicates that the tumor arises from the meninges. It is now generally accepted that meningiomas are of arachnoid cell origin. Meningiomas are most frequently found in relation to the superior sagittal, the cavernous, and the sphenoparietal venous sinuses. They are seen where clusters of arachnoidal cells are located. This explains the preponderance of sphenoidal ridge meningiomas among meningiomas of the skull base.[15,19,20] Arachnoidal granulations or villi are very small in children, but can be identified at 18 months of age. They increase in number and size with advancing age.

Meningiomas are tumors found in adults and are rare in children. They reach a peak incidence in individuals 40 to 50 years of age. They are more common in women, although the sex incidence varies in tumors at different sites. In the sellar region, they are three to four times more common in women. Meningiomas constitute approximately 15% of all intracranial neoplasms.

Meningiomas of the sellar and parasellar region may be located on the planum sphenoidale, tuberculum, diaphragma, or dorsum sellae. A meningioma may also appear within the cavernous sinus region or medial third of the sphenoid wing.[23,26,32] Meningiomas may extend to the nasal cavity, the frontal, sphenoidal, and maxillary sinuses.[39,42] They may penetrate into the orbit or they may be ectopic in the neck or parotid region. Hemangiopericytoma is a neoplasm originating from pericytes and should not be confused with any type of meningioma.[5,14] Hemangiopericytomas are usually located on the posterior aspect of the skull or near the superior longitudinal sinus.

Meningiomas in the sellar area are often small and rarely acquire a large size. In this area they may present as flattened masses or "en plaque," particularly over the sphenoid ridge. They have a notorious tendency to wrap themselves around nerves and blood vessels at the base of the brain, rendering complete surgical removal very difficult. Tuberculum sella and planum sphenoidale meningiomas are difficult to diagnose early. The majority of patients complain of visual difficulties, cranial nerve palsies, (the sixth nerve being the most commonly involved), and vascular occlusions which may produce cortical motor and sensory manifestations. Meningiomas probably increase in size during menstruation and pregnancy. The chiasmal syndrome can be produced by olfactory groove, sphenoidal ridge, and tuberculum sella meningiomas. Multiple meningiomas or the occurrence of a meningioma and a neurilemmoma in the same patient should always arouse the suspicion of neurofibromatosis (von Recklinghausen's disease).[1,11]

The natural history of the different histological types of meningiomas is quite similar, except for the angioblastic papillary and malignant varieties, where the rate of recurrence and even extracranial metastases are much higher.[45] Meningiomas are well demarcated, encapsulated, solid and firm tumors which invaginate but usually do not invade the brain. They characteristically compress and displace rather than infiltrate the neural tissue. They are generally attached to the dura mater. Occasionally, they may originate from clusters of meningothelial cells in the choroid plexus. Some contain calcific deposits and infrequently cavitation is seen. The bone in close contact with the meningiomas is usually hyperostotic, and often infiltrated with the replacement of the bone marrow by meningothelial clusters and foci of meningioma.

The microscopic appearance is quite variable. These histological types have been described: meningothelial (syncytial), fibroblastic, psammomatous, papillary, transitional (mixed), angioblastic, vascular, and malignant. Meningiomas are in general characterized microscopically by "whorls," indistinct cellular borders, uniform, round nuclei, psammoma bodies, and abundant cytoplasm (Figs. 2A, B). Mitotic figures and necrosis are rare except in the malignant meningiomas, in which there is also invasion of CNS tissue. Occasional foci of metaplastic bone and cartilage may be found in meningiomas. Ultrastructural studies demonstrate elongated interlocking cytoplasmic processes and desmosomes (Fig. 3). Intranuclear pseudo-inclusions may be present.

Chondrosarcomas

Primary bone, cartilagenous, chondroid, and soft tissue tumors may arise in the middle fossa region usually in young adults.[18] Clinical presentation of this group of lesions is most often related to involvement of the visual pathways, the parapituitary area, and the middle cranial fossa. As a mass extends upward to the foramen of Monro, obstructive hydrocephalus and its resultant signs and symptoms occur. Compression of the brain stem may be caused by retrosellar extension. The gross morphological features consist of a multilobulated, ovoid, firm, and reddish-brown tumor, infiltrat-

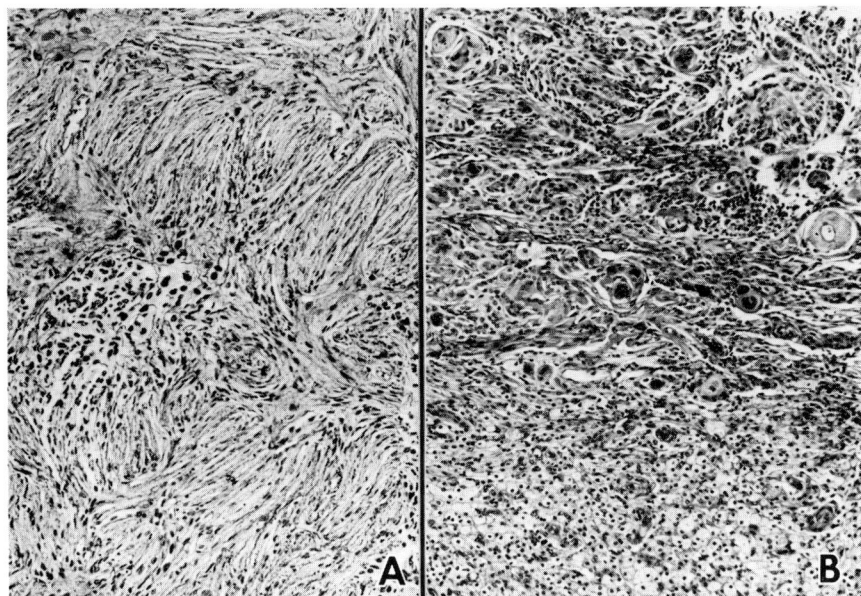

Figure 2: A: Fibroblastic meningioma composed of long, spindle-shaped cells arranged in streams and occasionally in whorls. A dense network of reticulin fibers can be detected between groups of cells. (Wilder Reticulin, original magnification X125.) **B:** Meningothelial meningioma formed of uniform cells with spherical and uniform nuclei encompassed by abundant cytoplasm with indistinct cellular borders. Some groups of cells have a whorled pattern. Occasional psammoma bodies and hyalinized blood vessels are seen. Areas of retrogressive changes are seen containing numerous macrophages. (H&E, original magnification X125.)

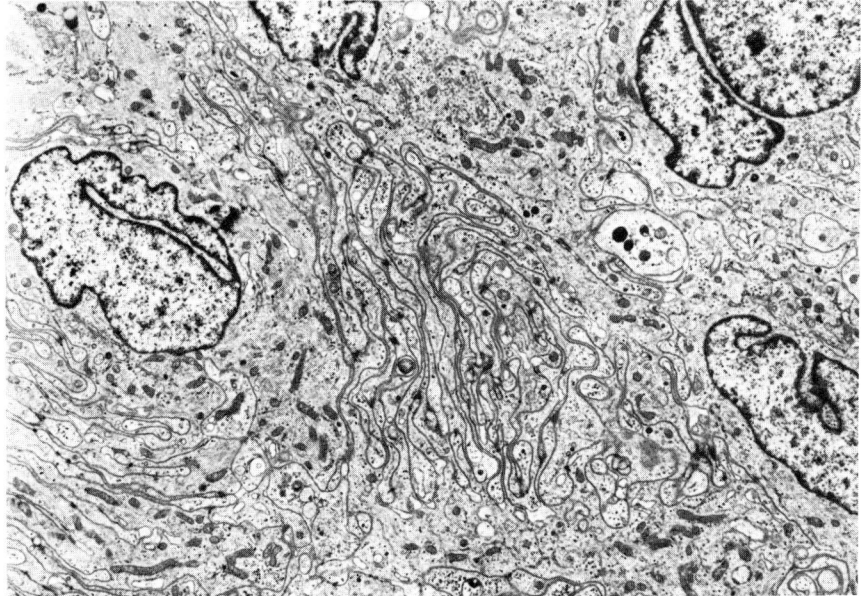

Figure 3: Electron micrograph of a meningioma showing the typical interdigitating cellular processes, desmosomes, and intracytoplasmic intermediate filaments. (Original magnification X5,000.)

ing locally the posterior and anterior clinoids and the cavernous sinuses. Mesenchymal chondrosarcoma consists of densely packed cellular areas, alternating with myxoid, chondroid, and embryonic cartilagenous tissue (Fig. 4). Foci of calcification may be present. This tumor must be differentiated from chondrosarcoma and from chondroid chordoma. There are overlapping histological features in these neoplasms. The natural history and topographical localizations help in the differential diagnosis. In the chondrosarcoma the neoplastic cells are most anaplastic, they are larger with greater pleomorphism, and the chondroid component is more anaplastic.

Paragangliomas

These tumors appear to arise from the neural crest or neuroectoderm along with other elements of the autonomic nervous system. They also contain conspicuous mesodermal components. They are also called apudomas. They include glomus jugulare tumors, carotid body tumors, glomus tympanicum tumors, and others located elsewhere in the body. Paraganglionic tissue has been found in the adventitia of the jugular vein, within the jugular foramen (glomus jugulare), and also along the tympanic branch of the glossopharyngeal nerve and along the postauricular branch of the vagus nerve. These two sites give rise to the glomus tympanicum tumors. Carotid body paragangliomas and the others in the neck can infiltrate the base of the skull or arise in the sellar region[7] or in the middle and inner ear. They are usually encapsulated, but the capsule is ill-defined and they may be locally aggressive and difficult to remove completely. Paragangliomas have similar morphological features of a normal carotid body. Histological features include an alveolar pattern separated by rich reticulin network with abundant capillaries. Ultrastructurally the cells are ovoid or polyhedral with many mitochondria, lysosomes, and numerous "secretory" dense core granules and vesicles.

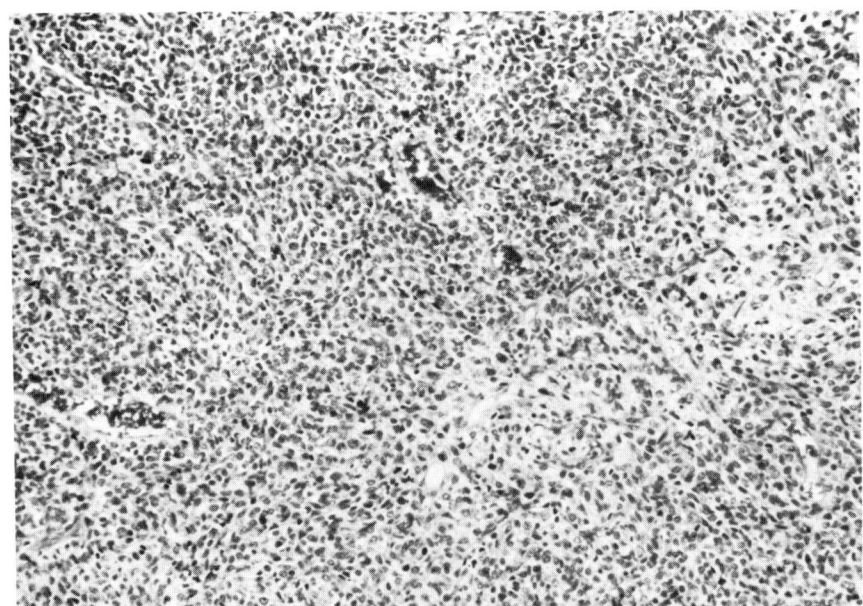

Figure 4: Mesenchymal chondrosarcoma. This is a densely cellular neoplasm. The nuclei are large, pleomorphic, hyperchromatic, and surrounded by scant cytoplasm. Mitotic figures usually are abundant. (H&E, original magnification X150.)

Fibromas, Sarcomas, Osteomas, Chondroma, Lipoma, Liposarcoma, Angiomas, Hemangiomas, and Angiosarcomas

These tumors occur in the cranial base, and the parasellar and suprasellar areas, but they are rare.[33]

Ectodermal Tumors

Craniopharyngiomas

Craniopharyngiomas are benign tumors arising from squamous epithelial remnants of the hypophyseal duct (Rathke's pouch). Craniopharyngiomas are the most common tumors in childhood and adolescence in the suprasellar region. Their incidence has a second peak during middle age. They are more common in young men. In elderly patients, the possibility of craniopharyngioma is often overlooked.

Children with craniopharyngiomas present with headache (due to increased intracranial pressure associated with obstruction of the lateral ventricles), short stature, and poor sexual development. Visual symptoms and diabetes insipidus may be present.

The majority of craniopharyngiomas arise above the sella turcica, but some are intrasellar. An infrasellar tumor is exceedingly rare. The walls of the tumor tend to adhere to the adjacent brain rendering its separation difficult. The solid part of the tumor may invade or infiltrate the brain and in this respect behave like a malignant neoplasm. Some of them have a tendency toward cystic degeneration. The fluid within the cyst is often yellow-brown, looking almost like fresh lubricating oil. It is rich in cholesterol crystals which give it a characteristically glittering appearance. The craniopharyngiomas in the adult do not contain calcification as frequently as is seen in childhood.[34,36]

Craniopharyngiomas are composed of squamous epithelial cells with intercellular bridges and keratin pearls (Fig. 5). Necrosis is uncommon. Calcific deposits are

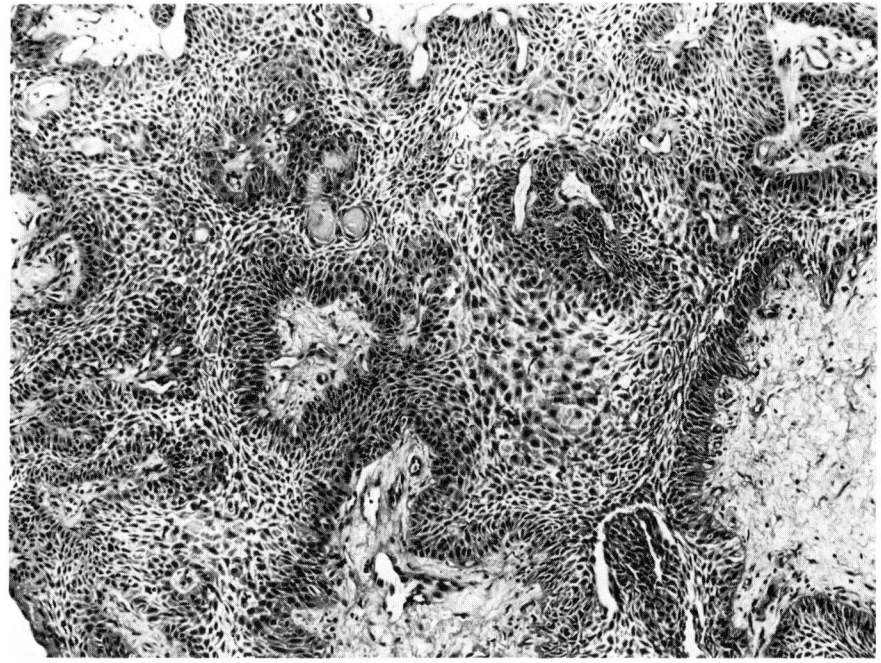

Figure 5: Craniopharyngioma. Squamous epithelial cells with isolated island of loose connective tissue. Occasional keratinized and calcific areas are seen. (H&E, original magnification X125.)

also seen. The immunoperoxidase stain reveals intracytoplasmic keratin in epithelial cells.[4] Ultrastructural features are characteristics showing intercellular connections, desmosomes, and tonofilaments (Fig. 6).

Pituitary Adenomas

Pituitary adenomas are the second most frequently encountered intracranial tumor among the nonglial neoplasms. Pituitary adenomas may grow beyond the confines of the sella turcica and extend into the suprasellar, parasellar, and infrasellar regions. With it there is often a rupture or invasion of the dura and bony erosions. The chromophobe adenomas are frequently larger, with extrasellar expansions. Occasionally necrosis and bleeding into the tumor occurs (pituitary apoplexy) and calcification may be seen. Pituitary adenomas become symptomatic by secreting excessive quantities of one or more hormones, by compressing normal pituitary tissue, by compression of the optic apparatus in the suprasellar region, or by invasion of parasellar structures.[40]

The traditional classification of pituitary adenomas has been into acidophil, basophil, mixed acidophil-basophil, and the chromophobe varieties. A modern classification based on functional, ultrastructural features, and immunocytochemical characteristics is current: i.e., prolactin-secreting adenomas or prolactinomas, growth hormone cell adenomas, ACTH-producing adenomas, gonadotropic adenomas, and undifferentiated or nonfunctional pituitary adenomas. The last group is subdivided into oncocytic tumors (oncocytomas) and nononcocytic tumors on the basis of ultrastructural features.

Differential Diagnosis of Pituitary Adenomas

Pituitary adenomas are grossly pink-gray, soft, and friable. Microscopically they may be difficult to diagnose using hematoxylin and eosin (H&E) stains (Fig. 7A). They may mimic ependymomas,

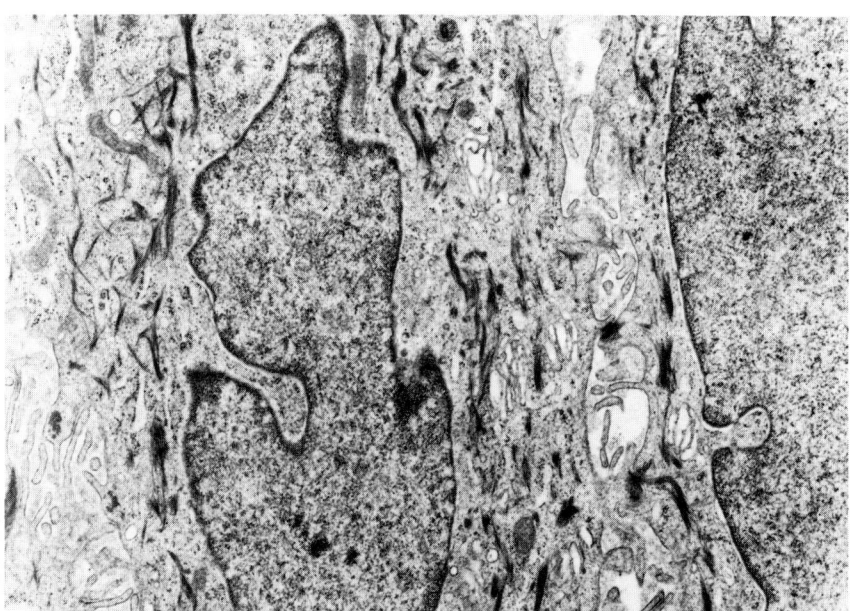

Figure 6: Electron micrographs of a craniopharyngioma showing the typical ultrastructural characteristics consisting of bundles of tonofilaments and intercellular desmosomal junctions. (Original magnification X10,000.)

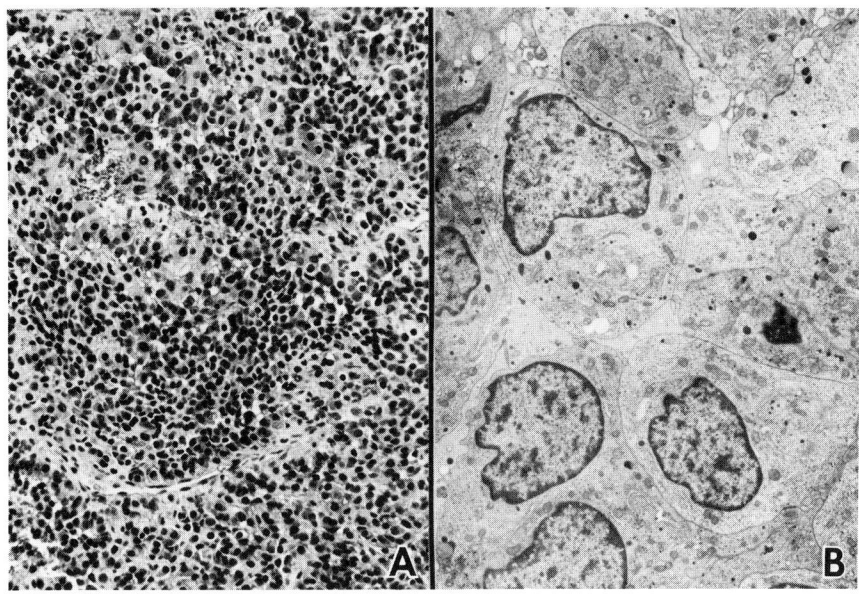

Figure 7: A: Pituitary adenoma, chromophobe, composed of a patternless sheet of cells with rounded nuclei and indistinct cytoplasmic borders. (H&E, original magnification X150.) **B:** Electron microscopy of a nonsecretory, nononcocytic pituitary adenoma demonstrating few, small secretory granules, scant number of mitochondria, and evenly dispersed nuclear chromatin. (Original magnification X15,000.)

oligodendrogliomas, metastatic adenocarcinomas, lymphomas or plasma cell neoplasms. The histopathological patterns consist of sinusoidal, papillary, diffuse, or mixed types. There is no relationship between the cytological features and the size of the adenoma. There is no correlation between the histological pattern and the biological behavior of the adenoma. Wilder reticulin stain reveals lack of reticulin fibrils between adenomatous, epithelial cells, and clusters of cells. In contrast, normal or compressed adenohypophysis is rich in reticulin fibrils. PAS Orange G is also useful in differentiating the chromophobic, basophilic, and eosinophilic cells. Touch preparations stained with H&E are useful for rapid intraoperative diagnosis of pituitary adenomas. This technique is more reliable than frozen sections.[28] Electron microscopic (Fig. 7B) and immunocytochemical techniques using antisera for pituitary hormones are essential for the precise diagnosis.

Myoblastoma (Granular Cell Myoblastoma, Choristoma, "Pituicytoma")

The granular cell myoblastoma is a benign tumor occurring within the striated muscle of the tongue but it has also been reported in the subcutaneous tissue, the gastrointestinal tract, omentum, retroperitoneum, bladder, larynx, breast, and peripheral nerves.[9,37,41] A Schwann cell origin has been associated. It may also occur in the region of the pituitary gland (usually pars nervosa), infundibulum, and hypothalamus. Some authors consider this tumor a hamartoma, meaning a mass of tissue histologically normal for an organ or part of the body but disordered in arrangement. Macroscopically, it is a well-demarcated, homogenous, firm and pinkish-gray nodular mass. Microscopically, the lesion consists of large, regular polygonal cells with abundantly granular cytoplasm. Ultrastructurally, the neoplastic cells contain abundant lysosomes, mitochondria, and a prominent basement membrane. This supports an origin of this tumor from Schwann cells.

Congenital, Embryonic, and Malformative Tumors

Epidermoid Cyst (Pearly Tumor; Cholesteatoma)

Epidermoid cysts are usually found in young adults and are often associated with pilonidal sinuses, spina bifida, and diastematomyelia. Epidermoid tumors are formed of epithelial tissue only, whereas dermoid tumors contain epidermis, sebaceous glands, and dermal appendages. These slow-growing tumors may occur in the anterior third ventricular region. Signs of hypothalamic dysfunction, ventricular obstruction, or visual abnormalities may be present. If the contents of these cysts are spilled and disseminated into the subarachnoid space during the surgical procedure, an aseptic or chemical leptomeningitis may develop with possible ependymitis.

Epidermoid cysts represent malformative and displaced embryonic nests.[44] They occur preferentially in the cerebellopontine angle ("parapontine"), the parasellar region, the quadrigeminal plate, the posterior and anterior corpus callosum, the Sylvian fissure, the lateral ventricles, the third ventricle, the fourth ventricle, and the spinal cord. They may also occur in the petroclival bony region. Because of the glistening silvery appearance, this tumor has been called "pearly tumor." Usually they are well-encapsulated, containing a friable, leafy, brittle and soft white material. Histologically they are composed of squamous epithelium lining a laminated "keratinaceous" debris.

Dermoid Cysts

Dermoid cysts are more frequently found in children. This tumor develops from germ cell displaced during early embryonic development.[44] These have a predilection for the suprasellar and parapontine areas, for the midline of the posterior cranial fossa, and for the sacrum. Occasionally they are found in the maxillo-orbital closing line and grow in the direction of the orbit. Usually the dermoid cysts are encompassed by a firm capsule filled with a pale gray soft, greasy mass which contains hairs and rarely teeth. Histologically, they are composed of epidermis, sebaceous and sweat glands, and hair follicles. They are frequently calcified. Severe inflammatory reaction may develop in the surrounding CNS tissue if they become fragmented.

Arachnoid Cysts

Arachnoid cysts in the region of the sella turcica are rare but should be included in the differential diagnosis of space-occupying lesions within or above the sella. Histologically, they are composed of membranes of collagenous-connective tissue lined by flattened, hyperplastic arachnoid. Cerebrospinal fluid may be found within the cavitary structures.[44]

Teratomas

Teratoma, by definition, contains tissue from more than one germinal layer. This lesion occurs more frequently in younger age groups and in men.[29] The presenting clinical symptoms are visual disturbances, diabetes insipidus, and hypopituitarism. Teratomas are frequently found in the pineal region, the pituitary region, the white matter of the cerebral hemispheres, and the lateral ventricles. Teratomas are knotty, well-encapsulated, firm, occasionally calcified, or interspersed with bone, cartilage, hair, and teeth. The different components include mature, immature, and embryonic tissue of all three germ layers.

Chordomas

Chordomas are neoplasms arising from remnants of the notochord.[10,17] The majority are seen between 30 to 50 years of age. One peculiar feature of these tumors is that they are very rare in the dorsal and lumbar parts of the vertebral column which contain the largest portion of the nucleus pulposus, the remains of the notochord. In spite of their embryonic origin, chordomas are rare in children. Most of the chordomas arise in the sacrococcygeal region, followed by the base of the skull and few occur in the cervical, lumbar, and thoracic vertebral column. Most intracranial chordomas occur in the midline in the clivus and rarely in the middle fossa region. The most frequent clinical symptoms of clivus chordoma are headache, visual disturbances, nasal obstruction, and neck pain. Cranial nerve palsies may occur.

From an historical point of view, this tumor was first reported by Luschka who in 1856 described small mucus-containing excrescences which protruded from the basisphenoid and perforated the dura mater. Virchow saw similar nodules and designated them "ecchordosis physaliphora" (derives from the Greek words: *ek* = out, *chordo* = cord, *osis* = a disease process, and *physallis* = bubble). In 1838 Muller suggested that these masses originated from remnants of the notochord which they resembled histologically, and also traced the notochord up to the sella turcica.

A chordoma is soft, lobulated, and jelly-like. It may be colorless or grayish-white depending on its cellularity and mucin content. Areas of hemorrhage and calcification may be present. The tumor is

It cannot be totally removed. Intracranially, it usually arises from the midline of the clivus, but may extend entirely to one side. It may grow upward toward the sella turcica, forward into the nasopharynx, or backward toward the brain stem.

It is known that in some cases the histological features of chordomas are simulated by a variant of mesenchymal chondrosarcoma (also called chondroid chordoma) that has some immature myxoid elements, a few cells, and much fibrous-connective and bony tissues.

Histologically, chordomas are characterized by lobulation and a cord-like arrangement of the tumor cells (Fig. 8). The most characteristic feature is the presence of mucin inside the neoplastic cells or in the extracellular space. Because of the high content of glycosaminoglycans, they stain strongly with Alcian blue. Ultrastructurally, the neoplastic cells are characterized by desmosomes and prominent stalks of rough endoplasmic reticulum (Fig. 9).

Colloid Cysts

The colloid cyst of the third ventricle is a true cyst, most commonly found at the anterior third of the third ventricle and producing obstruction of the foramina of Monro (synonyms: *paraphysial* or *neuroepithelial* cyst).[44,49] There is no sex predominance. Histologically the colloid cyst is formed by ciliated columnar epithelial cells resting on a thin fibrous capsule (Fig. 10A). The cyst is filled with a "colloid," dense hyaline substance which stains positive for mucin and with PAS-H. Ultrastructurally, the cells contain cilia and microvilli (Fig. 10B).

Aneurysms and Other Vascular Tumors

Aneurysms, angiomas, hemangiomas, angiosarcomas, and glomus tumors are vascular lesions that may be present in the sellar and parasellar regions. Aneurysms of the cavernous portion of the internal carotid artery may cause erosion and enlargement of the sella turcica and may appear as parasellar or suprasellar masses. Common symptoms include retro-orbital and periorbital pain, extraocular muscle palsies, and facial hypesthesia. Exophthalmos may be seen with involvement of the orbit. Rarely hypopituitarism secondary to pituitary compression is seen with significant medial extension. Visual loss is most commonly seen with aneurysms of the ophthalmic artery, fusiform enlargement of the intradural portion of the internal arotid artery, or large aneurysms of the

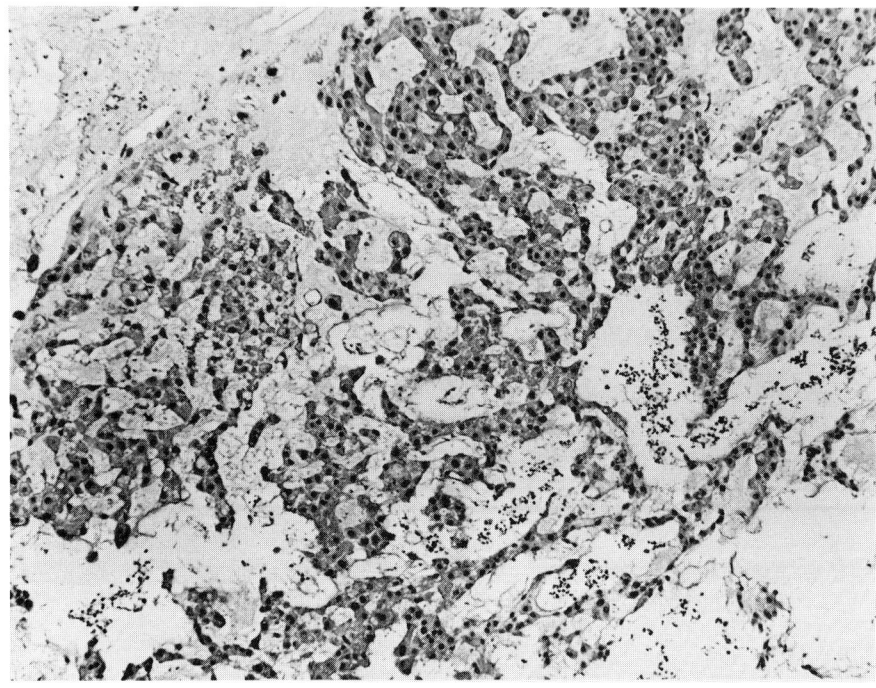

Figure 8: Chordoma. The neoplastic cells are arranged in clusters and cords separated by abundant extracellular mucinous material. The nuclei are round, hyperchromatic, and uniform, encompassed by cells with the characteristic of bubbly cytoplasm (physaliphorous). Abundant extracellular proteinaceous material is present. (H&E, original magnification X125.)

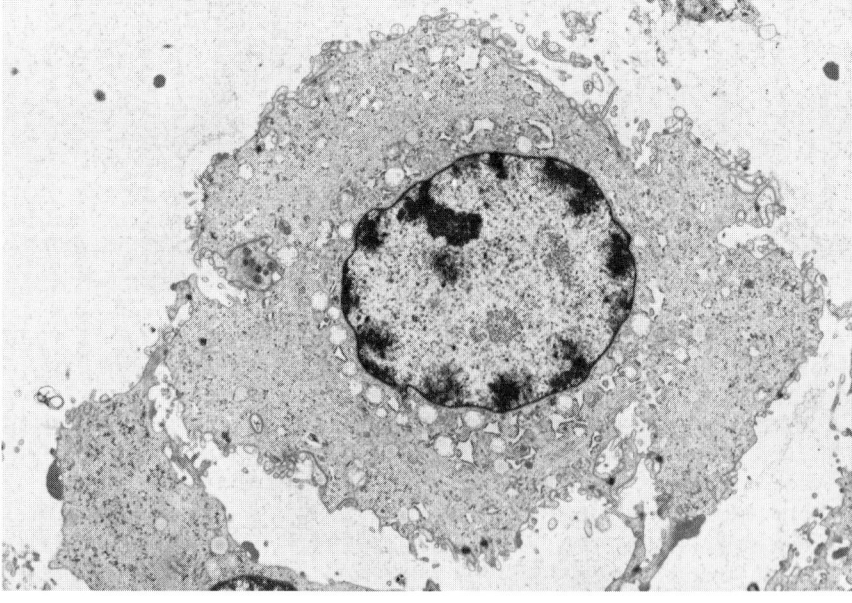

Figure 9: Chordoma. Ultrastructural features of a chordoma cell. The nucleus is surrounded by prominent stalks of rough surface endoplasmic reticulum sometimes forming parallel arrays. Desmosomes may be seen at the periphery. (Original magnification X25,000.)

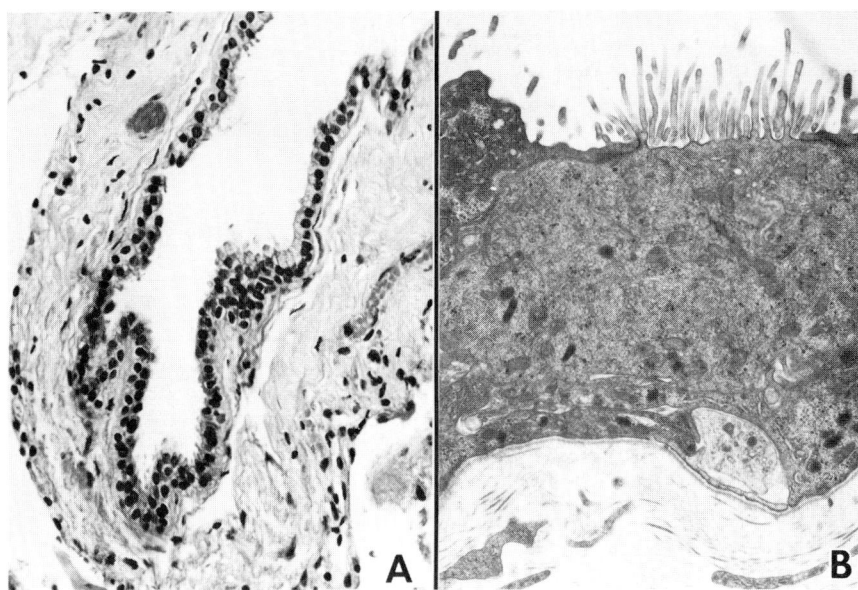

Figure 10: A: Colloid cyst of the third ventricle. It is composed of a layer of fibrous-connective tissue, lined by ciliated cuboidal epithelial cells. Focal areas of pseudostratified epithelium are seen. The cystic cavity usually is filled with "colloid" material. (H&E, original magnification X315.) **B:** Electron micrograph from the wall of a colloid cyst showing the ciliated cell with short microvilli. (Original magnification X25,000.)

anterior communicating artery. Angiography is diagnostic but may reveal only a portion of larger aneurysms. If the aneurysmal dilatation is occupied by an organized thrombus, then it fails to opacify by angiography.

Mucocele of the Sphenoid Sinus

Mucoceles of the sphenoidal sinus occur when the sinus openings become occluded with subsequent accumulation of mucous secretions, usually from minor salivary glands. As mucoceles expand toward the sellar floor, cavernous sinus, or orbit, headache, throbbing orbital pain, extraocular muscle palsies, and abnormalities of vision evolve. However, signs and symptoms are nonspecific and they may suggest a retrobulbar mass. A soft tissue mass within an expanded sphenoidal sinus and destruction of the adjacent bone may be seen on skull films and x-ray tomography. Histologically, they are characterized by mucosal epithelial lining, forming a cyst and containing abundant mucous secretion.

Germinomas and Intracranial Germ Cell Tumors

Germinoma, ectopic pinealoma, and other intracranial germ cell tumors are tumors occurring in younger age groups, mainly in men.[21,27] Germinomas of the suprasellar region have also been called ectopic pinealomas, atypical teratomas, or dysgerminomas. These tumors are histologically similar to seminomas. Usually the tumors of the pineal gland region cause paralysis of upward gaze (Parinaud's syndrome) due to pressure on the colliculi and tectum of the midbrain. Diabetes insipidus and hypopituitarism may be seen in the ectopic variety.

Germinomas have a distinctive histological appearance. They are composed of two types of cells: large polygonal cells with well-defined membrane, pale, and scant cytoplasm, and conspicuous central nuclei and mucleoli (Fig. 11A); and groups of small darkly staining cells; presumably lymphocytes, usually distributed along the vascular connective tissue stroma of the tumor. A true teratoma containing many kinds of tissue of endodermal, mesodermal, and ectodermal origin in the sellar region is rare, but they are known to occur in the pineal region. Ultrastructurally, the cells are poorly differentiated with round nucleus and prominent nucleoli (Fig. 11B).

Hypothalamic Hamartoma or Infundibuloma

This is a developmental tumor also called pituicytoma, often located in the posterior part of the hypothalamus, behind the dorsum sellae, the neurohypophysis, and closely related to the floor of the third ventricle and interpenduncular fossa. Neurosecretory activity of hamartoma has been suggested.[7] The majority occur in male children and the main presenting clinical feature is precocious puberty both in physical and sexual development, associated with mental retardation and occasionally acromegaly. Macroscopically, this neoplasm is encapsulated, well circumscribed and firm and has a coarsely lobulated, smooth glistening surface. Histologically, it is basically a pilocytic astrocytoma composed of a haphazard assembly of astrocytes, bundles of glial fibers and glial tissue and neurons.[2,22]

Rathke Cleft Cyst (Rathke's Pouch Cyst)

These cysts are lined by a single layer of mucus-secreting, ciliated cuboidal-columnar epithelium. These lesions are considered derivatives of the Rathke's pouch remnants. They probably arise from the pars intermedia of the pituitary gland. These cysts have occurred twice as often in women as in men. Usually they are asymptomatic until they reach a sufficient size to produce compressive symptoms in the optic pathway and the hypothalamus.[6] These lesions are filled with a viscid, clear, mucoid fluid. Histologically cellular debris, foci of calcification, and fragmented columnar or cuboidal epithelial cells may be found

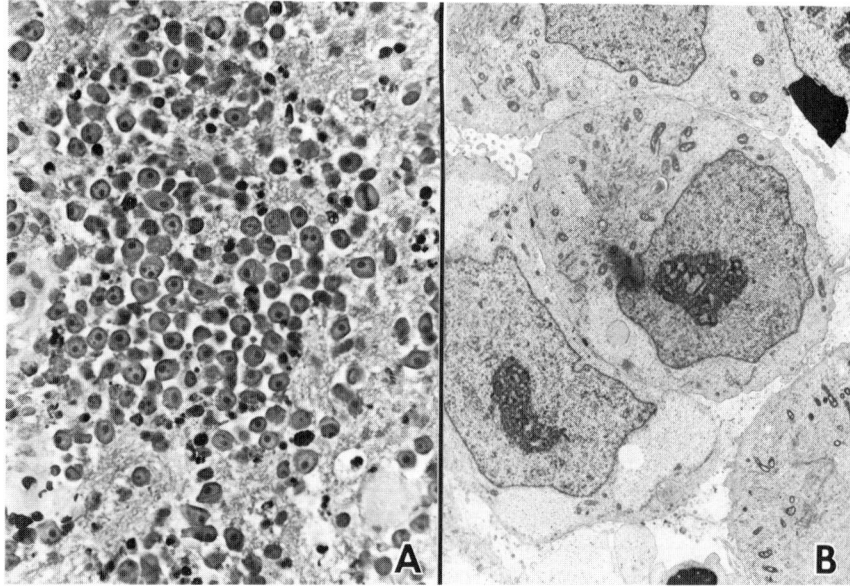

Figure 11: A: Ectopic germinoma of the suprasellar region composed of polygonal and spherical "epithelioid" cells with large, round nuclei, and prominent nucleoli. The cytoplasm is scant. (H&E, original magnification X400.) **B:** Electron micrograph of this ectopic germinoma showing large cells with big nuclei, conspicuous nucleoli, few cytoplasmic organelles, abundant glycogen, and rare junctional complexes. (Original magnification X20,000.)

with multinucleated giant cell reaction and cholesterol clefts.

Inflammatory Lesions

Granulomas

The main granulomatous lesions that may affect the pituitary-hypothalamic area are: tuberculosis, sarcoidosis, histiocytosis, meningovascular syphilis, and cryptococcus neoformans (*Torula histolytica*). However, involvement in coccidiodomycosis, histoplasmosis, blastomycosis, sporotricosis, candidiasis, and aspergillosis may also occur.[46,50]

Tuberculomas

Tuberculomas are the most frequent intracranial lesions in some countries where tuberculosis is still a common disease. They may be single or multiple and are more frequent in the posterior fossa. In the Western hemisphere, the form that is more likely to be seen is tuberculous meningitis, sometimes leading to hydrocephalus. The possibility of a tuberculoma should always be considered in the differential diagnosis of intracranial space-occupying lesions in patients with tuberculosis. Histologically the lesion is characterized by chronic granulomatous inflammation (Fig. 12). Special stains for acid-fast bacilli rarely demonstrate the organism.

Sarcoidosis

Sarcoidosis affects the central nervous system very rarely. The lesions may involve: the cranial nerves (facial, optic, glossopharyngeal, and vagus); the spinal nerves; the meninges; and the brain and the spinal cord. Intracranially the most frequent site of involvement is the base of

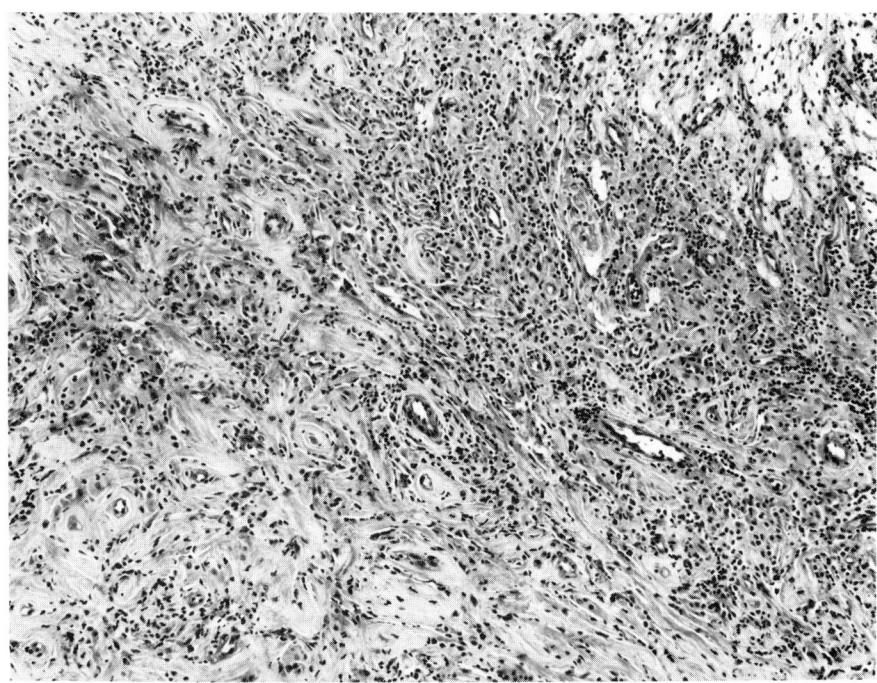

Figure 12: Tuberculoma from the suprasellar region characterized by fibrous-connective tissue heavily infiltrated by lymphocytes and plasma cells and profuse vascularity. (PAS-H, original magnification X125.)

the brain, in the form of granulomatous or adhesive arachnoiditis, or an invasion of the floor of the third ventricle in which case the optic nerves and chiasm may be involved. Macroscopically, the lesions may be too small to be visible, or rarely, they may occur as a circumscribed large tumor. Microscopically, sarcoidosis is characterized by a chronic granulomatous inflammation with multinucleated giant cells.

Gumma

This rare granulomatous lesion is caused by spirocheta pallidum.

Pituitary Abscess

Intrasellar pituitary abscess is an uncommon lesion that may arise in a preexisting Rathke cleft cyst or in an adenoma. Surgical treatment is essential and effective. Pre-existing CSF rhinorrhea and paranasal sinusitis are predisposing causes.

Hypophysitis or Lymphoid Hypophysitis

The anterior lobe of the pituitary gland can be involved in an inflammatory reaction mediated by lymphocytes that enlarge the volume of the gland and can lead to various degrees of dysfunction. Autoimmunity has been implicated as the pathogenetic mechanisms of this chronic inflammatory response.[3,12,35]

Parasitic Lesions

Cysticercosis

Cysticercus cellulosae is the larva of the *taenia solium* or pork tapeworm. They may be located in the suprasellar region and third ventricle producing obstruction of the cerebrospinal fluid pathways. In the "racemose" form, the cysts form groups like a bunch of grapes.

Ecchinococcal Cyst

Echinococci are the larva of the hydatis tapeworm *Echinococcus granulosus*. Occasionally the vesicles may produce symptoms of increased intracranial pressure if they are located near the ventricles, the foramina, or the aqueduct.

Fungal

Cryptococcosis (Torulosis)

Cryptococcus neoformas is a fungus that is known for its predilection for the central nervous system (CNS). The organism has been cultured from the skin and mucous membrane of normal healthy individuals and has been isolated from the soil; it is also frequently associated saprophytically with pigeon droppings. Man and animal frequently acquire the fungi by inhalation of yeasts. CNS invasion occurs by hematogenous seeding from a primary pulmonary focus. When the natural resistance is diminished man is liable to acquire the disease, but cryptococcosis may also occur in healthy individuals. The pathological features may consist of chronic cryptococcal leptomeningitis with a thick, opaque, and gelatinous appearance of the leptomeninges, mainly at the base of the brain. The cerebral cortex and basal ganglia often disclose "soap-bubble" spaces. Occasionally, the disease is manifested as space-occupying masses or "cryptococcomas" which may be present in the suprasellar or parasellar regions. Histologically, the lesions are well-circumscribed granulomas with chronic inflammatory reaction and Langhan giant cells. Intracellular yeast may be seen within giant cells.

Metastatic Tumors

Carcinoma and Other Malignant Neoplasms

Metastasis may be found in the parasellar region in 25% of the cases with malignant tumors.[8,16,24,25,30,38,48] Lytic lesions of bone in and around the sella turcica may be evident radiologically. CT scans may reveal the suprasellar or parasellar extent of metastatic lesions. Usually this clinical situation is seen in the "end-stage" of the malignant tumors in patients who have a short life expectancy. Carcinoma of the breast is the most common tumor that may be metastatic to the sellar and parasellar region, usually involving the pituitary gland. Other metastatic tumors include carcinomas of the lung, colon, prostate, and kidney. Visual symptoms with or without hypopituitarism may be present. Melanoma, plasma cell myeloma, and lymphoma may also produce metastatic foci in the parasellar or suprasellar regions and within the pituitary gland.

The Empty Sella Syndrome

This is a syndrome that was originally described in patients who had had chiasmal pressure symptoms and upon surgical exploration have an "empty sella." Now the term is also applied to patients in whom chiasmal symptoms recur some years after treatment of the original pituitary tumor. The recrudescence of symptoms in these cases is due to kinking and distortion of the optic nerves and chiasm as they are pulled down into the sella. This syndrome should be considered in the differential diagnosis of suprasellar and parasellar lesions because it can produce sellar enlargement and visual field defects.[13]

If there is an enlarged opening in the diaphragma sellae or congenital absence of the diaphragma sellae, an arachnoid diverticulum may extend into the sella turcica, compressing the pituitary gland. This disease entity is called primary empty sella syndrome. A secondary empty sella syndrome is seen following surgery for pituitary tumors, following radiotherapy directed to the sellar region, following pituitary infarction, in pseudotumor cerebri, and in other conditions causing atrophy of the pituitary gland. Patients with the empty sella syndrome may present with headache, visual disturbance, and spontaneous cerebrospinal fluid rhinorrhea.

Occasionally, a sella is described as "empty" when its cavity is largely occupied by ballooned recesses of the third ventricle. Usually this finding has no pathological significance, but there are cases in which thinning of the sellar floor may lead to the escape of CSF into the sphenoid sinus or to headache and visual impairment.

ACKNOWLEDGMENT: *My sincerest thanks to Miss Karen Perkins for typing and retyping the manuscript and to Dr. David Engle for valuable suggestions during the preparation of the manuscript.*

References

1. Arieti S: Multiple meningioma and meningiomas associated with other brain tumors. *J Neuropathol Exp Neurol* 3:255, 1944.
2. Asa SL, Bilbao JM, Kovacs K, et al: Hypothalamic neuronal hamartoma associated with pituitary growth hormone cell adenoma and acromegaly. *Acta Neuropathol* 52:231, 1980.
3. Asa SL, Bilbao JM, Kovacs K, et al: Lymphocytic hypophysitis of pregnancy resulting in hypopituitarism: a distinct clinicopathologic entity. *Ann Intern Med* 95:166, 1981.
4. Asa SL, Kovacs K, Bilbao JM, et al: Immunohistochemical localization of keratin in craniopharyngiomas and squamous cell nests of the human pituitary. *Acta Neuropathol* 54:257, 1981.
5. Begg Ch F, Garrett R: Hemangiopericytoma occurring in the meninges. *Cancer* 7:602–6, 1954.
6. Berry RG, Schlezinger NS: Rathke-cleft cysts. *Arch Neurol* 1:62-72, 1959.
7. Bilbao JM, Horvath E, Kovacs K, et al: Intrasellar paraganglioma associated with hypopituitarism. *Arch Pathol Lab Med* 102:95-98, 1978.
8. Bitoh S, Hasegawa H, Fujiwara M, et al: Nasopharyngeal malignancies causing abducens palsy. *Neurol Med Chir (Tokyo)* 23:571-576, 1983.
9. Campbell JAH: Adamantinoma containing tissue resembling granular-cell myoblastoma. *J Pathol Bacteriol* 71:45-49, 1956.
10. Carty CS, Beabout JW: Chordomas and cartilaginous tumors of the skull base. *Cancer* 32:410, 1973.
11. Castellano F, Guidetti B, Olivecrona H: Pterional meningiomas "en plaque." *J Neurosurg* 9:188-196, 1952.

12. Cebelin MS, Velasco M, de las Mulas JM, et al: Galactorrhea associated with lymphocytic adenohypophysitis: case report. *Br J Obstet Gynaecol* 88:675, 1981.
13. Evans DC, Netsky MG, Allen VE, et al: Empty sella secondary to suprasellar colloid cyst of foregut (respiratory) origin: Case report. *J Neurosurg* 5115-5117, 1979.
14. Goellner JR, Laws ER, Soule EH, et al: Hemangiopericytoma of the meninges: Mayo Clinic experience. *Am J Clin Pathol* 70:375, 1978.
15. Grant FC, Hedges TR: Ocular findings in meningiomas of the tuberculum sellae. *Arch Ophthal* 56:163-170, 1956.
16. Greenberg HS, Deck MDF, Vikram B, et al: Metastasis to the base of the skull: clinical findings in 43 patients. *Neurology* 31:30-37, 1981.
17. Heffelfinger MJ, Dahlin DC, MacCarty CS, et al: Chordomas and cartilaginous tumors at the skull base. *Cancer* 32:410-420, 1973.
18. Heros RC, Martinez AJ, Ahn HS: Intracranial mesenchymal chondrosarcoma. *Surg Neurol* 14:311-317, 1980.
19. Ho K-L: Primary meningioma of the nasal cavity and paranasal sinuses. *Cancer* 46:1442-1447, 1980.
20. Jane JA, McKissock W: Importance of failing vision in early diagnosis of suprasellar meningiomas. *Br Med J* 2:5-7, 1962.
21. Jennings MT, Gelman R, Hochberg F: Intracranial germ-cell tumors: Natural history and pathogenesis. *J Neurosurg* 63:155-167, 1985.
22. Judge DM, Kulin HE, Page R, et al: Hypothalamic hamartoma: A source of luteinizing-hormone-releasing factor in precocious puberty. *N Engl J Med* 296:7, 1977.
23. Karp LA, Zimmerman LE, Borit A, et al: Primary intraorbital meningiomas. *Arch Ophthalmol* 91:24-26, 1974.
24. Kistler M, Pribram HM: Metastatic disease of the sella turcica. *AJR* 123:13-21, 1975.
25. Leramo OB, Booth JD, Zinman B, et al: Hyperprolactinemia, hypopituitarism, and chiasmal compression due to carcinoma metastatic to the pituitary. *Neurosurgery* 8:447, 1981.
26. Majoros M: Meningioma of the paranasal sinuses. *Laryngoscope* 80:640-645, 1970.
27. Marcovitz S, Guyda HJ, Finlayson MH, et al: Intrasellar germinoma associated with hyperprolactinemia. *Surg Neurol* 22:387-396, 1984.
28. Martinez AJ, Moossy J: Cytological diagnosis of pituitary adenomas (Abst). *J Neuropathol Exp Neurol* 42:307, 1983.
29. McGrath P: Cysts of sellar and pharyngeal hypophyses. *Pathology* 3:123-131, 1971.
30. Mills RP, Insalaco SJ, Joseph A: Bilateral cavernous sinus metastasis and ophthalmoplegia: case report. *J Neurosurg* 55:463-466, 1981.
31. Myerson PG: Multiple tumors of the brain of diverse origin. *J Neuropathol Exp Neurol* 1:406, 1942.
32. Nager GT: Meningioma involving the temporal bone. Springfield, IL: Charles C. Thomas, 1964.
33. Pardo-Mindan FJ, Guillen FJ, Villas C, et al: A comparative ultrastructural study of chondrosarcoma, choroid sarcoma, and chordoma. *Cancer* 47:2611-2619, 1981.
34. Petito CK, DeGirolami U, Earle KM: Craniopharyngiomas: A clinical and pathological review. *Cancer* 37:1944, 1976.
35. Portocarrero CJ, Robinson AG, Taylor AL, et al: Lymphoid hypophysitis: An unusual cause of hyperprolactinemia and enlarged sella turcica. *JAMA* 246:1811, 1981.
36. Randall RV, Laws ER, Abboud CF: Clinical presentation of craniopharyngiomas: A brief review of 300 cases. Year Book Medical Publishers, 1984, 321-323.
37. Rhodes RH, Dusseau JJ, Boyd AS, et al: Intrasellar neural-adenohypophyseal choristomâ: a morphological and immunocytochemical study. *J Neuropathol Exp Neurol* 41:267, 1982.
38. Roessmann U, Kaufman B, Friede RI: Metastatic lesions in the sella turcica and pituitary gland. *Cancer* 25:478-480, 1970.
39. Rosalki SB, McGee LE: Meningioma representing as nasopharyngeal tumor. *J Laryngol* 76:133-139, 1962.
40. Sakalas R, Harbison JW, Vines FS, et al: Chronic sixth nerve palsy. *Arch Ophthalmol* 93:186-190, 1975.
41. Scheithauer BW, Kovacs K, Randall RV, et al: Hypothalamic neuronal hamartoma and adenohypophyseal neuronal choristoma: their association with growth hormone adenoma of the pituitary. *J Neuropathol Exp Neurol* 42:648-663, 1983.
42. Shah RP, Leavens ME, Samaan NA: Galactorrhea, amenorrhea, and hyperprolactinemia as manifestations of parasellar meningioma. *Arch Intern Med* 140:1608-1612, 1980.
43. Sherwin RP, Grassi JE, Sommers SC: Hamartomatous malformation of the posterolateral hypothalamus. *Lab Invest* 11:89, 1962.
44. Shuangshoti S, Netsky MG, Nashold BS:

Epithelial cysts related to sella turcica: Proposed origin from neuroepithelium. *Arch Pathol* 90:444-450, 1970.
45. Simpson D: The recurrence of intracranial meningiomas after surgical treatment. *J Neurol Psychiatry Neurosurg* 20:20-39, 1957.
46. Taylon C, Duff TA: Giant cell granuloma involving the pituitary gland: Case report. *J Neurosurg* 52:584-587, 1980.
47. Thomas JE, Yoss RE: The parasellar syndrome: problems in determining etiology. *Mayo Clin Proc* 45:617-623, 1970.
48. Unsold R, Safran AB, Safran E, et al: Metastatic infiltration of nerves in the cavernous sinus. *Arch Neurol* 37:59-61, 1980.
49. Verkijk A, Botts GT: An intrasellar cyst with both Rathke's cleft and epidermoid characteristics. *Acta Neurochirurgica* 51:203-207, 1980.
50. Viale GL: Giant cell tumours of the sella region. *Acta Neurochirurgica* 38:259-268, 1977.

2

The Biology of Skull Base Tumors

James T. Rutka, M.D.
Mark L. Rosenblum, M.D.

Introduction

The biological behavior of tumors located at the base of the skull is largely dependent on two interactive factors: the proximity to critical areas of the brain and brainstem and the characteristics of the tumor itself, such as the cell kinetics, tissue of origin, and invasive potential. Because skull base tumors of equal volume can theoretically produce equivalent neurological symptoms regardless of histological type, we have decided to stress the biology of the individual tumors rather than their behavior as determined by location. Since Bingas' comprehensive review of skull base tumors in 1974,[9] much progress has been made in the fields of tumor cell biology and immunology. In this chapter, we will review some of these advances and describe other factors that reflect clinical behavior, including the etiology, epidemiology, natural history, metastatic potential, tumor radiosensitivity, and patient survival. The text focuses on nasopharyngeal carcinomas, esthesioneuroblastomas, chordomas, glomus tumors, meningiomas, and chondrosarcomas. Whenever possible, the distinction will be made between the behavior of these tumors in general and their behavior when located at the skull base. A synopsis of the chapter is provided in Table I.

Nasopharyngeal Carcinoma

Although rare in most countries, nasopharyngeal carcinoma has become an epidemiological curiosity largely because of its high prevalence among the Chinese. In China, nasopharyngeal carcinoma is a major cancer problem, occurring in 20/100,000 persons compared with less than 1/100,000 persons in North America and Europe.[5,29,39,66] For this reason and because the tumor is associated with the Epstein-Barr virus, the etiology of nasopharyngeal carcinoma is one of the most intriguing issues in cancer research today.

The highest frequency of nasopharyngeal carcinoma occurs in southern China, among the Cantonese.[66] Native

---

From: Sekhar LN, Schramm VL Jr, eds: *Tumors of the Cranial Base: Diagnosis and Treatment*. Mount Kisco, New York, Futura Publishing Co, Inc, © 1987.

Dr. Rutka was supported by the Medical Research Council of Canada.

Dr. Rosenblum is the recipient of NIH grants CA 13525 and CA 31882 and Teacher Investigator Development Award 1K07NS00604NSPA from the National Institute of Neurological and Communicative Disorders and Stroke.

Table I.
Characteristics of Skull Base Tumors

Tumor	Frequency	M:F Ratio	Genetics	Age at Onset (years)	X-ray Appearance	Survival	Metastases	Radiosensitivity	Other
Meningioma	8% of all intracranial tumors	1:3	Von Recklinghausens	20–60	hyperostosis	less than normal population at 15 years	rare	probably radiosensitive	sex steroid hormones
Chordoma	1% of all intracranial tumors	2:1	—	40	erosion of bone tumor Ca++ sphenoid mass	30–50% 5-year	10%	unknown	chondroid chordoma variant
Nasopharyngeal Carcinoma	25% of NPCs affect skull base	3:1	HLA A2, BW46,D,DR	45	destruction of bone	20–40% 5-year	55%	radioresistant except lympho-epithelioma	Chinese, EBV
Chondrosarcoma	6% of all skull base tumors	1:1	—	30–40	erosion of bone tumor Ca++	40–60% 5-year	rare	radioresistant	—
Esthesioneuroblastoma	3% of all nasal tumors	2:1	—	bimodal: 20–30; 50–60	erosion of cribiform plate	40% 5-year	20–40%	radiosensitive	long survival with RT
Glomus jugulare	1% of all intracranial tumors	1:6	familial clustering	55	destruction of bone	93% 10-year	rare	local control frequent	—

EBV = Epstein-Barr virus; NPC = nasopharyngeal carcinoma; Ca++ = calcification; RT = radiation therapy.

Chinese living in other countries have a greater risk of developing nasopharyngeal carcinoma than the population of the country to which they have moved; and the prevalence of this tumor among Chinese born in the United States is slightly higher than in the general population.[29,66] Elevated rates of nasopharyngeal carcinoma have also been reported among Eskimos, Vietnamese, and Indonesians.[45,66] It is because the Chinese are more susceptible to acquiring nasopharyngeal carcinoma that certain etiological factors have been implicated, including inhaled carcinogens in the home, ingestion of salted fish (which contain dimethylnitrosamines), and prior noncancerous disease of the oronasopharynx.[29,34] Age distribution curves are compatible with the hypothesis that exposure to an environmental carcinogen must occur early in life to cause nasopharyngeal carcinoma,[66] but no specific agent has been isolated.

Males are two to three times more commonly affected than females in many large series.[29,39,66] Recently, some familial clustering and HLA associations have been reported in patients with nasopharyngeal carcinoma; HLA-A2, BW46, D, and DR haplotypes have been shown to occur more frequently than other determinants.[29,66,83] The best interpretation of the epidemiological and etiological data is that probably no single factor can account for the development of nasopharyngeal carcinoma in a given patient; rather, persons with certain physical characteristics that are determined by multiple genes or associated with a simple gene marker may be at higher risk, especially when exposed to a triggering environmental carcinogen.[29]

The average age of patients with nasopharyngeal carcinoma at the time of presentation is approximately 45 years.[39,56] The interval between the appearance of symptoms and the time of diagnosis is approximately 7 months.[5] Tumor within the nasal fossae, palate, and tonsils usually produces local symptoms initially.[75] However, because of its proximity to the brain and to a high density of regional lymphatic channels, nasopharyngeal carcinoma tends to spread quickly and can involve the skull base in up to 25% of cases.[2,56,77] With invasion of the skull base, cranial nerve palsies are the most frequently seen neurological symptoms; the Vth nerve is involved most often.[5,75] By the time of diagnosis, approximately 55% of patients have regional cervical lymph node metastases.[5] Distal skeletal and visceral metastases have also been reported.[75]

The duration of survival among patients with nasopharyngeal carcinoma depends in part on the histological subtype of the tumor. Generally, patients with squamous cell carcinoma do more poorly than those with nonkeratinizing or undifferentiated carcinoma.[3,66] Overall, the 5-year survival rate is 20–40%.[2,5,22,75] Undifferentiated carcinoma gives rise to a peculiar variant known as lymphoepithelioma, which is associated with a better prognosis than other types of nasopharyngeal carcinoma.[3,39,66] The possible reasons for this will be considered below.

The only factor that has been linked consistently with nasopharyngeal carcinoma is the Epstein-Barr virus, a herpes-type virus that has been found in tumor cells of nasopharyngeal carcinoma patients throughout the world.[5,29,45,47,55,66,83] An association between nasopharyngeal carcinoma and certain Epstein-Barr related antigens has also been noted. Serological evaluation of the antibody to the diffuse (D) component of the induced early antigen (EA) and the IgA antibody to viral capsid antigens (VCA) have been shown to have the highest specificity for nasopharyngeal carcinoma.[55] Some data show a correlation between increasing Epstein-Barr viral titers and decreased survival in patients with nasopharyngeal carcinoma.[29] Patients who have been in remission for 3 or more years or who have clinically inactive disease tend to have lower viral titers.[5,55] These serological findings and the presence of viral DNA in tumor cells, which has been demonstrated by electron microscopy, suggest that exposure to the Epstein-Barr virus and the subsequent host immune response are important factors in the development of nasopharyngeal carcinoma.[3,5,66]

The abundance of lymphoid elements in nasopharyngeal carcinomas of various histological subtypes is now thought to represent an immunological response to the tumor.[3] In one such subtype, lymphoepithelioma, the lymphocytic component is predominant.[3,47] Patients who have this tumor tend to present at an earlier age and live longer than patients with other types of nasopharyngeal carcinoma.[3,39] The normal nasopharynx contains tonsillar tissue and forms part of the lymphoepithelial organ system, which also includes the thymus.[61] A recent study has linked the Epstein-Barr virus with thymic carcinoma,[46] providing further evidence of the oncogenic potential of herpes viruses in cells and organs that mount an immune response. Research on the interactions between the immune system and nasopharyngeal carcinoma should increase our understanding of the basic biology of this tumor.

Esthesioneuroblastoma

Esthesioneuroblastoma, or olfactory neuroblastoma, is a rare tumor arising from the olfactory epithelium high in the nasal cavity near the cribiform plate. These lesions account for approximately 3% of all intranasal neoplasms.[40] First described by Berger[6] in 1924, esthesioneuroblastoma has recently been reported extensively in the literature, largely because of its characteristic histological features and poorly understood embryogenesis.

Histochemical, biochemical, and structural evidence now suggests that esthesioneuroblastomas arise from cells of neural crest derivation and that this tumor strongly resembles the classic childhood neuroblastoma.[12,14,25,33] The presence of neurosecretory granules, demonstrated by electron microscopy,[78] and biogenic amines, detected by formaldehyde fume-induced fluorescence,[41] within the tumor has linked esthesioneuroblastoma with other neoplasms of neural crest origin that travel ventrad to the neural tube during embryogenesis and that are biochemically similar to tumors belonging to the amine precursor and decarboxylation (APUD) system, such as carcinoid, chemodectoma and pheochromocytoma.

Esthesioneuroblastomas occur predominantly during the third decade of life,[25,40] although a bimodal incidence with a later peak occurrence at 50 to 60 years has been described.[65] The tumor is twice as common in males as it is in females.[12] No familial clustering has been reported.

Unilateral nasal obstruction and epistaxis, thought to be produced by the location and intrinsic vascularity of the tumor, are among the earliest and most common presenting symptoms.[14,25] As the tumor enlarges and fills the neighboring paranasal sinuses, it may invade the cribiform plate and extend upward into the anterior cranial fossa, resulting in complete anosmia.

The natural history of esthesioneuroblastoma is marked by a slow and insidiously malignant course.[14] Death results from local recurrences, intracranial invasion, or metastatic disease.[14,25,40,65,80] Overall 5-year survival rates of more than 50% have been reported;[53,78,80] but when the anterior skull base is involved, the 5-year survival rate decreases to 40%.[25] Unfortunately, patients who survive 5 years are not necessarily cured, for the tumor often recurs 10 to 20 years after the original diagnosis and treatment. In fact, the tendency toward persistent local recurrences is a hallmark of esthesioneuroblastoma.[14,65,80]

The metastatic potential of esthesioneuroblastoma is thought to be 20–40%.[14,25,65] The most common metastases are to regional cervical lymph nodes, lungs, and bone. Although there is some correlation between tumor stage and the duration of patient survival—the 5-year survival is 75% among patients with tumors confined to the nasal cavity and 41% among those with skull base involvement and distant metastases[25]—the biological and clinical behavior of esthesioneuroblastomas cannot be determined from the histological findings. In one study, discriminant analyses showed that advanced regional tumor extensions, recurrence of tumor, metastatic disease, and old age were all poor prognostic features.[37]

Unlike many skull base tumors, esthesioneuroblastoma responds to radiation therapy and is potentially curable.[14,53] Total radiation doses of 5000–6000 rads are needed to achieve tumor regression and control.[25] Objective response rates have also been obtained by adjuvant chemotherapy with cyclophosphamide, vincristine, and doxorubicin.[80]

Esthesioneuroblastoma has been induced with nitrosodiethylamine in hamsters. This may provide an adequate animal model with which to study the biological behavior of this skull base tumor.[35]

Chordomas

Chordomas are histologically benign, slow-growing tumors that occur most frequently at the cranial and sacral ends of the axial skeleton.[7,32,36] Approximately 30–40% of all chordomas are localized to the cranium;[42,79] of these, the vast majority extensively involve the skull base, resulting in neurological symptoms and a slow, inexorable course that is nearly always fatal.

The similarities in histological appearance between the typical chordoma and the fetal notochord were discovered by pathologists more than a century ago. Thought to be derived from the endoderm, the notochord is the intitial axial structure in human embryogenesis.[7,33] Except for its contribution to the nucleus pulposus, the notochord almost completely disappears by the sixth week of gestation. However, ecchordoses, or small rests of ectopic notochordal tissue that persist into adult life, can be found incidentally in approximately 2% of autopsies.[72] It has been thought, but not proven, that chordomas may arise from these aberrant notochordal nodules.[27,33,57]

Chordomas account for approximately 1% of all intracranial malignancies.[42,57] They are found predominantly in adults and usually occur at about 40 years of age, approximately 10 years earlier than the sacral chordomas.[72] The results of several large series suggest that intracranial chordomas affect males twice as often as females.[33,42,79] There does not appear to be a genetic predisposition to the development of chordoma.

Chordomas are preferentially located over an extensive area of the skull base, including the clivus, sellar and perisellar regions, the basal middle cranial fossa, the cerebellopontine angle, and occasionally extending as far anteriorly as the olfactory groove.[26,27,72] Chordomas are generally expansile lesions that erode bone and often form a soft-tissue mass.[32,33,42] Tumors arising from the rostral clivus have been classified as basisphenoidal chordomas, while those arising from the caudal clival margin, at or below the spheno-occipital synchondrosis, have been classified as basioccipital. By virtue of their proximity to the pons and diencephalon, basisphenoidal chordomas tend to cause upper cranial nerve palsies and endocrine disturbances.[72] Basioccipital chordomas generally produce lower cranial nerve palsies and long tract signs.[53] Lateral extension of the tumor usually gives rise to unilateral signs. In approximately one-third of cases, basisphenoidal and basioccipital chordomas extend ventrally into the nasal cavities, the paranasal sinuses, and the pharynx.[2,7,32,42] Rarely, craniocervical chordomas will present extracranially as exophthalmos in patients with orbital invasion[26] or as a mass in the parotid region in patients with extensive ventral tumor spread from the clivus.[7]

The biological behavior of cranial chordomas is reflected in their x-ray appearance. Erosion of bone at the base of the skull is seen in 75–95% of cases, intratumoral calcification in 30–50%, a soft-tissue tumor mass in the sphenoid sinus in 40%, and evidence of bilateral destruction of bone in approximately 60%.[27,42,72,79] Sclerosis of bone is rare.[42]

Although patients with cranial chordoma survive longer than those with nasopharyngeal carcinoma or chrondrosarcoma of the skull base, there are probably no real cures in patients with chordoma in the sense that their survival rate becomes equal to that of the general population.[32] There appears to be little success in delaying the progression of the disease, and most patients die of uncontrolled, recurrent local tumor growth.[18] The 5-year survival rate for the classic form of chordoma is 30–50%.[7,18,27]

The chondroid variant of chordoma has an unusual biological behavior. Its histological appearance is similar to that of the classic chordoma, except for the conspicuous presence of cartilaginous foci intertwined with tumor cells. Unlike the typical chordoma, the chondroid chordoma appears in younger patients (average age, 35 years), is equally common among men and women, has a preference for the basiocciput, and is associated with a far better 5-year survival rate. Many patients live for two to three decades after diagnosis.[33,72,76]

The metastatic potential for cranial chordomas is about 10%.[27,32,33] Blood-borne metastases have been found in the lung, liver, lymph, bone, skin, and peritoneum. As the duration of patient survival increases, so does the metastatic potential.[33] It has been suggested that the malignant and metastatic potentials of chordomas are lower when cartilaginous foci are present.[33] Some evidence also suggests that the more anaplastic the chordoma, the more likely it is to metastasize.[79] In later stages of growth, chordomas can invade and transgress the dura and leptomeninges, which may explain the rare dissemination of chordomatous nodules in the subarachnoid space.[1,57]

Biochemical studies have shown that the mucinous, metachromatically staining matrix of the chordoma contains a concentration of glycosaminoglycan that is more similar to the fetal notochord than to mature, adult intervertebral disks.[74] Since cartilaginous matrix is primarily composed of glycosaminoglycans and has been found to modulate the growth and proliferation of tumor cells, further biochemical studies may help to delineate more fully the biology of chordoma.

Glomus Tumors

Glomus tumors, or chemodectomas, are the most common tumor of the middle ear and, after neurilemmoma, the second most common tumor of the temporal bone.[10,54,60] In general, glomus tumors arise from nests of chemoreceptor tissue, which normally responds to changes in arteriolar partial pressure of oxygen and carbon dioxide and to changes in pH.[60] It is thought that during embryogenesis, foci of cells (glomera) that have developed chemoreceptor activity become localized to the vicinity of the major vessels in the head and neck.[10] While the evidence is not conclusive, the ability of these cells to synthesize catecholamines implies a neural crest origin.[10,38] Normal glomus tissue may be found in the adventitia of the jugular bulb beneath the floor of the middle ear (glomus jugulare), in the bony walls of the tympanic canals that transmit the tympanic branches of the IXth and Xth cranial nerves (glomus juxtavole), and in the bone of the promontory close to the mucosal lining of the middle ear (glomus tympanicum).[10]

In 1941, Guild described the perivascular localization of solid masses containing epithelioid (glomus) cells in the temporal bone.[31] However, it was not until 1945, when Rosenwasser[62] reported the strong similarities between unusually vascular tumors of the middle ear and the normal glomus jugulare tissue, that the association was made between the two.

Glomus tumors affecting the skull base account for 0.03% of all malignancies.[60] The average age at the time of the initial diagnosis is approximately 55 years.[54] These tumors are reported most frequently in patients between the second and sixth decades[10] and are rare in childhood. For some unexplained reason that might relate to their biology, these tumors are six times more common in women than in men.[10,54,67] Familial clustering and the increased prevalence of glomus tumors among the children of patients with these lesions suggest at least a genetic predisposition.[60]

The biological behavior of glomus tumors is predictable. They grow slowly and progressively, extending multidirectionally along the planes of least resistance.[24,54,60] Glomus jugulare tumors at the base of the skull can extend intracranially, following the carotid artery within the intracranial carotid canal to the middle cranial fossa, the temporal bone air cell system to the petrous apex, and the jugular foramen and the hypoglossal canal into the posterior fossa. Although histologically benign, glomus tumors may exhibit clinically malignant behavior, such as local invasiveness, destruction of bone, intracranial extension into the cerebellopontine angle and brain stem, and a marked propensity for intratumoral hemorrhage.[24]

The early clinical signs and symptoms of glomus tympanicum tumors include a conductive hearing loss, pulsatile tinnitus, and a detectable mass in the external auditory canal.[10,38,82] Lower cranial nerve dysfunction is an early clinical sign of glomus jugulare tumors. Approximately one-half of all patients with glomus tumors present with cranial nerve symptoms;[10,54] the facial nerve is most commonly involved.[10,54,70] Advanced disease and extensive tumor are heralded by Vth and VIth nerve symptoms, hydrocephalus, and long tract signs.[70]

Widespread destruction of the temporal bone, widening and destruction of the jugular foramen, and a soft-tissue mass in the middle ear space may be seen on computerized tomography scans.[10] Because glomus tumors are composed of many thin-walled blood vessels between cords of epithelioid cells, angiography may demonstrate marked tumor vascularity.[10,19,38]

The natural history of glomus tumors is generally long.[10,67] A patient may survive without treatment for more than 20 years, even when there is intracranial extension of the tumor.[10] As with esthesioneuroblastomas, 5-year survival does not mean a cure has been achieved. Glomus tumors recur within 3 years of the initial treatment in 10–70% of patients.[10,60] Metastases occur in less than 1% of cases and have been found in cervical lymph nodes, liver, spleen, lungs, and bone.[10,24,71] Dissemination of tumor along CSF pathways has been reported after transgression of the dura by a glomus tumor that had extended intracranially.[82] Most patients with glomus tumors die from advanced intracranial extension of tumor or from intercurrent disease.[67]

Radiation therapy induces fibrosis of tumor vessels in some cases,[19,60,67] usually without histologic and radiographic evidence of decreased tumor vascularity or size. However, symptomatic improvement is usually seen and tumor size frequently remains stable over many years.[19,67] This has led to the suggestion that local control of chemodectomas can be achieved with radiation therapy.

Meningiomas

Meningiomas, which constitute 15% of all intracranial tumors, are thought to be tumors of arachnoid cells.[43,58,63] Their prevalence in the general population has been estimated from autopsy series, which quote a rate of about 1.5%.[59] Many of the tumors, however, were found incidentally at autopsy and had caused no symptoms. This underscores the major biological features of meningiomas—their slow growth and limited invasiveness. Although meningiomas of the skull base are seldom life-threatening, they may pose special problems to the neurosurgeon because of their critical location and the often extensive involvement of neighboring bone.[23]

Approximately 40–50% of all meningiomas affect the skull base.[20,58] Approximately 35% of basal meningiomas are in the sphenoid ridge, 20% are in the olfactory groove, 20% are suprasellar, 20% are in the posterior fossa, and 5% are in Meckel's cave.[28,43] Skull base meningiomas, like meningiomas in other locations, are more common in females by a ratio of about 2.5:1.[11,58] The well-documented susceptibility of patients with von Recklinghausen's neurofibromatosis to the development of meningiomas and the commonly observed deletion of chromosome 22 in cells cultured from meningiomas suggest that genetic factors are involved in tumor formation.[43] Several cases of familial clustering of meningioma have been reported in patients without neurofibromatosis.[28]

Although governed in part by intrinsic cell kinetics, the biological behavior of skull base meningiomas also depends upon location. For example, sphenoid ridge meningiomas tend to produce an exuberant hyperostotic reaction in neighboring bone, which can cause symptoms by impinging on neurovascular foramina.[23,43,48] Olfactory groove meningiomas grow to very large sizes before detection and are associated with local hyperostosis in approximately one-half of patients.[58] Clival meningiomas, though rare, cause symptoms similar to basilar insufficiency and, because of their critical location, carry an extremely poor prognosis.[15,58]

The hyperostosis seen frequently with meningiomas largely represents stippling of bone and enlargement of meningeal vascular grooves near tumor neovascularity.[23,63] However, there is evidence that pathological bone is produced where meningiomatous cells invade haversian canals.[43] In patients with meningiomas that grow as a carpet (en plaques) along the sphenoid ridge, it is this hyperostosis that frequently causes clinical symptoms.

The overall 15-year survival for patients with meningiomas is just below that of the normal population.[48] Meningioma patients with the worst prognosis are those with skull base tumors; their average survival time depends greatly on tumor location and the treatment undertaken. Although slow to appear, recurrence of tumor after subtotal surgical resection is the rule for skull base meningiomas.[13,23,58,68] Despite their local invasiveness of bone, skull base meningiomas seem to share with meningiomas in other locations a relatively low incidence of metastasis. With the exception of the hemangiopericytic meningioma and malignant variants, which have an increased metastatic potential, meningiomas metastasize rarely to lungs, liver, lymph, bones, pleura. and kidney.[43,63] Distant metastases are diagnosed an average of 10–18 years after the initial operation on the primary tumor.[43]

Hormonal factors have been implicated in the growth and development of meningiomas for several reasons, including the preponderance of female patients, clinical worsening of symptoms during pregnancy,[8] and the association of meningiomas with breast cancer.[69] Estrogen and progesterone receptors have been found with varying frequency in meningioma specimens and in the normal leptomeninges.[11,49] It is still uncertain whether steroid hormones affect tumor cell promotion or extracellular edema formation.[43] Nonetheless, the evidence strongly implies that hormones exert an influence on the biological behavior of some meningiomas.

Chondrosarcomas

Chrondrosarcomas account for approximately 8% of all primitive bone tumors.[16] While seemingly rare in comparison to osteogenic sarcoma, chondrosarcomas have a predilection for the base of the skull: roughly 6% of all skull base tumors are chondrosarcomas, and 75% of cranial chondrosarcomas are found at the skull base.[16] These facts, and the dismal prognosis associated with skull base chondrosarcomas, have made endeavors to understand the biological behavior and to find better treatment modalities of paramount importance.

The predilection of chondrosarcomas for the skull base may in part be explained embryologically. Unlike the skull vault, which is formed by intramembranous ossification, the skull base is derived from a cartilaginous matrix through a process known as endochondral calcification.[52] It is thought that chondrosarcomas may arise from a primitive mesenchymal stem cell within this matrix[21,30] or, in the case of ectopic tumors, within cartilaginous rests other than at the base of the skull.[4] In support of this hypothesis is a rare congenital condition of mesodermal dysplasia known as Maffucci's syndrome in which multiple benign tumors of cartilage (enchondromata) undergo malignant degeneration.[17] A common feature of many histological variants of chondrosarcoma is the presence of elements that resemble the cells and matrix of cartilage.[50]

The average age of patients at the time of presentation is 40 years for chondrosarcomas in all locations and 30 years for those in the head and neck region.[16,81] The most common location for skull base chondrosarcomas is the middle cranial fossa (63.4%), followed by the anterior fossa (14.3%) and the posterior fossa (7.1%).[16] Of all locations, the most common site of origin is the parasellar region.[4,30] Except for the variant known as intracranial mesenchymal chondrosarcoma, which occurs slightly more often in females, chondrosarcomas appear to be equally distributed between males and females.[44]

Chondrosarcomas of the skull base are slow-growing, locally recurrent, aggressively destructive tumors that expand and cause symptoms through intracranial mass effect.[4,30,81] Parasellar lesions have been reported to compress the optic nerves and the hypothalamic-pituitary axis, resulting in various visual acuity and field defects and endocrine dysfunction.[30] There have been reports of chondrosarcomas that arise from the nasal and paranasal sinuses and penetrate the skull base, but these rarely result in neurological symptoms.[81] Radiographs show erosion of bone and intratumoral calcification in up to 60% of cases.[30,81]

Although it is often difficult to predict the biological behavior from the degree of histological anaplasia, some data show 5- and 10-year survival rates for chondrosarcomas that decrease with increasing tumor grade—the 5-year survival is 90% for grade 1 tumors and 40% for grade 3 tumors.[81] Nevertheless, the failure rate for treatment of chondrosarcomas localized to the base of the skull is almost 100%.[73] This probably reflects the relative inaccessibility of these tumors compared with chondrosarcomas elsewhere in the body and the tumor's resistance to radiation therapy.[81] Metastasis from skull base chondrosarcomas to distant visceral and osseous locations is uncommon.[4,44,64]

Recent biochemical studies on the chemical composition of human chondrosarcomas may illuminate what has previously been a rather dark page in the treatment of skull base chondrosarcomas. Mankin et al.[50,51] described the histological and biochemical heterogeneity of chondrosarcomas and identified by extracellular matrix analysis a hyaline subtype of chondrosarcoma, which is least malignant, and myxoid and fibrous subtypes that behave much more malignantly. The chemical constitution of chondrosarcomas was similar to immature cartilage, indicating a possible reversion by the chondrocytes to an embryonal state. Knowledge of the phenotype of chondrosarcomas may prove useful in predicting survival and planning future therapies.

References

1. Aleksic S, Budzilovich GN, Nirmel K, et al: Subarachnoid dissemination of thoracic chordoma. *Arch Neurol* 36:652-654, 1979.
2. Amornmarn R, Prempree T, Sewchand W: Radiation management of advanced nasopharyngeal cancer. *Cancer* 52:802-807, 1983.
3. Applebaum EL, Mantravadi P, Haas R: Lymphoepithelioma of the nasopharynx. *Laryngoscope* 92:510-514, 1982.
4. Bahr AL, Gayler BW: Cranial chondrosarcomas. *Radiology* 124:151-156, 1977.
5. Baker SR: Carcinoma of the nasopharynx in childhood. *Otolaryngol Head Neck Surg* 89:555-559, 1981.
6. Berger L: L'esthesioneuroepitheliome olfactif. *Bull Assoc Franc Etude Cancer* 13:410-421, 1924.
7. Berryhill BH, Armstrong BW: Extracranial presentation of craniocervical chordoma. *Laryngoscope* 94:1063-1065, 1984.
8. Bickerstaff ER, Small JM, Guest IA: The relapsing course of certain meningiomas in relation to pregnancy and menstruation. *J Neurol Neurosurg Psychiatry* 21:89-91, 1958.
9. Bingas B: Tumors of the base of the skull. In Vinken PJ, Bruyn GW (eds): *Handbook of Clinical Neurology*, Vol 17, New York, Holland-North Publishing Co., 1974, pp 136-232.
10. Brown JS: Glomus jugulare tumors revisited: a ten year statistical follow-up of 231 cases. *Laryngoscope* 95:284-288, 1985.
11. Cahill DW, Bashirelahi N, Solomon LW, et al: Estrogen and progesterone receptors in meningiomas. *J Neurosurg* 60:985-993, 1984.
12. Cantrell RW, Ghorayeb BY, Fitz-Hugh GS: Esthesioneuroblastoma: diagnosis and treatment. *Ann Otol* 86:760-765, 1977.

13. Carella RJ, Ransohoff J, Newall J: Role of radiation therapy in management of meningioma. *Neurosurgery* 10:332-339, 1982.
14. Chaudhry AP, Haar JG, Koul A, et al: Olfactory neuroblastoma. *Cancer* 44:564-579, 1979.
15. Cherington M, Schneck SA: Clivus meningiomas. *Neurology* 16:86-92, 1966.
16. Cianfriglia F, Pompili A, Acchipinti E: Intracranial malignant cartilaginous tumors: Report of two cases and review of the literature. *Acta Neurochir* 45:163-175, 1978.
17. Cook PL, Evans PG: Chondrosarcoma of the skull in Maffucci's syndrome *Br J Radiol* 50:833-836, 1977.
18. Cummings BJ, Hodson I, Bush RS: Chordoma: the results of megavoltage radiation therapy. *Int J Radiation Oncol Biol Phys* 9:633-643, 1983.
19. Cummings BJ, Beale FA, Garrett PG, et al: Treatment of glomus tumors in the temporal bone by megavoltage radiation therapy. *Cancer* 53:2635-2640, 1984.
20. Cushing HW, Eisenhardt L: *Meningiomas: Their Classification, Regional Behavior, Life Histology and Surgical End Result*, New York, Heffner Publishing Co., 1938.
21. Dabska M, Huvos AG: Mesenchymal chondrosarcoma in the young. *Virchows Arch* 399:89-104, 1983.
22. Decker DA, Drelichman A, Al-Sarraf M, et al: Chemotherapy for nasopharygeal carcinoma. *Cancer* 52:602-605, 1983.
23. Derome PJ, Buiot G: Bone problems in meningiomas invading the base of the skull. *Clin Neurosurg* 25:435-451, 1978.
24. El-Fiky FM, Paparella MM: Metastatic glomus jugulare tumor. *Am J Otol* 5:197-200, 1984.
25. Elkton D, Hightower SI, Lim ML, et al: Esthesioneuroblastoma. *Cancer* 44:1087-1094, 1979.
26. Ferry AP, Haddad HM, Goldman JL: Orbital invasion by an intracranial chordoma. *Am J Ophthalmol* 92:7-12, 1981.
27. Firooznia J, Pinto RS, Lin JP, et al: Chordoma: radiological evaluation of 20 cases. *AJR* 127:797-805, 1976.
28. Gaist G, Piazza G: Meningiomas in two members of the same family. *J Neurosurg* 16:110-113, 1959.
29. Gastpar J, Wilmes E, Wolf H: Epidemiologic, etiologic, and immunologic aspects of nasopharyngeal carcinoma. *J Med* 12:257-284, 1981.
30. Grossman RI, Davis KR: Cranial CT appearance of chondrosarcoma of the base of the skull. *Radiology* 141:403-408, 1981.
31. Guild SR: A hitherto unrecognized structure: the glomus jugularis in man. *Anat Rec* (Suppl 2) 79:28-42, 1941.
32. Harwick RD, Miller AS: Craniocervical chordomas. *Am J Surg* 138:512-516, 1979.
33. Heffelfinger MJ, Dahlin DC, MacCarty CS, et al: Chordomas and cartilaginous tumors at the skull base. *Cancer* 32:410-420, 1973.
34. Henderson BE, Louie E, Jing JSH, et al: Risk factors associated with nasopharyngeal carcinoma. *N Engl J Med* 295:1101-1106, 1976.
35. Herrold KM: Induction of olfactory neuroepithelial tumors in Syrian hamsters by diethylnitrosamine. *Cancer* 17:114-121, 1964.
36. Higinbotham NL, Phillips RF, Farr HW, et al: Chordoma: thirty-five year study at Memorial Hospital. *Cancer* 29:1841-1850, 1979.
37. Homzie MJ, Elkon D: Olfactory esthesioneuroblastoma: Variables predictive of tumor control and recurrence. *Cancer* 46:2509-2513, 1980.
38. Hosoda S, Suzuki J, Kito J, et al: Tumor of glomus jugulare: Report of a case. *Acta Pathol Jpn* 589-597, 1975.
39. Hsu MM, Juang SC, Lynn TC: The survival of patients with nasopharyngeal carcinoma. *Otol Head Neck Surg* 90:289-295, 1982.
40. Jobst SB, Ljung BM, Gilkey FN, et al: Cytologic diagnosis of olfactory neuroblastoma. *Acta Cytologica* 27:299-305, 1983.
41. Judge DM, McGarvon MJ, Trapukdi S: Fume-induced fluorescence in the diagnosis of nasal neuroblastoma. *Arch Otolaryngol* 102:97-98, 1976.
42. Kendall BE, Lee BCP: Cranial chordomas. *Br J Radiol* 50:687-698, 1977.
43. Kepes JJ: Meningiomas: biology, pathology, and differential diagnosis. In Steinberg SS (ed): *Masson Monographs in Diagnostic Pathology*, New York, Masson, 1982, pp 10-57.
44. Kubota T, Hayashi M, Yamamoto S: Primary intracranial mesenchymal chondrosarcoma: Case report with review of the literature. *Neurosurgery* 10:105-110, 1982.
45. Lanier A, Bender T, Talbot M, et al: Nasopharyngeal carcinoma in Alaskan Eskimos, Indians and Aleuts. *Cancer* 46:2100-2106, 1980.
46. Leyvraz S, Henle W, Chahinian AP, et al: Association of EBV with thymic carcinoma. *N Engl J Med* 312:1296-1299, 1985.
47. Lynn TS, Hsu MM, Tu SM: Prognosis of nasopharyngeal carcinoma by Epstein-

Barr virus antibody titers. *Arch Otolaryngol* 103:128-132, 1977.
48. MacCarty CS, Piepgras DS, Ebersold MJ: Meningeal tumors of the brain. In Youmans JR (ed): *Neurological Surgery*, Philadelphia, WB Saunders, 1982, pp 2936-2966.
49. Magdelenat H, Pertuiset BF, Poisson M, et al: Estrogen and progesterone receptors found in normal human leptomeninges: Biochemical characterization, clinical and pathological correlations in 42 cases. *Acta Neurochir* 64:199-213, 1982.
50. Mankin HJ, Cantley KP, Lippiello L, et al: The biology of human chondrosarcoma. I. Description of the cases, grading, and biochemical analyses. *J Bone Joint Surg (Am)* 62A:160-176, 1980.
51. Mankin JH, Cantley KP, Schiller AL, et al: The biology of human chondrosarcoma. II.Variation in chemical composition among types and subtypes of benign and malignant cartilage tumors. *J Bone Joint Surg (Am)* 62A:176-188, 1980.
52. Moore KL: *The Developing Human.* Toronto, WB Saunders, 1973, pp 288-290.
53. Newbill ET, Johns ME, Cantrell RW: Esthesioneuroblastoma: diagnosis and management. *South Med J* 78:275-282, 1985.
54. Ogura JH, Spector GJ, Gado M, et al: Glomus jugulare and vagele. *Ann Otol* 87:622-629, 1978.
55. Pearson GR, Weiland LH, Neel HB, et al: Application of Epstein-Barr virus serology to the diagnosis of North American nasopharyngeal carcinoma. *Cancer* 51:260-268, 1983.
56. Petrovich Z, Juisk H, Jose L: Advanced carcinoma of the nasopharynx: treatment results. *Acta Radiol Oncol* 20:245-251, 1981.
57. Peese JPP, Borges JM, Nudelman M, et al: Unusual subarachnoid metastasis of an intracranial chordoma in infancy. *Childs Brain* 4:251-256, 1978.
58. Quest DO, Meningiomas: An update. *Neurosurgery* 3:219-225, 1978.
59. Rausing A, Ybo W, Stenflo J: Intracranial meningioma: A study of 10 years. *Acta Neurol Scand* 46:102-110, 1970.
60. Reddy EK, Mansfield C, Hartman GV: Chemodectoma of glomus jugulare. *Cancer* 52:337-340, 1983.
61. Rosai J: "Lymphoepithelioma-like" thymic carcinoma: another tumor related to Epstein-Barr virus? *N Engl J Med* 312:1320-1321, 1985.
62. Rosenwasser H: Carotid body tumor of the middle ear and mastoid. *Arch Otolaryngol* 41:64, 1945.
63. Rubinstein LJ: *Tumors of the CNS: Atlas of Tumor Pathology*, Washington, DC, Armed Forces Institute of Pathology, 1972, fascicle 6, pp 169-204.
64. Scheithauer BW, Rubinstein LJ: Meningel mesenchymal chondrosarcoma. *Cancer* 42:2744-2752, 1978.
65. Shah JP, Feghali J: Esthesioneuroblastoma. *CA-A Cancer Journal For Clinicians* 33:154-159, 1983.
66. Shanmugaratnam K: Nasopharyngeal carcinoma: epidemiology, histopathology, and etiology. *Ann Acad Med (Sing)* 9:290-295, 1980.
67. Simko TG, Griffin TW, Gerdes AJ, et al: Role of radiation therapy in the treatment of glomus jugulare tumors. *Cancer* 42:104-106, 1978.
68. Simpson D: The recurrence of intracranial meningiomas after surgical treatment. *J Neurol Neurosurg Psychiatry* 20:22-39, 1957.
69. Smith FP, Slavik M, MacDonald JS: Association of breast cancer with meningioma. *Cancer* 42:1992-1994, 1978.
70. Spector GJ, Sobol S: Surgery for glomus tumors at the skull base. *Otolaryngol Head Neck Surg* 88:524-530, 1980.
71. Spector GJ, Ciralsky RH, Ogura JH: Glomus tumors in the head and neck. III. Analysis of clinical manifestations. *Ann Otol* 84:73-79, 1975.
72. Spoden JE, Bumsted RM, Warner ED: Chondroid chordoma: case report and literature review. *Ann Otol* 89:279-285, 1980.
73. Suit HD, Goitein M, Munzenrider J, et al: Definitive radiation therapy for chordoma and chondrosarcoma of the base of the skull and cervical spine. *J Neurosurg* 56:377-385, 1982.
74. Sweet MBE, Thonar EJMA, Berson SD, et al: Biochemical studies of the matrix of craniovertebral chordoma and a metastasis. *Cancer* 44:652-660, 1979.
75. Tan BC, Khor TH, Chia KB: Radiotherapy in the treatment of nasopharyngeal carcinoma. *Ann Acad Med (Sing)* 9:347-349, 1980.
76. Valderrama E, Kahn LB, Lipper S, et al: Chondroid chordoma: electronmicroscopic study of two cases. *Am J Surg Pathol* 7:625-632, 1983.
77. Vita HCV, Mendiondo OA, Shaw DL, et al: Nasopharyngeal cancer in the second decade of life. *Radiology* 148:2153-256, 1983.
78. Vollrath M, Altmannsberger M, Hunneman DH, et al: Esthesioneuroblastoma: ul-

trastructural, immunohistochemical, and biochemical investigation of one case. *Arch Otorhinolaryngol* 239:133-144, 1984.
79. Volpe R, Mazabraud A: A clinicopathologic review of 25 cases of chordoma. *Am J Surg Pathol* 7:161-170, 1983.
80. Wade PM Jr, Smith RE, Johns ME: Response of esthesioneuroblastoma to chemotherapy. *Cancer* 53:1036-1041, 1984.
81. Waga S, Tochio H, Yamagiwa M, et al: Chondrosarcoma of the ethmoid sinus extending to the anterior fossa. *Surg Neurol* 16:324-328, 1981.
82. Welsh LW, Welsh JJ, Huck GF Jr: Glomus jugulare tumor: disseminated form in the CNS. *Arch Otolaryngol* 102:507-510, 1976.
83. Wolf H, Seibl R: Benign and malignant disease caused by Epstein-Barr virus. *J Invest Derm* 83:88s-95s, 1984.

II

Radiological Diagnosis and Embolization Techniques

3

Imaging of Tumors at the Base of the Skull: The Sphenoid Bone

Richard E. Latchaw, M.D.

Introduction

The sphenoid bone is a complex portion of the bony skull base that has as its center the sphenoid body which contains the sella turcica. It extends anteriorly (planum sphenoidale), laterally (greater and lesser wings), and postero-inferiorly (the clivus). Many demands are made upon imaging techniques which must not only define a neoplastic mass, but more importantly must demonstrate the involvement of this complex bony anatomy. Many vascular structures and cranial nerves are contiguous to portions of the sphenoid bone, and appropriate preoperative evaluation requires an assessment of the involvement of these important structures by the tumor.

Numerous imaging techniques are available today for evaluation of the bony and soft tissue anatomy of the skull base. These techniques include plain films, computed tomography (CT), magnetic resonance imaging (MRI), cerebral angiography, and digital subtraction angiography (DSA). Two less common techniques to be discussed are CT cisternography, the CT examination performed after the movement of intrathecally deposited water-soluble contrast material into the intracranial subarachnoid cisterns, and cerebral blood flow determination as performed with CT during the inhalation of stable xenon during a test occlusion of an internal carotid artery.

Following an evaluation of the various advantages and disadvantages of these imaging techniques for the evaluation of lesions involving the sphenoid bone and contiguous structures, there will be a discussion of specific parameters that must be evaluated in attempting to predict preoperatively the histology of the neoplasm present and to determine the extent of skull base involvement. These parameters include the type of bone involvement; the location and extent of the soft tissue mass and its apparent point of origin; the presence of calcification within the soft tissue mass; CT enhancement patterns with intravenous contrast material, such as the homogeneity or irregularity of enhancement; MRI relaxation parameters

From: Sekhar LN, Schramm VL Jr, eds: *Tumors of the Cranial Base: Diagnosis and Treatment*. Mount Kisco, New York, Futura Publishing Co, Inc, © 1987.

that may predict the presence of fat or blood, and that may give some degree of specificity of histology; the relationship of the mass to vascular structures and nerves; and finally, the angio-architecture as determined with cerebral angiography.

The differential diagnosis of a neoplasm depends to a large extent upon the portion of the sphenoid bone involved. The last part of this chapter will discuss neoplasms that typically involve each portion of the sphenoid and parasphenoidal tissues, emphasizing specific features that may allow a determination of the type of neoplasm present.

Techniques of Radiographic Examination

Plain Films

Plain skull films are important only for a gross overview of the bony anatomy. Large amounts of calcification can be detected as can gross bone destruction. However, skull films lose their value because of the complexity of the bony anatomy, multiple overlying densities, and inability to demonstrate intracranial soft tissue involvement.

Computed Tomography

Both axial and direct coronal scanning are necessary for appropriate evaluation of the complexities of the sphenoid bone (Fig. 1). We prefer to obtain axial scans parallel to the planum sphenoidale in all patients, in order to decrease the artifact from bony structures and to reduce partial volume artifact caused by scanning at an angle through dense bones such as the tuberculum sellae. Such scanning is, therefore, perpendicular to the infundibulum and optic chiasm, and allows excellent visualization of the parasellar regions. Scanning parallel to the planum, or even at a negative angle relative to the planum, gives the best visualization of the brain stem. Coronal scans are extremely important for evaluation of the pituitary, cavernous sinuses with the enclosed cranial nerves, and the cribiform plate. In order to decrease artifacts, direct coronal scans should be obtained with the gantry angled so that the beam does not pass through the teeth. Computer-reformatted coronal images are of much lower quality relative to direct coronal scanning. Not only must soft tissue axial and coronal views be obtained, but bone algorithms should be utilized for the optimum evaluation of bony structures (Fig. 1). Simply changing the window and level to visualize bone produces images of lesser quality relative to those employing a bone algorithm.

The thickness of the slices in either the axial or coronal projection depends upon the size of the structures or lesion to be evaluated. Slices of 1.5, 3, or 5 mm should be available, along with 10 mm cuts performed above and below the level of the lesion to evaluate the rest of the head. Lesions of the sella turcica, cavernous sinuses, optic chiasm, and cribiform plate generally require slice thicknesses of 1.5 to 3 mm. Because multiple high photon thin cuts must be obtained which produce a significant heat load on the x-ray tube, dynamic scanning cannot be used; dynamic scanning, however, is particularly valuable for evaluating intravascular flow or the relationship of a mass to vascular structures. Reformatted images may be of value in demonstrating an aneurysm at the base of the skull (Fig. 2), but are of lesser quality for evaluating bony structures than direct views.

It goes without saying that evaluation of the complex bony and soft tissue anatomy at the base of the skull requires a high resolution CT scanner. Excellent spatial and contrast resolution is necessary if appropriate preoperative evaluation of the small and vital structures at the base of the skull is to be made.

Computed tomography is excellent for demonstrating bony and soft tissue anatomy (Figs. 3, 4).[1] It has the finest spatial resolution of all imaging techniques, has very good contrast resolution of soft tissue structures, and is very fast and very accurate. CT is the best modality for defining bony detail (Figs. 1, 3, 4), and for de-

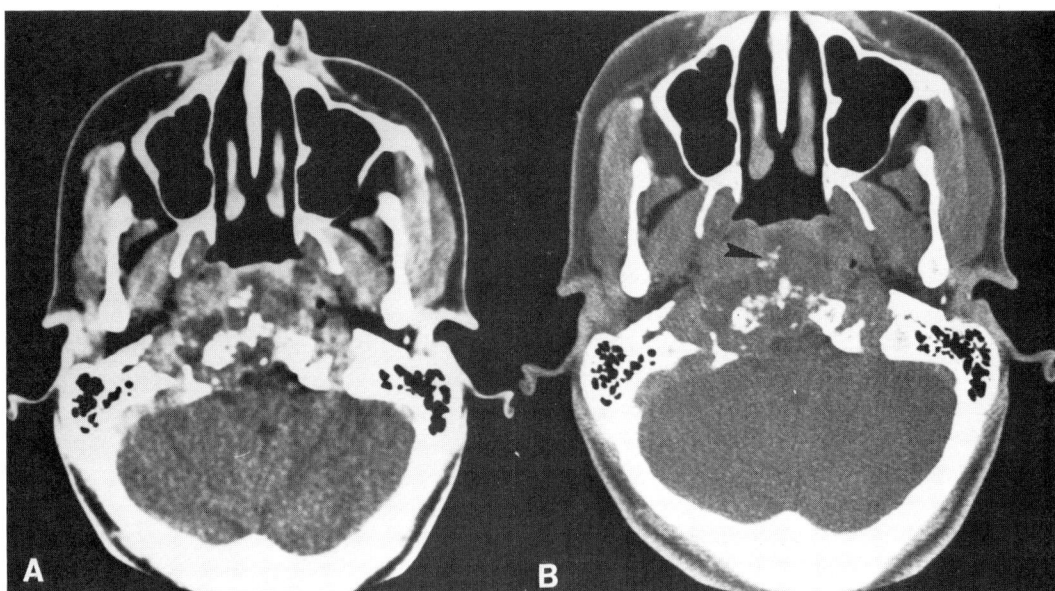

Figure 1A, B: Chordoma of the lower clivus. CT scanning in the axial projection utilizing soft tissue **(A)** and bone **(B)** algorithms, along with direct coronal scanning **(C)**, demonstrate a large inhomogeneously enhancing soft tissue mass extending into the nasopharynx. The extensive bone destruction of the lower clivus and contiguous petrous bones is well demonstrated with the bone algorithm **(B)**. There are areas of calcification within the neoplasm (B and C, arrowheads). MRI imaging in the sagittal plane **(D)** nicely demonstrates the site of origin of the tumor and its relationship to the brain stem and nasopharynx. This image was obtained utilizing a partial saturation technique (GE 1.5 T Scanner, T_R600 ms, T_E25 ms) so that the image is relatively T_1-weighted. The neoplasm has a longer T_1 than does normal brain. The third echo of an MRI axial spin echo series **(E)** is a relatively T_2-weighted image (GE 1.5 T Scanner, T_R2500, T_E75 ms). The high intensity of the neoplasm indicates a long T_2. Its extension laterally into the petrous bones and posteriorly towards the spinal cord is well demonstrated. Right common carotid angiography **(F)** demonstrates an avascular mass which displaces the cavernous portion of the right internal carotid artery (arrowhead) laterally to a mild degree.

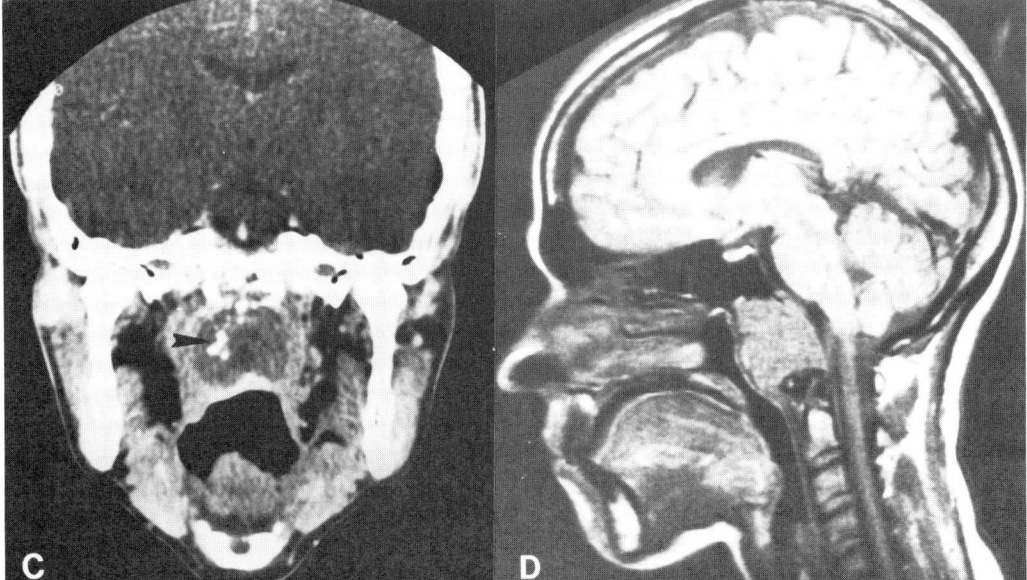

Figures 1C, D.

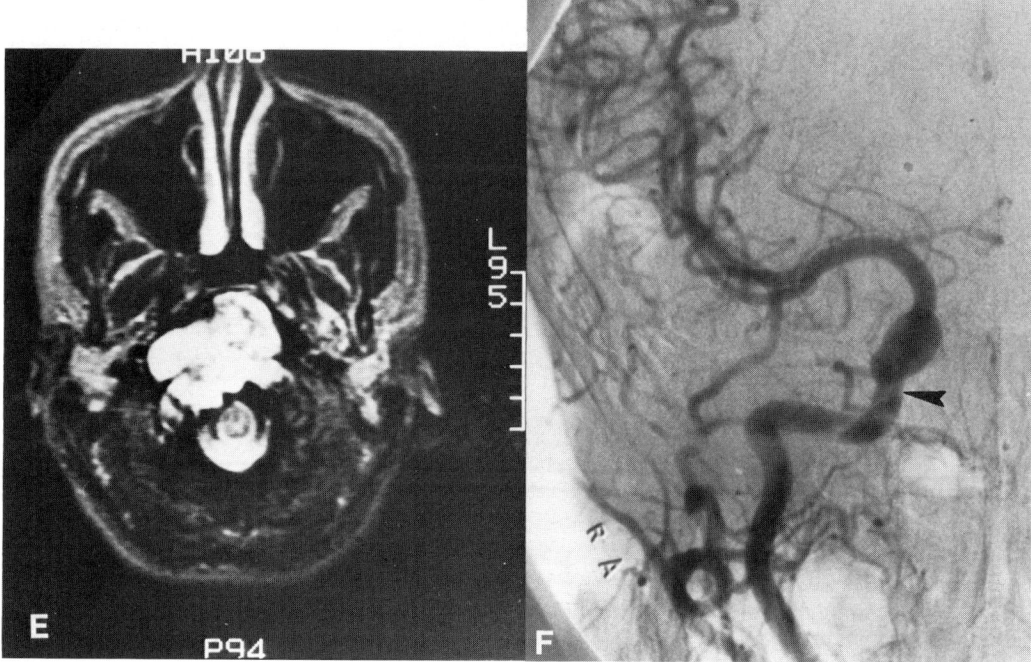

Figures 1E, F.

tecting the presence of calcium either within a tumor mass or in the wall of an aneurysm (Fig. 2). Occasionally, however, CT is unable to resolve tiny soft tissue structures or lesions. A water-soluble contrast material such as metrizamide may be placed into the thecal sac, run into the intracranial subarachnoid cisterns, with subsequent CT scanning in the axial and/or coronal projections. Such a technique may allow the evaluation of a subtle mass involving the optic chiasm, determination of the position of the cerebellar tonsils, visualization of the relationship of a neoplasm to the brain stem, or the demonstration of a small isodense mass such as a hamartoma involving the tuber cinereum. CT cisternography may also demonstrate the confines of an encephalocele.[1]

CT scanning may also be used for a volumetric determination of a soft tissue mass for subsequent radiation therapy (Fig. 5). Such volumetric determination by CT is equal to or greater in accuracy than intracystic radionuclide deposition at the time of stereotactic cyst puncture.[2]

Magnetic Resonance Imaging

Magnetic resonance imaging has quickly become the best modality for demonstrating soft tissue anatomy. There is no question that MRI has the best contrast resolution of all imaging techniques for intracranial work and is therefore the best method for evaluating and characterizing the soft tissue components of a skull base neoplasm (Figs. 1, 3). It is excellent for demonstrating structures in which there is flowing blood, and allows for multiple projections, particularly the coronal and sagittal projections, without the need for reformatted images (Figs. 1, 3).[3] MRI is not as good as CT for the spatial resolution of small structures, and because of its inability to detect a strong signal from bony structures, it is not as good as CT for definition of the bony anatomy of the skull base. MRI will not detect any but the largest accumulations of intratumoral calcium, and it is impossible to angle the gantry for unusual projections.

We believe that the best MRI is provided by a magnet with high field

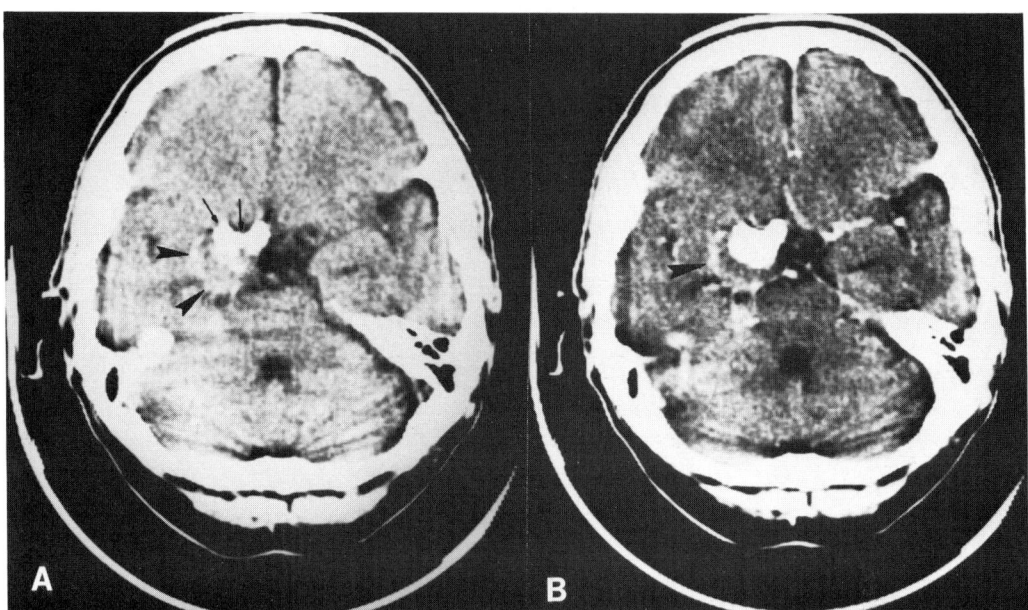

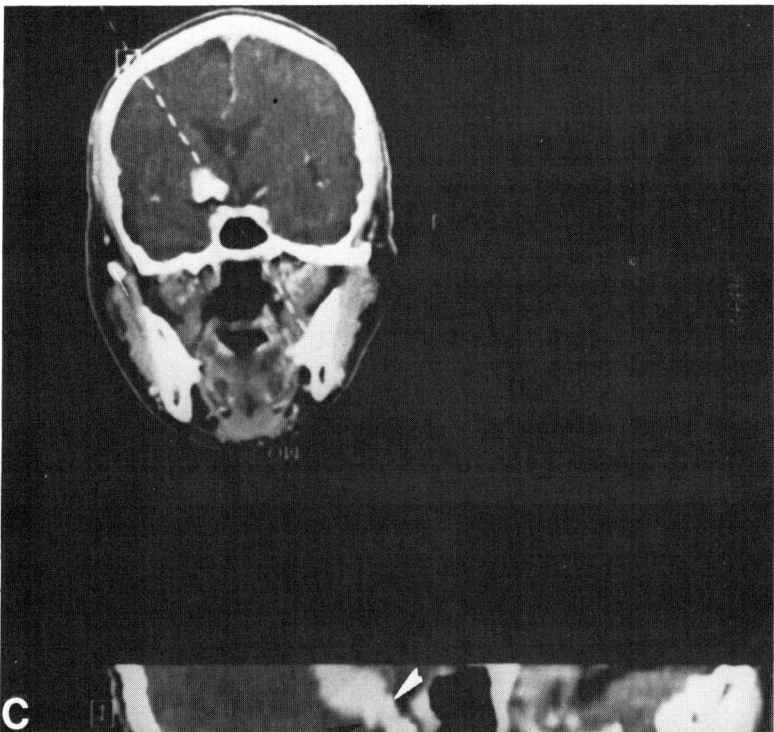

Figure 2A, B: Partially thrombosed, calcified right parasellar internal carotid artery aneurysm. CT scanning in the axial projection without **(A)** and with **(B)** contrast enhancement demonstrates the right parasellar aneurysm. Calcification is present (A, arrows), and there is enhancement in the medial portion of the aneurysm (B) indicating the residual lumen. The dense outer wall of the aneurysm (A and B, arrowheads) is separated from the lumen by thrombus. A direct coronal scan was utilized to produce an oblique coronal reformatted image **(C)**. This reformatted image allows visualization of the tortuous neck of the aneurysm and the demonstration of calcification within that neck (arrowheads).

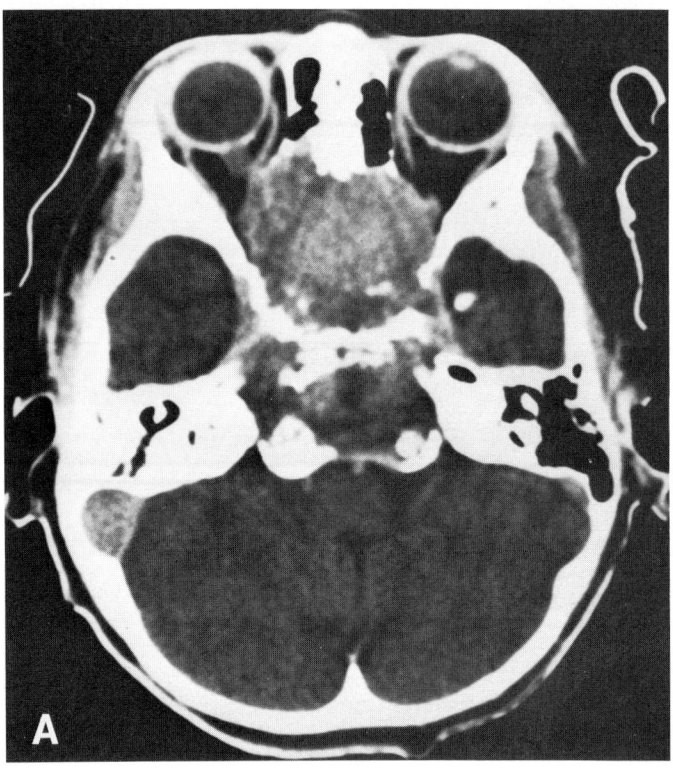

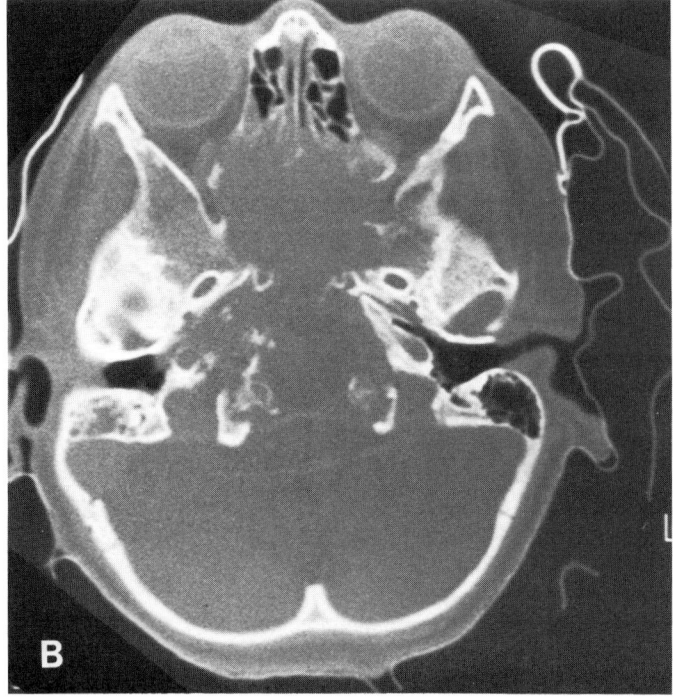

Figure 3A, B: Chordoma of the body of the sphenoid in a 3-year-old child. CT scanning in the axial plane with contrast enhancement was performed, with both soft tissue **(A)** and bone **(B)** algorithms utilized. The large inhomogeneous soft tissue mass extends anteriorly into the face (A), and the extensive bone destruction of the base of the skull is well demonstrated with the bone algorithm (B). (continued)

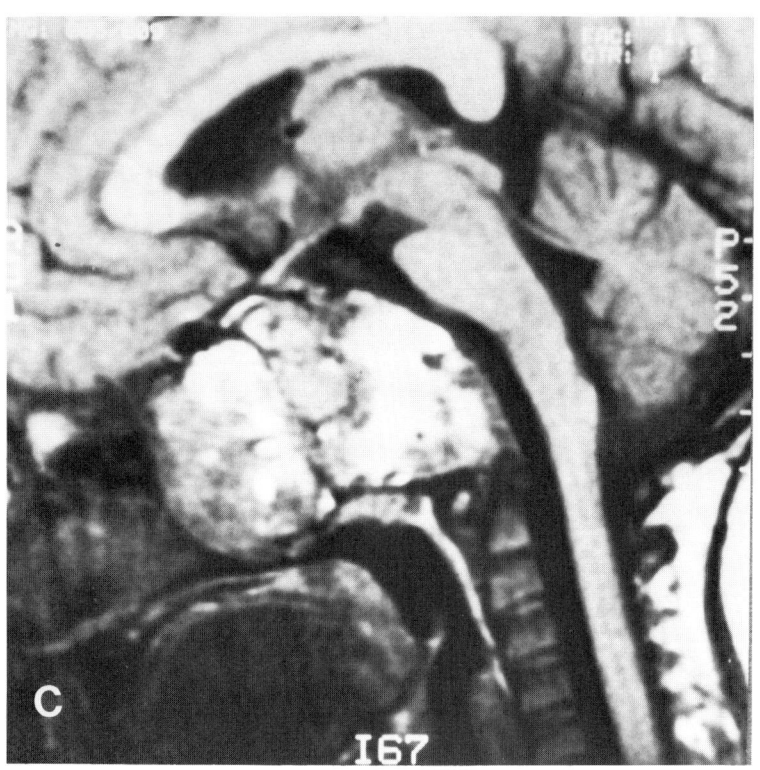

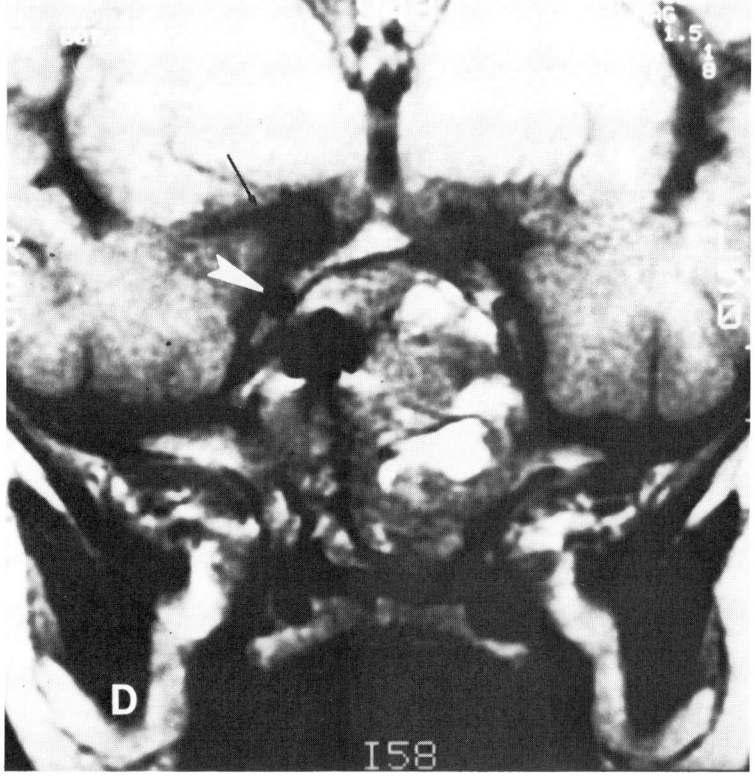

Figure 3C, D: MRI images utilizing the partial saturation technique (GE 1.5 T Scanner, T_R600 ms, T_E25 ms) have been obtained in both the sagittal **(C)** and coronal **(D)** projections. The large neoplasm is inhomogeneous, with the high intensity portions representing mucoid material, not blood, at the time of surgery. There is excellent demonstration of the extent of the tumor anteriorly and posteriorly. The intracavernous right internal carotid artery (D, arrowhead) and internal carotid bifurcation (D, arrow) are well demonstrated.

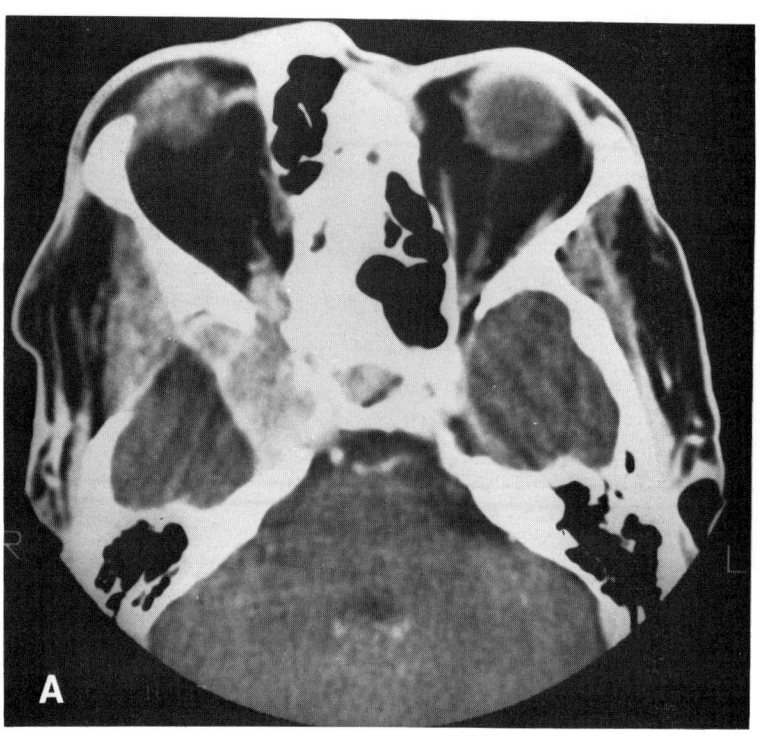

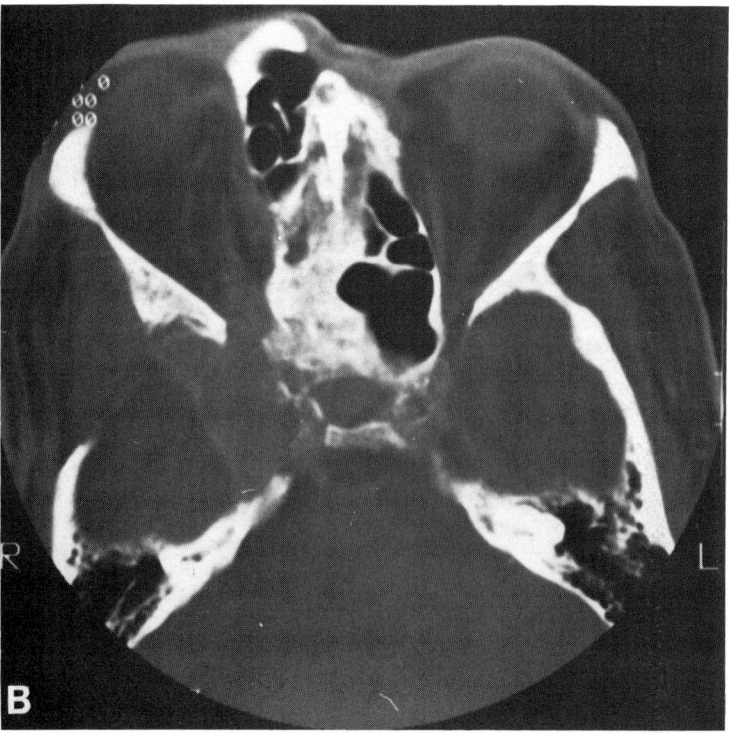

Figure 4A, B: Right parasellar meningioma with intra-orbital extension and bony hyperostosis. Enhanced CT scanning in the axial projection was obtained with both soft tissue **(A)** and bone **(B)** algorithms utilized. The large homogeneously enhancing soft tissue mass extends medially into the sella and anteriorly into the orbit through a widened right superior orbital fissure (A). The extensive bony hyperostosis of all of the contiguous bony structures is well demonstrated (B).

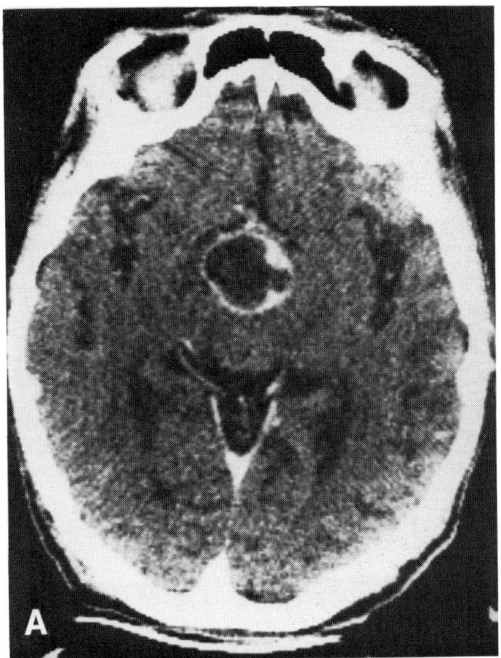
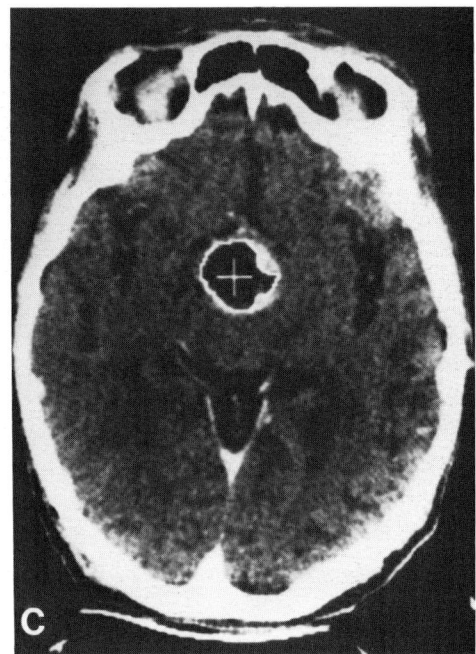

Figures 5A, 5C.

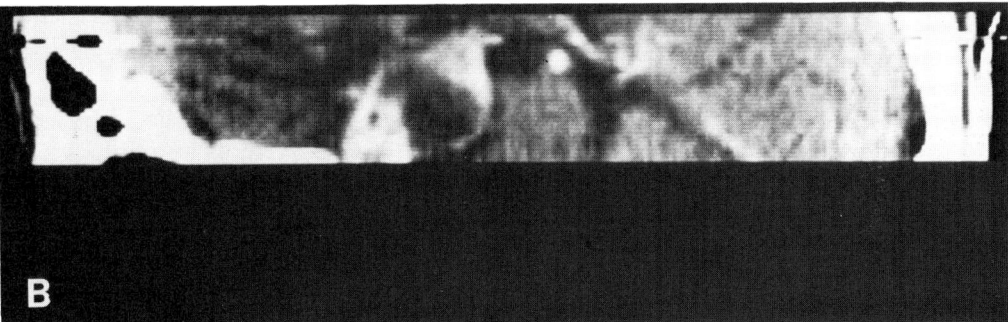

Figure 5B: Cystic craniopharyngioma with volumetric determination. Axial enhanced CT scanning **(A)** demonstrates the large cystic craniopharyngioma in the suprasellar space. Coronal reformatted imaging **(B)** could be utilized to determine the cyst volume. For greater accuracy, however, each contiguous 3 mm axial image through the mass is used, with the trackball method of encircling the cyst employed **(C)**. The cyst area in each slice is plotted and multiplied by the slice thickness to give volume; summation of these volumes results in the total cyst volume.

strength. All of the work at our institution is performed on 1.5 Tesla unit. Evaluation of neoplasms of the skull base requires thin slices such as 3 mm cuts with 1 mm of space between each cut, or contiguous slices with an interleaving technique. Relatively T_1-weighted images are obtained utilizing the partial saturation technique. Multi-echo, multi-level slices are obtained with four spin echos for appropriate determination of T_1 and T_2 characteristics (Fig. 6). The T_1 and T_2 characteristics allow for the distinction of fat versus other soft tissue components within a lesion, CSF-like fluid versus cystic or necrotic regions, and the presence of both static and flowing blood.[3] A major question continues, however, as to the

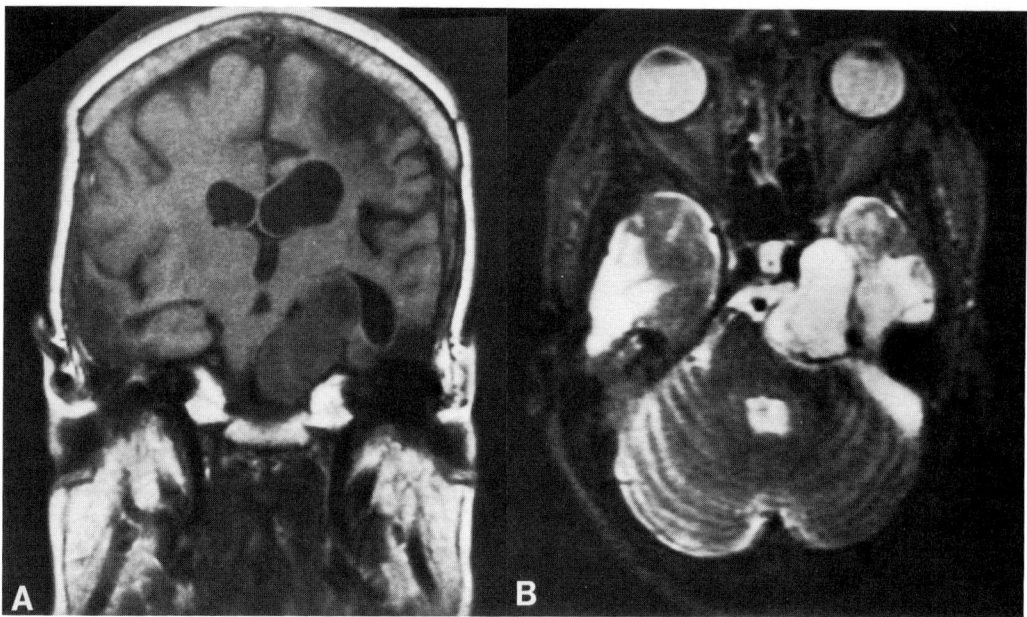

Figure 6A, B: MRI of trigeminal schwannoma. Coronal imaging **(A)** was performed using the partial saturation technique (GE 1.5 T Scanner, T_R600 ms, T_E25 ms). The fourth echo of a spin echo axial series (GE 1.5 T Scanner, T_R3500 ms, T_E100 ms) is shown in **B**. The images nicely demonstrate the sharp margintion of the left parasellar trigeminal schwannoma. The T_1 of the lesion is longer than brain but shorter than CSF (A), while the T_2 of the lesion (B) is almost as long as CSF.

specificity of relaxation parameters in the determination of histology. Morphologic characteristics remain the major parameter for preoperative histologic assessment, as in CT.

While MRI is a relatively difficult technique, requires relatively long scanning times, and is expensive, its greatest sensitivity to the presence of soft tissue abnormalities has quickly made it of immense value in the evaluation of neoplasms at the base of the skull. Today, we utilize MRI for soft tissue evaluation of skull base tumors, followed by CT to demonstrate bony anatomy.

Cerebral Angiography

Cerebral angiography has three major roles in evaluating lesions at the skull base. The first is to define the relationship of the mass to major vascular structures such as the carotid (Fig. 1) and basilar arteries and their branches, and the cavernous sinuses. The second role is the exclusion of an aneurysm as an etiology of an enhancing mass on a CT scan. However, angiography may be supplanted by dynamic CT in which rapid filling of an aneurysm by a bolus of contrast material may be seen, and by MRI which may differentiate an aneurysm from a neoplasm by the presence of flowing blood. The third role is the definition of the angio-architecture of the soft tissue mass. For example, many meningiomas exhibit a typical vascular pattern and vascular supply that confirms the CT or MRI diagnosis (Fig. 7). Angiographic evaluation of the blood supply is also necessary for preoperative embolization, as discussed in Chapter 5.

The techniques of standard cerebral angiography are well known. For lesions at the base of the skull, high quality angiography with subtraction views are necessary, and selective injections into the internal, external, and vertebral arteries are preferred.

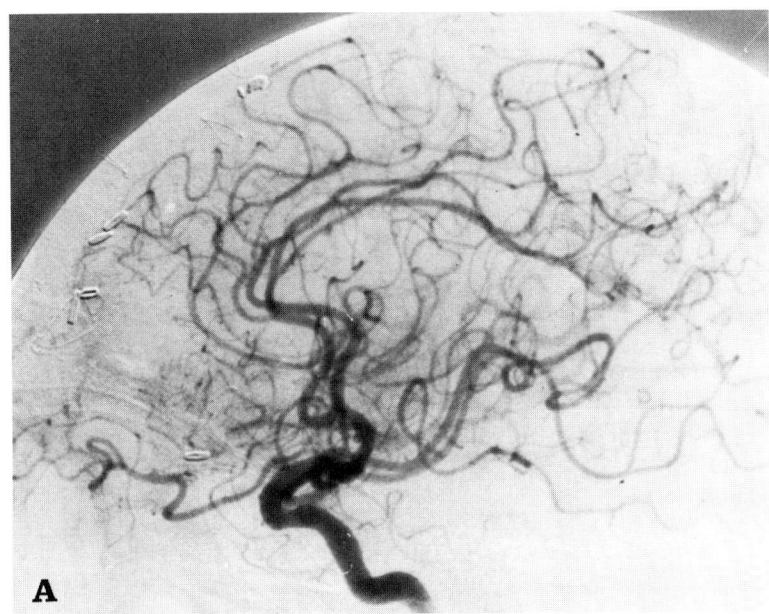

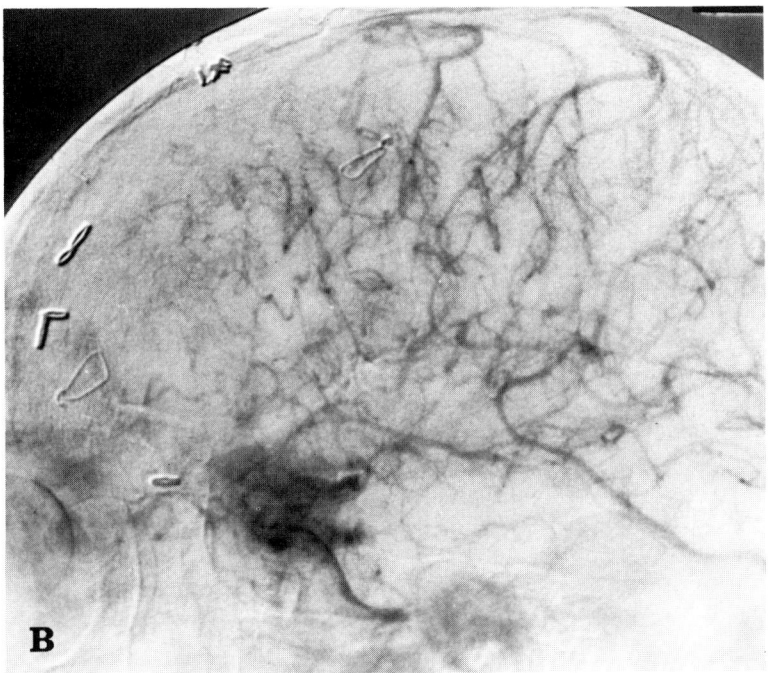

Figure 7A, B: Cerebral angiography of a planum sphenoidale meningioma. Lateral views of an internal carotid artery injection are shown in the mid-arterial **(A)** and mid-venous **(B)** phases. There are small perforating branches of the ethmoidal arteries which come from the ophthalmic artery (A), resulting in a dense, homogeneous stain (B). The findings are typical of meningioma.

A film/screen combination gives the best detail of fine vascular structures. Digital subtraction angiography is a technique that avoids the use of a film/screen combination in favor of a solid-state detector system and computerized manipulation of digitized data.[4] Venous DSA is performed by the injection of contrast material into the venous system with subsequent movement of that contrast into the arterial structures of the head and neck. Because of the dilution of the contrast material by the time it reaches the head, and the overlap of vessels, venous

DSA produces a much lower quality of angiographic detail than does a film/screen combination during selective arterial injection. Venous DSA, however, is satisfactory for the exclusion of a large aneurysm and the demonstration of the vascular structures in relation to the mass. Arterial DSA uses the same technology but with an intra-arterial injection. While not having as high a spatial resolving power as a good film/screen combination, this is certainly a better technique than venous DSA for precise anatomic detail. In our opinion, the complexity of tumors at the base of the skull requires a good film/screen combination for the best evaluation, particularly before undertaking an embolization procedure.

Test Occlusion of Vascular Structures With or Without Xenon/CT Cerebral Blood Flow Determination

It may become necessary during surgery on a complex tumor at the base of the skull to temporarily occlude or sacrifice one of the internal carotid arteries. Some patients may not tolerate such vascular compromise because of an incompetent circle of Willis. Because of this, we routinely perform a test occlusion of the internal carotid artery on the side of the mass during angiographic evaluation of tumors involving the sphenoid and parasphenoidal regions.

A Swan-Ganz catheter is placed into one of the internal carotid arteries after the patient has been systemically heparinized. The balloon is inflated for a 15 minute period of time during which neurological examinations are frequently performed. If there is any suggestion of a neurological deficit, the balloon is deflated and the catheter removed. Stump pressures are also measured through the Swan-Ganz catheter to determine the change in intra-arterial pressures before and after balloon inflation. This is a further check into the possible compromise of cerebral blood flow during surgical compromise of an internal carotid artery.

The production of a neurological deficit during balloon inflation requires an extreme degree of change of cerebral perfusion. The lack of such a deficit, however, does not mean that significant changes in flow reserve are not occurring. If these were to be combined with postoperative hypotension or decreased cardiac output following carotid ligation, cerebral infarction might occur. An additional method of evaluation of the adequacy of cerebral blood flow is provided by the xenon/CT cerebral blood flow (CBF) technique. The xenon/CT CBF analysis is a technique that allows for the rapid determination of the adequacy of cerebral blood flow secondary to vascular compromise.[5]

After the test occlusion with the Swan-Ganz catheter, the balloon is deflated and the patient moved to the CT scan suite. He breathes a 31% concentration of stale xenon, mixed with 68% oxygen and 1% CO_2. This inhalation over a 4 minute period of time is performed while the patient is scanned at two or three levels. Multiple scans are obtained at each level during the 4 minutes, utilizing dynamic scanning techniques. A computer program utilizes the end-tidal xenon concentration as an approximation of the intra-arterial concentration, along with the change of attenuation coefficients of the brain during the perfusion of xenon into the cerebral parenchyma. A blood flow map is produced that shows flow to each cubic centimeter of brain scanned (Fig. 8). The study is then repeated with the balloon inflated to show the change of cerebral perfusion with the temporary carotid occlusion (Fig. 8). This serves as a further evaluation of the degree of blood flow compromise from carotid ligation and gives evidence for the degree of risk which arterial ligation may produce.[6]

General Radiographic Findings

There are a number of radiographic features that can be evaluated with the imaging techniques previously discussed. These radiographic parameters allow the

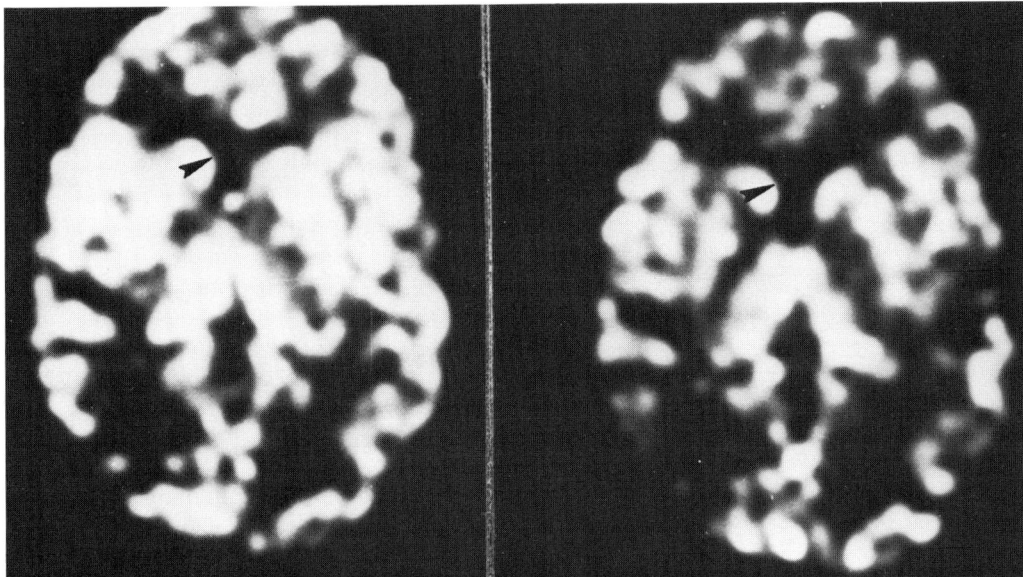

Figure 8: Xenon/CT blood flow maps before and after temporary carotid occlusion. Axial xenon/CT blood flow maps were obtained at the level of the frontal horns (arrowheads). The image on the left was performed before temporary carotid occlusion and demonstrates normal flows to both cerebral hemispheres, with mean blood flows of 50–60 cc/100 gm/min. The image on the right was obtained during temporary carotid occlusion utilizing a Swan-Ganz balloon catheter in the right internal carotid artery. The blood flow to both cerebral hemispheres has dropped to mean values of 40–45 cc/100 gm/min. The equal flow to both hemispheres is indicative of patent communicating arteries.

evaluation of the location and extent of the neoplasm, along with a preoperative histologic characterization of the lesion in many cases.

Location and Extent of Soft Tissue Mass

Even when a mass is extensive, the apparent point of origin or epicenter can frequently be determined. This will establish the appropriate differential diagnosis and lead to better preoperative histological characterization. For example, one may be able to determine whether a mass appears to have started in the nasopharynx or within the sphenoid bone proper. It may be possible to distinguish a mass that has started within the sella turcica because of a "ballooned" sella from one that has originated within the sphenoid sinus or the nonaerated sphenoid bone (Fig. 9).

Bone Destruction

Irregular bone destruction generally indicates that the lesion is aggressive and is probably malignant (Figs. 1, 3). A smooth contour of bone erosion is more commonly associated with a benign lesion. A "ballooned" or "exploded" appearance of residual bony margins suggests a slow-growing benign lesion such as a mucocele of the sphenoid sinus (Fig. 10) or an intrasellar pituitary tumor (Fig. 9). These statements are generalizations, however, and it must be stressed that slow-growing malignant lesions may produce a smooth contoural change of bone, whereas some benign lesions such as nasopharyngeal angiofibroma are sufficiently aggressive to give irregular bone destruction.[1]

An osteoblastic response is characteristically associated with meningioma (Fig. 4).[1] Some metastatic tumors, such as

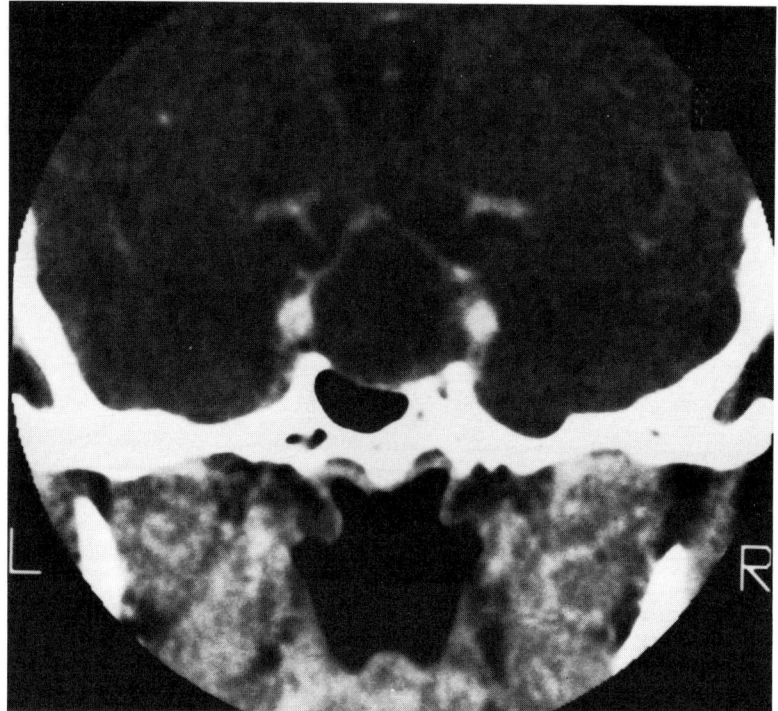

Figure 9A, B: Intrasellar pituitary tumor. A large intrasellar pituitary tumor pushes the diaphragma superiorly and deforms the floor of the sella. Old blood was found within the tumor at the time of surgery, accounting for the low density of the expansion.

prostatic carcinoma, may also produce an osteoblastic response. A focal malformation such as a hypoplastic or atretic segment of bone would suggest the presence of a congenital lesion such as an encephalocele (Fig. 11). A dermal sinus tract with associated bony lesion is frequently found with an intracranial dermoid. Multifocal bony lesions are most typically associated with metastatic tumors, histiocytosis, and hematopoietic neoplasms.

Calcification

The character of calcification within a mass lesion may suggest a particular histological diagnosis. Aneurysms (Fig. 2) and epidermoid cysts commonly have calcification within their walls. Chunks of calcium may be present within a chordoma (Fig. 1), dermoid cyst, or craniopharyngioma (Fig. 12). Confluent calcification may be present in the cartilaginous cap of an osteochondroma, whereas multiple "popcorn-like" calcifications are frequently present in a chondrosarcoma (Fig. 13). Finally, tiny (psamommatous) calcifications are characteristic of a meningioma.[1]

Patterns of Contrast Enhancement on CT

Certain patterns of CT contrast enhancement are characteristic of specific lesions.[1] Homogeneous enhancement is usually present with meningioma (Fig. 4), germinoma, and the hematopoietic tumors including lymphoma and plasmocytoma. Irregular enhancement is the rule with chordoma (Fig. 1). Schwannoma may have either a homogeneous or irregular type of enhancement pattern (Fig. 14). Very intense degrees of enhancement are present with meningioma and angiofibroma, while no enhancement is present with arachnoid, dermoid or epidermoid cysts, or with a mucocele (Fig. 10).

MRI Relaxation Parameters

Most neoplasms have a moderate-to-long T_1 and a long T_2 (Figs. 1, 6),[3] al-

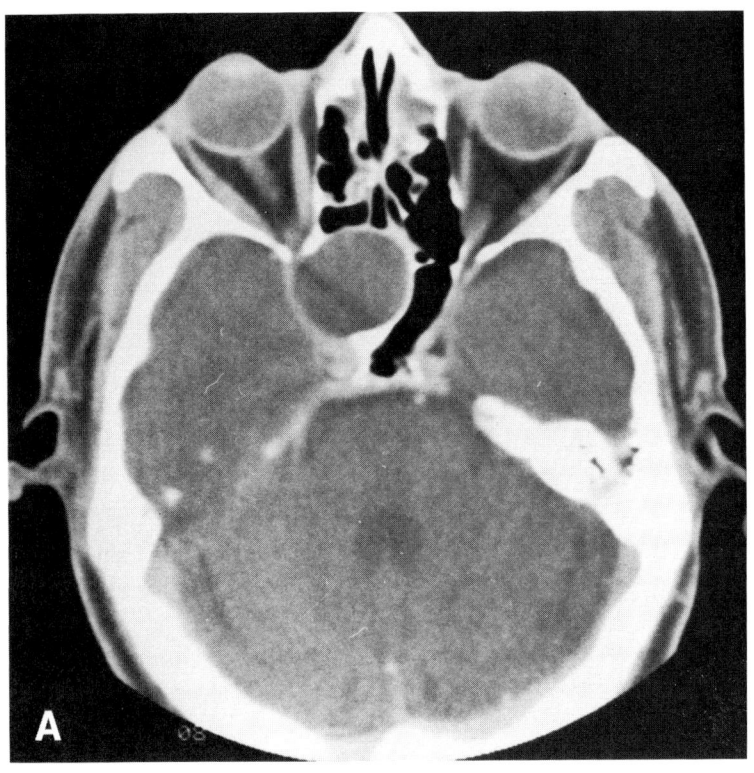

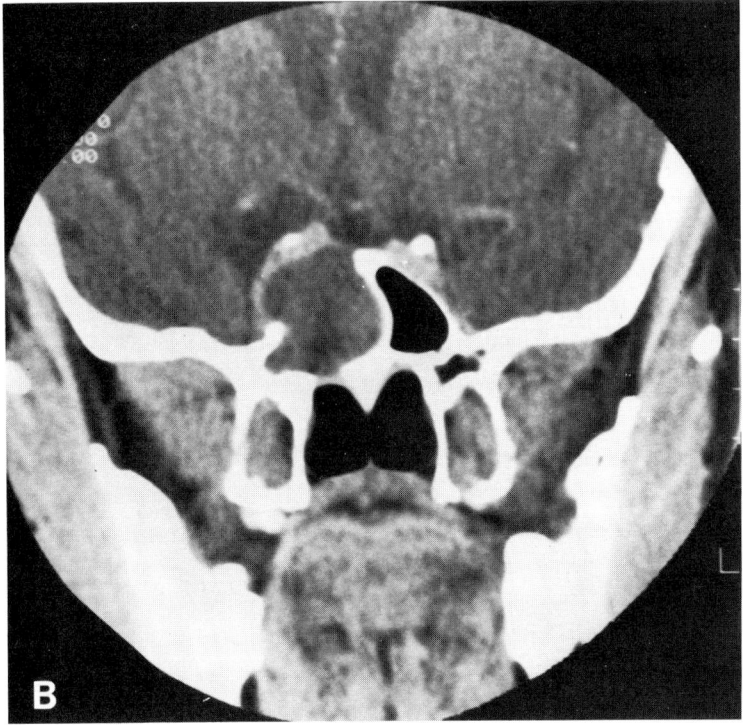

Figure 10A, B: Mucocele of the sphenoid sinus. Axial **(A)** and direct coronal **(B)** enhanced CT images demonstrate the expansion involving the sphenoid sinus. The sphenoid septum and anterior wall of the sphenoid sinus are thinned and bowed, characteristic of a slow expansion. While it might be difficult to determine on one view whether the lesion has begun within or outside of the sphenoid sinus, the combination of views supports an origin within the sinus. The bowing of the bony structures and superior and lateral displacement of the overlying dura further supports this concept. The density of a typical mucocele is equal to that of cerebral parenchyma.

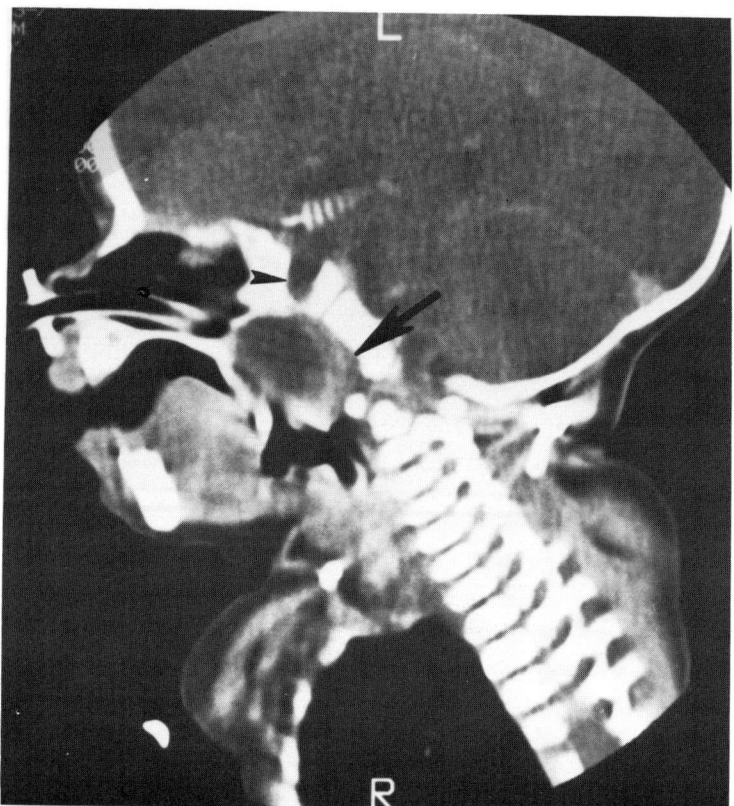

Figure 11: Trans-sphenoidal encephalocele. Direct sagittal CT scanning of a tiny infant demonstrates a soft tissue mass in the nasopharynx (arrow) and a bony defect in the sphenoid bone (arrowhead) all of which are characteristic of trans-sphenoidal encephalocele.

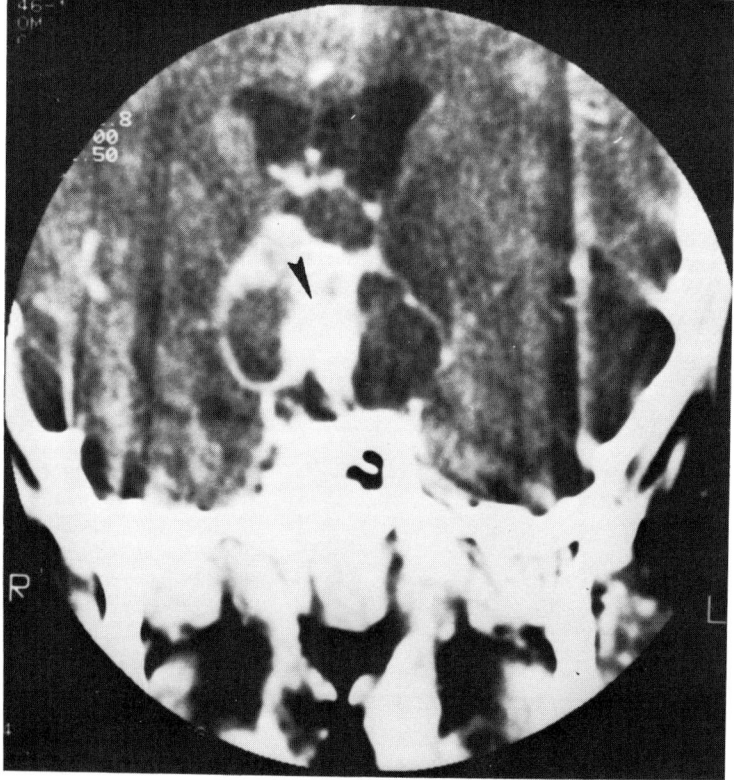

Figure 12: Cystic and calcified craniopharyngioma. Direct coronal enhanced CT imaging demonstrates the classic appearance of a craniopharyngioma having cystic, calcified (arrowhead), and solid components.

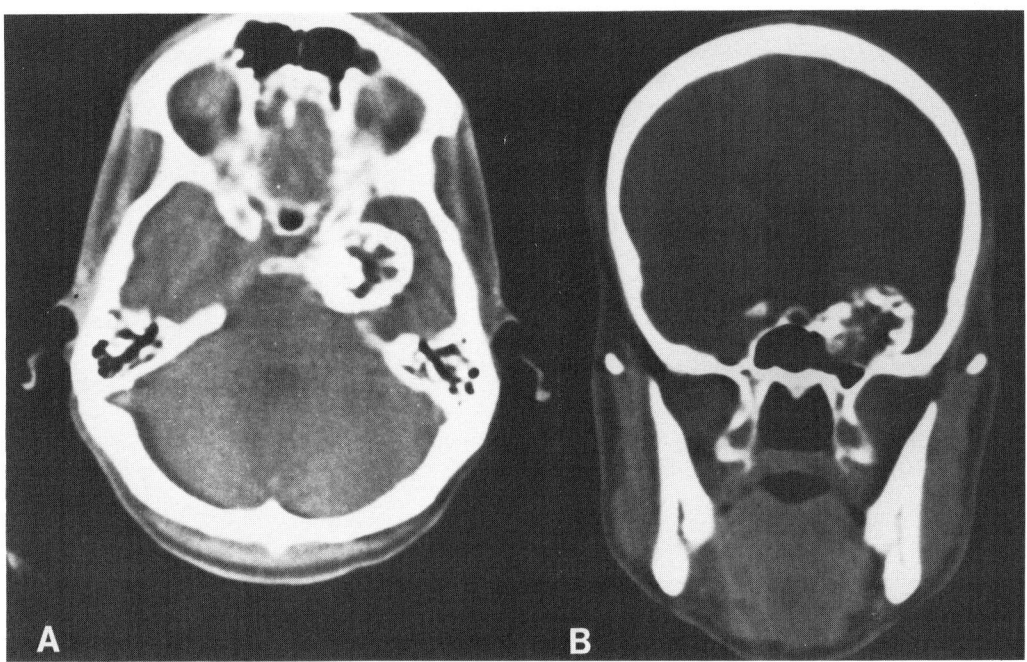

Figure 13A, B: Embryonal chondrosarcoma. CT scanning in the axial (A) and direct coronal (B) projections, utilizing bone windowing, demonstrates the classic location of an embryonal chondrosarcoma originating at the junction of the left petrous and sphenoid bones. There is extensive calcification along the periphery and within this cartilaginous neoplasm.

though a short T_1 may be present with some tumors. While meningiomas are said to have relaxation parameters close to the brain, we have found some meningiomas to differ from cerebral parenchyma in both T_1 and T_2 parameters. In addition, the use of paramagnetic contrast agents such as gadolinium DTPA will make many tumors such as meningiomas much more apparent.

Moving blood is characterized by a long T_1 and a short T_2 with an unchanging character on the multi-echo sequence (Fig. 3). Fat is characterized by both a short T_1 and a short T_2. Water and cerebrospinal fluid have long T_1 and T_2 values, whereas intratumoral cysts and/or necrosis have shorter T_1 and T_2 values.[3]

While it was initially hoped that specific T_1 and T_2 relaxation parameters might be present with certain histological types of neoplasms, such specificity has not been found to date. General characteristics of long or short T_1 or T_2 values are cited for most neoplasms, but there is sufficient overlap to discount the value of specific numerical values. Patterns of T_1 and T_2 relaxation parameters plus morphologic characteristics remain the major criteria for the MRI prediction of histology.

Angio-Architecture and Relationship to Vascular Structures: This has previously been discussed under Cerebral Angiography.

Differential Diagnosis by Area

Planum Sphenoidale, Tuberculum Sellae, Olfactory Groove, and Cribiform Plate

Meningioma

Meningiomas characteristically have dense homogeneous enhancement on CT scanning (Fig. 4).[1] Their extra-axial loca-

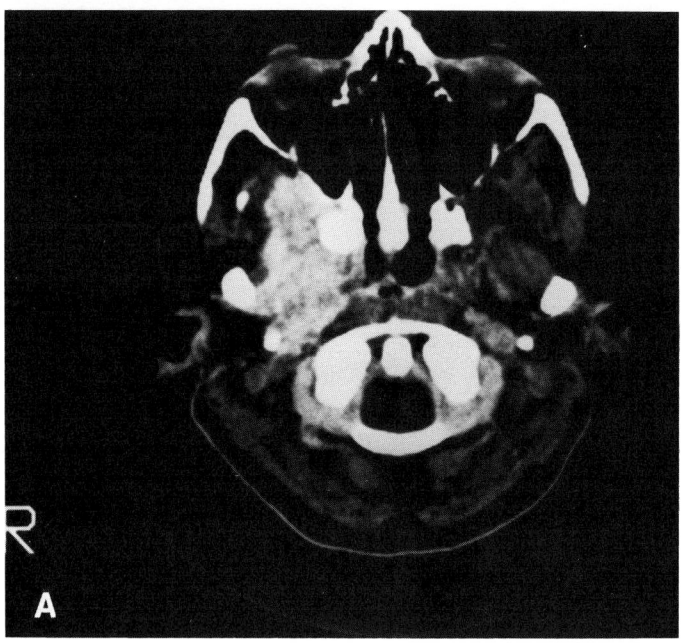

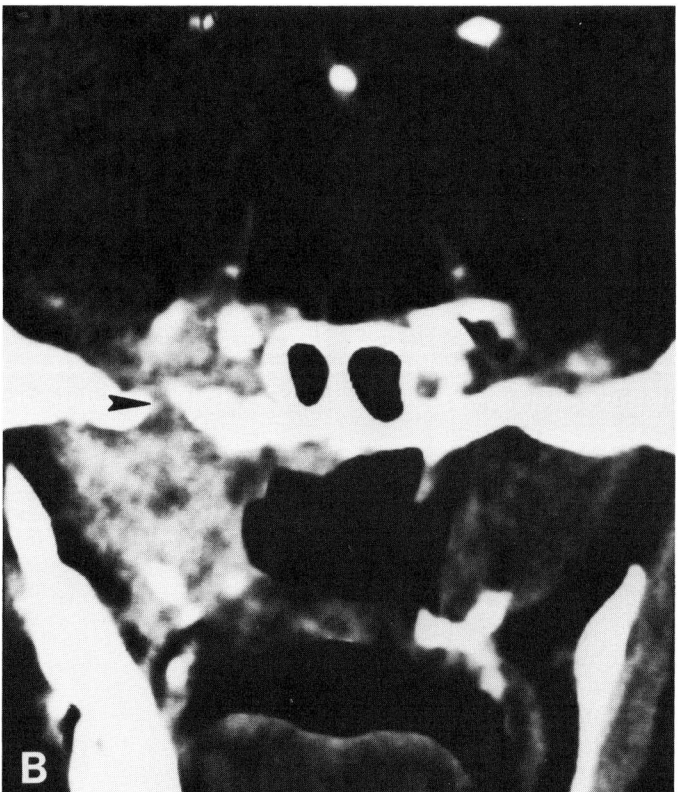

Figure 14A, B: Parasellar schwannoma extending into the parapharyngeal space. Axial **(A)** and direct coronal **(B)** CT scanning demonstrates the large right parasellar schwannoma which has inhomogeneous enhancement, best seen on the coronal view **(B)**. There is enlargement of the right foramen ovale (B, arrowhead), and the mass extends deeply into the right parapharyngeal region.

tion in the anterior fossa is best appreciated on coronal CT and coronal and/or sagittal MRI. Bony change may be present, such as either hyperostosis (Fig. 4) or a "scalloped" deformity of the underlying bone. The angiographic blood supply is generally from ethmoidal perforators, which are second order branches of the ophthalmic artery (Fig. 7). The intense, prolonged stain into the venous phase of the angiogram is characteristic. MRI relaxation parameters similar to cerebral parenchyma are frequent and strongly suggest meningioma.[3]

Esthesioneuroblastoma and Other Nasal Tumors

Esthesioneuroblastoma is a tumor arising in the ganglion cells below the cribiform plate. The mass produces irregular bone destruction throughout the upper nose and cribiform plate. Other malignant nasal tumors may produce the same type of bone destruction. The mass may extend intracranially but remains in an extra-axial location. There may be spread to other portions of the nose or paranasal sinuses.

CT characteristics are that of homogeneous enhancement. Angiography of esthesioneuroblastoma generally demonstrates a mild increase of vascularity or stain. Other nasal tumors are usually avascular.

Tumors of Bony Origin

Osteochondroma has the characteristic appearance of a sharply marginated lesion with a densely calcified cap. Chondrosarcoma produces irregular bone destruction and contains chondroid calcification with a "popcorn" configuration (Fig. 13).[1] Other bony sarcomas may simply produce bone destruction, while osteogenic sarcoma may produce irregular new bone formation.

Encephalocele

An encephalocele in this region generally involves the cribiform plate, producing a soft mass near the glabella. Evaluation of the bony structures reveals a focal bony abnormality best characterized as nondevelopment of that portion of bone. A soft tissue mass is seen extending into the nose and/or intra-orbital region. CT cisternography may be utilized to demonstrate the filling of the meningeal sac and to determine if there is cerebral parenchyma within that sac.[1] However, MRI has now become the procedure of choice for evaluating the soft tissue components of an encephalocele.

Intrasellar/Suprasellar Masses

Pituitary Tumors

This discussion excludes tumors confined to the pituitary gland such as a microadenoma. Tumors extending beyond the confines of the sella, whether into the suprasellar or parasellar regions, or into the sphenoid sinus, are called "invasive" tumors (Fig. 15). The best method of evaluation is coronal scanning with CT or MRI, with better detail of small structures provided by CT but MRI giving better soft tissue differentiation. Axial scanning is also useful to determine parasellar and/or retrosellar extension of the mass. It has long been difficult to differentiate on CT the enhancing pituitary tumor from the dense enhancement of the cavernous sinus. MRI, however, is better able to define the margin of the tumor relative to the flowing blood within the cavernous sinuses and carotid arteries.

The differentiation of a large intrasellar tumor from tumors of other origin is afforded by determination of the epicenter of the expansion (Fig. 15). A ballooned sella strongly suggests that the mass began within the sella rather than within the sphenoid sinus, even though much of the mass may be within the sinus.

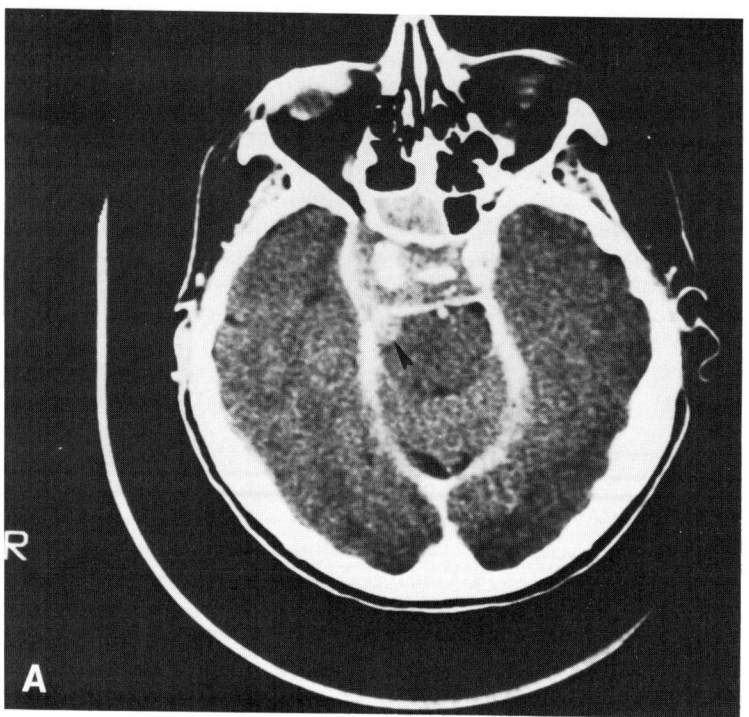

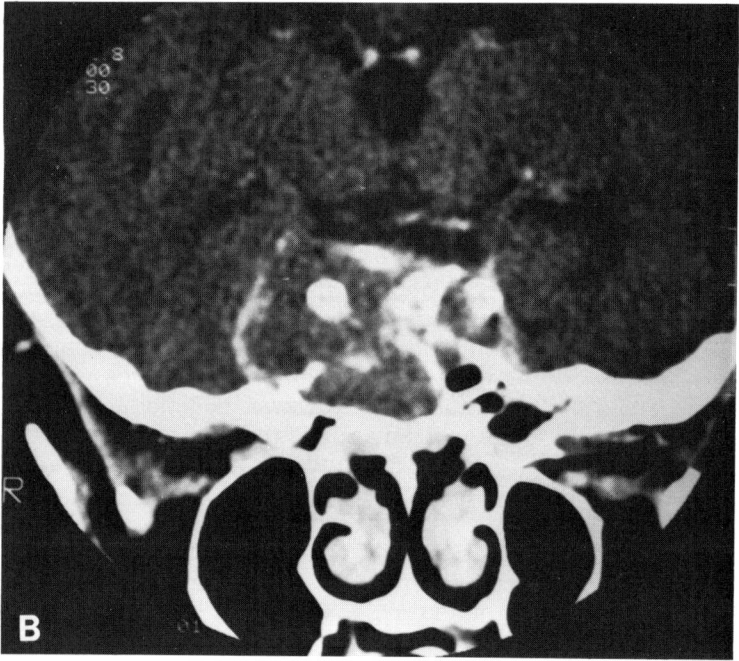

Figure 15A, B: Invasive pituitary adenoma. The large pituitary adenoma has produced extensive destruction of the sphenoid bone, as seen on axial **(A)** and direct coronal **(B)** enhanced CT scans. There is lateral, superior, and posterior displacement of dural structures, along with extension of tumor to course along the right side of the brain stem (A, arrowhead). Such extensive bone destruction, along with the deep extension into the sphenoid sinus, makes it difficult to determine whether this tumor has started within the sella, within the sphenoid sinus, or within the nonaerated sphenoid bone.

Angiographically, there is usually no stain with a pituitary tumor, although cavernous carotid displacement may indicate the extension of the mass laterally (Fig. 1). A densely CT-enhancing aneurysm that extends into the sella may be indistinguishable from a pituitary tumor; venous DSA is an excellent technique for the exclusion of an aneurysm and a determination of the relationship of the mass to contiguous vascular structures.[4] CT may demonstrate calcification within the wall of an aneurysm (Fig. 2). Dynamic CT may demonstrate rapid filling of an aneurysm relative to the slow enhancement of a pituitary tumor. MRI, however, provides all of these benefits except definition of calcification and is noninvasive. In addition, MRI is the only technique that adequately defines a thrombosed aneurysm. Slow enhancement in the wall of the thrombosed aneurysm may produce a parasellar density indistinguishable from a parasellar neoplasm. Slow filling of the aneurysm, as defined by the high intensity signals of slow moving blood on MRI, will give the appropriate diagnosis, thereby excluding meningioma and schwannoma.

Craniopharyngioma

The most common appearance of craniopharyngioma is that of a suprasellar mass containing chunk-like calcification and both cystic and solid components (Figs. 5, 12). Craniopharyngioma may also be purely solid and may have no calcium. CT and MRI are excellent for evaluating the extent of the cyst and defining the relationship of the mass to the infundibulum, optic chiasm, and vascular structures. Volumetric CT analysis of the cyst may aid in the deposition of a radionuclide into the cyst cavity for cyst wall irradiation (Fig. 5). Cerebral angiography is usually of no value.

Meningioma

A meningioma of the diaphragma sella has CT scan characteristics similar to the tuberculum sella meningioma. An aneurysm of the carotid or basilar arteries may be positioned immediatley above the diaphragma sella, mimicking a meningioma. MRI for visualization of flowing blood, DSA, or dynamic CT are helpful in excluding aneurysm.

Other Suprasellar Masses

The differential diagnosis of other suprasellar masses includes optic and hypothalamic glioma, with the characteristic bulbous expansion of the chiasm on coronal CT and/or MRI and the extension into optic nerves and/or optic tracts; germinoma, with an intense homogeneous enhancement on CT; arachnoid cyst, which has a CSF-like density without enhancement on CT; suprasellar dermoid which frequently contains fat, calcium, or sebaceous debris, all of which have characteristic appearances on CT and MRI; histiocytosis, which has an intense homogeneous enhancement pattern on CT and may produce multifocal bone destruction involving the sella, orbits, and petrous bones; hamartoma, which is a disorganized accumulation of otherwise normal tissue and, therefore, is usually isodense to brain; and metastasis, which produces irregular bone destruction and/or a rapidly growing mass.[1]

All of these tumors are best evaluated with CT and/or MRI of the region of the sella and orbits. CT cisternography may be necessary for the evaluation of a subtle abnormality of the optic chiasm or the demonstration of a small isodense lesion such as a hamartoma of the tuber cinereum.[1]

Parasellar Masses

Meningioma

Like most meningiomas, the parasellar varieties have intense homogeneous enhancement on CT scanning (Figs. 4, 16). While most have MRI relaxation parameters similar to cerebral paren-

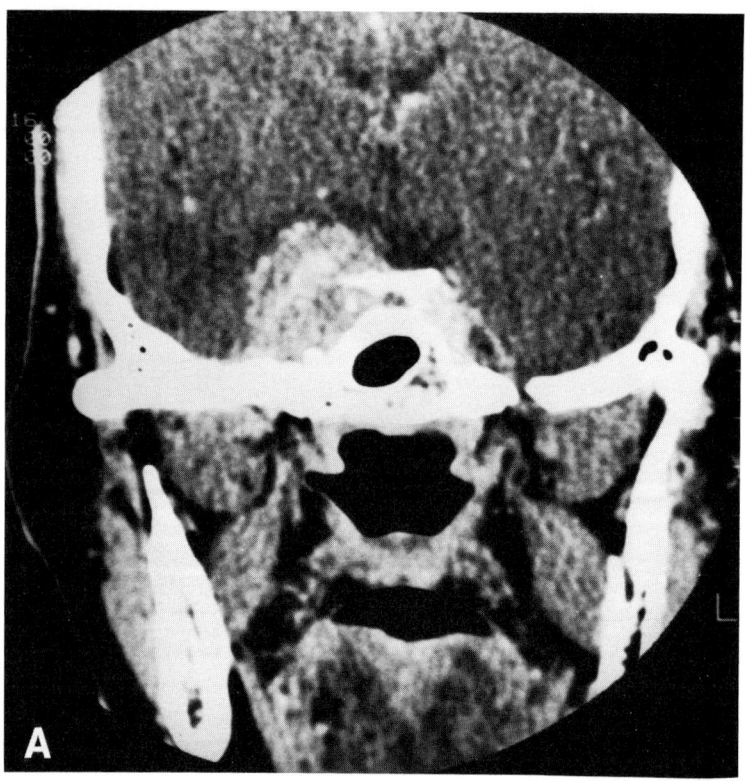

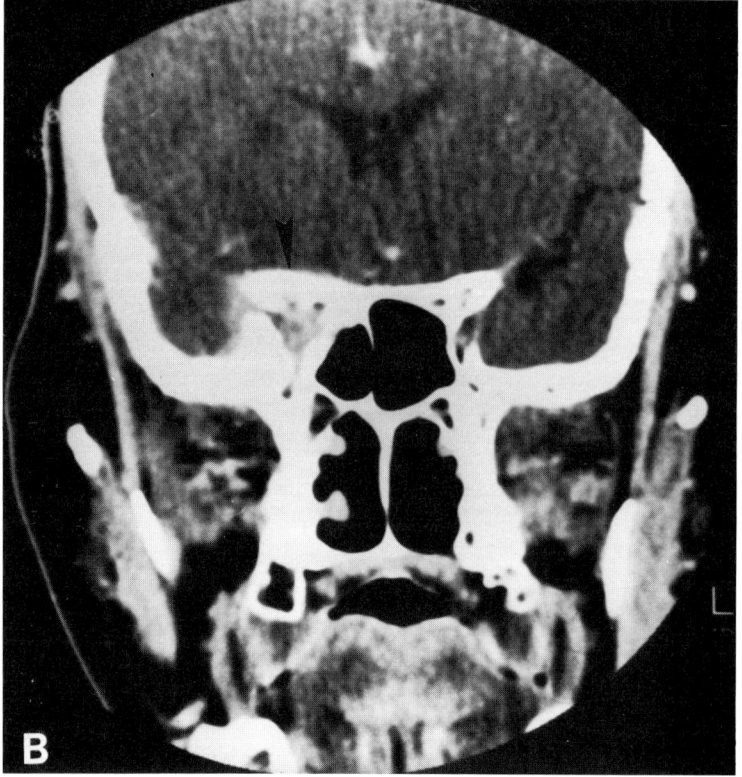

Figure 16A, B: Right parasellar meningioma with bone destruction and intra-orbital extension. Direct coronal enhanced CT scanning demonstrates a large right parasellar meningioma which produces destruction of the right side of the dorsum sella (A). There is extension into the superior orbital fissure (B) with secondary hyperostosis of the lesser wing of the sphenoid (arrowhead).

chyma, variations are not infrequent. Paramagnetic contrast agents will make these tumors even more apparent.

It is necessary to evaluate the extent of the spread of meningioma with CT and/or MRI. Extension along the sphenoid wing may produce bony hyperostosis (Figs. 4, 16). The mass may extend into the orbit through the sphenoidal fissure (Figs. 4, 16), with or without secondary bony involvement, and may even extend deeply into the face similar to a schwannoma (Fig. 14). Involvement of the cavernous sinus is best evaluated with MRI which will define the blood pool within the cavernous sinus relative to the tumor.

Similar CT characteristics are present for both schwanomma (Fig. 17) and aneurysm (Fig. 2).[1] Cerebral angiography, dynamic CT scanning, or MRI will evaluate the possibility of aneurysm and demonstrate the relationship of the mass to the vascular structures. The blood supply to a parasellar meningioma is usually from branches of the meningohypophyseal trunk, and a tumor stain is also characteristic. A schwannoma may have a similar degree of vascularity and stain on cerebral angiography, with blood supply frequently from the external carotid circulation. However, many parasellar schwannomas are relatively avascular as opposed to the hypervascularity of most parasellar meningiomas. Thus, angiography may be useful in differentiation.

Schwannoma

Most patients with a parasellar schwannoma present with face pain. The CT characteristics are similar to parasellar meningioma (Figs. 16, 17), as discussed above. The angiographic features have also been described previously. Schwannoma may spread along any or all of the three divisions of the fifth nerve, producing either enlargement of these structures within the cavernous sinus, or evidence of enlargement of bony foramina (Fig. 14). MRI defines these tumors exquisitely (Fig. 6). While experience is limited, the T_1 and T_2 relaxation parameters appear to be longer than most meningiomas.

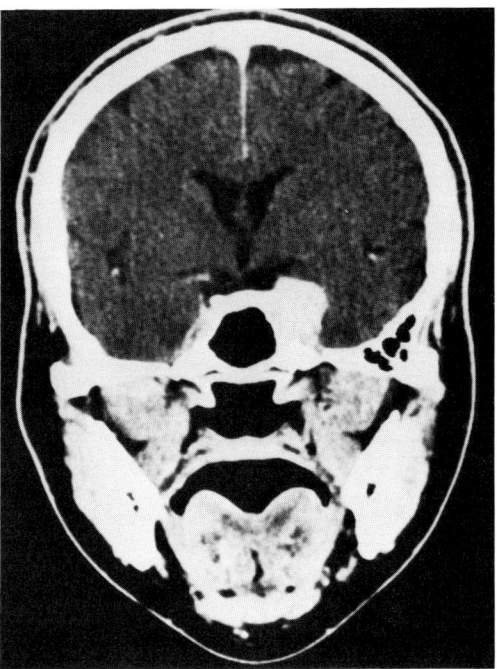

Figure 17: Left parasellar trigeminal schwannoma. A densely enhancing left parasellar trigeminal schwannoma is demonstrated on this direct coronal enhanced CT scan. The lesion has a similar appearance to a parasellar meningioma (Fig. 16), and cerebral angiography or MRI would be necessary for differentiation, if that is possible.

Aneurysm

While CT characteristics may be similar to schwannoma and meningioma, the presence of calcification in the wall of the aneurysm may suggest its appropriate diagnosis (Fig. 2).[1] Some form of angiography, or dynamic CT scanning, will usually allow its differentiation from solid neoplasm. MRI defines both the blood pool in the aneurysm and its relationship to other structures.

Lateral Extension of Pituitary Tumor

Some pituitary tumors have a prominent lateral extension, mimicking the presence of a parasellar meningioma, schwannoma, or aneurysm. Suspicion may be raised by the presence of both ballooning of the sella and bony erosion of the lateral wall of the sella. Angiography to exclude both meningioma and aneurysm is usually definitive.

Metastasis

Most metastases in the parasellar region represent local extension of a nasopharyngeal tumor such as carcinoma or rhabdomyosarcoma, or perineural extension of adenocarcinoma of a paranasal sinus into the cavernous sinus. Evidence of multifocal involvement, with or without bone destruction, is the key to appropriate preoperative histological characterization.

Tumors of the Sphenoid Body and Sinus

Chordoma

Chordoma is a slow-growing bulky lesion that usually presents with inhomogeneity of enhancement on the CT scan (Fig. 1).[1] MRI reveals a mixed pattern of long and short T_1 and T_2 relaxation parameters (Figs. 1, 3). The mass generally produces irregular and extensive bone destruction. Because of slow growth and the late appearance of symptoms, the mass is often large at the time of presentation. The tumor commonly extends into the nasopharynx, and may spread as far caudally as the upper spinal canal (Figs. 1, 3). Multiple calcifications are common, and the lesion is generally avascular on angiography (Fig. 1).

Mucocele

A mucocele represents an obstructed sinus, either because of inflammatory disease or a mass lesion obstructing the sphenoid ostium, such as osteoma of the ethmoid sinus. This produces a "ballooning" of bone, and the appearance of and eggshell of bone surrounding a soft tissue mass is characteristic of mucocele (Fig. 10). The lesion has a CT density equal to cerebral parenchyma and does not enhance unless infected (pyocele).[1] This lack of enhancement destinguishes the mass from most soft tissue tumors arising in the sphenoid sinus such as carcinoma or plasmocytoma.

Encephalocele

The characteristic of the transsphenoidal or sphenoethmoidal encephalocele is the presence of a bony defect extending through the body of the sphenoid (Fig. 11). This well-marginated bony defect contains the tract of the encephalocele which may or may not contain cerebral parenchyma. There may be a low-lying optic chiasm or other abnormalities of the suprasellar tissues, or more extensive midline parenchymal anomalies such as agenesis of the corpus callosum.

A mass is usually present in the nasopharynx (Fig. 11). MRI nicely defines the CSF-containing mass and the presence or absence of brain tissue in the sac. CT cisternography in multiple views may aid in the demonstration of the meningeal sac relative to the bony lesion if MRI is not available.

Osteochondroma and Chondrosarcoma

The characteristics of osteochondroma have been previously discussed, including thick bone with a calcified cartilaginous cap. Chrondrosarcoma presents with irregular bone destruction and multiple "popcorn" areas of calcification. Embryonal chondrosarcoma has a propensity to begin in the junction between the petrous and sphenoid bones, and may have a rim of enhancement and/or calcification (Fig. 13).[1]

Sphenoid Sinus Carcinoma

The unusual tumor begins within the sinus and produces destruction of the sellar floor but without ballooning of the sella turcica, unlike a pituitary tumor which produces sellar enlargement and extension into the sphenoid sinus. There is irregular bone destruction but without the presence of calcification so typical of chordoma.

Hematopoietic Tumors

These tumors include plasmocytoma, lymphoma, and chloroma (leukemic deposit). They all present with a homogeneous enhancement pattern on CT, and they may all extend into the paranasal sinuses and/or orbits. The knowledge of systemic disease may be necessary to make an appropriate preoperative diagnosis.

Metastasis

Hematogenous metastasis to the sphenoid bone may come from any source. A particularly common source in the child is neuroblastoma. Direct extension of neoplasm may come from tumors of the paranasal sinuses or nasopharynx. Rhabdomyosarcoma is a typical neoplasm in the child, while carcinoma is the typical adult tumor.

Angiofibroma of the nasopharynx presents an extremely intense enhancement pattern on CT and is markedly vascular on angiography. This lesion may occupy the sphenoid sinus as extension from the nasopharynx, and may break through the walls of the sphenoid and/or temporal bones to become intracranial in location.

Clival and Foramen Magnum Tumors

Chordoma: See previous discussion.

Meningioma

There is a similar appearance to meningiomas in other locations. Multiple areas of calcification may mimic a chordoma. However, the clivus is usually deformed in a "scalloped" manner, without the irregular bone destruction of chordoma. Angiographically, meningioma is usually vascular, while chordoma generally is avascular. A giant basilar artery aneurysm may occasionally mimic a meningioma and will be demonstrated with angiography. CT cisternography may be helpful in demonstrating the relationship of the meningioma to the contiguous brain stem and/or spinal cord, particularly with a foramen magnum meningioma. MRI, however, gives exquisite demonstration of these relationships and should obviate the need for any further examination.[3]

Chondrosarcoma

Chondrosarcoma of the clivus has a similar appearance to chondrosarcoma in other locations. Particularly noteworthy are the multiple calcifications in the chondroid matrix and the irregular bone destruction.

Metastasis

Nasopharyngeal carcinoma and rhabdomyosarcoma may spread superiorly and posteriorly to involve the clivus. Irregular bone destruction may also be produced by a more benign tumor such as a chemodectoma (glomus tumor). Angiography is of value in defining the relationship of the tumor to vascular structures such as the basilar artery. MRI, however, demonstrates very nicely the relationship of the basilar artery with its flowing blood, and the brain stem, to the soft tissue mass and underlying bone destruction; of particular value is the sagittal view on MRI for all of these structural relationships.

References

1. Latchaw RE (ed): *Computed Tomography of the Head, Neck, and Spine*, Chicago, IL, Year Book Medical Publishers, 1985.
2. Lunsford LD, Levine G, Gumerman LW: Comparison of computerized tomographic

and radionuclide methods in determining intracranial cystic tumor volumes. *J Neurosurg* 63(5):740-744, 1985.
3. Newton TH, Potts DB (eds): *Modern Neuroradiology, Vol. 2, Advanced Imaging Techniques*, San Anselmo, CA, Clavadel Press, 1983.
4. Price RR, Rollo FD, Monhahn WG, et al. (eds): *Digital Radiography: A Focus on Clinical Utility*, New York, NY, Grune & Stratton, 1982.
5. Yonas H, Good WF, Gur D, et al: Mapping cerebral blood flow by xenon-enhanced computed tomography: Clinical experience. *Radiology* 152:435-442, 1984.
6. Horton JA, Erba SM, Latchaw RE, et al: Xenon/CT cerebral blood flow mapping before and after temporary carotid occlusion. *AJNR*, submitted.

4

Radiology of Skull Base Lesions

Hugh D. Curtin, M.D.

Introduction

New imaging techniques have greatly increased our ability to define precisely the extent of pathology involving the skull base. This new capability has been combined with advancements in surgical fields to allow much more aggressive approaches to tumors, raising hopes of changing palliative procedures into possible cures.

The imaging tools currently available include plain films, pluridirectional (complex motion) tomography, computed tomography, magnetic resonance, and angiography. These have been described in Chapter 3 with the exception of pluridirectional tomography, which though replaced almost entirely by computed tomography, is still occasionally useful. Pluridirectional tomography provides very high spatial resolution combined with the ability to image in almost any projection or view.[20] This, however, requires very high density differences. For instance, pluridirectional tomography gives very good images of bony structures but almost no information about soft tissue.

Computed tomography is currently the primary tool showing soft tissues as well as giving excellent spatial resolution (bony detail). Magnetic resonance may well replace CT eventually but is currently somewhat limited in skull base analysis by relatively thick slices and lower spatial resolution as well as the inability to reliably image cortical bone and air. The ability to provide sagittal and easily obtained coronal images, however, represents a definite advantage over CT.

Often the specific characteristics of a lesion along with the identification of the site of probable origin of a lesion can narrow the differential diagnosis to a few possibilities. Choosing the precise histologic diagnosis is becoming less of a priority for the radiologist whose role is turning to definition of the exact margins of the lesion and the relationship of the tumor to vital structures. In this, the radiologist must work closely with the skull base surgeon whose varying approach to a certain location may require precise anatomical information which would not be helpful to someone else.

In this section, differential diagnosis is covered briefly but emphasis will be placed on radiologic approaches to tumor evaluation in various regions. Further discussion of differential diagnosis, especially in the region of the sphenoid and sella, can be found in Chapter 3.

From: Sekhar LN, Schramm VL Jr, eds: *Tumors of the Cranial Base: Diagnosis and Treatment.* Mount Kisco, New York, Futura Publishing Co, Inc, © 1987.

Temporal Bone

External Ear Canal

Tumors of the external auditory canal are very accessible to biopsy. The radiologist tries primarily to define the margin of the disease. CT with bone algorithm is used to detect erosion of the external auditory canal and extension into the mastoid, temporomandibular joint, or into and possibly through the middle ear[1,14] (Fig. 1). The sagittal orientation can be very helpful in questionable cases (Fig. 2). This is difficult, if not impossible, to achieve with CT, so this is one of the few times pluridirectional tomography is helpful.

Tumors can also spread inferiorly. The region inferior to the external auditory canal contains well-defined fat planes and so is easily evaluated with CT.[3]

Malignant neoplasms are the first consideration when a mass is seen with bone destruction but so-called "malignant external otitis" has a very similar appearance (Fig. 3). This chronic pseudomonas infection in elderly diabetics can present with soft tissue swelling, bone destruction, opacification of the mastoid, and extension into the area beneath the temporal bone as well as with cranial nerve palsies.[4] The cranial nerves are often involved as the indolent infection progresses medially through the soft tissue beneath the temporal bone. The process reaches the area inferior to the temporal bone by passing through narrow fissures between bony and cartilaginous external canal. These are called the fissures of Santorini.

Middle Ear and Jugular Bulb Region

Again, in this area, the diagnosis has usually been made before the radiologist sees the patient. Usually the "tumor" is either a cholesteatoma or a vascular lesion such as a paraganglioma (glomus tumor).

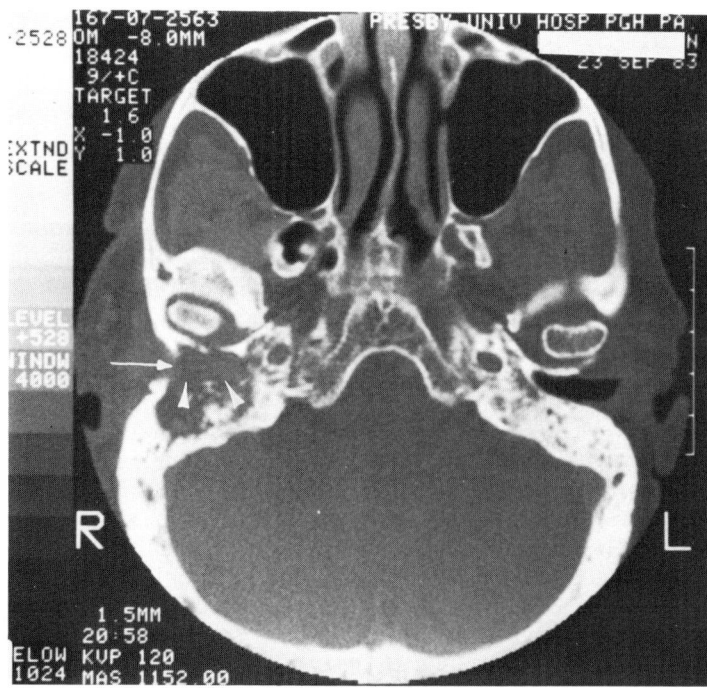

Figure 1: Carcinoma of the external auditory canal. Soft tissue fills the external auditory canal (white arrow). There is bone erosion of the posterior wall (arrowheads) with tumor extending into the mastoid. Note the air-filled external canal on the opposite side.

Radiology of Skull Base Lesions • 67

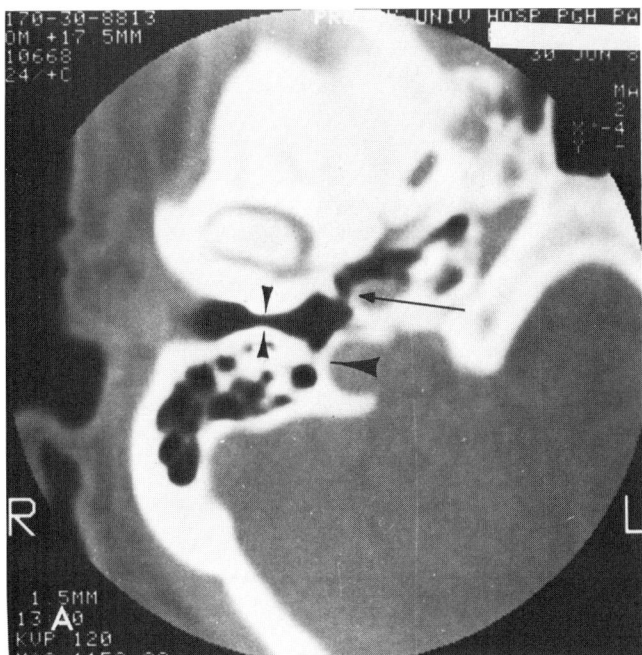

Figure 2A: Exostosis of the external canal. Axial slice shows narrowing of the anterior posterior dimension of the external auditory canal (small arrowheads). Other bony landmarks include the bony wall of the carotid canal (long arrow) separating the carotid artery from the middle ear and the lateral bony wall of the jugular canal (large black arrowhead) separating the vein from the middle ear. (Used with permission.[1])

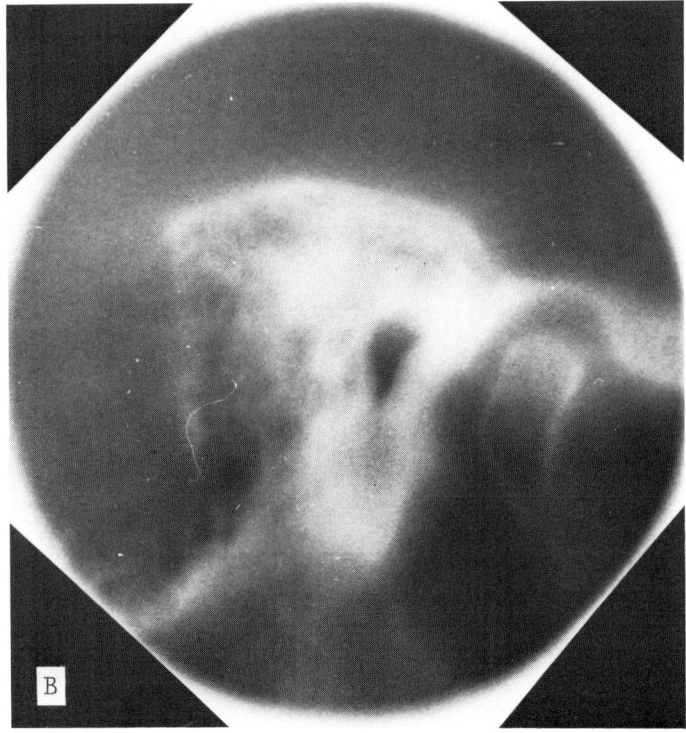

Figure 2B: Tomographic lateral view gives the sagittal section of the external auditory canal which is a true cross-section showing the narrowing of the canal rather than its usual oval configuration. This orientation would be very difficult to obtain with CT scanning. (Used with permission.[1])

68 • TUMORS OF THE CRANIAL BASE: DIAGNOSIS AND TREATMENT

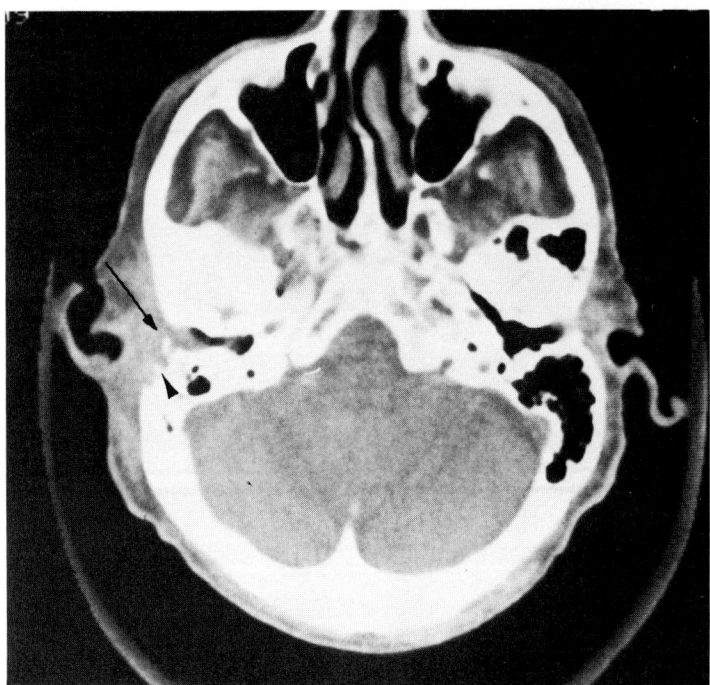

Figure 3A: Malignant external otitis. Soft tissue density in the external canal (black arrow) with erosion of the bony margin (black arrowhead).

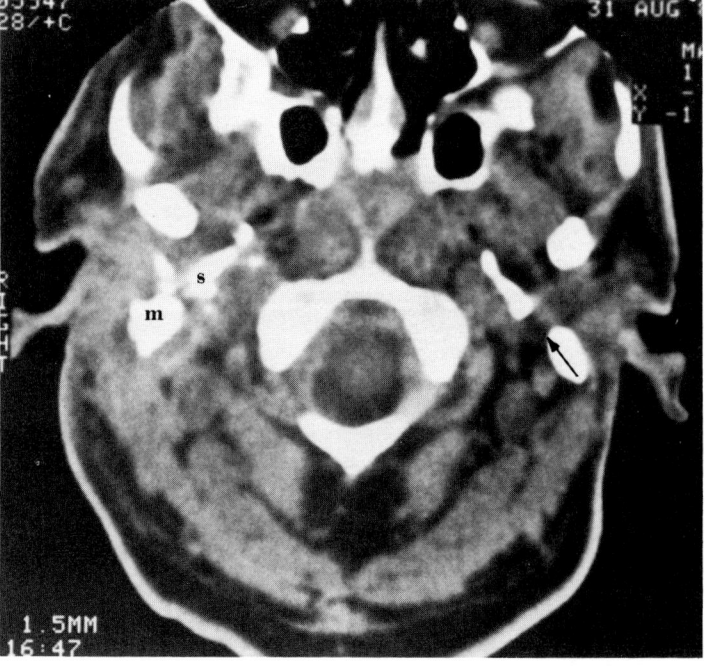

Figure 3B: Lower slice shows soft tissue density obliterating fat planes around mastoid tip (M) and styloid (S). Compare with normal side noting the fat density (black arrow). This is immediately below the stylomastoid foramen. This patient had a facial paralysis on the affected side.

This differentiation has often been made by visual inspection through the otoscope. Other tumors, such as primary malignancies, middle ear adenomas, etc., are extremely rare.

If the diagnosis is cholesteatoma, then the radiologist looks for erosion of the semicircular canals, facial nerve, and tegmen tympani and excludes anomalies such as an abnormal course of the facial nerve which may lead to complications at surgery.[22] Though tomography can answer many of these questions, CT is preferred because of the good differentiation between air and soft tissue as well as the good demonstration of bony structures. The actual margin of the cholesteatoma can often be defined (Fig. 4). Without bone erosion, small cholesteatoma cannot reliably be differentiated from granulation tissue or mucosal thickening by CT.

Encephaloceles must be considered when evaluating masses in the attic or upper middle ear especially in a postmastoidectomy patient. The radiologist must carefully search for defects in the tegmen tympani or posterior wall of the mastoid.

Unfortunately, the tegmen tympani can be very difficult to evaluate. Even in the normal situation, apparent defects are frequent due to the thin bone, even with 1.5 mm slices. The clinician, as well as the radiologist, must realize that both false negatives and false positives will occur. Any defect, especially associated with a contiguous soft tissue mass, must be considered suspicious.

Evaluation of vascular lesions brings us to a brief discussion of two very important bony landmarks, the bony walls separating the jugular bulb and the carotid artery from the middle ear. The integrity of these is the key finding in evaluation of vascular middle ear masses. If the bony wall of the jugular bulb is smooth and not eroded, then a lesion seen in the middle ear is not a glomus jugulare tumor (paraganglioma) but a glomus tympanicum tumor which requires much less surgical dissection to remove (Fig. 5). This determination must be done carefully as these paragangliomas can cause a moth-eaten subtle destruction rather than a large sharply marginated hole (Figs. 6,

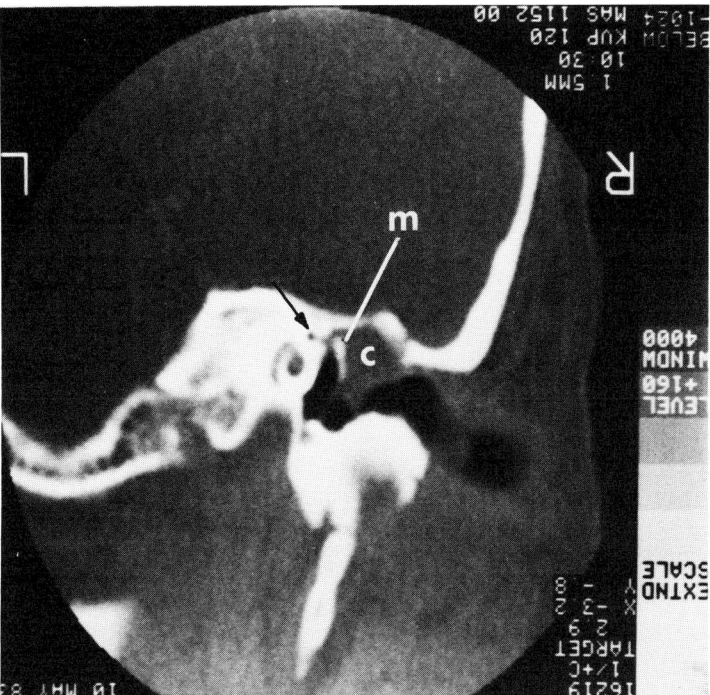

Figure 4A: Cholesteatoma. Coronal section. Cholesteatoma (C) erodes the scutum and fills the attic displacing the malleus (M) medially. Note the two small holes representing the facial nerve (black arrow). (Used with permission.[1])

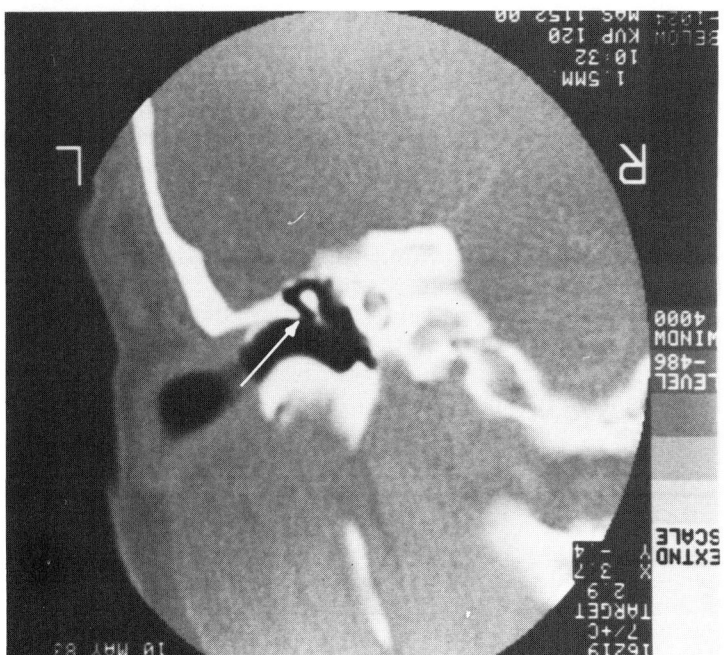

Figure 4B: Compare with opposite side showing the relationship of the head of the malleus surrounded by the air in the attic. The scutum (arrow) represents the junction of the roof of the external auditory canal and the lateral wall of the attic. (Used with permission.[4])

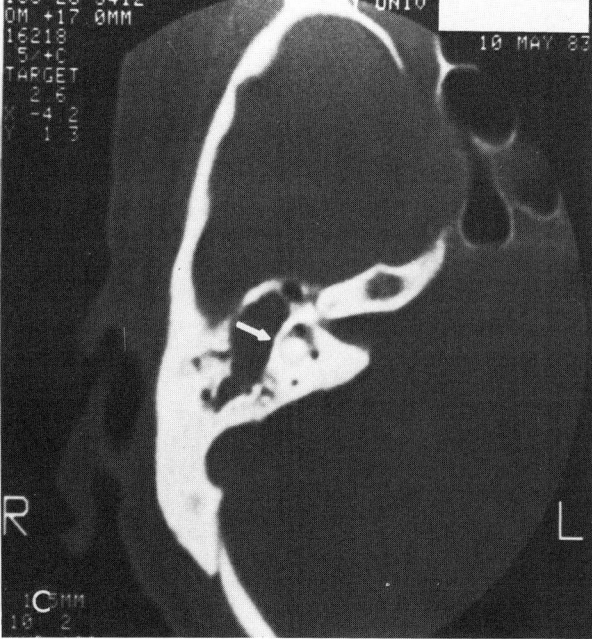

Figure 4C: Axial slice through the attic shows smoothly marginated enlargement of the attic and antrum which is characteristic of cholesteatoma. Note that the bony wall (arrow) separating the horizontal semicircular canal from the cholesteatoma is intact.

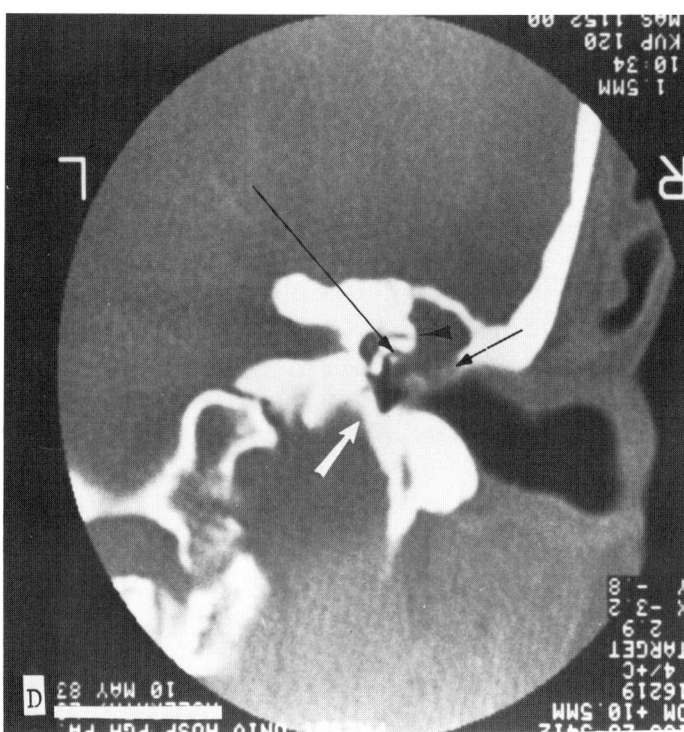

Figure 4D: Coronal view shows eroded scutum (short black arrow). Facial nerve is intact (long arrow). Bone covers the horizontal semicircular canal (arrowhead). Wall of jugular canal (white arrow).

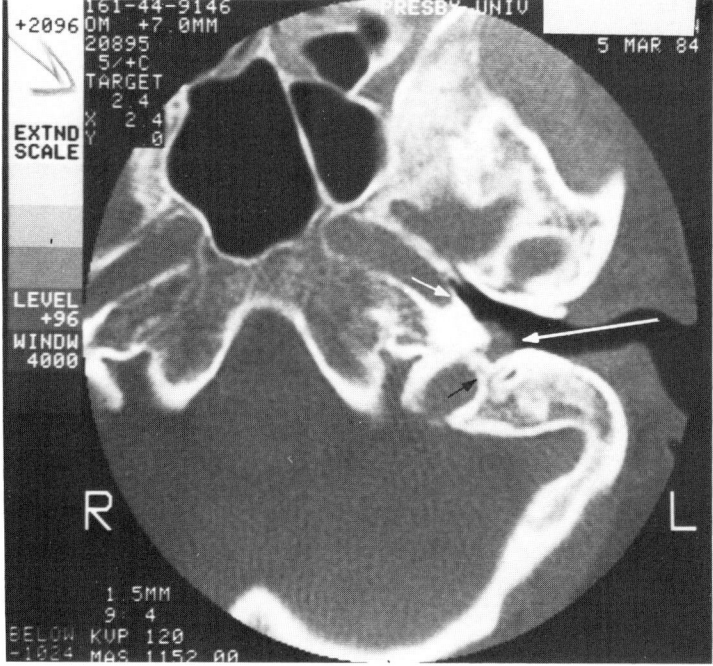

Figure 5: Glomus tympanicum tumor. Small nodular lesion in the middle ear without bone erosion (long white arrow). The lateral bony wall of the jugular foramen (black arrow) separating the vein from the middle ear is smooth and intact. The lateral wall of the carotid canal (short white arrow) separating the artery from middle ear is intact and in normal position. The lesion was confined to the middle ear.

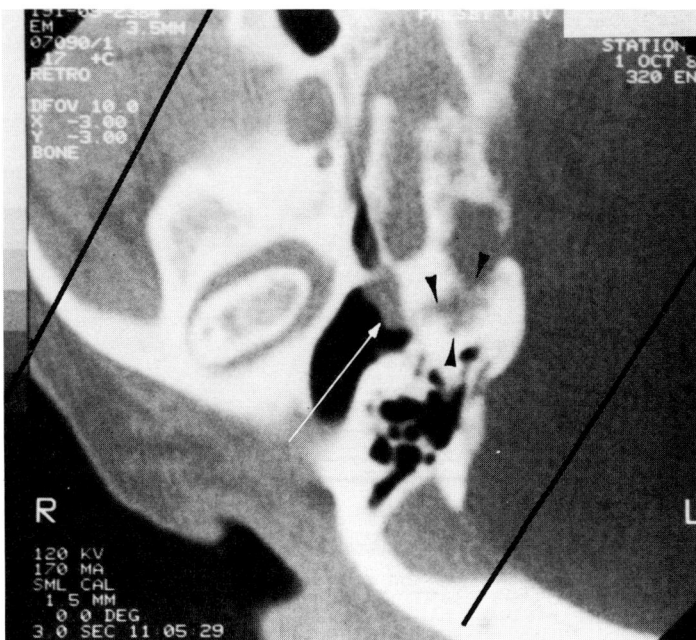

Figure 6A: Glomus jugulare tumor. Nodular mass in the middle ear (long white arrow). Here the lateral wall of the jugular bulb and the bone lateral to it (arrowheads) is indistinct and eroded.

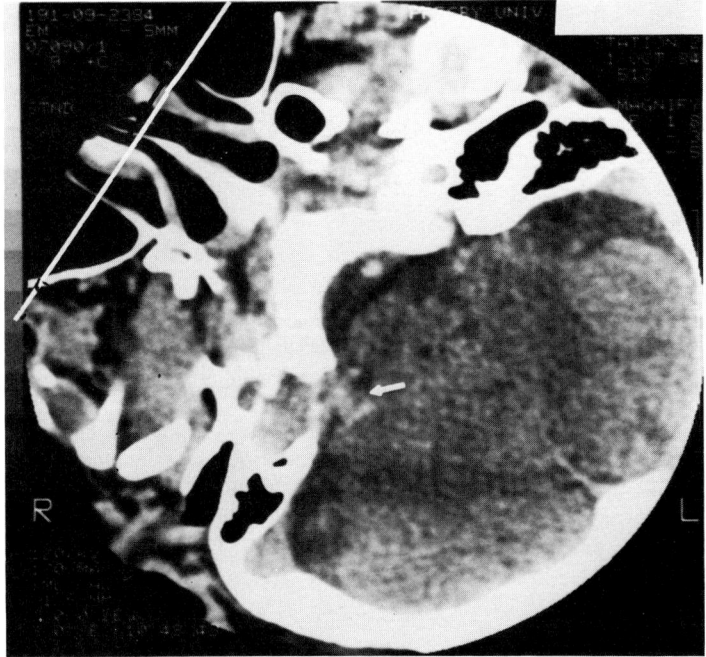

Figure 6B: Slightly more inferior slice than 6A. Tumor extension into the posterior fossa (white arrow).

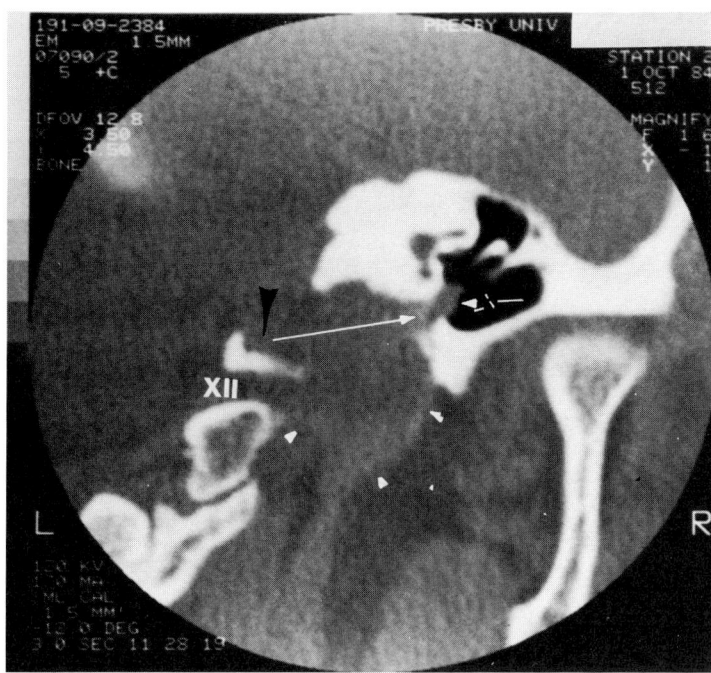

Figure 6C: Coronal view. Nodular tumor (short arrow) which could be seen through the tympanic membrane represented the tip of a glomus jugulare. The lateral wall of the jugular foramen is eroded (long arrow). The tumor mass extends below the temporal bone (small arrowheads). There is also erosion of the jugular tubercle (black arrowhead) just above the hypoglossal canal (XII).

7). If the bony wall is destroyed, then arteriography is done to evaluate the inferior extension and blood supply of this tumor. Some feel digital subtraction angiography is adequate. If the bony wall of the jugular bulb is intact, then arteriography is not necessary. Digital subtraction angiography may still be performed as multiple lesions occur in approximately 10% of cases (see Fig. 18). This is probably not necessary if CT scanning down to the hyoid is normal. If a tumor is involving the jugular bulb and, therefore, represents a glomus jugulare type paraganglioma, certain other landmarks become key. These landmarks are best defined by high resolution CT. The relationship of the tumor to the cochlea, internal auditory canal, and especially the internal carotid artery are very important. The medial extent can be defined by erosion of bone past the pars nervosa and at times into the clivus. Often large tumors will extend intracranially and this component must be measured for surgical planning.

The lateral wall of the carotid canal that separates the artery from the middle ear is also important. If the lateral wall is in normal position, inferior to the cochlea, and is intact, then an aberrant carotid artery present in the middle ear is effectively excluded. This anomaly can mimic a glomus tumor with catastrophic consequences[10] (Fig. 8). In this anomaly, there is a defect in the lateral wall of the carotid canal and the soft tissue representing the artery can often be seen extending into the middle ear. Often the foramen spinosum is absent because of an associated anomaly, the persistent stapedial artery. Here the middle meningeal artery derives its blood supply from the aberrant carotid via a vessel through the middle ear and facial nerve canal rather than from the external carotid via the foramen spinosum.

In summary, if a vascular mass is seen in the middle ear, CT is used to define the lateral walls of the jugular bulb and the carotid canal. If these are eroded or not present, then a vascular study is done.

Petrous Apex[1,20,21]

Lesions of the petrous apex are again best evaluated by CT. These may be primary or may represent an extension of neoplasm from surrounding structures.

74 • TUMORS OF THE CRANIAL BASE: DIAGNOSIS AND TREATMENT

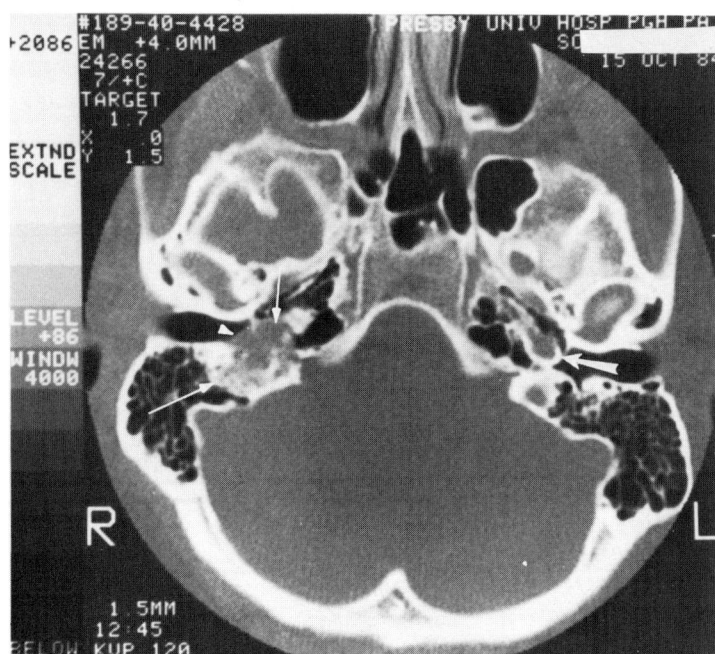

Figure 7: Glomus jugulare tumor. Mass visible through the external auditory canal (arrowhead). Moth-eaten erosion between white arrows. The wall of the jugular foramen was eroded. The wall of the carotid artery was also indistinct representing erosion by glomus tumor. Compare with opposite side (large white arrow).

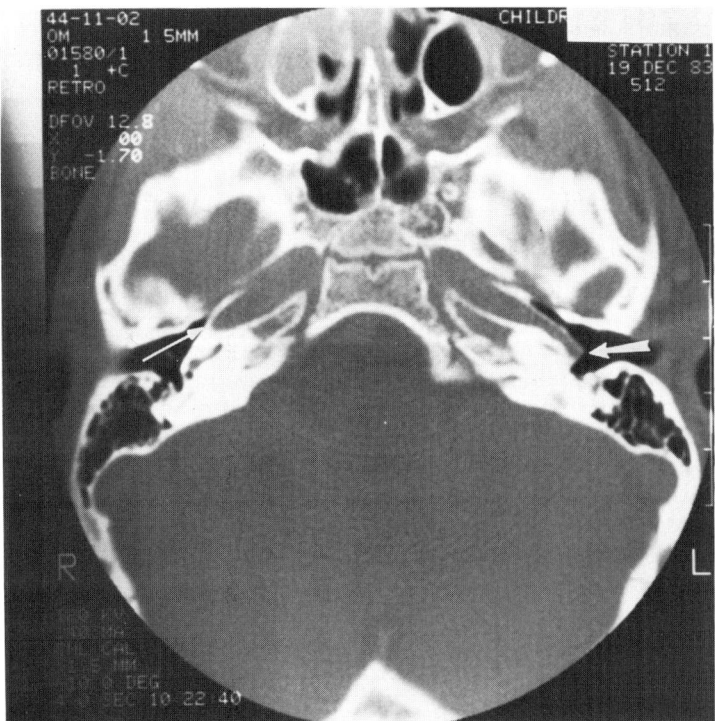

Figure 8: Aberrant carotid artery left side. The carotid artery extends further laterally than usual extending into the middle ear (large white arrow). Here the artery can be visualized as a red mass deep to the tympanic membrane. Compare to the normal position of the carotid artery on the right side (small white arrow).

Here there are two considerations. These lesions are not readily accessible to biopsy or direct visualization, so the radiologist does try to define the nature and the extent of the disease. The location of the lesion is helpful in the differential diagnosis. As stated in the previous section, most paragangliomas erode the lateral wall of the jugular bulb. Indeed the most common presentation of glomus jugulare tumors is as a mass in the middle ear. Lesions involving more medial portions of the jugular foramen are most likely to be neurilemmomas. These often have a more sharply marginated bone defect. Both neurilemmomas and paragangliomas tend to enhance with intravenous contrast.

Lesions with very low attenuation are usually epidermoids (Fig. 9), but cholesterol cysts, mucoceles, and arachnoid cysts must also be considered.[11] Lesions that involve the facial nerve include neurilemmomas, meningiomas, hemangiomas, and ossifying hemangiomas (Fig. 10).

The facial nerve is easy to evaluate with CT if thin sections are used. Lesions arising within the canal, such as neurilemmomas, widen the canal. Those outside erode the sharp margin of the canal. If the sharp margins are identified and the canal is not widened in any section (labyrinthine, tympanum, or mastoid), then the radiologist can be confident that no tumor is present. However, if a section is not sharply seen, the radiologist must equivocate rather than state that no tumor is found. Areas where the facial nerve can be "lost" by CT include the pyramidal or second turn, and occasionally the geniculate ganglion, especially if this area is not covered by bone. Occasionally coronal CT or even pluridirectional tomography can help answer the question in problem cases.

The facial nerve canal passing through the temporal bone is very reliably evaluated by high resolution CT. However, the portion of the facial nerve in the internal auditory canal must be evaluated in the same fashion as an acoustic neuroma (see below). Tumor of the parotid region can also cause facial paralysis and this must be considered during CT evaluation.

Lesions of the extreme apex close to the petro-occipital suture are often chondromatous lesions or are lesions arising in

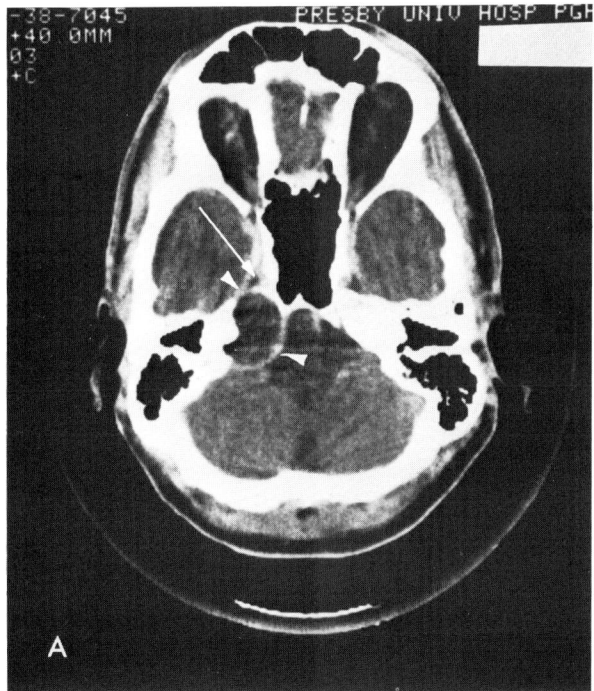

Figure 9A: Epidermoid of the petrous apex showing low density area between arrowheads extending up to Meckel's cave (long arrow).

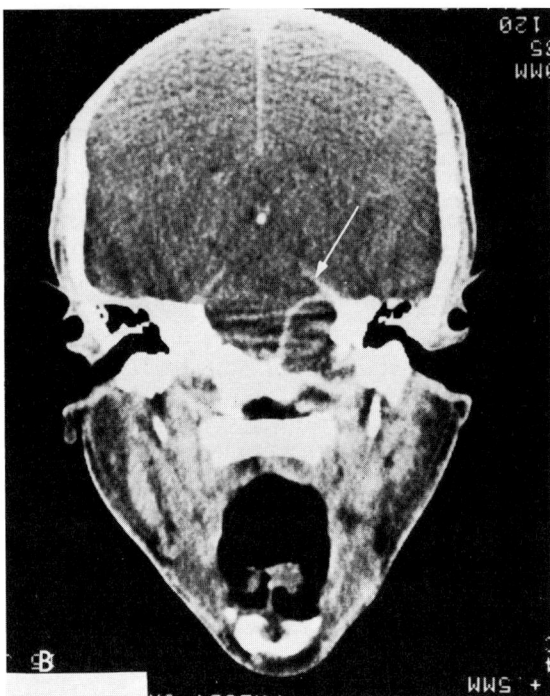

Figure 9B: Coronal view shows relationship of the low density epidermoid to the tentorium (long arrow). (Used with permission.[1])

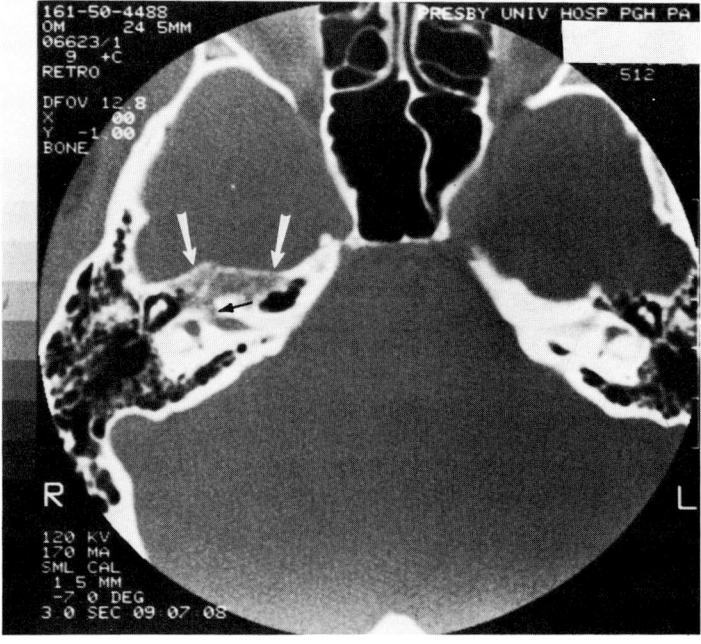

Figure 10: Ossifying hemangioma of the temporal bone shows indistinct expanding lesion with demineralization of the cortex of the temporal bone (white arrows). There is enlargement of the labyrinthine segment of the facial nerve canal (black arrow).

the trigeminal ganglion or nasopharynx extending into the region of the suture (Figs. 11, 12). The relationship of the lesion to the important structures in the petrous bone can best be demonstrated by axial and coronal CT. This usually requires very thin 1.3 mm sections with bone algorithm reformation. As with glomus jugulare tumors (paragangliomas), important landmarks to be evaluated are the cochlea and internal auditory canals, and most importantly, the carotid artery and facial nerve. It is also very important to determine if the lesion of the petrous apex or jugular foramen extends into the posterior fossa, and if so, the dimensions of the intracranial component become important.

Internal Auditory Canal and Cerebellopontine Angle

The internal auditory canal and cerebellopontine angle are currently evaluated by CT with intravenous contrast or, if this is equivocal, by CT with intrathecal air (air cisternogram) (Fig. 13). Acoustic neuromas represent most of the lesions of the internal auditory canal. Virtually all enhance but many have areas of decreased attenuation. Most, but not all, enlarge the internal auditory canal (Fig. 14). To exclude an acoustic neuroma entirely, the nerves must be followed into and through the internal auditory canal. This requires the air cisternogram but it is hoped that magnetic resonance will decrease the necessity for this procedure in the near future (Fig. 15). Already magnetic resonance is being used as an initial screening procedure in many acoustic neuroma suspects.

Wherever there is a meningeal covering, meningiomas must be considered and this includes the surfaces of the petrous bones, cerebellopontine angle, and internal auditory canal. Meningiomas tend to enhance more uniformly than acoustic neuromas and may cause hyperostosis or calcification (Fig. 16). They tend to have a flat appearance with an obtuse junction with the petrous bone unlike the acoustic neuroma which usually makes an acute angle (see Fig. 14). This last finding, however, only indicates that the lesion arises from the posterior surface of the temporal bone rather than the internal auditory ca-

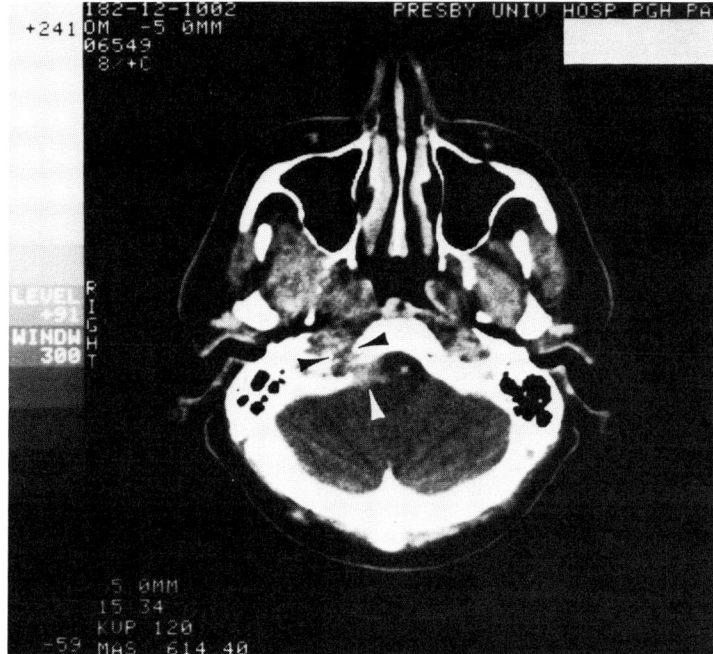

Figure 11: Tumor of the nasopharynx extending through the petro-occipital suture (black arrowheads) (petroclival). A small nodule of tumor extends intracranially (white arrowhead).

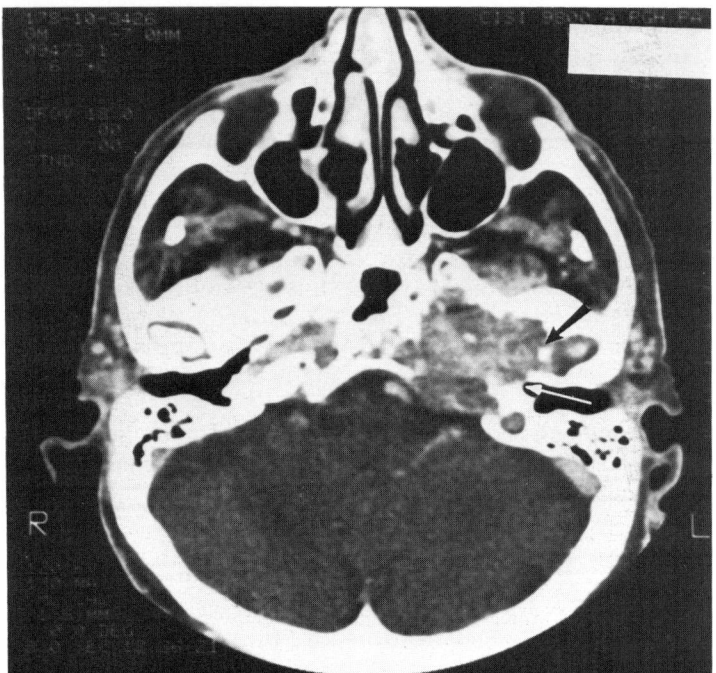

Figure 12A: More extensive tumor extending from nasopharynx through the petroclival region with considerable erosion of the temporal bone. Erosion extends to the TMJ (black arrow) and middle ear (white arrow).

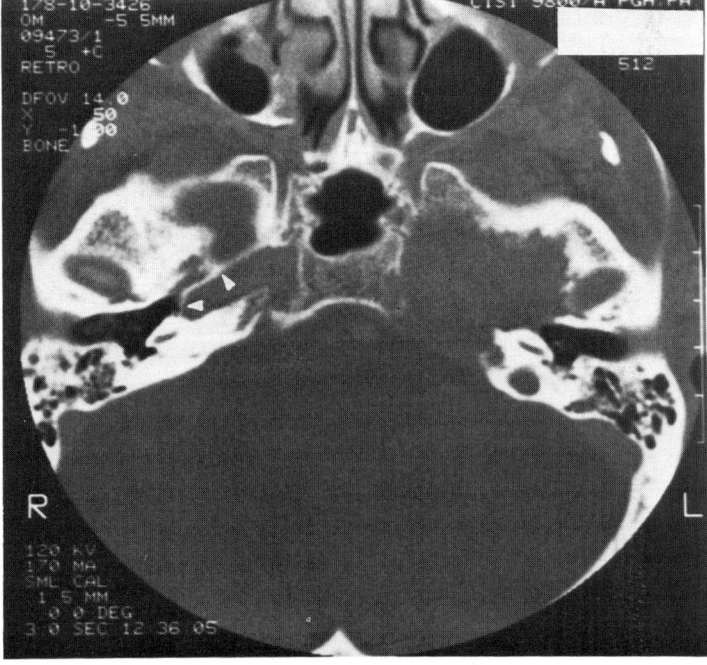

Figure 12B: Bone algorithm to better define a complete erosion of the bony walls of the carotid canal. Compare to normal opposite side (arrowheads).

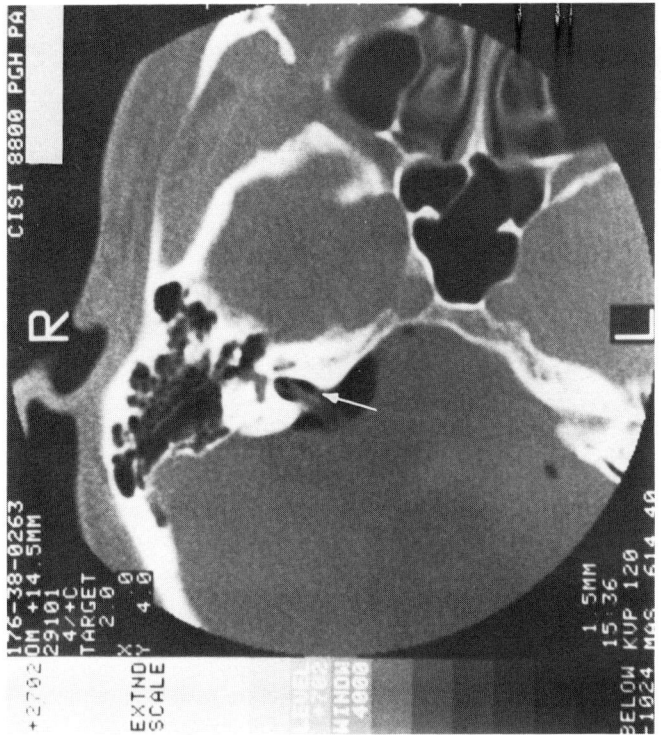

Figure 13: Air cisternogram shows air in the CPA cistern extending into the internal auditory canal. The cochlear nerve can be seen just anterior to the vestibular nerve in the intracanalicular portion. The image has been rotated 90° to give the usual axial orientation of the internal auditory canal. The examination was done with the right ear up.

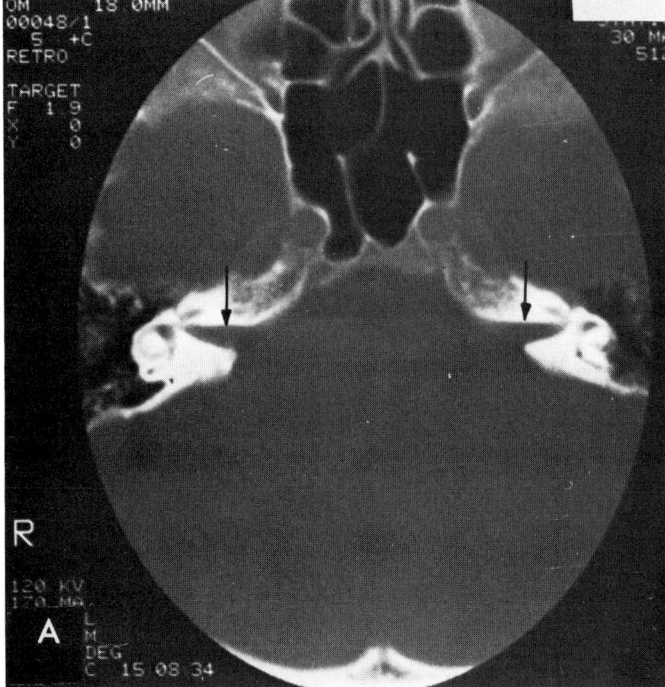

Figure 14A: Atypical acoustic neuroma with no actual enlargement of the internal auditory canal (black arrows). (Used with permission.[1])

80 • TUMORS OF THE CRANIAL BASE: DIAGNOSIS AND TREATMENT

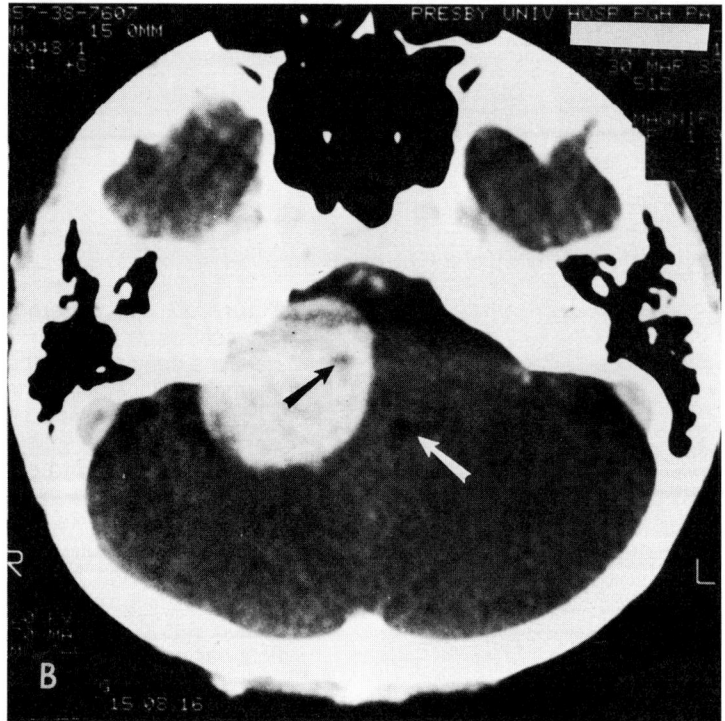

Figure 14B: In spite of the lack of erosion of the IAC, there is a large enhancing tumor with a small low density area (black arrow). There is deviation of the brain stem and the 4th ventricle (white arrow). Note how the tumor has an acute angulation with the petrous bone reflecting its origin in the internal auditory canal.

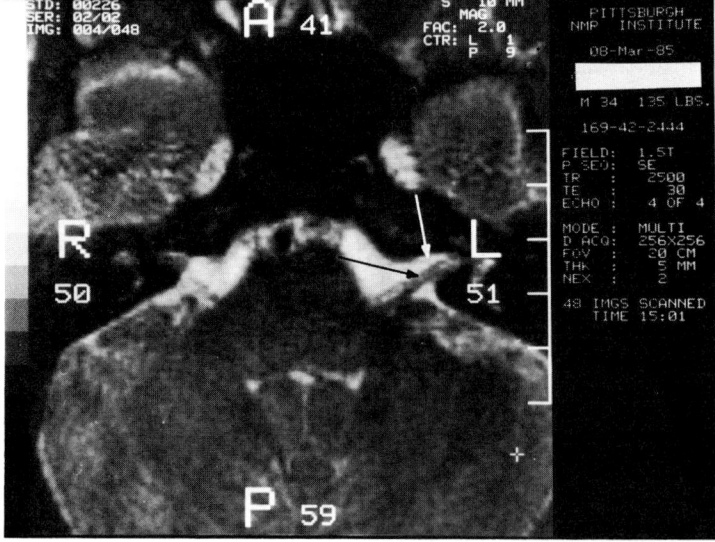

Figure 15: Magnetic resonance imaging through the internal auditory canal. The cerebrospinal fluid in the IAC can be well visualized (white arrow) as can the nerves extending from the brain stem through the IAC (black arrow).

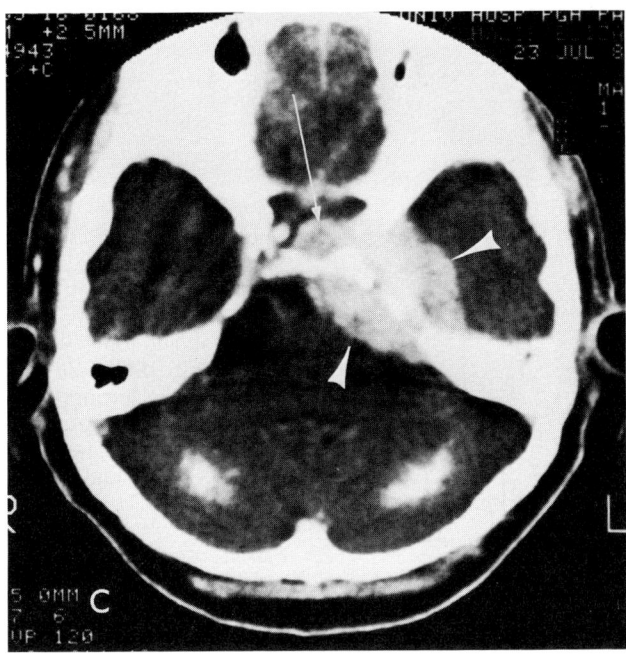

Figure 16: Meningioma of the petrous apex (white arrowheads) extending into the sella (long white arrow). Note the lesion's obtuse angle at its junction with the petrous bone. (Used with permission.[1])

nal. Occasionally a meningioma arises within the internal auditory canal and this would have an acute angle.

Other lesions of the cerebellopontine angle, which can involve the internal auditory canal, are epidermoids (low density), facial neurilemmomas, and intraaxial tumors. Aneurysms of the vertebral basilar system could also be occasionally mistaken for an acoustic neuroma.

Clivus, Sphenoid, and Sella

These areas are discussed in Chapter 3.

Parapharyngeal Space/Infratemporal Fossa[5,12,15,16,18]

The area deep to the zygomatic arch and superficial to the pharyngeal mucosa is very accessible to CT evaluation but very difficult to examine clinically. The region contains two very distinct groups of muscles. The deglutitional muscles form a partial ring around the nasopharyngeal airway (Fig. 17). In the nasopharyngeal region, on CT the soft tissue density associated with this ring is made up mostly by the levator veli palatini as well as the eustachian tube and pharyngobasilar fascia. Posteriorly the prevertebral muscles appear to close this "ring." Laterally the masticator muscles are in the region of the mandible and include pterygoid, masseter, and temporalis muscles. The masticator group of muscles is separated from the deglutitional muscles by the parapharyngeal fat which is the key to the evaluation of this area. The parapharyngeal fat is in turn separated by a thin layer of fascia to pre- and poststyloid compartments. This layer of fascia extends from the styloid process and muscles to fuse with the fascia of the tensor veli palatini. The poststyloid compartment is sometimes called the carotid or vascular space because the carotid artery, jugular vein, and their accompanying nerves are found in this space.[17] The pre- and poststyloid spaces are actually anterolateral and posteromedial to one another. Poststyloid lesions tend to have a component extending posterior to the styloid and extend anterior and medial

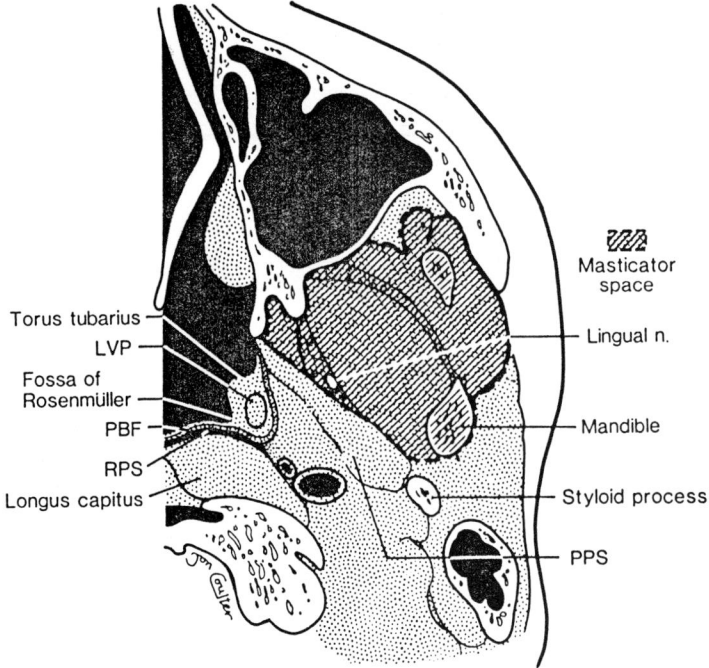

Figure 17: The pharyngeal and parapharyngeal region. PPS represents the parapharyngeal space. The line extending roughly from the styloid obliquely anteromedially through the parapharyngeal space is the approximate differentiation pre- and post-styloid compartments. LVP represents levator veli palatini. PBF represents the pharyngobasilar fascia and RPS is the retropharyngeal space. (Used with permission.[5])

from this point. Prestyloid lesions pass anterior to the styloid between the styloid and mandible following the protrusion of the deep lobe of the parotid gland.[18] Almost all prestyloid lesions are salivary gland origin (Fig. 18). This is especially true if they can be separated from the masticator muscles. The origin of a tumor can usually be identified on CT by the characteristic effect on the parapharyngeal fat.

Poststyloid lesions arise from the structures associated with the jugular and carotid and include cranial nerves IX-XII. Most primary lesions are paragangliomas (glomus tumors) or neurilemmomas, and they push the parapharyngeal fat anteriorly and laterally. They can be differentiated by angiography where the paraganglioma has a very characteristic vascular pattern (Fig. 19).

Paragangliomas at the level of the nasopharynx may be glomus vagale tumors or inferior extensions of glomus jugulare tumors. Thus the jugular foramen must be very carefully examined by CT, looking for small erosions, or for possible extension into the posterior fossa or middle ear.

Retropharyngeal lymphadenopathy can also be seen in the poststyloid region. However, these lymph nodes do not usually enhance but rather have peripheral enhancement with central decreased attenuation after intravenous contrast is given (Fig. 20).

If a lesion is confined to the masticator space region, the histology is unlikely to be related to the salivary gland. These are sarcomas, undifferentiated tumors, etc.[9] Again the effect on the parapharyngeal fat is very important. The parapharyngeal fat is now pushed posteriorly and medially. Tumors arising in this location may follow the third division of the trigeminal nerve through the foramen ovale which should be evaluated, as well as the floor of the middle cranial fossa (Fig. 21).

Tumors arising medial to the parapharyngeal fat and pushing it laterally are usually of mucosal origin, the most significant being squamous cell carcinoma. In these cases, the bony margin of the skull base and floor of the sphenoid sinus and clivus must be carefully examined. Adenoid cystic carcinomas, lymphomas, neuromas, and other lesions can also occur here.

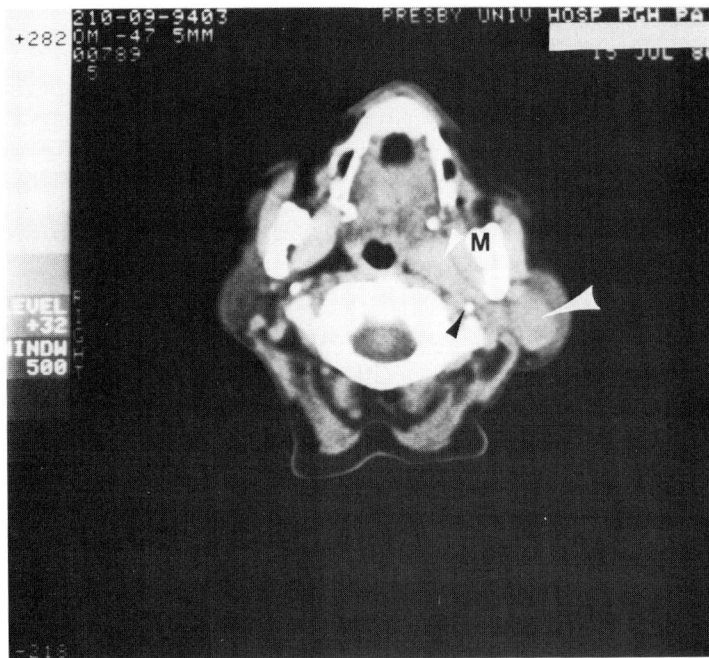

Figure 18: Prestyloid Warthin's tumor (arrowheads). Typical dumbbell-shaped tumor "squeezes" between styloid (black arrowhead) and mandible (M). Parapharyngeal (small white arrowhead) and more superficial (large white arrowhead) components are identified. (Used with permission.[5])

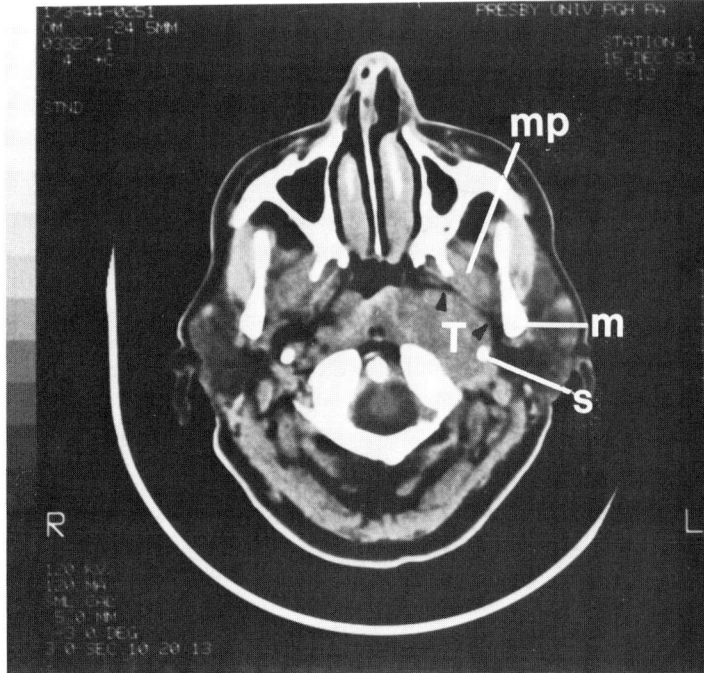

Figure 19A: Paraganglioma (glomus intravagale). the tumor extends posterior to the styloid (S) rather than between the styloid and mandible (M). Medial pterygoid (MP). Tumor (T) pushes parapharyngeal fat anteriorly and laterally.

carotid especially if there is extension posteriorly into basisphenoid.

The parapharyngeal/infratemporal fossa region can be evaluated with magnetic resonance imaging which can differentiate tumor from muscle (a frequent failing of CT) and also can determine the position of vessels with respect to the tumor better than CT.

Sinuses and Nasal Cavity[6,15,19]

In dealing with tumor of the sinuses, the radiologist's role is often one of staging rather than actually making the diagnosis. The air and bone interfaces lend themselves to evaluation by high resolution computed tomography (HRCT). As this discussion relates primarily to skull base surgery, principles related to the upper sinuses are emphasized. Here carcinomas, meningiomas, and esthesioneuroblastomas (olfactory neuroblastomas) are considered.

With tumors of the upper nasal cavity and sinuses, it is most important to evaluate their superior margin, especially if the lesion extends through the cribiform plate or roof of the ethmoid (Fig. 22). This information is most easily obtained in coronal imaging usually using HRCT with bone algorithms. This defines the integrity of the bony plates or identified tumor above the bony margin (Fig. 23). Usually the tumor enhances somewhat differently than the brain (Fig. 24).

Tumors of the nasal cavity tend to obstruct the outflow of sinuses rendering them opaque on plain film. This can be difficult to differentiate from actual tumor involvement of the sinuses or air cells. If they have the characteristic low density of an obstructed sinus on CT, one can be fairly confident that this is an obstructive phenomenon. However, if there is secondary infection, the sinus may not have the decreased attenuation. Even a little mucosal swelling in the ethmoid may fill an entire air cell with "enhancement" mimicking tumor involvement. In this case, if the septations of the ethmoid are intact, the opacification is more likely due to obstruction but this principle cannot be considered absolute (Fig. 22).

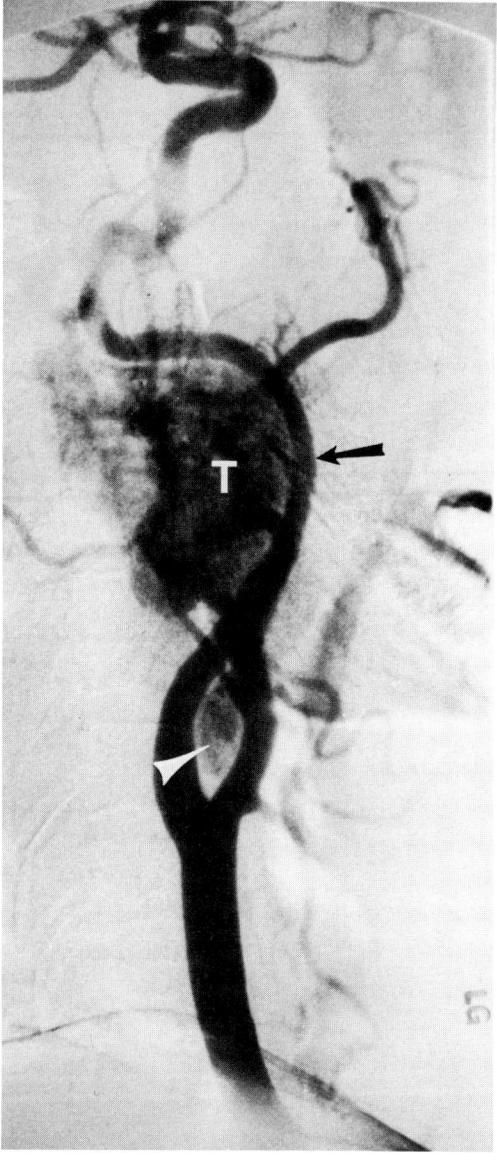

Figure 19B: Arteriogram showed tumor (T) pushing the internal carotid (arrow) anteriorly. Note also the small carotid body tumor (white arrowhead) at the bifurcation.

Juvenile angiofibroma involves the posterior nasal cavity and nasopharynx in adolescent males. Most involve and enlarge the pterygopalatine fossa. Their extent is best defined by CT, but angiography is necessary to define blood supply which is predominantly from external carotid but can be partially from internal

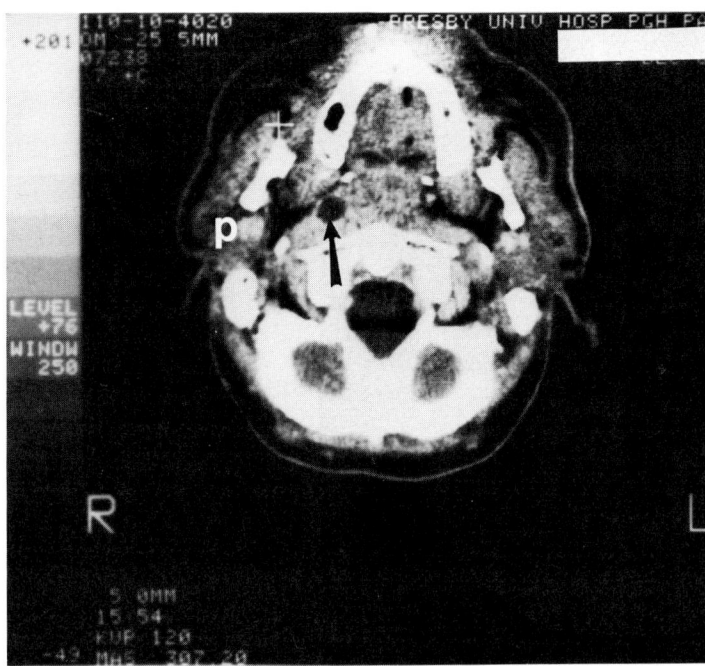

Figure 20: Post-styloid parapharyngeal mass with chronic center (black arrow). Again, the lesion appears to be medial and slightly posterior to the styloid rather than passing anterior to the styloid towards the parotid (P). (Used with permission.[5])

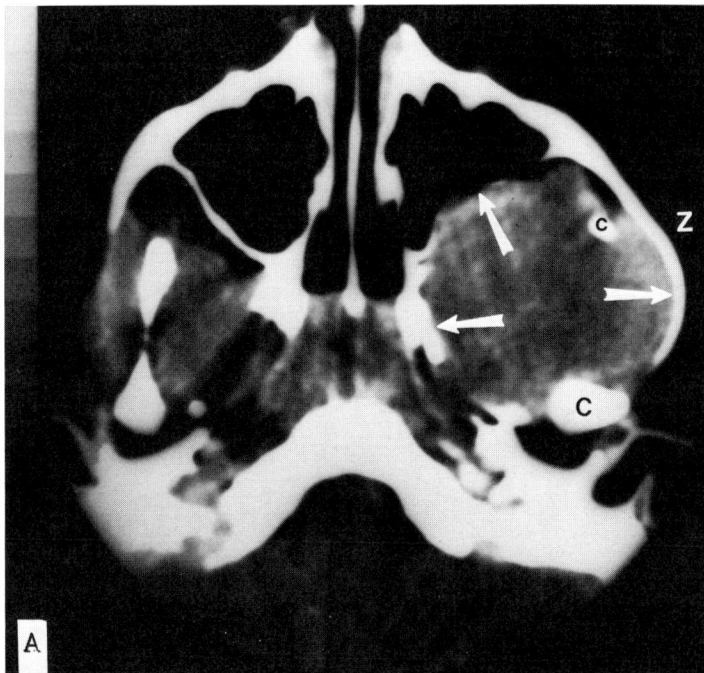

Figure 21A: Synovial sarcoma. Tumor of the masticator space (white arrow). The Zygomatic (Z) arch is pushed laterally and the lesion extends anterior to the condyle (C). Coronoid process (c). (Used with permission.[5])

86 • TUMORS OF THE CRANIAL BASE: DIAGNOSIS AND TREATMENT

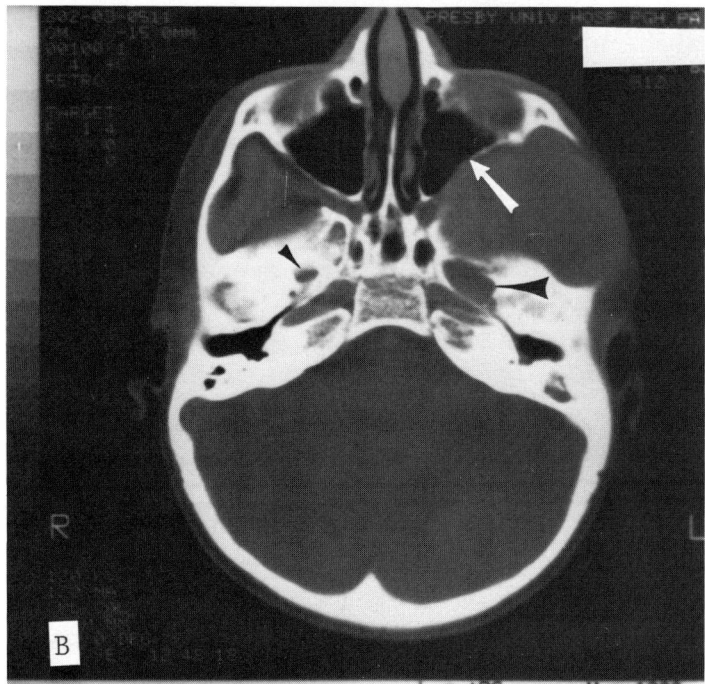

Figure 21B: Higher axial view shows bowing. There is enlargement of the foramen ovale (large black arrowhead). Compare to the normal side (small black arrowhead).

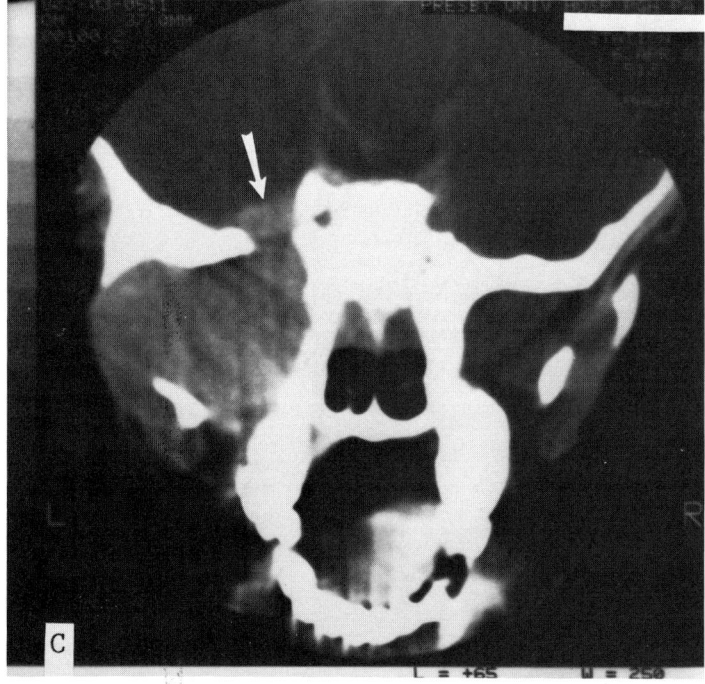

Figure 21C: Coronal view shows lesion of the masticator space extending through the foramen ovale (white arrow).

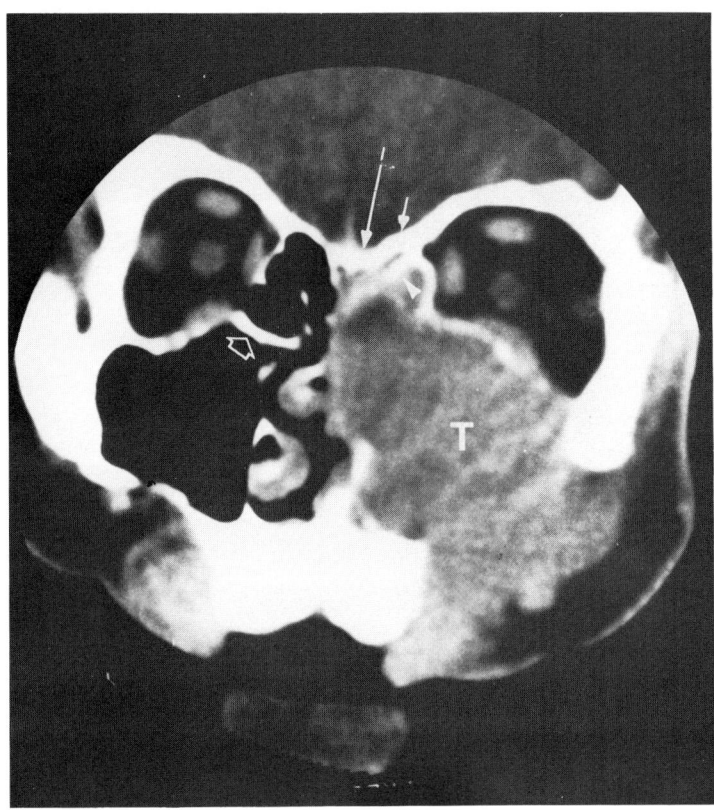

Figure 22: Lesion of the maxillary sinus extending through the maxillary-ethmoid plate into the lower ethmoid. Some septations (arrow) in the ethmoid remain intact. The roof of the ethmoid (short white arrow) and the cribiform plate region (long white arrow) are intact indicating the tumor had not reached the intracranial area. The area around the small white arrowhead may well represent obstructive phenomenon in one of the ethmoid air cells rather than tumor. Tumor (T). Maxillary-ethmoid plate on the normal side (open arrow). (Used with permission.[6])

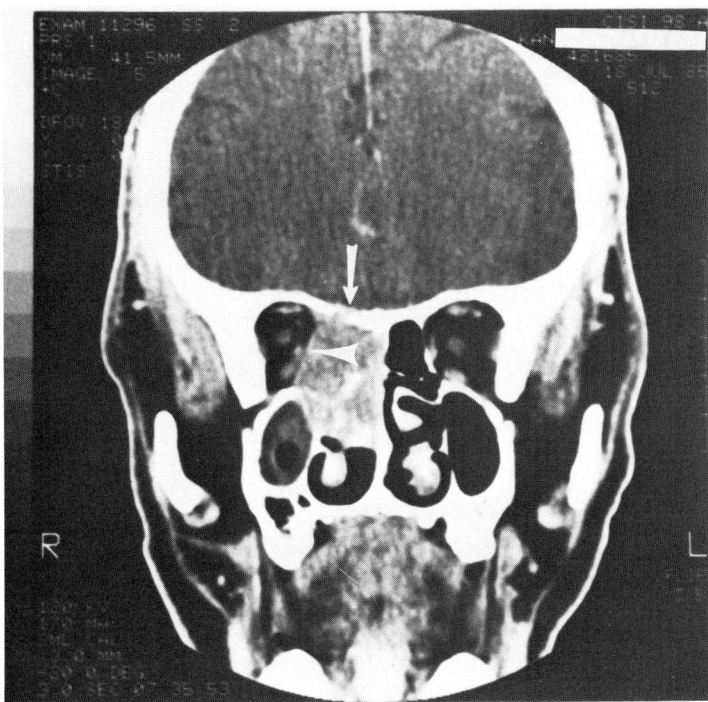

Figure 23: Tumor of the ethmoid with minimal erosion of the roof of the ethmoid (white arrow). Also note involvement of the orbital wall on the right side most likely limited by the periorbita (white arrowhead).

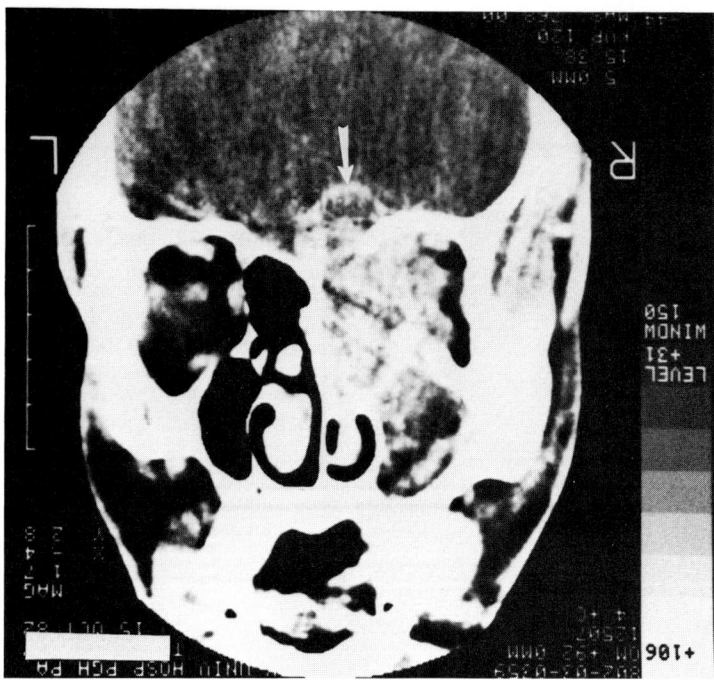

Figure 24: Rhabdomyosarcoma of orbit, ethmoid cells, and cribiform plate. The margin of the tumor in the intracranial area can be easily defined (white arrow). (Used with permission.[6])

Prolonged obstruction of a sinus can cause a mucocele or expansion of the sinus. This is usually caused by an inflammatory obliteration of the ostium but occasionally can be produced by tumorous obstruction. Early mucocele formation, which may be seen in tumors, can cause demineralization of the bone without expansion. This is, of course, very difficult to differentiate from actual bone destruction caused by the tumor.[6]

In a benign type mucocele (not associated with malignancy), the extent is the key information sought by the radiologist with CT. Again, the interface with the intracranial contents is most important (Fig. 25). Demonstration of an intact bone interface is very reassuring to the surgeon.

Although tumors and mucoceles are the most common "masses" confronting the radiologist, encephaloceles must also be considered, especially in the younger population. These are usually seen in the anterior sphenoid, posterior ethmoid, or in the anterior cribiform plate, crista galli area (Fig. 26). Often other midline anomalies are present.

Perineural Extension/ Pterygopalatine Fossa

Tumors of the head and neck and thus the skull base region often tend to follow nerves preferentially.[2,7,8] The tumors grow into a nerve and follow through a foramen to resurface in a deeper region even intracranially (Fig. 27). This is especially characteristic of adenocystic carcinoma which arises predominantly in the minor salivary glands that are found in sinuses and in the nasal and pharyngeal mucosa. Squamous cell carcinoma and lymphoma can also do this.

Any nerve can be involved. Therefore the nerve extending centrally from a region of a tumor must be carefully evaluated including their neural foramina and their potential destinations intracranially.

Tumors of the nasal cavity, sinuses, and palate may spread along the trigeminal nerve eventually reaching the foramen rotundum and Meckel's cave in the middle fossa. Tumor reaching the foramen rotundum must first pass through the pterygopalatine fossa (PPF). This is a

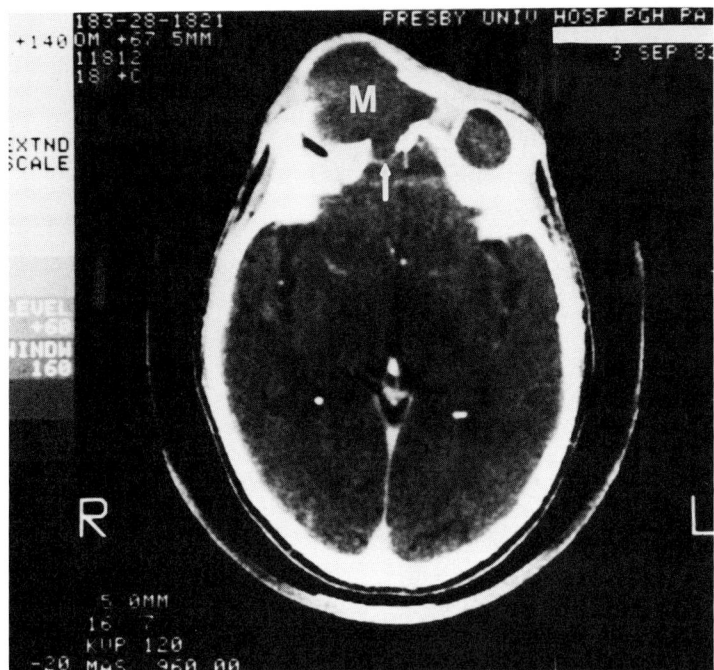

Figure 25: Mucocele of the frontal sinus. Mucocele (M). Note absence of bone along the posterior wall (white arrow). (Used with permission.[6])

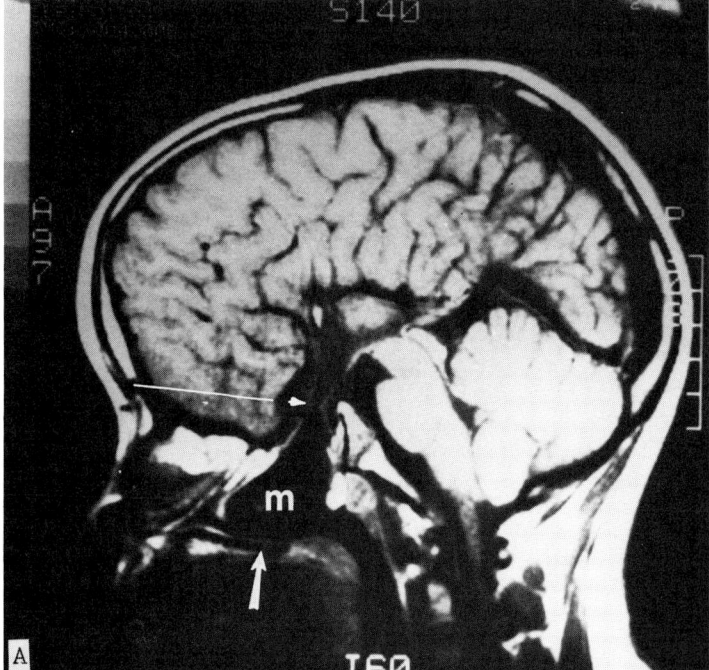

Figure 26A: Meningoencephalocele (M). Extends down to the hard palate (large white arrow). Note its point of communication (long white arrow) area going through the region of the anterior sella.

90 • TUMORS OF THE CRANIAL BASE: DIAGNOSIS AND TREATMENT

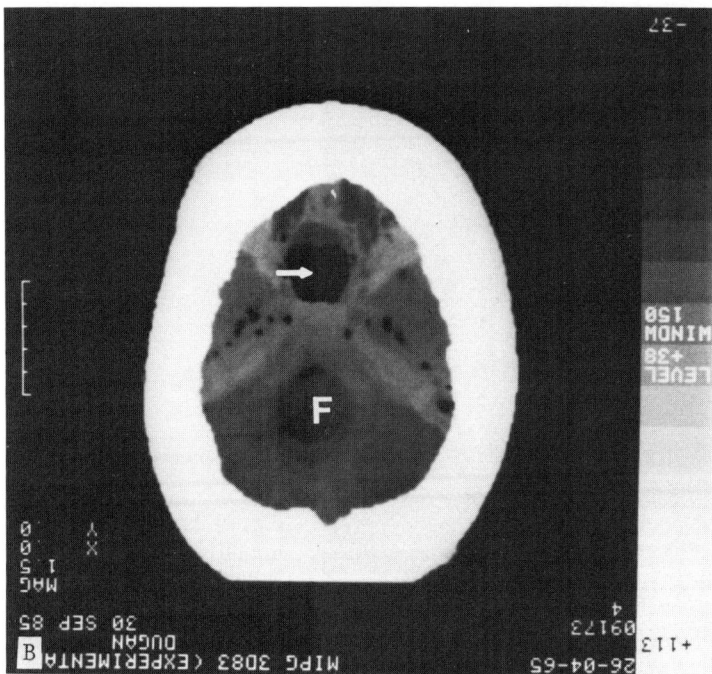

Figure 26B: 3-D reconstruction from CT scan from above shows a large bony defect (white arrow) which is almost as large as the foramen magnum (F).

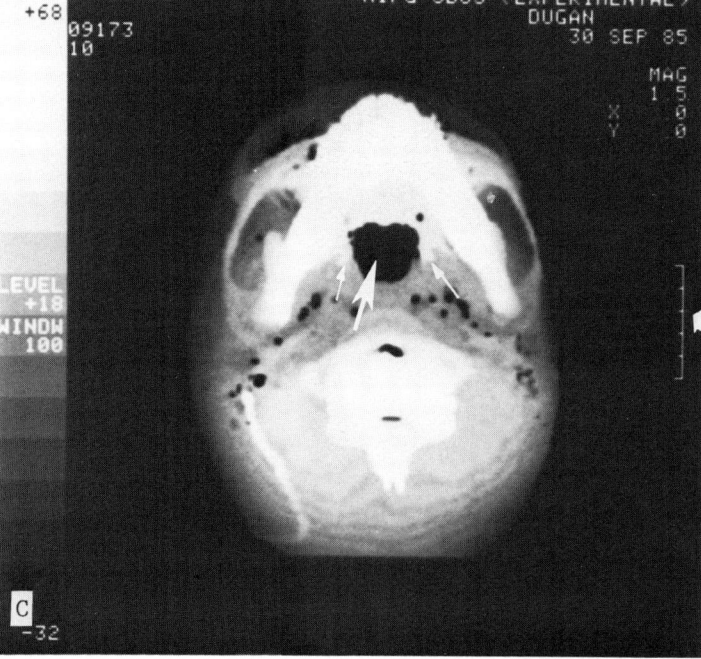

Figure 26C: View from below. The defect (large white arrow) is seen above the pterygoid plate (small arrows).

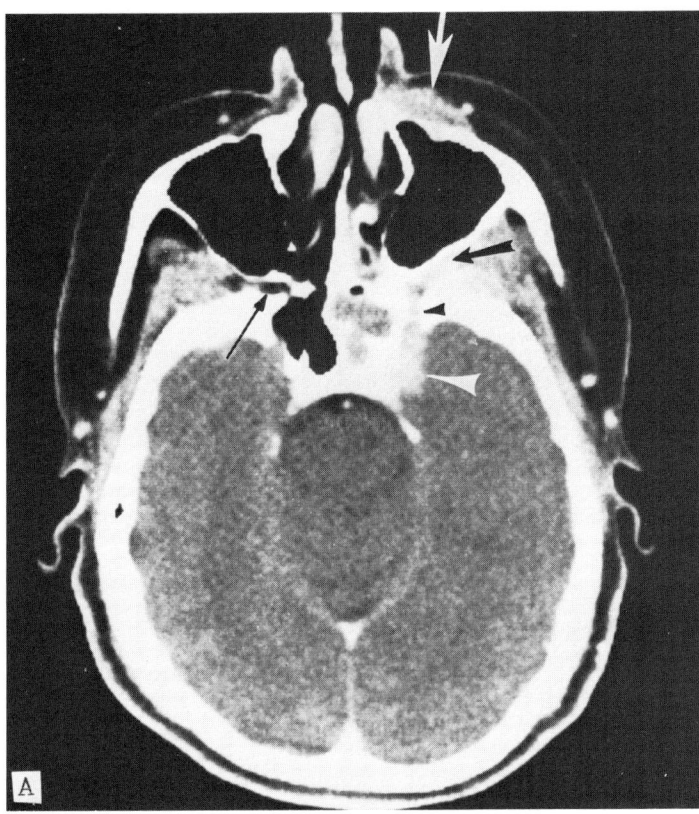

Figure 27A: Perineural extension of tumor along the maxillary division of the trigeminal nerve. Tumor of the malar region (white arrow) with tumor of the pterygopalatine fossa and pterygomaxillary fissure (large black arrow). Tumor also extends through the foramen rotundum (black arrowhead) to the region of the middle cranial fossa (white arrowhead). Compare the obliteration of the fat in the pterygopalatine fossa on the affected side with the normal fat density in the pterygopalatine fossa of the normal side (black arrow). (Figures 27A–C used with permission.[8])

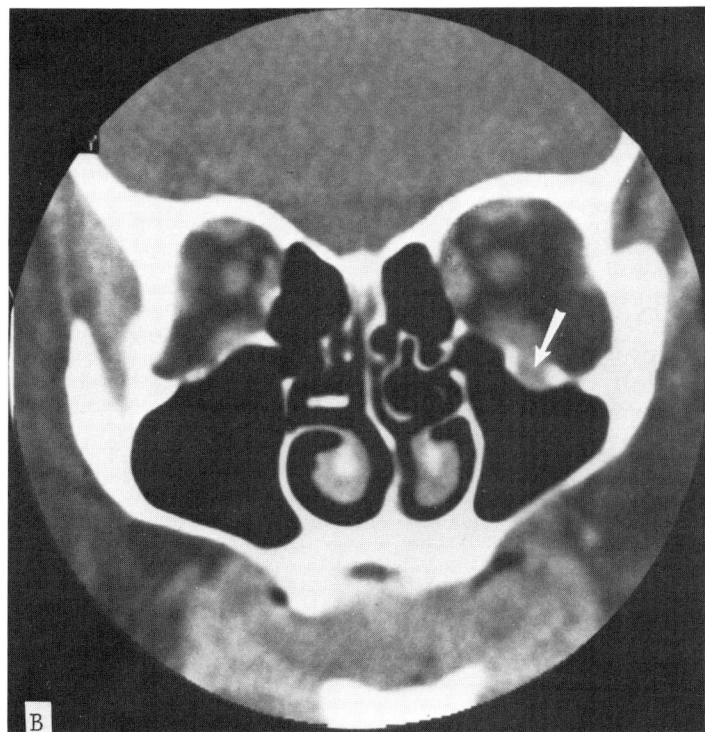

Figure 27B: The connection between the pterygopalatine fossa and the malar region tumor is completed by the enlarged infraorbital canal seen on the coronal view (white arrow).

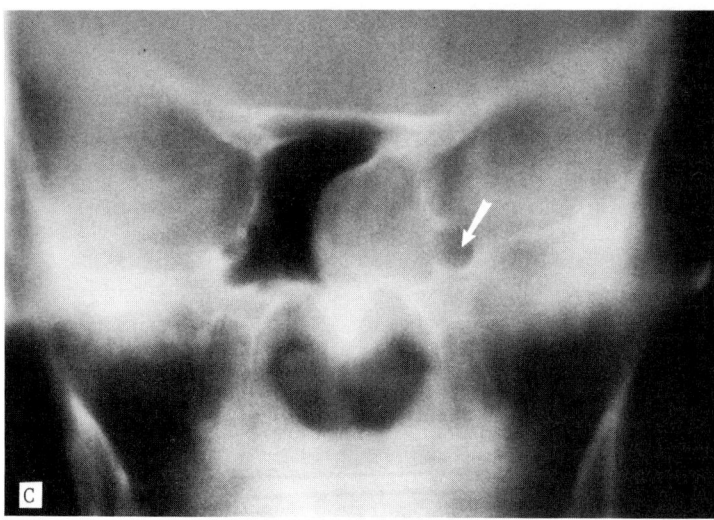

Figure 27C: Pluridirectional tomogram confirms the enlargement of the foramen rotundum (white arrow). Compare with normal opposite side.

branching point of the maxillary division of the trigeminal nerve (V$_2$). The PPF is a small fat-filled space between the posterior wall of the maxillary sinus and the pterygoid plates. Tumor passing through the PPF following the nerves obliterates the fat.[8] This obliteration of the fat is a very sensitive sign in detection of tumor extension along the trigeminal nerve even though the fossa is very narrow.

Summary

Although the actual tumor type may be suggested by the radiologist, definition of the precise position and extent of the tumor, as well as the relationships of the tumor to various vital structures, is usually the more significant role of the radiologist. As surgical approaches change, the radiologist and the skull base surgeon work closely together so the radiologist can precisely define the structures that are important to the particular surgeon. Currently, high resolution computed tomography is the key tool of the skull base radiologist but magnetic resonance is making rapid strides and imaging approaches to the skull base may be very different in the near future.

References

1. Curtin HD: CT of acoustic neuroma and other tumors of the ear. *Radiol Clin North Am* 22(1):77-105, 1984.
2. Ballantyne AJ, McCarten AB, Ibanez ML: The extension of cancer of the head and neck through peripheral nerves. *Am J Surg* 106:651-667, 1963.
3. Curtin HD, Wolfe P, Snyderman N: The facial nerve between the stylomastoid foramen and the parotid: Computed tomographic imaging. *Radiology* 149(1):165-169, 1983.
4. Curtin HD, Wolfe P, May M: Malignant external otitis: CT Evaluation. *Radiology* 145:383-388, 1982.
5. Curtin HD: Nasopharynx, intratemporal fossa and skull base. In Carter B (ed): *Contemporary Issues in Computed Tomography: Computed Tomography of the Head and Neck.* New York, Churchill Livingstone, 1985, pp 59-83.
6. Curtin HD: Nose, paranasal sinuses, and facial bones. In Latchaw RE (ed): *Computed Tomography of the Head, Neck & Spine.* Chicago, Year Book Medical Publishers, 1985, pp 517-550.
7. Dodd GD, Dolan PA, Ballantyne AJ, et al: The dissemination of tumors of the head and neck via the cranial nerves. *Radiol Clin North Am* 8(3):445-461, 1970.
8. Curtin HD, Williams R, Johnson J: CT of perineural tumor extension: Pterygopalatine fossa. *AJNR* 5:731-737, 1984.

9. Hardin CW, Harnsberger HR, Osborn AG, et al: Infection and tumor of the masticator space: CT evaluation. *Radiology* 157:413-417, 1985.
10. Lo WWM, Solit-Bohman LG, McElveen JJ: Aberrant carotid artery: Radiologic diagnosis with emphasis on high-resolution computed tomography. *Radiographics* 5(6):985-993, 1985.
11. Lo WWM, Solit-Bohman LG, Brachmann DE, et al: Cholesterol granuloma of the petrous apex: CT diagnosis. *Radiology* 153:705-711, 1984.
12. Mancuso AA, Hanafee WN: Nasopharynx and parapharyngeal space. *Computed Tomography and Magnetic Resonance Imaging of the Head and Neck*. Baltimore, Williams & Wilkins, 1985, pp 428-497.
13. Mancuso AA, Hanafee WN: *Computed Tomography and Magnetic Resonance Imaging of the Head and Neck*, Chapters 1 and 2. Baltimore, Williams & Wilkins, 1985.
14. Shaffer KA: CT in otolaryngology: The temporal bone. In Latchaw RE (ed): *Computed Tomography of the Head, Neck and Spine*. Chicago, Year Book Medical Publishers, 1985, pp 489-516.
15. Silver AJ, Mawad ME, Hilal SK, et al: Computed tomography of the nasopharynx and related spaces. Part I. Anatomy. *Radiology* 147:725-731, 1983.
16. Silver AJ, Mawad ME, Hilal SK, et al: Computed tomography of the nasopharynx and related spaces. Part II. Pathology. *Radiology* 147:733-738, 1983.
17. Silver AJ, Mawad ME, Hilal SK, et al: Computed tomography of the carotid space and related cervical spaces. *Radiology* 150:723-728, 1984.
18. Som SP, Biller HF, Lawson W: Tumors of the parapharyngeal space (preoperative evaluation, diagnosis, and surgical approaches). *Ann Otol Rhinol Laryngol* 90:3-15, 1981.
19. Som P: Paranasal sinuses and pterygopalatine fossa. In Carter B (ed): *Contemporary Issues in Computed Tomography: Computed Tomography of the Head and Neck*. New York, Churchill Livingstone, 1985, pp 101-130.
20. Valvassori GE, Buckingham RA: Tomography of the temporal bone. In Valvassori GE, et al. (ed): *Radiology of the Ear, Nose and Throat*. Philadelphia, W.B. Saunders Co., 1982, pp 12-29.
21. Valvasorri G, Mafee MF: The temporal bone. In Carter B (ed): *Contemporary Issues in Computed Tomography: Computed Tomography of the Head and Neck*. New York, Churchill Livingstone, 1985, pp 171-205.
22. Wright JW, Taylor CC: *Polytomography of the Temporal Bone*. St. Louis, Warren H. Green, Inc., 1973.

5

Embolization and Balloon Occlusion Techniques in the Management of Cranial Base Tumors

P. Lasjaunias, M.D. Ph.D.
K. Ter Brugge, M.D.
M. Chiu, M.D.
L. Lopez Ibor, M.D.

Introduction

Therapeutic angiography has been and still is largely synonymous with embolization procedures. Acute cellular damage can be observed following embolization; however, fibrotic transformation is the expected long-term outcome of satisfactory microembolization.

When a tumor is present at the base of the skull, embolization may improve most of the symptoms by decreasing the tumor mass and reducing arterial flow, and the benefits of embolization before biopsy or radical removal are well known to surgeons. For many of the classic skull base tumors, the rate of recurrence has decreased tremendously with combined embolization and surgery. However, to date, embolization, infusion, or chemoembolization alone are not adequate for the management of a lesion that is amenable to surgical resection.

Nevertheless, with improvements in anatomic knowledge, control of blood flow, and embolization materials, embolization has become an important therapeutic step that should not be overlooked, even by those not accustomed to using it. Obviously, if the operability of a lesion depends more on the surgeon than on the lesion itself, whether or not it may be embolized depends upon the availability of an angiographer. A multidisciplinary approach, with decisions being made by a team to harmonize individual skills, will be the best possible strategy in a given situation. The approach described in this chapter has been discussed in detail by Lasjaunias and Berenstein.[1]

Effects of Embolization

Pathology

Depending on the type of embolus, several reactions may be observed, some

From: Sekhar LN, Schramm VL Jr, eds: *Tumors of the Cranial Base: Diagnosis and Treatment.* Mount Kisco, New York, Futura Publishing Co, Inc, © 1987.

of them related to the inflammatory changes induced locally by the agent, and others related to the effects of ischemia.

Certain general effects can be expected: occlusion of large arteries in the periphery of the tumor, occlusion of arteries within the tumor bed, necrosis of the tumor, irreversible cellular damage, and secondary venous thrombosis (Figs. 1A and B). As a long-term effect, microparticle embolization can induce a fibrotic transformation of a vascular tumor such as a paraganglioma (Fig. 2).

Therefore, the most appropriate embolic agent is chosen according to the alterations in tumor anatomy to be achieved and the timing of the embolization in relation to the overall plan of treatment of the tumor. The smaller the agent, the most distal is its migration and the better its effect; fluid emboli will usually travel to the capillary network, whereas particle emboli will reach vessels 50 to 1000 microns in caliber, according to the size of the emboli. In our experience, the effect of the embolization on the tumor cells depends more on the completeness of the embolization than on the type of embolic agent used; therefore, control of the flow to the tumor and a thorough study of the vascular anatomy of the tumor as well as the potential sources of collateral circulation are essential to achieve the best results from embolization.

In general, fistulae in tumors occur as direct results of mechanical changes in the vascular architecture (surgery, trauma). Therefore, although a rapid venous return is observed in some lesions (paragangliomas), there is always a capillary barrier which will allow the use of small particles (160 microns) for embolization.

Clinical Symptoms

The symptoms of a tumor at the base of the skull are related to either the mass effect or the vascular character of the tumor, and include: (1) airway obstruction (nasal fossa, eustachian tube) cranial nerve palsies (II to XII), (2) pulsatile tinnitus (sometimes associated with conductive deafness), and (3) bleeding (epistaxis or otorrhagia).

These symptoms can be regrouped into topographic syndromes suggesting a particular type of lesion for a specific population group. Relief of the symptoms is obtainable by embolization, but the stability of the results will depend on the long-term character of the agent used and on the pathological effects induced.

Commonly, embolization produces rapid (24-hour) shrinkage of vascular tumors, particularly if the vascular stroma is prominent (juvenile angiofibroma). Therefore, rapid relief of airway obstruction may be observed following proper

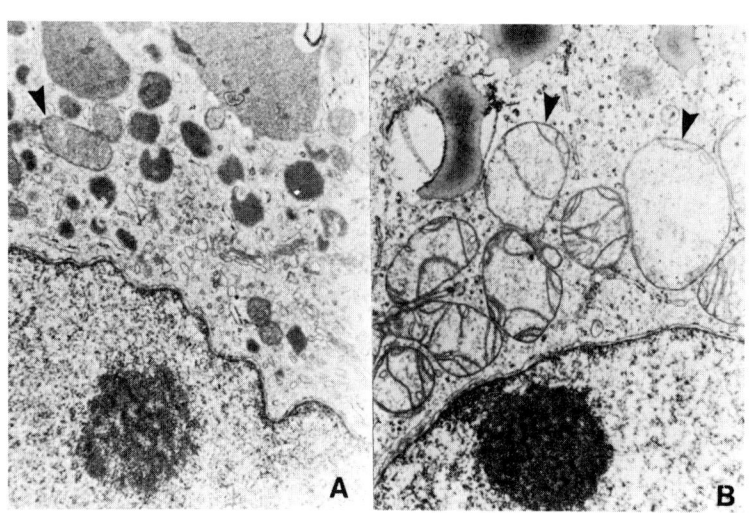

Figure 1: Electron microscopic view of surgically removed paraganglioma. **A:** Without embolization; **B:** 48 hours following embolization (microparticles). Note mitochondrial (arrowhead) swelling and lipidic vacuolization on the embolized lesion, testifying to the aggressiveness of the tumor cells. (Courtesy of Dr. Bock; unpublished data.)

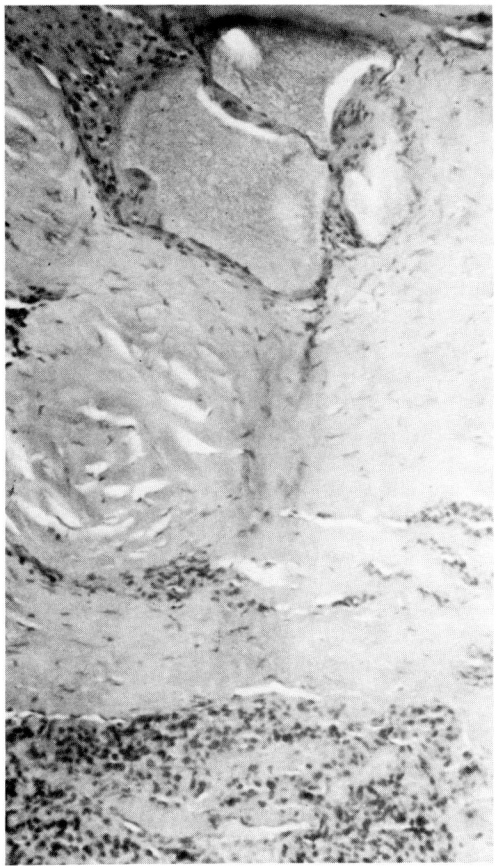

Figure 2: Pathological specimen of paraganglioma removed 1 year after tumor microparticle embolization. Note the dramatic fibrotic changes that have occurred in the lesion, even though it retains some cellular loci.

embolization of this kind of lesion. In our experience, reduction by up to 30% in the tumor size can be obtained in a 48-hour period. For less vascularized lesions, shrinkage will be related to cellular damage, and is observable usually in 2 to 4 weeks; it will affect a lower percentage of the tumor mass.

Metastases can respond dramatically to embolization since they often exist in a subischemic state; extensive necrosis will then occur very rapidly. In these situations, staged procedures in which macroparticles are used may be considered, if too rapid and extensive necrosis would be undesirable.

Most cranial nerve palsies are related to mechanical compression. Decrease of the tumor mass will, therefore, improve this deficit. However, in some instances, although no change in the effects of the tumor mass is noted (cavernous sinus meningioma), the cranial nerve symptoms will regress following microparticle embolization. Two types of mechanisms may be implicated: arterial steal and "venous" congestion. In our experience, arterial steal occurs only with vascular malformations, and occasionally with paragangliomas during a stage in their evolution. Usually, the cranial nerve palsies related to such arterial steals are intermittent. The venous ischemic mechanisms, on the contrary, produce stable cranial nerve palsies which may not be transient but can be reversed with treatment. Therefore, embolization may reverse all three possible mechanisms (mass effects, arterial and venous effects).

An exceptional means by which embolization may relieve tumor symptoms is also due to relief of congestion of the surrounding tissues (venous?) close to the tumor. Such congestion is thought to be due to angiogenetic activity induced by the tumor. Such activity disappears with the cure of the lesion, with simultaneous relief of the related symptoms and normalization of the angiographic picture. If the lesion recurs, congestion may not reappear if the biological behavior of the tumor is not the same. We have encountered this phenomenon in only two types of tumors (hemagiopericytomas and paragangliomas).

Bleeding and pulsatile tinnitus are obviously related to the vascular nature of the lesion; they will be instantaneously relieved if complete embolization is achieved. Their persistence is definitive proof that embolization has been too proximal, or that a feeder was not embolized.

Treatment

Knowing what can be achieved clinically and pathologically, a decision to undertake embolization will depend on the therapeutic goal to be achieved and the type of risks that can reasonably be taken, considering the natural history of the disease.

At the pretherapeutic stage, embolization may be indicated if a highly vascularized lesion is suspected from an enhanced computerized tomography study. During the initial angiography, resorbable macroparticle embolization can be carried out as a safe means of performing diagnostic biopsy. These indications are rare; they may only be present with lesions having a high suspicion of malignancy, when neither surgery nor embolization is the desired treatment.

Presurgical embolization is most commonly used to manage tumors at the base of the skull that are likely to bleed excessively during operative excision. However, the vascularity of the lesion at operation depends as much on the surgeon as on the lesion itself. This emphasizes the need for a multidisciplinary approach and a common therapeutic strategy, more than strict rules of behavior. The effects of embolization on preoperative bleeding, duration of hospitalization, and the patient's postoperative course are well-known economic advantages of this combined approach. Surgery is usually planned for 2 to 15 days after the embolization, depending on the technique and the quality of the embolization achieved.

Palliative embolization is indicated when the lesion is thought to be surgically unresectable (as a result of the patient's status or the extent of the lesion), or is known to be unresponsive to chemo- or radiation therapy. Specific symptomatic relief will then be the goal of the procedure (to relieve bleeding, mass effect, pulsatile tinnitus, etc.). The portion of the tumor causing the symptoms will be identified and selectively treated with the best permanent agent possible, under the safest conditions (avoiding dangerous vessels or anastomoses). Ideally, an attempt to stabilize the entire lesion should be considered first, then successive compromises between this ideal goal and the risks to obtain it should be made. Thus the final therapeutic strategy may be to limit intervention in some cases.

Is embolization curative? For the time being, one cannot guarantee that with the available methods a cure can be obtained. Conceptually, a cure is anatomic and functional disappearance of the disease; however, we do not remove the lesion, we merely erase its image(s) and symptom(s) in the best cases. Although we have histopathological evidence that the tumor can become fibrotic, we can never be sure that a potentially active residue of tumor cells has not been left behind. For this reason, and considering what can be achieved at present, we think that *any surgically removable lesion should still be operated upon.* Embolization can make a lesion easier to operate upon, and even turn what was considered to be an inoperable lesion into an operable one. To this extent, embolization may be a necessary part of overall treatment aimed at cure.

Tumor recurrences should be treated like primary tumors if they are surgically resectable. In fact, combined embolization and surgery have brought the rate of recurrence to below 5% for lesions such as paragangliomas and juvenile angiofibromas.

For all the reasons just expressed, we believe that no benign tumor should *a priori* be irradiated unless an endovascular approach has proven to be not feasible. In addition, radiation and chemotherapy may induce their effects on tumors on the basis of vascular damage. It is our experience that embolization does not compromise the response of a tumor sensitive to radiation therapy, except when postradiation endarteritis is the dominant mechanism of tumor response.

Infusion

In the few cases in which a malignant lesion is inaccessible at the base of the skull, infusion may be used. Cytotoxic agents or ethanol are rarely used, as yet, in such cases. However, control of blood flow or redistribution of the supply at the base of the skull may transform a multiple feeder area into a single feeder target. Successive occlusion of each arterial source of supply, except one, makes the latter the unique source of vascularization for the entire lesion. At this point, infusion of the appropriate drug will have maximal efficacy with minimal side effects. The final feeder vessel must be carefully chosen from the beginning to be the most reachable and safest (no anastomoses and not in a dangerous region) for final catheterization and infusion.

Chemoembolization

Chemoembolization corresponds to microencapsulation of a drug, which is then released from the capsule by spontaneous dissolution of the capsule. Different types of capsules, dissolving at different rates and containing the same drug or combination of drugs, should allow long-lasting impregnation of the target. However, this technique has not yet been used at the cranial base. At present, only cytotoxics and steroids have been incorporated in capsules, but further research is being done in Europe, North America, and Japan to perfect the use of this technique, and a method of chemoembolization of cranial base tumors may be developed.

Technical Strategies and Indications

Anterior Cranial Fossa, Ethmoid Cells, Nasal Fossa

Tumors in this region are always supplied by the same vessels: ethmoid arteries and sphenopalatine branches. In our experience, esthesioneuroblastomas, capillary hemangiomas, meningiomas, and hemangiopericytomas can easily be reached if the distal internal maxillary artery can be catheterized. Bilateral embolization is *always* necessary, even if the lesion is located in one nasal fossa or ethmoid cell.

Control of blood flow in this region is the key to making the lesion more easily accessible. The ethmoid blood supply may need to be interrupted in some cases before embolization. Two methods can be used: (1) reversal of the flow in the ophthalmic artery, by a balloon catheter transiently inflated into the internal carotid siphon; or (2) intraorbital surgical clipping of the ethmoid arteries. Both techniques have proven to be equally effective. However, they require, from the angiographer, a perfect knowledge of the arterial supply to the orbits and its collateral circulation patterns.

Sellar Region and Cavum

Three arteries are usually involved in the supply to this area (six if it reaches the midline): internal maxillary branches, anterior division of the ascending pharyngeal artery, and intrapetrous and intracavernous internal carotid artery collaterals.

Most lesions in the cavum will be seen with selective injection of each of these arteries. However, blood supply from the internal carotid artery siphon does not necessarily indicate intracranial extension of the lesion: therefore, the injected arteries must be studied carefully since the lesion may be thought to be inoperable if the results of injection are misinterpreted. Juvenile angiofibroma is the disease most typical of this area, and embolization in this particular disease has been most successful in the past 15 years. Again, these tumors should be surgically removed whenever possible.

Embolization of individual feeders is usually sufficient, but redistribution of the flow is sometimes necessary for very invasive lesions or recurrences; the usual indication for redistribution of flow is intracavernous or epidural middle cranial fossa extension of the tumor. In these instances, transient inflation of a balloon catheter in the internal carotid artery siphon increases the area of the intracranial branches of the internal maxillary artery or of the ascending pharyngeal artery (Figs. 3A–E). Microparticle embolization at this time can more easily reach the distal tumoral capillary bed intracranially.

If the internal carotid artery (ICA) must be permanently occluded, proper functional testing of the patency of the

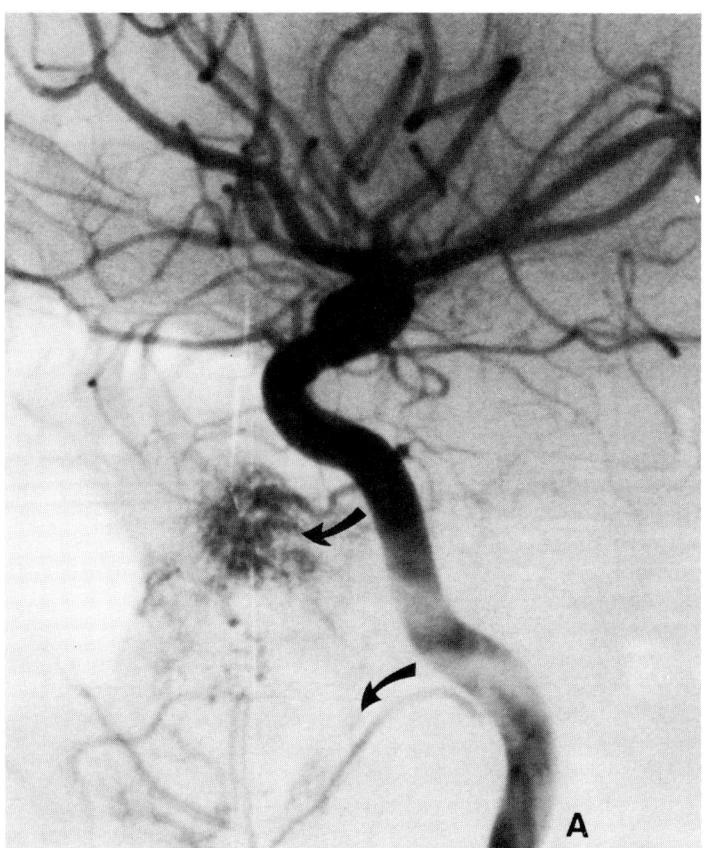

Figure 3A: Juvenile angiofibroma with epidural intracranial extension (curved arrows) is well demonstrated on the internal carotid artery (ICA) injection.

circle of Willis must be performed prior to any definitive procedure. One should remember that anatomical patency is not a guarantee of functional patency: the blood pressure at which the artery is functionally patent may be the minimum for functional efficiency. If, for any reason, blood pressure drops within the 2 or 3 days following occlusion of the ICA, the circle of Willis may not be able to ensure blood supply to the distal ipsilateral cerebral hemisphere. Therefore, patients must be carefully monitored. A delayed progressive deficit may be reversible by raising the blood pressure to a higher level.

Intolerance to internal carotid artery occlusion during the functional test would lead to extra-intracranial vascular anastomosis, if sacrifice of the internal carotid artery is mandatory to remove the tumor. In our experience, some lesions in this area have been treated that way: cavernous meningiomas, juvenile angiofibromas, paragangliomas, and metastases. In all cases the entire therapeutic strategy was discussed by a multidisciplinary team before embolization.

Temporal and Pharyngeal Region

Embolization of paragangliomas, as well as juvenile angiofibromas, has been extensively reviewed in the literature during the past 10 years. Some surgeons still operate successfully without embolization; however, the rate of recurrence and the quality of cranial nerve preservation is better when embolization precedes surgical removal. The protocol for embolization differs depending on the extensions of the tumor. However, when dominant vertebral and ipsilateral internal carotid angiograms are performed properly, internal carotid canal and cerebellopontine angle extensions can be excluded.

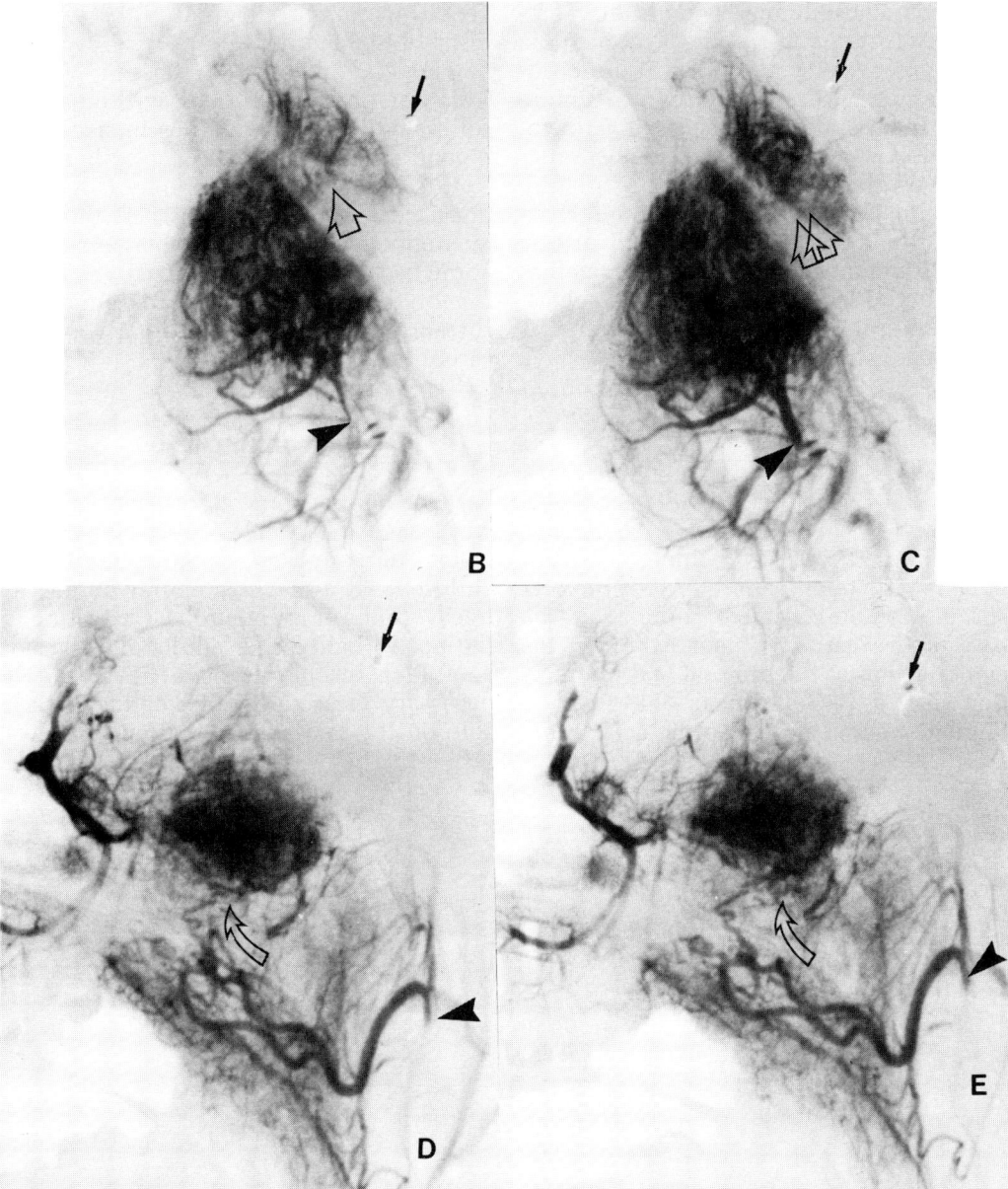

Figure 3: B–E: In order to reach the blood supply from the ICA, a balloon has transiently been inflated in front of both vessels (arrow) during selective accessory meningeal artery (AMA) angiography (arrowheads in **B** and **C**) and anterior division of the ascending pharyngeal artery (APA) (arrowheads in **D** and **E**). Straight open arrows show increases in the area of the tumor following inflation of the balloon during AMA injection (double open arrow); however, the area of the APA remained the same (double and single open curved arrows).

The venous phase of the dominant vertebral artery reliably gives a morphological and functional picture of the ipsilateral jugular vein.

Next, the internal maxillary, posterior auricular, occipital, and posterior division of the ascending pharyngeal arteries are studied successively, and with most temporal paragangliomas sequentially embolized (Figs. 4A–E). Flow control is rarely necessary, as the monocompartmental nature of tympanic tumors makes them particularly accessible to embolization. For extensive tumors, proper flow control may be achieved by inflating a balloon transiently or permanently in the intrapetrous internal carotid artery; this permits satisfactory devascularization of the entire lesion. Meningiomas, metastases, and schwannomas benefit from this combined approach; however, we have not yet needed to use any flow control technique in such cases.

Embolic Material

Since 1979, we have chosen polyvinyl alcohol foam (PVA) for the presurgical embolization of tumors at the base of the skull. We usually follow the embolization of the tumoral bed by injection of strips of Gelfoam soaked in thrombin and gamma-aminocaproic acid to devascularize the surgical field with a resorbable material.

For palliative or long-lasting effects, Gelfoam powder with or without PVA calibrated to be 160 microns in size gives a good response and satisfactorily stable results. Isobutyl cyanoacrylate (IBCA) is not used for tumors unless it is the only technique available in an emergency situation; because it may produce rapid swelling of the tumor, its use for enlarging intracranial lesions should always be carefully discussed.

Balloon Occlusion

For balloon procedures, we have always used detachable Latex devices (Ingenor Company, Paris) for both adults and children; the usual size employed for intracavernous or intrapetrous ICA testing is the no. 16 balloon for adults and the no. 17 for children. We have never felt it necessary to use any other balloon available on the market. The balloon that we

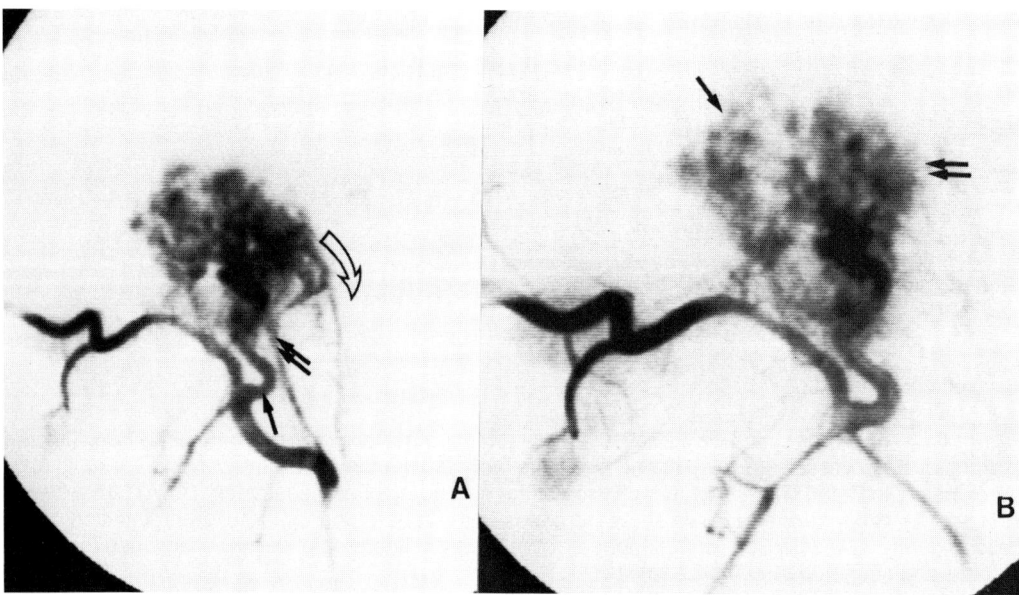

Figure 4A: Embolization of the pharyngo-occipital trunk supplying a temporal paraganglioma through a mastoid (arrow), stylomastoid (double arrow), and ascending pharyngeal artery opacified by reflux through the tympanic nidus (open curved arrow). **B:** Selective occipital artery injection permitted visualization of most of the nidus (arrow and double arrow); selective injection of the mastoid branch could not be achieved but distal occipital artery injection was. (Continued)

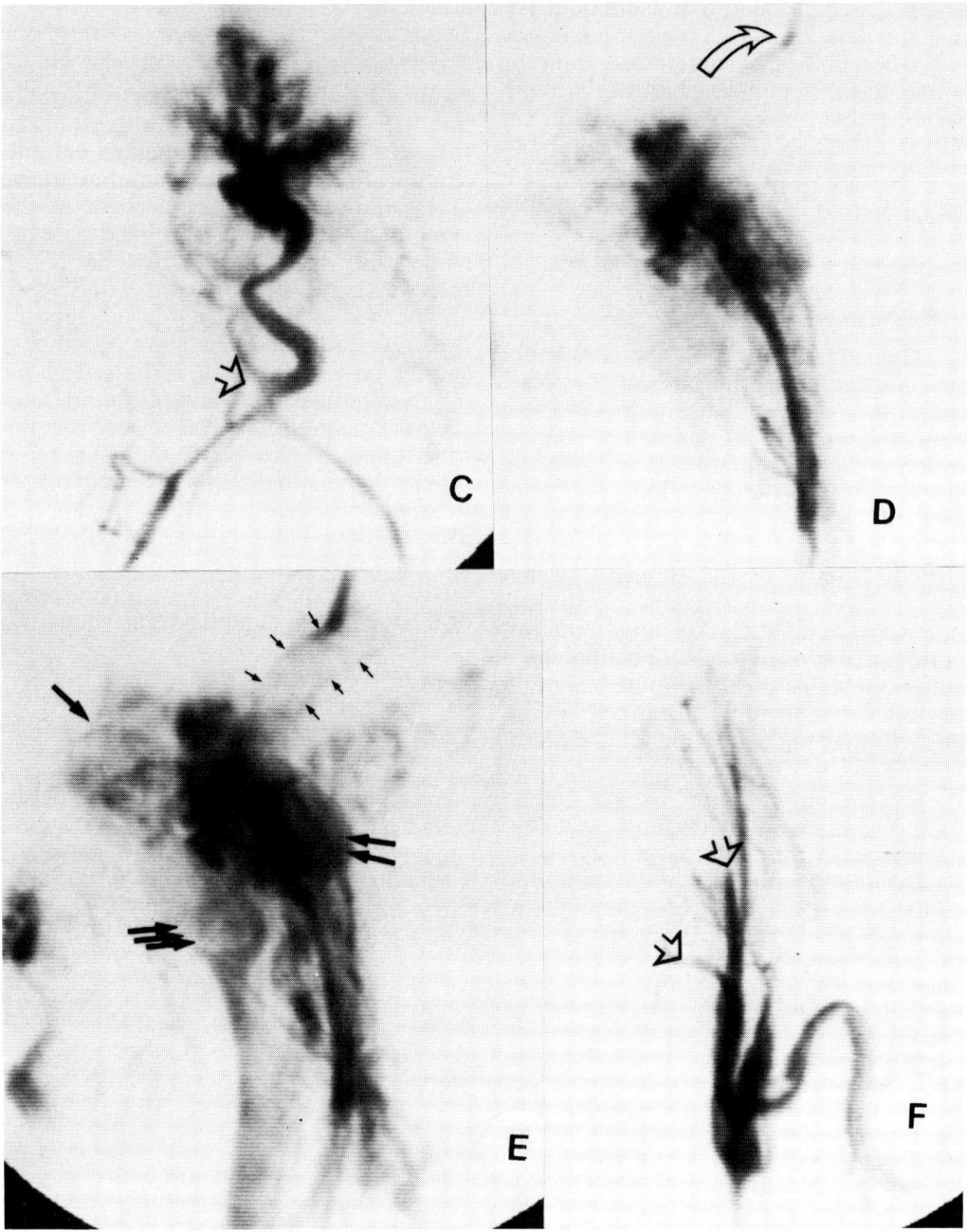

Figure 4C: Protective embolization was first achieved (open arrow), then microparticles could be used to reach the tumor nidus. **D:** Ascending pharyngeal artery early and (**E**) late in embolization. Note the arteriovenous shunt (open curved arrow) draining into the pericarotid venous plexus (small arrows), the mastoid (arrow), the tympanic vein (double arrow), and the intraluminal jugular vein (triple arrow) extensions. **E:** Control after embolization (open arrows).

use is ligated, inflated with isotonic material, and detached. We have never had any indication that a measurable leak from the balloon occurred into the base of the skull. We feel that there is no indication for either detachable balloon catheters or Silastic bids or coils to be used for management of tumors in the external carotid system.

Complications

Over 150 tumors of the head and neck area, extending to the base of the skull, have been embolized in the last 8 years, and we have seen no permanent complication related to the procedure. However, as already pointed out, we have noted one progressive hemiparesis following a secondary drop in blood pressure in a patient with occlusion of the internal carotid siphon who had satisfactory results of preoperative functional testing. Other occurrences included transient cranial nerve palsies, which are known to be one of the hazards of using this approach in that area. Proper choice of embolic material and proper evaluation of the anatomy of the area by radiology are obviously necessary. We have never had any premature detachment of a balloon or early secondary deflation with intracranial migration.

Conclusions

Therapeutic angiography can be extremely helpful in the surgical removal of tumors at the base of the skull. All of the tumors that had been embolized in children were successfully operated upon, and did not recur. Ten percent of the tumors in adults were embolized only because they were inoperable. Radiation therapy should only be considered when an endovascular approach is not feasible because irradiated vessels are fragile and cannot be satisfactorily catheterized for microembolization. State-of-the-art neurosurgery entails removal of any resectable tumor; however, in some cases, it seems unreasonable to resect a tumor without embolization. Arterial ligation is unnecessary when proper embolization has been done. Diagnostic and therapeutic angiography should be done if recurrence or postoperative complications occur.

Reference

1. Lasjaunias P, Berenstein A (eds): *Interventional Neuroradiology: (Craniofacial) Embolization*, Vol. I, *Anatomy and Angiographic Protocols*, Vol. II, *Techniques and Results*, New York, Springer-Verlag, 1986.

III

Anesthetic and Monitoring Techniques

6

Anesthesia for Cranial Base Tumor Operations

Karen B. Domino, M.D.

Introduction

The major goals of our anesthetic management are to maintain perioperative hemodynamic stability, prevent increases in intracranial pressure, enhance surgical exposure and removal of the tumor, and allow appropriate neurophysiological monitoring of cranial nerve functioning. The choice of particular anesthetic agents depends upon the patient's general medical and surgical condition. Anesthetic considerations for the resection of pituitary adenomas, acoustic neuromas, cavernous sinus tumors with carotid artery involvement, and glomus jugulare tumors are all different and are subjects of individual reviews.[23,30,39,69] This chapter will review pertinent neurophysiology, cerebral metabolic and vascular effects of anesthetic agents, and discuss the anesthetic considerations for cranial base tumor surgery in general.

Review of Pertinent Physiology

Cerebral Blood Flow

Cerebral blood flow (CBF) is dependent upon the cerebral perfusion pressure (CPP). CPP is equal to the mean arterial pressure minus the cerebral venous pressure, which is best approximated by the intracranial pressure (ICP).

The cerebral vasculature of normal brain autoregulates to changes in mean arterial pressure from 60 mmHg to 130–150 mmHg.[54] Within this range, the vessels dilate at low blood pressures and constrict at high blood pressures to maintain a constant CBF. Above and below the limits of autoregulation, CBF becomes passively dependent on cerebral perfusion pressure. Autoregulation is shifted to the right in patients with chronic hypertension, although long-term antihypertensive

From: Sekhar LN, Schramm VL Jr, eds: *Tumors of the Cranial Base: Diagnosis and Treatment.* Mount Kisco, New York, Futura Publishing Co, Inc, © 1987.

therapy may reverse the shift.[47] Autoregulation is abolished by hypercapnia, hypoxia, high concentrations of volatile anesthetics, trauma, and focal ischemia, so that perfusion is pressure-dependent.[108]

Normal cerebral vessels dilate in response to increases in $PaCO_2$ and constrict in response to decreases in $PaCO_2$.[70] CBF varies linearly with $PaCO_2$ between 20 and 80 mmHg in normal persons. The mechanism involves changes in CSF and periarteriolar pH, which gradually normalize by changes in CSF bicarbonate levels over 4–36 hours.

Other factors that alter CBF include hypoxia, cerebral metabolism, hematocrit, and body temperature.[70] CBF increases when the PaO_2 is reduced below 50 mmHg. CBF varies directly with cerebral metabolism, which is altered by brain activity. Hence, seizures increase CBF. Cerebral metabolic rate and CBF are reduced by decreasing body temperature. Hematocrits over 50 reduce CBF by increasing viscosity, and hematocrits under 30 increase CBF by decreasing viscosity.[70,123]

Vasomotor paralysis, in which the cerebral vessels do not normally autoregulate to changes in blood pressure or changes in $PaCO_2$, may occur within ischemic areas, around a tumor or infarction, or distal to vascular occlusions.[53,70] In these cases, flow is passively dependent upon perfusion pressure. Blood pressure control, with avoidance of hypertension and hypotension, is key in patients with significant vasomotor paralysis.

Intracranial Pressure

The rigid cranium is composed of three tissue compartments: brain, cerebrospinal fluid (CSF), and blood. Increases in volume of any one of these compartments must be compensated by decreases in volume of the others or else ICP increases. Brain tissue is relatively noncompressible and its volume is relatively constant. CSF and cerebral blood volume (CBV) may be displaced out of the cranial cavity with slow-growing tumors, such that an increase in intracranial volume causes little change in ICP. As the space-occupying lesion expands and the compensatory mechanisms fail, small increases in intracranial volume cause large increases in ICP. This generates the typical pressure-volume curve illustrated by Langfitt and associates (Fig. 1).

Since we rarely know where our patient is on the intracranial pressure-volume curve, we usually assume that any patient with a space-occupying intracranial mass has reduced intracranial compliance. Our anesthetic management aims mostly to alter CBF and CBV, with CSF and brain interstitial volumes altered to a limited degree.

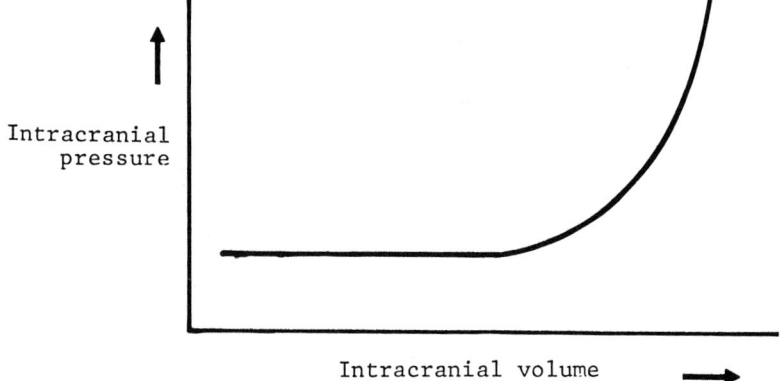

Figure 1: This figure illustrates the typical intracranial pressure-volume curve generated by Langfitt and associates. Initial increases in intracranial volume cause little change in intracranial pressure (ICP). As the space-occupying lesion expands and the compensatory mechanisms fail, small increases in intracranial volume cause large increases in ICP.

Anesthetic Effects

The effects of the commonly used anesthetic agents on cerebral metabolic rate, CBF, and CSF dynamics are discussed below and are summarized in Figure 2.

Inhalation Anesthetics

All currently used inhalation anesthetics, including nitrous oxide, are cerebrovasodilators to varying degrees. The vasodilation can be minimized by use of low concentrations and hyperventilation.

Halothane

Halothane is the oldest and the prototype of the currently available volatile anesthetics. It is a cerebrovasodilator that decreases cerebrovascular resistance (CVR) and increases CBF in a dose-dependent fashion.[8,65,115,121] Low doses (0.5 MAC*) have little effect (Fig. 3). The increase in CBF is transient, since CBF decreases to close to normal levels after 150 minutes in goats.[7] Cerebral blood volume, however, remains elevated by 11–12% over 3 hours.[11]

Halothane reduces the cerebral metabolic rate ($CMRO_2$) by 17 to 33 percent.[8,65,113] The cerebral metabolic rate for glucose is also reduced by halothane in proportion to the reduction in $CMRO_2$, with the primary reduction occurring in occipital cortex, cerebellar cortex and white matter, brain stem nuclei, and the anterior commissure.[107]

The cerebral vasculature remains responsive to changes in arterial PCO_2,[9,33,74,121] so that the cerebral vasodilation can be attenuated by prior hyperventilation for 10 minutes before halothane is added.[4] Halothane in high concentrations (2.0 MAC), abolishes autoregulation of the cerebral circulation in response to changes in mean arterial blood pressure.[74,81,115] Halothane alters blood-brain barrier permeability since it enhances the extravasation of plasma proteins into normal brain during acute hypertension.[38]

Halothane reduces CSF formation by 30% in dogs,[10] but increases the resistance of reabsorption of CSF.[13] Since ICP is determined by cerebral blood volume, CSF volume, and brain tissue volume, it is not surprising that ICP increases with halothane.[11,28,48,115] Peak increases are observed in 3–13 minutes, although the increase persists over 3 hours.[11] The increase in ICP in patients with intracranial mass lesions can be attenuated by the es-

EFFECTS OF ANESTHETIC AGENTS ON CEREBRAL CIRCULATION, ICP, AND CSF DYNAMICS

Anesthetic	CBF	$CMRO_2$	Autoregulation	CO_2 Responsiveness	ICP	CSF Production	Resistance to absorption of CSF	Seizures
INHALATION								
Halothane	↑↑	↓	Abolishes	Yes	↑[b]	↓	↑	no
Enflurane	↑	↓	Abolishes	Yes	↑[b]	↑↑	↑	yes[c]
Isoflurane	-↑[a]	↓↓	Preserves, unless high dose	Yes	↑[b]	-	↓	no
INTRAVENOUS								
Thiopental	↓	↓↓	Preserves	Yes	↓	-	-	no
Fentanyl (low dose)	-	-	Preserves	Yes	-	-	↓	very high doses
Etomidate	↓	↓	Preserves	Yes	↓	unknown	unknown	rare

Figure 2: Effects of anesthetic agents on cerebral circulation, ICP, and CSF dynamics. a = Dose-related increase in CBF; b = Increase in ICP blunted by hyperventilation; c = Seizures occur with high concentrations and hyperventilation.

---

*MAC is the minimum alveolar concentration required to prevent 50% of patients from moving in response to a surgical stimulus.

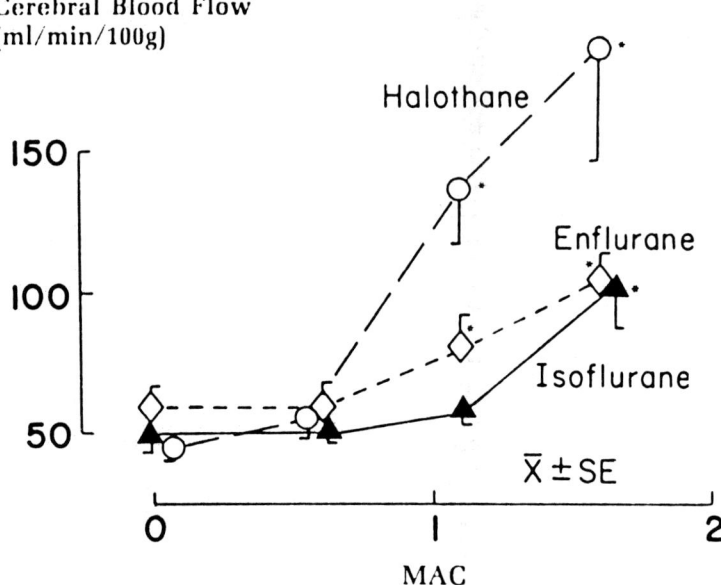

Figure 3: Effects of halothane, enflurane, and isoflurane on cerebral blood flow in human volunteers (data from Murphy et al., 1974). The volunteers were paralyzed with d-tubocurarine and their $PaCO_2$ and systemic blood pressure were kept at normal levels. All three agents had little effect on CBF at 0.5 MAC and all increased CBF at 1.6 MAC. The largest increases in CBF occurred with halothane. Reproduced with permission from Lippincott.

tablishment of hyperventilation for 10 minutes prior to the introduction of halothane.[4] Halothane can cause excessive brain protrusion if PCO_2 is not reduced.[34]

Enflurane

Enflurane does not increase CBF as much as halothane does, with a maximum increase in CBF of 12–37% observed at higher concentrations (Fig. 3).[72,86,102] Enflurane increases CBV[11] and reduces $CMRO_2$[72,102] similar to halothane. Like halothane, it disrupts autoregulation in high concentrations,[74] but it does not alter the responsiveness of the cerebral circulation to changes in PCO_2.[72,74]

Two properties of enflurane which make it undesirable in neuroanesthesia are its ability to increase the rate of CSF production and to induce seizure-like activity. In contrast to other anesthetics, enflurane causes a 50% increase in the rate of CSF production in dogs.[16] Enflurane also increases the resistance to reabsorption of CSF to a greater degree than halothane,[12] which leads to large late-occurring increases in ICP during prolonged anesthesia with enflurane.[11] Thus, ICP may increase during enflurane anesthesia due to its effects on both CBF and CSF volume.[11,18,82]

Another disadvantage of enflurane is its ability to induce seizure-like EEG activity (high voltage spike waves with burst suppression) when it is administered in high concentrations (2.0 MAC).[56,72,88] Hyperventilation increases the frequency and magnitude of high voltage spike activity at even lower alveolar enflurane concentrations.[56,72] Low doses of enflurane do not cause EEG abnormalities during hyperventilation.

Isoflurane

Isoflurane has become quite popular in neuroanesthesia because it is less of a cerebrovasodilator than halothane and it does not possess the undesirable properties of enflurane. Low concentrations of isoflurane (0.5 and 1.0 MAC) have little effect on CBF (Fig. 3).[58,60,86,115] Intermediate concentrations increase CBF,[25] particularly to cerebellar, limbic system, and brain stem structures, while high concentrations (2 MAC) increase CBF uniformly.[58] Isoflurane decreases $CMRO_2$ by 30%[91] and it causes an isoelectric EEG at 2 MAC concentrations.[36,91] It is unique among the volatile agents in that it preserves normal cerebral energy states and aerobic metabolism at very low blood pressures (40 mmHg), in contrast to halothane, enflurane, trimethaphan, and nitroprusside.[91,92] Like the barbiturates, it provides some degree of cerebral protection by increasing the survival time of mice exposed to 5% oxygen and increased cerebral energy stores in dogs with incomplete global cerebral ischemia, presumably by depressing cortical electrical activity and cerebral metabolism.[90] It is not protective in regional cerebral ischemia.[116]

The CO_2 responsiveness of the cerebral circulation is intact[25] and is enhanced during administration of 1.0 MAC isoflurane (with 75% nitrous oxide) compared to halothane-nitrous oxide and nitrous oxide alone.[33] Cerebral autoregulation is less affected by isoflurane than by halothane.[115]

Cerebrospinal fluid production is not affected by isoflurane[14] and the resistance to reabsorption of CSF is reduced.[12] Brain protrusion following isoflurane is significantly less than is observed with halothane.[34] Isoflurane can increase ICP[3,43,115] due to an increase in CBV.[15] The increase in ICP can be blunted by the simultaneous initiation of hyperventilation,[3] in contrast to halothane, which requires 10 minutes of prior hyperventilation to prevent the increase in ICP.[4] However, dangerous increases in ICP may still occur in patients who have a midline shift evident on CT scan.[43]

Nitrous Oxide

Nitrous oxide (N_2O) is a weak cerebrovasodilator whose effects are offset by hyperventilation and barbiturate anesthesia. The variable effects of N_2O on CBF and ICP are due to differences in species and background anesthesia. In many animals, N_2O in subanesthetic doses (60–70%) causes excitement and cerebral metabolic stimulation, with an accompanying increase in CBF.[94,100,113] Since N_2O is not an adequate anesthetic in the absence of other inhalational or intravenous anesthetics, the modification of the cerebral effects of N_2O by the background anesthesia is particularly important. Seventy percent N_2O does not cause a change in CBF and it reduces $CMRO_2$ by 15 to 20% during barbiturate and narcotic anesthesia.[100,122] However, when N_2O is added to a volatile anesthetic such as isoflurane[60] or halothane,[101] both CBF and $CMRO_2$ increase. The cerebral vascular responses to changes in PCO_2 and mean arterial pressure (MAP) are preserved during N_2O anesthesia.[109] ICP may increase in patients with intracranial mass lesions and reduced intracranial compliance.[46,83,95] The increase in ICP with N_2O is readily reversible by diazepam and barbiturate anesthesia and simultaneously initiated hyperventilation.[95] N_2O is used extensively in neuroanesthesia because it is safe and it is eliminated rapidly, permitting a rapid emergence from anesthesia.

Intravenous Anesthetics

Thiopental

Thiopental has been the mainstay of induction agents in neuroanesthesia. When the EEG is isoelectric, CBF, CBV, and $CMRO_2$ decrease by about 50%.[8,71,96] Autoregulation and the cerebral vascular response to changes in PCO_2 are intact during barbiturate anesthesia.[110] The rate of CSF formation and the resistance to reabsorption of CSF are not altered by barbiturates.[59] Intracranial pressure can be acutely reduced by barbiturates.[106] Thiopental may also be used as a continuous infusion, since it is short-acting as a bolus drug.

Etomidate

Etomidate is a valuable induction agent in the patient with cardiovascular disease due to the stability of blood pressure, heart rate, cardiac output, and systemic vascular resistance. It reduces CBF (34%), CMRO$_2$ (45%), and ICP and preserves the CO$_2$ responsiveness of the cerebral circulation.[84,98] Myoclonus has been reported after a prolonged continuous infusion of etomidate.[55]

Narcotics

Fentanyl is a short-acting synthetic narcotic that is commonly used in anesthesia. Sufentanil is a newer, more potent short-acting narcotic that has a shorter elimination half-life than fentanyl.[19] These drugs are used more frequently in neuroanesthesia than the longer-acting narcotics, morphine and meperidine. Morphine tends to be overly sedative and meperidine may be associated with hypertension and tachycardia.

Narcotics in low doses have little effect on CBF, CBV, an ICP unless respiration is depressed and PCO$_2$ is increased.[77,80,85] Fentanyl, when combined with N$_2$O, decreased CBF (47%) and CMRO$_2$ (18%).[73] Autoregulation and CO$_2$ responsiveness of the cerebral circulation are not altered.[66] Fentanyl does not alter the rate of CSF formation[10] and it reduces the resistance to reabsorption of CSF by 50%.[13]

Lidocaine

Lidocaine in nontoxic doses decreases CBF, increases CVR, and reduces the increase in MAP, HR, and ICP associated with endotracheal intubation.[31,45,103]

Muscle Relaxants

Most muscle relaxants have little effect on cerebral blood volume and ICP. Large doses of curare may release histamine, which can cause cerebrovasodilation and increase ICP.[112] Succinylcholine may also increase ICP if muscle fasciculations occur.[63] Atracurium and vecuronium have no effect on ICP.[78,79] They may be advantageous in patients with intracranial disease, since they have clinically insignificant cardiovascular effects compared to pancuronium. They have an intermediate duration of action and may be useful in cases where facial or extraocular muscle EMG monitoring is planned.

Anesthetic Management

Preoperative Assessment/Premedication

The preoperative assessment of the patient with a cranial base tumor is similar to other presurgical patients, with special emphasis paid to the neurological exam. The patients may have reduced intracranial compliance, cranial nerve deficits, or endocrinologic abnormalities. Many are receiving steroids, which may cause glucose intolerance, and anticonvulsants, particularly phenytoin, which causes resistance to neuromuscular blockade with nondepolarizing relaxants.[93] Although many of these patients are anxious, nonsedative premedications are used. Standard doses of sedative premedications may make these patients very drowsy postoperatively and obscure the neurological examination. Narcotics are avoided in patients with reduced intracranial compliance, since increases in PaCO$_2$ may increase ICP. Antihypertensives, anticonvulsants, thyroid replacement, steroids, and other critical medications are given on the morning of surgery with small sips of water.

Routine Monitoring

Standard monitoring for cranial base tumor surgery involves monitoring the electrocardiogram, temperature, heart tones, and respiration by an esophageal stethoscope, blood pressure via an arterial line, central venous pressure, neuromuscular blockade by a twitch monitor, end-tidal carbon dioxide tension, urine output by Foley catheter, Doppler ultrasound, and intermittent serum electrolytes, glucose, osmolality, and arterial blood gases.

Choice of Anesthetic Agents

The presence of overt or potential intracranial hypertension requires an anesthetic technique that will avoid increasing the intracranial blood volume, while maintaining adequate cerebral perfusion. Hypoxia, hypercarbia, hypertension, coughing, straining, or bucking can increase cerebral blood volume and should be avoided. Hypotension may reduce CPP and cause cerebral ischemia, especially in areas of vasomotor paralysis.

While selection of anesthetic agents that decrease $CMRO_2$, CBF, and CBV (e.g., narcotics, barbiturates, etomidate) is desirable, volatile agents may be used depending upon the patient's general medical and surgical condition. They are necessary when intraoperative EMG monitoring is required so that neuromuscular blockers can be avoided. Cerebral vasodilation induced by the volatile anesthetics can be minimized by hyperventilation and use of low concentrations. A "light" anesthetic technique is usually desirable, so that the patient awakens promptly at the conclusion of the surgical procedure. This permits early assessment of the neurological exam and allows prompt diagnosis of subsequent changes. Intravenous anesthetics need to be given in low doses to accomplish this goal. Prolonged sedation and respiratory depression may result from doses that do not sedate patients undergoing noncraniotomy procedures. Hemodynamic control, while avoiding relative overdosage of anesthetic drugs, can be achieved by infiltration of the wound with a long-acting local anesthetic and use of vasodilators and beta blockers.

Fluid Management

Preoperative fluid deficits and intraoperative losses are replaced in sufficient quantities to allow hemodynamic stability without increasing cerebral edema. Many of the patients are hypovolemic due to poor oral intake, administration of radiological contrast, diuretics, and supine diuresis.[61,118] Hypovolemia is particularly problematic during the induction of anesthesia and initiation of positive pressure ventilation because it may lead to hypotension, hypoxemia, and the compromise of cerebral perfusion.[111] Hypovolemia may be also associated with a decrease in CBF despite a presence of normal blood pressure.[27] Administration of isotonic solutions (normal saline, Plasmalyte®, or lactated Ringer's) is preferred since hypotonic solutions may increase brain water.[111] Replacement of fluid deficits by colloid-containing solutions (plasma protein fraction, 5% albumin, or Hetastarch) is also helpful. In the presence of an intact blood-brain barrier, these molecules stay in the intravascular space longer than isotonic crystalloid solutions. Studies in normal rabbits suggest that increases in brain water and intracranial pressure are reduced when colloids are used for hemodilution instead of crystalloid solutions.[117]

Administration of glucose-containing solutions should be avoided in patients at risk for focal cerebral ischemia (e.g., those with cerebrovascular disease, during brain retraction, and with use of deliberate hypotension).[52,89] Hyperglycemia exacerbates cerebral injury in global[97] and regional eschemia animal models.[52,97] A poorer outcome was noted at blood glucose levels as low as 160–180 mg/100 ml.[52] Since hypoglycemia rarely develops during anesthesia, especially in patients given steroids, it is prudent to avoid glucose-containing solutions and check intraoperative blood glucose levels periodically.

Improving Surgical Exposure

Surgical exposure of cranial base tumors may be enhanced by shrinkage of the brain by hyperventilation, administration of diuretics, removal of cerebrospinal fluid, and careful control of blood pressure. PCO$_2$ is generally maintained at 25–30 mmHg intraoperatively to reduce CBF and cerebral blood volume. Acute reductions in PCO$_2$ to 20 mmHg or less are avoided since it may reduce CBF to the point of ischemia.[70]

Furosemide and/or mannitol may be used to shrink the brain. Mannitol induces an osmotic gradient between the plasma and normal brain, in areas of intact blood-brain barrier. It decreases brain water content by drawing the water from the brain into the plasma. Lower (0.25 gm/kg) doses of mannitol may be as effective as higher doses (0.5–1.0 gm/kg).[64] Beneficial effects are seen in 60–90 minutes. The initial increase in intravascular volume may increase CVP, blood pressure, and ICP. A small (5–10 mg) dose of furosemide may be given prior to mannitol to avoid this problem. Larger doses of furosemide may cause severe volume depletion and electrolyte derangements (hyperosmolality, hyponatremia, hypochloremia, hypokalemia).[105] Reports of the effectiveness of furosemide alone in the treatment of intracranial hypertension have been conflicting.[22,120] Small doses (5–10 mg) of furosemide may induce a large diuresis under general anesthesia. Therefore, it is best to start with low doses and give supplemental doses if adequate diuresis and decreases in ICP are not obtained. Patients with brain tumors also occasionally have a spontaneous profound diuresis upon induction of anesthesia.[67]

Withdrawal of CSF through a lumbar subarachnoid catheter is used to reduce brain retraction and the need for diuretic agents. An #18 gauge subarachnoid catheter can be inserted after the patient is anesthetized. Since CSF is formed at a rate of 0.35 to 0.4 ml/min with a total CSF volume of 150 ml, slow withdrawal of 20–60 ml of CSF usually results in excellent brain conditions.

Surgical excision of the tumor can also be enhanced by reduction of cerebral venous pressure with a slight head-up position and careful control of blood pressure. Hypertension not only increases CBF and subsequent edema formation, but it also increases blood loss, reduces visibility, and may increase surgical time. Systemic blood pressure is generally maintained at low normal levels during surgical dissection, except in the case where carotid artery clamping is required (see complications section). Deliberate hypotension may be useful in selected patients who have intact cerebral vasomotor autoregulation and the absence of major cardiopulmonary disease.[35] Deliberate hypotension reduces blood loss and the number of transfusions and the clearer surgical field can improve surgical conditions and reduce surgical time.[104,114] This can be particularly helpful in resection of glomus jugulare tumors and vascular meningiomas which are associated with a large blood loss.

Neurophysiologic Monitoring

Another goal of the anesthetic management is to allow the desired neurophysiological monitoring of cranial nerve function (see Chapter 7 for details). Monitoring of cranial nerves III, IV, VI, and VII is performed by recording EMG potentials. Therefore, neuromuscular blockers are avoided during monitoring of the facial muscle and extraocular movements. Volatile anesthetics, such as isoflurane, are used to immobilize the patient. Brain stem auditory evoked potentials are monitored during operations in which the auditory nerve is at risk. They can also provide information concerning compression and perfusion of the brain stem. They are not measurably affected by anesthetic agents, although changes in temperature, blood pressure, arterial tensions of respiratory gases, and intracranial pressure may alter them.[21,44] Because cortical visual evoked responses are exquisitely sensitive to premedicants and anesthetic agents,[29] techniques to measure responses recorded directly from the optic nerve are being developed (see Chapter 7).

Intraoperative Complications

Cranial Nerve Stimulation

Abrupt cardiovascular alterations commonly occur because of surgical manipulation of the cranial nerves or brain stem during posterior fossa surgery.[5,51,68,75,99,119] Bradycardia occurs in up to 25% and supraventricular tachycardia in 23% of posterior fossa cases.[5] Stimulation of the trigeminal nerve may elicit bradycardia, ventricular arrhythmias, and hypertension. Vagal nerve stimulation may cause bradycardia and hypotension. PVCs, ventricular tachycardia, ST segment depression,[99] conduction abnormalities,[87] sinus arrhythmias,[32] and severe hypotension[87] have also been reported.

The surgeon should be immediately notified of any arrhythmia or hemodynamic aberration so that the source of the stimulus can be identified and removed. In most cases, the cardiovascular change is transient and disappears once the surgical stimulation is terminated. Treatment with antiarrhythmic drugs is unnecessary unless the arrhythmia is life-threatening. Prophylactic treatment is not advised since it reduces the warning of deleterious surgical stimulation.

Air Embolism

Another important complication associated with craniotomies in general, and posterior fossa surgery in particular, is air embolism. Although air embolism is more commonly associated with sitting craniotomies, an 8% incidence (5 of 60 patients) detected by Doppler ultrasound has been reported with posterior fossa surgery in the lateral position.[6] Air embolism can occur because of the presence of noncollapsible venous channels such as diploic venis and dural sinuses. Venous air embolism may increase dead space, impair gas exchange, causing hypercarbia, hypoxia, and reflex pulmonary vasoconstriction with slow, continuous entrainment of air. Larger volumes may obstruct the right ventricular outflow tract and reduce venous return and cardiac output, which can result in cardiac arrhythmias, hypotension, and cardiovascular collapse. Attention has been recently focused on the rare possibility of paradoxical or arterial air embolism, which may pass via an intracardiac defect (probe patent foramen ovale occurs in 25% of the population)[24,42] or due to pulmonary shunting.[62] The most sensitive readily available method for the detection of venous air embolism is the precordial Doppler ultrasound.[37,40] Because of its sensitivity, it can detect as little as 0.1 ml of air and microbubbles within a saline flush, but it fails to reflect embolus size. Larger, clinically significant air emboli, are detected by decreases in end-tidal PCO_2 and increases in pulmonary artery pressure.[37,40] Hypotension, ECG changes indicative of right heart strain, cardiac arrhythmias, and the Millwheel murmur are late-occurring manifestations of large amounts of air.[37,40] Thus, end-tidal PCO_2 monitoring in combination with the Doppler provide a combination of sustained, sensitive, and reliable detection of air embolism and a quantitative indication of embolus size. Newer methods of detection, such as end-tidal N_2 analysis and transesophageal echocardiography are currently being investigated.[23,24]

Treatment of the air embolism involves notifying the surgeon of its occurrence so that its source can be identified, discontinuing nitrous oxide (to slow the increase in size of air bubbles), elevation of venous pressure by a Valsalva maneuver, or jugular venous compression to aid the surgeon in detecting the source, withdrawal of air through a central venous catheter, and maintenance of hemodynamic stability by volume infusion and vasopressors. The use of positive end-expiratory pressure (PEEP) to prevent further emboli is controversial.[23] PEEP increases right atrial pressure resulting in right-to-left shunt in a patient with a probe-patent foramen ovale, and thereby may increase the likelihood of a paradoxical air embolus.[17]

Carotid Arterial Occlusion

During the resection of cavernous sinus tumors, the carotid artery may require cross-clamping. Adequacy of collateral blood flow is assessed preoperatively by a balloon occlusion test during arteriography (see Chapter 12). Intraoperative EEG monitoring may be useful to detect cortical cerebral ischemia with carotid clamping in all cases and to reduce cerebral metabolic rate by barbiturate loading when collateral flow is known to be inadequate.

The key to reducing a neurological deficit during carotid artery clamping is the maintenance of adequate CPP. Collateral blood flow is especially dependent upon perfusion pressure. Systemic blood pressure should be elevated to or slightly above the upper level of the patient's normal pressure, with the use of volume infusion and vasopressors if necessary. Increases in cardiac output and reduction in viscosity with volume loading may improve regional cerebral perfusion.[27]

The choice of the ideal PCO_2 is controversial. There is a theoretical concern that collateral blood flow to ischemic zones could be reduced by hyperventilation, since hypocapnia causes cerebral vasoconstriction. However, an "inverse steal" or "Robin Hood" syndrome, in which only the normal vessels constrict and shunt blood flow into the ischemic area which has vasomotor paralysis, may occur.[54] Since there is no practical way of predicting what will actually happen to regional CBF in a given patient, most anesthesiologists maintain normocapnia for patients undergoing surgery for cerebrovascular insufficiency. Thus, the advantages of hyperventilation to reduce brain bulk must be weighed against the benefits of normocapnia in patients subject to regional cerebral ischemia.

Anesthetic agents may be helpful in reducing cerebral metabolic rate and thus protect the brain against regional cerebral ischemia. Barbiturates, in doses which cause burst suppression on the EEG, improve neurological outcome in acute focal ischemia.[110,116] Although isoflurane also reduces brain metabolism,[115] causes an isoelectric EEG,[91] prolongs hypoxic survival,[90] and preserves normal brain metabolism during hypotensive anesthesia,[92] it is not protective against neurological injury in temporary focal cerebral ischemia, in contrast to barbiturates.[116]

Massive Blood Transfusion

Blood loss may be extensive in cranial base surgery, especially with vascular tumors and extensive reconstruction of the cranium. Massive transfusion may be associated with coagulation disorders due to dilutional thrombocytopenia, deficiencies of labile factors V and VIII, and disseminated intravascular coagulation (DIC).[20,76] Thrombocytopenia is usually the most important cause of bleeding.[20,76] Two units of fresh frozen plasma and platelet concentrates should be given every 10 units of blood to restore dilute factors.[20] Other complications of blood transfusions include hypothermia, transfusion reactions (hemolytic, febrile, and allergic), disease transmission (viral hepatitis in 7% of blood recipients,[1] AIDS[26]), hyperkalemia, citrate intoxication with hypocalcemia, acid-base imbalance, and microaggregate deposition.[20]

Postoperative Complications

Cranial Nerve Deficits

Postoperative loss of cranial nerve function may occur following removal of cranial base tumors. The manipulation or stretching of the IX, X, XII cranial nerves is particularly important to the anesthesiologist. Injury to cranial nerves IX and XII may be associated with impaired pharyngeal sensation, swallowing discoordination, and aspiration, while injury to cranial nerve X may result in a unilateral vocal cord paresis. The patient should remain intubated in the immediate postoperative period if trauma to pharyngeal or laryngeal nerve supply occurs.[41]

Tension Pneumocephalus

Tension pneumocephalus has been reported as a cause of postoperative neurological dysfunction, particularly with posterior fossa operations in the seated position, although it may occur in cranial base surgery. As the CSF leaks out of the subarachnoid space, the cerebral hemispheres collapse and air accumulates over the cortex. A tension pneumocephalus can occur since CSF accumulates faster than the air can be absorbed.[50,57] It may occur very rarely during posterior fossa surgery in the lateral position and should be included in the differential diagnosis of postoperative coma.

Other Complications

Airway obstruction may occur in patients with IX nerve palsies; it may occur following transphenoidal hypophysectomies, in which nasal packs are inserted, or after cranial base reconstruction procedures where a muscular flap is placed in the neck. Edema, venous infarction, and hemorrhage into these flaps may cause postoperative upper airway obstruction. Aspiration is a particular concern in patients with IX and X cranial nerve palsies and hypothyroid patients, who may be unusually sensitive to narcotics and sedatives.

Arterial hypertension occurs frequently after craniotomies, especially posterior fossa surgery. It should be treated aggressively with vasodilators and beta-blockers to prevent risk of intracranial bleeding and brain edema. Nausea and vomiting are also frequent complications of anesthesia, posterior fossa surgery, and in procedures where blood drains into the stomach. If the patient is not sedated, low doses (1.25 mg) of droperidol is an effective antiemetic.[2]

References

1. Aach RD, Kahn RA: Post-transfusion hepatitis: Current perspectives. *Ann Int Med* 92:539-546, 1980.
2. Abramowitz MD, Oh TH, Epstein BS, et al: The antiemetic effect of droperidol following outpatient stabismus surgery in children. *Anesthesiology* 59:579-583, 1983.
3. Adams RW, Cucchiara RF, Gronert GA, et al: Isoflurane and cerebrospinal fluid pressures in neurosurgical patients. *Anesthesiology* 54:97-99, 1981.
4. Adams RW, Gronert GA, Sundt TM, et al: Halothane, hypocapnia, and cerebrospinal fluid pressure in neurosurgery. *Anesthesiology* 37:510-517, 1972.
5. Albin MS, Babinski M, Maroon JC, et al: Anesthetic management of posterior fossa surgery in the sitting position. *Acta Anaesth Scand* 20:117-128, 1976.
6. Albin MS, Carroll RG, Maroon JC: Clinical considerations concerning the detection of venous air embolism. *Neurosurgery* 3:380-384, 1978.
7. Albrecht RF, Miletich DJ, Madala LR: Normalization of cerebral blood flow during prolonged halothane anesthesia. *Anesthesiology* 58:26-31, 1983.
8. Albrecht RF, Miletich DJ, Rosenberg R, et al: Cerebral blood flow and metabolic changes from induction to onset of anesthesia with halothane or pentobarbital. *Anesthesiology* 47:252-256, 1977.
9. Alexander SC, Wollman H, Cohen PJ, et al: Cerebrovascular response to $PaCO_2$ during halothane anesthesia in man. *J Appl Physiol* 19:561-565, 1964.
10. Artru AA: Effects of halothane and fentanyl on the rate of CSF production in dogs. *Anesth Analg* 62:581-585, 1983.
11. Artru AA: Relationship between cerebral blood volume and CSF pressure during anesthesia with halothane or enflurane in dogs. *Anesthesiology* 58:533-539, 1983.
12. Artru AA: Effects of enflurane and isoflurane on resistance to reabsorption of cerebrospinal fluid in dogs. *Anesthesiology* 61:529-533, 1984.
13. Artru AA: Effects of halothane and fentanyl anesthesia on resistance to reabsorption of CSF. *J Neurosurg* 60:252-256, 1984.
14. Artru AA: Isoflurane does not increase the rate of CSF production in the dog. *Anesthesiology* 60:193-197, 1984.

15. Artru AA: Relationship between cerebral blood volume and CSF pressure during anesthesia with isoflurane or fentanyl in dogs. Anesthesiology 60:575-579, 1984.
16. Artru AA, Nugent M, Michenfelder JD: Enflurane causes a prolonged and reversible increase in the rate of CSF production in the dog. Anesthesiology 57:255-260, 1982.
17. Bedford RF, Perkins NAK: Hemodynamic consequences of PEEP in seated neurological patients. Implications for paradoxical air embolism. Anesth Anal 63:429-432, 1984.
18. Boop WC, Knight R: Enflurane anesthesia and changes of intracranial pressure. J Neurosurg 48:228-231, 1978.
19. Bovill JG, Sabel PS, Blackburn CL, et al: The pharmacokinetics of sufentanil in surgical patients. Anesthesiology 61:502-506, 1984.
20. Brzica SM: Complications of transfusion. In Stehling LC (ed): *Techniques of Blood Transfusion*, Int Anesth Clinics, Boston, Little Brown, Co., 20:171-193, 1982.
21. Clark DL, Rosner BS: Neurophysiologic effects of general anesthetics: I. The electroencephalogram and sensory evoked responses in man. Anesthesiology 38:564-582, 1973.
22. Cottrell JE, Robustelli A, Post K, et al: Furosemide- and mannitol-induced changes in intracranial pressure and serum osmolality and electrolytes. Anesthesiology 47:28-30, 1977.
23. Cucchiara RF: Monitoring and management of the anesthetized patient in the sitting position. In Hershey SG (ed): *ASA Refresher Courses in Anesthesiology*, Philadelphia, Lippincott, 12:63-72, 1984.
24. Cucchiara RF, Nugent M, Seward JB, et al: Air embolism in upright neurosurgical patients: Detection and localization by two-dimensional transesophageal echocardiography. Anesthesiology 60:353-355, 1984.
25. Cucchiara RF, Theye RA, Michenfelder JD: The effects of isoflurane on canine cerebral metabolism and blood flow. Anesthesiology 40:571-574, 1974.
26. Curran JW, Lawrence DN, Jaffe H, et al: Acquired immunodeficiency syndrome (AIDS) associated with transfusions. NEJM 310:69-75, 1984.
27. Davis DH, Sundt TM Jr: Relationship of cerebral blood flow to cardiac output, mean arterial blood pressure, blood volume, and alpha and beta blockade in cats. J Neurosurg 52:745-754, 1980.
28. DiGiovanni AJ, Goodrick J, Neigh JL, et al: The effect of halothane anesthesia on intracranial pressure in the presence of intracranial hypertension. Anesth Analg 53:823-827, 1974.
29. Domino EF: Effects of preanesthetic and anesthetic drugs on visually evoked responses. Anesthesiology 28:184-191, 1967.
30. Donegan JH: Anesthesia for patients with ischemic cerebrovascular disease. In Hershey SG (ed): *ASA Refresher Courses in Anesthesiology*, Philadelphia, Lippincott, 10:63-74, 1982.
31. Donegan MF, Bedford RF: Intravenously administered lidocaine prevents intracranial hypertension during endotracheal suctioning. Anesthesiology 52:516-518, 1980.
32. Drummond JC, Todd MM: Acute sinus arrhythmia during surgery in the fourth ventricle: An indication of brainstem irritation. Anesthesiology 60:232-235, 1984.
33. Drummond JC, Todd MM: The response of the feline cerebral circulation to $PaCO_2$ during anesthesia with isoflurane and halothane and during sedation with nitrous oxide. Anesthesiology 62:268-273, 1985.
34. Drummond JC, Todd MM, Toutant SM, et al: Brain surface protrusion during enflurane, halothane, and isoflurane anesthesia in cats. Anesthesiology 59:288-293, 1983.
35. Edwards MW: Complications of deliberate hypotension. In Orkin FK, Cooperman LH (eds): *Complications in Anesthesiology*, Philadelphia, pp 613-623, 1983.
36. Eger EI, Stevens WC, Cromwell TH: The electro-encephalogram in man anesthetized with Forane. Anesthesiology 35:504-508, 1971.
37. English JB, Westenskow D, Hodges MR, et al: Comparison of venous air embolism monitoring methods in supine dogs. Anesthesiology 48:425-429, 1978.
38. Forster A, VanHorn K, Marshall LF, et al: Anesthetic effects on blood-brain barrier function during acute arterial hypertension. Anesthesiology 49:26-30, 1978.
39. Ghani GA, Sung YF, Per-Lee JH: Glomus jugulare tumors: origin, pathology, and anesthetic considerations. Anesth Analg 62:686-691, 1983.
40. Gildenberg PL, O'Brien RP, Britt WJ, et al: The efficacy of Doppler monitoring for

the detection of venous air embolism. *J Neurosurg* 54:75-78, 1981.
41. Gorski DW, Rao TLK, Scarff TB: Airway obstruction following surgical manipulation of the posterior cranial fossa, an unusual complication. *Anesthesiology* 54:80-81, 1981.
42. Gronert GA, Messick JM, Cucchiara RF, et al: Paradoxical air embolism from a patent foramen ovale. *Anesthesiology* 50:548-549, 1979.
43. Grosslight K, Foster R, Colohan AR, et al: Risk factors for increases in intracranial pressure. *Anesthesiology* 63:533-536, 1985.
44. Grundy BL: Intraoperative monitoring of sensory-evoked potentials. *Anesthesiology* 58:72-87, 1983.
45. Hamill JF, Bedford RF, Weaver DC, et al: Lidocaine before endotracheal intubation: Intravenous or laryngotracheal? *Anesthesiology* 55:578-581, 1981.
46. Henriksen HT, Jorgensen PB: The effect of nitrous oxide on intracranial pressure in patients with intracranial disorders. *Br J Anaesth* 45:486-492, 1973.
47. Hoffman WE, Miletich DJ, Albrecht RF: Cerebrovascular response to hypotension in hypertensive rats: Effect of antihypertensive therapy. *Anesthesiology* 58:326-332, 1983.
48. Jennett WB, Barker J, Fitch W, et al: Effect of anesthaesia on intracranial pressure in patients with space-occupying lesions. *Lancet* 1:61-64, 1969.
49. Jobes DR, Kennell EM, Bush GL, et al: Cerebral blood flow and metabolism during morphine-nitrous oxide anesthesia in man. *Anesthesiology* 47:16-18, 1977.
50. Kitahata LM, Katz JD: Tension pneumocephalus after posterior fossa craniotomy, a complication of the sitting position. *Anesthesiology* 44:448-450, 1976.
51. Lall NG, Jain AP: Circulatory and respiratory disturbances during posterior cranial fossa surgery. *Br J Anaesth* 41:447-449, 1969.
52. Lanier WL, Stangland KJ, Scheithauer BW, et al: The effects of dextrose infusion and head position on neurologic outcome after complete cerebral ischemia in primates: Examination of a model. *Anesthesiology* 66:39-48, 1987.
53. Lassen NA: The luxury-perfusion syndrome and its possible relation to acute metabolic acidosis localized within the brain. *Lancet*, 2:1113, 1966.
54. Lassen NA, Christensen MS: Physiology of cerebral blood flow. *Br J Anaesth* 48:719-734, 1976.
55. Laughlin TP, Newberg LA: Prolonged myoclonus after etomidate anesthesia. *Anesth Analg* 64:80-82, 1985.
56. Lebowitz MH, Blitt CD, Dillon JB: Enflurane-induced central nervous system excitation and its relation to carbon dioxide tension. *Anesth Analg* 51:555-565, 1972.
57. Lunsford LD, Maroon JC, Sheptak PE, et al: Subdural tension pneumocephalus: Report of two cases. *J Neurosurg* 50:525-527, 1979.
58. Maekawa T, Tommasino C, Shapiro HM, et al: Local cerebral blood flow and glucose utilization during isoflurane anesthesia in the rat. *Anesthesiology* 65:144-151, 1986.
59. Mann JD, Mann ES, Cookson SL: Differential effects of pentobarbital, ketamine hydrochloride, and enflurane anesthesia on CSF formation rate and outflow resistance in the rat (abstract). *Neurosurgery* 4:482, 1979.
60. Manohar M, Parks C: Regional distribution of brain and myocardial perfusion in swine while awake and during 1.0 and 1.5 MAC isoflurane anaesthesia produced without or with 50% nitrous oxide. *Cardiovasc Res* 18:344-353, 1984.
61. Maroon JC, Nelson PB: Hypovolemia in patients with subarachnoid hemorrhage: Therapeutic implications. *Neurosurgery* 4:223-226, 1979.
62. Marquez J, Sladen A, Gendell H, et al: Paradoxical cerebral air embolism without an intracardiac septal defect. *J Neurosurg* 55:997-1000, 1981.
63. Marsh ML, Dunlop BJ, Shapiro HM, et al: Succinylcholine: Intracranial pressure effects in neurosurgical patients. *Anesth Analg* 59:550-551, 1980.
64. Marshall LF, Smith RW, Rauscher LA, et al: Mannitol dose requirements in brain-injured patients. *J Neurosurg* 48:169-172, 1978.
65. McDowall DG: The effects of clinical concentrations of halothane on the blood flow and oxygen uptake of the cerebral cortex. *Br J Anaesth* 39:186-196, 1967.
66. McPherson RW, Traystman RJ: Fentanyl and cerebral vascular responsivity in dogs. *Anesthesiology* 60:180-186, 1984.
67. Mehta MP, Gergis SD, Sokoll M: Paradoxical diuresis in some neurosurgical patients under balanced anesthesia. *Anesthesiology* 59:585-587, 1983.
68. Meridy HW, Creighton RE, Humphreys

RP: Complications during neurosurgery in the prone position in children. *Canad Anaesth Soc J* 21:445-453, 1974.
69. Messick JM, Laws ER, Abboud CF: Anesthesia for transsphenoidal surgery of the hypophyseal region. *Anesth Analg* 57:206-215, 1978.
70. Michenfelder JD: The cerebral circulation. In Prys Roberts C (ed): *The Circulation in Anesthesia: Applied Physiology and Pharmacology*, Oxford, Blackwell Scientific Publications, 209-225, 1980.
71. Michenfelder JD: The interdependency of cerebral functional and metabolic effects following massive doses of thiopental in the dog. *Anesthesiology* 41:231-236, 1974.
72. Michenfelder JD, Cucchiara RF: Canine cerebral oxygen consumption during enflurane anesthesia and its modification during induced seizures. *Anesthesiology* 40:575-580, 1974.
73. Michenfelder JD, Theye RA: Effects of fentanyl, droperidol, and Innovar on canine cerebral metabolism and blood flow. *Br J Anaesth* 43:630-635, 1971.
74. Miletich DJ, Ivankovich AD, Albrecht RF, et al: Absence of autoregulation of cerebral blood flow during halothane and enflurane anesthesia. *Anesth Anal* 55:100-109, 1976.
75. Millar RA: Neurosurgical anaesthesia in the sitting position. *Br J Anaesth* 44:495-505, 1972.
76. Miller RD: Complications of massive blood transfusions. *Anesthesiology* 39:82-93, 1973.
77. Miller R, Tausk HC, Stark DCC: Effect of Innovar, fentanyl and droperidol on the cerebrospinal fluid pressure in neurosurgical patients. *Canad Anaesth Soc J* 22:502-508, 1975.
78. Minton MD, Stirt JA, Bedford RF, et al: Intracranial pressure after atracurium in neurosurgical patients. *Anesth Analg* 64:1113-1116, 1985.
79. Minton MD, Stirt JA, Bedford RF: Vecuronium and intracranial pressure in man (abstract). *Anesth Analg* 65:5101, 1986.
80. Misfeldt BB, Jorgensen PB, Spotoff H, et al: The effects of droperidol and fentanyl on intracranial pressure and cerebral perfusion pressure in neurosurgical patients. *Br J Anaesth* 48:963-968, 1976.
81. Morita H, Nemoto EM, Bleyaert AL, et al: Brain blood flow autoregulation and metabolism during halothane anesthesia in monkeys. *Am J Physiol* 233:H670-H676, 1977.
82. Moss E, Dearden NM, McDowall DG: Effects of 2% enflurane on intracranial pressure and cerebral perfusion pressure. *Br J Anaesth* 55:1083-1088, 1983.
83. Moss E, McDowall DG: ICP increases with 50% nitrous oxide in oxygen in severe head injuries during controlled ventilation. *Br J Anaesth* 51:757-761, 1979.
84. Moss E, Powell D, Gibson RM, et al: Effect of etomidate on intracranial pressure and cerebral perfusion pressure. *Br J Anaesth* 51:347-352, 1979.
85. Moss E, Powell D, Gibson RM, et al: Effects of fentanyl on intracranial pressure and cerebral perfusion pressure during hypocapnia. *Br J Anaesth* 50:779-784, 1978.
86. Murphy FL, Kennell EM, Johnstone RE, et al: The effects of enflurane, isoflurane, and halothane on cerebral blood flow and metabolism in man (abstract). Abstracts of Scientific Papers, Annual meeting of American Society of Anesthesiologists, 1974, pp 61-62.
87. Nagashima C, Sakaguchi A, Kamisasa A, et al: Cardiovascular complications on upper vagal rootlet section for glossopharyngeal neuralgia. *J Neurosurg* 44:248-253, 1976.
88. Neigh JL, Garman JK, Harp JR: The electroencephalographic pattern during anesthesia with Ethrane: Effects of depth of anesthesia, $PaCO_2$ and nitrous oxide. *Anesthesiology* 35:482-487, 1971.
89. Newberg LA: Use of intravenous glucose solutions in surgical patients. *Anesth Analg* 64:558, 1985.
90. Newberg LA, Michenfelder JD: Cerebral protection by isoflurane during hypoxemia or ischemia. *Anesthesiology* 59:39-45, 1983.
91. Newberg LA, Milde JH, Michenfelder JD: The cerebral metabolic effects of isoflurane at and above concentrations that suppress cortical electrical activity. *Anesthesiology* 59:23-28, 1983.
92. Newberg LA, Milde JH, Michenfelder JD: Systemic and cerebral effects of isoflurane-induced hypotension in dogs. *Anesthesiology* 60:541-546, 1984.
93. Ornstein E, Matteo RS, Young WL, et al: Resistance to metocurine-induced neuromuscular blockade in patients receiving phenytoin. *Anesthesiology* 63:294-298, 1985.
94. Pelligrino DA, Miletich DJ, Hoffman WE, et al: Nitrous oxide markedly increases cerebral cortical metabolic rate and blood flow in the goat. *Anesthesiology* 60:405-412, 1984.
95. Phirman JR, Shapiro HM: Modification of nitrous oxide-induced intracranial

hypertension by prior induction of anesthesia. *Anesthesiology* 46:150-151, 1977.
96. Pierce EC, Lambertsen CJ, Deutsch S, et al: Cerebral circulation and metabolism during thiopental anesthesia and hyperventilation in man. *J Clin Invest* 41:1664-1671, 1962.
97. Pulsinelli WA, Waldman S, Rawlinson D, et al: Moderate hyperglycemia augments ischemic brain damage: A neuropathologic study in the rat. *Neurology* 32:1239-1246, 1982.
98. Renou AM, Vernhiet J, Macrez P, et al: Cerebral blood flow and metabolism during etomidate anaesthesia in man. *Br J Anaesth* 50:1047-1051, 1978.
99. Rubin RC, Frost EAM: Posterior cranial fossa surgery. In Frost EAM (ed): *Clinical Anesthesia in Neurosurgery*, Boston, Butterworth, 1984, Chapter 7, pp 155-185.
100. Sakabe T, Kuramoto T, Inoue S, et al: Cerebral effects of nitrous oxide in the dog. *Anesthesiology* 48:195-200, 1978.
101. Sakabe T, Kuramoto T, Kumagae S, et al: Cerebral responses to the addition of nitrous oxide to halothane in man. *Br J Anaesth* 48:957-962, 1976.
102. Sakabe T, Maekawa T, Fujii S, et al: Cerebral circulation and metabolism during enflurane anesthesia in humans. *Anesthesiology* 59:532-536, 1983.
103. Sakabe T, Maekawa T, Ishikawa T: The effects of lidocaine on canine cerebral metabolism and circulation related to electroencephalogram. *Anesthesiology* 40:433-441, 1974.
104. Schaberg SJ, Kelly JF, Terry BC, et al: Blood loss and hypotensive anesthesia in oral-facial corrective surgery. *J Oral Surg* 34:627-629, 1976.
105. Schettini A, Stahurski B, Young HF: Osmotic and osmotic-loop diuresis in brain surgery: Effects on plasma and CSF electrolytes and ion excretion. *J Neurosurg* 56:679-684, 1982.
106. Shapiro HM, Galindo A, Wyte SR, et al: Rapid intraoperative reduction of intracranial pressure with thiopentone. *Br J Anaesth* 45:1057-1062, 1973.
107. Shapiro HM, Greenberg JH, Reivich M, et al: Local cerebral glucose uptake in awake and halothane anesthetized primates. *Anesthesiology* 48:97-103, 1978.
108. Siesjo BK: *Brain Energy Metabolism*. New York, John Wiley and Sons, 1978.
109. Smith AL, Neigh JL, Hoffman JC, et al: Effects of general anesthesia on autoregulation of cerebral blood flow in man. *J Appl Physiol* 29:665-669, 1970.
110. Smith AL, Wollman H: Cerebral blood flow and metabolism: Effects of anesthetic drugs and techniques. *Anesthesiology* 36:378-400, 1972.
111. Smith DS: Fluid management in neurosurgical anesthesia. In Hershey SG (ed): *ASA Refresher Courses in Anesthesiology*, Philadelphia, Lippincott, 11:205-216, 1983.
112. Tarkkanen L, Laitinen L, Johansson G: Effects of d-tubocurarine on intracranial pressure and thalamic electrical impedence. *Anesthesiology* 40:247-251, 1974.
113. Theye RA, Michenfelder JD: The effect of nitrous oxide on canine cerebral metabolism. *Anesthesiology* 29:1113-1118, 1968.
114. Thompson GE, Miller RD, Stevens WC, et al: Hypotensive anesthesia for total hip arthroplasty: A study of blood loss and organ function (brain, heart, liver, and kidney). *Anesthesiology* 48:91-96, 1978.
115. Todd MM, Drummond JC: A comparison of the cerebrovascular and metabolic effects of halothane and isoflurane in the cat. *Anesthesiology* 60:276-282, 1984.
116. Todd MM, Hehls DG, Drummond JC, et al: A comparison of the protective effects of isoflurane and thiopental in a primate model of temporary focal cerebral ischemia (abstract). *Anesthesiology* 63:A412, 1985.
117. Todd MM, Tommasino C, Moore S, et al: The effects of acute isovolemic hemodilution on the brain: A comparison of crystalloid and colloid solutions (abstract). *Anesthesiology* 61:A122, 1984.
118. VanBeaumont W, Greenleaf JE, Julos L: Disproportional changes in hematocrit, plasma volume, and proteins during exercise and bed rest. *J Appl Physiol* 33:55-61, 1972.
119. Whitby JD: Electrocardiography during posterior fossa operations. *Br J Anaesth* 35:624-630, 1963.
120. Wilkinson HA, Rosenfeld S: Furosemide and mannitol in the treatment of acute experimental intracranial hypertension. *Neurosurgery* 12:405-410, 1983.
121. Wollman H, Alexander SC, Cohen PJ, et al: Cerebral circulation of man during halothane anesthesia. *Anesthesiology* 24:180-184, 1964.
122. Wollman H, Alexander SC, Cohen PJ, et al: Cerebral circulation during general anesthesia and hyperventilation in man. *Anesthesiology* 26:329-334, 1965.
123. Wood JH, Snyder LL, Simeone FA: Failure of intravascular volume expansion without hemodilution to elevate cortical blood flow in region of experimental focal ischemia. *J Neurosurg* 56:80-91, 1982.

7

Electrophysiological Monitoring of Cranial Nerves in Operations in the Skull Base

Aage R. Møller, Ph.D.

Introduction

Electrophysiological monitoring is justified when it can reduce the risk of complications or when it can aid the surgeon during the operation by providing information that is valuable for performing the procedure. It is important that information that has relevance is made available at the time when it is valid, and that the methods that are used interfere minimally with other activities in the operating room. Also, it is important that the methods used do not increase electrical hazards.

Electrophysiological monitoring of the cranial nerves that may be subjected to surgical manipulation can help to avoid injury to those nerves. During neurosurgical operations of the skull base, such monitoring can also aid the surgeon in identification of the nerves when the anatomy is distorted, e.g., by tumors.

During skull tumor operations, it is important to monitor the cranial nerves innervating the extraocular and the facial muscles. However, the optic nerve and the auditory nerve may also be at risk in such operations, and therefore it is important to monitor these nerves as well. We have previously described methods for monitoring auditory evoked potentials during neurosurgical operations, and showed the usefulness of such monitoring in reducing the incidence of postoperative hearing loss.[4] Recently, we have described a method for recording visual evoked potentials that is suitable for use during neurosurgical operations.[8] Monitoring auditory evoked potentials can also provide valuable information about compression of the brain stem, since changes in these potentials may often occur before there is any detectable change in the vital signs.

Monitoring of NIII, NIV, NVI, and NVII

The nerves that innervate the extraocular muscles may most easily be monitored by recording compound action potentials from the muscles that are inner-

From: Sekhar LN, Schramm VL Jr, eds: *Tumors of the Cranial Base: Diagnosis and Treatment*. Mount Kisco, New York, Futura Publishing Co, Inc, © 1987.

vated by these three nerves while the nerves are stimulated electrically.

However, the facial nerve is monitored by recording the compound action potentials (EMG) from several groups of facial muscles. This is especially important to identify fascicles of the facial nerve when they have been spread apart by tumors. If monitoring was based upon recording the EMG from muscles innervated by a single branch of the facial nerve alone, stimulation of parts of the nerve that innervate other muscles would go unnoticed and this may result in damage to those parts of the nerve.

Electrode Placement

Figure 1 shows a schematic drawing of the placement of the various electrodes for recording muscle EMGs. The extraocular muscles can be reached by inserting needle electrodes through the skin. However, it must be pointed out that safe insertion of recording needles requires a thorough knowledge of the anatomy of the extraocular muscles and the eye. For monitoring the spontaneous or stimulated activity of the extraocular muscles, it is not necessary that the recording needle electrodes actually be placed in the respective muscles—being close to the muscles is sufficient to obtain a satisfactory recording. We use subdermal platinum electrodes (Grass Instrument Co.,* type E2), but other similar electrodes will give satisfactory results.

The lateral rectus (innervated by NVI) can be reached by inserting a needle electrode in the lateral corner of the eye, and the superior oblique muscle (NIV), which is the most difficult one to reach externally, by inserting a needle in the medial upper corner of the orbit, aiming medially and upward. NIII can be monitored by recording from any of the muscles that are innervated by NIII. We have been recording from the medial rectus muscle, which can be reached by inserting a needle

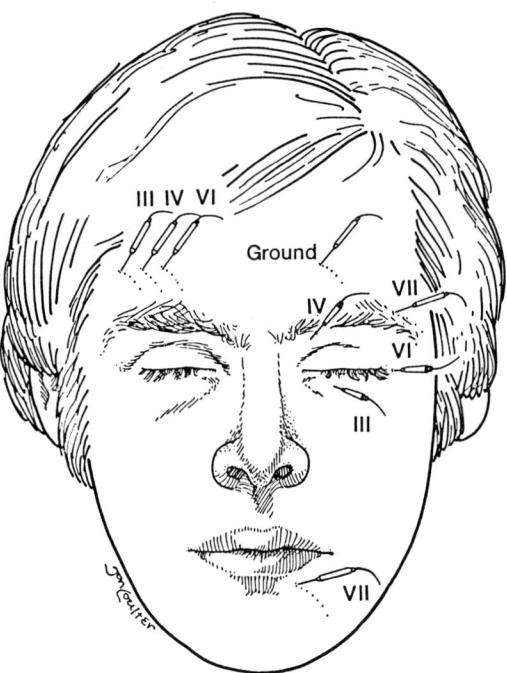

Figure 1: Schematic drawing of electrode placement for differential recording from the muscles innervated by cranial nerves III, IV, VI, and VII. Reference electrodes for recording from the extraocular muscles are not critical but should be placed on the contralateral side to avoid recording facial muscle activity on the operated side.

through the skin in the lower medial portion of the orbit, aiming away from the globe. Reference electrodes are placed on the forehead on the opposite side and a ground electrode is likewise placed on the forehead. Monitoring of the facial nerve is done by placing one needle electrode in the orbicularis oris muscle, and the other in the obicularis oculi superior and the frontalis muscle. A ground electrode is placed on the forehead. All the electrodes are secured in place by adhesive plastic tape (3M Company,** Blenderm®). It is especially important that the electrodes used to record from the extraocular muscles be bent and secured in such a way that pressure, e.g., from the drape, cannot change

---

*Grass Instrument Company, 101 Old Colony Avenue, P.O. Box 516, Quincy, Massachusetts 02169.
**3M Company, Minnesco Division/3M, 224-4 N.W., 3M Center, St. Paul, Minnesota 55144.

their direction to cause injury to the eye. Finally, the electrode wires are secured to the headholder with plastic tape.

The advantages of the needle electrodes used are that they provide a very stable electrical contact and do not come loose as easily as surface electrodes. When removed carefully they leave no noticeable marks on the skin. Needle electrodes, however, have a small surface area, and therefore the risk of burns (should the return connection to the electrocoagulator be insufficient) is greater than when surface electrodes having a larger area are used. Such surface electrodes will provide equally good results, and may be used when there is any doubt about the return connection of the electrocoagulator.

Amplifiers and Display

The recorded EMG potentials can be amplified by any good quality amplifier (we use Grass Instrument Co., type P511J or Grass Instrument Co., model 12), and the responses displayed on an oscilloscope (preferably four-channel). The bandwidth of the amplifier is set to 0.3 to 3000 Hz. This low highpass limit (0.3 Hz) minimizes the extension of the stimulus artifact, but if the stimulus artifact is of a small amplitude, a higher cutoff frequency (e.g., 10 or 30 Hz) can be used without interfering with the EMG recording. The electrodes are connected to the amplifiers via special probes that have a solid-state, current-limiting device built in (e.g., Grass Instrument Co., type IG3 P511).

Figure 2 shows examples of responses recorded from the extraocular muscles, and from the orbicularis oculi and oris muscles when their respective nerves are electrically stimulated intracranially.

In addition to displaying the responses on an oscilloscope, it is useful to have the responses made audible through a loudspeaker, so that the surgeon can directly hear the responses, rather than having an assistant communicate the results to the surgeon. Earlier we showed the usefulness of this when facial muscle re-

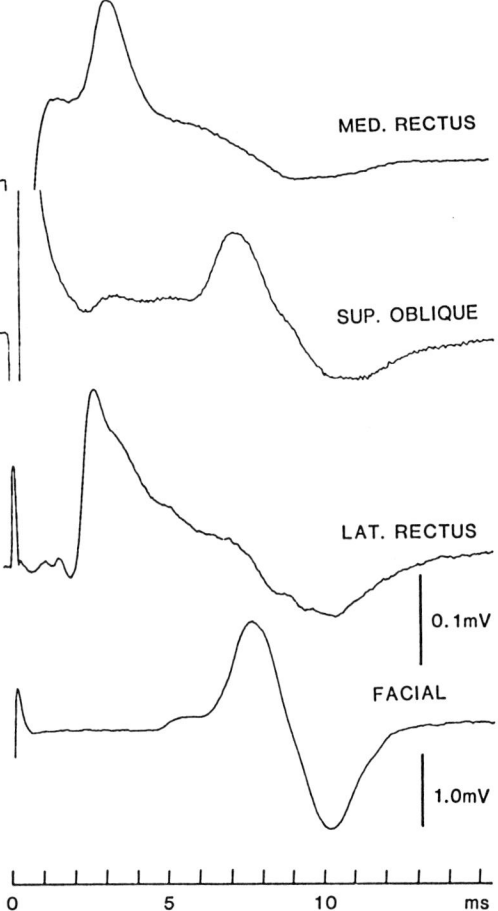

Figure 2: Examples of responses recorded from extraocular muscles and from the orbicularis oculi and mental muscles in response to electrical stimulation of the respective motor nerves. The vertical calibration is the same for the three recordings from extraocular muscles.

cordings were used to help preserve the facial nerve during removal of acoustic tumors. However, because the stimulus artifact is often very large, it is necessary to include a circuit that suppresses the stimulus artifact between the physiological amplifier and the audio amplifier.[5] This not only enables the surgeon to hear when the nerve in question is electrically stimulated, but also makes it immediately evident when the nerve has been manipulated or heated (by electrocoagulation or laser) to an extent that would injure the nerve. Mild injury to any one of the motor nerves may result in injury potentials that can be recorded from the respective muscles. When using the technique described above, such injury potentials become audible even in the absence of electrical stimulation.

Stimulation

The nerves are stimulated electrically using a hand-held monopolar electrode (Fig. 3). It has a Teflon-insulated malleable wire with an uninsulated gold-plated tip about 2 mm long. The return electrode is a 25-gauge, all-metal hypodermic needle that is placed in the wound near the craniotomy. The stimulator used should be capable of delivering 100- to 200-μs long rectangular pulses with a balanced charge (bipolar). Since the effective stimulus is a cathodal impulse, it is important that the stimulating electrode always be connected to the negative terminal of the stimulator. The stimulator must have a stimulus isolation unit of good quality in order to minimize stimulus artifacts and for safety reasons. Units that contain the amplifier and loudspeaker as well as the stimulator, including an oscilloscope, are available commercially (e.g., Facial Nerve Locator, Grass Instrument Co.).

Anesthesia

Since cranial nerve function is monitored by recording EMG potentials, the patient cannot be paralyzed during the time when recordings are being made. This, however, usually does not cause any major problems and anesthesia of these patients has been satisfactorily maintained by administration of Forane® (isoflurane) and nitrous oxide throughout the operation. Occasionally, it is beneficial to administer a small amount of a narcotic (e.g., Fentany ®). In our institution, anesthesia is induced for these operations with pentothal and succinylcholine together with a small dosage of tubocurarine (3 mg) or a short-duration end-plate blocking agent (Atricurium®) for intubation. The effects of these agents have disappeared by the time monitoring of muscle potentials is required (see Chapter 6).

Monitoring of NVIII

The monitoring of brain-stem auditory evoked potentials (BAEP) is of value in preventing hearing loss. Because of the wide extension of the ascending auditory pathway in the brainstem, the BAEP will change if the brainstem is compressed. Therefore, BAEP may provide one of the earliest signs of increased intracranial pressure.

For the purpose of monitoring the integrity of the auditory nerve, direct recording from the eighth cranial nerve is superior to recording farfield potentials, i.e., BAEP. This is because the NVIII response is large enough that it can be viewed directly on an oscilloscope, or only a few responses need to be averaged in order to obtain a response that can be interpreted.[4] This makes it immediately evident when an injury to the nerve has occurred. On the other hand, when BAEP are used, the need to average a large number of responses to obtain an interpretable recording delays the recognition of nerve injury. In addition, since the pro-

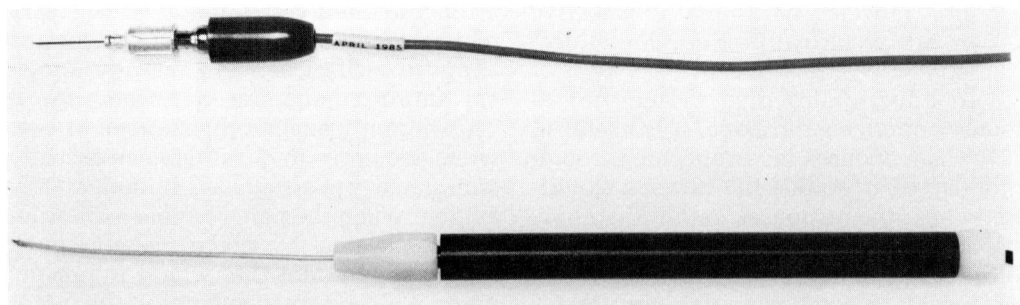

Figure 3: Hand-held electrode (Grass Instrument Co) for intracranial nerve stimulation.

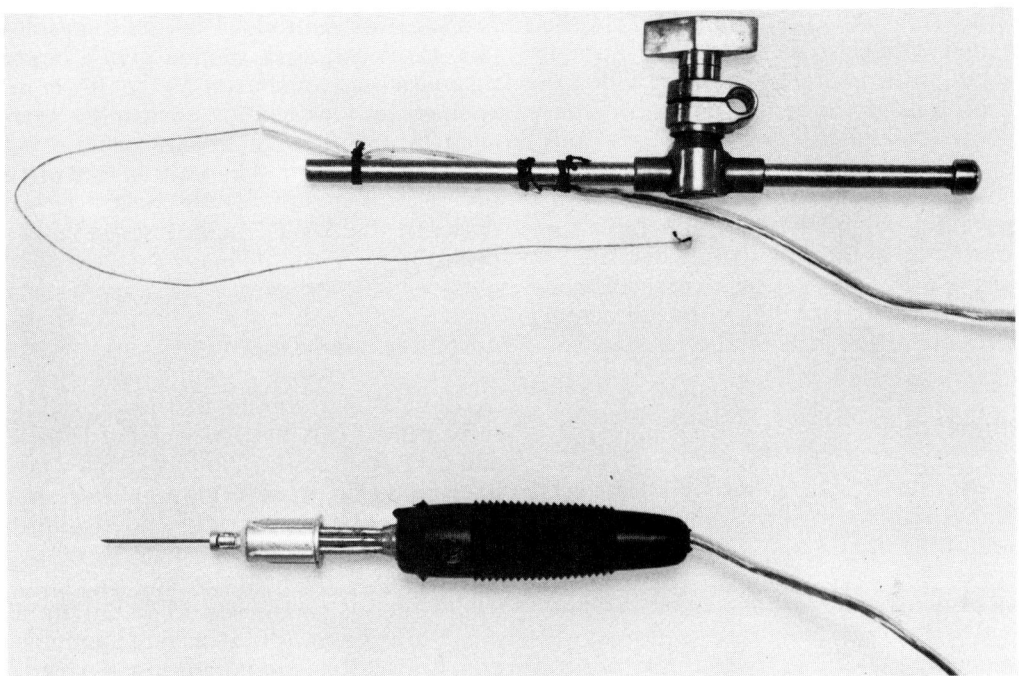

Figure 4: The electrode used to record compound action potentials from the eighth nerve intracranially.

cess of averaging many responses to enhance a signal that is buried in noise relies on the assumption that the response does not change during the averaging process, results obtained over a period of time become meaningless when the response changes as a result of nerve injury. Recording directly from the eighth cranial nerve, however, only reflects injuries to the part of the auditory pathway that is peripheral to the location of the recording electrode. Such direct recording has been shown to be efficient in reducing the risk of damage to the auditory nerve during microvascular decompression operations for hemifacial spasm, tic douloureux, and disabling positional vertigo.[1,4]

Electrode Placement

BAEP can be recorded from electrodes placed on the scalp. Traditionally, BAEP are recorded differentially between one electrode placed on the vertex and another electrode placed on the ipsilateral mastoid. If the latter position is not possible because of the surgical approach to be used, a position in front of the pinna or in the earlobe may be used. If a recording is being made from both ears, one electrode is placed on each mastoid. A ground electrode is placed on the forehead near the hair line.

We use the same type of subdermal platinum needle electrodes as used to record muscle EMG (Grass Instrument Co., type E2) placed subcutaneously and secured in place with adhesive plastic tape (3M Co., Blenderm®).

We use Teflon-insulated silver wires (Medwire Corporation,* types AG 10T, or AG 7/40T) for recording the compound action potentials (CAP) from the eighth cranial nerve directly.[4] The insulation is removed from the tip for about 5 mm and the tip is bent over and a cotton wick is sutured to the uninsulated tip using 5-0 silk. The wick is trimmed using microscissors and all loose cotton is removed. This electrode is connected to a conventional insulated copper wire that is connected to the input of the amplifier. The electrode is secured to a rod of the retractor (see Fig. 4), or a retractor blade

---

*Medwire Corporation, 121 S. Columbus Avenue, Mt. Vernon, New York 10553.

using 3-0 silk. The cotton wick is then wetted with saline and brought into contact with the neural tissue from which the recordings are to be made. The reference electrode is a 25-gauge, all-metal hypodermic needle that is placed in the wound nearby and connected to another insulated copper wire, which is in turn connected to the other input terminal of the recording amplifier. This electrode can be gas sterilized or, if the connecting wires are of adequate quality, autoclaved.

Stimulation

Sound is generated by insert earphones (Fig. 5) fitted with standard Lucite earmolds (Microsonic*). Five sizes of earmolds for each ear are available, so it is possible to obtain an adequate fit for practically any ear. We use earphones designed for masking in audiometry, and supplied by a manufacturer of audiometers (Madsen Electronics**). However, any hearing aid earphone (for body hearing aids) that is of good quality can be used. Either tonebursts or click sounds can be used as stimuli. The response to tonebursts is probably more sensitive to small changes in neural conduction of the auditory nerve than are the responses to click sounds. Tonebursts also offer the advantage that the resulting BAEP are affected very little by any hearing loss that originates in the cochlea such as noise-induced hearing loss, presbyacusis, or a hearing loss caused by ototoxic antibiotics. However, click sounds give a larger response than tonebursts, so that fewer responses to click sounds need to be averaged in order to obtain a recording that can be interpreted. A repetition rate of 10 per second is suitable for recording all peaks in the BAEP, including the earlier peaks.

Amplifiers and Display

Amplifiers similar to those used to record EMG can be used to record BAEP and CAP from NVIII. We have used Grass Instrument Co., type P511J amplifiers, but any differential amplifier of a good quality can be used.

The potentials recorded from electrodes placed on the scalp (BAEP) are of much lower amplitude than are spontaneous brain electroencephalograms and other nonauditory potentials, while the CAP recorded directly from the eighth cranial nerve are usually large enough to be viewed directly on an oscilloscope.

When recording BAEP, it is necessary to average a large number of responses in order to obtain a recording that can be interpreted. Suitable filter settings are 150 to 300 Hz for low cutoff, and 1000 to 1500 Hz for high cutoff. This introduces a certain degree of distortion, and because of the frequency-dependent phase shift in such electronic filters, a change in the waveform (e.g., a broadening of a peak) may give rise to a change in the latency of one or more peaks. To avoid this problem, we use digital filters instead of conventional electronic filters.[2] In the operating room in our institution, averaging is done using a LSI 11/73 microprocessor that also performs the digital filtering. This is updated at every 500 sweeps, and a baseline is displayed together with the current recording, making it easy to detect small changes. Printouts of latencies and amplitudes of each peak are also provided by the same computer system.

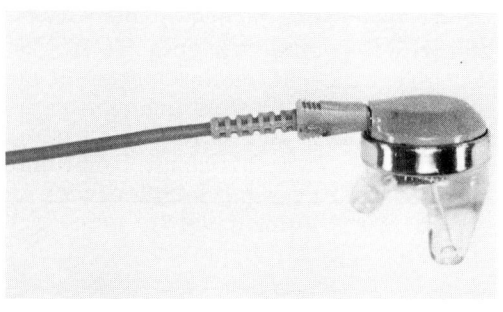

Figure 5: Insert earphone with Lucite earmold.

---

*Microsonic, Full Service Earmold Laboratory, P.O. Box 184, 1421 Merchant Street, Ambridge, Pennsylvania 15003.
**Madsen Electronics, P.O. Box 535, 1074 S. Service Road, Oakville, Ontario, Canada.

Anesthesia

There are no restrictions as to the type of anesthesia that can be used when recording BAEP or CAP from the eighth nerve. These potentials are not influenced by muscle relaxants nor are they affected by inhalation anesthetics or barbiturates but body temperatures below 34.5° Celsius increase the latencies noticeably.[9]

Interpretation

Knowledge about the origin of the individual peaks in the BAEP makes it possible to estimate the site of injury.[3,4,6] Thus, disappearance of all peaks is a sign of injury to the ear, most likely due to interruption of its blood supply to the inner ear. Disappearance or delay of peak II or peak III and the later peaks is indicative of injury to the auditory nerve, while disappearance or delay of peak V with preservation of earlier peaks is a sign of injury to the superior olivary complex or the contralateral lateral lemniscus.

As has been mentioned earlier, signal enhancement by averaging of many responses relies on the assumption that the signal (response) does not change during the time over which responses are averaged. Thus, if the individual responses change in such a way that the latencies of one or more of the peaks changes during the time that the potentials are averaged, then the resultant averaged response becomes meaningless because it is the sum of a series of potentials with different latencies. When there is a gradual change in the latency, the resultant averaged potentials will change in appearance, but such averaged potentials do not provide any direct information about the magnitude or the character of the change. Until the effect of injury that caused the change in the potentials stabilizes, it will not be possible to interpret the averaged potentials. It is often seen that as the potentials change, the amplitude of the averaged potentials becomes low. This is a result of the fact that potentials with different latencies are added together. When the pathological condition becomes stable, the amplitude of the potentials increases[4] (Fig. 6). However, this increase in amplitude should not be taken as an indication that the potentials have improved.

Compound action potentials recorded directly from the eighth nerve are easier to interpret than are BAEP, but the former potentials provide information mainly about the integrity of the ear and the portion of the auditory nerve distal to the location of the electrode.

The potentials that are recorded directly from the eighth nerve have a triphasic shape with an initial small positive deflection followed by a large negative deflection, which again is followed by a small positivity (Fig. 7). Injury to the nerve will result in prolongation of the latency and, if injury is severe and causes a

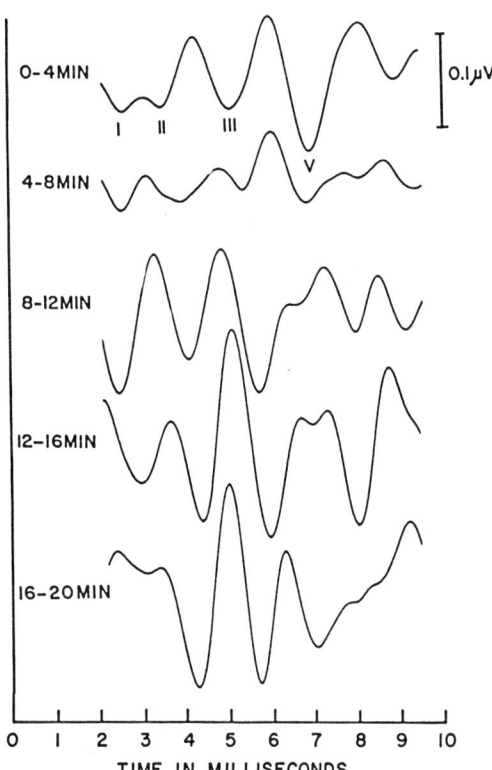

Figure 6: Brain stem auditory evoked responses obtained at intervals of four minutes before, during, and after injury to the eighth nerve (used with permission[4]).

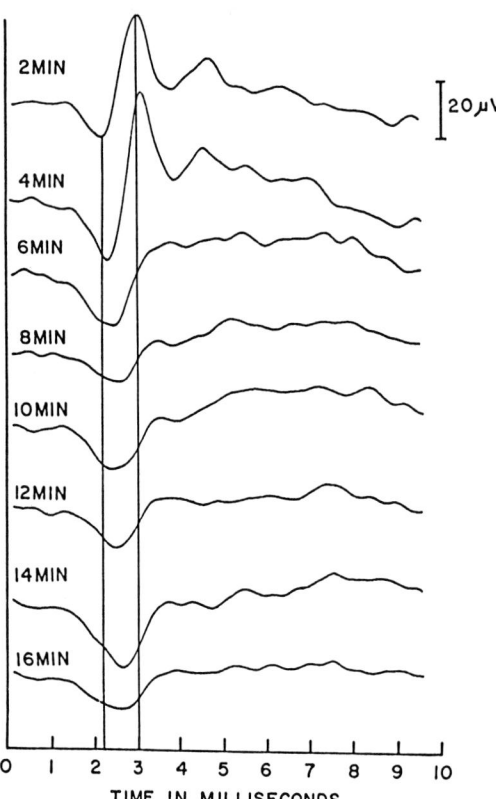

Figure 7: Recordings directly from the eighth nerve made simultaneously with the recordings shown in Figure 6 (used with permission[4]).

partial conduction block, a decrease in the amplitude of the negative peak. A total conduction block results in total disappearance of the negative peak if the recording electrode is located close to the site of injury (Fig. 7). Injury to the portion of the nerve that is immediately proximal to the recording site also causes the amplitude of the negative peak to decrease, thus leaving a response that is dominated by the intitial positivity. The changes in the CAP from the eighth nerve thus provide information about neural conduction in the auditory nerve also in the case when the injury affects a portion of the nerve that is located immediately proximal to the location of the recording electrode.

Monitoring of NII

Monitoring visual evoked potentials (VEP) is more difficult than monitoring auditory potentials and extraocular muscle activity (EMG) for several reasons. The most efficient form of stimulation to elicit VEP is the pattern-reversal checkerboard which is used clinically; however, such stimuli cannot be used intraoperatively. During surgery only flash stimulation is practical, and further, the stimulator must be so small that it does not interfere with the operation, but large enough to elicit a stable response. Light stimulation through the closed eyelid has been used. Recently, light stimulators consisting of light-emitting diodes attached to contact lenses have been developed for intraoperative use[8] (see Fig. 8). These contact lenses can be placed directly on the eye and they provide a light source for recording VEP that does not interfere with the operative procedure.

However, a second problem with using intraoperatively recorded VEP to monitor optic nerve function is the relatively sparse knowledge about the origin of these potentials. The potential that is used clinically is the P_{100}, which is a positive deflection that occurs about 100 msec after the reverse of a checkerboard pattern is presented. A similar potential is seen after a brief light flash. Since this potential most likely is generated in the visual cortex, it is affected by inhalation anesthetics and possibly also by analgesics such

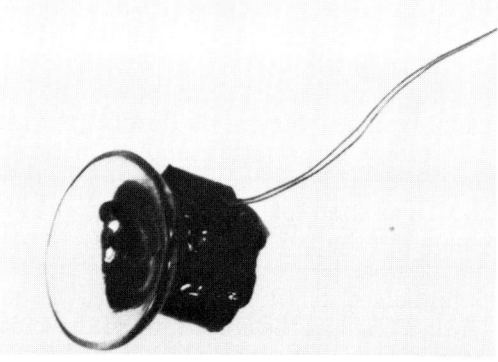

Figure 8: Contact lens with light-emitting diodes.

as Fentanyl®. While it is unusual to record directly from the optic nerve, this can be done using a technique similar to that used to record evoked potentials from the eighth cranial nerve.[8] Examples of recordings from the optic nerve in a patient undergoing a neurosurgical operation are shown in Figure 9. As was the case for the auditory potentials, recording potentials directly from the optic nerve may offer advantages over farfield potentials that can be recorded from electrodes placed on the scalp in that the former are more robust and can more rapidly signal injury to the optic nerve. However, so far, little experience has been gained with this technique.

Electrode Placement

VEP can be recorded by using scalp electrodes similar to those used to record brain stem auditory evoked potentials. Traditionally, electrodes are placed at O_z, with the reference electrode either on C_z or a noncephalic site. Responses can be recorded directly from the optic nerve and optic tract using electrodes similar to those described above for recording from the eighth cranial nerve (Fig. 4).

Electrical Safety in the Operating Room

Whenever electrodes that are in contact with line-powered electronic equipment (or, for that matter, any equipment that has electrical power) are placed in contact with a patient, there is a potential hazard from leaking current. The situation in an operating room is particularly risky in this respect and every precaution must be taken to minimize the risks.

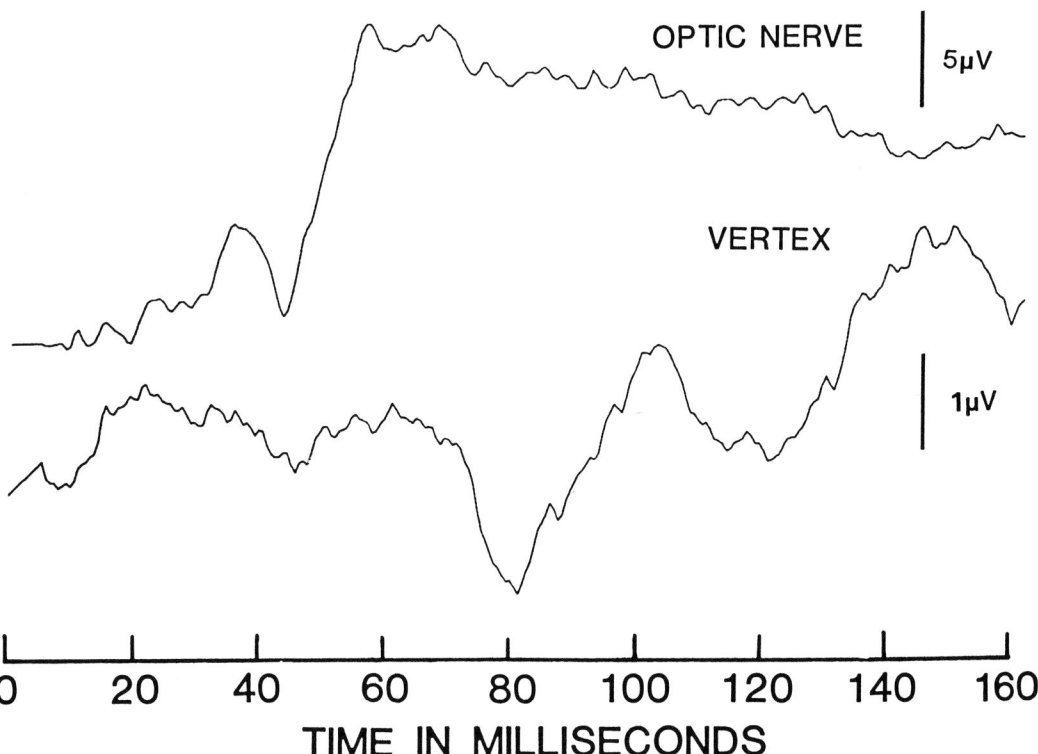

Figure 9: Recordings made from electrodes placed on the scalp (C_z) with a reference on the shoulder and directly from the optic nerve in response to a light flash delivered by the device illustrated in Figure 8.

We use capacitance-coupled interfaces between the patient and the electronic equipment, which in addition contain solid-state devices that instantaneously increase the input impedance to very high values in case the leaking current exceeds 4 µA (Grass Instrument Co., type IG3 P511). These devices thus effectively disconnect the patient from the electronic equipment that is connected to the electrodes in case of a current leak. Ground electrodes should also be attached through similar devices. These considerations are, of course, even more important when electrodes are placed intracranially, in which case utmost caution must be exercised to avoid current leaks.

Precautions must also be taken when operating the electronic equipment that is connected to such electrodes. Thus, it is important to turn on the equipment before the patient is connected to it, and to disconnect the patient from the equipment before the equipment is turned off. The reason for this is that switching the electronic equipment on or off may generate transients that could affect the patient, and the safety switches mentioned above are designed to be functional only when the equipment is switched on.

Whenever electrophysiological recordings are made from electrodes placed on the skin and the electrocoagulator is used, there is a risk that the high-frequency current used in coagulation may return through the recording electrodes. This can cause skin burns and since the surface area of needle electrodes is smaller than that of surface electrodes, such burns will be more severe if needle electrodes are used. The risk of such burns depends upon the type of coagulator that is used and, particularly, on whether the return electrode from the coagulator to the patient has a sufficiently low impedance. The greatest risk for such burns will occur when the electrocautery equipment is used in its cutting mode, and it is least likely to occur when bipolar coagulation is used. Modern high-quality electrocautery equipment is less likely to cause such problems than older equipment.

When electrical stimulation of nervous tissue is done, it is important that the stimulator have an efficient isolation unit. An electrical stimulator must never be connected to a patient without such a unit placed between the equipment and the patient. In addition, precautions must be taken to assure that no direct current is applied, and only a balanced-charge type of stimulation is acceptable. Some nerve stimulators deliver a direct current instead of rectangular pulses and many stimulators can deliver large enough currents to cause injury. Thus, it is preferable to avoid using stimulators that are capable of delivering direct current or large current pulses, or to build in protocol safeguards against applying such currents as the result of operator mistakes.

References

1. Jannetta PJ, Møller MB, Møller AR: Disabling positional vertigo. N Engl J Med 310:1700-1705, 1984.
2. Møller AR: Improving brain stem auditory evoked potential recordings by digital filtering. Ear and Hearing 4:108-113, 1983.
3. Møller AR, Jannetta PJ: Auditory evoked potentials recorded intracranially from the brainstem in man. Exp Neurol 78:144-157, 1982.
4. Møller AR, Jannetta PJ: Monitoring auditory functions during cranial nerve microvascular decompression operations by direct recording from the eighth nerve. J Neurosurg 59:493-499, 1983.
5. Møller AR, Jannetta PJ: Preservation of facial function during removal of acoustic neuromas: Use of monopolar constant-voltage stimulation and EMG. J Neurosurg 61:757-760, 1984.
6. Møller AR, Jannetta PJ, Møller MB: Neural generators of brain stem evoked potentials: Results from human intracranial recordings. Ann Otol Rhinol Laryngol 90:591-596, 1982.
7. Møller MB, Møller AR, Jannetta PJ, Sekhar LN: Diagnosis and surgical treatment of disabling positional vertigo. J Neurosurg 64:21-28, 1986.
8. Møller AR, Burgess JE, Sekhar LN: Potentials evoked from the optic nerve in monkeys and man. Electroenceph Clin Neurophysiol 1986.
9. Stockard JJ, Sharbrough FW, Tinker JA: Effect of hypothermia on the human brain stem auditory response. Ann Neurol 3:368-370, 1978.

IV

Specialized Treatment Modalities

8

Use of the Laser for Resection of Cranial Base Tumors

John M. Tew, Jr., M.D.
William D. Tobler, M.D.
Myles L. Pensak, M.D.
Gary Jacobson, Ph.D.

Introduction

The introduction of lasers to clinical surgery has expanded the abilities of surgeons to remove tumors of the skull base.[1,9,10,16,19,25] Continued development of surgical techniques and refinement of laser systems allow surgeons to further improve treatment methods of these difficult lesions. Since 1981 the carbon dioxide laser has been routinely used on skull base tumors at our institution. Beginning in 1984, the Nd:YAG laser has been available for selected vascular tumors. We routinely use evoked potentials in posterior fossa laser surgery. In this chapter we will describe the basic functions and applications of currently available laser systems which will be followed by a discussion of evoked potential monitoring during laser surgery. A review of the basic neurotological approaches to skull base tumors will be followed by selected cases where lasers played a significant role in removal of these tumors. We will close with a discussion of our results.

Laser Systems and Function

Laser energy is composed of electromagnetic radiation of a selected wavelength. It is produced by electrical stimulation of a chosen substance called the active medium which results in excitation and subsequent emission of photons from these excited molecules. Capture of these photons yields a beam of powerful energy that can be manipulated for surgical applications. Focusing the beam creates a fine point with the power to incise tissue. Diffusing or defocusing the beam creates a larger spot of less intense energy that can vaporize and coagulate tissue.[30]

There are a multitude of lasers that have been created for business, military, industrial, and biological applications.[11,15] Carbon dioxide, Nd:YAG, and Argon lasers have been adapted to surgical use. However, the carbon dioxide laser is the only laser in widespread clinical application in neurological surgery. Use of the Nd:YAG laser requires an Investigational Device Exception from the Food

From: Sekhar LN, Schramm VL Jr, eds: *Tumors of the Cranial Base: Diagnosis and Treatment.* Mount Kisco, New York, Futura Publishing Co, Inc, © 1987.

and Drug Administration, thus experience with this laser is limited to carefully designed protocol studies. Inadequate power has restricted the acceptance of the Argon laser for ablative purposes.

The specific tissue effects of any laser are an intrinsic property of the specific wavelength of the laser. A varying combination of absorption, scatter, transmission, and reflection imparts the characteristics of each surgical laser when applied to biological tissue (Fig. 1). The optical properties of the target tissue also determine the reaction of the laser. More detailed discussion of these factors can be found elsewhere.[5,8,20-22,26]

The active medium of the carbon dioxide laser is carbon dioxide gas. This invisible laser beam has a wavelength of 10.6 microns which is located in the far infrared region of the electromagnetic spectrum and therefore it requires a coaxial helium-neon pilot beam for visualization in surgery. Carbon dioxide laser energy is absorbed at the surface of application and its absorption is independent of tissue pigmentation. These properties enable the carbon dioxide laser to vaporize mass lesions rapidly with precision. The heat of the carbon dioxide laser seals capillary vessels as it vaporizes so that it functions to aid hemostasis. However, larger vessels greater than approximately 1.0 mm may be incised rather than sealed by laser energy. Since carbon dioxide laser energy is superficially absorbed, precise dissection of thin layers of tumor from critical neurovascular structures may be accomplished when expertise in laser techniques has been gained. However, heat conduction to adjacent structures, and unintentional injury to neurovascular structures are potential severe complications even in the most experienced hands. The carbon dioxide laser may be used freehand, or may be attached to the microscope for microsurgical use. This laser is the most widely used laser for skull base tumors.[1,19,25,28,30]

The Nd:YAG laser also produces an invisible beam in the near infrared region of the electromagnetic spectrum with a wavelength of 1.06 microns and use also requires a coaxial helium-neon guiding beam. This energy is characterized by deep tissue scatter with minimal surface absorption. It is preferentially absorbed by heme-pigmented tissue. These combined properties make the Nd-YAG laser a powerful coagulative device which functions

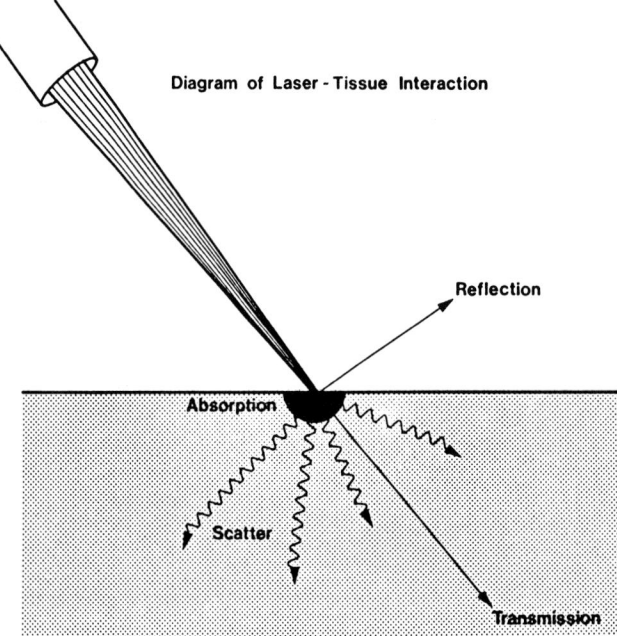

Figure 1: Diagram of laser tissue interaction. The intrinsic properties of a laser's wavelength determine the amount of absorption, scatter, transmission, and reflection. The optical properties of the tissue further determine the laser's effect.

mainly to coagulate highly vascular tumors and vascular malformations.[31] Application of this laser to such a tumor results in coagulation and shrinkage, but minimal vaporization of tissue. A coagulated, vascular tumor may then be vaporized with carbon dioxide energy, or removed by other methods.[2,29] Because of the deep scatter of 6–8 mm or more below the surface of application, use of this laser in critical areas has been associated with more serious risk than with the carbon dioxide laser.[18] This laser should be used with extreme caution; because of deep scatter, it is less precise than the carbon dioxide laser. Its role in the surgery of skull base tumors is primarily as a coagulative instrument, whereas the carbon dioxide laser is principally an ablative tool.

The Argon laser is a visible blue-green laser with a wavelength of 0.488–0.514 microns. Its properties are intermediate between the carbon dioxide and the Nd:YAG lasers. It possesses both moderate scatter and absorption properties.[23] It does not vaporize as efficiently as the carbon dioxide laser nor does it coagulate as well as the Nd:YAG laser. Current Argon lasers are not capable of generating sufficient wattage for efficient vaporization of tissue and therefore they have not gained more acceptance in tumor surgery. Table I compares the properties of these lasers.

Laser Heat and Evoked Potentials

Evoked potentials are routinely recorded in many centers during posterior fossa surgery. (This topic is reviewed in Chapter 9.) The brain stem auditory evoked potential (i.e., BAEP) has been shown to be useful in the detection of perioperatively induced hearing loss and pontine level brain stem damage.[12-14,24] The median nerve somatosensory evoked potential also has been useful in the detection of brain stem compromise when the BAEP could not be recorded because of the presence of significant preoperative hearing loss.[14] The blink reflex has been used successfully at our institution for the perioperative monitoring of facial nerve function. Although the effects of variables such as blood pressure, O_2/CO_2 tension, hemodilution, anesthesia, retraction (i.e., of cerebellum, brain stem, cranial nerves, arteriovenous supply) have been amply documented in the scientific literature,[12,14,24] the effects of laser heat on the normal electrophysiology of the brain have not been investigated.

The effects of Argon laser irradiation of the dorsal column in cats have recently been reported.[32] Changes in the sciatic nerve cortical SEP were observed with a mean radiant exposure of 2698 J/cm², i.e., radiant exposure was defined by the investigators as: power (w)/cross-sectional area of laser beam (cm²) × time of exposure (seconds). A significant change was defined as the absence of the early cortical SEP.[31] These investigators did not measure the heat diffusion of the laser.

Changes in cellular electrophysiology may be detected when the body temperature is reduced to below 32° C or is raised to greater than 40° C. For example, the BAEP P1–P5 interwave latency shows a statistically significant increase when the body temperature is reduced to 32° C (i.e.,

Table I
Characteristics of Neurosurgical Lasers

	CO_2	Nd:YAG	Argon
Wavelength (mm)	10.6	1.06	0.488–0.514
EM Spectrum	Far Infrared	Near Infrared	Visible (Blue-Green)
Absorption	High	Low	Moderate
Scatter	Low	High	Moderate
Transmission	No	Yes	Yes
Pigment Dependence	No	Yes	Yes

esophageal temperature), and may show significant latency increases if the body temperature is raised to above 40° C.[27] Accordingly, it might be expected that laser-generated heat would alter neuronal transmission, and thus the evoked potential.

The heat from the laser impact size may be conducted to nearby tissue. This occurs because the intracellular fluids within adjacent tissue act as a thermal conductor. The heat generated by a CO_2 laser at the impact site easily exceeds 100° C during extended periods of tissue vaporization. The degree of heat transfer occurs as a function of: (1) the duration of tissue exposure to the laser beam; (2) the power density of the beam; and (3) the absorption properties of the involved tissue.[4,22] It is not surprising then that evoked potentials that originate from within sensory pathways that are in proximity to the site of laser surgery are often transiently disrupted, particularly during extended bursts of the laser. The frequent use of irrigating media, we have found, serves to cool the tissue and to restore normal electrical conduction. Examples of transient laser heat effects on the median nerve brain stem somatosensory evoked potentials for two subjects are shown in Figure 2. It is our opinion that the recording of evoked potentials during laser surgery enable or permit detection of transient heat-induced changes in nerve/brain stem function that, if undetected, might lead to permanent postoperative brain stem deficits.

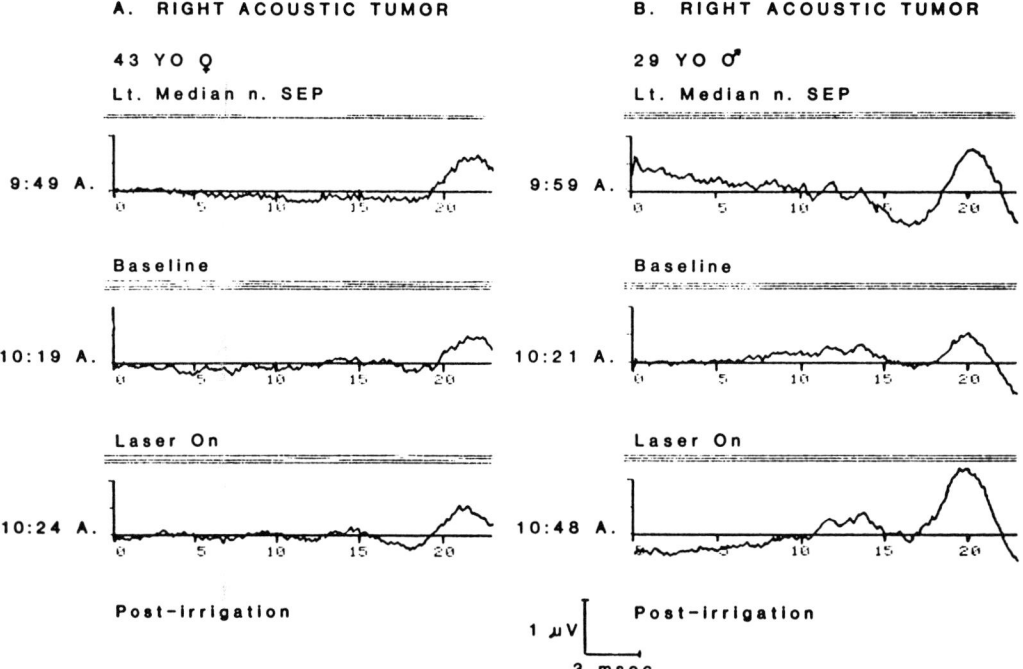

Figure 2: The effects of laser heat on the median nerve cortical somatosensory evoked potential of two patients who underwent laser surgery for the removal of acoustic neuromas. The top tracings show the SEP prior to the introduction of the laser. The middle tracings show the effects of heat diffusion on the SEP that is derived from electrical transmission through the medial lemniscal pathway. The bottom tracings illustrate the restorative effects of irrigating media on the SEP. The laser heat effects a temporary increase in SEP latency and a temporary reduction in SEP amplitude. Stimuli consisted of .150 ms electrical square pulses that were delivered superficially to the median nerve at the left wrist at a presentation rate of 9/sec. Each tracing represents the average of 256 samples. Grid one positivity is represented by an upward deflection in this figure.

Neurotological Approaches to Skull Base Tumors[3,6,9,17]

The complex irregular osteology of the skull base provides numerous preformed pathways for the growth of tumors. While vital neurovascular structures traverse and exit the skull base, it is not unusual for a lesion to have grown to significant proportion before it begins to compromise function and is detected. The neurotological approaches to the skull base reflect an attempt by surgeons to design approaches that will optimize visualization and allow for manipulation of lesions with the least intra- and postoperative morbidity.

Translabyrinthine Approach

This procedure was advocated in the early 20th Century by Panse but fell into disfavor in the premicrosurgical era, being condemned by both Dandy and Cushing.[9] Reintroduced in the 1960s by House, it has become the standard neurotological approach to lesions of the cerebellopontine angle for small to moderate sized tumors and is used in conjunction with a standard suboccipital approach for larger lesions.[3]

With the patient in the supine position and head turned, an extended postauricular incision is made. A cortical mastoidectomy with facial recess exposure is obtained. An organized labyrinthectomy is performed and the region of the lamina cribrosa superioris is noted (Mike's dot). The sigmoid sinus is skeletinized to the level of the jugular bulb. From the cribriform region superiorly to the cochlea aqueduct inferiorly, the internal auditory canal is thinned and opened. Removing the bone overlying the posterior fossa dura allows for dural opening to the level of the sigmoid sinus, thus giving visualization of the posterior fossa contents and cerebellopontine angle. Following tumor removal, the eustachian tube is obliterated with proplast and the wound packed with harvested abdominal fat and closed in layers.

Combined Translabyrinthine Suboccipital Approach

For large lesions of the cerebellopontine angle and posterior fossa, this approach provides optimal exposure. As described above, the contents of the internal auditory canal are identified laterally. The bone over the occipital region is removed, allowing surgeons to work anterior and posterior to the bridge created by the undisturbed sigmoid sinus.

Middle Cranial Fossa Approach

This procedure, which is principally an extradural approach, affords visualization of the petrous apex and access to the internal auditory canal for small intracranial lesions.

The affected side is faced upward with the patient in the supine position and the surgeon seated at the head of the table. An incision is made from the zygomatic root superiorly approximately 6–8 cm. Soft tissue is divided and a craniectomy is done on the squamosa portion of the temporal bone. The middle fossa dura is reflected from the floor of the cavity and the temporal lobe is held with a House-Urban® retractor. The middle meningeal artery is identified anteriorly. Two important landmarks are the greater superficial petrosal nerve exiting from the facial hiatus and the arcuate eminence identifying the superior semicircular canal. The geniculate ganglion is identified and the internal auditory canal may be opened with preservation of cochlea and/or vestibular function. The defect is closed with muscle packing and a layered closure.

Transcochlear Approach

This approach gives added exposure to the internal auditory canal (anteriorly), the petrous apex, and midline structures including the clivus. A translabyrinthine approach is undertaken with bone being removed from the retrosigmoid region.

The entire temporal bone path of the facial nerve is exposed and the chorda tympani and greater superficial petrosal nerve branches are divided. The facial nerve is then mobilized from the fallopian canal and transposed posteriorly. The middle ear contents are removed and the cochlea is opened exposing the intratympanic portion of the internal carotid artery. The dura is then opened from the level of the superior petrosal sinus to the jugular bulb and internal auditory canal. Following tumor removal, the wound is packed with abdominal fat and closed in layers.

Retrolabyrinthine Approach

This approach gives limited exposure to the posterior fossa. The labyrinth is exposed following facial recess cortical mastoidectomy. Bone overlying the sigmoid sinus is removed and the dura is opened between the posterior semicircular canal and the sigmoid sinus. Superiorly, the superior petrosal sinus defines the upper limit while the jugular bulb limits the field inferiorly. Care must be taken to avoid injury to the endolymphatic sac. The wound is closed in similar fashion to that employed in the translabyrinthine approach.

Infratemporal Fossa Approach

This technique introduced by Fisch[6] and modified by Glassock[9] gives exposure to the midline structures including the parasellar region, clivus, and parasphenoid area.

With the affected side upward and the patient in the supine position, an extended S-shaped or C-shaped incision is made to give exposure to the temporal-parietal region of the skull as well as the upper neck. The auricle is reflected anteriorly with a broad flap. The external auditory canal is transected and oversewn. A limited superficial parotidectomy is performed and the facial nerve is identified. Neck dissection exposes the common carotid artery, internal jugular vein, and the 9th, 10th, 11th, and 12th cranial nerves. A radical mastoidectomy is performed with exposure of the facial nerve which may be mobilized and reflected or transposed to a newly created anterior niche. To optimize exposure, the facial nerve may need to be divided. The sigmoid sinus is packed off after proximal control and ligation of the internal jugular vein is obtained and the inferior and superior petrosal sinuses are occluded. An organized labyrinthinectomy is performed and the internal auditory canal is opened. The internal carotid artery is identified from the carotid bulb through its intra-tympanic portion and may be followed from the middle ear to the foramen lacerum. For added exposure, the mandibular condyle may be mobilized or divided for additional exposure in the area of the glenoid fossa. Fisch reports exposure to the pterygoid process and plates anteriorly through this exposure. In some cases the bone overlying the middle fossa dura is removed and the temporal lobe must be retracted for added visualization.

Tumor removal is accomplished both intracranially and extracranially in one or more staged procedures. The wound is closed by means of a rotated temporalis muscle flap with or without abdominal fat. With intracranial involvement, a Pudenz® shunt may be placed prior to flap closure.

Pathology

A wide variety of lesions may be encountered at the skull base. While recent reports by Fisch have begun to extend the indications for surgery to include squamous cell carcinoma, most of the lesions that are amenable to removal are benign histologically.[7] Commonly encountered lesions include: neuromas, especially acoustic schwannomas (neurilemmomas), meningiomas, chordomas, paragangliomas (glomus jugulare and glomus vagale), cholesteatomas, juvenile nasopharyngeal angiofibromas, and primary nasopharyngeal tumors. Less commonly reported are hemangiomas, lipomas, bony and cartilaginous tumors. A report of an adenocarcinoma invading the skull base, temporal bone, and foramen magnum successfully debulked with the carbon dioxide laser can be found elsewhere.[9]

Selected Cases

Our cumulative experience with lasers in neurosurgery is approaching 300 cases. Many of these applications have been in the treatment of basal tumors. Included in this series are basal meningiomas, craniopharyngiomas, acoustic neuromas, clivus chordomas, and glomus jugulare tumors. The following case histories represent the various types of lesions encountered.

Suprasellar Meningioma

A 25-year-old woman developed rapidly failing vision in her third trimester of pregnancy. She presented with finger counting only in the left eye and a partial temporal cut in the right eye. CT scan (Fig. 3) and angiogram were consistent with a suprasellar meningioma. She underwent caesarean section at the 37th

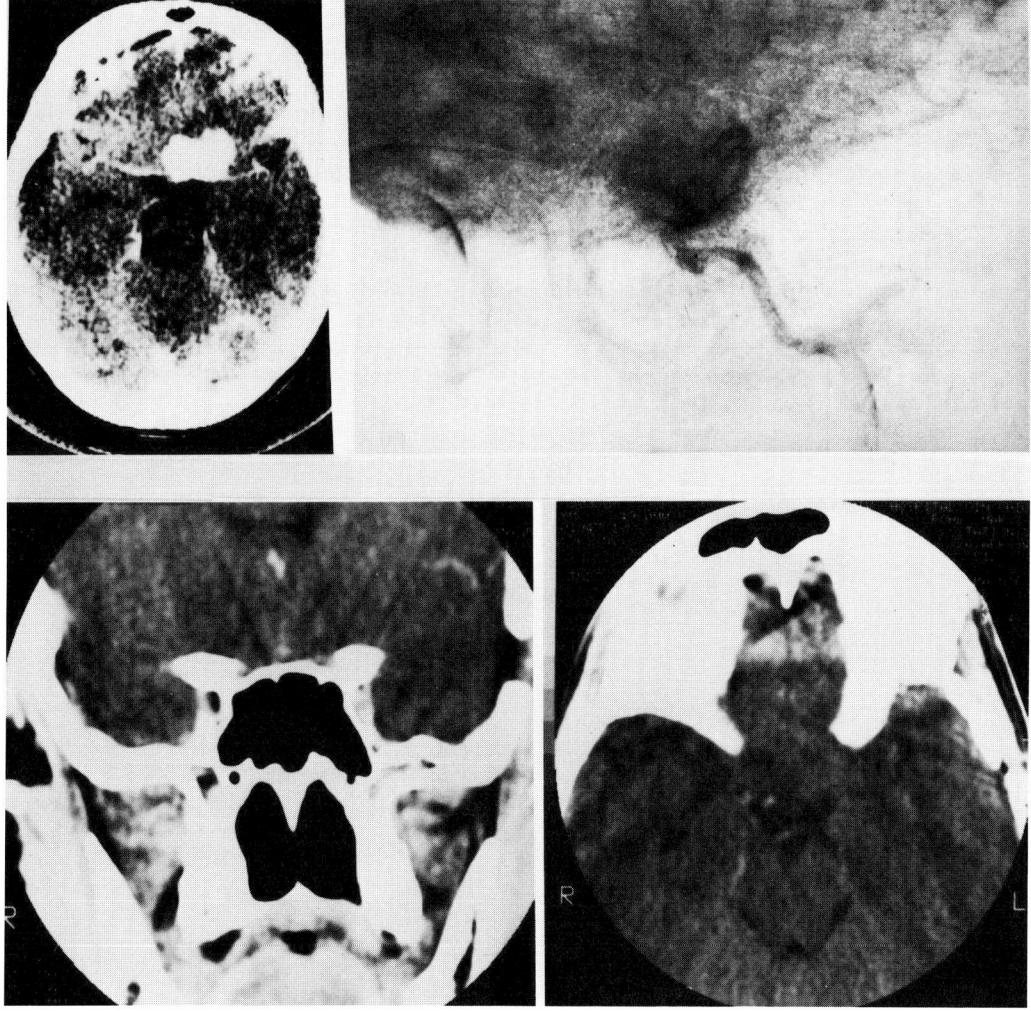

Figure 3: Top left: Tuberculum sella meningioma. Top right: Angiogram shows vascular blush. Bottom left and right: Coronal and axial CT show no residual tumor.

week of gestation followed by craniotomy one week later. The tumor was exposed through a left pterional craniotomy and its attachment was to the tuberculum sella. This firm tumor was vaporized with the carbon dioxide laser and complete excision was obtained. Her visual acuity returned to 20/20 in the right eye and 20/25 in the left eye and CT shows no residual tumor (Fig. 3). The value of the carbon dioxide laser here is its ease of use in critical areas and its ability to vaporize the dural origin of meningiomas.

Pituitary Adenoma: Post Radiation

An elderly woman underwent transphenoidal hypophysectomy followed by radiation therapy for a pituitary adenoma some years prior to her return to us with progressive visual loss and recurrence (Fig. 4). This fibrotic tumor was tenacious and attempted decompression or removal with standard microdissection techniques would have resulted in significant risk to the patient. Careful use of the carbon dioxide laser allowed a safe debulking of this unyielding mass with decompression of the otpic apparatus and improved visual function. She remains without symptomatic tumor progression at three years now.

Craniopharyngioma

A young 10-year-old child underwent a frontal craniotomy for resection of a craniopharyngioma but the intrasellar portion could not be excised because of a pre-fixed chiasm (Fig. 5). The remaining portion of tumor was removed with laser-assisted vaporization through a transphenoidal approach. The postoperative scan shows the operative defect filled with a fat graft (Fig. 5).

Whether a transcranial or transsphenoidal approach is chosen for these difficult lesions, the laser has become a valuable adjunct for vaporizing adherent calcified portions of these tumors. In spite of the increased capabilities of the experienced laser neurosurgeon, the risks of dissecting tissue from the optic apparatus, hypothalmic region, and other eloquent

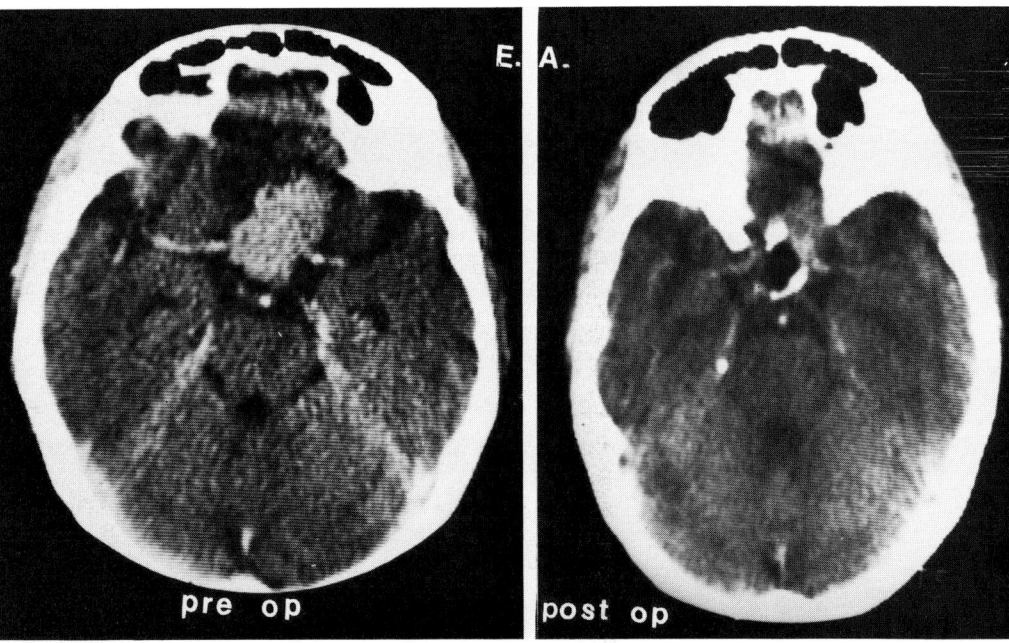

Figure 4: Radiated, recurrent pituitary adenoma. Left: Preoperative. Right: Postoperative decompression.

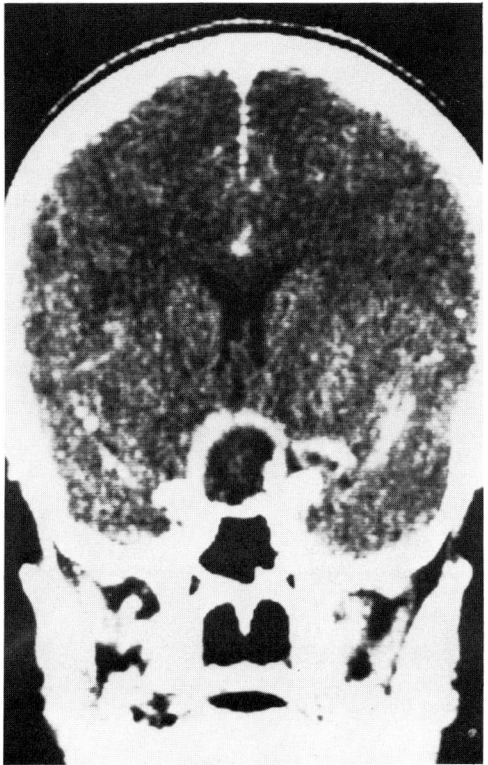
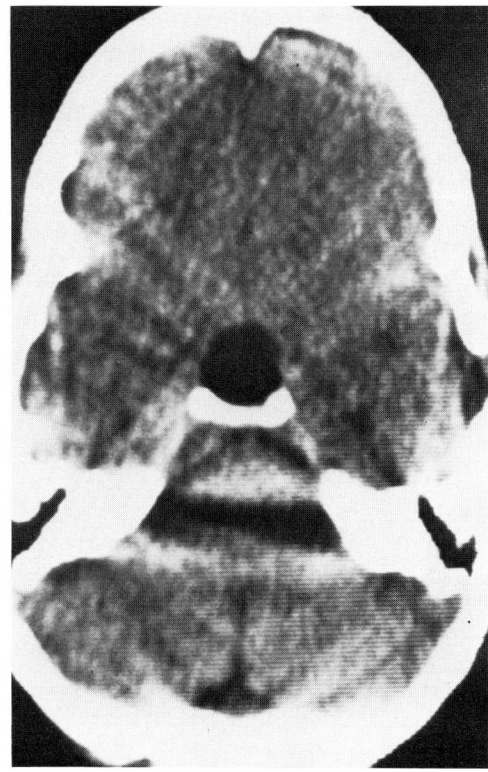

Figure 5: Calcified craniopharyngioma. Left: Preoperative. Right: Postoperative; operative site filled with fat.

structures remain unchanged. The laser does not substitute for sound surgical judgment under these difficult circumstances.

Parasellar Hemangiopericytoma

A 19-year-old woman presented with an incomplete cavernous sinus syndrome and was found to have a highly vascular mass-lesion invading the right cavernous sinus (Fig. 6). This fungating mass in the temporal fossa bled heavily when biopsied. With low power Nd:YAG energy (10–15 watts), the lesion was coagulated and shrunk. Its attachment site at the cavernous sinus was treated with the Nd:YAG laser until further lasing was judged unsafe. Hemostasis was satisfactorily obtained, and after a course of radiation therapy, the patient's neurological abnormalities have resolved and CT scan shows no evidence of tumor (Fig. 7).

Clivus Chordoma

A 54-year-old woman presented to us with upper cranial nerve palsies and a large mass with destruction and invasion of the clivus consistent with the diagnosis of chordoma. This tumor was exposed via the transsphenoidal approach. An incomplete but radical debulking of this vascular lesion was achieved with the carbon dioxide laser (Fig. 8). At the time we operated on this patient, we did not have the Nd:YAG laser, and retrospectively realize the value of the Nd:YAG laser for this type of lesion.

Foramen Magnum Meningioma

A 25-year-old woman with headaches and intermittent paresthesias was found to have a lesion in the lateral and anterior foramen magnum region most consistent

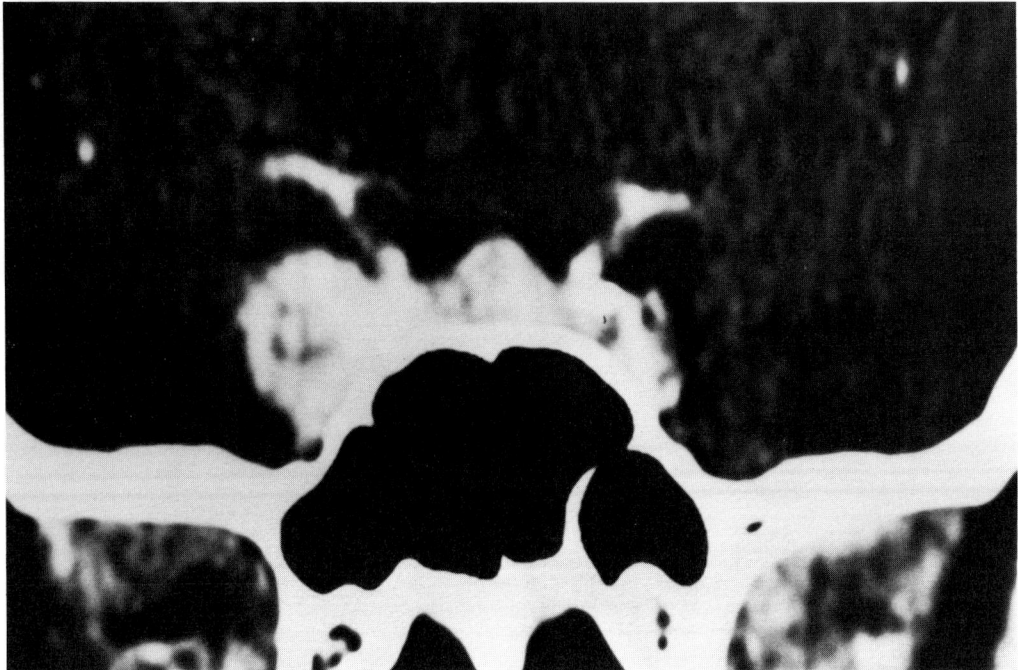

Figure 6: Hemangioperiocytoma invading the right cavernous sinus.

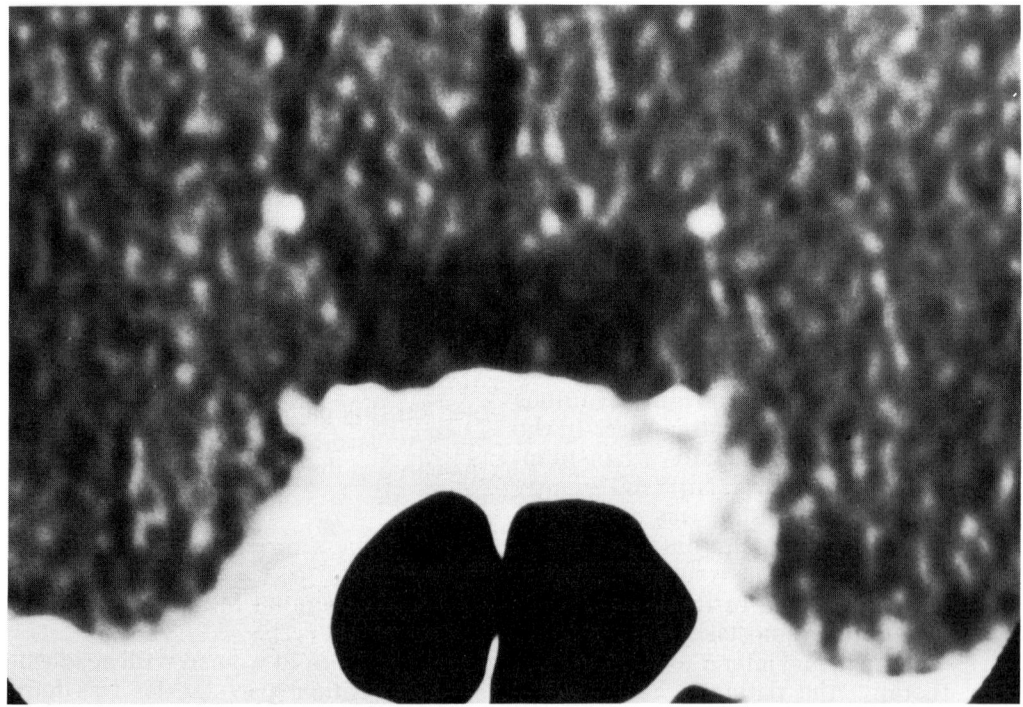

Figure 7: Postoperative CT scan shows no residual tumor.

with meningioma (Fig. 9). this lesion was exposed by a lateral suboccipital craniotomy and cervical laminectomy. The access to this critically located lesion was very narrow, and safe removal with conventional microtechniques would have been difficult. The encased vertebral artery was sacrificed, and with low powers of 3 to 5 watts in a focused mode, this lesion was vaporized. Its firm anterior foramen magnum dural attachment was safely and completely vaporized. The laser provides a significant margin of safety in the removal of this type of lesion because it permits constant visualization of the target; there is no obscuration of the tumor bed by the various instruments one might need to remove this tumor. This additionally minimizes any traction or compression of these critical structures. The patient's symptoms resolved and postoperative CT scan shows no residual tumor (Fig. 9).

Glomus Jugulare Tumor

A 57-year-old woman with a known glomus tumor operated on in 1957 returned with progressive headaches and new fifth nerve findings in 1984. She already had complete cranial nerve palsies, seven through twelve. CT scan disclosed a large angle lesion with the typical vascular pattern of a glomus tumor (Fig. 10). In surgery this tumor was coagulated with the Nd:YAG laser and the entire posterior fossa mass was removed. Its basal attachments were also vaporized with the Nd:YAG laser. Postoperative scan shows no residual tumor (Fig. 10). This highly vascular tumor is the ideal lesion for treatment with the Nd:YAG laser. Application of Nd:YAG energy in this case was safer because of the total loss of function of the lower cranial nerves which were not at risk of injury from the unpredictable scatter effect of Nd:YAG energy.

Acoustic Neuroma

A 29-year-old man with von Recklinghausen's disease and bilateral acoustic neuromas had previously undergone two incomplete resections of the right acoustic tumor which had progressed to a very large size at the time of referral to us

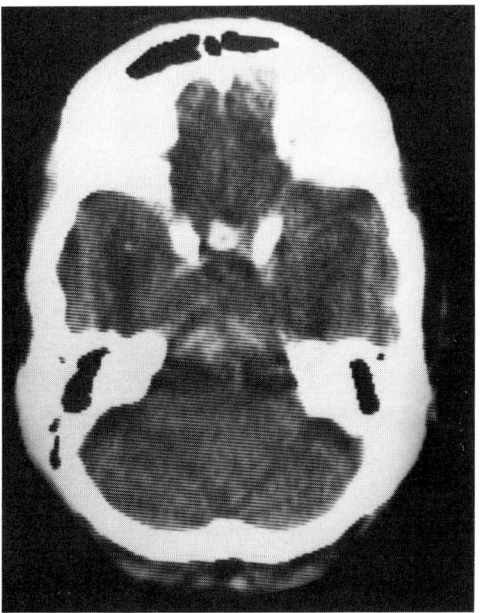
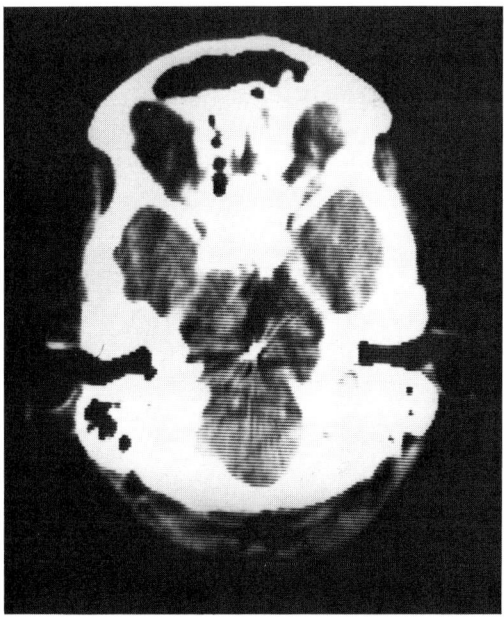

Figure 8: Preoperative CT scan shows destruction of the clivus and large enhancing mass. Postoperative scan shows decompression and artifact from metallic clips.

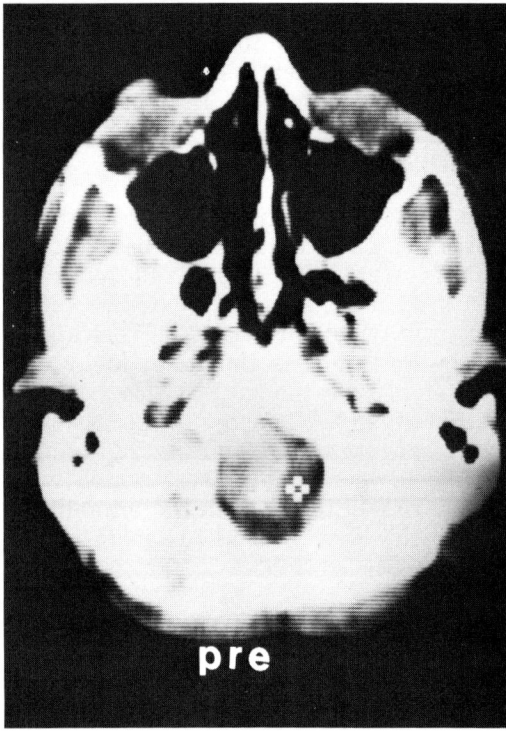
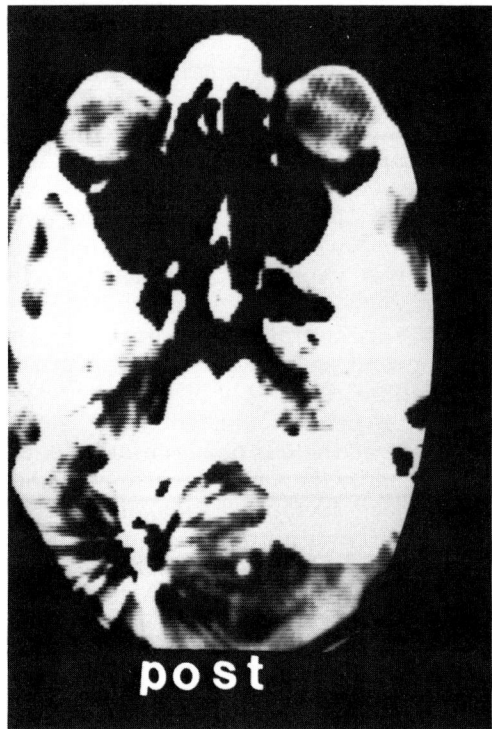

Figure 9: Pre- and postoperative films of foramen magnum meningioma. Scatter artifacts from metallic clips are noted on the postoperative scan.

(Fig. 11). Examination of the patient demonstrated nystagmus, hearing loss, and severe ataxia. At surgery the tumor was removed with the carbon dioxide laser employing a central coring technique. The adherent capsule was vaporized from the brain stem using low powers of focused energy. This case, as in five others in our series, illustrates a major role for the carbon dioxide laser; safe removal of an adherent capsule from the brain stem can be accomplished which could not be

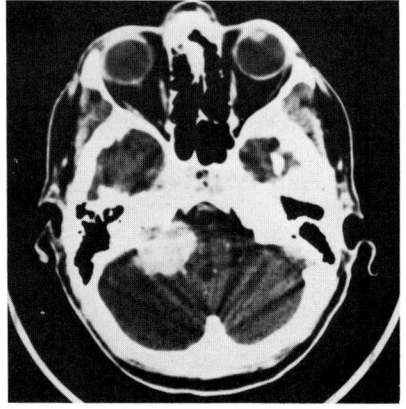
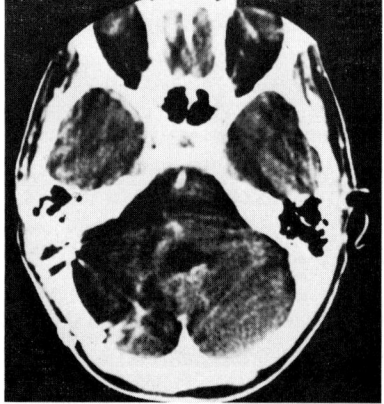

Figure 10: Pre- and postoperative CT scans of highly vascular glomus jugulare tumor.

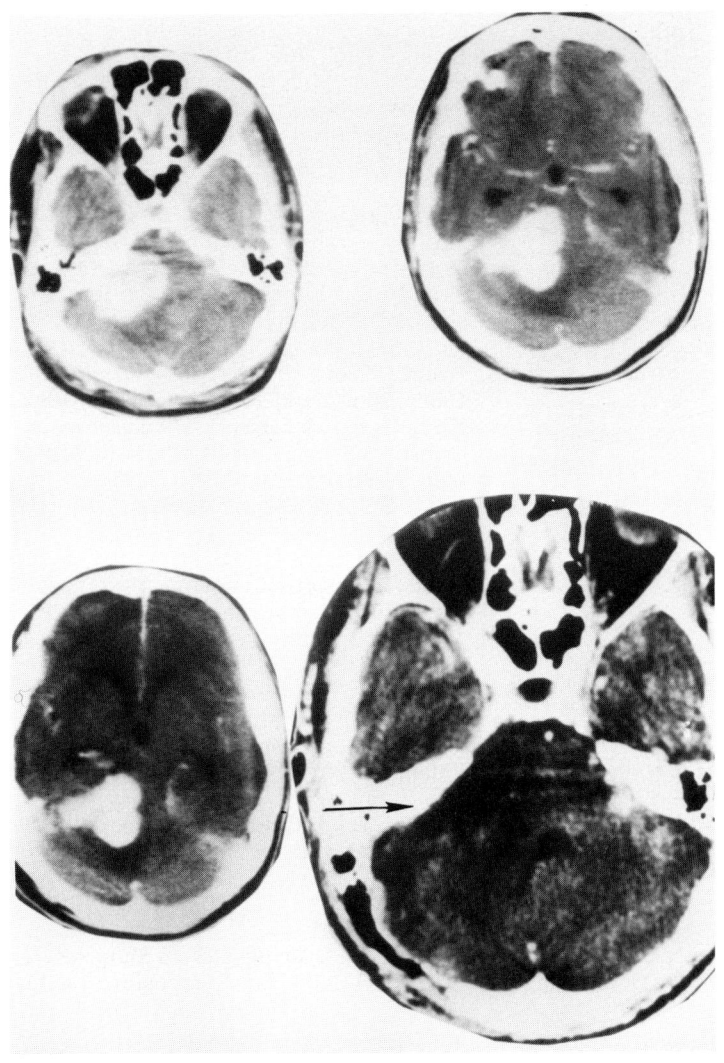

Figure 11: Postoperative CT of large right acoustic neuroma. Postoperative CT (arrow) shows no residual tumor.

removed by instrument microdissection. Postoperative CT scan shows no residual tumor (Fig. 11). The patient's ataxia improved considerably prior to discharge.

Conclusion

Since the introduction of lasers into our surgical armamentarium, we have drawn certain conclusions. In meningioma surgery, more complete removal of inaccessible lesions can be accomplished. More complete excision of the dural attachment, especially in deep midline locations, or in the cavernous sinus region can be achieved. In our series of 33 basal meningiomas, we have had two recurrence/progressions after an average follow-up of 3 years. The long-term recurrence rates will not be known for several years.

In our series of 66 acoustic neuromas, 33 in which the carbon dioxide laser was used, we have found no change in our ability to preserve seventh and eighth nerve function with the laser. However, we have noted a marked decrease in incidence in complications of exposure (i.e., cerebellar infarction, hematoma, and brain stem injury). We attribute this to an improved ability to expose and vaporize these tumors with less cerebellar retraction. Additionally, the laser has enabled us to remove residual tumor capsule adherent to the brain stem which could not be removed in prior surgery by conventional techniques in six cases.

The ability to remove radiated, recurrent adenomas, fibrous and calcified meningiomas, or other calcified lesions has improved with the carbon dioxide laser. Experience with Nd:YAG energy is still anecdotal, but our impression is that its coagulative properties in vascular tumors provide the surgeon with a significant therapeutic advantage. However, one's enthusiasm for lasers, as with any new surgical tool, must be tempered by the perilous risks of this form of energy when misapplied.

References

1. Bartal AD, Heilbronn VD, Avram J, et al: Carbon dioxide laser surgery of basal meningiomas. Surg Neurol 17:90, 1982.
2. Beck OJ: The use of the Nd:YAG and the CO_2 laser in neurosurgery. Neurosurg Rev 3:261-266, 1980.
3. Brackman DE (ed): Neurological Surgery of the Ear and Skull Base, NY, Raven Press, 1982.
4. Dagan J: The Sharplan family of CO_2 lasers for surgery. Neurosurg Rev 7:113-121, 1984.
5. Edwards MSSB, Boggan JE, Fuller TA: The laser in neurological surgery. J Neurosurg 59:555-566, 1983.
6. Fisch U: Infratemporal fossa approach to tumors of the temporal bone and base of skull. J Laryngol Otol 92(II):949-967, 1978.
7. Fisch U, Kumar A: Infratemporal Surgery of the Skull Base in Microneurosurgery, Third Edition, Rand RW (ed), St. Louis, MO, Mosby, 1985.
8. Fuller TA: The physics of surgical lasers. Lasers Surg Med 1:5-14, 1980.
9. Glassock ME, III, Pensak ML, Gulya AJ: Surgery of the Skull Base in Microneurosurgery, Third Edition, Rand RW (ed), St. Louis, MO, Mosby, 1985.
10. Glassock ME, Jackson CG, Whitaker SR: The argon laser in acoustic tumor surgery. Laryngoscope 71:1405-1416, 1981.
11. Goldman L, Rockwell RJ, Jr: Lasers in Medicine, New York, Gordon & Breach Science Publ., Inc., 1971.
12. Grundy BL, Lina A, Procupio T, et al: Reversible evoked potential changes of the eighth cranial nerve. Anesth Analg 60:835-838, 1981.
13. Grundy BL, Jannetta PJ, Procupio BA, et al: Intraoperative monitoring of brain stem auditory evoked potentials. J Neurosurg 57:674-681, 1982.
14. Grundy BL: Intraoperative monitoring of sensory evoked potentials. Anesthesiology 58:72-87, 1983.
15. Hecht J, Teresi D: Laser, Super Tool of the 1980s, New York, Ticknor & Fields, 1982.
16. Hudgins RW, Jacques D: The Laser in Microneurosurgery, Third Edition, Rand RW (ed), St. Louis, MO, Mosby, 1985.
17. Jackson CG: Skull base surgery. Am J Otol 3:161-171, 1981.
18. Jain KK: Complications of the use of the neodymium:yttrium-aluminum garnet laser in neurosurgery. Neurosurgery 16:759-762, 1985.
19. Mattos Pimenta LH, Mattos Pimenta A, Martins JL: The use of the CO_2 laser for the removal of awkwardly situated meningiomas. Neurosurg Rev 4:53-55, 1981.
20. Polani TG: Physics of the surgical laser. Int Adv Surg Oncol 1:205-215, 1978.
21. Polanyi TG: Physics of surgery with the CO_2 laser. In: Microscopic and Endoscopic Surgery with the CO_2 Laser. Andrews AH, Polanyi TG (ed), London, John Wright, 1982, pp 26-72.
22. Polanyi TG: Laser physics. In Simpson GT, Shapshay SM (eds): Symposium on the Use of Lasers. Otolaryngol Clin N Am 16:753-774, 1983.
23. Powers SK, Edwards MSB, Boggan JE, et al: Use of the argon surgical laser in neurosurgery. J Neurosurg 60:523-530, 1984.
24. Raudzens RA, Shetter AG: Intraoperative monitoring of brainstem auditory evoked potentials. J Neurosurg 57:341-348, 1982.
25. Robertson JH, Clark WC, Robertson JT, et al: Use of the carbon dioxide laser for acoustic tumor surgery. Neurosurgery 12:286-290, 1983.
26. Stellar S, Polanyi TG, Bredemeier HC: Lasers in surgery. In: Laser Applications in Medicine and Biology, New York, Plenum Press, 1974, pp 241-293.
27. Stockard JJ, Stockard JE, Sharbrough FW: Brainstem auditory evoked potentials in neurology: Methodology, interpretation, clinical application. In Aminoff M (ed):

Electrodiagnosis in Clinical Neurology, New York, Churchill Livingstone, 1980, pp 370-413.
28. Straight TA, Robertson JH, Clark WC: Use of the carbon dioxide laser in the operative management of intracranial meningiomas: A report of twenty cases. *Neurosurgery* 10:464-467, 1982.
29. Takeuchi J, Handa H, et al: The Nd:YAG laser in neurological surgery. *Surg Neurol* 18:140-142, 1982.
30. Tew JM, Tobler WD: The laser: History, biophysics, and neurosurgical applications. *Clin Neurosurg* 341:506-549, 1984.
31. Wharen RE, Jr, Anderson RE, Scheithauer B, et al: The Nd:YAG laser in neurosurgery. Part I. Laboratory investigations: dose-related biological response of neural tissue. *J Neurosurg* 60:531-539, 1984.
32. Yoshihiko Y, Egashira T, Maki Y: Use of evoked responses to measure laser photoradiation tissue effects. *Neurosurgery* 14:131-134, 1984.

9

Stereotactic Methods for Diagnosis and Treatment of Skull Base Lesions

L. Dade Lunsford, M.D.

Introduction

Stereotactic surgery refers to the usage of a guiding device that is attached to the head and is capable of reaching the depths of the brain or skull base with one millimeter precision. Originally developed in the earlier part of the 20th Century for animal physiology studies, stereotactic devices were first used in patients in the late 1940s for the treatment of intractable movement disorders. Resurgent usage of stereotactic systems was mandated by the development of advanced imaging tools such as computed tomography (CT). The recognition of intracranial mass lesions earlier in disease states prompted the need for accurate and safe guiding devices capable of reaching lesions previously felt to be unapproachable or unresectable. The combination of stereotactic devices with CT has increased the accuracy of diagnostic brain biopsy to as high as 96% of cases.[14] Surgical mortality after brain biopsy has declined from as high as 33% to less than 1%.[12] Dedicated stereotactic CT systems have been developed for the operating room and have been used for both diagnosis and therapy of unresectable brain tumors.[8,12] More recently, the combination of stereotactic devices with magnetic resonance imaging (MRI) promises the possibility of increased contrast resolution and multiplanar imaging to provide superior target definition.[11]

Multiple stereotactic devices are now commercially available; which device is selected by each individual surgeon usually reflects the goals and needs of that particular surgeon as well as prior training. Each device has its own merits and deficiencies. Both rectilinear coordinate system devices such as the Leksell stereotactic frame (AB Elekta Instruments, Stockholm, Sweden) (Fig. 1) and spherical coordinates system (e.g., The Brown Robert-Wells device) represent modern adaptations of stereotaxy to advanced imaging tools. Both devices allow intraoperative craniotomy and resection of tumors under certain circumstances, as well as a multipurpose approach to various lesions of the skull base.

Diagnostic Biopsy

Histological diagnosis remains of paramount importance in all patients har-

From: Sekhar LN, Schramm VL Jr, eds: *Tumors of the Cranial Base: Diagnosis and Treatment.* Mount Kisco, New York, Futura Publishing Co, Inc, © 1987.

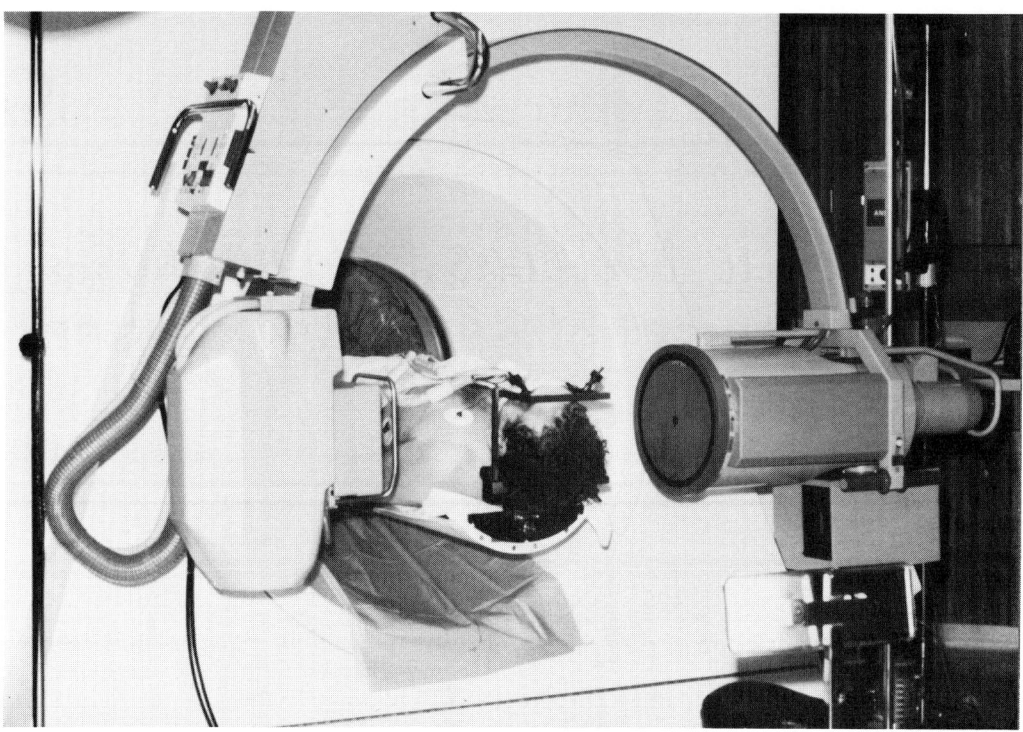

Figure 1: A CT-NMR compatible stereotactic guiding device. Intraoperative angiography can be performed during surgery if needed. (Reproduced with permission.[14])

boring skull base neoplasms. Despite recent advances in imaging, no one test or combination of tests has proven to be a sufficiently accurate method of histological diagnosis upon which to base subsequent therapy. From February 1981 to June 1985 at the University of Pittsburgh, stereotactic biopsy combined with CT was performed in 250 patients with intracranial masses. No patient has sustained permanent neurological morbidity or mortality. Definitive histological diagnosis was obtained by biopsy in more than 96% of patients. Lesions of the skull base were referred for stereotactic biopsy when the lesion itself was throught to be surgically unresectable, when viable alternative therapeutic techniques such as radiation therapy were under consideration, or when the patient was too old or too infirm to undergo a major surgical resection. At our hospital, surgery was performed in a dedicated stereotactic operating room containing an advanced generation CT scanner (GE 8800 CT scanner, GE Medical Systems, Milwaukee, Wisconsin) (Fig. 2). After intravenous contrast infusion, serial axial CT examination of the brain was obtained with the stereotactic coordinate frame applied to the head. Three-dimensional rectilinear coordinates (X, Y, and Z) were determined for the biopsy target using standard software available on the CT scanner. Multiplanar reformatted images were used to define an anatomically safe trajectory (Fig. 3). Serial samples of the lesion were taken at selected biopsy points using a spiral (corkscrew) biopsy instrument as well as by aspiration.[12,14] Serial sampling of the entire lesion using a single trajectory was designed to minimize trauma and to allow accurate histopathological study of various areas of the neoplasm (Fig. 3). Frozen sections were not routinely performed unless specific queries indicated rapid treatment plans, i.e. infections. Specimens were routinely fixed for light microscopic study and reviewed the day after surgery in conjunction with the

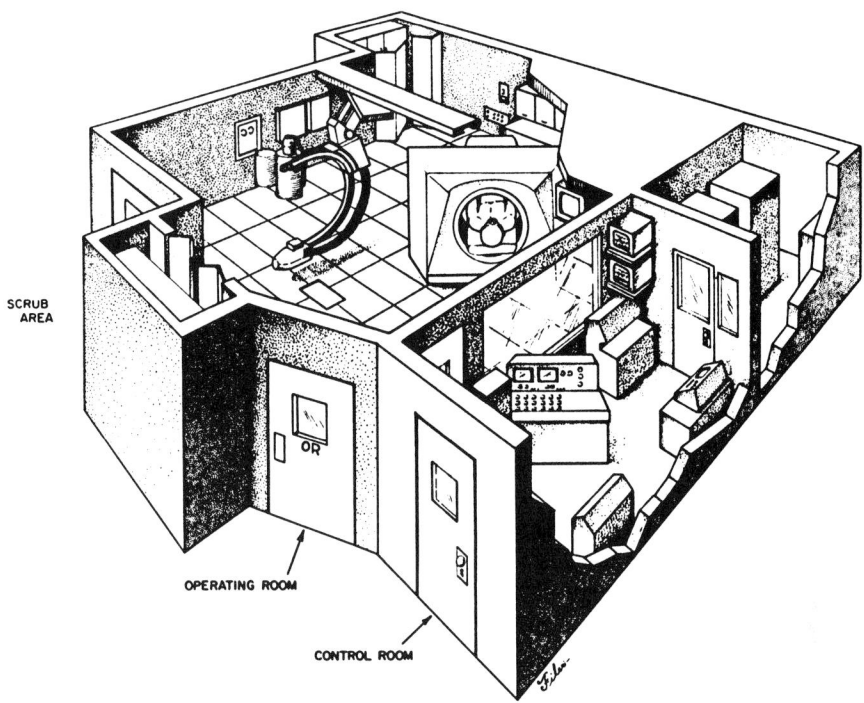

Figure 2: A dedicated operating room for stereotactic surgery that permits intraoperative CT imaging. Both conventional stereotactic procedures as well as craniotomy can be performed with intraoperative CT. (Reproduced with permission from Lunsford LD, Parrish R, Albright L: Intraoperative imaging with a therapeutic CT scanner: Technical note. *Neurosurgery* 15:559-561, 1984.)

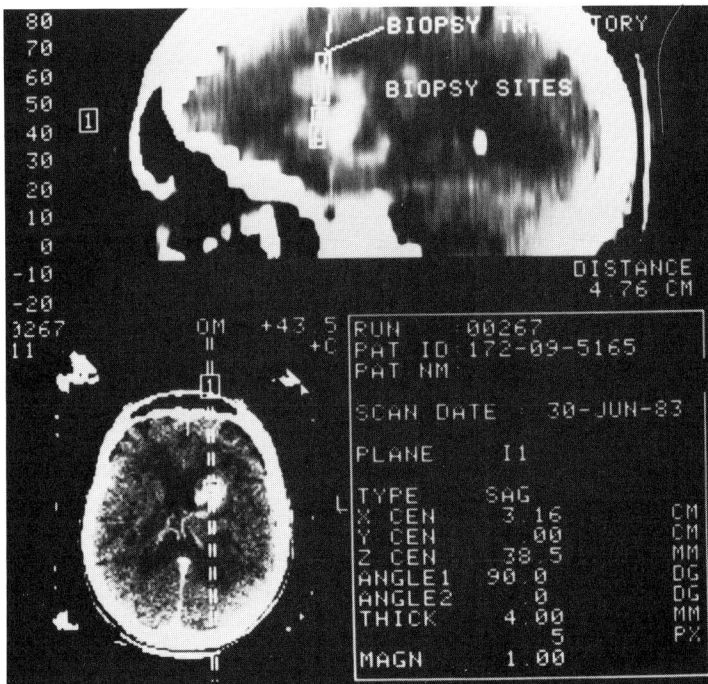

Figure 3: Reformatted CT images permit preoperative depiction of the probe pathway and biopsy target sites in the tumor. (Reproduced with permission.[14])

diagnostic images performed before and during surgery.

The surgical biopsy itself was performed under local anesthesia in most patients. Preoperative cerebral angiography was mandatory in most patients with skull base lesions, so that the relationship of the mass to the major cerebral vessels was assessed prior to final selection of a target trajectory for stereotactic biopsy.

Intracavitary Irradiation

Cystic tumors arising from or near the skull base can be treated by intracavitary placement of radioisotopes designed to provide a tumoricidal dose to the cyst wall. Initially described in the early 1950s by Wycis[19] and subsequently by Leksell,[10] intracavitary irradiation has been used almost exclusively for cystic craniopharyngiomas. Craniopharyngiomas can be divided into those tumors that are (1) solitary cysts, (2) multicystic, or (3) predominantly solid tumors.[2,3] Cystic craniopharyngiomas are suitable for intracavitary irradiation by installation of a beta-emitting isotope that has the advantage of relatively short penetrance of the emitted energy. Radioactive phosphorus (^{32}P) was initially used, and remains the only available isotope in the United States. In Europe and Asia ^{99}yttrium and ^{186}rhenium have been used. Only two isotopes are strictly beta-emitting, and each has a variable range of penetrance of the beta-emitting ray. ^{32}P has a half value tissue penetrance of 0.8 mm. The radioactive isotope in colloidal suspension is injected into the cyst and subsequently coats the cyst wall. A minimum target dosage to the cyst wall is set at 20,000 rads to be delivered over the effective lifetime (i.e., five half-lives) of the isotope. Because of the short penetrance of the beta emission, surrounding structures such as the hypothalamus, optic chiasm, and the pituitary receive virtually no irradiation. Backlund has demonstrated virtually total regression and involution of the cyst after successful treatment. In his series of more than 100 patients with cystic craniopharyngiomas followed for up to 15 years, more than 90% are alive and well.[4] Solid craniopharyngiomas have been treated by Backlund and colleagues by stereotactic irradiation using the gamma unit,[1] as described below.

In our hospital, the volumes of cystic lesions were estimated by preoperative CT imaging, after which the isotope (^{32}P) was ordered. Accurate estimation of the cyst volume was mandatory for accurate dosimetry. After application of the stereotactic coordinate frame to the patient's head, serial axial CT scan images of the brain were performed with high resolution technique after intravenous contrast infusion. With our scanning technique, we have found that 5 mm slice thicknesses incremented by 3 mm table movement provided the most accurate method for volume determination.[13] The areas of all portions of the cyst seen on the axial CT scan image were summed to provide a volume estimation. In six patients, we performed a radioisotope (^{99m}technetium) dilution technique for volume estimation and compared these results to the values obtained by CT (Fig. 4). Radioisotope dilution technique, as described by Backlund,[3] was performed after stereotactic puncture of the cyst. After withdrawing 1 ml of cyst fluid for microscopic analysis (including analysis for cholesterol crystals), the cyst volume was replaced with 1 ml of ^{99m}technetium in colloidal suspension. After repeated aspiration and flushing of the needle, two one-half (0.5 ml) samples were taken for measurement on a dose calibrator, after which the actual volume of the cyst was determined.[13] In our six cases, no significant differences were found between radioisotope and CT estimations. Subsequently we have abandoned the radioisotope technique, solely relying now on CT for volume estimations. Radiation dosimetry was calculated so that the volume of ^{32}P injected provided a dosage of 20,000–25,000 rads of irradiation to the cyst wall over five half-lives (70 days) of the isotope. It was considered crucial to maintain the preoperative volume of the cyst both before and after puncture of the cyst and placement of the ^{32}P. Early reduction in the volume of the cyst posed the

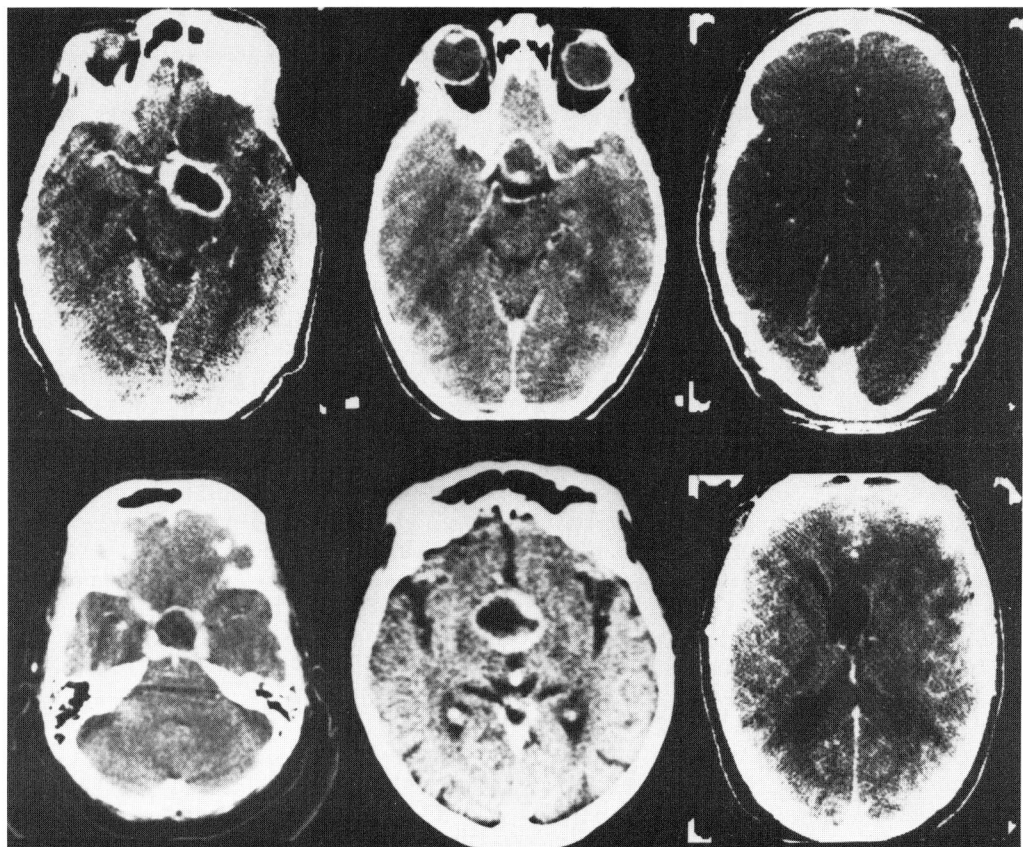

Figure 4: CT of six patients with cystic lesions of the cranial base treated by intracavitary placement of ^{32}P. All but one patient had craniopharyngioma; this patient had a cystic glioma (right lower corner).

risk that portions of the cyst wall could "deflate" and not receive radiation. Therefore the total volume of the cyst at the conclusion of the procedure was kept equal to the volume prior to stereotactic puncture of the cyst. When early reduction of the cyst wall was necessary because of mass effect resulting in hypothalamic or optic nerve compression, repuncture of the cyst was performed between 14 and 35 days after the initial isotope placement. Virtually no isotope was recovered from the second puncture since the colloidal suspension vigorously adhered to the internal cyst wall.

Leakage of isotope from the cyst proved to be of little practical significance; initial blood samples failed to disclose any evidence of isotope after intracystic placement. It was important to use a small sized needle (0.9 mm outer diameter) to puncture the cyst wall, so that leakage of the isotope was not likely. The trajectory of the puncture needle to a basal cystic tumor was usually transfrontal after skull trephination near the ipsilateral coronal suture. One patient underwent transsphenoidal placement of the isotope. This technique was suboptimal because of the risk of leakage of the isotope through a puncture needle traversing the sphenoid sinus.

Serial follow-up examinations in our patients have shown gradual involution of the cyst wall with collapse of the cyst occurring from 3 to 12 months after isotope treatment. During this time, preoperative visual field defects frequently stabilized or improved, and new endocrinological deficits were not encountered. In comparison to direct surgical attack on such lesions, the risk of diabetes insipidus using this technique was very low, and the vast majority of patients continued to have a stable or improving endocrinological function in accordance with the observations of Backlund.[4] Other cystic tumors can be treated in this way providing that the cyst wall is relatively thin. We have treated three cystic gliomas successfully in the same fashion; these patients had reduction in the cyst and no regrowth.

Interstitial Brachytherapy

Implantation of radioactive isotopes into unresectable tumors was first employed in 1901 at the recommendation of Pierre Curie.[5] Radiation therapy itself has been demonstrated to be an effective treatment for malignant primary brain tumors, significantly prolonging life. Interstitial irradiation has been suggested as a means of local, relatively long-term, low dose rate, high dose radiation therapy. When properly implanted, interstitial radiation sources will spare surrounding normal brain and vasculature. Interstitial radiation utilizing ^{222}radon, ^{125}iodine, ^{192}irridium, ^{198}gold, and other radioactive sources implanted into tumor tissue have been reported and recognized to provide tumor growth control. The major advantage of interstitial irradiation using removable sources (brachytherapy) are noted to be its focal intratumoral placement compared to conventional external beam treatment (teletherapy).

In the last 20 years, extensive experience has been gained with stereotactic implantation of radioisotopes, especially in severeal European centers.[15] This form of treatment has been used primarily to treat low grade gliomas, but more recent extensive experience in the United States has begun to evaluate prospectively the treatment of malignant gliomas by providing an "interstitial boost" of radiation therapy to the tumor in combination with external beam therapy. Although not widely used at the present time, these techniques are also being explored in the treatment of recurrent skull base tumors. Integration of stereotactic systems with CT has resulted in earlier recognition and expanded abilities to implant such lesions.

Implantation of radioisotopes can be done by two techniques: (1) after open surgery with direct inspection of the tumor and implantation of the isotope, and (2) by stereotactic implantation of the tumor visualized by CT or MRI. Two methods of implantation can be selected: (1) permanent implantation of low dose radioactive isotopes arranged in a volumetric fashion to provide continued dose rate over prolonged periods of time, or (2) interstitial implantation with a removable isotope placed within the tumor delivering a relatively high dose rate (approximately 1000 rads per day) over a 5 to 7 day period. Recent experience suggests that ^{125}I is the superior radioactive source and has certain attractive features such as less risk to health care personnel.[5]

Stereotactic Technique

We have chosen to use high dose rate implantable radioactive ^{125}I sources which were afterloaded and removed between 5 and 7 days after implantation. Patients referred for treatment after histological diagnosis undergo high resolution CT scanning of the brain. The target area to be implanted was selected on the basis of an intravenous contrast enhanced scan and more recently compared to MRI (Fig. 5). Multiplanar reformatted images were used to define the volume of the lesion to be implanted. These measurements were subsequently used in a computer dosimetry program that allowed the plotting of various seed strengths in various geometric arrangements in order to optimize the radiation dose. Target dosages of 6000 rads to the enhancing tumor margin were selected. With this technique, central dosages within the tumor were considerably higher. However, with the fall-off of radiation by the inverse square law, radiation at 1 cm beyond the tumor margin was well within brain tolerance levels. After completion of the radiation dosimetry planning, the patient was admitted to the hospital for stereotactic implantation.

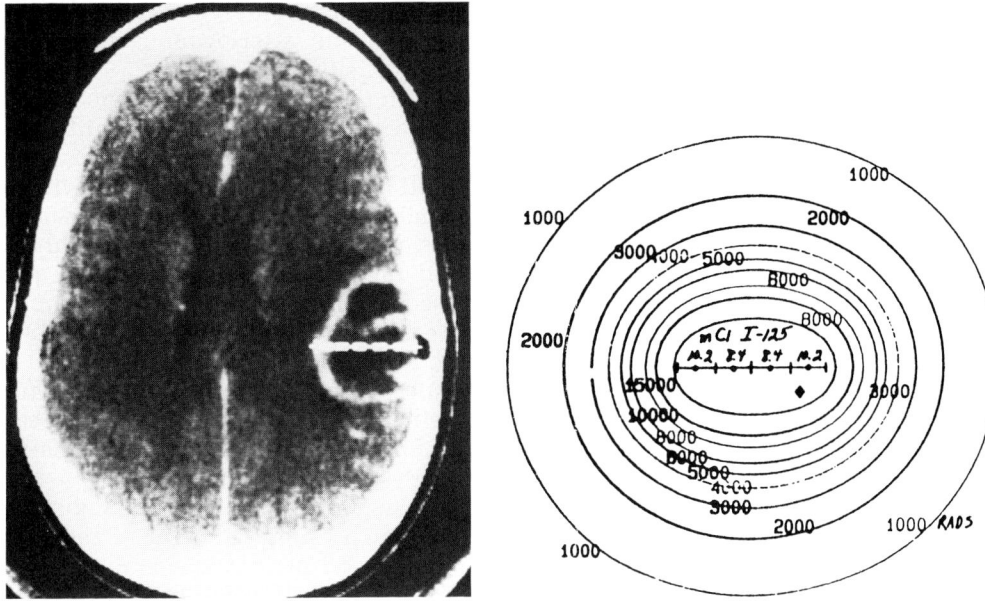

Figure 5: Left: Target volume of parenchymal brain lesion undergoing brachytherapy (^{125}I) implantation. Right: Isodose planning of lesion for ^{125}I brachytherapy.

A stereotactic instrument was applied to the head under local anesthesia, and repeat CT scan images of the brain were performed after contrast infusion. These CT images were compared to the original CT images and the targets were selected on the CT images chosen for implantation of the isotopes. One or more catheters were implanted at the target area using stereotactic technique and twist drills through the skull. An outer catheter was placed at the target area after which the preloaded inner catheters containing the radioactive iodine sources were afterloaded into the outer catheters. The catheters were sutured to the scalp. Repeat CT scan images immediately after implantation confirmed appropriate placement of the catheters. The patients wear a lead-lined helmet during the time of implantation to reduce radiation exposure to health care workers. At the conclusion of the prescribed radiation dosage, the afterloaded catheters were removed and the incisions closed. The patients generally tolerated implantation very well and were ambulatory with no significant complaints during the time of implantation.

Unanswered Questions

At the present time, interstitial brachytherapy for both benign and malignant skull base tumors is under investigation. Many questions remain unanswered. The radiation sensitivity of these lesions varies considerably and the appropriate dosimetry and total dosage to be given to the tumor is yet unknown. Because of the intimate relationship of the important structures of the brain, its vascular supply, and other cranial nerves and adjacent structures, the implantation itself must be done with great care and precision. Injury to vascular structures such as the carotid artery runs the risk of radiation necrosis and catastrophic hemorrhage. Because many skull base lesions tend to be infiltrative in nature, it seems unlikely that anything other than tumor palliation will be achieved by such an approach in the future. While at the present time interstitial brachytherapy appears to be a useful adjunctive treatment of malignant gliomas of the brain, the role and usefulness for skull base tumors as yet remain undefined.

Stereotactic Radiosurgery

The ability to focus radiation on a target by stereotactic technique led to the development of the field of stereotactic radiosurgery. With such techniques, an overwhelming dosage of radiation can be focused on a target and delivered rapidly without the need for a surgical incision. At the present time, three techniques are in clinical usage: (1) a stereotactic radiosurgical unit (Fig. 6) consisting of a multisource radioactive cobalt unit that cross-fires onto a target area; this is the "gamma knife" developed at the Karolinska Hospital in Stockholm, Sweden by Professor Leksell[2]; (2) the proton beam unit which utilizes the Bragg peak effect of the proton beam and has been pioneered by Kjellberg using the Harvard University cyclotron[9]; (3) linear accelerator units cross-fired at a target by stereotactic technique as recently proposed by Heifetz[7] and utilized by Patil.[17]

Between 1968 and 1985 approximately 1500 patients have been treated by radiosurgical technique at the Karolinska Hospital in Stockholm. Indications for stereotactic radiosurgery included pituitary adenomas, craniopharyngiomas, pineal region tumors, meningiomas, acoustic tumors, and arteriovenous malformations. The proton beam has been used almost exclusively for pituitary adenomas and arteriovenous malformations by Kjellberg.[9]

Both units have several attractive features which warrant their continued usage and development in the treatment of skull base tumors. First, an overwhelming and potentially tumoricidal dosage of radiation can be collimated and highly focused on the lesion, delivering a prescribed dosage of radiation, for example 6000 rads, to the tumor mass in a brief period of time, perhaps between 10 and 90 minutes. This is in contrast to fractionated radiation therapy given by external beam technique, with 200 rads per fractionation and treatment programs lasting 5 to 6 weeks. In addition, the radiobiological effect of such a large amount of radiation given at one time is considerably greater than that of fractionated treatments. Second, the radiation can be focused with very steep isodose curves and minimal effective radiation delivered to surrounding vital structures of the brain or skull base. Third, integration with stereotactic technique has allowed precise radiation doses without the need to make a surgical incision. At the present time, proton beam cyclotron units are being used at the Massachusetts General Hospital, Boston, Massachusetts, and in Berkeley, California. Stereotactic radiosurgical units ("the

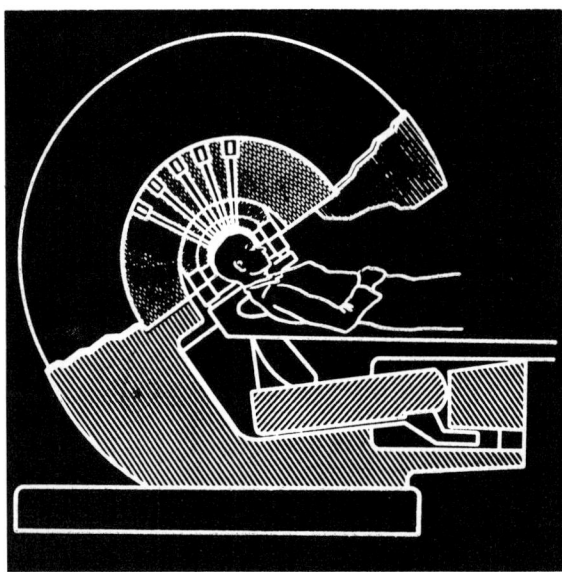

Figure 6: Line drawing of stereotactic radiosurgical unit ("the gamma knife") with 179 ^{60}cobalt sources collimated at a target volume specified by CT. (Reproduced with permission from AB Elekta Instruments, Stockholm, Sweden.)

gamma knife") are being used at the Karolinska Hospital in Stockholm, Buenos Aires, Argentina, and in Sheffield, England. In the United States, stereotactic radiosurgical units are under development in several centers, including the University of Pittsburgh. Because of the author's own experience and interest in the usage of the gamma knife, this unit will be described in more detail.

Stereotactic Radiosurgery Unit ("Gamma Knife")

In the late 1940s, Professor Lars Leksell developed a stereotactic system for guided deep brain surgery. With this principle, the target was placed at the center of a semicircular arc and this target could be reached by any radius. Leksell suggested that radiation could be crossfired at a target area without the need for a surgical incision. The first stereotactic radiosurgical unit was installed in Stockholm in 1968 and was used primarily for the creation of lesions in the brain for functional neurosurgery, including the treatment of intractable pain, trigeminal neuralgia, Parkinson's disease, and psychoneuroses. In 1975, the second gamma unit was installed at the Karolinska Institute, and redesigned for tumor treatment. The Leksell gamma unit consists of 179–201 cobalt 60 sources positioned in a hemispherical pattern and oriented towards a common focal point. Radiation sources are enclosed by heavy lead shielding which provides adequate external radiation protection. The individual beams are collimated towards the target and directed through a helmet located on a sliding table. When the table is moved into the central body containing the cobalt 60 sources, the collimation helmet is engaged, giving a beam channel accuracy of more than 10 one-hundredths of a millimeter.

The sliding table moves on parallel rails and is moved in and out of the radiation sources by means of a hydraulic system. Different collimator helmets are used to provide different aperture lesions (4, 8, and 14 mm in diameter). By plugging certain beam channels, lesion configuration can be varied to change the isodose characteristics depending on the tumor dimensions. The dose distribution and calculations are performed by means of a computerized dose planning system.

The intracranial target is determined by stereotactic technique. Visualization of a target and determination of its locations (coordinates) are done by preoperative CT, MRI, or angiography. The entire radiation treatment can frequently be done in approximately 1 hour. Since no surgical incision is necessary, patients in Sweden have even been treated as outpatients or with minimal hospitalization of 2 days. In the more than 1000 patients operated on with this technique, over 15 years in Sweden, there has been no operative mortality and no postoperative infection.

Clinical Applications for Skull Base Lesions

Pituitary Adenoma

Both secretory and nonsecretory adenomas have been treated by stereotactic radiosurgery, especially in patients not considered suitable for transsphenoidal resection. Treatment can be considered if the tumor volume can be enclosed within a 50% isodose curve of the gamma unit using the large collimator. Lesions greater than approximately 3 cm in size are not generally considered treatable by this technique. Therefore, the technique has been especially useful in patients with smaller or even microadenomas including those patients with Nelson's syndrome, acromegaly, and especially Cushing's disease. Rähn detailed the results of a large series of patients with Cushing's disease treated by stereotactic radiosurgery.[8] In his series, 86% of the patients have been successfully treated with resolution of the hypercortisolism. Further development of the technique might be especially useful in the treatment of patients with invasive adenomas localized within the cavernous sinus area.

Craniopharyngioma

Backlund has reported the usage of the gamma knife for solid craniopharyngiomas of the skull base.[1] Cystic portions of the tumor are treated by intracavitary radiation as described above. Solid tumors are subsequently treated by stereotactic radiosurgical technique. When the lesion can be enclosed within the 50% isodose curve, progressive involution and shrinkage of the lesion occurs between 6 months and 1 year after treatment. Increasingly, radiation therapy has been reported to be an effective means of treating craniopharyngiomas. The results frequently surpass open total surgical excision both in terms of reduction of postoperative endocrinological deficits as well as preservation of intellectual function.[6]

Acoustic Neurinoma

Norén has pioneered treatment of acoustic neurinomas with stereotactic radiosurgery.[16] These benign tumors are not ordinarily felt to be radiation-sensitive lesions, but have been found to respond well to radiosurgical treatment using the gamma unit. At the present time, acoustic tumors of less than 3 cm in size are preferentially treated in Stockholm by radiosurgical technique. Usually, two lesions are given, one larger lesion to the body of the tumor mass which extends intracranially, and a smaller lesion tailored to fit the configuration of the tumor that enters the porus acousticus (Fig. 7). From 1967 to 1984, 128 patients with acoustic tumors have been treated at the Karolinska Institute. Only eight patients with continued growth were documented by serial follow-up examinations with CT. During this time, 23 patients with bilateral acoustic tumors were treated. Stereotactic lesions have been given after subtotal resection, and especially in patients with neurofibromatosis, who have bilateral lesions with preserved hearing. Hearing preservation has been maintained in many patients with useful hearing prior to

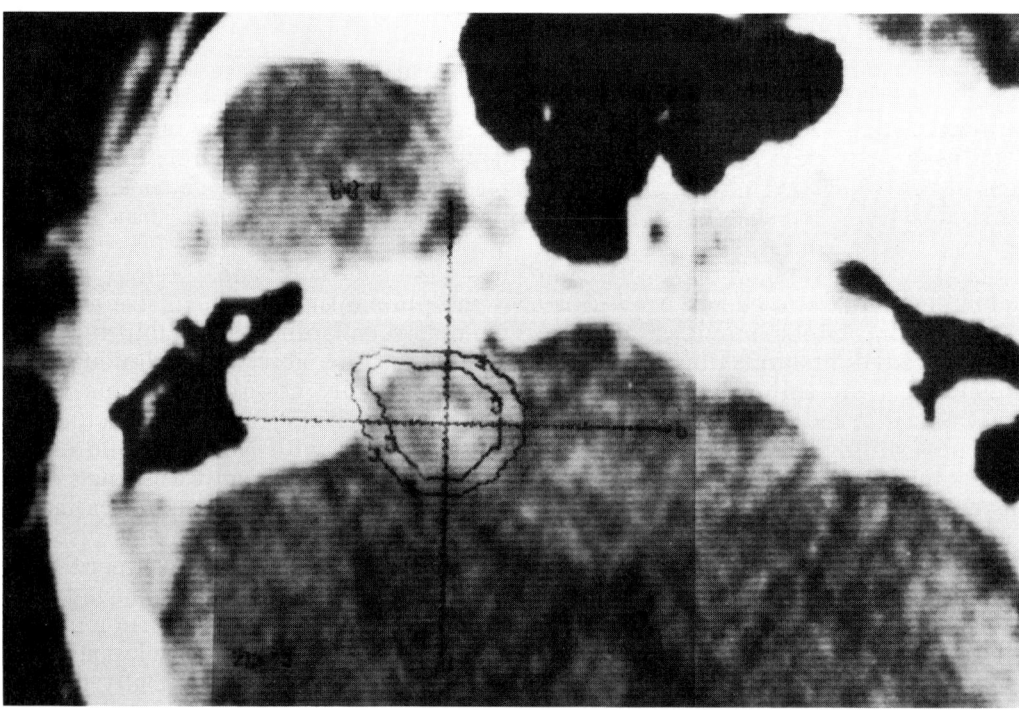

Figure 7: Acoustic neurinoma demonstrated by CT scan. Isodose planning for stereotactic radiosurgical treatment is demonstrated. (Photograph courtesy of Georg Norén.)

surgery. Transitory facial palsies developed 6 to 12 months after surgery in 9% of the patients but in only 2% of patients treated by improved technique in the last 7 years. Serial follow-up CT examinations usually showed either no further growth, central cavitation, reduction in contrast enhancement, and in many cases slow involution of the tumors. Longer-term follow-up will be necessary to clearly define the advantages of stereotactic radiosurgery over microsurgical excision. Nonetheless, those patients who are either too elderly or too frail to undergo craniotomy and removal because of associated medical conditions can be candidates for radiosurgery.

Other lesions that have been felt suitable for stereotactic radiosurgery include meningiomas of the skull base and rarer lesions such as chordomas and chondrosarcomas. It is possible that skull base metastases, if found early enough, may be suitable candidates in the future, obviating the need for extensive cranial base surgery.

Future of Stereotactic Surgery for Cranial Base Tumors

Stereotactic surgery has been firmly integrated as a valuable component of modern neurological surgery in the same way as the operating microscope. Stereotactic technique can be considered as a primary or an alternative treatment for many lesions of the skull base. Diagnostic biopsy is possible to achieve histological definition, especially when total resection is not deemed possible or wise, and effective alternative treatment such as radiation therapy exists. Cystic neoplasms of the skull base can be treated by intracavitary placement of beta-emitting radiation isotopes frequently with progressive involution of the cyst. Interstitial implantation by brachytherapeutic technique allows the possibility of focal radiation to be given in overwhelming amounts to a tumor margin and to spare the surrounding brain. Technical limitations exist as to the route and ability to implant various skull base lesions. Many patients may be suitable for stereotactic radiosurgical technique, especially using such units as the "gamma knife." Increasingly, these techniques will be used to combat tumors of the cranial base.

Acknowledgments: Phyllis Shoemaker and Mary Ann Vincenzini aided in the preparation of the manuscript.

References

1. Backlund EO: Solid craniopharyngiomas treated by stereotactic radiosurgery. INSERM Symposium No. 12, *Stereotactic Cerebral Irradiation*, Elsevier, North Holland Biomedical Press, 1979, pp 271-277.
2. Backlund EO: Stereotactic radiosurgery in intracranial tumors and vascular malformations. In Krayenbuhl H (ed): *Advances and Technical Standards in Neurosurgery*, Springer Verlang, Wien, NY. 6:1-37, 1979.
3. Backlund EO: Stereotaxic treatment of craniopharyngiomas. *Acta Neurochir* (Suppl) 21:177-183, 1974.
4. Backlund EO: Stereotactic treatment of craniopharyngiomas: 15 years experience. Presented at the 32nd Scandinavian Neurosurgical Society Meeting, September 1980, Linkopping, Sweden (abstract).
5. Bernstein M, Gutin PH: Interstitial irradiation of brain tumors: A review. *Neurosurgery* 9:741-750, 1981.
6. Fischer EG, Welch K, Belli JA, et al: Treatment of craniopharyngiomas in children, 1972-1981. *J Neurosurg* 62:496-501, 1985.
7. Heifetz MD, Wexler M, Thompson R: Single-beam radiotherapy knife: A practical theoretical mode. *J Neurosurg* 60:814-818, 1984.
8. Kelly PJ, Alker GJ, Kall BA, et al: Method of computed tomography-based stereotactic biopsy with arteriographic control. *Neurosurgery* 14:172-177, 1984.
9. Kjellberg RN, Kliman B: Bragg peak proton hypophysectomy for hyperpituitarism, induced hypopituitarism, and neoplasms. *Prog Neurol Surg* 6:295-325, 1975.
10. Leksell L, Backlund EO, Johansson L: Treatment of craniopharyngiomas. *Acta Chir Scand* 133:345-350, 1967.
11. Leksell L, Leksell D, Schwebel J: Stereotaxis and nuclear magnetic resonance. *J Neurol Neurosurg Psychiat* 48:14-18, 1985.

12. Lunsford LD: Stereotaxy and the role of CT in morphological and functional surgery of the human brain. In Latchaw RE (ed): *Computed Tomography of the Head, Neck and Spine*, Chicago, Year Book Medical Publishers, 1985, pp 743-764.
13. Lunsford LD, Levine J, Gumerman LW: A comparison of computed tomographic and radionuclide methods to determine intracranial cystic tumor volumes. *J Neurosurg* 17:12-18, 1985.
14. Lunsford LD, Martinez AJ: Stereotactic exploration of the brain in the era of computed tomography. *Surg Neurol* 22:222-230, 1984.
15. Mundinger F: Implantation of radioisotopes (Curie-therapy). In Schaltenbrand G, Walker AE (eds): *Stereotaxy of the Human Brain*, 2nd Edition, New York, Thieme-Stratten, Inc., 1982, pp 410-435.
16. Norén G, Arndt J, Hindmarsh J: Stereotactic radiosurgery in cases of acoustic neurinomas: Further experiences. *Neurosurgery* 13:12-22, 1983.
17. Patil A: Isocentric placement of targets in the linear accelerator using CT stereotaxis. Presented at the 36th Annual Scandinavian Neurosurgical Society Meeting, Stockholm, Sweden, September 14, 1984 (abstract).
18. Rähn T, Thorén M, Hall K, et al: Stereotactic radiosurgery in Cushing's syndrome: Acute radiation effects. *Surg Neurol* 14:85-92, 1980.
19. Wycis H, Robbins R, Spiegel-Adolph M, et al: Studies in stereoencephalotomy III: Treatment of a cystic craniopharyngioma by injection of radioactive ^{32}P. *Confin Neurol* 14:193-202, 1954.

10

Radiation Therapy in the Treatment of Tumors of the Cranial Base

Melvin Deutsch, M.D.

Introduction

The successful use of radiotherapy to treat a tumor necessitates delivery of an adequate dose to the entire tumor volume. Conversely, the causes of local failure are: an inadequate dose to the tumor and/or tumor beyond the irradiated volume. The treatment of skull base tumors by radiotherapy involves the precise determination of the extent of the tumor. This is not a region where one can safely increase the irradiated volume by large increments just to be on the "safe side." Once the volume to be irradiated and dose to be delivered have been determined, a technique of delivery must be devised which delivers the dose as homogenously as possible to the tumor.

Tumors of the skull base can be divided into those arising from the floor of the cranium and those invading into the skull base from adjacent areas such as the paranasal sinuses, nasopharynx, and middle ear–mastoid region (Table I).

Effects of Radiation on Normal Tissue

Treatment planning for skull base tumors must take into account the sensitivity of adjacent normal tissues. The volume of normal tissue irradiated, the maximum administered dose,* daily fraction size, number of fractions, and the sensitivity of the particular tissue are the factors associated with radiation damage.

Obviously it is difficult to avoid irradiation of adjacent brain when treating base of skull neoplasms. Sheline[99] in 1980 did an extensive review of the literature on radiation damage to the brain. Acute reactions, those occurring during the course of radiotherapy, are generally mild unless one is using very large daily doses, e.g., 750–1000 rad. During the 10 weeks following completion of radiotherapy, transient signs and symptoms suggesting tumor progression may occur but usually resolve spontaneously and probably are representative of demyelination. Of major

---

*The rad is the currently accepted unit of absorbed dose of radiation. However, in the past, other terms such as "roentgen," "R," and "r" have been used to express dose and these different terms have been retained when used in referenced material.

From: Sekhar LN, Schramm VL Jr, eds: *Tumors of the Cranial Base: Diagnosis and Treatment*. Mount Kisco, New York, Futura Publishing Co, Inc, © 1987.

Table I
Base of Skull Tumors

I. Arising from Floor of Cranium
   A. Meningioma
   B. Chordoma
   C. Pituitary adenoma
   D. Craniopharyngioma
II. Extending into Base of Skull from Adjacent Sites
   A. Tumors of nasal fossa and paranasal sinuses
      1. Squamous cell carcinoma
      2. Adenocarcinoma—adenocystic
      3. Esthesioneuroblastoma
      4. Lymphoma
   B. Tumors of Nasopharynx
      1. Squamous cell carcinoma
      2. Soft tissue sarcoma—rhabdomyosarcoma
      3. Lymphoma
      4. Juvenile angiofibroma
   C. Tumors of Middle Ear, Mastoid, External Auditory Canal
      1. Squamous cell carcinoma
      2. Soft tissue sarcoma—rhabdomyosarcoma
   D. Tumors of orbit
      1. Lymphoma
      2. Rhabdomyosarcoma
   E. Chemodectoma—glomus jugulare
   F. Metatasis

concern is the possibility of late damage occurring several months to years after completion of radiotherapy. Of 83 cases summarized by Sheline, 45 had received a total dose ⩾7000 R. Of 22 patients whose total dose was equal to or less than 5000 rad, 14 had daily fractions greater than 250 rad. This still leaves a small group of patients who had therapy regimens considered to be "safe." Using data from patients treated for craniopharyngioma and pituitary tumors, Sheline et al.[98] estimate the incidence of brain necrosis from a therapy regimen administering 5200 rad/26 fractions at 200 rad/day to be 0.04–0.4%. Marks et al.[71] reported cerebral necrosis in 7/139 patients (5%) irradiated for primary brain and pituitary tumors. Necrosis was not seen in patients who received doses biologically equal to or less than 5400 rad/30 fractions over 42 elapsed days. For most base of skull neoplasms, whole brain irradiation will not be necessary. Still, it is important to limit as much as possible the amount of normal brain included in the high dose volume. On the basis of the above-cited data indicating an increased likelihood of brain necrosis with increasing the size of daily fractions, therapy should be administered at ⩽200 rad per day except in situations where long-term survival is extremely unlikely, such as patients with metastatic disease. For such patients who have limited survival, the use of high daily doses, 250–300 rad, is justified.

Cranial nerve injury is a rare complication of radiotherapy.[58] Shukovsky and Fletcher[101] evaluated 15 long-term survivors after radiotherapy for cancer of the nasal fossa and ethmoid sinuses. Three patients developed blindness between 4 or 5 years post-radiotherapy and one also had olfactory nerve damage. All had received doses of greater than 7000 rad to the affected optic nerves. Parsons et al.[83] studied patients treated with radiotherapy for neoplasms either involving or close to the orbit. Doses of 6000–7300 rad at 165–190 rad fractions produced optic nerve damage in 2/24 (8%) long-term survivors. The same total doses at ⩾195 rad fractions produced injury in 7 of 17 patients (41%). Aristizabal et al.[5] reviewed 122 patients with pituitary adenomas treated with radiotherapy using various fractionation schemes and total doses. Five of the 122 patients showed evidence of radiation damage either to the brain (1 patient) or the optic tracts (4 patients). The likelihood of complications seemed to be related to fraction size. Of 106 patients treated with ⩽220 rad per fraction, there were only three complications (3%) compared to 2 of 16 patients having complications when the treatment fraction was ⩾220 rad. There was a 15% incidence of complications in patients treated 4 days per week with 250–280 rad per fraction. The total dose was also related to the incidence of complications with all five patients having received over 4600 rad.

There is a similarity between damage to cranial nerves and brain in that the incidence and likelihood of radiation damage is related to total dose and also to individual fraction size.

Whenever possible, the eyeball should be shielded since doses to the lens as low as 400 rad can cause cataract.[75] Also, the retina is not as radio-resistant as once thought. Retinal damage leading to blindness usually appears 2–2½ years after radiotherapy doses biologically equivalent to 7000 rad/35 fractions.[101] Parsons et al.[83] reported only one patient with retinal injury who had received less than 5000 rad and this patient also had chemotherapy. Above 6000 rad administered in 25–38 fractions, 8 of 9 patients had severe retinal injury.

The external and internal auditory structures occasionally are included in the radiation portals used to treat skull base neoplasms. When the ears are included in the irradiated volume, symptoms of otitis media such as hearing loss, earache, and the sensation of fullness frequently occur during treatment.[14-16] Hearing loss following radiotherapy for nasopharyngeal malignancy has been reported and seems to be related to dose.[79] However, the exact incidence of damage to the auditory mechanism is not known since in most reported series, patients were probably tested because of decreased hearing complaints. It is also not known what effect coexisting factors such as age, infection, and chemotherapy may have on the incidence of radiation-induced hearing loss.

In the course of irradiation of skull base neoplasms, the pituitary gland is likely to be included in the high dose volume. There are conflicting reports in the literature concerning the likelihood of endocrine dysfunction following irradiation of the pituitary gland. Differences in reported incidences of pituitary dysfunction following radiotherapy are probably related to the thoroughness with which patients were tested. There have been reports of little or no pituitary dysfunction in children and adults who had radiotherapy directed to the pituitary gland in the course of treating nasopharynx cancer and brain tumors.[9,17,20,32] By contrast, there have been many reports describing a high incidence of pituitary dysfunction especially in children receiving radiotherapy for tumors not involving the hypothalamus or pituitary gland.[31,46,95,96,117] The most common abnormality noted was suppression of growth hormone secretion. The likelihood of growth hormone dysfunction is related to dose and age. There seems to be a critical dose level between 2000 and 3000 rad at 200 rad/day below which growth hormone abnormalities would not occur. In addition, the younger the child, the greater the risk of pituitary dysfunction following radiotherapy.

Bone and dermis are unavoidably irradiated whenever tumors in the skull are treated. Because of the relatively small volume of bone and marrow irradiated, clinical sequelae are most unlikely. However, in the child, radiotherapy can interfere with normal bone growth causing cranial-facial deformity. The severity of the hypoplasia correlates with high dose and young age at the time of treatment. Occasionally, osteoradionecrosis is seen following high dose radiotherapy for neoplasms of the paranasal sinuses and temporal bone region. However, this complication is probably related not only to the radiation but to other coexisting factors such as the surgical procedure, presence of infection, and pre-treatment involvement of bone by the tumor. Skin changes such as erythema and limited moist desquamation are usually self-limiting and of little clinical significance. However, alopecia can be permanent with skin doses above 5000–6000 rad. Whenever possible, treatment should not be administered just by parallel opposed fields since by this technique, the dose to the skin and subcutaneous tissues can be higher than the actual dose to the tumor, especially when cobalt-60 or 4 MV x-rays are used.

Radiation can be tumorogenic, but fortunately this complication is so rare that it should not be considered a contraindication to radiotherapy. Sporadic cases of fibrosarcoma have been reported years after radiation for brain tumor and pituitary adenoma.[81,100,114] Also, brain tumors have been noted in children treated with radiotherapy for tinea capitus[22,77,91] and acute lymphocytic leukemia.[3]

Meningioma

Meningiomas frequently arise from base of skull structures such as the olfactory groove, orbit, sphenoid ridge, parasellar region, and posterior fossa. Meningiomas from base of skull sites account for approximately 50% of all meningiomas.[1,25,76,116,121] Total resection is the treatment of choice. The rate of complete resection in various reported series varies from 44–83%.[1,25,76,116,121] The extent of resection is related to the site of the tumor. For meningiomas involving the convexity, Mirimanoff et al.[76] reported a 96% incidence of complete resectability. For orbit and olfactory groove meningiomas, the rates of complete resectability were 80% and 77%, respectively. Meningiomas in the parasellar region had a 57% complete excision rate whereas for meningiomas arising in the posterior fossa and sphenoid ridge, the complete resection rate was 32% and 28%, respectively. In other large series, the likelihood of complete resection was higher for meningiomas involving the parasagittal region and convexity than for lesions involving base of skull regions.[25,121]

For meningiomas of all sites treated by total excision, Mirimanoff et al.[76] reported actuarial recurrence free survival rates of 93%, 80%, and 68% for 5, 10, and 15 years, respectively. In their series, sphenoid ridge meningiomas had the highest risk of recurrence or progression at 5 and 10 years (34% and 54%, respectively). Parasellar meningiomas had a 19% and 35% progression rate at 5 and 10 years. Interestingly, olfactory groove meningiomas with a total resection rate of 77% still had a 30% and 41% probability of recurrence at 5 and 10 years.

Wara et al.[116] also reported that of 84 patients undergoing total resection of meningioma, none had a recurrence. However, only 57% had been observed for six years or more. Chan and Thompson[25] reported a recurrence rate of 37% following partial removal of meningioma with an average follow-up of 9 years. For recently diagnosed cases with computerized tomography (CT) follow-up, the average time to detection of tumor recurrence was 2.9 years. In the pre-CT scan era, the average time to detection of tumor recurrence was 5.7 years.

Wara et al.[116] reported a retrospective series comparing patients undergoing subtotal removal of meningioma who did not receive postoperative radiotherapy with those that did. Follow-up ranged from 2 to 32 years. Of 58 patients not receiving postoperative radiotherapy, the recurrence rate was 74%. Thirty-four patients underwent subtotal resection of tumor followed by radiotherapy and there was a 29% recurrence rate. Administered doses ranged from 3000 to 5500 rad. Two of the patients with recurrence had less than 5000 rad, which is considered a low dose by today's standards. Of the 22 irradiated patients without recurrence, 14 had been observed for 6 or more years and 10 for 11–30 years following surgery.

Carella et al.[23] also reported on a series of 43 patients with meningiomas who received postoperative radiotherapy. Forty-two patients had known residual tumor and one had a malignant meningioma which had been totally excised. During a follow-up period of 1–10 years, only two patients died and two others deteriorated. Patients were treated with a minimum of 5000 rad. The likelihood of control did not correlate with dose past 5000 rad. In addition to maintaining at least a stable neurological status, all patients were evaluated by CT scanning and/or nucleotide brain scanning at least 1 year after therapy and did not have growth of the residual tumor.

The above-cited studies, although not randomized in a way that would have allowed a direct comparison of surgery alone versus surgery plus radiotherapy for meningioma, do suggest that there may be a role for radiotherapy in such a setting. Friedman[41] has reported on patients treated for postoperative residual tumor with dosages of 7000–8860 rad delivered to small volumes. Of seven such patients, four were alive and doing well 3–29 years after treatment. However, such doses are associated with a high incidence of brain necrosis. Also, lower doses in the range of 5000–6000 rad seem to be effective especially for small amounts of postoperative residual tumor. If it is possible to treat the region of the tumor with a technique that does not administer high doses to a large portion of the normal brain, then 5500 rad in 30 fractions to 6000 rad in 35 fractions is suggested.

For patients with recurrent meningioma, the prognosis is worse than for newly diagnosed meningioma. Mirimanoff et al.[76] reported 58% and 44% survival at 5 and 10 years, respectively, without subsequent surgery in 28 patients operated on for recurrent tumor. Wara et al.[116] reported 43 patients with recurrence following subtotal resection. Of 16 subsequently treated with radiation, seven were alive and well (1–9 years). Two had died of intercurrent disease at 8 and 18 years following radiotherapy for the recurrence. Of 27 treated with a second surgical procedure, only five were alive and well (1–23 years). Seventeen had died of tumor and five others were alive with tumor. Carella et al.[23] reported 14 patients with recurrent meningioma following initial surgery. All were treated with radiotherapy. Five patients showed neurological improvement and seven showed deterioration. Friedman[41] has also reported on the use of radiation for recurrent meningioma again using relatively high doses with two patients doing well for prolonged periods. Recurrent meningioma may show a more aggressive pathological picture and behave more aggressively clinically. Dosages of 6000 rad in 7 weeks administered to a relatively localized area are suggested (Figs. 1, 2).

There are a small number of patients with meningioma who are treated just with radiotherapy either because of the hazards of attempted resection or patient refusal to undergo surgery. In such cases, the diagnosis is usually made on clinical and radiographic evidence. Eleven patients reported by Carella et al.[23] who received radiotherapy alone as their initial management were alive for periods ranging from 3 to 6 years. Nine showed neurological improvement while two remained unchanged. The authors also presented CT scans showing residual mass following radiotherapy but with areas of central lucency suggestive of necrosis of the tumor. In those cases where radiotherapy is used as the primary modality, doses of 6000 rad/35 fractions should be administered to the localized tumor volume using a technique that spares the normal tissues. Occasionally, we have used radiotherapy as a primary modality for orbital meningioma when the surgeon has felt that resection would entail loss of vision (Figs. 1, 2).

A small percentage of patients have malignant characteristics by histological examination. In the series by Carella et al.,[23] there were 11 patients with malignant meningioma. Eight of the 11 were alive and stable 1–10 years following treatment, whereas three died. In contrast, Solan and Kramer[103] reported seven patients with malignant meningioma treated by surgery and radiotherapy and only two were alive without evidence of disease after 8½ years and 7 years, respectively, whereas five had died at 3–36 months (average 6.6 months) from treatment. Because of the small numbers of malignant meningioma in any series, it is hard to make a definitive statement as to the precise role of radiotherapy for this lesion. It is suggested that they be treated in the same manner as one would treat a benign meningioma, except that postoperative radiotherapy should be administered in all cases where there is any doubt at all as to completeness of the resection.

Cranial Chordoma

Arising in the spheno-occipital synchondrosis, the tumor may extend to the sella, parasella, clivus, retronasopharynx, sphenoid sinus, and even superiorly into the cranium. Symptoms will depend upon the sites of extension. The rarity of this tumor precludes meaningful comparisons concerning treatment modalities. With the realization that total extirpation of cranial base chordoma is unlikely, if not impossible, there were many early attempts at using radiotherapy alone or after surgery.

Occasional reports indicated benefit from radiotherapy. Wood and Himadi[120] in 1950 reported a patient who received

168 • TUMORS OF THE CRANIAL BASE: DIAGNOSIS AND TREATMENT

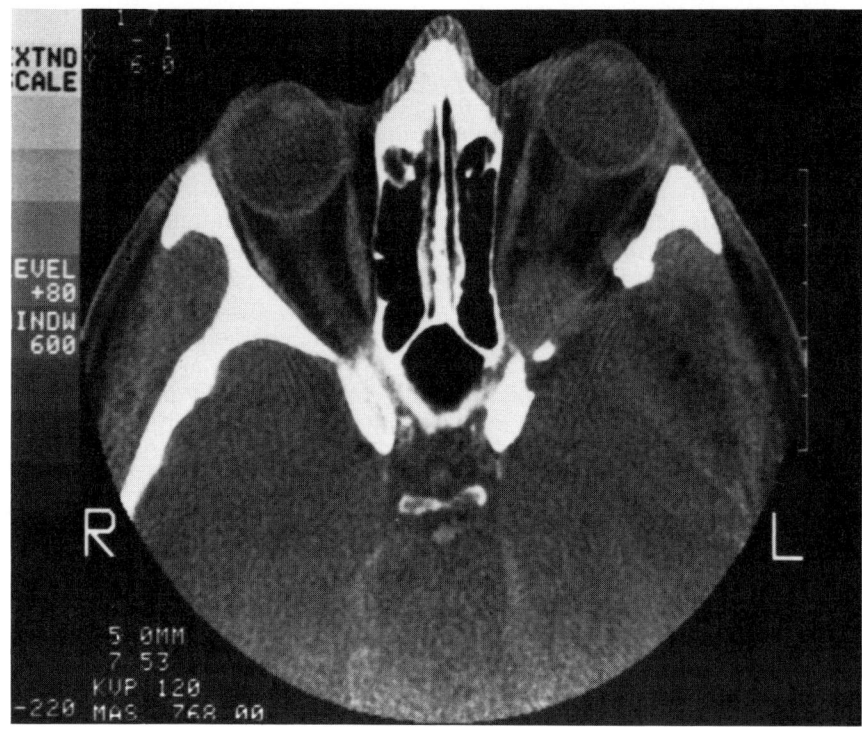

Figure 1: Forty-three-year-old male with recurrent meningioma in the orbit after gross total resection.

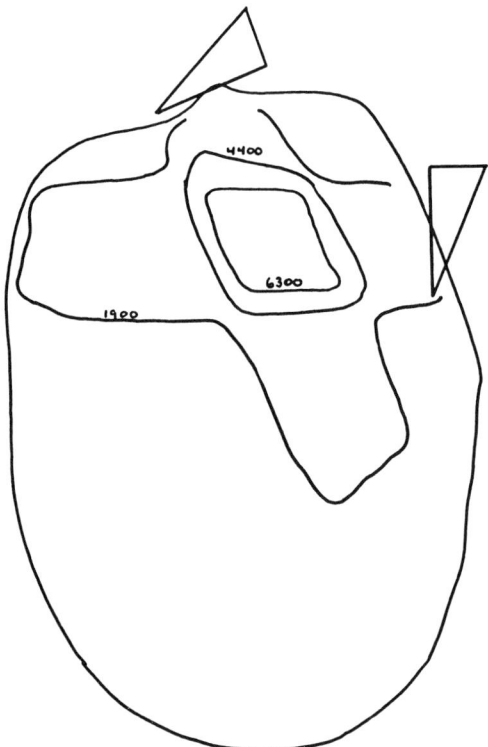

Figure 2: Patient in Figure 1 treated with anterior oblique and left lateral wedged fields (8 mV). The region of high dose is confined to the tumor.

1000 r in courses at repeated intervals over a 9 year period to a total dose of 8000 r and the patient was without symptoms at the time of report. Another one of their cases had "almost" complete regression after 2300 r.

Ormerod[82] in 1960 reported a case of clivus chordoma treated with 6157 r/10 weeks with good regression over a 1 year period. A second course of 4175 r was given 2 years later for recurrence and the patient was reported to be alive and well 4 years later. Boyle[18] also reported a chordoma which rapidly responded to "6500–5000 r" in 35 days. The patient did well for over 4 years but was retreated 5 years later for recurrence with another 5000 r. Again, he had a good symptomatic response but there was progression of tumor within 1 year.

In 1964, Kamrim[56] reported on 16 cases of cranial base chordoma of which 13 received postoperative radiotherapy. After an initial course of 3000–5000 r, additional courses of radiotherapy were usually repeated as necessary for recurrence. There were two long-term survivors at 11 and 14 years who had received 16,000 and 17,500 r, respectively. They noted that higher doses, 5000 r per course, produced more prolonged remissions.

Dahlin in 1952[30] reported on 15 chordomas of the clivus and stated that radiotherapy did not seem to alter the course of the disease. A subsequent report from the same institution by Heffelfinger et al.[48] in 1973 concerned 55 patients with cranial chordomas. They pointed out that chordomas with a chondroid component similar to chondrosarcoma or chondroma had a better prognosis than the "typical" chordoma. For all 55 patients, the average survival time from primary therapy was 7.4 years but only 14 patients had a longer survival. The average survival time for 36 patients with typical chordoma was 4.1 years compared to an average survival time of 15.8 years for the 19 patients with chondroid chordomas. Only 1 of the 36 patients with typical chordoma survived greater than 10 years but 9 of 19 patients with a chondroid chordoma survived over 10 years. Of the 36 typical chordoma patients, 9 were treated with surgery and radiation, 20 with radiation alone, 3 with surgery, and 4 had no therapy. The average survival times were 5.2, 4.8, 1.5, and 0.9 years, respectively. Of the 19 chondroid chordoma patients, 6 were treated with surgery and radiotherapy and their average survival was 24.9 years. Four patients treated with radiation alone had an average survival of 3.6 years and 9 patients treated with surgery alone had an average survival of 17.4 years. The authors stated that most patients had long symptom-free periods following therapy. Data were not given as to the doses employed. This large retrospective review points out the importance of the histological subdivisions as related to prognosis. It indicates that histological characteristics may be more important in determining prognosis than the administered treatment.

Richter et al.[89] in 1975 reported a 69-year-old male with a typical nonchondroid chordoma of the clivus causing multiple cranial nerve neuropathies treated with 6630 rad. The patient had a gradual but complete response and was well approximately 10 years later.

Becker et al.[8] reported a 23-month-old child with an extensive chordoma treated by subtotal resection and 5264 rad administered by bilateral fields. Further details of the radiotherapy were not given. The child was well 2 years later with no evidence of tumor.

Wold and Laws[119] reported a series of 12 children aged 8–19 years seen at the Mayo Clinic over an 8-year period. Two patients died postoperatively and two others died from tumor. Eight patients were alive and well 1 month to 21 years after surgery and radiotherapy.

There are very little data in the literature as to a dose response curve for radiotherapy in the treatment of chordomas. Since a complete extirpation of a cranial chordoma is unlikely, it seems reasonable to administer radiotherapy postoperatively in hopes of destroying residual tumor and at least prolonging remission. Recurrence after surgery and/or radiotherapy seems to be the rule. For any chance of permanent sterilization of the tumor, doses of at least 6000 rad in 7 weeks are suggested and 7000 rad over 7½ weeks to 8 weeks probably should be administered for gross residual tumor following surgery or for those cases which are just biopsied. Care should be taken to limit the dose to the adjacent brain stem and spinal cord as much as possible.

Craniopharyngioma

Craniopharyngiomas are histologically benign tumors but their location makes complete extirpation difficult. Up until the 1950s, surgery for craniopharyngioma was associated with an operative mortality of 20–40%.[22,43,66,74,107] Overall survival was also disappointing. Gordy et al.[43] in 1949 had only 12 of 51 patients (23.5%) who were living at 10 months to 10 years. Eleven of these 12 patients had undergone a "complete" resection of their tumor. Six other patients who underwent total excision died of recurrence. In the large series from the Serafimer Hospital in Stockholm, Sweden, covering 106 patients who underwent surgery for craniopharyngioma from 1924 to 1958, 26 died in the early postoperative period.[107] Of the 80 patients who survived the operative procedure, only 30 were alive with a minimum follow-up of about 3 years. Forty-three patients died from recurrent tumor at intervals of 2 months to 23 years following surgery.

By the 1930s, radiotherapy was occasionally employed. Carpenter et al.[24] in 1937 reported four patients with craniopharyngioma treated with radiotherapy. All four patients had undergone craniotomy, with evacuation of a cyst in three. The fourth patient had a solid tumor without a cyst. Orthovoltage equipment was used. Two patients received single courses with an estimated tumor dose of 1782 and 2844 r, respectively. A third patient had two courses separated by 3 months. Each course delivered 2743 r. The fourth patient had three courses of radiotherapy separated by 5 month intervals receiving 1371 r in the first course, then 2032 r and then 3464 r. All four patients were alive and well an average of 25 months following treatment. Of eight patients treated with just surgery, only one was alive 30 months following operation.

Leddy and Marshall[66] had six patients who received radiotherapy following surgery and five were alive more than 5 years after surgery. Of 35 patients who did not receive any radiotherapy, only 16 (45.7%) were alive 5 or more years. In this group, radiotherapy was also administered with orthovoltage equipment. Tumor doses of 800–2000 r were usually administered and sometimes repeated several months later.

Kramer et al.[61] in 1960 reported on 10 consecutive patients with craniopharyngioma treated with minimal surgery (biopsy and/or aspiration) followed by high dose radiotherapy. One patient died of coronary occlusion 2 years after radiotherapy but without evidence of recurrence. The remaining nine patients were alive and well over 6 years. Kramer et al.[62] later reported that the six children from this series were all alive over 13½ years following treatment. Of the initial four adult patients, two others subsequently died of intercurrent disease 10 and 14 years post-therapy but without evidence of recurrence. Children were treated with approximately 5500 rad in 7 weeks and adults were treated with 7000 rad in 7 weeks. A rotational technique with small fields was used in order to avoid high doses to the normal tissues. They also reported a second series of 16 patients (6 children and 10 adults) treated with radiotherapy following biopsy and/or aspiration of cyst.[62] Four of the six children and seven of the ten adults were alive and well up to 8 years after treatment. One adult patient died with necrosis of the brain and another of intercurrent disease. Both had no residual tumor at postmortem examination. It was the conclusion of these authors that craniopharyngioma should be treated by aspiration of any cyst and biopsy, if feasible, followed by radiotherapy.

In 1966, McKissock and Ford[74] reported on 100 patients wtih craniopharyngioma. Fifty-five were treated with radical excision and 12 (22%) were alive and well. Of 45 patients treated with minor surgery and radiotherapy, 33 (77%) were alive and well at the time of report. Details of the administered radiotherapy were not presented.

Petito et al.[84] reviewed 245 cases of craniopharyngioma from the files of the AFIP. In this retrospective review, the size of the tumor (under 3 cm), normal CSF protein, and absence of calcification in adult patients were associated with improved survival rates. In addition, patients diagnosed after 1955 and those who received radiotherapy after 1955 did better. However, only 31 patients in this retrospective series had received radiotherapy.

Lichter et al.[70] reported 10 patients treated with surgery and postoperative radiotherapy. There were two recurrences in this group. One patient had an extremely large tumor and the second had radiotherapy discontinued at 3450 rad. The eight patients alive free of disease 3–15.5 years (average 10 years) received 5000–5675 r. Eighteen patients were treated with surgery alone. There was one postoperative death. Eight patients had a total resection and three developed recurrent tumor at 5, 6, and 8 years, respectively. Five patients were alive free of disease at 3–5 years. Five of nine patients in the subtotally resected group without postoperative radiotherapy had recurrence of tumor 6–36 months. Three of these patients were retreated by surgery and radiotherapy (two patients) or just radiotherapy (one patient) and all were alive at 3.5, 8, and 16 years, respectively.

In 1980, Bloom[10] reported a series of 122 patients treated with radiotherapy for craniopharyngioma. One hundred and twelve were newly diagnosed patients and ten were referred for treatment of recurrence following previous surgery. Surgery was usually confined to aspiration or limited excision, with radical excision attempted in only 14 patients. For children, 5 and 10 year survival rates were 85% and 74%, respectively. For adults, the 5 and 10 year survival rates were 74% and 60%, respectively. Among the more recently treated patients in whom 6–8 MeV x-rays were used, (doses and other details not given) the projected 5 and 10 year survival rates for 16 children were 100% and 89%, respectively, and for 35 adults, 94% and 81%.

Sung et al.[105] also demonstrated the value of radiotherapy after incomplete excision of craniopharyngioma. For children undergoing total resection (14 patients) 5 and 10 year survivals were 100% and 100%, respectively. None of these patients had postoperative radiotherapy. For adults undergoing total resection (23 patients) without postop radiotherapy, the 5 and 10 year survivals were 58.6% and 24.4%, respectively. In children undergoing subtotal excision without radiotherapy, the 5 and 10 year survival rates were 71.4% and 52.1% compared to 92.6% and 79.4% 5 and 10 year survival rates in children having subtotal or minimal surgery followed by radiotherapy. Of the adults undergoing subtotal resection without radiotherapy, 5 and 10 year survival rates were 36.9% and 30.7%, respectively. In adults who had subtotal or minimal surgery plus radiotherapy, the 5 and 10 year survival rates were 81.2% and 73.1%, respectively. Children were treated with doses of 5000–6000 rad (mean dose of 5500 rad in 44 days). Adults were treated with 4000–6900 rad (mean dose of 5700 rad in 46 days). Dose increments were 200 rad per day except in a few children who received 150–180 rad per day. The authors state that their present regimen is to treat children with 5500 rad in 6–6½ weeks and adults with 6500 rad in 6½–7½ weeks using 360° rotational technique and 6 MV x-rays.

Shapiro et al.[97] reported 60 children with craniopharyngioma treated by one of four methods: (1) cyst aspiration followed by "deep x-ray therapy," presumably orthovoltage radiation, (2) radical excision, (3) incomplete tumor excision, or (4) incomplete excision followed by deep x-ray therapy. Radiotherapy was delivered to a total dose of 4000–5500 rad. Among the group undergoing gross total excision, there was a recurrence rate of 23% but the mean follow-up for this group of patients was only 6.8 years. Patients treated with drainage of the cyst and radiotherapy had a 50% recurrence rate with a mean follow-up of 9.4 years. In patients treated with incomplete removal and deep radiotherapy, there were no recurrences for a mean follow-up of 3.3 years. For the group having partial excision without radiotherapy, the recurrence rate was about 80%. Presumably, incomplete excision implies more than drainage of a cyst. These relatively short-term follow-up results indicate that incomplete excision followed by radiotherapy may be as effective as gross total removal of craniopharyngioma in children.

Richmond et al.[88] have shown that in children with craniopharyngioma, subtotal resection plus radiotherapy seems to be as good as total removal. Administered doses were usually in the range of 4900–5700 rad over 6 weeks.

Fischer et al.[36] demonstrated that children treated initially with radiotherapy after biopsy or cyst aspiration do as well as patients subjected to attempted total resection. Of 14 patients in the latter group, 11 required radiotherapy either for recurrence or because of incomplete excision. Twenty-three patients had primary radiotherapy and only one has had "suspected" asymptomatic tumor growth. Four have required re-aspiration of cysts.

Advances in neurosurgical technique have made radical excision of craniopharyngioma a less hazardous procedure than in the past. Still it is hard to show by retrospective reviews that attempted total resection provides better control and survival than subtotal resection and radiotherapy. In those cases where radical excision cannot be safely performed, it is recommended that patients be treated with aspiration of any cyst present followed by radiotherapy. It is suggested that children be treated with doses of 5500 rad delivered in 30 fractions and adults be treated with 6500–7000 rad in 35 fractions. It is important that these doses be limited to just the tumor, and either a rotational technique or a multiple field technique is suggested in order to minimize the dose delivered to normal structures (Fig. 3).

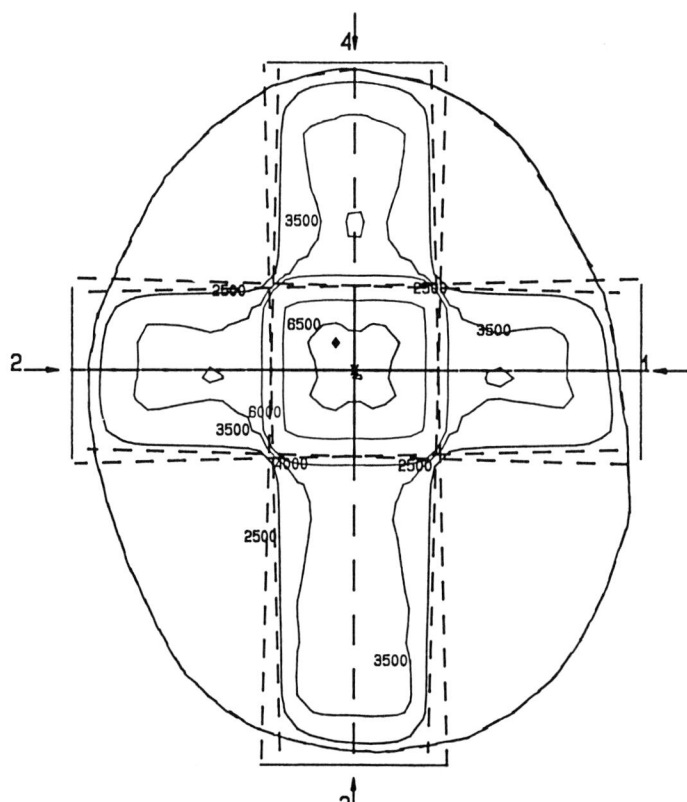

Figure 3: Four-field treatment technique (6 mV x-ray) used to treat craniopharyngioma.

Pituitary Tumors

Pituitary tumors can be considered in two broad categories, hormone-producing and nonhormone-producing. Tumors that secrete hormone produce symptoms mainly due to the excess of a particular hormone or group of hormones. Nonsecreting tumors do not produce an excess of hormone and symptoms are due mainly to mass effect. As the tumor increases, it compresses adjacent normal tissue and hypopituitarism may develop. As the tumor grows out of the sella to compress the optic chiasm, visual problems may arise. Headache is also a common feature of both secreting and nonsecreting tumors. Because secreting pituitary adenomas are symptomatic mainly due to excess hormone production, they often can be detected at a much smaller size than the nonsecreting tumor.

Since the beginning of this century, radiotherapy has been used in the treatment of pituitary adenomas. The large series of Harvey Cushing's patients operated upon from 1913 to 1933 was reviewed by Henderson in 1939. Slightly less than one-half of the tumors considered to be chromophobe adenoma had postoperative radiotherapy. For patients undergoing transsphenoidal surgery for chromophobe adenoma, recurrence-free survival at 5 years was 32.8% (22/67). For patients undergoing transsphenoidal resection plus postoperative radiotherapy, the recurrence-free survival at 5 years was 65.3% (32/49). Five-year recurrence-free survival was 57.5% (23/40) for patients undergoing transfrontal surgery alone. For those having transfrontal surgery and postoperative radiotherapy, the 5 year recurrence-free survival was 87.1% (27/31). Radiotherapy was administered in a series of three or four treatments and patients had one or two series but sometimes they were treated at 3 or 6 month intervals for about 1 year. Considering the physical factors of the therapy, each series of three or four treatments probably delivered a tumor dose of less than 1000 rad. In Cushing's series there were also 14 cases of recurrent adenoma after surgery alone who were subsequently treated with radiation. Four patients had return of vision for follow-up periods of 7–12 years. Six had stabilization of their vision, and in four patients there was no effect. This early series strongly suggested that radiotherapy could have a beneficial effect on pituitary adenomas.

Kerr in 1948[57] reported a series of 50 patients with pituitary adenoma treated by orthovoltage radiotherapy (200 kV). Radiotherapy was delivered in a single course which delivered an estimated tumor dose of 2400–3600 R. By clinical criteria, "excellent and good results" were obtained in 70% of patients. It was noted that cystic tumors were unlikely to respond favorably to radiotherapy.

Poppen in 1963[86] reported on a large series of 110 patients treated primarily with orthovoltage irradiation for pituitary adenomas. Patients were treated in one to three series, each of several treatments, which would deliver approximately 800–900 roentgens per series by his estimate. Of this group of 110 patients treated primarily with radiotherapy, 50% improved and did not require further therapy. Poppen also reported on 119 patients treated with 4000 roentgens in 20 fractions administered with 2 mV radiation. This included 73 patients treated primarily with radiotherapy. The remainder were adenomas progressive or recurrent after orthovoltage radiotherapy or surgery. One hundred patients (84%) improved and did not require further treatment. The author suggested radiotherapy as the first line of treatment for pituitary adenomas.

In 1962, Correa and Lampe[28] showed that the success rate of radiotherapy for pituitary adenoma could be correlated with dose. For patients receiving doses of 2000–2500 rad, only 12 of 27 (44.4%) showed improvement when treated with radiotherapy alone. With doses of 2900–3500 rad, 20 of 33 (60.6%) showed improvement. In those patients treated with cobalt or cesium teletherapy to doses of 4000 rad, there was success in 23 of 27 patients (79.3%).

Ray and Patterson[87] reported on a series of 106 patients treated by craniotomy for pituitary adenoma. Approximately one-half had radiotherapy and there was an 8% recurrence rate in the limited period of follow-up compared to a 22% recurrence rate in patients who did not have postoperative radiotherapy.

Urdaneta et al.[112] compared 34 patients with chromophobe adenoma treated by surgery and postoperative radiotherapy with 32 patients treated with primary radiotherapy. Twelve of the latter 32 patients had subsequent surgery because of failure to control the disease. These patients had received 4500–5500 rad at 200 rad per day. The overall survival and control rates were similar for the two groups in spite of a higher relapse rate following initial radiotherapy since surgery was able to salvage some of the radiotherapy failures.

Pistenma et al.[85] compared 33 patients with chromophobe adenoma treated by surgery and postoperative radiotherapy with 29 patients treated just by radiotherapy. Patients were treated with relatively high doses, the average equivalent dose being 5700 rad in 6 weeks. Of the 29 patients treated just with radiotherapy, there were 12 failures (41.4%). Eight of these patients were salvaged by further surgery and were alive 2–16 years subsequently. Two patients had control following craniotomy and a second course of radiotherapy. Of 33 patients treated initially with surgery and postoperative radiotherapy, only six (18.2%) have failed. The overall 5 year control rate for the radiotherapy alone group was 86.5% counting the salvage surgery, and for the postoperative radiotherapy group, 81.5%. Four patients in the entire group who had invasive adenomas died of disease or complications. Interestingly, 9 of the 12 failures in the group treated by radiotherapy alone had cystic tumors and 9 of these 12 failures occurred within 3 months. The authors recommend surgical decompression followed by 5000 rad in 5 weeks in patients with "more than minimal depression of peripheral visual fields," corrected visual acuity of less than 20/30 in either eye or more than 1 cm suprasellar extension of tumor. Radiotherapy alone was recommended for small adenomas accompanied by less extensive or no visual abnormalities.

It should be remembered that the above-cited studies were from the era before the use of CT scanning, modern surgical techniques, and sophisticated endocrine evaluations. These early series probably contained more patients with advanced large tumors producing visual problems and hypopituitarism than one would see in comparative series today. However, there is little doubt that radiotherapy was frequently beneficial for these patients with advanced lesions.

Pituitary adenomas producing ACTH (Cushing's disease) have been successfully treated by radiotherapy. Lamberts et al.[64] reported 18 patients with Cushing's disease treated with unilateral adrenalectomy followed by pituitary irradiation to a dose of 4500 rad. Nine patients (50%) had a remission determined by the clinical picture and a normal cortisol secretion rate. Four patients with radiographic abnormalities of the sella did not respond.

Better results were obtained by Jennings et al.[54] who treated 15 children with pituitary irradiation for Cushing's disease. Patients were treated between January 1957 to June 1976. All received 4000–4950 rad except for one patient who had only 3500 rad. Twelve were considered cured of their Cushing's disease within 1–18 months after radiotherapy. A patient was considered cured when urinary hydroxy corticosteroid secretion was less than 70 mg per g of creatinine and plasma cortisol was normal or subnormal. Interestingly, the pituitary irradiation did not cause deficiency in other pituitary hormone secretions. However, all were over age 12 years at time of radiotherapy. There were normal growth hormone responses to hypoglycemia or arginine in 11 of 12 patients and the twelfth patient did have a level of 5 μg/ml in response to stimulus which indicates that there was still growth hormone reserve present. Pituitary ACTH secretion following irradiation was adequate to maintain normal cortisol levels and steroid replacement was not necessary. The authors concluded that irradiation of the pituitary with 4000–4500 rad at 200 rad per day was safe and effective treatment for children with Cushing's disease.

Growth hormone-secreting tumors

(acromegaly) also have been successfully treated by radiotherapy. Ellis in 1949[35] reported improvement in 59% of 47 patients with eosinophilic adenoma treated with radiotherapy in varying dosages. This was before the availability of serum growth hormone level determinations and improvement was determined on a clinical basis. Twenty-four of these patients had received estimated tumor doses of only 1200–1500 r and 18 had shown some improvement and in 11 cases, there was "marked" improvement. Ellis suggested doses of 3000 r.

Urdaneta et al.[112] reported on 13 patients with eosinophilic adenoma producing acromegaly. Of seven who had radiotherapy alone, four were alive without *clinical* evidence of disease progression 1 year, 2 years, and two at 10 years following treatment. Two died of disease at 3 and 6 months following treatment and one was alive with evidence of disease 7 years following therapy. Of three additional patients who received surgery and postoperative radiotherapy, two were alive without evidence of disease 4 and 5 years later and one was alive with disease 3 years later. Three patients had radiotherapy and then subsequent surgery because of progression and one was alive without disease at 7 years but two had died within 2 years.

Lawrence et al.[65] evaluated 28 patients following pituitary irradiation for acromegaly. Sixteen patients were irradiated prior to 1965 and therefore did not have a pretreatment baseline growth hormone determination available. Of these 16 patients, 13 (81%) had post-therapy basal growth hormone levels in the normal or near normal range (≤ 10 ng/ml). Twelve patients treated since 1965 had pretherapy baseline serum growth hormone levels. Nine patients (75%) had lowering of the basal serum growth hormone level into the normal range within 6 months to 4 years after irradiation. Lowering of growth hormone levels was also associated with disappearance of clinical and laboratory findings of acromegaly. Six of the total group of 28 patients still had active disease with elevated growth hormone levels 2–9 years after radiotherapy. For all patients, administered doses to the pituitary ranged from 1680 rad to 6600 rad. Interestingly, in the early group of 16 patients, only seven received ≥ 4000 rad. In the latter group of 12 patients, only two received less than 5000 rad and they each received 3500 rad. Within the range of doses used for these patients, there did not seem to be a definite correlation between dose and good result. The authors suggested 5000 rad as adequate.

Lamberg et al.[63] in 1976 reported on 31 patients treated with pituitary irradiation for acromegaly. Administered doses ranged from 1500 rad to 8000 rad. Seventeen received ≥ 4000 rad. Thirty of the 31 patients had improvement or arrest of disease. However, within 2–5 years, a definite relapse occurred in 12 patients and seven were given a repeat course of radiotherapy. Five of the seven patients experienced benefit from the second course of radiotherapy. At the time of evaluation (1–21 years after treatment), 21 of the original 31 patients were considered to have their disease under control. Only 12 patients (39%) had a growth hormone basal level below 5 ng/ml. Sixteen (52%) had a level below 10 ng/ml. The authors noted a trend towards improved control rates with higher doses.

Roth et al.[93] evaluated 20 patients who received radiotherapy to the pituitary for acromegaly. Post-therapy plasma growth hormone levels were decreased in 19 of 20 patients. Between 1 and 2 years after radiotherapy, the mean fall in plasma hormone concentration for the entire group was 51% (range 0–88%). In seven patients who were restudied between 2½ and 4 years after radiotherapy, the mean decrease was 76% (60–89). A further report from the same institution[33] reviewed 47 patients with acromegaly treated with radiotherapy. By 5 years after treatment, the mean fall in growth hormone concentration was 77% and the growth hormone level was less than 10 ng/ml in 73% of cases. Interestingly, there was a continued fall in growth hormone in the majority of patients over the subsequent 5 year period. Thus, by 10 years, plasma growth hormone levels were ≤ 10 ng/ml in 81% and ≤ 5 ng/ml in 69% of patients. Improvement in the clinical and objective effects of acromegaly roughly paralleled the fall in growth hormone concentration. Patients received 4000–5000 rad. The authors emphasize the fact that patients may show a very slight decrease in growth hormone levels within the first 2 years following radiotherapy but may thereafter show substantial reductions in growth hormone levels. The converse situation also occurred whereby patients would have a substantial fall in growth hormone levels during the first 2 years and then have little or no further fall subsequently.

The above-cited results of radiotherapy for treatment of acromegaly certainly demonstrate the value of radiotherapy in this disease. There are less data as to the effect of radiotherapy on prolactin-secreting tumors in terms of the effect on prolactin levels. Gomez et al.[42] reported eight patients with galactorrhea and elevated prolactin levels who also had an abnormal sella turcica. These eight patients were treated by radiotherapy to the pituitary with a multiple field technique using cobalt-60. Forty-five hundred rad were administered in 20 fractions. In three patients in whom prolactin levels were measured at the end of therapy, there was a decrease observed in all of them followed by a return towards the pretreatment high level. Six patients followed for more than 2 years had a gradual decline of prolactin levels with time but only one patient maintained normal levels. Menstruation did resume in three patients within 3 months after radiation and in the fourth patient after about 3½ years, but the prolactin levels were still elevated in all four patients.

When radiotherapy is used either as the primary treatment or post surgery, 4500–5000 rad at 180 rad/day is suggested. The higher dose is for larger lesions. Either a rotational or a multiple field technique should be used in order to minimize the dose delivered to the temporal lobes (Figs. 4, 5).

Tumors of the External Auditory Canal, Middle Ear, and Mastoid

Cancers arising in the external auditory canal, middle ear, or mastoid are extremely rare tumors. Few institutions see more than one to three cases per year. The great majority of these cancers are squamous cell carcinoma. They are usually discovered in an advanced stage with involvement of the temporal bone. Surgery alone, surgery with pre- or postoperative radiotherapy, and radiotherapy alone have been used for treatment of carcinoma but the rarity of these lesions makes valid comparison of treatment modalities difficult. Most authors recommend a combination of surgery and radiotherapy for the treatment of these lesions.[40,55,67,69,78,104,111,115]

Boland[12] advocated supervoltage radiotherapy as the treatment of choice for carcinoma of the middle ear. He recommended that surgery be limited to just a biopsy. Using four MV x-rays, a 5 year cure rate of 56% (10/18) was obtained compared to 22% (6/27) with the use of orthovoltage irradiation.[11]

Lederman[67] recommended radiotherapy alone only for those early lesions in which there was absence of bone involvement. For more advanced cases, surgery and radiotherapy was recommended. Overall 5 year survival for external auditory canal carcinoma was 24% (6/25) and for the middle ear and mastoid 30.7% (12/39). The majority of patients were treated with surgery followed by radiotherapy with dosages of 6000–8000 rad in 6–8 weeks.

Frew and Finney[40] recommended "limited surgical excision" for the purposes of draining necrotic material followed by supervoltage irradiation using oblique wedged fields to administer 6500 r in 6 weeks. The authors specifically recommended against doing a radical temporal bone resection. Of 11 patients treated, six were alive and well more than 2 years from diagnosis. There were no survivors among 11 patients treated with orthovoltage irradiation.

Tucker[111] reviewed 89 cases of middle ear cancer. Eighty-nine percent were carcinoma. Most were treated with mastoidectomy and supervoltage radiotherapy, and for such patients, the 3 year cure rate was 26%. This is similar to the results of Lewis[69] who had a 5 year survival of

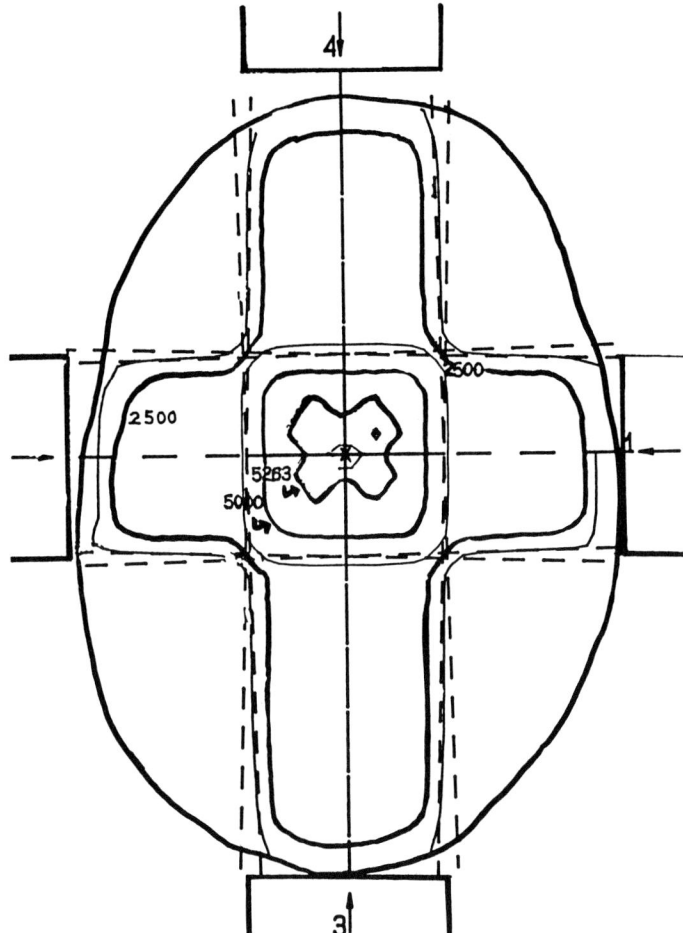

Figure 4: Pituitary adenoma treated with a four-field technique (6 mV). Note the relatively low dose delivered to the temporal lobes and scalp.

25% for squamous cell carcinoma. Lewis advocated preoperative radiotherapy with doses of 3500–5000 rad. If margins were in doubt, additional postoperative radiotherapy was given.

Sorensen[104] reported five of 12 patients alive and well 5 years after surgery and radiotherapy (in some patients intracavitary radium) for middle ear carcinoma. An additional patient died 2½ years from diagnosis free of disease. The five deaths from tumor were all due to intracranial extension.

Johns and Headington[55] reported on 20 patients with squamous cell carcinoma of the external auditory canal. Half were considered "early" lesions, and of these 10, five were alive from 26 months to 15 years following treatment. Of 10 patients with advanced lesions, one was alive at 18 months. All of the survivors were treated with combined surgery and radiotherapy except for one patient in the "early" group who was treated with surgery alone.

Wang[115] reported on 23 patients treated with combined surgery and radiotherapy for squamous cell carcinoma of the external auditory canal, mastoid, or middle ear. Three patients treated with preoperative irradiation received 4000 rad in 4 weeks. All of the postoperative cases received at least 5000 rad in 5 weeks and three received greater than 7000 rad. Of the total group, 11 (48%) were alive and well 5 years. However, there were five cases of osteoradionecrosis, all of whom had received doses biologically equivalent to 7800 rad/39 to part of the irradiated volume due to "faulty radiotherapeutic technique." Wang recommended 6000 rad

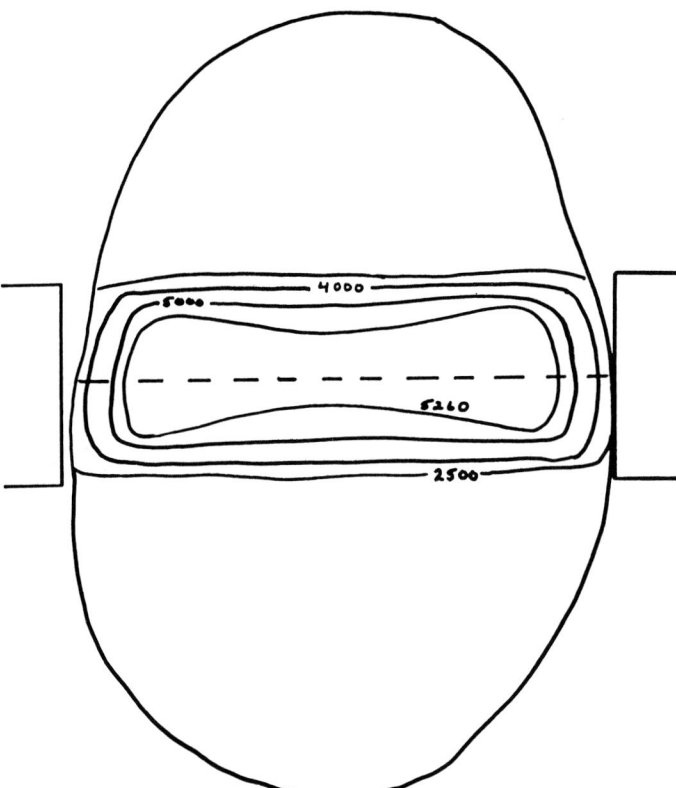

Figure 5: Same patient as in Figure 4. Dose distribution if only two lateral fields were used. Note the rather large area receiving ≥ 5000 rad.

in 6 weeks with no portion of the temporal bone receiving doses equivalent to over 7000 rad/35 fractions.

Because of the advanced nature of most carcinomas of the external auditory canal, middle ear, and mastoid, it would seem that the combination of surgery and radiotherapy has the best chance for providing long-term control. Most such cases will have associated infection requiring drainage prior to initiating radiotherapy. From a limited number of cases reported in the literature, it is difficult to state whether or not extensive surgery (temporal bone resection) provides much more benefit than limited resection followed by postoperative radiotherapy. In all cases where radiotherapy is used, it is essential that care be taken to insure that the entire tumor volume is adequately irradiated. At least 6000–7000 rad in 6–7 weeks should be administered. Oblique wedged fields provide an adequate dose distribution and limit the amount of brain irradiated (Fig. 6). As pointed out by Wang,[115] dosages above 7000 rad in 7 weeks to large portions of the temporal bone must be avoided in order to prevent osteoradionecrosis.

Glomus Jugulare Tumors (Chemodectoma)

Glomus jugulare tumors are histologically benign but locally invasive vascular neoplasms arising from the glomus jugulare. Tumors may grow to invade the middle ear and mastoid. They frequently involve cranial nerves 7–12 inclusively and may extend into the petrous bone and further into the intracranial cavity or even extracranially into the nasopharynx. Tumors confined to the middle ear and mastoid (glomus tympanicum) can often be effectively treated by radical mastoidectomy. For more advanced cases, those involving the petrous bone and extending intracranially, complete extirpation is seldom possible. Several reviews

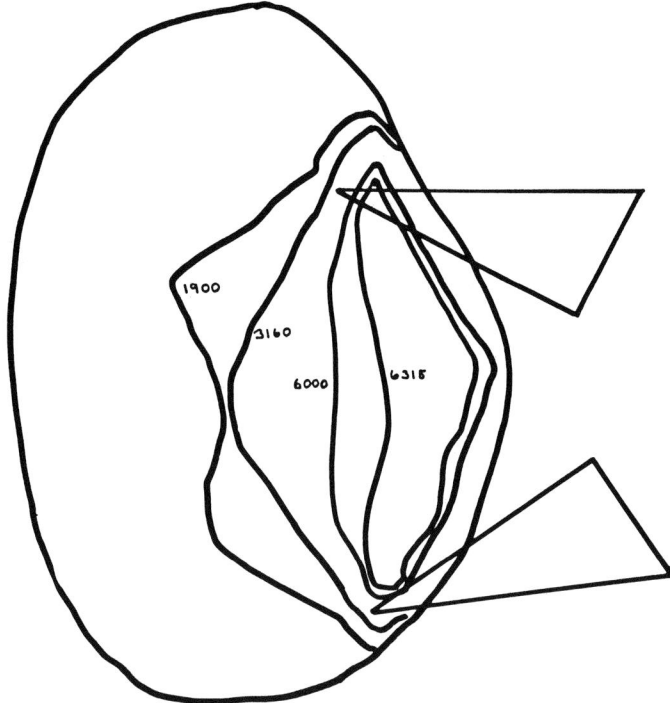

Figure 6: Oblique wedged fields (CO-60) used to treat squamous cell carcinoma of the middle ear.

have indicated the value of radiotherapy for inoperable cases or those with residual tumor following surgery.

Rosenwasser,[92] who first described this tumor in 1945, had a patient with residual tumor postoperatively who was treated with radiation (5500 r, 200 kV, over 30 days) and the patient was alive and well without clinical or radiographic evidence of recurrent tumor 30 years later. Rosenwasser recommended radiotherapy for tumors not completely excised, and for those recurrent after surgery.

Silverstone[102] reported six cases treated by radiotherapy after biopsy or incomplete resection. Doses of 4000-5000 rad over 3½–7 weeks were administered. All patients were alive and well 6 months to 8 years after treatment. The author recommended 4000–5000 rad over 4–6 weeks for all patients with tumor extension beyond the middle ear and mastoid and also for those cases with recurrence after surgery. McCabe and Fletcher[73] also recommended that early tumors be treated by surgery (radical mastoidectomy) followed by radiation therapy if excision was incomplete. They recommended radiotherapy after biopsy for tumors extending into the petrous bone and beyond. Recommended doses were not given. Hatfield et al.[89] also showed very good results when radiotherapy was administered either alone or after surgery. None of 16 patients who received greater than 4000 rad either alone or after surgery had a recurrence with a minimum follow-up period of 5 years. They recommended 4500 rad following radical mastoidectomy as the treatment of choice. For patients with multiple cranial nerve deficits and bone destruction, radiotherapy alone was recommended. Similarly, Tidwell and Montague[110] treated 17 patients with radiotherapy and 16 were alive and well 4–18 years later. One patient died of brain necrosis at 37 months and there was microscopic residual tumor at autopsy. They also recommended 4500–5000 rad over 4½–5 weeks. The above-cited studies indicate a definite role for radiation therapy in the management of patients with glomus jugulare tumors.

In summary, radiation in moderate doses, 4500–5000 rad over 5 weeks, seems to be adequate for extensive inoperable lesions and probably would also be effective for the localized cases involving just the middle ear and mastoid. However, results with radical mastoidectomy are good for tumors which can be encompassed by the surgical procedure.[92] In all cases treated by surgery, radiotherapy should be administered postoperatively if there is likelihood of incomplete excision.

The author recommends 5000 rad in 25 fractions either alone or postoperatively. Radiation should be administered using a field set-up which keeps the 5000 rad isodose confined, as much as possible, to the involved area.

Cancer of the Nasal Cavity and Paranasal Sinuses

Malignancies of the nasal cavity and paranasal sinuses may involve the base of skull by direct growth. These tumors are often extensive when first seen and sometimes it is difficult to ascertain the exact site of origin since there may be involvement of multiple sinus regions. Among a group of 39 patients with squamous cell carcinoma of the maxillary antrum, without lymph node or distant metastasis, there were 30 patients (77%) who had base of skull involvement. In twenty-four patients (62%), it had spread into the ethmoid sinuses and in 15 (38%), there was involvement of the sphenoid sinus. The orbit was involved by contiguous growth in 28 patients (72%).[91] The majority of cancers of the paranasal sinuses and nasal cavity are squamous cell carcinoma. Adenocarcinoma accounts for less than 10% of malignancies. Nonepithelial cancers such as rhabdomyosarcoma and esthesioneuroblastoma account for a smaller percentage of malignancies arising from the nasal cavity–paranasal sinuses.[13]

Carcinoma of the sphenoid sinus is extremely rare and accounts for approximately 0.3% of all sinus cancer.[45] Harbison et al.[45] reported three cases of sphenoid sinus carcinoma and reviewed 39 cases identified in the English language literature. Practically all patients with sphenoid sinus carcinoma have neuro-ophthalmological symptoms due to extension of the tumor through the roof of the sinus into the skull base. Their review of the literature revealed a 93% mortality by 2 years.

Cancer of the nasal cavity and ethmoid sinus has a better prognosis. A series of 30 patients with cancers of the ethmoid sinus and nasal cavity were treated with high doses of radiation by Shukovsky and Fletcher.[101] Minimum tumor doses of 6000 rad were delivered in 6 weeks. The dose to the main bulk of the tumor was 7000–7500 rad. For 30 patients with various malignancies, 21 had local control (70%). For 24 patients at risk more than 4 years, the disease-free survival was 63%. If only squamous cell carcinomas are considered, the local control rate was 87% and the disease-free survival was 67% at a minimum of 4 years. However, severe complications resulted when the orbits had to be included. Retinal damage and optic nerve injury resulted when these structures received doses in excess of 6800 rad in 6 weeks. Unfortunately, because of the pathways of likely spread from ethmoid sinus carcinomas, it is frequently necessary to deliver high doses to the ipsilateral orbit.

Ellingwood and Million[34] treated 32 patients with cancer of the nasal cavity and ethmoid–sphenoid sinuses using high doses of radiation (6091–7972 rad over 6–9 weeks). Fifteen patients had involvement of the cranial contents, nasopharynx, or base of skull. Local control was achieved in 95% of the nasal cavity cases and 71% of the ethmoid–sphenoid sinus patients with 2 years of follow-up. Local recurrence was detected within 6 months of the end of treatment in five of nine therapeutic failures. Three patients developed local recurrence 3½–5½ years from treatment and all had adenoid-cystic carcinoma of the ethmoid–sphenoid sinus region. In five cases of failure, recurrence occurred within the treated volume. The authors suggest that insufficient dose may have been a contributing factor in four patients (less than 6500 rad). Four other cases had local recurrence at the edge of the treatment fields. The ipsilateral eye was irradiated in 15 patients because of tumor extension. Nine patients free of disease more than 2 years following treatment had complete loss of vision and in every case the eye had received 6500 rad or more. There was no difference in local control rates according to histology.

Cheng and Wang[26] reviewed 66 patients with carcinomas of the paranasal sinuses. With radiation alone, 6000–7000 rad, the absolute 3 year NED survival was only 18% (6/34). With preoperative radiotherapy followed by radical surgery, the NED 3 year survival was 57% (8/14). Preoperative radiation was administered in doses of 4000–6000 rad over 4–6 weeks. Eleven patients received postoperative radiotherapy with doses of 6000 rad in 6–6½ weeks and the 3 year NED survival was 33% (6/18). Sixty-seven percent of the patients not cured had local failure. Of 40 patients with maxillary sinus tumors, the 3 year NED survival was 42.5% (17/40). Of 11 patients with ethmoid sinus tumors, only two were alive free of disease at 3 years and both were treated with surgery followed by radiotherapy.

Similar results were reported by Bush and Bagshaw.[21] For 38 patients with carcinoma of the paranasal sinuses treated with radiotherapy alone or in combination with surgery, the relapse-free survival at 5 years was 37%. For those treated with radiotherapy alone, the 5 year absolute survival was 22.7% (5/22). The dose of radiation varied from 5562 rad/37 days to 8050 rad/46 days. There did not seem to be a difference in survival between patients receiving more or less than 6600 rad to the primary site. The authors point out that five of six patients who developed recurrent disease within the orbit had evidence of orbital involvement at presentation but the globe was blocked during treatment. This points out the necessity of treating the ipsilateral orbit without shielding when there is penetration of tumor into the orbit.

Hintz et al.[50] reported local control in only four of 14 patients (28%) treated with radiotherapy alone for paranasal sinus carcinoma. For patients treated with combination surgery and radiation, either postop or preop, the local control was 7/13 or 53.8%. None of five patients with adenoidcystic carcinoma had local control regardless of the treatment regimen. The authors recommend preoperative radiotherapy for paranasal sinus carcinoma. They emphasize the importance of accurate localization and treatment planning to be sure that the entire tumor volume is adequately irradiated.

Therapy will depend upon extent of disease at presentation. Early well-localized tumors involving the nasal cavity and especially the infrastructure of the maxillary sinus can probably be adequately controlled by either surgery or radiation alone. For extensive tumors involving the suprastructure of the maxillary sinus, ethmoid sinus, and sphenoid sinus, either radiation alone or the combination of radiation and surgery will be necessary. For carcinomas, whether squamous cell or adenocarcinomas, high doses of radiation are necessary. For the pre- or postsurgical patient, doses of at least 6000 rad administered in 6 weeks are suggested. When radiotherapy is used alone, 6500–7000 rad in 6½–7 weeks is suggested. Treatment planning must insure that the tumor is adequately irradiated and "hot spots" in the brain must be avoided. Often, it will be necessary to irradiate the ipsilateral eye because of orbital involvement.

Esthesioneuroblastoma is a rare tumor arising in the nasal olfactory mucosa. Sixty percent of patients will have extension to the cribiform plate, orbit, intracranial sites, or have metastasis at presentation.[94] Shah and Feghali[94] suggested surgery and postoperative radiotherapy as the treatment of choice for advanced lesions. They pointed out that many patients may have a slowly progressive course manifested by recurrent tumor, and in their series of 31 patients, only eight had a single surgical procedure for the primary tumor. Of 31 patients, 16 were alive at 5 years (52%). Fourteen of these sixteen patients had recurrence at the primary site or neck nodes requiring further salvage therapy. Bailey and Barton,[6] from their review of the literature, also suggested that surgery and radiation provided the best chance for 5 year disease free survival.

Nasopharynx Carcinoma

Carcinoma of the nasopharynx may extend to the base of skull by direct growth superiorly. In the era prior to the use of CT scans, invasion into the base of skull was detected either radiographically or clinically in at least 25% of newly diagnosed patients.[7,38] The actual incidence of skull base involvement by nasopharynx carcinoma is likely to be much higher. For all carcinomas of the nasopharynx, the treatment volume must include the posterior ethmoid sinuses, sphenoid sinus, cavernous sinus, and base of skull including the foramen ovale, carotid canal, and foramen spinosum. For those patients with demonstrable extension into the base of skull, fields must be enlarged to include the base of the brain and the suprasellar area and the middle cranial fossa base. Doses of 6500–7000 rad over 7–7½ weeks are recommended.

Juvenile Nasopharyngeal Angiofibroma

Juvenile nasopharyngeal angiofibroma is a highly vascular, nonmetastasizing tumor of the nasopharynx which occurs predominantly in pubescent males. Extension into the sphenoid sinus is extremely common, occurring in over 80% of cases.[19,52] Extension into the ethmoid sinuses and maxillary sinuses occurs in over 50% of cases.[19] Intracranial extension of the tumor was reported by Jafek et al.[53] in 15 of 42 patients (35.7%). Ward et al.[118] reported seven of 35 patients (20%) with intracranial extension.

Surgical treatment is a formidable undertaking especially when intracranial extension is present. The average blood loss reported by Jafek et al.[52] was 3160 cc when carotid ligation was not carried out. In those cases that did have ipsilateral carotid ligation, there was still an average blood loss of 2490 cc. In his series, the average blood loss in patients with intracranial extension was 3390 cc. Neel et al.[80] had a 9% mortality among 56 patients undergoing lateral rhinotomy for juvenile angiofibroma. Jafek et al.[53] had one operative death among 15 patients with intracranial extension of juvenile angiofibroma. Ward et al.[118] also had an intraoperative death in a patient with intracranial extension of juvenile angiofibroma leading them to suggest that surgery be avoided in favor of radiotherapy for cases with intracranial extension.

Briant et al.[19] reported 45 cases of juvenile nasopharyngeal angiofibroma treated with moderate doses of radiotherapy (3000–3500 rad in 15 fractions over 3 weeks.). In 10 cases, radiotherapy was administered after surgical failure. Of the total 45 patients, there was control of the tumor in 35 (77.8%). Of the 10 failures, seven were considered due to tumor beyond the irradiated volume, usually in the sphenoid sinus. One additional failure had less than the intended dose. Seven of the failures were controlled with a second course of radiotherapy.

Ward et al.[118] claimed poor results in four patients treated with 3000 rad. However, it is not stated whether or not failure was due to inadequate technique. He had good results in two patients who received 4500–5500 rad over 4½–5½ weeks and recommends such doses for patients with intracranial extension as the preferred treatment.

Cummings[29] has compared radiotherapy with surgery in the treatment of juvenile nasopharyngeal angiofibroma in terms of the risk of death associated with each treatment. By his calculations, the risk of death associated with surgery, including the risks from anesthesia and blood transfusions, is about equal to the one potential fatal complication of radiotherapy, namely induction of malignancy. As he points out, the risk of death from surgery is an immediate complication whereas death from a radiation-induced malignancy, if it occurs, will be many years after treatment. Conley et al.[27] reported an extensive squamous cell carcinoma of the face and orbit which developed 18 years after the delivery of

"12,000 roentgens" for a juvenile nasopharyngeal angiofibroma. Fitzpatrick[37] also reported a case of a squamous cell carcinoma of the nasopharynx which developed 40 years after treatment of a juvenile nasopharyngeal angiofibroma. Radium tubes inserted into the nose and nasopharynx had delivered an estimated minimum tumor dose of 60,000 rad at 0.5 cm from the mucosal surface over a 6 month period. In each of these two reported cases, the dose administered was well in excess of what is currently recommended for juvenile nasopharyngeal angiofibroma. There have not been any cases of thyroid carcinoma reported following radiotherapy for juvenile nasopharyngeal angiofibroma. Cummings[29] calculates a lifetime risk of developing thyroid carcinoma to be 1 in 150 for patients under 18 years of age and 1 in 400 for patients over 18 years of age following treatment with 3000 rad.

Radiation deserves to be considered as the primary mode of therapy for all cases of juvenile nasopharyngeal angiofibroma. Doses of 3000–3600 rad in 15–18 treatments are suggested. Doses of this magnitude should produce only mild and transient skin and mucosal reactions. It is imperative that the extent of tumor be accurately delineated prior to treatment in order to avoid geographical misses. Even those authors who advocate surgery as the primary treatment admit to the necessity of postoperative radiotherapy for those patients with intracranial extension. In the series reported by Jafek et al.,[53] 11 of their 15 cases with intracranial extension had postoperative radiotherapy. The only contraindication to radiation therapy is the possibility of developing a radiation-induced malignancy. However, this risk certainly seems offset by the morbidity and mortality associated with surgery.

Miscellaneous Tumors

Lymphomas

Non-Hodgkin's lymphoma occasionally arises in the nasopharynx. Base of skull involvement is not a common feature as it is with carcinomas of the nasopharynx. Treatment with radiation and/or chemotherapy will depend upon the histologic subtype and extent of dissemination. Doses of 3000–5000 rad over 3–6 weeks should be adequate for local control. Dissemination to regional nodes and distant sites is more likely than persistence or recurrence of tumor in the nasopharynx.

Lymphoma occasionally arises in the paranasal sinuses. Of 156 patients with non-Hodgkin's lymphoma of head and neck extranodal sites, 20 patients (12.8%) had paranasal sinus involvement. In this series reported by Jacobs and Hoppe,[51] the 5 year survival was only 12% for paranasal lymphoma versus 36% for lymphoma of the nasopharynx. Six patients with paranasal lymphoma had relapse in the central nervous system (CNS) prompting the authors to suggest consideration of CNS prophylaxis.

Lymphoma and pseudolymphoma tumors may arise in the orbit. Occasionally, it is difficult for the pathologist to differentiate malignant lymphoma from benign lymphoid hyperplasia especially if the biopsy specimen is small. Spread into the cranial cavity is rare and treatment needs to be directed just to the orbit. Doses of 2000–3000 rad over 2–3 weeks will provide local control in over 90% of patients. Distant dissemination occurs in about 20% of cases.

Rhabdomyosarcomas

Rhabdomyosarcoma is the most common soft tissue sarcoma occurring in parameningeal sites such as the paranasal sinuses, orbit, middle ear, and nasopharynx. Most patients are under age 21. Rhabdomyosarcoma of the orbits accounts for approximately 26% of head and neck rhabdomyosarcomas. The nasopharynx, middle ear, nasal fossa, and paranasal sinuses account for about 40% of head and neck rhabdomyosarcomas.[106] Tefft et al.[109] have pointed out the importance of meningial extension as a cause of therapeutic failure in the treatment of rhabdomyosarcoma from these parameningeal sites other than the orbit. Orbital rhabdomyosarcoma rarely extends into the cranial cavity.[106,109] However, of 57 patients with rhabdomyosarcoma of the nasopharynx, paranasal sinuses, or middle ear, 10 had meningial involvement at diagnosis and 10 others developed meningial spread during their clinical course.[109] Most of the patients were considered to be inadequately irradiated in terms of volume and/or dose. It is extremely important to assess accurately the extent of these lesions and to irradiate the tumor with an adequate margin covering a broad area of the adjacent meninges. Doses of 5000 rad over 6 weeks are recommended. All patients with rhabdomyosarcoma also received chemotherapy.

Other Soft Tissue Sarcomas

Soft tissue sarcomas other than rhabdomyosarcoma may occur in the head and neck region. Unfortunately, they are not as responsive to chemotherapy. High doses of radiation either alone or with surgery should be administered. The author has treated two children with soft tissue sarcoma of the skull base. The first was a 2½-year-old male with a malignant fibrous histiocytoma of the clivus and retropharyngeal area. He developed local recurrence 1½ years after resection and radiotherapy. The second patient was a 7-year-old female with an infratemporal fossa synovial sarcoma extending into the foramen ovale. She is alive and well 2 years after surgery and radiotherapy.

Bone Tumors

Fortunately, malignant bone tumors involving the skull are exceedingly rare. Usually, complete surgical removal will be impossible and the treatment of choice will be radiation ± chemotherapy. At least 6000 rad over 6 weeks should be administered but chances of control will be much better with doses of 7000 rad or even higher. Obviously, with such high doses, care should be taken to use a treatment plan which will avoid, as much as possible, high dose irradiation of normal brain.

Metastasis

Metastatic involvement of the skull base occasionally is seen as part of disseminated malignancy. Metastasis may involve bone, paranasal sinuses, orbit, pituitary gland, and brain either alone or in combinations.

Bone

Carcinoma of the breast is the most common malignancy to metastasize to the osseous base of the skull.[44,90] However, carcinoma of the prostate was the most common primary malignancy in a small series of base of skull metastasis reported by Kistler and Pribraun[59] from a VA Hospital. Pain and cranial nerve involvement are the most common symptoms of base of skull involvement. Greenberg et al.[44] reported on 43 patients with base of skull metastatic involvement and described five syndromes based on the location of the lesion: orbital, parasellar, middle fossa, jugular foramen, and occipital condyle. The middle fossa was the most commonly involved site with 15 patients followed by the jugular foramen and occipital condyle area with nine patients each. Seven patients presented with parasellar syndrome and only three with orbital syndrome. Sixty-seven percent of the patients had metastatic involvement to other sites. All were treated with radiotherapy usually with 3000 rad administered in 10 treatments to the skull base via two lateral fields. The overall symptomatic response to radiotherapy was 86%. There was an objective response rate of 53% (37% partial, 16% complete). Patients with a duration of symptoms less than 1 month had a much better chance of response than if symptoms were present longer than 1 month. There seemed to be an increased response rate with higher doses (3600 rad/12 versus 2400 rad/8). The authors stressed the fact that most patients had relief of symptoms until death. They emphasize that treatment should be administered if the clinical picture is strongly suggestive of metastatic involvement even if radiological studies are negative.

Radiotherapy is the usual treatment for symptomatic osseous metastasis. Chemotherapy and/or hormone manipulation is also used for those malignancies which are sensitive to systemic therapy such as carcinoma of the breast, small cell carcinoma of the lung, etc. In view of the limited survival of patients with metastatic tumor, the standard radiotherapeutic approach for treatment of osseous metastasis is to administer large daily fractions over a relatively short total period. Most patients with base of skull osseous metastasis will have metastatic involvement elsewhere and the aim of radiotherapy is palliation for the duration of the patient's limited survival. Doses of 3000 rad in 10 treatments to 4000 in 15 treatments are probably adequate for such patients. Radiotherapy should be limited to the site of involvement using two lateral fields. For the patient with concomitant cerebral metastatic disease or leptomeningial dissemination, whole-brain radiotherapy is indicated. For the rare patient with solitary metastatic involvement of the skull base either from an unknown primary or from a "controlled primary" where long-term survival is possible, higher doses should be considered with care to avoid normal tissues. In such cases, 5000 rad in 5 weeks or even higher should be administered. The experience of Vikram and Chu[113] suggests that very few patients with base of brain involvement will subsequently need whole-brain irradiation and there is no reason to administer whole-brain irradiation for the usual patient with base of skull bone involvement.

Orbit

Metastatic involvement of the orbit is extremely rare, occurring about one-tenth the frequency of metastatic involvement of the eye. Carcinoma of the breast is the most common primary involvement. As with metastatic disease in general, the prognosis is poor with a median survival of 15.6 months.[39] Palliative radiotherapy to the involved orbit 3000/10–3900/13 is suggested using a single lateral field arrangement. Even an anterior field can be used for the patient with widespread metastasis and limited expected survival.

Pituitary Metastasis

Symptomatic involvement of the pituitary gland by metastatic cancer is rare. In a review of the English literature from 1912–1979, Max et al.[72] were able to find only 28 symptomatic cases with histological proof of metastatic tumor. Breast carcinoma was the most common primary involvement accounting for 16 cases. In an autopsy series of 500 cases, 27 asymptomatic pituitary tumors were identified. Nine were adenomas and 18 were metastatic tumors. All cases with metastatic involvement of the pituitary had widespread systemic metastatic disease. Metastatic involvement of the pituitary and pituitary adenoma can often be separated by clinical presentation. Metastasis to the pituitary usually involves the posterior lobe and causes diabetes insipidus as an early symptom. Less frequently, ocular motor palsies result from metastatic involvement. These two symptoms are rare signs of adenoma. However, metastasis can also involve the anterior lobe mimicking primary adenoma.[68] Likewise, it should be remembered that pituitary adenoma can occur in patients with other primary carcinomas.

The propensity for metastatic carcinoma to involve the posterior lobe of the pituitary gland has also been noted by Tears and Silverman.[108] As in other series, breast cancer was the most frequent site of the primary tumor in women and lung cancer was the most common primary site in men.

Kovacs[60] found 18 cases of pituitary metastasis in an autopsy cancer series of 1857 patients (1.0%). In all cases, widespread metastases were found in other organs and breast carcinoma was the most common primary tumor. Yap et al.[122] also reported on 39 breast cancer patients who had diabetes insipidus secondary to metastatic involvement of the neurohypophysis. All had evidence of advanced metastatic breast cancer. The median interval from the primary diagnosis of carcinoma of the breast to the diagnosis of diabetes insipidus was 29 months with a range of 0–180 months. The median interval from first evidence of metastasis to the diagnosis of diabetes insipidus was 7 months with a range of 0–39 months. Interestingly, in 27% of their patients, diabetes insipidus was among the initial signs of recurrent breast carcinoma. Eighty-seven percent of the patients had osseous involvement. Fifty-four percent of patients had evidence of metastasis in the central nervous system besides the hypothalamic pituitary axis. About one-half of those patients were suspected of having meningial carcinomatosis. However, confirmation of meningial carcinomatosis by spinal fluid examination was carried out in only two patients. Among 15 autopsied patients, there was also metastatic involvement of the sella. Five of those patients also had evidence of meningial carcinomatosis. The authors emphasize the fact that the majority of their patients with diabetes insipidus had CNS involvement either simultaneously or subsequently and they suggest that prophylactic cranial irradiation should be considered in these patients.

Therapy depends on the clinical situation. Max et al.[72] suggest treatment with corticosteroids and local radiation therapy (4000 rad in 3 weeks) unless there is cerebral or meningial spread. Yap et al.[122] suggest that the entire brain should be treated prophylactically in patients with breast cancer and pituitary metastasis. In a patient with disseminated metastasis and a limited life expectancy, symptomatic pituitary metastasis can be treated with radiotherapy to just the involved volume with a dose of 3000 rad/10 to 3900/13 via two lateral fields. In the rare patient where metastastic tumor in the pituitary is the only evidence of dissemination or where life expectancy is greater than 1 or 2 years, higher doses of at least 5000 rad over 5 weeks should be administered. Also, appropriate systemic therapy should be considered for those patients whose malignancies are likely to be responsive to chemotherapy and/or hormone manipulation.

References

1. Adegbite AB, Khan MI, Paine KWE, et al: The recurrence of intracranial meningiomas after surgical treatment. J Neurosurg 58:51-56, 1983.
2. Albert RE, Omran AR, Brauer EW, et al: Follow-up study of patients treated by x-ray for tinea capitis. Am J Public Health 56:2114-2120, 1966.
3. Albo V, Miller D, Leiken S, et al: Eight brain tumors as a late effect in children "cured" of acute lymphoblastic leukemia from a single protocol study (abstr). Proc. ASCO, 1985.
4. Amendola BE, Eisert D, Hazra TA, et al: Carcinoma of the maxillary antrum: Surgery or radiation therapy? Int J Radiat Oncol Biol Phys 7:743-746, 1981.
5. Aristizabal S, Caldwell WL, Avila J: The relationship of time-dose fractionation factors to complications in the treatment of pituitary tumors by irradiation. Int J Radiat Oncol Biol Phys 2:667-673, 1977.
6. Bailey BJ, Barton S: Olfactory neuroblastoma. Arch Otolaryngol 101:1-5, 1975.
7. Baker SR: Nasopharyngeal carcinoma: Clinical course and results of therapy. Head Neck Surg 3:8-14, 1980.
8. Becker LE, Yates AJ, Hoffman HJ, et al: Intracranial chordoma in infancy. J Neurosurg 42:349-352, 1975.
9. Bloom HJG, Wallace ENK, Henk JM: The treatment and prognosis of medulloblastoma in children; a study of 82 verified cases. Am J Roentgenol 105:43-61, 1969.
10. Bloom HJG: Intracranial tumors: Response and resistance to therapeutic endeavors, 1970–1980. Int J Radiat Oncol Biol Phys 8:1083-1113, 1982.
11. Boland J, Paterson R: Cancer of the middle ear and external auditory meatus. J Laryngol Otol 69:468-478, 1955.
12. Boland J: The management of carcinoma of the middle ear. Radiology 80:285, 1963.
13. Boone MLM, Harle TS, Higholt HW, et al: Malignant disease of the paranasal sinuses and nasal cavity: Importance of precise localization of extent of disease. Am J Roentgenol 102:627-636, 1968.
14. Borsanyi SJ: The effects of radiation therapy on the ear; with particular refer-

ence to radiation otitis media. *South Med J* 55:740-743, 1962.
15. Borsanyi SJ, Blanchard CL: Ionizing radiation and the ear. *JAMA* 181:134-137, 1962.
16. Borsanyi SJ, Blanchard CL, Thorne B: The effects of ionizing radiation on the ear. *Ann Otol Rhinol Laryngol* 70:255-262, 1961.
17. Bouchard J, Peirce CB: Radiation therapy in the management of neoplasms of the central nervous system, with a special note in regard to children; twenty years experience, 1939–1958. *Am J Roentgenol Radiat Ther Nucl Med* 84:610-628, 1960.
18. Boyle TM, Frank HG: The management of nasopharyngeal chordoma by repeated irradiation. *J Laryngol* 80:533-535, 1966.
19. Briant TDR, Fitzpatrick PJ, Berman J: Nasopharyngeal angiofibroma: A twenty year study. *Laryngoscope* 88:1247-1251, 1978.
20. Broadbent VA, Barnes ND, Wheeler MB: Medulloblastoma in childhood: long term results of treatment. *Cancer* 48:26-30, 1981.
21. Bush SE, Bagshaw MA: Carcinoma of the paranasal sinuses. *Cancer* 50:154-158, 1982.
22. Campbell JB, Hudson FM: Craniobuccal origin, signs, and treatment of craniopharyngiomas. *Surg Gynecol Obstet* 183-191, 1960.
23. Carella RJ, Ransohoff J, Newall J: Role of radiation therapy in the management of meningioma. *Neurosurgery* 10:332-339, 1982.
24. Carpenter RC, Chamberlin GW, Frazier CH: The treatment of hypophyseal stalk tumors by evacuation and irradiation. *Am J Roentgenol* 38:162-177, 1937.
25. Chan RC, Thompson GB: Morbidity, mortality and quality of life following surgery for intracranial meningiomas. *J Neurosurg* 60:52-60, 1984.
26. Cheng VST, Wang CC: Carcinomas of the paranasal sinuses. *Cancer* 40:3038-3041, 1977.
27. Conley J, Healey WV, Blaugrund SM, et al: Nasopharyngeal angiofibroma in the juvenile. *Surg Gynecol Obstet* 825-837, 1968.
28. Correa JM, Lampe I: Radiation treatment of pituitary adenomas. *J Neurosurg* 19:626-631, 1962.
29. Cummings BJ: Relative risk factors in the treatment of juvenile nasopharyngeal angiofibroma. *Head Neck Surg* 3:21-26, 1980.
30. Dahlin DC, MacCarty CS: Chordoma: A study of fifty-nine cases. *Cancer* 5:1170-1178, 1952.
31. Danoff BF, Cowchock SF, Marquette C, et al: Assessment of the long-term effects of primary radiation therapy for brain tumors in children. *Cancer* 49:1580-1586, 1982.
32. DeSchryver A, Ljunggren JG, Baryd I: Pituitary function in long-term survival after radiation therapy of nasopharyngeal tumors. *Acta Radiol Ther Phys Biol* 12:497-508, 1973.
33. Eastman RC, Gorden P, Roth J: Conventional supervoltage irradiation is an effective treatment for acromegaly. *J Clin Endocrinol Metabol* 48:931-940, 1979.
34. Ellingwood K, Million R: Cancer of the nasal cavity and ethmoid/sphenoid sinuses. *Cancer* 43:1517-1526, 1979.
35. Ellis F: Radiotherapy in the treatment of pituitary basophilism and eosinophilism. *Proc R Soc Med* 42:853-860, 1949.
36. Fischer EG, Welch K, Belli JA, et al: Treatment of craniopharyngiomas in children: 1972–1981. *J Neurosurg* 62:496-501, 1985.
37. Fitzpatrick PJ: The nasopharyngeal angiofibroma. *Can J Surg* 13:228-235, 1970.
38. Fletcher GH, Million RR: Nasopharynx. In Fletcher GH: *Textbook of Radiotherapy*, Edition 3, Philadelphia, Lea & Febiger, 1980, pp 398-400.
39. Font RL, Ferry AP: Carcinoma metastatic to the eye and orbit. *Cancer* 38:1326-1335, 1976.
40. Frew I, Finney R: Neoplasms of the middle ear. *J Laryngol Otol* 77:415-421, 1963.
41. Friedman M: Irradiation of meningioma: A prototype circumscribed tumor for planning high-dose irradiation of the brain. *Int J Radiat Oncol Biol Phys* 2:949-958, 1977.
42. Gomez F, Reyes FI, Faiman C: Nonpuerperal galactorrhea and hyperprolactinemia. *Am J Med* 62:648-660, 1977.
43. Gordy PD, Peet MM, Kahn EA: The surgery of the craniopharyngiomas. *J Neurosurg* 6:503-517, 1949.
44. Greenberg HS, Deck MDF, Vikram B, et al: Metastasis to the base of the skull: Clinical findings in 43 patients. *Neurology* 31:530-537, 1981.
45. Hardison JW, Lessell S, Selhorst JB: Neuro-ophthalmology of sphenoid sinus carcinoma. *Brain* 107:855-870, 1984.
46. Harrop JS, Davies TJ, Capra LG, et al: Hypothalamic-pituitary function following successful treatment of intracranial

tumors. *Clin Endocrinol* 5:313-321, 1976.
47. Hatfield PM, James AE, Schulz MD: Chemodectomas of the glomus jugulare. *Cancer* 30:1164-1168, 1972.
48. Heffelfinger MJ, Dahlin DC, MacCarty CS, et al: Chordomas and cartilaginous tumors at the skull base. *Cancer* 32:410-420, 1973.
49. Henderson WR: Pituitary adenomata: A follow-up study of the surgical results of 338 cases. *Br J Surg* 26:811-921, 1939.
50. Hintz BL, Kagan AR, Wollin M, et al: Reassessment of technical and biological factors in paranasal sinus carcinoma. *J Surg Oncol* 27:59-66, 1984.
51. Jacobs C, Hoppe RT: Non-Hodgkin's lymphomas of head and neck extranodal sites. *Int J Radiat Oncol Biol Phys* 11:357-364, 1985.
52. Jafek BW, Nahum AN, Butler RM, et al: Surgical treatment of juvenile nasopharyngeal angiofibroma. *Laryngoscope* 83:707-720, 1973.
53. Jafek BW, Krekorian EA, Kirsch WM, et al: Juvenile nasopharyngeal angiofibroma: Management of intracranial extension. *Head Neck Surg* 2:119-128, 1979.
54. Jennings AS, Liddle GW, Orth DN: Results of treating childhood Cushing's disease with pituitary irradiation. *N Engl J Med* 297:957-962, 1977.
55. Johns ME, Headington JT: Squamous cell carcinoma of the external auditory canal. *Arch Otolaryngol* 100:45-49, 1974.
56. Kamrin RP, Potanos JN, Pool JL: An evaluation of the diagnosis and treatment of chordoma. *J Neurol Neurosurg Psychiat* 27:157-165, 1964.
57. Kerr HD: Irradiation of pituitary tumors. *Am J Roentgenol* 60:348-359, 1948.
58. Kinsella TJ, Weichselbaum RR, Sheline GE: Radiation injury of cranial and peripheral nerves. In Gilbert HA, Kagan AR (eds): *Radiation Damage to the Nervous System*, New York, Raven Press, 1980, pp 145-153.
59. Kistler M, Pribram HW: Metastatic disease of the sella turcica. *Am J Roentgenol* 123:13-21, 1975.
60. Kovacs K: Metastatic cancer of the pituitary gland. *Oncology* 27:533-542, 1973.
61. Kramer S, McKissock W, Concannon JP: Craniopharyngiomas—Treatment by combined surgery and radiation therapy. *J Neurosurg* 18:217-226, 1960.
62. Kramer S, Southard M, Mansfield CM: Radiotherapy in the management of craniopharyngiomas. Further experiences and late results. *Am J Roentgenol* 103:44-52, 1961.
63. Lamberg BA, Kivikangas V, Vartianen J, et al: Conventional pituitary irradiation in acromegaly. *Acta Endocrinol* 82:267-281, 1976.
64. Lamberts SW, deJong FH, Birkenhager JC: Evaluation of a therapeutic regimen in Cushing's disease: The predictability of the result of unilateral adrenalectomy followed by external pituitary irradiation. *Acta Endocrinol* 86:146-155, 1977.
65. Lawrence AM, Pinsky SM, Goldfine ID: Conventional radiation therapy in acromegaly. *Arch Intern Med* 128:369-377, 1971.
66. Leddy ET, Marshall TM: Roentgen therapy of pituitary adamantinomas (craniopharyngiomas) *Radiology* 56:384-393, 1951.
67. Lederman M: Malignant tumours of the ear. *J Laryngol Otol* 85-119, 1965.
68. Leramo OB, Booth JD, Zinman B, et al: Hyperprolactinemia, hypopituitarism, and chiasmal compression due to carcinoma metastatic to the pituitary. *Neurosurgery* 8:477-480, 1981.
69. Lewis JS: Squamous carcinoma of the ear. *Arch Otolaryngol* 97:41-42, 1973.
70. Lichter AS, Wara WM, Sheline GE, et al: The treatment of craniopharyngiomas. *Int J Radiat Oncol Biol Phys* 2:675-683, 1977.
71. Marks JE, Baglan RJ, Prassad SC, et al: Cerebral radionecrosis: incidence and risk in relation to dose, time, fractionation and volume. *Int J Radiat Oncol Biol Phys* 7:243-252, 1981.
72. Max MB, Deck MDF, Rottenberg DA: Pituitary metastasis: Incidence in cancer patients and clinical differentiation from pituitary adenoma. *Neurology* 31:998-1002, 1981.
73. McCabe BF, Fletcher M: Selection of therapy of glomus jugulare tumors. *Arch Otolaryngol* 89:156-159, 1969.
74. McKissock W, Ford RK: Results of treatment of the craniopharyngiomas (abstract). *J Neurol Neurosurg Psychiat* 29:475, 1966.
75. Merriam GR, Szechter A, Focht EF: The effects of ionizing radiations on the eye. *Front Radiat Ther Oncol* 6:346-385, 1972.
76. Mirimanoff RO, Dosoretz DE, Linggood RM, et al: Meningioma: Analysis of recurrence and progression following neurosurgical resection. *J Neurosurg* 62:18-24, 1985.
77. Modan B, Mart H, Baidatz D, et al: Radiation-induced head and neck tumours. *Lancet* 1:277-279, 1974.
78. Montague ED: Tumors involving the

middle ear and temporal bone. In Fletcher GH: *Textbook of Radiotherapy*, Edition 3, Philadelphia, Lea and Febiger, 1980, pp 398-400.
79. Moretti JA: Sensori-neural hearing loss following radiotherapy to the nasopharynx. *Laryngoscope* 86:598-602, 1976.
80. Neel HB, Whicker JH, Devine KD, et al: Juvenile angiofibroma. *Am J Surg* 126:547-556, 1973.
81. Noetzli M, Malamud N: Postirradiation fibrosarcoma of the brain. *Cancer* 15:617-622, 1962.
82. Ormerod R: Clinical Records—A case of chordoma presenting in the nasopharynx. *J Laryngol* 74:245-254, 1960.
83. Parsons JT, Fitzgerald CR, Hood CI, et al: The effects of irradiation on the eye and optic nerve. *Int J Radiat Oncol Biol Phys* 9:609-622, 1982.
84. Petito CK, DeGirolami U, Earle KM: Craniopharyngiomas: A clinical and pathological review. *Cancer* 37:1944-1952, 1976.
85. Pistenma D, Goffinet DR, Bagshaw MA, et al: Treatment of chromophobe adenomas with megavoltage irradiation. *Cancer* 35:1574-1582, 1975.
86. Poppen JL: Changing concepts in the treatment of pituitary adenomas. *Bull NY Acad Med* 39:21-36, 1963.
87. Ray BS, Patterson RH: Surgical experience with chromophobe adenomas of the pituitary gland. *J Neurosurg* 34:726-729, 1971.
88. Richmond IL, Wara WM, Wilson CB: Role of radiation therapy in the management of craniopharyngiomas in children. *Neurosurgery* 6:513-517, 1980.
89. Richter HJ, Batsakis JG, Boles R: Chordomas: Nasopharyngeal presentation and atypical long survival. *Ann Otol* 84:327-332, 1975.
90. Roessman U, Kaufman B, Friede RL: Metastatic lesions in the sella turcica and pituitary gland. *Cancer* 25:478-480, 1970.
91. Ron E, Modan B: Thyroid and other neoplasms following childhood scalp irradiation in radiation carcinogenesis; epidemiology and biological significance. In Boice J, Fraumeni J (eds): *Radiation Carcinogenesis*, New York, Raven Press, 1984, pp 139-151.
92. Rosenwasser H: Long-term results of therapy of glomus jugulare tumors. *Arch Otolaryngol* 97:49-54, 1973.
93. Roth J, Gorden P, Brace K: Efficacy of conventional pituitary irradiation in acromegaly. *New Engl J Med* 282:1385-1391, 1970.
94. Shah JP, Feghali J: Esthesioneuroblastoma. *CA-A Cancer J Clin* 33:154-159, 1983.
95. Shalet SM, Morris-Jones PH, Beardwell CG, et al: Pituitary function after treatment for intracranial tumours in children. *Lancet* 2:104-107, 1975.
96. Shalet SM, Beardwell CG, Pearson D, et al: The effect of varying doses of cerebral irradiation on growth hormone production in childhood. *Clin Endocrinol* 5:287-290, 1976.
97. Shapiro K, Till K, Grant DN: Craniopharyngiomas in childhood. *J Neurosurg* 50:617-623, 1979.
98. Sheline GE, Wara WM, Smith V: Therapeutic irradiation and brain injury. *Int J Radiat Oncol Biol Phys* 6:1215-1228, 1980.
99. Sheline GE: Irradiation injury of the human brain: A review of clinical experience. In Gilbert HA, Kagan AR (eds): *Radiation Damage to the Nervous System*, New York, Raven Press, 1980, pp 39-58.
100. Shi T, Farrell MA, Kaufmann JCE: Fibrosarcoma complicating irradiated pituitary adenoma. *Surg Neurol* 22:277-283, 1984.
101. Shukovsky LJ, Fletcher GH: Retinal and optic nerve complications in a high dose irradiation technique of ethmoid sinus and nasal cavity. *Radiology* 104:629-634, 1972.
102. Silverstone SM: Radiation therapy of glomus jugulare tumors. *Arch Otolaryngol* 97:43-48, 1973.
103. Solan MJ, Kramer S: The role of radiation therapy in the management of intracranial meningiomas. *Int J Radiat Oncol Biol Phys* 11:675-677, 1985.
104. Sorensen H: Cancer of the middle ear and mastoid. *Acta Radiol* 54:460-468, 1960.
105. Sung DI, Chang CH, Harisiadis L, et al: Treatment results of craniopharyngiomas. *Cancer* 47:847-852, 1981.
106. Sutow WW, Lindberg RD, Gehan EA, et al: Three-year relapse-free survival rates in childhood rhabdomyosarcoma of the head and neck. *Cancer* 49:2217-2221, 1982.
107. Svolos DG: Craniopharyngiomas. *Acta Chir Scand* (Suppl) 403:1-44, 1969.
108. Teears RJ, Silverman EM: Clinicopathologic review of 88 cases of carcinoma metastatic to the pituitary gland. *Cancer* 36:216-220, 1975.

109. Tefft M, Fernandez C, Donaldson M, et al: Incidence of meningeal involvement by rhabdomyosarcoma of the head and neck in children. Cancer 42:253-258, 1978.
110. Tidwell TJ, Montague ED: Chemodectomas involving the temporal bone. Radiology 116:147-149, 1975.
111. Tucker WN: Cancer of the middle ear. Cancer 18:642-650, 1965.
112. Urdaneta N, Chessin H, Fischer JJ: Pituitary adenomas and craniopharyngiomas: Analysis of 99 cases treated with radiation therapy. Int J Radiat Oncol Biol Phys 1:895-902, 1976.
113. Vikram B, Chu FCH: Radiation therapy for metastases to the base of the skull. Radiology 130:465-468, 1979.
114. Waltz TA, Brownell B: Sarcoma: A possible late result of effective radiation therapy for pituitary adenoma. Report of two cases. J Neurosurg 24:901-907, 1966.
115. Wang CC: Radiation therapy in the management of carcinoma of the external auditory canal, middle ear, or mastoid. Radiology 116:713-715, 1975.
116. Wara WM, Sheline GE, Newman H, et al: Radiation therapy of meningiomas. Am J Roentgenol 123:453-458, 1975.
117. Wara WM, Richards GE, Grumbach MM, et al: Hypopituitarism after irradiation in children. Int J Radiat Oncol Biol Phys 2:549-552, 1977.
118. Ward PH, Thompson R, Calcaterra T, et al: Juvenile angiofibroma: A more rational therapeutic approach based upon clinical and experimental evidence. Laryngoscope 2181-2194, 1974.
119. Wold LE, Laws ER: Cranial chordomas in children and young adults. J Neurosurg 59:1043-1047, 1983.
120. Wood EH, Himadi GM: Chordomas: A roentgenologic study of sixteen cases previously unreported. Radiology 54:706-716, 1950.
121. Yamashita J, Handa J, Iwaki K: Recurrence of intracranial meningiomas with special reference to radiotherapy. Surg Neurol 14:33-40, 1980.
122. Yap H, Tashima CK, Blumenschein GR, et al: Diabetes Insipidus and breast cancer. Arch Intern Med 139:1009-1011, 1979.

11

The Role of Chemotherapy in Management of Tumors of the Cranial Base

Charles H. Srodes, M.D.
David G. Mayernik, M.D.

Introduction

The role of chemotherapy in the management of tumors of the cranial base is inchoate. Tumors in this region are uncommon and many are histologically rare. Therefore, there are no large series and no prospective random studies have been performed to establish the appropriate setting for the institution of chemotherapy or establishing the optimum regimen. Also, the critical location of these tumors makes local control of paramount importance even if there is a high risk of dissemination. Finally, it is often difficult to measure responses to chemotherapy because of previous treatments and the lack of standardized measurable response criteria. It is also clear that a wide variety of benign and malignant tumors may occur and each histologic subtype needs to be evaluated separately.

Nonetheless, there have been encouraging reports of objective and durable tumor regressions in advanced recurrent or metastatic nasopharyngeal carcinoma, juvenile angiofibroma, rhabdomyosarcomas, lymphomas, and squamous cell carcinomas. There are some preliminary reports that are beginning to look at the potential role of chemotherapy as an adjuvant in the management of some tumors in association with surgery and/or radiation therapy, in those circumstances with a high probability of distant metastases or local recurrence. All of these data are preliminary but do suggest that there will be a definite role for chemotherapy in the combined modality approach towards tumors of the cranial base.

Juvenile Nasopharyngeal Angiofibroma (JNA)

Juvenile nasopharyngeal angiofibroma is a benign tumor with a high propensity for local recurrence and destruction of adjacent structures by local invasion.[1,2] Surgery is felt to be superior to radiotherapy with excellent cure rates, especially in those patients who have

From: Sekhar LN, Schramm VL Jr, eds: *Tumors of the Cranial Base: Diagnosis and Treatment.* Mount Kisco, New York, Futura Publishing Co, Inc, © 1987.

preoperative arterial embolization to shrink the tumor and reduce blood flow.[1-6] Radiation therapy can then be reserved for those who fail surgery or for whom there is an unacceptable cosmetic defect with surgery.

There have been multiple reports of endocrine responsiveness in angiofibroma. Estrogen receptors have been documented[7] and clinical evidence of tumor responses to androgens[8] and estrogens[9,10] have been described. These responses have been unpredictable, however, and do not seem to justify the use of hormonal agents instead of surgery or radiation. These observations may help to explain the occasionally reported cases of spontaneous regression.[8]

Goepfert et al.[11] reported five patients with recurrent nasopharyngeal angiofibromas, all of whom had received radiation therapy, who were treated with doxorubicin and DTIC with courses repeated every 3 to 4 weeks (to a total doxorubicin dose of 480 mg/M^2). If patients required further systemic chemotherapy, a combination of vincristine, dactinomycin, and cyclophosphamide was used. All five patients reported showed objective regression of tumors within 1 to 2 months of initiating therapy. Objective responses were accompanied by new bone formation and marked reduction of tumor blood supply and decrease of the soft tissue mass, and in one patient, complete disappearance of all disease as proven by polytomography, angiography, and biopsy 6 months after chemotherapy. Two of the patients continued to have evidence of tumors. The remaining three patients were alive and free of disease, 3–10 years following chemotherapy.

These observations indicate a clear role for chemotherapy in JNAs not amenable to alternative therapies with a potential for durable regressions. The optimal chemotherapy schedule and duration cannot be determined nor are there any data to support the adjuvant use or primary use of chemotherapy. However, chemotherapy should be considered if there is recurrent disease after adequate local therapy, intracranial extension with involvement of vital structures, or if the tumor blood supply comes from major intracranial arteries occlusion of which by embolization or radiation therapy could have disastrous neurologic consequences.

Rhabdomyosarcomas

Rhabdomyosarcoma is the most common soft tissue sarcoma found in patients under the age of 16 years. By the use of multidisciplinary treatment programs, the 2-year survival approaches 70%.[209,210] In infants and children, rhabdomyosarcoma occurs most commonly in the head and neck regions, especially nasopharynx, middle ear, paranasal sinuses, intratemporal fossa, and pterygopalatine fossa.[205-209]

The therapy for rhabdomyosarcoma is truly a multidisciplinary exercise. The role and extent of surgery is dependent upon the size, location, and extent of the tumor.[211,212] Total surgical removal, if it can be performed without a major functional disability, can allow the elimination of postoperative radiation or reduction in dose field. In some cases of orbital or parameningeal rhabdomyosarcomas, biopsy only is probably appropriate, preferably including sampling of regional lymph nodes. Staging can be performed using the Intragroup Rhabdomyosarcoma Study (IRS) nomenclature.[213] It seems clear that patients in group I, those whose disease has been totally excised without any evidence of microscopic residual tumor, do not need postoperative radiation therapy.[214]

All other patients should be carefully treated with at least 5000 rads to any remaining gross residual disease, and with at least 4500 rads for microscopic residual disease. The necessity of treating pathologically negative regional lymph nodes is unknown at this time. Use of radiation doses less than those described results in a very high rate of local failure including tumor invasion into the CNS in those patients with parameningeal rhabdomyosarcomas. Radiation ports should definitely involve local contiguous extension sites. The need for central nervous system (CNS) prophylaxis in some patients remains to be further defined.

Unlike the recommendations for radiation therapy, all patients should receive adjuvant chemotherapy. There are multiple agents reported to have activity in rhabdomyosarcoma, but the most intensively studied have been actinomycin D, vincristine, and cyclophosphamide.[215-224] The experience with the IRS trials reveals that patients in group I (those who have no evidence of residual disease either grossly or microscopically), have an excellent 2-year relapse-free survival of 83% using a regimen of vincristine and actinomycin D. Postoperative radiation was not necessary in this group. Patients in group II who have no gross disease but have microscopic residual disease had an 81% 2-year relapse-free survival, with a slightly more intensive regimen of vincristine and actinomycin D.[225] Patients with stage II disease should be treated with radiation therapy as mentioned above. Those who fall into group III with gross residual disease and group IV with obvious metastatic disease are very difficult to cure. All, of course, should receive postoperative radiation therapy and adjuvant chemotherapy. The use of vincristine, actinomycin D, and cyclophosphamide and doxorubicin, however, results in a 3-year survival of approximately 40% in group IV patients. The majority of those patients achieving disease-free 2-year survival will remain in remission and are probably cured.[226] However, of those who do relapse, only about 6% will remain disease-free assuming they achieve a second complete response with aggressive chemotherapy and/or radiation therapy. Trials are in progress currently investigating the use of DTIC, VP-16, and cis-platinum in the treatment of rhabdomyosarcoma, but data and accrual are preliminary at this time.

Because rhabdomyosarcoma is eminently curable in all stages but especially with group I and group II disease, careful pretreatment planning is essential and discussion between the surgeon, radiation therapists, and medical oncologist should involve such issues as extent of surgery, need for postoperative radiation therapy, and whether the radiation therapy should be simultaneous with the adjuvant chemotherapy. The latter is an issue which is also not yet resolved. Finally, because many long-term survivors will be expected among patients with early stage rhabdomyosarcoma utilizing these newer techniques, these patients will have some risk of long-term sequelae such as CNS toxicity seen with prophylaxis and the possibility of secondary tumors, especially leukemias and lymphomas, due to chemotherapy. The use of more aggressive regimens to try to improve the cure rate must be balanced against risks.

Mid-Line Reticulosis, Polymorphic Reticulosis, and Lymphomatoid Granulomatosis

Mid-line reticulosis (MMR), polymorphic reticulosis (PMR) and lymphomatoid granulomatosis (LYG) are very similar histologic diseases with an atypical lymphoid infiltrate accompanied by plasma cells, eosinophils, histiocytes and angio-destruction.[231-237] All three of these are probably variants of the same disease and can involve the nose, paranasal sinuses, palate, and nasopharynx. The kidneys, central nervous system, peripheral nervous system, skin, lung, and gastrointestinal tract can also be involved. They may actually represent variants of peripheral T-cell lymphomas. Originally described as benign disorders, these are now clearly recognized as having a propensity to develop diffuse lymphomas of the large cell immunoblastic type. Survival in patients is often less than 2 years and their tendency to be locally invasive and destructive can produce severe functional deficits wherever they may be found.

The treatment of these is not well understood. The surgical approach should be one of biopsy only. Radiation therapy has been documented to provide rather durable responses with 75% of patients so treated being free of local or peripheral recurrence. Patients with LYG have been treated with cyclophosphamide and prednisone with rather prolonged durable responses being obtained up to 50% of the time.[230] The approach to those patients who progress despite radiation therapy and cytoxan and prednisone is unknown but aggressive multiagent chemotherapy such as that used for the diffuse aggressive lymphomas could be attempted. Historically, survival in such patients with recurrence or resistant disease has been poor. Because this may be a T-cell disorder, the use of a drug that has some specificity for T-cell malignancies, such as 2'deoxycorformycin, would seem to be an attractive alternative. There are no clinical data to support this but experience with 2'deoxycorformycin in other T-cell disorders would seem to suggest such a trial.[232-238]

Mucosal Malignant Melanoma

Mucosal malignant melanoma can rarely involve the cranial base as a primary site assuming that it is not bony metastasis from a previously recognized primary site or from an unknown primary.[12-16] Such involvement would have to arise as a consequence of a primary melanoma in the nasopharynx or paranasal sinuses. Such a location would account for less than 3% of all recorded melanomas.[17] It is clear from the literature that surgical treatment alone is effective in only a very small number of these patients. This appears to be true despite the less frequent occurrence of regional lymph node metastases that occurs with typical cutaneous melanoma. The majority of these patients suffer local recurrence at the primary site despite what are described as adequate surgical margins at the time of operation. Pathologically, many of these are found to have the presence of intralesional blood vessels and/or lymphatic invasion.[15]

Surgery with wide excision remains the cornerstone of intitial therapy with wide excision, but this approach is often hampered by anatomic constraints. No data exist concerning the efficacy of regional lymph node dissection in patients with mucosal melanomas.

Radiation therapy instead of surgery for curative intent is not effective[18,19] and should be reserved for those whose age or medical condition prevents excision. The use of adjuvant radiation either before or after surgery cannot be recommended with any enthusiasm at this time. In patients with clinically involved regional nodes, postoperative irradiation did not change survival or the local disease-free interval over that achieved with lymphadenectomy.[20] In a palliative setting, the response rate to radiation therapy is only modest. This is especially true of disease of the bone which has a low response rate, regardless of increasing fraction sizes.[21] Soft tissue disease may respond slightly better to radiation therapy at a lower total dose.

Dimethyl triazeno imidazole carboxamide (DTIC) remains the single most active agent for melanoma.[22] The overall response rate remains less than 25% with the mean time of response approaching 1 year. There have been multiple clinical trials which have demonstrated little, if any, antitumor activity with other single agents against melanoma.[23-41] DTIC, unfortunately, remains the drug of choice. There are no single agents or combinations of agents that have been demonstrated to produce a better response rate than DTIC alone.[42-77] The use of DTIC or any other drug in an adjuvant fashion pre- or postoperatively cannot be recommended. Using DTIC,[79,80] methyl-CCNU,[80] or DTIC with BCG[78] has failed to improve survival or disease-free survival over surgery alone. Likewise, levamisole or transfer factor appears ineffective in an adjuvant setting.[81,82] DTIC for the treatment of residual or recurrent disease is indicated but the results are relatively disappointing as outlined above. The use of more aggressive regimens involving multiple agents has likewise failed to improve the response rate significantly and toxicity has been increased. Principally among these combinations has been the vinblastine, bleomycin, and cis-platinum regimen which except on a protocol basis cannot be recommended for routine therapy at this time.[83-87]

Some melanomas may contain intracytoplasmic progesterone, androgen, estrogen, or steroid receptors.[88,97,108] A few studies have been done using tamoxifen,[98-107] diethystilbestrol,[109] estramustine,[110-111] orchectomy,[112] or hypophysiectomy[113] in an attempt to utilize these receptors in a therapeutic manner but without much success.

It has long been suggested that melanoma may significantly be affected by immunologic intervention by the host.[114-116] This would help explain the occasional spontaneous regression which has been described. Systemic treatment with BCG[117] or C. Parum[126] has resulted in equivocal and brief responses. A variety of other nonspecific immunotherapeutic approaches such as plasmaphoresis[119] viral oncolysate,[121] and autologous irradiated tumor cells[120] have likewise not proven to induce significant responses. The efficacy of interferon, monoclonal antibodies, and biologic response modifiers awaits completion of ongoing and future trials.[122]

In summary, melanomas of the cranial base are rare with very little information available from the literature concerning their management. It is clear, however, that the vast majority of them recur both locally and at a distant site, that the use of pre- or postoperative radiation therapy in an adjuvant fashion is not recommended and radiation therapy should be reserved for palliation only. Likewise, the use of chemotherapy, specifically DTIC, is not recommended adjuvantly. DTIC could be given systemically for recurrent disease but carries a very low response rate. The use of BCG or other conventional immunotherapy cannot be recommended for adjuvant use or metastatic and recurrent disease. Patients should, if possible, be entered into clinical trials of new chemotherapeutic and immunotherapeutic agents.

Meningiomas

Meningiomas are generally benign tumors arising from the arachnoid cells covering brain and spinal cord. In most cases these are surgically curable; however, those that may be located at the base of the cranium and those that are invasive may not lend themselves to complete surgical removal and multiple neurosurgical procedures are sometimes necessary.[136]

The chemotherapy experience with meningiomas is minimal with efficacy trials scattered and inconsistent. There have been reports over the past few years, however, documenting the presence of steroid receptors in human meningiomas.[123-126,128-132,134] Tilzer et al.[124] defined progesterone receptors in some meningiomas in amounts nearly as high as those found in breast carcinoma. These biochemical observations tend to explain the clinical phenomenons of enlargement of meningiomas during pregnancy,[125] their more frequent occurrence in women,[127] and their association in women with pre-existing breast cancer.[133]

Jay et al.[135] have demonstrated modulation of meningioma cell growth in vitro with sex-steroid hormones. They found estradiol stimulated the growth of tumor cells in culture in a subset of meningiomas demonstrating estradiol binding and that this growth stimulation could be significantly blocked by either the addition of tamoxifen or progesterone. When progesterone and tamoxifen were added separately to the cultures, meningioma cell growth was stimulated but to a lesser extent than with estradiol alone. Unfortunately, this information does not allow the clinician to predict effects in vivo of hormonal manipulations of meningiomas. Theoretically, the administration of progesterone or tamoxifen to a patient with a locally recurrent or surgically resectable meningioma could result in a beneficial response.[138] Markwalder et al. reported their experience using tamoxifen at 10 mg three times a day in six patients with no significant responses.[137] Progesterone agonists may be more promising, but there are no clinical trials that yet confirm this. In the absence of such data, we do not recommend hormonal manipulation except in instances of last resort in which a paradoxical response, such as tumor growth, would not be harmful.

Nasopharyngeal Carcinoma

Nasopharyngeal carcinomas are relatively uncommon in the Western world constituting less than 1% of all head and neck cancers. The incidence is 100 times more frequent in the Chinese population of Southern Asia. The overwhelming majority of these carcinomas arising in the nasopharynx demonstrate squamous differentiation, with nonkeratinizing carcinoma and lymphoepithelioma occurring less frequently.[239-244]

The association of nasopharyngeal carcinomas with a positive titre of Epstein-Barr virus exposure is prevalent in the Western countries and even more prevalent in the nasopharyngeal carcinomas in the Orient. Reports of the use of chemotherapy are sporadic but it remains clear that the nasopharyngeal carcinomas are responsive to a single agent or combinations with substantial remissions seen in advanced measurable disease.[244] Decker[240] reported the experience from Wayne State of 17 patients seen from 1971 to 1981. Fourteen patients had recurrent disease following radiation therapy and two patients had far advanced disease at the time of presentation. The majority had recurrent metastases within prior radiation fields. Four of the 17 had pulmonary metastases, seven had local bony extension, and five had distant metastases to bone, liver, and abdominal nodal sites. Three complete responses and six partial responses (53%) were seen primarily with the combination of 5-fluorouracil (5-FU) and cis-platinum. Other studies support the use of single agent chemotherapy for advanced nasopharyngeal carcinoma.[241] The single agents such as methotrexate, cyclosphamide, bleomycin, and cis-platinum have all shown approximately a 40% response rate with the responses being of relatively brief duration. However, occasional patients with advanced measurable disease will have major responses with significant prolongation of survival.

Because of the poor prognosis of nasopharyngeal carcinoma, particularly those with advanced local-regional diseases, and stages III and IV, chemotherapy may well be considered as initial therapy in conjunction with radiation and/or surgery. A pilot study of 12 patients with lymphoepithelioma treated with adriamycin, bleomycin, velban, and DTIC resulted in nine of 12 patients achieving measurable objective remission.[242] Chemotherapy was followed by radiation therapy. The medium duration of response exceeded 27 months.

Preliminary information on the use of human leukocyte interferon shows that interferon may be active in nasopharyngeal carcinoma as well. Of six patients treated, three had measurable tumor regression. However, there was no decrease in E-B virus titre and there were no complete responses.[243]

It is likely with the poor prognosis of this histologic subtype that chemotherapy will evolve into a primary mode of therapy in conjunction with radiation therapy and/or surgery. Additionally, because of the antigenic alterations in tumor cell differentiation that may be seen with exposure to the E-B virus, the possibility of monoclonal antibodies for diagnostic or therapeutic interventions offers promise for future research.

Plasmacytomas

Plasmacytomas are an unusual manifestation of plasma cell neoplasms. These will rarely present as solitary tumors in extramedullary sites such as bone, tonsil, paranasal sinuses, and nasopharynx.[139-143,153,154] Of all extramedullary sites, the upper respiratory tract is the most common, accounting for approximately 75% of all extramedullary plasma cell tumors.[166] Less commonly, plasma cell tumors can arise in the dura or in an extradural cranial location. Those that involve the base of the skull can compress cranial nerves and cause palsies and proptosis.[144-152] Those which arise in the bone most likely represent a very early stage of myeloma with progression to classic multiple myeloma being common. Progression to multiple myeloma occurs rarely in solitary extramedullary plasmacytomas of soft tissue unless there is adjacent bone involvement, and local therapy will often result in a long disease-free survival.[139-143,153,154]

The surgical treatment of extramedullary or solitary bone plasmacytoma of the cranial base should probably be one of biopsy only. Once the diagnosis of plasmacytoma is established, the patient should be aggressively staged to determine whether this is truly a solitary lesion with no evidence of systemic disease or if it represents a plasmacytoma occurring in a patient with wide-spread multiple myeloma.[155] A complete blood count with differential, serum calcium, BUN, creatinine, uric acid, total serum protein, serum electrophoresis, quantitative immunoglobulin determination, urine protein electrophoresis, and urine immunoelectrophoresis should be done to determine the presence or absence of anemia, hypercalcemia, renal disease, hyperuricemia, and the M-protein in serum or urine. Solitary extramedullary plasmacytomas may secrete M-protein which can be recovered in the serum or urine and their presence should not be interpreted as evidence of systemic disease. For that reason it is essential to perform a bone marrow biopsy and aspirate on these patients. In no case should the bone marrow aspirate contain more than 5 to 10% plasma cells. In addition, skeletal radiographs of the entire body should be normal with no evidence of other lytic defects. If the marrow contains an excess of plasma cells or if lytic defects are seen on the skeletal survey, then the distinction that this is a solitary lesion is not valid.

The therapy depends explicitly upon the results of the staging maneuvers discussed above. Patients who are found to have a plasmacytoma presenting as or complicating the more general systemic diagnosis of multiple myeloma should be treated for the systemic disease with the well-recognized combination of melphalan and prednisone.[156-158] The interval between subsequent treatments often must be lengthened and the dose of the alkylating agent often must be lowered depending upon the patient's subsequent blood counts. A variety of other agents and combinations have been and are currently being compared to melphalan and prednisone in the treatment of all stages of myeloma and as yet no combinations have shown to be consistently more effective.[157,165-169] This regimen will result in a response rate of approximately 50%. Those patients not responding and those who relapse can be treated with a variety of second-line regimens including prednisone, cyclosphamide, doxorubicin, methyl-CCNU, and vincristine in a variety of schedules.[159-165] Unfortunately, the majority of those patients who either failed initial therapy or have relapsed after an initial response will go on to die of their disease in less than 18 to 24 months.

Radiation therapy can play a very useful role in palliating a plasmacytoma occurring at the cranial base in patients with systemic myeloma. Tumoricidal doses of 1500 to 2000 rads are generally effective, eliminating symptoms locally.

Patients who have a solitary bone lesion and have no evidence of systemic multiple myeloma based on staging procedures discussed above should be treated more aggressively with radiation therapy. Tumoricidal doses of 3500 rads will generally be enough to totally eradicate the local disease. If a monoclonal protein was present prior to therapy, it should be absent following completion of the radiation. If it persists, it is likely that multiple myeloma is present and the patient should be treated with the systemic regimen as suggested above. Most of these patients with persistent M-protein will eventually go on to develop systemic myeloma[139-143] within 5 years.

Those soft tissue extramedullary plasmacytomas appearing in the paranasal sinuses and nasopharynx should likewise be treated aggressively with about 3500 rads of radiotherapy. The majority of these lesions will be very well controlled with this local therapy alone, but in some cases there may be persistence of the monoclonal protein in the serum and clinical evidence of a residual mass at the anatomic site. In some cases, surgical removal of nasopharyngeal or tonsillar masses several months after completion of radiotherapy resulted in disappearance of the protein.[141] The overall survival of these patients is very good with few going on to develop multiple myeloma and local recurrence occurring less than 10% of the time.[139-143] There currently appears to be no indication for the use of adjuvant chemotherapy in solitary extramedullary plasmacytomas without bone involvement unless the patient develops radiation therapy-resistant disease or multiple myeloma.

Lymphoma

Lymphomas can involve the cranial base as a result of their origin in the nose and paranasal sinuses, nasopharynx, maxillary antrum, and dura.[170-179] All of these sites represent a very small percentage of the lymphomas, but it is important to recognize their possible existence since they are eminently curable and their clinical appearance can easily mimic inflammatory or other nonlymphomatous neoplastic processes. In addition, many of these lymphomas will be stage I and II which improves their cure rate and makes early diagnosis that much more important. When classified according to the International Working Formulation, the majority of these lymphomas are of the intermediate or high-grade diffuse large cell type.[180] As is the case with most other extranodal lymphomas, few if any are of the follicular type. In the review by Frierson et al.,[171] over half were reported to be a high-grade type of lymphoma, the diffuse immunoblastic variety. These are thought to have a somewhat more aggressive natural history.[181-182]

The surgical therapy should be limited to that of a biopsy. Once a diagnosis of lymphoma is established, it becomes very important to stage the patient since ultimate therapy will depend on presence or absence of distant disease. An appropriate staging work-up would include a bone marrow biopsy and aspirate, and abdominal and pelvic computerized axial tomography.

The experience with these lymphomas has been somewhat limited given their rarity. Most series have used radiation therapy to the involved field with the addition of chemotherapy for patients with higher-stage disease.[170,171,179,183-186] Traditionally, a course of 5000 rads to include ipsilateral sinuses with or without elective nodal irradiation has been the approach. Unfortunately, the recurrence rate would appear to be in the 40–60% range with a majority of those patients dying eventually of disseminated disease. In most radiation therapy series, patients were not adequately staged, which by strict criteria requires a laparotomy to confirm stage I disease. Sweet, in his extensive review considering only diffuse histiocytic lymphomas which were laparotomy-staged, was able to effect a cure rate of 93% with stage I disease.[187] This represents all stage I disease and not only those with lymphomas of the head or neck. This contrasts sharply with an only 33% relapse-free rate in stage II patients. If one wishes to extrapolate the data from all stage I diffuse histiocytic lymphomas to those found in the extranodal sites of the paranasal sinuses and nasopharynx, then involved field radiation therapy would offer an excellent cure rate for those who have been staged by laparotomy. For the diffuse large cell variety, it is suggested that a dose in the vicinity of 5000 rads be given in 200 rads fractions. There are currently no data to suggest that radiation to clinically uninvolved contiguous lymph nodes is of value. For the nondiffuse large cell or immunoblastic varieties, a low total dose of approximately 3500 rads appears to be adequate.

Because of the high incidence of recurrent rates in nonlaparotomy clinically staged patients who are felt to have clinical stage I or contiguous stage II disease with diffuse histiocytic lymphoma, several groups have attempted to combine radiotherapy with systemic chemotherapy. Nissen et al.[188] treated the aggressive lymphomas with radiation therapy only or radiation followed by combination chemotherapy. Only 12% of the patients in a combined modality had subsequent relapse compared to 68% who received radiation alone. Comella et al.,[189] using cyclosphamide, vincristine, and prednisone or cyclosphamide, doxorubicin, vincristine, and prednisone (CHOP) combined with radiation therapy, achieved similar results. More importantly, Miller and Jones treated stage I and II aggressive lymphomas with CHOP alone or CHOP plus involved field radiation.[190] Overall survival between the two groups was virtually the same with 89% of the patients being disease-free in the follow-up at 29 months. These results were confirmed in a similar study performed by Cabanillas et al.[191] CHOP is a moderately aggressive chemotherapy regimen but is generally well tolerated by all but the more elderly patients or those with pre-existent cardiac disease. It is currently unclear whether patients with stage I diffuse histiocytic lymphoma should be treated with involved field radiotherapy or chemotherapy alone, but there seems to be little argument in the absolute necessity for chemotherapy either alone or in combination with radiation for patients with stage II disease. If it seems that patients who have stage I aggressive lymphomas have virtually the same survival rate when given chemotherapy as do those who receive radiation therapy, there would appear to be some advantages to the use of the chemotherapy alone. Most importantly, it eliminates the staging laparatomy. By then giving these clinical stage I patients systemic chemotherapy, there is no danger that they would get inadequate treatment as could occur with radiation alone. In the authors' own experience, we have had no recurrences (with a mean follow-up of 2 years) in five patients treated with CHOP for eight courses. We would therefore recommend the use of CHOP as primary therapy in patients with diffuse large cell (histiocytic), diffuse mixed, and diffuse poorly differentiated lymphoma. Stage III and IV patients are best treated with systemic chemotherapy. The use of chemotherapy alone cannot be recommended for any of the other histologic subtypes since there is so little experience with these rather rare types in the paranasal sinus and nasopharyngeal regions. For those patients presenting with clinical stage I and contiguous stage II disease who have follicular poorly differentiated, follicular mixed, and nodular histiocytic histologies, we would recommend involved field radiotherapy, with the use of chemotherapy alone only in those with recurrent disease or disease persisting after radiotherapy is complete.

Esthesioneuroblastoma

Esthesioneuroblastoma is a rare tumor of neural crest origin which arises from olfactory epithelium in the nasal cavity.[192,193] Despite treatment with curative intent with surgery and radiation therapy, a 5-year disease-free interval of less than 20% and an overall 5-year survival rate of 50% only has been reported with either modality.[192,193] Patients who are not cured of their disease will eventually die from distant metastases or regional recurrence with intracranial extension.

Objective responses of measurable advanced disease has been reported with chemotherapy in 8 of 13 patients for an overall response rate of 62%. Single drug activity has been reported for nitrogen mustard, cyclophosphamide, thiopeta, doxorubicin, and DTIC. Because of the response rates reported for childhood neuroblastoma,[195] Wade and associates have used cyclophosphamide and vincristine in the treatment of five patients with esthesioneuroblastoma.[192] Two patients were treated prior to definitive radiation therapy with a good objective response. One patient who failed to respond to radiation therapy responded to chemotherapy and two patients with recurrent disease responded to chemotherapy. One patient had died and one had persistent disease at the time of the report. Three patients remained free of disease from 6 months to a year following cessation of therapy.

It appears that esthesioneuroblastoma is a chemotherapy-sensitive tumor that has potential long-term responses.[192-196] The optimal chemotherapy regimen is unknown but it would seem reasonable to use a combination including vincristine, cyclophosphamide, and doxorubicin. Responses are often prompt and even minimal responses may produce palliation of pain, nasal obstruction, epistaxis, or diplopia. Because late recurrences are likely in this disease, the durability of even complete responses needs to be confirmed by longer follow-up. It is also unclear what the optimum duration of treatment should be. Based on current reports, 6 to 9 months of every 3 to 4 weeks of chemotherapy would seem reasonable.

Because of the high percentage of recurrent regional or distant metastatic disease, future considerations should look at adjuvant chemotherapy in conjunction with radiation therapy and surgery to increase the percentage of patients with extended disease-free survival.

Squamous Cell Carcinoma

Squamous cell carcinomas of the paranasal sinuses are most frequently found in the maxillary sinus. The analysis of 66 cases by St. Pierre and Baker[197] found that the majority of patients were stage III and IV with nodal involvement found in 10–20% at the time of diagnosis. Most patients were treated by combined radiotherapy and surgery with 5-year actuarial survivals of 75% for T2, 28.5% for T3, and 19.4% for T4 lesions. Chemotherapy was used for palliation only. However, recent experience with squamous cell carcinomas of other areas of the head and neck suggest that this is a highly chemotherapy-responsive malignancy. Protocols using methotrexate, bleomycin and cis-platinum, cis-platinum and 5-fluorouracil have shown response rates of greater than 65% with 20–30% complete responses and suggested that combination chemotherapy may afford palliation and may be able to increase the salvage with radiation and surgery.[198,199] Overall, malignant tumors of the paranasal sinuses have a notoriously poor prognosis. Standard treatments result in 5-year survivals of approximately 35%.[200] A higher 5-year survival rate was described by Sakai[201] and his associates with radiation therapy, surgery, interarterial 5-fluorouracil, and immunotherapy. Other reports by Konno et al.[202] and Sato et al.[203] confirm an improved 5-year survival with combined modality treatment.

If possible, such patients should be placed in a clinical trial using combined surgery, radiation, and chemotherapy. If no trials are available, a reasonable approach is as follows: patients with T1 and T2 disease should have surgery and no further therapy if margins are clear and no nodes are involved either clinically or pathologically. Those with T3 and T4 disease should be considered for preoperative chemotherapy with cis-platinum and 5-FU. Using this regimen, patients who are inoperable may become operable, and those who are operable will be more so. Postoperatively, these patients should probably receive radiation therapy. Those patients who relapse, and those who remain inoperative could continue to receive cis-platinum and 5-FU until progression, followed by methotrexate and 5-FU salvage. Virtually all such relapsing and residual disease patients will die of their disease. In some cases, they should be offered experimental drugs (i.e., interferon) when available.

It is important that prior to treatment, options of therapy are discussed among the surgeon, radiation therapist, and medical oncologist. The responsiveness of squamous cell of the head and neck region to cis-platinum, 5-FU, and methotrexate will prompt the use of these drugs in most future clinical trials.

Mucoepidermoid and Adenoidcystic Carcinomas

Mucoepidermoid carcinomas are both radiation therapy-resistant and chemotherapy-resistant with very few significant responses described in the literature. Adenoidcystic carcinomas, however, have responded to doxorubicin, 5-fluorouracil, and cis-platinum. Schramm et al.[204] reported 10 patients treated with cis-platinum alone, nine had objective responses, and two patients appeared to have been cured with chemotherapy (now greater than 4 years after stopping treatment with no measurable residual disease). The possibility that combined cis-platinum with doxorubicin could enhance the response and the number of complete responders and duration of response remains to be tested.

We would suggest the use of cis-platinum or adriamycin every 4 weeks in patients with residual or recurrent disease. Choice of drug would be dependent on cardiac status, age, and renal function.

Summary

The past decade has produced greater knowledge of the natural history and prognosis of tumors arising from the cranial floor. Better techniques of diagnosis and measurement have led to improved ability to monitor therapeutic responses. Techniques have evolved to combine the treatment modalities of neurosurgery, ENT surgery, reconstructive surgery, and radiation therapy, to improve the local control rates. Nonetheless, many of these uncommon tumors will recur either regionally or with evidence of distant metastases and will require systemic approaches to therapy. Clearly, the use of chemotherapy in combination with surgery and radiation offers the potential for prolongation of life and, in some cases, cure.

Directions for the future include:

1. Specific treatment for each histologic subtype.

2. The potential of a clonogenic assay to determine in vitro which tumors are likely to be sensitive to each chemotherapeutic agent.

3. Monoclonal antibodies which may have both diagnostic and therapeutic potential. Diagnostic potential is to distinguish areas of active tumor and therapeutic potential is to either interact with tumor cells by themselves or in conjunction with tagged chemotherapy or radioisotopes, to effect more specific tumoricidal activity, without affecting normal tissues.

4. Immunobiologic modifiers to augment the host's ability to recognize tumor cells as foreign and eliminate them through the physiologic immune mechanisms.

5. Establishment of optimal treatment schedules, both in terms of drugs, dosage, and administrative schedule.

6. The use of laser and other tools in combination with chemotherapy to augment the cytotoxic response.

7. Development of new chemotherapeutic agents with improved therapeutic/toxic ratios and the development of drugs that may act on different mechanisms of tumor cellular growth in contrast to those agents that are currently dependent on active cellular proliferation for their activity.

It will be difficult to mount a prospective randomized trial in these uncommon tumors, and it will therefore require close observation in those centers where concentration of these patients is seen to determine which developments are most likely to result in therapeutic advances.

References

Juvenile Nasopharyngeal Angiofibroma

1. Witt TR, Shah JP, Sternberg SS: Juvenile nasopharyngeal angiofibroma: A 30 year clinical review. *Am J Surg* 146:521-525, 1983.
2. Chandler JR, Moskowitz L, Goulding R, et al: Nasopharyngeal angiofibroma: Staging and management. *Am Otol Rhinol Laryngol* 93:322-329, 1984.
3. Fitzpatrick PJ, Briant DR, Berman JM: The nasopharyngeal angiofibroma. *Arch Otolaryngol* 106:234, 1980.
4. Jafek BW, Nahuon AM, Butler RM, et al: Surgical treatment of juvenile nasopharyngeal angiofibroma. *Laryngoscope* 83:707-720, 1973.
5. Biller HF: Juvenile nasopharyngeal angiofibroma. *Am Otol Rhinol Laryngol* 87:630-632, 1978.
6. Neel HB III, Whicker JH, Deuine KD, et al: Juvenile angiofibroma: Review of 120 cases. *Am J Surg* 126:547-556, 1973.
7. Lee DA, Rao BR, Meyer JS, et al: Hormonal receptor determination in juvenile nasopharyngeal angiomas. *Cancer* 46:547-551, 1980.
8. Martin H, Ehrlich HE, Abels JC: Juvenile nasopharyngeal angiofibroma. *Am Surg* 129:513-536, 1948.
9. John ME, MacLeod RM, Cantrell RW: Estrogen receptors in nasopharyngeal angiofibromas. *Laryngoscope* 90:628-639, 1980.
10. Walike JW, Mackay B: Nasopharyngeal angiofibroma: Light and electron microscopic changes after stilbesterol therapy. *Laryngoscope* 80:1109-1121, 1970.
11. Goepfert H, Cangir A, Lee Y: Chemotherapy for aggressive juvenile nasopharyngeal angiofibroma. *Arch Otolaryngol* 111:285-289, 1985.

Mucosal Malignant Melanoma

12. Shah JP, Hubos AG, Strong EW: Mucosal melanomas of head and neck. Am J Surg 134:53:535, 1977.
13. McCaffrey TV, Neel HB, Gaffey TA: Malignant melanoma of the oral cavity: Review of 10 cases. Laryngoscope 90:1329-1335, 1980.
14. Chaudhury AP, Hampel A, Gorlin RJ: Primary malignant melanoma of the oral cavity: A review of 105 cases. Cancer 11:923-928, 1958.
15. Cove H: Melanosis, melanocytic hyperplasia and primary malignant melanoma of the nasal cavity. Cancer 44:1424-1433, 1979.
16. Freedman HM, DeSanto LW, Devine KD, et al: Malignant melanoma of the nasal cavity and paranasal sinus. Arch Otolaryngol 97:322-325, 1973.
17. Jwerson K, Robins RE: Mucosal malignant melanomas. Am J Surg 139:660-664, 1980.
18. Cooper JS, Kopf AW, Bart RS: Present role and future prospects for radiotherapy in the management of malignant melanomas. J Dermatol Surg Oncol 5:134-139, 1979.
19. Kopf AW, Bart AS, Rodinquery-Sams RS, et al: *Malignant Melanoma*. New York, Mason Publishing USA, 1979, pp 197-199.
20. Creagon ET, Cupps RE, Irvins JC, et al: Adjuvant radiation therapy for regional nodal metastasis from malignant melanoma: A randomized prospective study. Cancer 42:2206-2210, 1978.
21. Katz HR: The results of different fractionation schemes in the palliative irradiation of metastatic melanoma. Int J Radiat Oncol Biol Phys 7:907-911, 1981.
22. Comis RL: DTIC (NSC-45388) in malignant melanoma: A perspective. Cancer Treat Rep 60:165-176, 1976.
23. Ramirez G, Wilson W, Grage T, et al: Phase II evaluation of 1,3-bis(2-chlorethyl-nitrosourea) (BCNU; NSC-409962) inpatients with solid tumors. Cancer Chemother Rep 56:787-790, 1972.
24. Lessner HE: BCNU (1,3-bis(2-chlorethyl)-1-nitrosourea). Effects on advanced Hodgkins's disease and other neoplasia. Cancer 22:451-456, 1968.
25. DeVita VT, Carbone PP, Owens AH, Jr, et al: Clinical trials with 1,3-bis(2-chloroethyl)-1-nitrosourea NSC-409962. Cancer Res 25:1875-1881, 1965.
26. Pugh R, Jacobs E, Bateman J, et al: CCNU versus CCNU + vincristine in disseminated melanoma. Proceedings of the 11th International Cancer Congress, Florence, Italy, pp 540-541, 1974.
27. Cruz AB, Jr, Armstrong DM, Aust JB: Treatment of advanced malignancy with CCNU (1-(2-chloroethyl)-3-cyclohexyl-1-nitrosourea, (NSC-79037): A phase II cooperative study. Proc Am Assoc Cancer Res 15:184, 1974.
28. Ahmann DL, Hahn RG, Bisel HF: A comparative study of 1-(2-chloroethyl)-3-cyclohexyl-1-nitrosourea (NSC-79037) and imidazole carbonxamide (NSC-45388) with vincristine (NSC-67574) in the palliation of disseminated malignant melanoma. Cancer Res 32:2432-2434, 1972.
29. Hoogstraten B, Gottlieb JA, Caoili E, et al: CCNU (1-(2-chloroethyl)-3-cyclohexyl-1-nitrosourea (NSC-7903)) in the treatment of cancer: Phase II study. Cancer 32:38-43, 1973.
30. Broder LE, Hansen HH: 1-(2-chloroethyl)-3-cyclohexyl-1-nitrosourea (CCNU, NSC-79037): A comparison of drug administration at four-week and six-week intervals. Eur J Cancer 9:147-152, 1973.
31. DeConti RC, Hubbard SP, Pinch P, et al: Treatment of advanced neoplastic disease with 1-(2-chloroethyl)-3-cyclohexyl-1-nitrosourea (CCNU, NSC-79037). Cancer Chemother Rep 57:201-207, 1973.
32. Perloff M, Muggia FM, Ackerman C: Role of a nitrosourea CCNU, (NSC-79037) in advanced non-hematologic cancer. Cancer Chemother Rep 58:421-429, 1974.
33. Wasserman TH, Slavik M, Carter SK: Review of CCNU in clinical cancer therapy. Cancer Treat Rev 1:131-151, 1974.
34. Young RC, Canellos GP, Chabner BA, et al: Treatment of malignant melanoma with methyl-CCNU. Clin Pharmocol Ther 15:617-622, 1974.
35. Tranum BL, Haut A, Rivkin S, et al: Methyl-CCNU in Hodgkins's disease and other tumors. Proc Am Assoc Cancer Res 15:171, 1974.
36. Firat D, Tekuzman G: Treatment of solid tumors and lymphomas with methyl-CCNU. Proc Am Assoc Cancer Res 15:5, 1974.
37. Wasserman TH, Slavik M, Carter SK: Methyl-CCNU in clinical cancer therapy. Cancer Treat Rev 1:251-259, 1974.
38. Van Amburg Al, Presant CA, Burns D: Phase II study of chlorozotocin in malig-

nant melanoma: A Southeastern Cancer Study Group report. *Cancer Treat Rep* 66:1431-1433, 1982.
39. Hoth DF, Schein PS, Winokur S, et al: A phase II study of chlorozotocin in metastatic melanoma. *Cancer* 46:1544-1547, 1980.
40. Houghton AN, Camacho FJ, Gralla RJ, et al: Phase II evaluation of chlorozotocin in patients with malignant melanoma. *Cancer Treat Rep* 65:705-706, 1981.
41. Silver BA, Barlock AL, Lippman ME, et al: Phase II trial of chlorozotocin in malignant melanoma, breast cancer and other solid tumors. *Cancer Treat Rep* 66:1229-1230, 1982.
42. Costanza ME, Nathanson L, Lenhard R, et al: Therapy of malignant melanoma with an imidazole carboxamide and bischloroethylnitrosourea. *Cancer* 30: 1457-1461, 1972.
43. Bellet RE, Mastrangelo MJ, Laucius JF, et al: Randomized perspective trial of DTIC (NSC-45388) alone vs BCNU (NSC-409962) plus vincristine (NSC-67574) in the treatment of metastatic malignant melanoma. *Cancer Treat Rep* 60:595-600, 1976.
44. Costanza ME, Nathanson L, Schoenfeld D, et al: Results with methyl-CCNU and DTIC in metastatic melanoma. *Cancer* 40:1010-1015, 1977.
45. Costani JJ, Vaitkevicus VK, Quagliana JM, et al: Combination chemotherapy for disseminated malignant melanoma. *Cancer* 35:342-346, 1975.
46. Beretta G, Bonadonna G, Cascinelli N, et al: Comparative evaluation of three combination regimens for advanced malignant melanoma: Results of an international cooperative study. *Cancer Treat Rep* 60:33-40, 1976.
47. Gardere SH, Cowan HD: Treatment of metastatic malignant melanoma with a combination of 5-(3,3-dimethyl-1-triazeno) imidazole-4-carboxamide (NSC-45388), cyclophosphamide (NSC-26271) and vincristine (NSC-67574). *Cancer Chemother Rep* 56:357-361, 1972.
48. Carmo-Pereira J, Costa FO, Pimental P: Combination cytotoxic chemotherapy for metastatic cutaneous malignant melanoma with DTIC, BCNU and vincristine. *Cancer Treat Rep* 60:1381-1382, 1976.
49. McKelvey EM, Luce JK, Talley RW, et al: Combination chemotherapy with bischloroethylnitrosourea (BCNU), vincristine and dimethyl-triazeno-imidazole-carboxamide (DTIC) in disseminated malignant melanoma. *Cancer* 39:1-4, 1977.
50. Einhorn LH, Furnas B: Combination chemotherapy for disseminated malignant melanoma with DTIC, vincristine and methyl-CCNU. *Cancer Treat Rep* 61:881-883, 1977.
51. Hill GJ II, Metter GE, Krementz ET, et al: DTIC and combination therapy for melanoma II. Escalating schedules of DTIC with BCNU, CCNU and vincristine. *Cancer Treat Rep* 1989-1992, 1979.
52. Luce JK, Torin LB, Price H: Combination dimethyl-triazeno-imidazole-carboxamide (NSC-45388; DIC), vincristine (NSC-67574; VCR) and 1,3-bis(2-chloroethyl)-1-nitrosourea (NSC-409962; BCNU) chemotherapy of disseminated melanoma. *Proc Am Assoc Cancer Res* 11:50, 1970.
53. Beretta G, Bonadonna G, Cascinelli N, et al: Comparative evaluation of three combination regimens for advanced malignant melanoma: Results of an international cooperative study. *Cancer Treat Rep* 60:33-40, 1976.
54. Cohen SM, Greenspan EM, Ratne LH, et al: Combinaton chemotherapy of malignant melanoma with imidazole carboxamide, BCNU and vincristine. *Cancer* 39:41-44, 1977.
55. Beretta G, Bojetta E, Bonadonna G, et al: Combination chemotherapy with 5-(3,3-dimethyl-1-triazeno) imidazole carboxamide (DTIC; NSC-45388), 1,3-bis(2-chloroethyl)-1-nitrosourea (BCNU; NSC-409962) and vincristine (VCR; NSC-67574) in metastatic malignant melanoma. *Tumor* 59:239-248, 1973.
56. Samson MK, Baker LH, Izbicki RM, et al: Phase I-II study of DTIC and cyclocytidine in disseminated melanoma. *Cancer Treat Rep* 60:1369-1371, 1976.
57. Carter RD, Krementz ET, Hill GJ, II, et al: DTIC (NSC-45388) and combination therapy for melanoma. I. Studies with DTIC, BCNU, CCNU, vincristine and hydroxyurea. *Cancer Treat Rep* 60:601-609, 1976.
58. Halpern J, Catane R, Biran S, et al: DTIC and actinomycin D with and without C. parvum immunotherapy in advanced malignant melanoma. *Tumor* 67:215-217, 1981.
59. Ramseur WL, Richards F II, Muss HB, et al: Chemoimmunotherapy for disseminated malignant melanoma: A prospec-

tive randomized study. *Cancer Treat Rep* 62:1085-1087, 1978.
60. Samson MK, Baker LH, Talley RW, et al: Phase I-II study of intermittent bolus administration of DTIC and actinomycin D in metastatic malignant melanoma. *Cancer Treat Rep* 62:1223-1225, 1978.
61. Ahmann DL, Edmonson JH, Frytak S, et al: Phase II study of ICRF-159 vs. combination cis-dichlorodiammineplatinum (II) and DTIC in patients with disseminated melanoma. *Cancer Treat Rep* 62:151-153, 1978.
62. Goodnight JE Jr, Moseley HS, Eilber FR, et al: Cis-dichlorodiammineplatinum (II) alone and combined with DTIC for treatment of disseminated malignant melanoma. *Cancer Treat Rep* 63:2005-2007, 1979.
63. Gerner RE, Moore GE, Dickey C: Combination chemotherapy in disseminated melanoma and other solid tumors in adults. *Oncology* 31:22-30, 1975.
64. Friedman MA, Kaufman DA, Williams JE, et al: Combined DTIC and cis-dichlorodiammineplatinum (II) therapy for patients with disseminated melanoma: A Northern California Oncology Group study. *Cancer Treat Rep* 63:493-495, 1979.
65. Karakousis CP, Getaz EP, Bjornsson S, et al: Cis-dichlorodiammineplatinum (II) and DTIC in malignant melanoma. *Cancer Treat Rep* 63:2009-2010, 1979.
66. Wittes RE, Wittes JT, Golbey RB: Combination chemotherapy in metastatic melanoma. *Cancer* 41:415-421, 1978.
67. Retsas S, Athanasiou A, Flynn MD, et al: Combined chemotherapy with vindesine and DTIC in advanced malignant melanoma. *Proc Am Soc Clin Oncol* 1:169, 1982.
68. Ahmann DL, Hahn RG, Bisel HF, et al: Comparative study of methyl-CCNU (NSC-95441) with cyclophosphamide (NSC-26271) and 5-(3,3-dimethyl-1-triazeno) imidazole-4-carboxamide (NSC-45388) with vincristine (NSC-67545) in patients with disseminated melanoma. *Cancer Chemother Rep* 59:451-453, 1975.
69. Ahmann DL, Hahn RG, Bisel HF: A comparative study of 1-(2-chloroethyl)-3-cyclohexyl-1-nitrosourea (NSC-79037) and imidazole carboxamide (NSC-45388) with vincristine (NSC-67574) in the palliation of disseminated malignant melanoma. *Cancer Res* 32:2432-2434, 1972.
70. Byrne MJ, Reynolds PM: Phase II study of cyclophosphamide, vincristine and DTIC + BCG in the treatment of malignant melanoma. *Aust NZ J Med* 12:263-266, 1982.
71. Samson MK, Baker LH, Cummings G, et al: Clinical trial of chloroztocin, DTIC, and dactinomycin in metastatic malignant melanoma. *Cancer Treat Rep* 66:371-373, 1982.
72. Costanzi JJ, Al-Sarraf M, Groppe C, et al: Combination chemotherapy plus BCG in the treatment of disseminated malignant melanoma: A Southwest Oncology Group study. *Med Pediatr Oncol* 10:251-258, 1982.
73. McKelvey EM, Luce JK, Vaitkevicius VK, et al: Bis-chloroethylnitrosourea, vincristine, dimethyltriazeno-imidazole carboxamide and chlorpromazine combination chemotherapy in disseminated malignant melanoma. *Cancer* 39:5-10, 1977.
74. Carey RW, Green MR, Anderson J: Vinblastine-dimethyltriazenoimidazole carboxamide (DTIC-cis-platinum (VDP): Active regimen in metastatic melanoma. *Proc Am Soc Clin Oncol* 2:237, 1983.
75. Seigler HF, Lucas VS, Pickett JN, et al: DTIC, CCNU, bleomycin and vincristine (BOLD) in metastatic melanoma. *Cancer* 45:2346-2348, 1980.
76. Ahn SS, Giuliano A, Kaiser L, et al: The limited role of BOLD chemotherapy for disseminated malignant melanoma. *Proc Am Soc Clin Oncol* 2:228, 1983.
77. Cohen SM, Ohnuma T, Cheung T, et al: Bleomycin, carmustine, vincristine and decarbazine in patients with metastatic melanoma. *Clin Treat Rep* 67:947-948, 1983.
78. Veronesi U, Adamus J, Aubert C, et al: A randomized trial of adjuvant chemotherapy and immunotherapy in cutaneous melanoma. *N Engl J Med* 307:913-916, 1982.
79. Hill GL, Moss SE, Golomb FM, et al: DTIC and combination therapy for melanoma: III. DTIC (NSC-45388) surgical adjuvant study COG protocol 7040. *Cancer* 47:2556-2562, 1981.
80. Terry WD, Hodes RS, Rosenberg SA, et al: Treatment of stage I and II malignant melanoma with adjuvant immunotherapy or chemotherapy: Preliminary analysis of a prospective randomized trial. In Terry WD, Rosenberg SA (eds.): *Immunotherapy of Human Cancer*, New York, Elsevier North Holland, 1982, pp 251-257.

81. Bukowski RH, Deodhar S, Hewlett JS, et al: Randomized controlled trial of transfer factor in stage II malignant melanoma. *Cancer* 51:269-272, 1983.
82. Spitler LE, Sagebiel R: Levamisole in the treatment of melanoma. In Terry WD, Rosenberg SA (eds.): *Immunotherapy of Human Cancer*, New York, Elsevier North Holland, 1982, pp 289-291.
83. Creagan ET, Ahmann DL, Schutt AJ, et al: Phase II study of the combination of vinblastine, bleomycin and cisplatin in advanced malignant melanoma. *Cancer Treat Rep* 66:567-569, 1981.
84. Nathanson L, Kaufman SD, Carey RW: Vinblastine, infusion bleomycin, and cis-dichlorodiammine-platinum chemotherapy in metastatic melanoma. *Cancer* 48:1290-1294, 1981.
85. Bajetta E, Rovej R, Buzzoni R, et al: Treatment of advanced malignant melanoma with vinblastine, bleomycin and cisplatin. *Cancer Treat Rep* 66:1299-1302, 1982.
86. York RM, Lawson DH, McKay J: Treatment of metastatic melanoma with vinblastine, bleomycin by infusion and cisplatin. *Cancer* 52:2220-2222, 1983.
87. Mechl Z, Nekulova M, Sopkova B, et al: The VBD regimen (vinblastine-bleomycin-cisplatinum) with high dose of cisplatinum in the therapy of advanced malignant melanoma. *Proc 13th Int Cong Chemother*, 246:22-25, 1983.
88. Fisher RI, Neifeld JP, Lippman ME: Estrogen receptors in human malignant melanoma. *Lancet* 2:337-338, 1976.
89. Rumke P, Persijn JP, Korsten CB: Oestrogen and androgen receptors in melanoma. *Br J Cancer* 41:652-656, 1980.
90. Stedman KE, Moore GE, Morgan RT: Estrogen receptor proteins in diverse human tumors. *Arch Surg* 115:244-248, 1980.
91. Chaudhuri PK, Walker MJ, Briele HA, et al: Incidence of estrogen receptor in benign nevi and human malignant melanoma. *JAMA* 244:791-793, 1980.
92. Neifeld JP, Lippman ME: Steroid hormone receptors and melanoma. *J Invest Dermatol* 74:379-381, 1980.
93. Creagan ET, Ingle JN, Woods JE, et al: Estrogen receptors in patients with malignant melanoma. *Cancer* 46:1785-1786, 1980.
94. Grill HJ, Benes P, Manz B, et al: Steroid hormone receptors in human melanoma. *Arch Dermatol Res* 272:97-101, 1982.
95. Bojar H, Stuhldreier B, Becher R, et al: Gradient centrifugation analysis of steroid-hormone binding in human malignant melanoma. *Anticancer Res* 2:245-250, 1982.
96. Bhakoo HS, Milholland RJ, Lopez R, et al: High incidence and characterization of glucocorticoid receptors in human malignant melanoma. *J Natl Cancer Inst* 66:21-25, 1981.
97. Thompson AJ, Cook MG, Gill PG: Immunofluorescent detection of hormone receptors in cutaneous melanocytic tumors. *Br J Cancer* 43:644-653, 1981.
98. Meyskens FL, Jr, Voakes JB: Tamoxifen in metastatic malignant melanoma. *Cancer Treat Rep* 64:171-173, 1980.
99. Karakousis CP, Lopez R, Bhakoo HS, et al: Steroid hormone receptors and tamoxifen treatment in malignant melanoma. *Proc Am Soc Clin Oncol* 21:345, 1980.
100. Papac RJ, Kirkwood JM: High-dose tamoxifen in metastatic melanoma. *Cancer Treat Rep* 67:1051-1052, 1983.
101. Leichman CG, Samson MK, Baker LH: Phase II trial of tamoxifen in malignant melanoma. *Cancer Treat Rep* 66:1447, 1982.
102. Masiel A, Buttrick P, Bitran J: Tamoxifen in the treatment of malignant melanoma. *Cancer Treat Rep* 65:531-532, 1981.
103. Creagan ET, Ingle JN, Green SJ, et al: Phase II study of tamoxifen in patients with disseminated malignant melanoma. *Cancer Treat Rep* 64:199-201, 1980.
104. Creagan ET, Ingle JN, Ahmann DL, et al: Phase II study of high-dose tamoxifen (NSC-180973) in patient with disseminated malignant melanoma. *Cancer* 49:1353-1354, 1982.
105. Wagstaff J, Thatcher N, Rankin E, et al: Tamoxifen in the treatment of metastatic malignant melanoma. *Cancer Treat Rep* 66:1771, 1982.
106. Telhaug R, Klepp O, Bormer O: Phase II study of tamoxifen in patients with metastatic malignant melanoma. *Cancer Treat Rep* 66:1437, 1982.
107. Reimer R, Costanzi J, Fabian C: Southwest Oncology Group experience with tamoxifen in metastatic melanoma. *Cancer Treat Rep* 66:1680-1681, 1982.
108. Beattie CW, Chaudhuri PK, Walker MJ, et al: Hormonal regulation of the growth and metastasis of human melanoma. *Cancer Treat Rep* 63:1199, 1979.
109. Fisher RI, Young RC, Lippman MC: Diethylstilbestrol therapy of surgical non-resectable malignant melanoma. *Proc Am Soc Clin Oncol* 19:339, 1978.

110. Lopez R, Karakousis CP, Didolkar MS, et al: Estramustine phosphate in the treatment of advanced malignant melanoma. Cancer Treat Rep 62:1329-1332, 1978.
111. Didolkar RC, Catane R, Lopez R, et al: Estramustine phosphate (estracyt) in advanced malignant melanoma. Proc Am Soc Clin Oncol 19:381, 1978.
112. Herbst WP: Malignant melanoma of the choroid with extensive metastases treated by removing secreting tissue of the testicles. JAMA 122:597, 1943.
113. Lawson DL, Nixon DW, Black ML, et al: Evaluation of transsphenoidal hypophysectomy in the management of patients with advanced malignant melanoma. Cancer 51:1541-1545, 1983.
114. Clark WH, Jr, Ainsworth AM, Bernardino EA, et al: The developmental biology of primary human malignant melanomas. Semin Oncol 2:83-103, 1975.
115. Cole WH: Spontaneous regression of cancer: The metabolic triumph of the host. Ann NY Acad Sci 230:111-141, 1974.
116. Bodurtha AJ: Spontaneous regression of malignant melanoma. In Clark WH, Goldman LI, Mastrangelo MJ (eds): Human Malignant Melanoma, New York, Grune & Stratton, 1979, pp 227-241.
117. Orefice S, Cascinelli N, Vaglini M, et al: Intravenous administration of BCG in advanced melanoma patients. Tumor 64:437-443, 1978.
118. Israel L, Edelstein R, Depierre A, et al: Daily intravenous infusions of Corynebacterium parvum in twenty patients with disseminated cancer. JNCI 55:29-33, 1975.
119. Israel L, Edelstein R, Mannori P, et al: Plasmapheresis in patients with disseminated cancer: Clinical results and correlation with changes in serum protein. Cancer 40:3146-3154, 1977.
120. Laucius JF, Bodurtha AJ, Mastrangelo MJ, et al: A phase II study of autologous irradiated tumor cells plus BCG in patients with metastatic melanoma. Cancer 40:2091-2093, 1977.
121. Murray DR, Cassel WA, Torbin AH, et al: Viral oncolysate in the management of malignant melanoma. Cancer 40:680-686, 1977.
122. Mastrangelo MJ, Berd D, Maguire H: The current condition and prognosis of tumor immunotherapy: A second opinion. Cancer Treat Rep 68:207-219, 1984.

Meningiomas

123. Donnell MS, Meyer GA, Donegan WL: Estrogen receptor proteins in intracranial meningiomas. J Neurosurg 50-1199-1202, 1979.
124. Tilzer LL, Plopp FV, Evans JP, et al: Steroid receptor proteins in human meningioma. Cancer 49:633-636, 1982.
125. Backerstaff ER, Small JM, Guest JA: The relapsing course of certain meningiomas in relation to pregnancy and menstruation. J Neurol Neurosurg Psychiatry 21:89-91, 1958.
126. Cahill DW, Bashirelahi N, Soloman LW, et al: Estrogen and progesterone receptors in meningiomas. J Neurosurg 60:985-993, 1984.
127. Rauzing A, Yho W, Stenflo J: Intracranial meningioma: A population study of ten years. Acta Neurol Scand 46:102-110, 1970.
128. Glick RP, Molteni A, Focs EM: Hormone binding in brain tumors. Neurosurgery 13:513-519, 1983.
129. Magdelenat H, Pertuiset BF, Poisson M, et al: Progestin and oestrogen receptors in meningioma: Biochemical characterization clinical and pathological correlation in 42 cases. Acta Neurochir 64:199-213, 1982.
130. Markurolder TM, Zarua DT, Goldhirsch A, et al: Estrogen and progesterone receptors in meningiomas in relation to chemical and pathologic features. Surg Neurol 20:42-47, 1983.
131. Murtuza RL, MacLaughlin DT, Ojemann RG: Specific estradiol binding in schwanommas, meningiomas, and neurofibromas, Neurosurgery 9:665-671, 1981.
132. Schnegg JF, Gomey F, LeMarchand-Besaud T, et al: Presence of sex-steroid hormone receptors in meningioma tissue. Surg Neurol 15:415-418, 1981.
133. Schoenberg BS, Christine BW, Uhisnant JP: Nervous system neoplasms and primary malignancies of other sites: The unique association between meningiomas and breast cancer. Neurology 25:705-712, 1975.
134. Yu ZY, Wrange O, Hagland B, et al: Estrogen and progesterone receptors in intracranial meningiomas. J Steroid Biochem 16:451-456, 1982.
135. Jay JR, Maclanglin DT, Riley KR, Murtuza RL: Modulation of meningioma cell growth by sex-steroid hormones in vitro. J Neurosurg 62:757-762, 1985.
136. Adeglite AB, Khan MJ, Paine KWB, et al: The recurrence of intracranial meningiomas after surgical treatment. J Neurosurg 58:57-56, 1983.

137. Markwalder TM, Seiler RW, Zara DT: Antiestrogenic therapy of meningiomas—a pilot study. Surg Neurol 24:245-249, 1985.
138. Markwalder TM, Markwalder RV, Zara DT: Steroid hormone receptors in meningiomas: Clinicopathological correlations. Clin Neuropharmacol 7:368-374, 1984.
139. Woodruff RK, Whittle JM, Malpas JS: Solitary plasmacytoma. I. Extramedullary soft tissue plasmacytoma. Cancer 43:2340-2343, 1979.
140. Woodruff RK, Malpas JS, White FE: Solitary plasmacytoma. II. Solitary plasmacytoma of bone. Cancer 43:2344-2347, 1979.
141. Knowling M, Harwood A, Bergsagel DE: A comparison of extramedullary plasmacytomas with multiple and solitary plasma cell tumors of bone. J Clin Oncol 1:255-262, 1983.
142. Wiltshaw E: The natural history of extramedullary plasmacytoma and its relation to solitary myeloma of bone and myelomatosis. Medicine 55:217-238, 1976.
143. Crowin J, Linberg RD: Solitary plasmacytoma of bone vs. extramedullary plasmacytoma and their relationship to multiple myeloma. Cancer 43:1007-1013, 1979.
144. Somersen A, Osgood CP Jr, Brylski J: Solitary posterior fossa plasmacytoma. J Neurosurg 35:223-228, 1971.
145. Atweh GF, Jabbour N: Intracranial solitary extraskeletal plasmacytoma resembling meningioma. Arch Neurol 39:57-59, 1982.
146. Stark RJ, Henson RA: Cerebral compression by myeloma. J Neurol Neurosurg Psychiatry 44:833-836, 1981.
147. Jakubowski J, Kendall BE, Symon L: Primary plasmacytoma of the cranial vault. Acta Neurochir 55:117-134, 1980.
148. Kohli CM, Kawazu T: Solitary intracranial plasmacytoma. Surg Neurol 17:307-312, 1982.
149. Soffer D, Siegal T: Solitary dural plasmacytoma with conspicuous cytoplasmic inclusions. Cancer 49:2500-2504, 1982.
150. Mancardi GL, Mandybur TI: Solitary intracranial plasmacytoma. Cancer 51:2226-2233, 1983.
151. Coppeto JR, Monteiro MLR, Collias J, et al: Foster-Kennedy syndrome caused by solitary intracranial plasmacytoma. Surg Neurol 19:267-272, 1983.
152. Pritchard PB III, Martinez RA, Hungerford GD, et al: Dural plasmacytoma. Neurosurgery 12:576-579, 1983.
153. Fu YS, Perzin KH: Nonepithelial tumors of the nasal cavity, paranasal sinuses and nasopharynx: A clinocopatholgic study. IX. Plasmacytomas. Cancer 42:2399-2406, 1978.
154. Castro EB, Lewis JS, Strong EW: Plasmacytoma of paranasal sinuses and nasal cavity. Arch Otolaryngol 97:326-329, 1973.
155. Durie BGM, Salmon SE: A clinical staging system for multiple myeloma: Correlation of measured myeloma cell mass with presenting clinical features, response to treatment and survival. Cancer 36:842-854, 1975.
156. Costa G, Engle RL, Schilling A, et al: Melphalan and prednisone: An effective combination for the treatment of multiple myeloma. Am J Med 54:589-599, 1973.
157. Alexanian R, Dreicer R: Chemotherapy for multiple myeloma. Cancer 53:583-588, 1984.
158. Bergsagel DE: Treatment of plasma cell myeloma. Ann Rev Med 30:431-443, 1979.
159. Alexanian R, Yap BS, Bodey GP: Prednisone pulse therapy for refractory myeloma. Blood 62:572-577, 1983.
160. Salmon SE, Shadduck RK, Schilling A: Intermittent high-dose prednisone (NSC-10023) therapy for multiple myeloma. Cancer Chemother Rep 51:179-187, 1967.
161. Bergsagel DE, Cowan DH, Hasselback R: Plasma cell myeloma: Response of melphalan-resistant patients to high-dose, intermittent cyclophosphamide. Can Med Assoc J 107:851-855, 1972.
162. Kyle RA, Pajak TF, Henderson ES, et al: Multiple myeloma resistant to melphalan: Treatment with doxorubicin, cyclophosphamide, carmustine (BCNU), and prednisone. Cancer Treat Rep 66:451-456, 1982.
163. Brandes L, Israels LG: Treatment of advanced plasma cell myeloma with weekly cyclophosphamide and alternate-day prednisone. Cancer Treat Rep 66:1413-1415, 1982.
164. Bonnet J, Alexanian R, Salmon S, et al: Vincristine, BCNU, doxorubicin and prednisone (VBAP) combination in the treatment of relapsing or resistant multiple myeloma: A Southwest Oncology Study Group. Cancer Treat Rep 66:1267-1271, 1982.
165. Abramson N, Lurie P, Mietlowski WL, et al: Phase III study of intermittent carmustine (BCNU), cyclophosphamide, and prednisone versus intermittent melpha-

lan and prednisone in myeloma. *Cancer Treat Rep* 66:1273-1277, 1982.
166. Kapadia SB, Desai U, Cheng VS: Extramedullary plasmacytoma of the head and neck. A clinicopathologic study of 20 cases. *Medicine* 61:317-329, 1982.
167. Salmon SE, Haut A, Bonnet JD, et al: Alternating combination chemotherapy and levamisole improves survival in multiple myeloma: A Southwest Oncology Group study. *J Clin Oncol* 1:453-461, 1983.
168. Cavagnaro F, Lein JM, Pavlovsky S, et al: Comparison of two combination chemotherapy regimens for multiple myeloma: Methyl-CCNU, cyclophosphamide and prednisone versus melphalan and prednisone. *Cancer Treat Rep* 64:73-79, 1980.
169. Ahre A, Bjorkholm M, Mellstedt H, et al: Intermittent high-dose melphalan/prednisone versus continuous low-dose melphalan treatment in multiple myeloma. *Eur J Cancer Clin Oncol* 19:499-506, 1983.

Lymphoma
170. Wilder WH, Harner SG, Banks PM: Lymphoma of the nose and paranasal sinuses. *Arch Otolaryngol* 109:310-312, 1983.
171. Frierson HF, Mills SF, Innes DJ: Non-Hodgkin's lymphomas of the sinonasal region: Histologic subtypes and their clinicopathologic features. *Am J Clin Pathol* 81:721-727, 1984.
172. Freeman C, Berg JW, Cutler SJ: Occurrence and prognosis of extranodal lymphomas. *Cancer* 29:252-260, 1972.
173. Catlin D: Surgery for head and neck lymphomas. *Surgery* 60:1160-1166, 1966.
174. Sofferman RA, Cummings CW: Malignant lymphoma of the paranasal sinuses. *Arch Otolaryngol* 101:287-292, 1975.
175. Eichel BS, Harrison EG, Jr, Devine KD, et al: Primary lymphoma of the nose including a relationship to lethal midline granuloma. *Am J Surg* 112:597-605, 1966.
176. Birt BD: Reticulum cell sarcoma of the nose and paranasal sinuses. *J Laryngol Otol* 84:615-630, 1970.
177. Fu YS, Perzin KH: Nonepithelial tumors of the nasal cavity, paranasal sinuses and nasopharynx: A clinicopathologic study. X. Malignant lymphomas. *Cancer* 43:611-621, 1979.
178. Kapadia SB, Barnes L, Deutsch M: Non-Hodgkin's lymphoma of the nose and paranasal sinuses: A study of 17 cases. *Head Neck Surg* 3:490-499, 1981.
179. Roblins KT, Fuller LM, Vlasak M, et al: Primary lymphomas of the nasal cavity and paranasal sinuses. *Cancer* 56:814-819, 1985.
180. The Non-Hodgkin's Lymphoma Pathologic Classification Project: National Cancer Institute sponsored study of classifications of non-Hodgkin's lymphomas: Summary and description of a working formulation of clinical usage. *Cancer* 49:2112-2135, 1982.
181. Levin AM, Taylor CR, Schneider DR, et al: Immunoblastic sarcoma of T-cell versus B-cell origin: I. Clinical features. *Blood* 58:52-61, 1981.
182. Lichtenstein A, Levine AM, Lukes RJ, et al: Immunoblastic sarcoma: A clinical description. *Cancer* 43:343-352, 1979.
183. Jones SE, Fuks Z, Kaplan HS, et al: Non-Hodgkin's lymphomas: Results of radiotherapy. *Cancer* 32:683-691, 1973.
184. Mill WB, Fransiska AL, Kaarle OF: Radiation therapy treatment of stage I and II: Extranodal non-Hodgkin's lymphoma of the head and neck. *Cancer* 45:653-661, 1980.
185. Bush RS, Gaspodarowicz M, Sturgeon J, et al: Radiation therapy of localized non-Hodgkin's lymphoma. *Cancer Treat Rep* 61:1129-1136, 1977.
186. Hellman S, Chaffey JT, Rosenthal DS, et al: The place of radiation therapy in the treatment of non-Hodgkin's lymphomas. *Cancer* 39:843-851, 1977.
187. Sweet DL, Kinzie J, Gaeke ME, Golomb HM, et al: Survival of patients with localized diffuse histiocytic lymphomas. *Blood* 58:1218-1223, 1981.
188. Nissen NI, Ersbll J, Hansen HS, et al: A randomized study of radiotherapy vs radiotherapy post-chemotherapy in stage I-II non-Hodgkin's lymphoma. *Cancer* 52:1-7, 1983.
189. Comella P, Scoppa G, Abate G, et al: Combination chemotherapy (CVP or CHOP) radiotherapy approach in early stage non-Hodgkin's lymphomas. *Tumor* 68:137-142, 1982.
190. Miller TP, Jones SE: Initial chemotherapy for clinically localized lymphomas of unfavorable histology. *Blood* 62:413-418, 1983.
191. Cabanillas F, Bodey GP, Freireich EJ: Management with chemotherapy only of stage I and II malignant lymphoma of aggressive histologic types. *Cancer* 46:2356-2359, 1980.

Esthesioneuroblastoma
192. Wade PM, Jr, Smith RE, Johns ME: Response to esthesioneuroblastoma to chemotherapy: Report of five cases and

review of the literature. *Cancer* 53:1036-1041, 1984.
193. Cantrell RS, Gorayeb BY, Fitz-Hugh GS: Esthesioneuroblastoma: diagnosis and treatment. *Ann Otol Rhinol Laryngol* 86:760-765, 1977.
194. Suen JY, Myers EN: *Cancer of the Head and Neck*, New York, Churchill, Livingstone, 1981, pp 673-677.
195. Green AA, Hayes FA, Hustu HO: Sequential cyclophosphamide and doxyrubicin for induction of complete remission in children with disseminated neuroblastoma. *Cancer* 48:2310-2317, 1981.
196. Hayes FA, Green AA, Casper J, et al: Clinical evaluation of sequentially scheduled cis-platinum and VM26 in neuroblastoma. *Cancer* 48:1715-1718, 1981.

Squamous Cell Carcinoma
197. St-Pierre S, Baker SR: Squamous cell carcinoma of the maxillary sinus: analysis of 66 cases. *Head Neck Surg* Jul/Aug, 1983.
198. LoVerme PJ, Rush BF, Legaspi A, et al: Combined therapy in advanced squamous cell carcinoma of the head and neck. *Am Surgeon* 48:197-201, 1982.
199. Decker DA, Drelichman A, Jacobs J, et al: Adjuvant chemotherapy with cis-diamminodichloroplatinum II and 120-hour infusion 5-fluorouracil in stage III and IV squamous cell carcinoma of the head and neck. *Cancer* 51:1353-1355, 1983.
200. Goldsmith MA, Carter SK: The integration of chemotherapy into a contained modality approach to cancer therapy vs squamous cell carcinoma of the head and neck. *Cancer Treat Rev* 2:137-138, 1975.
201. Sakai S, Hohki A, Fuchihata H, et al: Multidisciplinary treatment of maxillary sinus carcinoma. *Cancer* 52:1360-1364, 1983.
202. Konno A, Togawa K, Inoue S: Analysis of the results of our combined therapy for maxillary cancer. *Acta Otolaryngol* (Suppl):372, 1980.
203. Sato Y, Morita M, Takahashi H, Watanabe N, Kirikae I: Combined surgery, radiotherapy and regional chemotherapy in carcinoma of the maxillary sinus. *Auris Nasuarynxs L* 5:29-37, 1978.
204. Schramm VL, Srodes CH, Myers EN: Cisplatin therapy for adenoid cystic carcinoma. *Arch Otolaryngol* Vol 107, 1981.

Rhabdomyosarcoma
205. Mauer HM: The Intergroup Rhabdomyosarcoma study. *Cancer Bull* 34:108-110, 1982.
206. Miller RW, Dalager NA: Fatal rhabdomyosarcoma among children in the United States 1960-1969. *Cancer* 34:1897-1900, 1974.
207. Mahour GH, Soule EH, Mills SD, et al: Rhabdomyosarcoma in infants and children: A clinico-pathologic study of 75 cases. *J Pediatr Surg* 2:402-409, 1967.
208. Enziger FM, Shiraki M: Alveolar rhabdomyosarcoma: An analysis of 110 cases. *Cancer* 24:18-31, 1969.
209. Mauer HM, Donaldson MH, Gehan EA, et al: The Intergroup Rhabdomyosarcoma: Update, November 1978. *Natl Cancer Inst Monogr* 56:61-68, 1981.
210. Sutow WW, Lindberg RD, Gehan EA, et al: Three-year relapse-free survival rates in children rhabdomyosarcoma of the head and neck: Report from the Intergroup Rhabdomyosarcoma study. *Cancer* 49:2217-2221, 1982.
211. Kilman JW, Clatworthy HW, Jr, Newton WA, et al: Reasonable surgery for rhabdomyosarcoma: A study of 67 cases. *Ann Surg* 178:346-351, 1973.
212. Johnson DG: Trends in surgery for childhood rhabdomyosarcoma. *Cancer* 35:916-920, 1975.
213. Maurer HM, Moon TE, Donaldson M, et al: The Intergroup Rhabdomyosarcoma study. *Cancer* 40:2015-2026, 1977.
214. Tefft M, Lindberg R, Gehan EA: Radiation therapy combined with systemic chemotherapy of rhabdomyosarcoma in children: Local control in patients enrolled in the Intergroup Rhabdomyosarcoma study. *Natl Cancer Inst Monogr* 56:75-81, 1981.
215. Ghavimi F, Exelby PR, D'Angio GH, et al: Multidisciplinary treatment of embryonal rhabdomyosarcoma in children. *Cancer* 35:677-686, 1975.
216. Heyn RM, Holland R, Newton WA, et al: The role of combined chemotherapy in the treatment of rhabdomyosarcoma in children. *Cancer* 34:2128-2142, 1974.
217. Green DM, Jaffe N: Progress and controversy in the treatment of childhood rhabdomyosarcoma. *Cancer Treat Rev* 5:7-27, 1978.
218. Heyn R, Holland R, Joo P, et al: Treatment of rhabdomyosarcoma in children with surgery, radiotherapy, and chemotherapy. *Med Pediatr Oncol* 3:32, 1977.
219. Jaffe N, Murray J, Traggis D, et al: Multidisciplinary treatment for childhood sarcoma. *Am J Surg* 133:405-413, 1977.
220. Donaldson SS, Castro JR, Wilbur JR, et al: Rhabdomyosarcoma of the head and neck in children: Combination treatment by

surgery, irradiation, and chemotherapy. *Cancer* 31:26-35, 1973.
221. Wilbur JR: Combination chemotherapy for embryonal rhabdomyosarcoma. *Cancer Chemother Rep* 58:281-284, 1974.
222. Tefft M, Fernandez CH, Moon TE, et al: Rhabdomyosarcoma: Response to chemotherapy prior to radiation in patients with gross residual disease. *Cancer* 39:665-670, 1977.
223. Pratt CB, Hustu HP, Pinkel D: Coordinated treatment of childhood rhabdomyosarcoma. *Prog Clin Cancer* 6:87-94, 1975.
224. Tan CTC, Rosen G, Gharimi F, et al: Adriamycin (NSC-123127) in pediatric malignancy. *Cancer Chemother Rep* 6(3):359-366, 1975.
225. Maurer HM, Foulkes M, Gehan EA, et al: Intergroup Rhabdomyosarcoma Study (IRS): Preliminary report. *Proc Am Soc Clini Oncol* 2:70 (Abstr C-274), 1983.
226. Raney RB, Crist WM, Maurer HM, et al: Prognosis of children with soft tissue sarcoma who relapse after achieving a complete response. A Report from the Intergroup Rhabdomyosarcoma Study. *Cancer* 52:44-50, 1983.

Mid-Line Reticulosis,
Polymorphic Reticulosis, and
Lymphomatoid Granulomatosis

227. Kassel SH, Echevarria RA, Guzzo FP: Midline malignant reticulosis (so-called lethal midline granuloma). *Cancer* 23:920-935, 1969.
228. DeRemee RA, Weiland LH, McDonald TJ: Polymorphic reticulosis, lymphomatoid granulomatosis: Two diseases or one? *Mayo Clin Proc* 53:634-640, 1978.
229. Liebow AA, Carrington CB, Friedman RJ: Lymphomatoid granulomatosis. *Human Pathol* 3:457-558, 1972.
230. Fauci AS, Haynes BF, Costa J, et al: Lymphomatoid granulomatosis, prospective clinical and therapeutic experience over ten years. *N Engl J Med* 306:68-74, 1982.
231. Katzenstein A, Carrington CB, Liebow AA: Lymphomatoid granulomatosis: A clinico-pathologic study of 152 cases. *Cancer* 43:360-373, 1979.
232. Prentice HG, et al: Remission induction with adenosine-deaminase inhibitor 2'deoxycoformycin in Thy-lymphoblastic leukemia. *Lancet* 2:170, 1980.
233. Poplack DG, et al: Phase I study of 2'deoxycoformycin in acute lymphoblastic leukemia. *Cancer Res* 41:3343, 1981.
234. Grever MR, et al: The biochemical and clinical consequences of 2'deoxycoformycin in refractory lymphoproliferative malignancy. *Blood* 57:406, 1981.
235. Grever MR, et al: Deoxycorformycin the treatment of refractory chronic lymphocytic leukemia. *Proc ASCO* 22:487, 1981.
236. Wortmann RI, et al: Biochemical basis for differential deoxyadenos toxicity to T and B lymphoblasts: Role for 5'Nucleotiades. *PNAS* 76:2434, 1979.
237. Carson DA, et al: Biochemical basis for the enhanced toxicity of deoxyribonuclesides toward malignant human T-cell lines. *PNAS* 76:2430, 1979.
238. Spiers ASD, et al: T-cell chronic lymphocytic leukemia (T-CLL) with unique cell phenotype, intradermal bleeding and dramatic response to deoxycorformycin (DCF). *Blood* 58(1):153, 1981.

Nasopharyngeal Carcinoma

239. Lederman M: *Cancer of the Nasopharynx: Its Natural History and Treatment.* Springfield IL, Thomas CC, 1961, p 103.
240. Decker DA, Drelichman A, Al-Sarraf M, et al: Chemotherapy for nasopharyngeal carcinoma: A ten year experience. *Cancer* 52:602-605, 1983.
241. Dickson RI, Flores AD: Nasopharyngeal carcinoma: An evaluation of 134 patients treated between 1971-1980. Abstract presented at the 87th Annual Meeting of the American Laryngological Rhinological and Otological Society, Inc., Palm Beach, FL, May 8, 1984.
242. Haines IE, Schwarz MA, Hurley RA, Rundle HMP: Recurrent nasopharyngeal carcinoma: Two long-term disease-free remissions with non-cisplatinum based combination chemotherapy. *Aust NZ J Surg* 55:153-156, 1985.
243. Connors JM, Andiman WA, et al: Treatment of nasopharyngeal carcinoma with human leukocyte interferon. *J Clin Oncol* 3:6, 1985.
244. Neel HB: Nasopharyngeal carcinoma: Clinical presentation, diagnosis, treatment and prognosis. *Otolaryngol Clin North Am* 18:3, 1985.

V

Reconstruction After Cranial Base Tumor Resection

12

The Exposure, Preservation, and Reconstruction of Cerebral Arteries and Veins During the Resection of Cranial Base Tumors

Laligam N. Sekhar, M.D.

Introduction

The blood vessels supplying the brain are commonly involved by tumors of the cranial base. Injury to these vessels during or after operations to resect cranial base neoplasms may result in stroke and death. Prevention of injury to such vessels, and their reconstruction in the event of vascular occlusion or resection, may reduce such morbidity. Many advances have been made in the management of neoplastic involvement of both the basal cerebral arteries and the veins. However, many problems remain to be solved.

Determinants of Outcome After Vascular Occlusion

Many factors influence whether infarction will occur after the occlusion of cerebral arteries. Experimental evidence indicates that when cerebral blood flow (CBF) is reduced to 12–20 ml/100 gm/min, synaptic transmission ceases, with resultant loss of function. This, however, is a reversible state for several hours and infarction can be prevented if blood flow is elevated above 20 ml/100 gm/min. When flow is reduced below 10–12 ml/100 gm/min, disruption of the membrane potential occurs and, after a variable length of time, permanent cellular damage results. Between 40 ml and 20 ml/100 gm/min, no functional abnormalities can be detected. However, when the basal flow values are diminished in this range, the collateral flow reserve is lower so that vascular occlusion would be more likely to be followed by stroke. It has also been shown experimentally that surrounding an area of dense ischemia, there is a *penumbra* zone, with blood flow values just below the threshold for synaptic blockade. Minimal improvements of blood flow or oxygen availability may produce major functional improvements in this region.

From: Sekhar LN, Schramm VL Jr, eds: *Tumors of the Cranial Base: Diagnosis and Treatment.* Mount Kisco, New York, Futura Publishing Co, Inc, © 1987.

In practical terms, whether a blood vessel can be safely occluded without the production of stroke and how long it can be occluded depend on the following factors: the size of the artery being occluded, the collateral circulation available, blood pressure, hematocrit, viscosity of the blood, and the aggregability of platelets and other blood components.[2] The pathogenesis of stroke may also be conceived of as being due to diminished flow caused by the occlusion of a large blood vessel, or due to embolic occlusion of smaller vessels resulting from a thrombus in a large vessel. Thus, even if blood flow is not significantly reduced after occlusion of a major blood vessel, distal thromboembolism from clots within the lumen of the vessel may produce a stroke.[7]

Preoperative Studies

During the preoperative evaluation of large cranial base tumors, angiography of the cerebral and cervical vessels is important to determine whether the blood vessels are patent, whether there is any narrowing or displacement, and to determine the potential sources of collateral circulation, particularly with respect to the circle of Willis. If one or both of the internal carotid arteries (ICA) are anticipated to be temporarily or permanently occluded during the operation, a balloon occlusion test is performed.[9,12] After heparinization, the vessel is temporarily occluded for 10–15 minutes with monitoring of the patient's neurological condition and the postocclusion stump pressure before and during test occlusion. If the test occlusion is clinically well tolerated, the test is repeated in the computed tomographic (CT) scanner, with measurements of CBF by the stable xenon-CT technique. On the basis of this test, patients may be classified into four groups:

Group I: Those who develop neurological deficits during test ICA occlusion are at high risk for the development of a stroke if the vessel is permanently occluded. They may tolerate a short period of temporary occlusion with the use of protective anesthetic agents. If the patient's ICA may have to be excised during operation because of tumor encasement, the surgeon should consider the performance of an extracranial to intracranial vascular bypass prior to the cranial base tumor operation. Such a bypass should be preferably a long saphenous vein graft from the external carotid artery to a major branch of the middle cerebral artery,[1,9] since a superficial temporal to middle cerebral artery does not carry a large volume of blood acutely.[11] Unfortunately, such long saphenous vein grafts have a high complication rate.[14] A direct vein graft reconstruction of the ICA with an intraluminal shunt is a technically more difficult alternative.

Group II: Patients who tolerate the balloon occlusion test clinically but develop CBF reduction in the range of 15 to 30 ml/100 gm/min will tolerate prolonged temporary occlusion but are at high risk for developing a stroke especially if there is hypovolemia or hypotension during the procedure. If the ICA of a patient in this group has to be excised, direct vein graft reconstruction, usually using a short length of saphenous vein (<5 cm), is recommended. This vein graft passes from a large vessel to another large vessel, and will have a high flow rate. An end-to-end rather than an end-to-side anastomosis is feasible at both ends, reducing turbulence. Both factors favor the long-term patency of the graft.[6,8] The use of high-dose steroids during the operation, and of aspirin and dipyridamole on a long-term basis postoperatively appear to favor the patency of such grafts.[3,6,10]

Group III: Patients who tolerate the test ICA occlusion well clinically but develop CBF reduction in the range of 30 to 40 ml/100 gm/min will tolerate permanent occlusion without a stroke, provided hypotension and hypovolemia are carefully avoided after such occlusion. When the ICA is permanently occluded in such a patient during operation, such occlusion should be as close to the ophthalmic artery as possible to minimize distal thromboembolism from a stump. Direct vein graft reconstruction of the ICA is optional, but may be considered for patients with benign tumors.

Group IV: Patients whose CBF remains above 40 ml/100 gm/min during test ICA occlusion are at least risk for development of a stroke after permanent ICA occlusion, provided embolism from a stump is avoided. In this group also, direct vein graft reconstruction of the ICA may be considered for patients with benign tumors, when the ICA is occluded during the operation.

Besides angiography, magnetic resonance imaging (MRI) has been found to be an invaluable tool in assessing the relationship of basal blood vessels to neoplasms. When a blood vessel is encased by a neoplasm, its angiographic appearance may be entirely normal, with no narrowing or displacement. However, the MRI scan accurately delineates this relationship (Fig. 1A–E).

Anesthesia and Monitoring

Anesthetic considerations during cranial base tumor surgery are discussed in detail in Chapter 6. When vascular occlusion is possible during surgery, hypotension and dehydration must be avoided. The author prefers brain relaxation by cerebrospinal fluid drainage, using diuresis induced by furosemide or mannitol only for cases where drainage is not possible. During temporary occlusion of major blood vessels, the anesthesiologist is asked to raise the blood pressure 20 torr above the baseline, and the blood pressure is normalized when flow is resumed. If there is extensive blood loss during the operation, the blood volume should be maintained, preferably with colloid replacement, and the hematocrit maintained between 30 and 35.

Monitoring of cerebral electrical activity may be useful to determine when an intraluminal shunt is needed. Electroencephalography, brain stem evoked response, and central conduction time may be used for such monitoring.

General Principles of Arterial Preservation and Reconstruction

Cranial arteries may be merely adherent to the periphery of a neoplasm, or may run right through the tumor. The arterial wall appears to be resistant to neoplastic invasion and arteries larger than 2 mm in diameter may remain patent for a long time even when they are encased by a locally invasive neoplasm. While attempting to dissect the artery from the neoplasm, it is crucial to start in an area where the vessel is normal and work towards the pathological area. It is ideal to have both proximal and distal control prior to dissection of large vessels, or at least proximal control. Dissection is performed sharply close to the adventitia of the vessel, parallel to the artery. The author prefers the use of the Rosen dissector, the Cottle elevator, and microscissors for the dissection. Tumor removal near the artery is performed with bipolar cautery. The use of the CO_2 laser for vaporization of the tumor from the arterial wall is discouraged. It is surprising how often tumors can be dissected away from arteries that are encased. Temporary clipping and suture of any tears of the vessel may be sometimes necessary during such dissection.

When the neoplasm cannot be dissected from the arterial wall, there are four options.[12] The first is to leave some tumor behind. The second is to excise the pathological segment and directly reconstruct the artery either with end-to-end suture or with a short interposition vein graft. The third option is to excise the artery along with involved tumor, and not to attempt reconstruction. This is acceptable when the artery is 1 mm or less in diameter. When the vessel involved is the vertebral or the ICA, occlusion without reconstruction is acceptable if the patient tolerated balloon occlusion without changes in neurological status and with minimal changes of cerebral blood flow. The artery must then be occluded as close to its next branch as possible (just proximal to the ophthalmic artery in the case of the ICA) to reduce the occurrence of

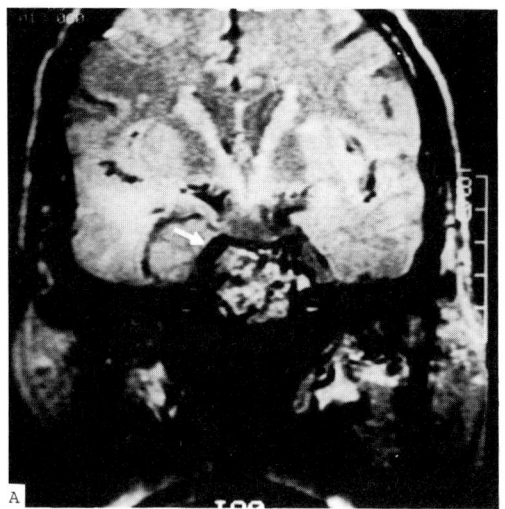
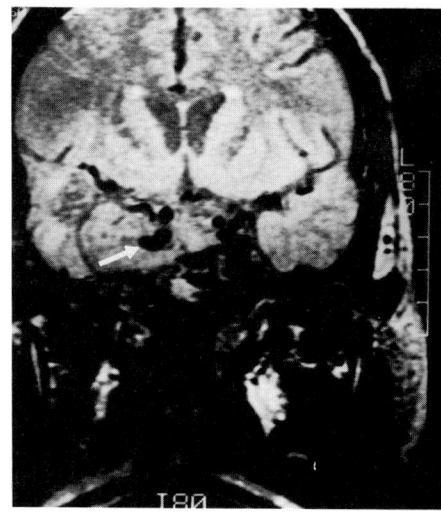
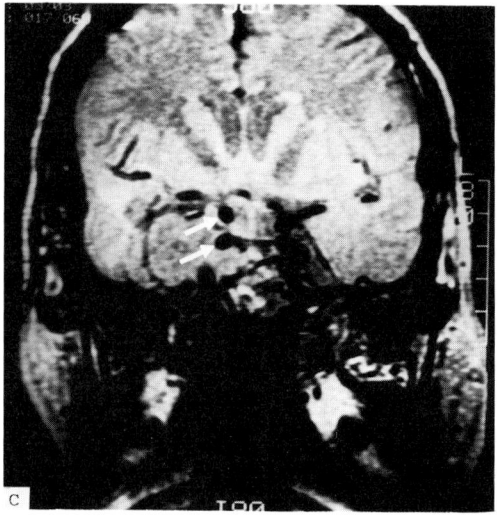

Figure 1: MRI images of a patient with middle fossa, cavernous sinus, and tuberculum sellae meningioma **(A, B, C)**. The relationship of the internal carotid artery and the middle cerebral artery to the neoplasm was not apparent from the CT scans **(D, E)** or from the cerebral angiogram, but is well shown by the MRI scans (arrows).

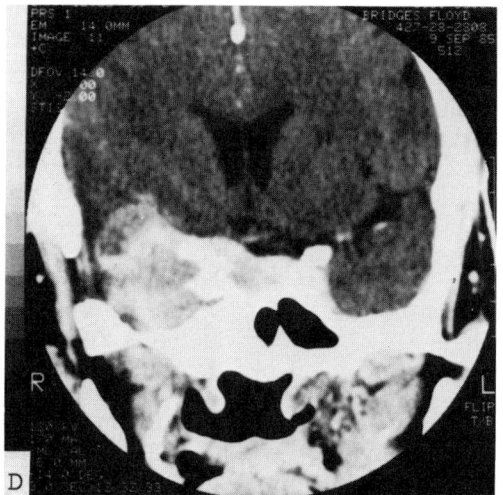
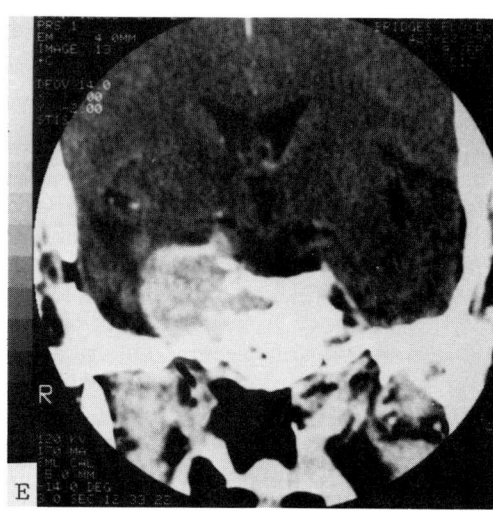

thromboembolism from a stump of the vessel. Hypovolemia and hypotension should be carefully avoided intraoperatively and postoperatively. The fourth option is to perform a long interposition vein graft or an arterial anastomosis to branch vessels well beyond the operative site. Examples are an external carotid to middle cerebral artery interposition vein graft, or a superficial temporal to middle cerebral artery branch (ST-MCA) anastomosis prior to occlusion of the ICA.[1,8,11] These options were discussed earlier in relation to the balloon occlusion test.

Preservation and Reconstruction of Veins

Cranial base neoplasms often involve venous sinuses and veins at the base of the brain such as the transverse and sigmoid sinus, the jugular bulb, the internal jugular vein, the cavernous sinus, the superior petrosal sinus, the inferior petrosal sinus, the sphenoparietal sinus, and the basilar venous plexus. Cerebral and orbital veins draining into these sinuses may be involved by neoplasm near their point of entry. Since the collateral circulation of the cerebral venous system is rich and will have developed further during the growth of the tumor into the venous system, the involved venous sinuses can generally be excised and the involved cerebral veins can be occluded near their point of entry into the venous sinus without major risk of venous infarction. The surgeon should try to preserve the venous collateral circulation as much as possible during the excision of the tumor. A careful study of the preoperative angiograms may reveal situations where the venous drainage of the temporal lobe (vein of Labbé, superficial middle cerebral vein, and deep middle cerebral vein) or of the cerebellum may be severely compromised by the neoplasm. In these cases, care should be taken to preserve existing venous drainage. Occasionally, reconstruction of the sagittal or the transverse sinus or of major cerebral veins is worthwhile. Because of a low flow rate, saphenous vein grafts used for venous sinus reconstruction are prone to thrombosis, but cerebral veins repaired by direct suture tend to remain open. The author has reconstructed two sagittal sinuses with saphenous vein grafts, and both were patent on postoperative angiography. Of two transverse sinuses reconstructed with vein grafts, one was patent and the other thrombosed, presumably due to a low flow rate, yet asymptomatic. Two major cortical veins were repaired with 9/0 nylon after intraoperative injury, and were both patent.

Exposure of Cerebral Arteries

The exposure of some basal cerebral arteries is discussed here since it is important for the management of cranial base neoplasms.

Upper Cervical and Petrous ICA

The upper cervical and petrous ICA often needs to be exposed during the resection of neoplasms of the petroclival and retropharyngeal areas. The method we prefer for the exposure of these vessels is outlined in Figures 2–7. An incision is started in the temporal region, and extended into the neck in front of the ear (Fig. 2). After reflecting the skin and subcutaneous flap forward, the facial nerve is dissected from the stylomastoid foramen through the parotid gland, to its distal branches in the face. The deeper portion of the parotid is mobilized as well. The ICA is exposed in the neck and dissected to the level of the styloid process (Fig. 3). The zygomatic arch is divided, and the temporalis muscle is reflected downward and forward. The mandibular condyle and the capsule of the temporomandibular joint are dissected free. For the exposure of the vertical segment of the petrous ICA, the condyle has to be merely displaced downwards, avoiding traction of the facial nerve. For optimal exposure of the segment of the ICA between the styloid process and the entrance into the carotid canal, resection of the condyle and neck of the mandible are essential (Fig. 4). Unila-

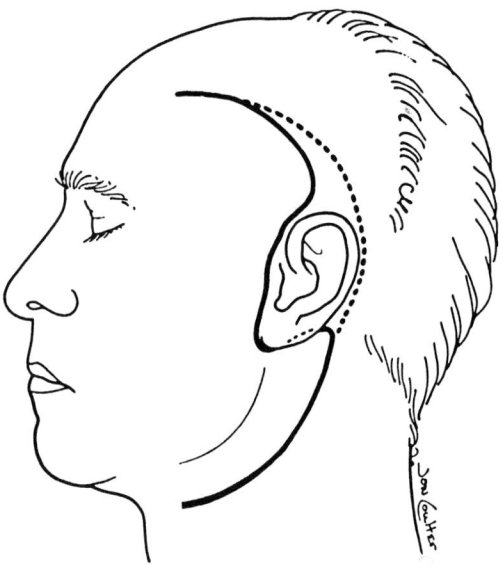

Figure 2: This figure illustrates the two types of incisions used for the exposure of the petrous and upper cervical ICA. The preauricular incision is preferred when the displacement of the facial nerve from the fallopian canal is not required. When the postauricular incision is used, the external ear canal is sutured shut as a blind sac and conductive hearing is sacrificed.

teral resection of the mandibular condyle does not cause any permanent disability.

A temporal craniotomy is performed along with the root of the zygomatic arch. About 50 cc of spinal fluid is withdrawn from the lumbar subarachnoid catheter to relax the brain. Under the microscope, the dura of the floor of the middle fossa is elevated to visualize the arcuate eminence, the greater superficial petrosal nerve (GSPN), the middle meningeal artery (MMA), and the mandibular nerve (V_3). The GSPN and MMA are divided, and the greater wing of the sphenoid bone rongeured to unroof V_3 (Figs. 5 and 6).

The petrous and tympanic bones deep to the temporomandibular joint are then drilled away starting near the floor of the middle fossa. The eustachian tube and tensor tympani muscle will be exposed and excised. The genu of the petrous ICA lies immediately deep to this region, and may be unroofed with curettes. The vertical segment of the petrous ICA may be unroofed with fine bone punches and the drill. At the entrance to the carotid canal, there is a dense fibrocartilaginous ring around the artery which has to be divided.

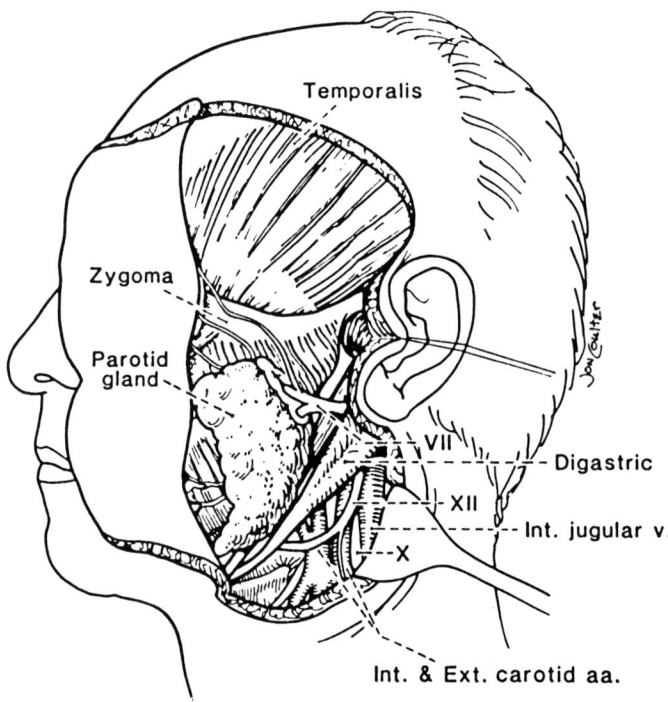

Figure 3: The skin and subcutaneous tissue flap has been reflected forward. The facial nerve has been dissected from the stylomastoid foramen through the parotid gland. The major vessels in the neck have been exposed. VII, X, XII = cranial nerves.

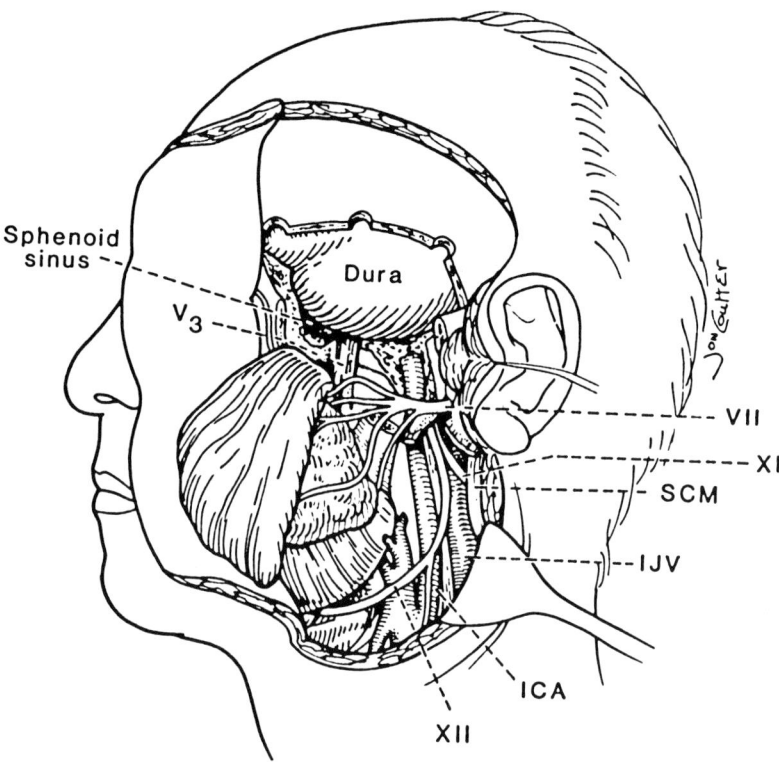

Figure 4: The temporalis muscle has been reflected down after division of the zygomatic arch, and a small craniotomy has been performed in the temporal area. The condyle of the mandible has been resected. When exposure of the upper cervical ICA between the styloid process and the carotid canal is not important, the condyle can be displaced inferiorly. The vertical segment of the ICA has been exposed after drilling away the petrous and the tympanic bone deep to the temporomandibular joint. The upper cervical ICA is being dissected. V_3 = mandilbular nerve; VII, XI, XII = cranial nerves; SCM = sternocleidomastoid muscle.

The upper cervical segment of the ICA is then dissected, working from above the facial nerve (Fig. 4). The styloid process is removed now, if not previously.

The horizontal segment of the ICA is then traced in an anteromedial direction (Fig. 6). V_3 has to be temporarily displaced to dissect the portion of the petrous ICA underlying the trigeminal ganglion, and V_3 may have to be divided for exposure of the ICA within the cavernous sinus. Care must be taken not to drill too much bone posterosuperior to the genu of the ICA, since the cochlea and the geniculate ganglion of the facial nerve are located here (Fig. 7).

A periosteal sheath and a venous plexus surround the petrous ICA. The periosteal sheath can be opened and the veins coagulated, if necessary. A Vidian branch and a caroticotympanic branch of the petrous ICA may rarely be encountered. 7/0 or 8/0 nylon sutures are appropriate for the repair of the petrous and the upper cervical ICA. When a vein graft repair is performed, the upper end is sutured first followed by the lower. After two stay sutures are placed at diametrically opposite points of the vein graft, a continuous suture is performed to complete the anastomosis.

When a retroauricular incision is used during operations for a glomus tumor, the external ear canal is divided and the flap reflected forward. The facial nerve may be unroofed in the fallopian canal entirely and reflected upward and forward. The remainder of the steps are as

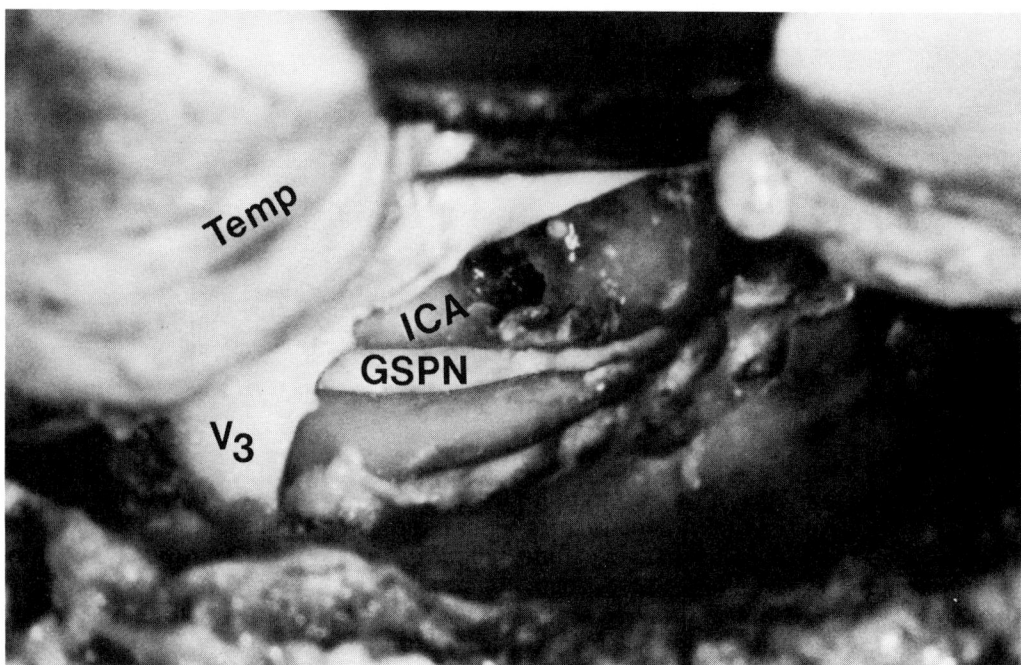

Figure 5: After cerebrospinal fluid drainage, the temporal dura has been elevated and held in place with a retractor. The important landmarks for the identification of the horizontal segment of the petrous ICA are shown. ICA = a small area of the carotid artery without a bony covering; GSPN = greater superficial petrosal nerve; V_3 = mandibular nerve.

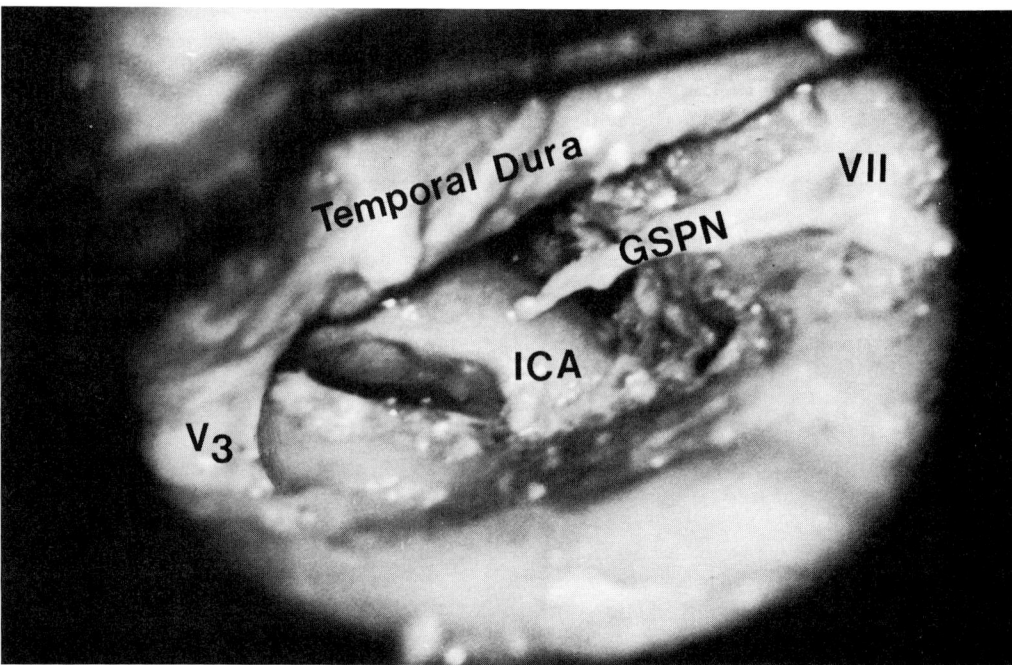

Figure 6: The horizontal segment of the petrous ICA lateral to the trigeminal ganglion has been exposed after removal of the bone with a drill and bone punches. The greater superficial petrosal nerve has been divided. The exposure of the geniculate ganglion and the facial nerve (VII) is not necessary but is shown to illustrate its relationship. V_3 = mandibular nerve.

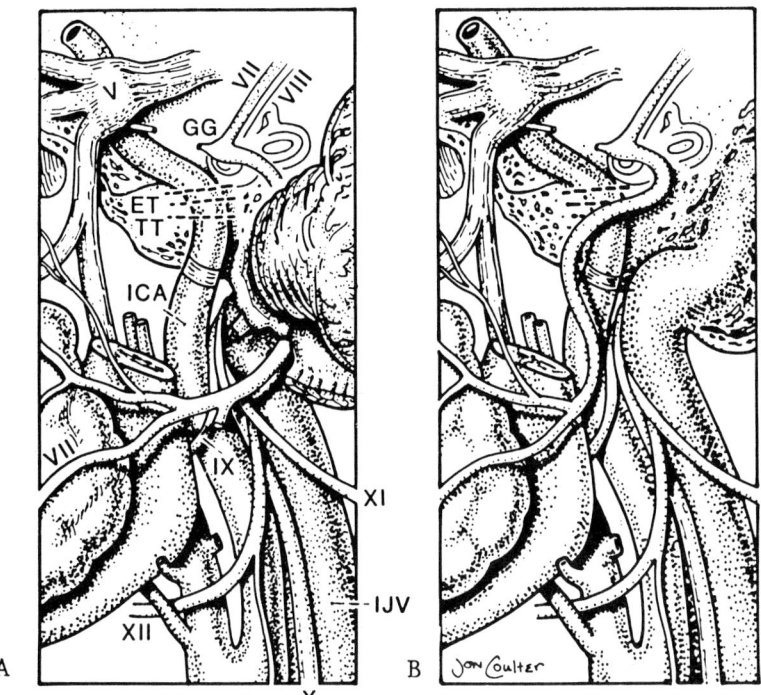

Figure 7: The entire upper cervical and petrous carotid artery area exposed except for the segment of the petrous ICA underlying the trigeminal ganglion. In order to expose this segment, one can displace the mandibular nerve temporarily forwards. Occasionally, it is necessary to divide it. Figure 7B shows the exposure when the retroauricular incision is used and the facial nerve is temporarily displaced upwards and forwards. The improved exposure of the facial recess, hypotympanic and jugular bulb area is illustrated. ET = eustachian tube; TT = tensor tympani muscle; GG =geniculate ganglion.

described above.[5] This technique provides slightly more room for work on the upper cervical and vertical petrous segment of the ICA, but is also associated with a prolonged facial paralysis, recovery may take up to 12 months (Fig. 7B).

When the petrous and upper cervical arteries are exposed to the nasopharynx or to the external surface after tumor resection, reconstruction using a rectus abdominis free flap or a myocutaneous flap is extremely important to prevent wound infection and arterial rupture postoperatively.

This author (along with V. Schramm, Jr., and N. Jones) has exposed and managed 29 upper cervical and petrous ICAs in 28 patients with cranial base neoplasms. The arteries were merely decompressed from the carotid canal in 12 patients, dissected free of encasing neoplasm in 13 patients, excised or occluded intentionally in three patients, and excised and reconstructed with vein grafts in four patients. One vein graft occluded asymptomatically in the early postoperative period, presumably due to an excessively swollen rectus abdominis muscle flap. Another patient whose artery was dissected free of neoplasm developed an occlusion 3 weeks later following an operation on the contralateral side. Unrecognized endothelial injury from the first operation, kinking of the artery due to excessive head turning, and perioperative hypercoagulability during the second operation may have all contributed to this occlusion. This patient suffered a right hemispheric stroke but recovered moderate function. Another patient suffered a delayed rupture of the ipsilateral upper cervical ICA 1 week postoperatively, and rupture of the contralateral petrous ICA 2 weeks postoperatively. The former was due to the exposure of the ICA to the nasopharynx, and was managed by excision of the bleeding segment of the artery and reanastomosis lateral to the facial nerve and a rectus abdominis muscle flap to isolate the nasopharynx. The contralateral ICA rupture was due to tumor erosion, and was managed by vascular occlusion. This patient was severely disabled, and died 2 months later from recurrent infection. All the other arteries are patent by cerebral angiography or by MRI scanning and the patients are asymptomatic.

Cavernous ICA

Exposure of the cavernous ICA is necessary during operations on cranial base neoplasms involving the cavernous sinus (CS).[4,13] There are three approaches for the exposure of the cavernous ICA (Fig. 8). The *inferior approach* is a continuation of the exposure of the horizontal segment of the petrous ICA. Division of V_3 may be necessary for this exposure, and the ICA can be followed to the crossing point of the abducens nerve. For the *lateral approach*, the cranial nerves in the lateral wall of the CS are dissected and the CS is entered between the trochlear and ophthalmic (V_1) nerves, or between the ophthalmic and maxillary nerves (V_2). Any bleeding from the cavernous venous plexus is controlled by packing with oxydized cellulose. Tumor removal is carried out piecemeal until the ICA is identified. The ICA can then be followed, removing tumor along the way. Alternately, when the meningohypophyseal branch of

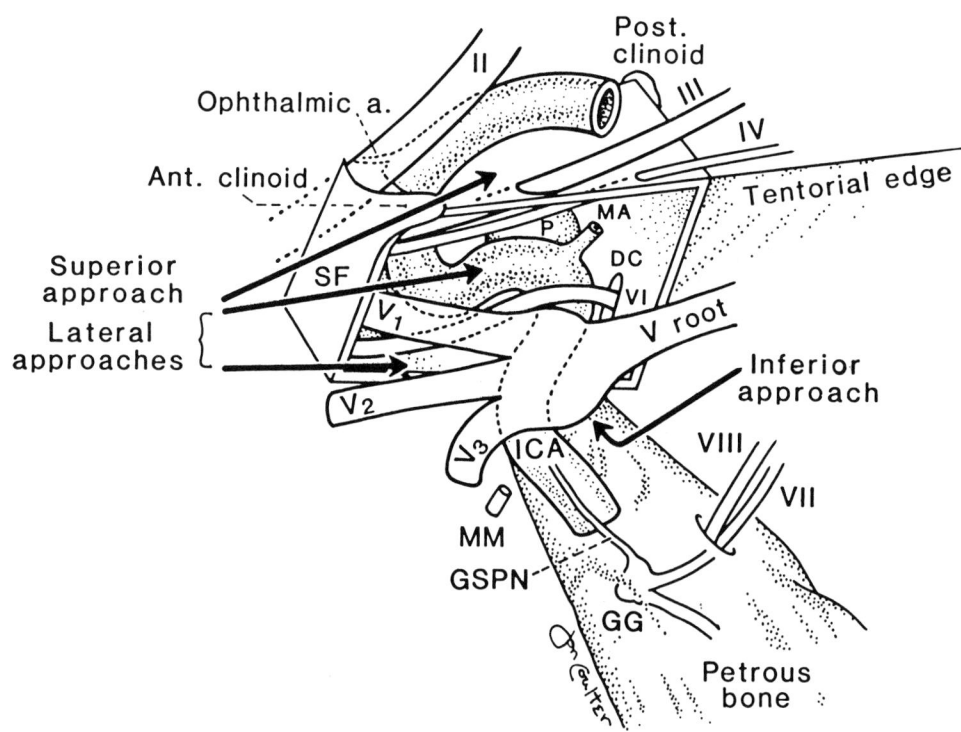

Figure 8: The operative approaches used for the exposure of the intracavernous carotid artery. The lateral approach enters the cavernous sinus between the fourth cranial nerve and ophthalmic (V_1) or between the ophthalmic and the maxillary (V_2) nerves. For the superior approach, the bony optic canal is unroofed and the anterior clinoid process is removed. The optic nerve is mobilized after opening the dural sheath. The superior wall of the cavernous sinus is then opened and the internal carotid artery is followed from above into the cavernous sinus. The inferior approach is from the infratemporal fossa and follows the internal carotid artery from the petrous apex region.

the ICA is identified, it can be followed to the ICA. For the *superior approach*, the anterior clinoid process is removed, the superior and lateral aspects of the optic canal are unroofed, and the dura around the optic nerve is opened to mobilize it. The superior wall of the CS is then opened, and the supraclinoid ICA is followed into the CS. There is often a dense dural band at the exit of the ICA from the CS. The ophthalmic artery usually arises just outside the CS, but may have its origin inside in some cases. Generally, in order to expose the entire cavernous ICA, a combination of approaches is needed. Tears of the artery can be repaired after temporary clipping. A saphenous vein graft to bypass the cavernous ICA (from the petrous ICA to the supraclinoid ICA) is possible, but has not been used by us.[13]

The author has exposed the cavernous ICA 16 times during operations on 16 patients with cavernous sinus neoplasma. Two arteries were intentionally occluded. The remaining arteries were preserved after tumor excision. Two arteries required suture of intraoperative tears after temporary clipping. Fourteen of 16 arteries were patent on postoperative angiography. None of these arteries ruptured postoperatively, and none of the patients suffered a postoperative stroke.

Intradural Internal Carotid Artery and Major Branches

When the intracranial ICA or its main branches are encased by neoplasm, the surgeon must first obtain proximal control of either the petrous or cervical segment. After opening the dura, the Sylvian fissure is opened from a lateral to medial direction (Figs. 9A, B, and 10). The middle cerebral artery (MCA) is then identified and followed to the ICA bifurcation. The tumor is then dissected from the vessels gradually (Fig. 11). Encasement of the ICA is common with medial sphenoid wing and parasellar meningiomas, and the anterior cerebral artery or its branches are often adherent to or encased by tuberculum sellae and olfactory groove meningiomas.

Vertebral and Basilar Artery

The extracranial vertebral artery may be encased by or be adherent to cranial

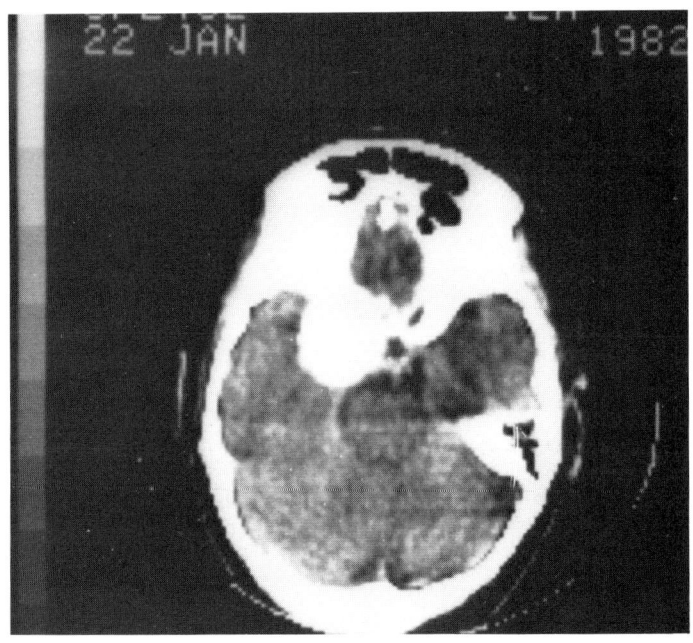

Figure 9A: Axial and coronal CT scans showing a medial sphenoid wing meningioma in a 67-year-old woman who presented with headaches, partial visual loss, and partial third nerve palsy.

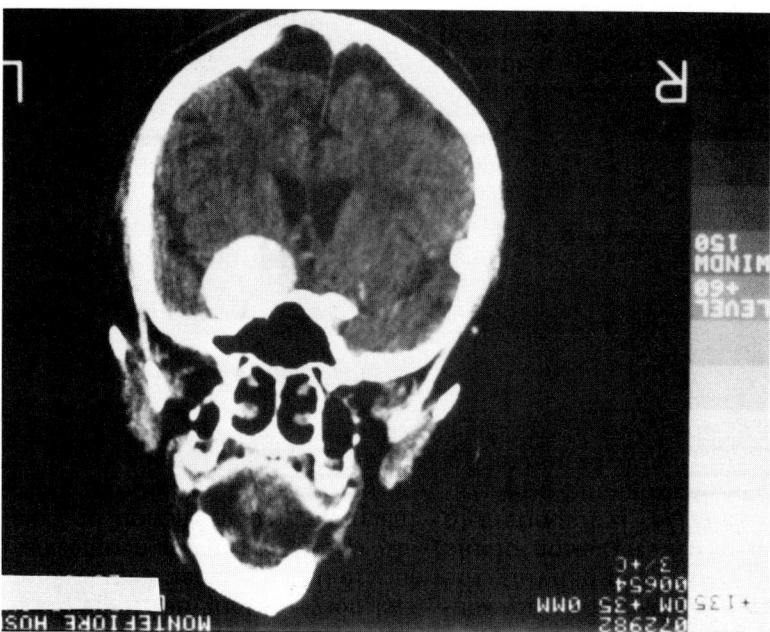

Figure 9B.

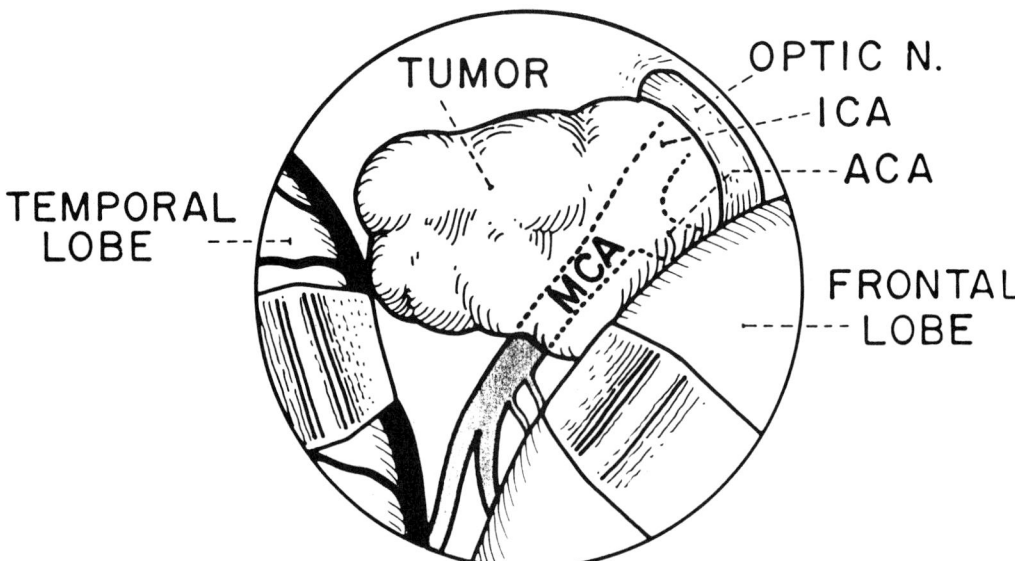

Figure 10: Operative exposure after a frontotemporal craniotomy and the splitting of the sylvian fissure. The proximal portion of the middle cerebral artery (MCA), the anterior cerebral artery (ACA), and the supraclinoid internal carotid artery (ICA) were totally encased by tumor. The optic nerve was stretched over the medial aspect of the tumor.

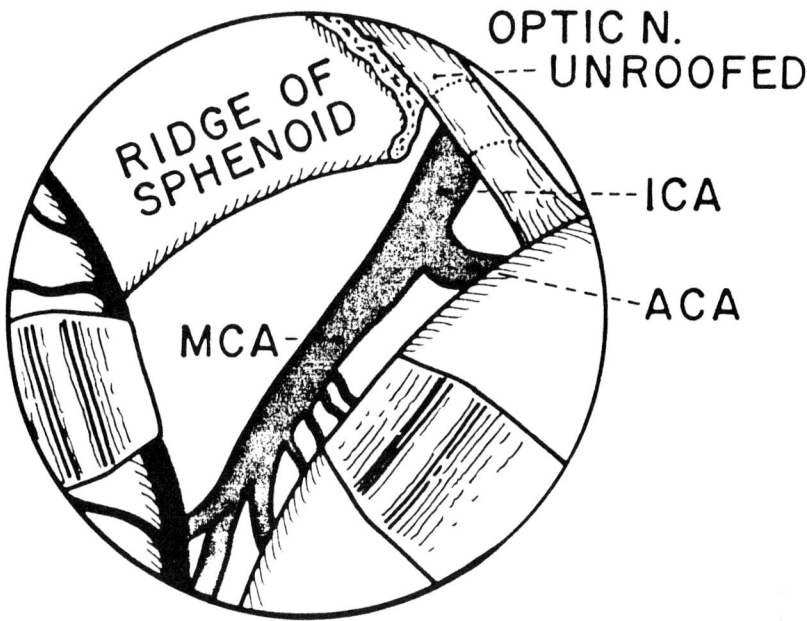

Figure 11: After unroofing the optic nerve in the bony and dural canal, the pressure on the nerve has been released. The middle cerebral, internal carotid, and anterior cerebral arteries have been dissected free of tumor, starting from the sylvian fissure and progressing toward the cavernous sinus region. The tumor was removed completely and the patient's postoperative course was uneventful.

base neoplasms after its exit from the foramen transversorium of the first cervical vertebra (C_1). The vertebral artery may also be encased by neoplasms after its entrance into the dura. Proximal control of the vertebral artery can be obtained in the former situation by unroofing the C_1 foramen, and in the latter situation by exposing the vertebral artery extradurally where it lies on the superior surface of the C_1 arch. Tumor encasement of the distal vertebral artery or of the basilar artery is difficult to manage and remains a problem to be solved. Major branches of the vertebrobasilar system such as the posterior inferior cerebellar artery or the superior cerebellar artery may be encased by meningiomas, and can generally be dissected free of neoplasm if the vessels are larger than 2 mm in diameter.

The author has dissected the vertebral artery free of encasing neoplasm in three patients, two extradurally, and one intradurally. The former two patients required suture of small tears with temporary clipping. All arteries are patent postoperatively and no one suffered a stroke.

Conclusion

Since damage to basal blood vessels is a major cause of morbidity and mortality after excision of cranial base neoplasms, the improved management of these vessels will improve our ability to resect more complex neoplasms and reduce the complications. Many problems in this area are likely to be solved by the application of the techniques of cerebrovascular surgery and a knowledge of the pathophysiology of stroke.

References

1. Ausman JI, Pearce JE, De Los Reyes RA, et al: Treatment of a high extracranial carotid artery aneurysm with CCA-MCA bypass and carotid ligation. *J Neurosurg* 58:421-424, 1983.

2. Countee RW, Vijayanathan T, Hubschmann OR, et al: Carotid ligation for recurrent ischemia due to inaccessible carotid obstruction. J Neurosurg 53:491-499, 1980.
3. Deen HG, Jr, Sundt TM, Jr: Mechanism of thrombotic occlusion of interposition vein grafts in the canine carotid artery: A role for combined aspirin and dipyridamole therapy. Presentation at the AANS Meeting, Atlanta, GA, April 24-29, 1985.
4. Dolenc V: Direct microsurgical repair of intracavernous vascular lesions. J Neurosurg 58:824-831, 1983.
5. Fisch UP, Oldring DJ, Senning A: Surgical therapy of internal carotid artery lesions of the skull base and temporal bone. Otolaryngol Head Neck Surg 88:548-554, 1980.
6. Fuster V, Chesebro JH, Steele PM: Concepts of platelet interaction with the development of cardiovascular pathology and interference with platelet inhibition. Cardiovasc Reviews Reports 6:65-76, 1985.
7. Landolt AM, Millikan CH: Pathogenesis of cerebral infarction secondary to mechanical carotid artery occlusion. Stroke 1:52-62, 1970.
8. Little JR, Furlan AJ, Bryerton B: Short vein grafts for cerebral revascularization. J Neurosurg 59:384-388, 1983.
9. Miller JD, Javad K, Jennett B: Safety of carotid ligation and its role in the management of intracranial aneurysms. J Neurosurg Psych 40:64-72, 1977.
10. Pearce J, Dujovny M, Ausman JI, et al: Vein grafts used as arterial replacements: Prevention of endothelial injury. Presented at the AANS Meeting, Atlanta, GA, April 24-29, 1985.
11. Samson DS, Newelt EA, Beyer CW, et al: Failure of extracranial-intracranial arterial bypass in acute middle cerebral artery occlusion: Case report. Neurosurgery 16:111-116, 1985.
12. Sekhar LN, Schramm Jr VL, Jones NF et al: Operative exposure and management of the petrous and upper cervical internal carotid artery. Neurosurgery 19:967-982, 1986.
13. Sekhar LN, Moller AR: Operative management of tumors involving the cavernous sinus. J Neurosurg 64:879-889, 1986.
14. Sundt TM, Jr, Piepgras DG, Houser OW, et al: Interposition vein grafts for advanced occlusive disease and large aneurysms in the posterior circulation. J Neurosurg 56:205-215, 1982.

13

Preservation and Reconstruction of Cranial Nerves During the Removal of Cranial Base Neoplasms

Laligam N. Sekhar, M.D.

Introduction

The preservation of cranial nerve function during operations on cranial base tumors greatly improves the quality of life postoperatively and may reduce mortality by preventing pneumonia and undernutrition. When such preservation is not possible, the reconstruction of the injured nerve or alternative methods of rehabilitation are important.

Principles of Cranial Nerve Preservation

The potential for preservation of the cranial nerves during operations on cranial base neoplasms is enhanced by the surgeon's knowledge of the pathological anatomy, microdissection techniques, intraoperative neurophysiological monitoring, and appropriate anesthetic management.

Neurophysiological monitoring helps the surgeon to locate cranial nerves when they are displaced by neoplasms and to avoid injury to them during dissection, or by retraction or coagulation. Occlusion of arteries supplying the nerve and delayed infarction is one mechanism of injury that may not be preventable by the use of monitoring. Details of the use of neurophysiological monitoring are discussed in Chapter 7. Anesthetic agents and techniques may need to be adjusted to facilitate the monitoring requirements. For instance, when motor function is being monitored, long-acting paralytic agents should be avoided.

During the removal of the neoplasm, the surgeon should be aware of the general location of the cranial nerve from the preoperative studies, previous experience, intraoperative observations, or intraoperative stimulation. The core of the neoplasm is then resected, working in an area removed from the cranial nerve to be preserved. The tumor is then dissected away from the cranial nerve, working with sharp microinstruments and magnification, and always dissecting from the normal to the abnormal area, and parallel to the nerve to be preserved. Careful

From: Sekhar LN, Schramm VL Jr, eds: *Tumors of the Cranial Base: Diagnosis and Treatment.* Mount Kisco, New York, Futura Publishing Co, Inc, © 1987.

neurophysiological observation and feedback to the surgeon are especially important during such dissection. It is also important to preserve the vascular supply of cranial nerves, especially that of the optic and the vestibulocochlear nerves. After the nerve has been dissected free, it is covered with nonadhesive material such as gel foam or a piece of rubber glove, rather than placing cotton patties directly on it. This prevents the injury to the nerve that may occur when cotton patties are removed at the end of the operation.

Principles of Cranial Nerve Reconstruction

When a cranial nerve cannot be preserved during an operation, those nerves which are sheathed by peripheral myelin should be reconstructed either by direct suture or by the use of an autologous nerve graft. The sural nerve is an ideal graft, but one may also use other nerves such as the great auricular or the medial antebrachial cutaneous. The nerve ends are stabilized over gel foam, and one or two sutures of 10/0 nylon are adequate to hold the ends in approximation. With respect to cranial nerves sheathed by central myelin, experimental evidence indicates that it may be possible to reconstruct them in the future, using peripheral nerve grafts.[1,12]

Olfactory Nerve

The olfactory nerve is very short and ends at the olfactory bulb. The surgeon must try to preserve at least one olfactory tract in patients with smaller olfactory groove meningiomas, and in all patients with tuberculum sellae meningiomas. Reconstruction of this nerve is not possible at this time.

Optic Nerve

The optic nerve is totally covered with central myelin, and its reconstruction may be possible in the future by using peripheral nerve grafts placed from the optic bulb to the lateral geniculate body. At present, preservation of function of the nerve is the only way to preserve vision after the excision of basal tumors. The blood supply of the optic nerve and chiasm are derived from the internal carotid artery, the anterior cerebral artery, and the ophthalmic artery. When the optic nerve is markedly bowed by a tumor underlying it, the nerve may be completely decompressed from the membranous and the bony optic canal prior to tumor resection. This maneuver releases the pressure on the nerve and also enables the identification of the ophthalmic artery. For the resection of tumors that are stretching both optic nerves and the chiasm, the use of a combination of approaches, such as the pterional and the unilateral subfrontal, may allow optimal visualization of all components of the nerve without much of a "blind spot." Intraoperative monitoring of visual evoked responses and direct optic nerve action potentials is in a state of evolution at present and needs to be further improved.[5] Occasionally, neoplasms such as craniopharyngiomas share their blood supply with the optic nerve or chiasm and the dissection of the capsule of the tumor may cause infarction of the nerve and visual loss. In the postoperative period, the use of high dose steroids and measures that improve the microcirculation may help to reverse visual deficits.

Oculomotor Nerve

The oculomotor nerve is the most important one for the control of ocular mobility and innervates many antagonistic muscles. It is commonly involved by neoplasms which invade the cavernous sinus, or the apex of the orbit. Neurophysiological monitoring is helpful to identify and preserve this nerve during the resection of such tumors.[10] Even if the ocular muscles are paralyzed at the end of the operation, a good functional recovery is possible if the nerve is anatomically well preserved. Such recovery occurs within 2 months in the event of neurapraxia, and within 8 months in the event of axonotmesis. Aberrant regeneration is common with axonotmetic lesions, but usually does not cause a functional disability.[3,4]

A functional recovery of ocular motility has been reported after oculomotor nerve suture in one patient by Yasargil, and an excellent quality of recovery was obtained after experimental suture in cats.[7,8,11] Graft reconstruction of the oculomotor nerve has not been performed to date in human patients, but should be tried under appropriate circumstances.[9]

Trochlear Nerve

The trochlear nerve is thin and easily damaged during the removal of cranial base neoplasms. Fortunately, its loss is associated with minimal functional disability. A good recovery of function has been reported after the suture of an injured trochlear nerve.[2]

Abducens Nerve

The abducens nerve has the longest course through the cavernous sinus (CS), and is very liable to be injured during the removal of neoplasms of the CS when it is totally encased. Preservation of the abducens nerve during the removal of neoplasma of the clivus and of the CS can be aided by neurophysiological monitoring. When the nerve is injured during the removal of CS tumors, it can be reconstructed with a graft from the posterior fossa to the orbit.[9] Since the nerve is purely motor and it supplies a single muscle, a good quality of recovery may be expected. When nerve reconstruction is not possible, ocular muscle surgery can be useful for rehabilitation.

Trigeminal Nerve

The trigeminal nerve is mainly sensory, its motor part accompanying the third division (V_3). Preservation of the ophthalmic division (V_1) is important to prevent corneal ulceration, and preservation of its motor division is important for the function of the jaw. In addition, sensory denervation may result in a disturbing dysethesiae and pain.

Because of its long course, the root, ganglion, and the divisions of the trigeminal nerve may be involved by many different types of cranial base neoplasms. Reconstruction of the peripheral divisions of the trigeminal nerve is possible and should be considered if there is an injury during the operation.[6]

Facial Nerve

A functioning facial nerve makes a great difference to the patient's quality of life. The intradural part of the nerve may be involved by lesions such as acoustic neurilemmomas and meningiomas, the intratemporal portion of the nerve by neoplasms such as squamous cell carcinoma, and the peripheral portion of the nerve by parotid gland neoplasms. Schwannomas of the facial nerve are rare, but may occur anywhere along the course of the nerve, usually in the intradural or the intratemporal portion. One should attempt to preserve the facial nerve physiologically during the removal of benign neoplasms except for facial nerve schwannomas. The functional preservation of the nerve rather than mere anatomical preservation is an advance in cranial base tumor surgery in recent years. This has been made possible by the use of monitoring of facial electromyographic activity, and the refinement of microsurgical techniques during the recent years (see Chapter 29). When function cannot be preserved, one must strive to preserve anatomical continuity of the nerve since recovery by regeneration usually follows within a year. Some degree of synkinesis is always associated with the latter.

With malignant neoplasms and facial nerve schwannomas, a segment of the facial nerve usually has to be resected. Injury to the nerve may also occur occasionally with other benign neoplasms. In such instances, reconstruction of facial nerve by direct suture or grafting must always be attempted, since the facial nerve regenerates vigorously, and the quality of function is always better than after a hypoglossal-facial nerve anastomosis. The sural nerve is ideal for grafting, but the greater auricular nerve may also be used. Facial nerve grafts may be placed from the brain stem to the mastoid segment through the temporal bone (Samii-Draf technique), or from the brain stem to the nerve at the stylomastoid foramen (Dott technique) after the resection of cerebellopontine angle lesions. A technique similar to the Dott procedure can also be used after the resection of temporal bone neoplasms (see Chapter 34). When the facial nerve is injured or resected during the removal of parotid gland neoplasms, the sural nerve and its branches may be used for reconstruction. Another alternative is to use facial-facial nerve anastomosis to reinnervate the uper face, and hypoglossal-facial anastamosis to reinnervate the lower face.

When a proximal stump of the facial nerve is not available for grafting, hypoglossal-facial nerve anastomosis is preferred over crossed facial-facial nerve anastomosis since the functional results are better with the former. After hypoglossal-facial nerve anastamosis, the ansa hypoglossi is sutured to the distal stump of the divided hypoglossal nerve. The hypoglossal nerve may also be divided into two fascicular groups, one being anastomosed to the facial nerve stump, with the preservation of tongue function (Sekhar LN, unpublished data).

Vestibulocochlear Nerve

The vestibulocochlear nerve is covered with central myelin from the brain stem to just within the porous acousticus, and is very easily damaged by operative manipulation. For the preservation of hearing, one needs to save not only the cochlear nerve, but also the internal auditory artery, which supplies the cochlea. Preservation of hearing should be attempted particularly in patients who have a hearing loss of 50 dB or less, and a speech discrimination score of 40% or more. If the patient has a hearing loss on the opposite side, maintenance of any hearing is worthwhile. Intraoperative monitoring of the brain stem evoked response, and of cochlear nerve action potentials with an electrode placed directly on the nerve, have proved very useful in the preservation of hearing. During the removal of acoustic neuromas and other lesions of the cerebellopontine angle, it is important to debulk the mass of the tumor initially and dissect the vestibulocochlear nerve subsequently. Sharp rather than blunt dissection along the direction of the nerve is also important. When the temporal bone is drilled for the exposure of the porous acousticus, one must be careful not to damage the posterior semicircular canal, since such damage may produce loss of hearing.

Successful reconstruction of the vestibulocochlear nerve has not been done to date. However, it may be possible to reconstruct it with a peripheral nerve graft placed from the part within the porous acousticus to the cochlear nucleus, which is very accessible in the floor of the lateral recess of the fourth ventricle.[1] In view of the extremely specific tonotopic organization within the cochlear nerve, it remains to be seen if useful hearing will result even if regeneration occurs through the graft.[12] Direct stimulation of the cochlear nucleus by implanted electrodes is being tried at present on an experimental basis in patients who have lost the vestibulocochlear nerve.

Glossopharyngeal and Vagus Nerves

The ninth and tenth cranial nerves are important for the function of the voice and swallowing. Bilateral denervation of the vagus does not seem to have any permanent effects on cardiac or gastrointestinal function, but greatly affects phonation, coughing, and deglutition. Unilateral damage to the glossopharyngeal and vagus nerve usually causes temporary dysphagia and dysphonia. A tracheostomy is occasionally needed to guard against aspiration pneumonia during this period. If problems persist, Teflon injection of the vocal cord function is adequate to restore function. Bilateral injury to the recurrent laryngeal nerves, however, is extremely difficult to manage. Recurrent laryngeal nerve resuture, ansa hypoglossi to recurrent laryngeal nerve anastomosis, and phrenic to recurrent laryngeal anastomosis have been tried experimentally in animals, and in humans. However, these techniques have not proven satisfactory at present and further experience is needed.[6]

Accessory Nerve

The cranial portion of the accessory nerve contributes to pharyngeal and laryngeal function, while the spinal portion supplies the sternomastoid and trapezius muscles. However, damage to the spinal accessory nerve does not invariably result in atrophy of these muscles, since the second and third cervical roots appear to be able to compensate for the loss in some patients. When this does not occur, reconstruction of the accessory nerve should be attempted at any level since it regenerates very vigorously. In addition to peripheral accessory nerve reconstruction, successful recovery has been observed after placing a sural nerve graft from the intracranial spinal accessory nerve to the extracranial portion (Sekhar LN, unpublished data).

Hypoglossal Nerve

The hypoglossal nerve is commonly involved by neoplasms in the clivus and jugular foramen area. It is also commonly used for facial nerve reconstruction. Unilateral loss of hypoglossal nerve function is generally well tolerated by the patient. When there is an associated paralysis of the glossopharyngeal and vagus nerves, the dysphagia may be quite marked. In the rare situation where the opposite hypoglossal nerve has been previously damaged, it would be crucial to preserve or to reconstruct the nerve.

Since the hypoglossal nerve is purely motor and is well known for its vigorous regenerative capability, a good recovery may be expected after reconstruction. I have resutured the nerve in one patient at the hypoglossal foramen, and in another patient, reconstructed it with a sural nerve graft in the neck. The former patient has not recovered function, while the latter has.

The Author's Series

The author's experience with cranial nerve reconstruction is summarized in Table I. The majority of these were performed in patients with cranial base neoplasms. From this limited experience, it

Table I
Cranial Nerve Reconstruction Series

Cranial Nerve	Type of Procedure	Total	Good	Fair	Poor	Too Early
Oculomotor	Resuture	1	—	—	—	1
Trigeminal (mandibular)	Graft reconstruction	3	2	1	—	—
Facial	Resuture	1	1	—	—	—
	Intra-extracranial graft	9	4	—	1	4
	Hypoglossal-facial	4	—	4	—	—
Spinal accessory	Intra-extracranial graft	1	1	—	—	—
	Extracranial graft	2	1	1	—	—
Hypoglossal	Resuture	1	—	—	1	—
	Extracranial graft	1	1	—	—	—
Total Number		23	10	6	2	5

appears that reconstruction of damaged cranial nerves should be attempted whenever possible.

Conclusion

Cranial base neoplasms pose several challenges to surgeons for the preservation and reconstruction of cranial nerves. An improved performance in this area will greatly reduce the morbidity of these operations.

ACKNOWLEDGMENT: The author gratefully acknowledges the inspiration provided by Prof. M. Samii.

References

1. Freed WJ, Medinacelli L, Wyatt RJ: Promoting functional plasticity in the damaged nervous system. Science 227:1544-1552, 1985.
2. Grimson BS, Ross MJ, Tyson G: Return of function after intracranial suture of the trochlear nere. J Neurosurg 61:191-192, 1984.
3. Hamer J: Incidence and prognosis of oculomotor palsy after subarachnoid hemorrhage due to ruptured aneurysms of the posterior communicating artery. In Samii M, Jannetta PJ, eds: The Cranial Nerves. New York, Springer-Verlag, 1981, pp 237-240.
4. Kerns JM, Smith DR, Jannotta FS, et al: Oculomotor nerve regeneration after aneurysm surgery. Am J Ophthalmol 87:225-233, 1979.
5. Moller AR, Burgess J, Sekhar LN: Potentials evoked from the optic nerve in monkeys and man. Electroencephalography Clin Neurophysiol (in press).
6. Samii M, Jannetta PJ, eds: The Cranial Nerves, New York, Springer-Verlag, 1981, p 649.
7. Sandvoss G, Cervos-Navarro J, Yasargil MG: Intracranial repair of oculomotor nerve in cats. Neurochirurgia (in press).
8. Sandvoss G, Smith RD, Yasargil MG: Experimentelle microchirurgische freileguarg der Lirnnerver III, IV and VI bei der Katse. Neurochirurgia 27:129-132, 1984.
9. Sekhar LN, Burgess J, Akin O: An anatomical study of the cavernous sinus with special reference to the operative approaches and reconstruction. Unpublished manuscript.
10. Sekhar LN, Moller A: Operative management of neoplasms involving the cavernous sinus. J Neurosurg 64:879-889, 1986.
11. Yasargil MG: Personal communication, 1985.
12. Zakon H, Capranica RR: Reformation of organized connections in the auditory system after regeneration of the eighth nerve. Science 213:242-244, 1981.

14

Methods of Cranial Base Reconstruction

Neil Ford Jones, M.D.

Introduction

Tumors involving the cranial base continue to pose a challenge to the neurosurgeon, ENT surgeon, and plastic surgeon. With refinements in CT scanning and NMR scanning, preoperative localization of these tumors and appreciation of their intracranial and extracranial extension is more easily accomplished. Craniofacial surgical techniques have allowed better visualization of tumors of the anterior cranial fossa[20-23] and the development of the infratemporal fossa approach has permitted better exposure of tumors of the middle and posterior fossa.[15-18]

Apart from preoperative localization and operative exposure, the other major problem is the close proximity of the paranasal sinuses and the nasopharynx to the exposed dura of the frontal and temporal lobes and posterior fossa following wide resection of these cranial base tumors. CSF leakage through the site of a dural repair may allow infection to ascend from the nasopharynx or paranasal sinuses into the extradural space to produce fulminant meningitis. It has been estimated that persistent CSF leakage is associated with meningitis in approximately one-third of postoperative cases. With better visualization of the tumor ensuring its complete intra- and extracranial resection, reconstruction of the resultant defect becomes crucial to reducing morbidity and mortality by (1) sealing any CSF leaks to prevent meningitis, (2) obliterating any open paranasal sinuses, (3) restoring continuity to the lateral and posterior pharyngeal walls, and (4) covering any exposed dural repair or dural graft with well-vascularized tissue.

Dural repair must be as secure as possible and preferably should be covered by transposition of well-vascularized tissue. Should a segment of dura need to be resected along with the en bloc excision of the tumor, the resulting dural defect should first be reconstructed using autogenous fascia lata or lyophilized dura and the graft covered with vascularized tissue.

As with reconstructive surgery in other areas of the body, the various options available may be considered as a reconstructive hierarchy consisting of (1)

From: Sekhar LN, Schramm VL Jr, eds: *Tumors of the Cranial Base: Diagnosis and Treatment*. Mount Kisco, New York, Futura Publishing Co, Inc, © 1987.

split-thickness skin grafts, (2) local flaps of skin, galeal-pericranial tissue or muscle, (3) distant pedicled musculocutaneous flaps—pectoralis major, latissimus dorsi, or extended trapezius musculocutaneous flaps, and (4) free flaps. Local flaps are segments of tissue adjacent to the defect in the cranial base that may be mobilized and transposed to cover this defect. The scalp flap, forehead flap, galeal-pericranial flap, and the temporalis muscle are all examples of local flaps that may be used in cranial base reconstruction. The pectoralis major, latissimus dorsi, and extended trapezius flaps are examples of distant flaps in which an island of skin is vascularized by musculocutaneous perforators from the underlying muscle which is itself mobilized to allow transposition of the muscle and the overlying skin island to a distant site. A free flap or free tissue transfer is an island of skin or a specific muscle which is specifically supplied by an identifiable artery and vein. The skin island or muscle is transferred from one area of the body to reconstruct a defect in another area of the body, and is immediately revascularized by microsurgical anastomoses of its arterial and venous pedicle to an artery and vein in the vicinity of the defect.

Reconstruction of the cranial base may be classified according to the location of the surgical defect and may most logically be divided into reconstruction of the anterior, middle, and posterior cranial base corresponding to the anterior, middle, and posterior cranial fossae. However, Jackson[20,23] has published another classification dividing the cranial base into anterior and posterior areas. The anterior area is synonymous with the anterior cranial fossa but the posterior area is divided into three segments: an anterior segment extending from the posterior wall of the orbit to the anterior border of the petrous temporal bone, a central segment consisting of the petrous temporal bone itself, and a posterior segment extending from the posterior border of the petrous temporal bone to the midline of the posterior cranial fossa.

Anterior Cranial Base

The frontal bones, frontal ethmoid and sphenoid sinuses, nasopharynx, nasal septum, and orbital contents are directly related to the anterior cranial fossa. Tumors of the maxilla, maxillary antrum, and skin of the midface may spread aggressively to invade the ethmoid sinuses, the cribriform plate, dura, and the frontal lobes in the anterior cranial fossa. Non-malignant tumors that may involve the anterior cranial fossa include osteomas, chondromas, parotid tumors, and neurofibromas. Malignant tumors include squamous cell carcinomas, basal cell carcinomas, malignant melanomas, and adenocarcinoma, adenoidcystic and mucoepidermoid carcinomas of the parotid.

A combined facial and intracranial resection of an ethmoid sinus carcinoma was described in 1954.[40] Ketcham,[25] utilized this combined approach for en bloc resection of paranasal sinus tumors in 19 patients. The exposed dura in the floor of the anterior cranial fossa was covered by a split-thickness skin graft. In their follow-up analysis of 31 patients, Ketcham et al.[26,43] reported that in only eight patients was there 100% take of the skin graft over the exposed dura of the anterior fossa defect and re-epithelialization was often delayed. Fifteen patients developed CSF leakage, and four patients developed meningitis, two of whom had split-thickness skin grafts applied over dural patch grafts. Two of these patients with meningitis subsequently died. Finally, one patient developed hemorrhaging from the carotid artery due to failure of the split-thickness skin graft to take over this area. These studies revealed the extreme importance of adequate coverage of the exposed dura and brain following removal of cranial base tumors. Skin grafts would appear to be inadequate in this situation, especially when large dural defects have required fascia lata grafting. Flap reconstruction would therefore appear to be mandatory. Split-thickness skin grafts have also been applied directly to the dura following radical cranio-orbital resection for recurrent orbital tumors but these were later replaced by tubed pedicle flap reconstruction.[29]

Millar et al.[28] described the use of a contralaterally based forehead scalp flap to reconstruct the defect of the anterior cranial base following en bloc excision of an ethmoid sinus carcinoma. Eight weeks postoperatively the flap was divided at the level of the orbital margin and the proximal flap returned to its original position. A temporal scalp flap and an ipsilateral forehead flap have also been described for coverage of the exposed dura following radical resection of the orbit, orbital roof, and dura.[14,42] Westbury et al.[45] have described four patients with tumors of the anterior cranial fossa who underwent reconstruction using a large ipsilateral-based frontal scalp flap. A second contralateral-based scalp flap was then rotated forward to cover the frontal craniotomy that remained uncovered by the first flap.

A local pedicle flap of pericranium or periosteum separated off a bicoronal scalp flap based on the supratrochlear or supraorbital vessels may be used to reconstruct a defect in the floor of the anterior cranial fossa and a split-thickness skin graft then applied to the pericranial flap from below.[39] Despite advocating the application of split-thickness skin grafts alone to exposed dura in anterior skull base defects, Schramm et al.[36,37] also described the use of a local flap of galea vascularized by the supraorbital artery to cover a dural patch graft and so prevent the complications usually resulting from the application of a skin graft immediately on top of a dural graft (Fig. 1). A series of 38 galeal flaps has recently been reported, 11 of these being used to separate the anterior cranial fossa from the nasopharynx, after resection of tumors of the anterior skull base.[1]

Other local flaps described to reconstruct the anterior cranial base to isolate the cranial cavity from the nasopharynx are the extended glabellar flap and a midline forehead flap. Jackson[21,23] has successfully used an extended glabellar skin flap vascularized by vessels in the supra-

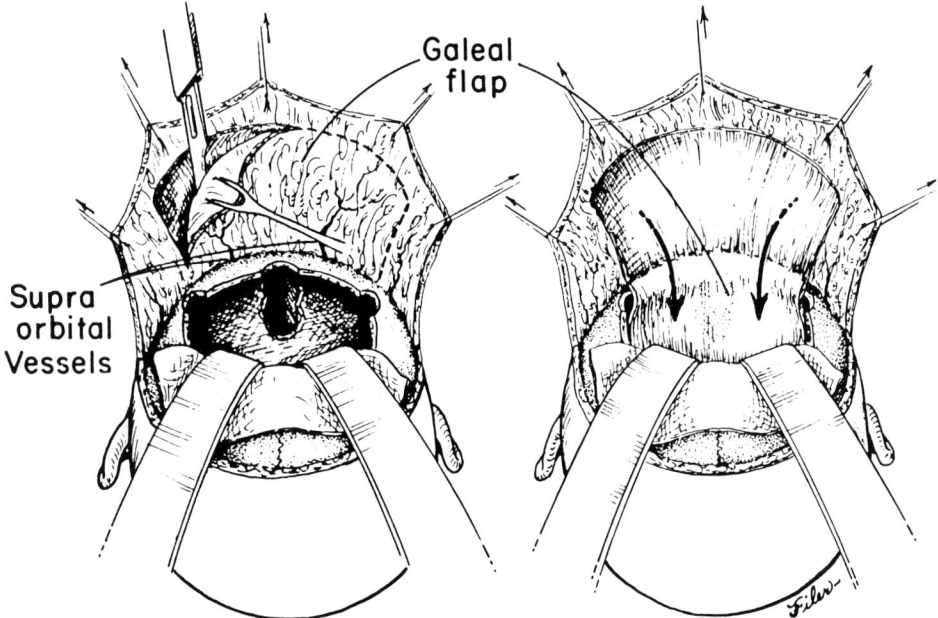

Figure 1: Galeal flap for reconstruction of midline defects of the anterior cranial base.

orbital area to cover the deficient floor of the anterior cranial fossa in 14 patients. A similar technique using a midline forehead flap has also been reported for closure of large cribriform plate defects in six patients.[30] The skin flap is transposed through a bony window in the glabellar area and positioned so that the epithelial surface faces towards the nasal cavity.

For lateral defects of the anterior cranial fossa, the temporalis muscle may be utilized and transposed medially[10,19] (Fig. 2). The temporalis muscle is innervated by the deep temporal nerve from the mandibular division of the trigeminal nerve. Its blood supply originates from the superficial temporal artery and the internal maxillary artery. Through a coronal incision, the muscle may be elevated together with periosteum deep to it. The superficial fascial attachments to the zygomatic arch are then divided transversely to facilitate anterior and medial transposition of the muscle. The large fan-shaped muscle converges on its insertion into the coronoid process and this becomes the point of rotation. Originally the temporalis muscle flap was described for coverage of the orbit by transposing the muscle through a fenestration in the lateral orbital wall taking great care to avoid strangulation of the muscle. The temporalis muscle may also be used to isolate the exposed dura of the anterior cranial fossa from the paranasal sinuses but its reliability becomes questionable for more medial defects.

More extensive defects of the anterior cranial fossa require utilization of distant flaps such as the pectoralis major and extended trapezius musculocutaneous flaps. An additional advantage of these musculocutaneous flaps is that they may provide greater protection against bacterial invasion when compared with conventional skin flaps.[8] Musculocutaneous flaps permit a one-stage reconstruction and essentially eliminate the need for split-thickness skin grafts or secondary division of flap pedicles. These flaps may also be used in areas that have been previously irradiated and can also tolerate large doses of postoperative irradiation.

The pectoralis major muscle is supplied by the thoracoacromial artery, and through musculocutaneous perforators, a paddle of skin based over the medial and inferior aspects of the muscle may be transposed with an arc of rotation at the middle third of the clavicle. Ariyan[2-5,7,35] has described eight patients in whom the pectoralis major musculocutaneous flap has been used to reconstruct the defect of the anterior skull base following resection of orbital and cranio-orbital tumors. Jaskson[21] has also reported using the pectoralis major musculocutaneous flap for reconstruction of

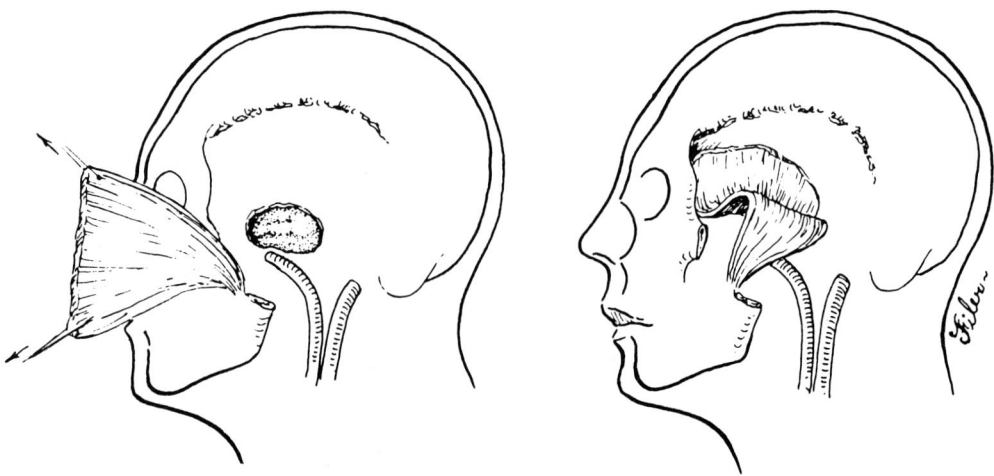

Figure 2: Temporalis muscle transposition for coverage of lateral defects of the anterior or middle cranial base.

the anterior cranial base in a patient where an extended glabellar flap could not be used. A possible disadvantage of the pectoralis major musculocutaneous flap is that in order to reach the supraorbital rim reliably, the muscle pedicle may have to be left external to the neck skin and the flap secondarily divided and inset about 2 weeks later.

An extended trapezius musculocutaneous flap has recently been described for coverage of the orbito-anterior cranial base region. The primary blood supply of the posterior trapezius muscle originates from the descending branch of the transverse cervical artery.[27] A skin island may be designed over the muscle with its long axis centered between the vertebral column and the medial border of the scapula and its distal end extending 10 to 15 cm beyond the tip of the scapula. A large arc of rotation is obtained by placing the distal half of the skin island beyond the edge of the trapezius muscle thus making its blood supply random and by totally mobilizing the trapezius muscle, thus sacrificing its function. However, this allows the muscle pedicle and skin island to be tunneled beneath the neck skin so that it may reach well beyond the supraorbital rim and across the midline. Rosen[33] has described the extended trapezius musculocutaneous flap to reconstruct dural defects of the anterior cranial base or to separate the dura from the nasopharynx and paranasal sinuses in four patients (Fig. 3). The supraorbital region and anterior cranial base, the temporal fossa, the maxillary sinus, the lateral nasal wall and nasopharynx, the ethmoid sinuses and intraorbital space, and the frontal sinus can all be reliably reached with a posterior extended trapezius flap provided the skin island is positioned with its distal half beyond the trapezius muscle and the muscle totally mobilized to the anterior neck. The disadvantage of the extended trapezius musculocutaneous flap is the sacrifice of trapezius muscle function. Furthermore, the flap must be raised in the prone position prior to the cranio-facial resection and requires repositioning the patient. A further possible disadvantage is that the muscle pedicle

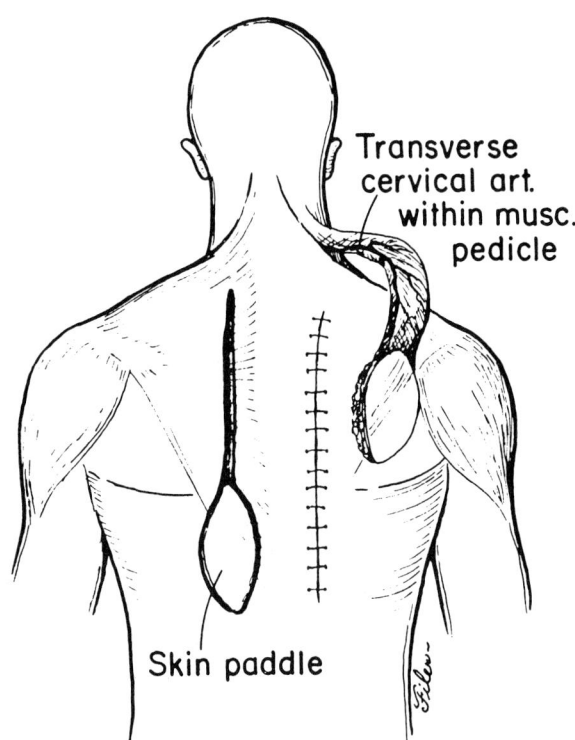

Figure 3: Extended trapezius musculocutaneous flap for coverage of the anterior cranial base.

beneath the neck and facial skin may be cosmetically unsatisfactory.

The latissimus dorsi musculocutaneous flap based on its reliable blood supply from the thoracodorsal artery and vein has become the work horse of reconstructive surgery. This flap has been advocated for reconstruction of massive facial defects around the orbit.[31,32,38] However, when the skin island with its muscle pedicle is passed through a subcutaneous tunnel into the neck, the skin paddle has an insufficient arc of rotation to reach the anterior cranial base for effective reconstruction in this area. A further disadvantage of the latissimus dorsi musculocutaneous flap for reconstruction in this area is that the patient must be placed in a lateral position to harvest the flap, otherwise the patient must be turned and redraped following the resection part of the procedure. Like the trapezius flap, the muscle pedicle may produce excessive bulk to the contour of the neck.

Finally, with the increasing reliability of microsurgical free tissue transfer, musculocutaneous and cutaneous flaps may be transferred into this area especially for reconstruction of massive cranio-orbito-maxillary defects. Despite requiring personnel experienced in microvascular surgery, these flaps have the great advantage that large areas of tissue are available and may easily be positioned anatomically in three dimensions, the only provision being that a suitable recipient artery and vein are available in the vicinity of the defect for the vascular anastomoses. The latissimus dorsi musculocutaneous flap has been described for closure of large orbito-maxillary defects,[11,12] and we have also used the latissimus dorsi for similar indications. The scapular flap, a free cutaneous flap based on the circumflex scapular artery and vein, and the radial forearm flap, a free fasciocutaneous flap based on the radial artery and cephalic vein, could also be used effectively in this area.[41] The greater omentum on the right gastro-epiploic vessels has also been described recently as a free tissue transfer for coverage of the chronically infected open frontal sinus and for reconstruction of the anterior skull base following tumor resection.[13]

Summary

For reconstruction of lateral defects of the anterior skull base, the temporalis muscle appears to be the method of choice. For medial and midline defects, a galeal flap is the most effective choice. For larger defects, the pectoralis major musculocutaneous flap and especially the extended trapezius musculocutaneous flap are most suitable. Finally, for massive defects in this region, free tissue transfer may occasionally be indicated.

Middle Cranial Base

The middle cranial fossa extends from the posterior wall of the orbit to the posterior aspect of the petrous temporal bone and has been divided into anterior and central segments by Jackson.[20,23] The anterior segment extends from the posterior wall of the orbit to the anterior edge of the petrous temporal bone. Within this segment, the second division of the trigeminal nerve (the maxillary nerve) exits through the foramen rotundum and the third division of the trigeminal nerve (the mandibular nerve) exits through the foramen ovale. The internal carotid artery enters the middle cranial fossa through the foramen lacerum and the middle meningeal artery enters the middle cranial fossa through the foramen spinosum. The central segment is the petrous temporal bone itself through which the internal carotid artery passes from the neck into the skull. The petrous temporal bone also contains the internal acoustic meatus through which pass the facial nerve and the acoustic nerve. Tumors of the middle cranial fossa may extend through any of these foramina into the pterygoid space and then further extend into the temporal fossa, the parapharyngeal area, or through the inferior orbital fissure into the orbit.

Tumors that involve the middle cranial fossa skull base include basal cell carcinomas and squamous cell carcinomas originating in the skin of the external ear and the adjacent scalp and neck skin, and carcinomas of the middle ear. Tumors originating more deeply include glomus jugulare tumors, meningiomas, chordomas of the clivus, nasopharyngeal carcinomas and parotid tumors.

Tumors originating externally and invading the temporal bone usually require a temporal bone resection with excision of the external ear and adjacent skin. Parotidectomy, excision of a portion of the mandible, and a radical neck dissection may be required in addition. Traditional methods of reconstructing the defect following temporal bone resection have included the use of large rotation or transposition scalp flaps elevated in the plane between the galea and the pericranium.[45] The donor site almost always requires a split-thickness skin graft. The deltopectoral flap described by Bakamjian, an axial pattern flap based on the anterior intercostal perforating branches of the internal mammary artery, also proved useful for reconstruction of this area although the distal portion of the flap often required a preliminary delay procedure and after transfer of the flap, secondary division of the pedicle and insetting was required.[45] With the advent of musculocutaneous flaps in the 1970s, the latissimus dorsi musculocutaneous flap,[31,32] the posterior trapezius musculocutaneous flap based on the transverse cervical artery,[27] and especially the pectoralis major musculocutaneous flap based on the thoracoacromial artery[3,9] have proved extremely efficacious in reconstruction of this area. They provide well-vascularized muscle to seal the dura against CSF leaks and large islands of skin that will withstand postoperative irradiation. Furthermore, the reconstruction may be completed in one stage.

More deeply situated tumors such as glomus tumors, clivus chordomas, nasopharyngeal carcinomas, and extracranial meningiomas may be adequately exposed by the infratemporal fossa approach of Fisch.[15-18] Through a hemicoronal incision with either a postauricular or preauricular extension, the facial nerve is exposed from the stylomastoid foramen to the geniculate ganglion and transposed anteriorly. The mandibular condyle is resected and the zygomatic arch displaced inferiorly. After drilling away the glenoid fossa, the middle meningeal artery and mandibular division of the trigeminal nerve are transected at the foramen spinosum and foramen ovale, respectively. Through a temporal craniotomy, the particular foramen through which the tumor is passing may be identified and that segment of the skull base from the foramen to the craniotomy excised as a wedge. The large defect following resection of the tumor has been reconstructed by Fisch using an inferior transposition of the temporalis muscle augmented by free grafts of abdominal fat. In a series of 51 patients, only three developed a CSF leak. Jackson[20] has used the sternomastoid muscle based superiorly on its vascular pedicle from the occipital artery for obliteration of dead space after removal of tumors of the anterior segment.[6,34]

However, with more medially situated tumors, and especially in those whose resection results in a communication between the nasopharynx and the dural repair, transposition of the temporalis muscle or the pectoralis major musculocutaneous flap to separate the nasopharynx from the exposed dura may be unreliable. Free muscle flaps have recently been described for reconstruction of the nasopharynx and middle cranial base following resection of tumors by the infratemporal fossa approach.[24] The rectus abdominis muscle has been transferred into the defect and its vascularity immediately restored by microsurgical anastomosis of the deep inferior epigastric artery and vein to the occipital artery and internal jugular or external jugular veins (Fig. 4). The internal surface of the muscle lining the lateral and posterior walls of the nasopharynx has not required skin grafting but rapidly mucosalizes. The disadvantage of this technique is the fact that microsurgical expertise is required and monitoring of these completely invisible free flaps is impossible. The major advantage of this technique is the fact tion is that the highly vascularized muscle may be positioned to reconstruct the posterior and lateral walls of the nasopharynx. Tongues of muscle may be used to obliterate the paranasal sinuses and the remainder of the muscle draped to cover the tenuous dural repair or dural graft and, if necessary, wrap around a saphenous vein graft reconstruction of the inter-

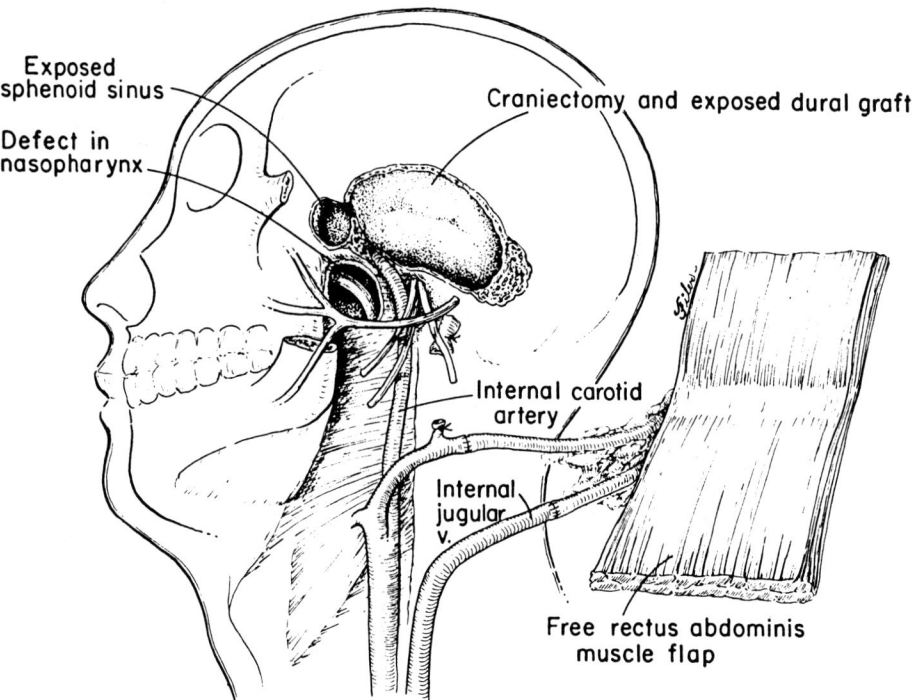

Figure 4: Free rectus abdominis muscle flap for reconstruction of defects of the middle or posterior cranial base.

nal carotid artery. Harvesting of the muscle does not require any repositioning or redraping of the patient.

Summary

For reconstruction of small defects and laterally situated defects, transposition of the temporalis muscle is the method of choice. For larger defects, the distant pedicled musculocutaneous flaps, the pectoralis major and the extended trapezius flap are more suitable. With the availability of microsurgical expertise, free rectus abdominis muscle flap transfer may be indicated for large medially situated defects.

Posterior Cranial Base

The posterior skull base or posterior segment as described by Jackson extends from the posterior aspect of the petrous temporal bone to the midline of the posterior skull. It contains the jugular foramen through which pass the glossopharyngeal nerve, vagus nerve, and spinal accessory nerve, and the internal jugular vein. The hypoglossal nerve exits from the skull through the separate hypoglossal canal or anterior condylar canal. Intracranial tumors may extend through the jugular foramen and involve the last four cranial nerves. Glomus tumors and schwannomas are the most common tumors of the posterior cranial base. Tumors of the jugular foramen may be approached through the infratemporal fossa exposure of Fisch[15-18] and en bloc resection usually requires resection of bone around the carotid artery and around the sigmoid sinus together with a retromastoid craniectomy.

Tenuous dural repairs and fascia lata grafts may be protected by inferior transposition of the temporalis muscle or superior transposition of the sternomastoid muscle based on its superior vascular supply from the occipital artery.[20,34] Pectoralis major and trapezius musculocutaneous flaps have also been used in this region for obliteration of the radical mastoid cavity and following radical resection of the temporal bone.[9,27] Finally, free rectus abdominis muscle flaps have recently been reported for reconstruction of massive defects of the posterior cranial base.[24]

Very aggressive squamous cell carcinomas or basal cell carcinomas of the skin of the posterior scalp may invade the posterior skull base and occasionally the underlying dura. This may require radical resection of a wide margin of skin, an occipital craniectomy and, if necessary, excision of involved dura. Split-thickness skin grafts will not take over bare skull and are unreliable for coverage of exposed dura. Conventional reconstruction would require a fascia lata graft or pericranial graft to the dural defect covered by a large rotation or transposition scalp flap. Walton and Krizek[44] have demonstrated, however, that dural defects themselves may be reconstructed by direct application of the galea of a scalp flap to the edges of the dural defect. A more reliable reconstruction can now be guaranteed using a dural graft and coverage by a well-vascularized musculocutaneous flap such as the trapezius or latissimus dorsi musculocutaneous flap. The trapezius musculocutaneous flap is especially indicated in this posterior skull base territory because of its close proximity and because the spinal accessory nerve is frequently sacrificed as part of the tumor resection. Finally, extensive ablation of scalp and soft tissues overlying the posterior skull base may require the use of a free flap for reconstruction. The flap of choice would be a free latissimus dorsi muscle flap covered by a split thickness skin graft.

Summary

Reconstruction of small defects of the posterior skull base may be accomplished by inferior transposition of the temporalis muscle, or superior transposition of the sternomastoid muscle. For larger laterally situated defects, the pectoralis major or trapezius musculocutaneous flaps are the method of choice. A free rectus abdominis muscle flap may be indicated for reconstruction of a large medial defect of the posterior cranial base and a free latissimus dorsi muscle flap would be the most effective choice for a massive laterally situated defect.

References

1. Adham MN, Jackson IT, Marsh WR: The use of the galeal frontalis flap in craniofacial surgery. *Plast Surg Forum* VIII:24-26, 1985.
2. Ariyan S: The pectoralis major myocutaneous flap: A versatile flap for reconstruction in the head and neck. *Plast Reconst Surg* 63:73-81, 1979.
3. Ariyan S: The pectoralis major for single stage reconstruction of the difficult wounds of the orbit and pharyngoesophagus. *Plast Reconstr Surg* 72:468-477, 1983.
4. Ariyan S: *Surgery of the Skull Base.* Sasaki CT, McCabe BF, Kirchner JA, eds. Philadelphia, J.B. Lippincott Co., 1984, p 227-243.
5. Ariyan S: Pectoralis major, sternomastoid and other musculocutaneous flaps for head and neck reconstruction. *Clin Plast Surgery* 7(1):89-109, 1980.
6. Ariyan S: One stage reconstruction for defects of the mouth using a sternomastoid myocutaneous flap. *Plast Reconstr Surg* 63:618-625, 1979.
7. Ariyan S, Cuono CB: Use of the pectoralis major myocutaneous flap for reconstruction of large cervical, facial or cranial defects. *Am J Surg* 140:503-506, 1980.
8. Ariyan S, Marfuggi RA, Harder G, et al: An experimental model to determine the effects of adjuvant therapy on the incidence of postoperative wound infection: I. Evaluating preoperative radiation therapy. *Plast Reconst Surg* 65:328-337, 1980.
9. Ariyan S, Sasaki CT, Spencer D: Radical en bloc resection of the temporal bone. *Am J Surg* 142:443-447, 1981.
10. Bakamjian VY, Souther SG: Use of the temporal muscle flap for reconstruction after orbito-maxillary resections for cancer. *Plast Reconstr Surg* 56:171-177, 1975.
11. Baker SR: Closure of large orbital maxillary defects with free latissimus dorsi

myocutaneous flaps. *Head Neck Surg* 6:828-835, 1984.
12. Baker SR: Surgical reconstruction after extensive skull base surgery. *Otolaryngol Clin North Am* 17(3):591-599, 1984.
13. Barrow DL, Nahai F, Tindall GT: The use of greater omentum vascularized free flaps for neurosurgical disorders requiring reconstruction. *J Neurosurg* 60:305-311, 1984.
14. Campbell HH: Surgery of lesions of the upper face. *Am J Surg* 87:676-687, 1954.
15. Fisch U: Infratemporal fossa approach to tumors of the temporal bone and base of the skull. *J Laryngol Otol* 92:949-967, 1978.
16. Fisch U: Infratemporal fossa approach to lesions in the temporal bone and base of skull. *Laryngoscope* 93:36-44, 1983.
17. Fisch U, Fagan P, Valavenis A: The infratemporal approach for the lateral skull base. *Otolaryngol Clin North Am* 17(3)513-552, 1984.
18. Fisch U, Pillsbury HC: The infratemporal fossa approach for nasopharyngeal tumors. *Arch Otolaryngol* 105:99-107, 1979.
19. Holmes AD, Marshall KA: Uses of the temporalis muscle flap in blanking out orbits. *Plast Reconstr Surg* 63:336-342, 1979.
20. Jackson IT, Hide TAH: A systematic approach to tumors of the base of the skull. *J Maxillofacial Surg* 10:92-98, 1982.
21. Jackson IT, Laws ER, Martin RD: A craniofacial approach to advanced recurrent cancer of the central face. *Head Neck Surg* 5:474-488, 1983.
22. Jackson IT, Marsh WR: Anterior cranial fossa tumors. *Ann Plast Surg* 11:479-489, 1983.
23. Jackson IT, Marsh WR, Hide TAH: Treatment of tumors involving the anterior cranial fossa. *Head Neck Surg* 6:901-913, 1984.
24. Jones NF, Sekhar LN, Schramm VL, et al: Free rectus abdominis muscle flap reconstruction allowing radical resection of cranial base tumors. *Plast Surg Forum* VIII:148-149, 1985.
25. Ketcham AS, Wilkins RH, Van Buren JM, et al: A combined intracranial facial approach to the paranasal sinuses. *Am J Surg* 106:698-703, 1963.
26. Ketcham AS, Hoye RC, Van Buren JM, et al: Complications of intracranial facial resections for tumors of the paranasal sinuses. *Am J Surg* 112:591-596, 1966.
27. McCraw JB, Magee WP, Kalwaic H: Uses of the trapezius and sternomastoid myocutaneous flaps in head and neck reconstruction. *Plast Reconstr Surg* 63:49-57, 1979.
28. Millar HS, Petty PG, Wilson WF, et al: A combined intracranial and facial approach for excision and repair of cancer of the ethmoid sinuses. *Aust NZ J Surg* 43:179-183, 1973.
29. Murray JE, Matson DD, Habal MB, et al: Regional cranio-orbital resection for recurrent tumors with delayed reconstruction. *Surg Gynecol Obstet* 134:437-47, 1972.
30. Ousterhout DK, Tessier P: Closure of large cribriform defects with a forehead flap. *J Maxillofacial Surg* 9:7-9, 1981.
31. Quillen CG, Shearin JC, Georgiade NG: Use of the latissimus dorsi myocutaneous island flap for reconstruction in the head and neck area. *Plast Reconstr Surg* 62:113-117, 1978.
32. Quillen CG: Latissimus dorsi myocutaneous flaps in head and neck reconstruction. *Plast Reconstr Surg* 63:664-670, 1979.
33. Rosen HN: The extended trapezius musculocutaneous flap for cranio-orbital facial reconstruction. *Plast Reconstr Surg* 75:318-324, 1985.
34. Sasaki CT: The sternocleidomastoid myocutaneous flap. *Arch Otolaryngol* 106:74-76, 1980.
35. Sasaki CT, Ariyan S, Spencer D, et al: Pectoralis major myocutaneous reconstruction of the anterior skull base. *Laryngoscope* 95:162-166, 1985.
36. Schramm VL: *Surgery of the Skull Base.* Sasaki CT, McCabe BF, Kirchner JA, eds. Philadelphia, J.B. Lippincott Co., 1984, pp 43-61.
37. Schramm VL, Myers EN, Maroon JC: Anterior skull base surgery for benign and malignant disease. *Laryngoscope* 89:1077-1091, 1979.
38. Schuller DE: Latissimus dorsi myocutaneous flaps for massive facial defects. *Arch Otolaryngol* 108:414-417, 1982.
39. Shah JP, Galicich JH: Craniofacial resection for malignant tumors of the ethmoid and anterior skull base. *Arch Otolaryngol* 103:514-517, 1977.
40. Smith RR, Klopp CT, Williams JM: Surgical treatment of cancer of the frontal sinus and adjacent areas. *Cancer* 7:991-994, 1954.
41. Swartz WM, Banis JC, Newton D, et al: Applications of the scapular osteocutaneous flap for maxillo-facial reconstruction. *Plast Reconstr Surg* (in press).
42. Thompson HG: Reconstruction of the orbit after radical exenteration. *Plast Reconstr Surg* 45:119:123, 1970.

43. Van Buren JM, Ommaya AK, Ketcham AS: Ten years experience with radical combined craniofacial resection of malignant tumors of the paranasal sinuses. J Neurosurg 28:341-350, 1968.
44. Walton RL, Krizek TJ: The scalp flap only onlay: a method for managing large dural defects. Plast Reconstr Surg 66:684-689, 1980.
45. Westbury G, Wilson JSP, Richardson A: Combined craniofacial resection for malignant disease. Am J Surg 130:463-469, 1975.

VI

Anterior Cranial Base

15

Anterior Cranial Base Anatomy

Johannes Lang, M.D.

Introduction

Postnatal enlargement of the skull base is mainly the result of endochondral bone growth in the area of the spheno-occipital and spheno-ethmoid synchondroses, and to a lesser extent of sutural growth and processes of remodeling (bone apposition and resorption). In our specimens, the distance between the foramen cecum and the internal occipital protuberance in newborns was 9.7 cm, in 1-year-old children it was 11.5 cm (range 10.9–12.1 cm), in 2- to 3-year-olds it was 12.8 cm (range 11.6–13.9 cm), in 4- to 5-year-old children it was 13.3 cm (range 11.9–14.3 cm), in 9- to 11-year-old children it was 13.5 cm (range 12.9–13.9 cm), and in adults it was 14.05 cm (range 12.7–15.9 cm). It should be noted that the maximal length between the nasion and the inion in our specimens was 16.48 cm (range 15.2–18.2 cm).[9]

The internal skull width was estimated between the inner surfaces of the skull in the area of the middle temporal gyrus. In newborns it was 6.8 cm, in 1-year-old children it was 10.2 cm (range 8.6–11.8 cm), in 4- to 5-year-old children it was 12 cm (range 11.2–13.2 cm), and in adults it was 12.9 cm (range 11.1–14.5 cm). The so-called auricular width (the distance between the two auricles measured from the middle of the external auditory meatus over the supramastoid crest) was measured in adults to be 12.4 cm (range 11.7–13.9 cm) (Fig. 1).

On the outer skull base, we measured distances between the anterior border of the external auditory meatus and different landmarks on the orbital rim, and distances between the posterior border of the external auditory meatus and the opisthocranion. The measurements in the area of the outer skull base show that anterior growth of the skull between birth and 2 years of age occurs mainly in the area of the ectoconchion and to a lesser extent in the nasomaxillofrontale. Between the second and fourth years of life we found that less growth occurs, and between the fourth and sixth years, in particular, growth is focused in the medial orbital area. Between 17 years of age and adulthood we found further increases in these values.

Between the external auditory meatus and the opisthocranion, little growth is measurable in the first 2 years of life, although greater growth occurs between the second and sixth years of life (Fig. 2).[11,14]

The sphenoid-clivus angle (between the planum sphenoidale and the clivus) measures 117.68° in adults (range 96–

From: Sekhar LN, Schramm VL Jr, eds: *Tumors of the Cranial Base: Diagnosis and Treatment.* Mount Kisco, New York, Futura Publishing Co, Inc, © 1987.

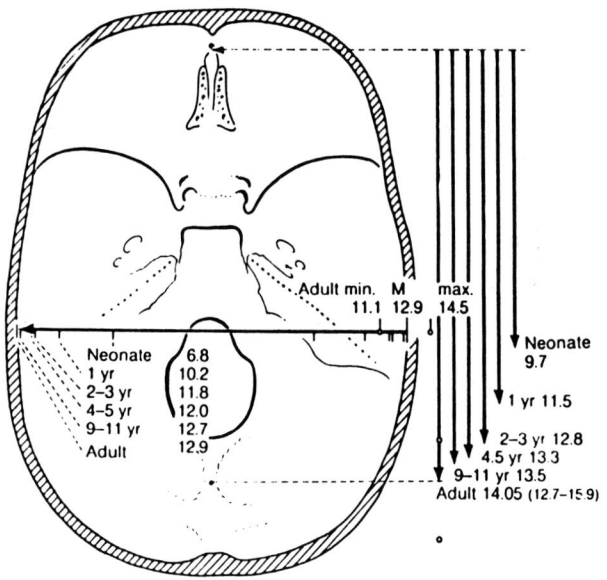

Figure 1: Mean internal cranial lengths and widths in centimeters.

143°). Figure 3 shows the postnatal changes in the mean values for this angle.[5] According to Bergerhof and Stilz, this angle is 117° in women and 118° in men 20 to 49 years old.[2] If the skull base angle is flattened beyond 140°, the condition is known as platybasia.

Terracing of the skull base was estimated on the inner skull base between the level of the Frankfort horizontal plane and different landmarks on the skull. The planum sphenoidale is situated in adults 23.8 mm (range 17.8–32.2 mm) above this plane. The deepest point of the posterior cranial fossa was estimated to be 23 mm (range 13–34 mm) below the Frankfort plane. Figure 4 shows our measurements of the arcuate eminence, the internal auditory meatus, the floor of the sella turcica, the lamina cribrosa, and the endofrontal eminence. In adults, the deepest point of the middle cranial fossa was found to be 0.45 mm below the Frankfort plane (range 6 mm above and 8 mm below this plane).[9]

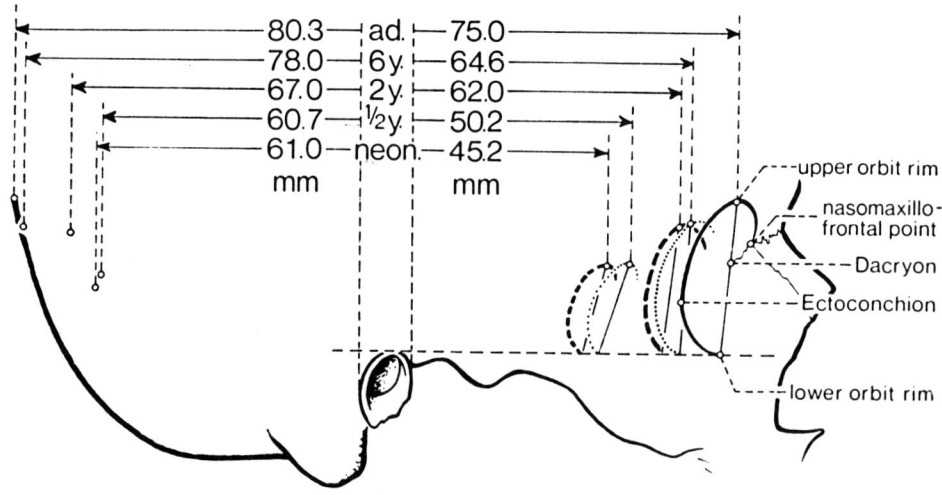

Figure 2: Postnatal growth of the exterior cranial base.

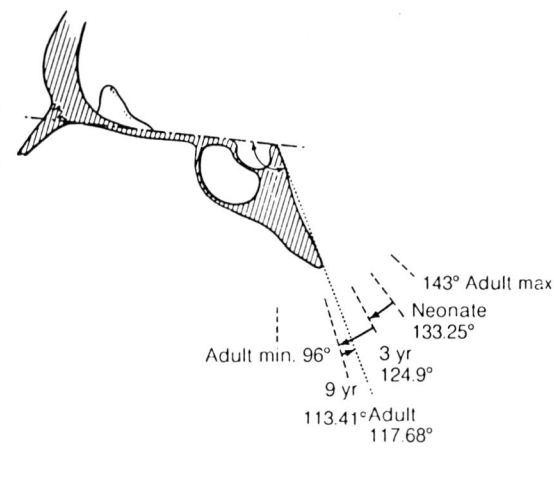

Sphenoidal-clivus angle, postnatal change ($\bar{x}$)		
Age	Degrees	n
Newborn	133.25	6
2 + 3 months	130.42	7
4–7 months	130.90	5
1 year	127.66	3
2 years	126.00	4
3 years	124.90	5
4 years	117.10	5
5 years	115.16	6
6 + 7 years	113.37	4
8 years	113.50	4
9–11 years	113.41	6
16–17 years	112.00	4

Figure 3: Mean sphenoid-clivus angle, measured in degrees at different postnatal ages.

Anterior Cranial Base Anatomy

Bone Anatomy

The anterior cranial base is shown in Figure 5. The floor of the anterior cranial fossa (and the roof of the orbit) is composed of the frontal bone (part of the squama), the ethmoid bone (lamina cribrosa and crista galli), and the sphenoid bone (anterior upper part of the body of the sphenoid and the lesser wing). The foramen cecum is situated in front of the crista galli, and in the skulls of children it is apparent that its posterior and lateral borders are formed by the ethmoid bone, and its anterior margin is the frontal bone. In most instances, this foramen is filled with a small extension of dura mater that is traversed by small blood vessels. Rarely, and only in young children, we found veins that connected the superior sagittal sinus with nasal veins. In very

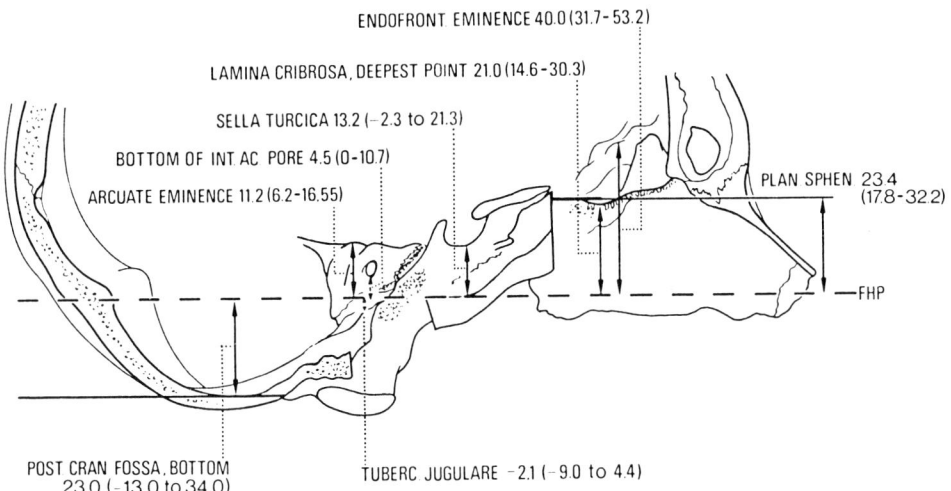

Figure 4: Contour of the inner skull base, with measurements given in millimeters (range). FHP, Frankfort horizontal plane.

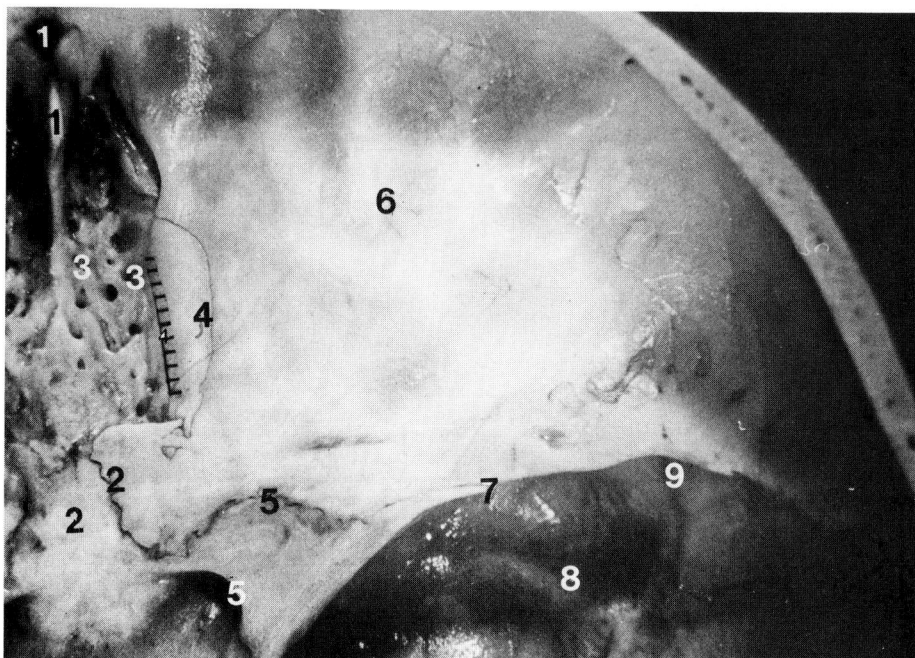

Figure 5: Anterior cranial fossa (15-year-old child). 1. Foramen cecum and crista galli. 2. Planum sphenoidale, comprised partly by the frontal bone (var.). 3. Lamina cribrosa. 4. Superior border of the superior ethmoid cells (on occasion composed of ethmoid bone); millimeter scale. 5. Frontosphenoid suture and roof of the optic canal. 6. Middle part of anterior cranial fossa. 7. Lateral tip of the lesser wing of the sphenoid bone. 8. Middle cranial fossa, floor. 9. Groove of frontal branch of the middle meningeal artery.

rare circumstances encephaloceles or nasal gliomas may pass through an opening in the area of the foramen cecum.[26] The cribriform plate on each side contains about 44 (range 26–71) foramina, and anterolaterally includes the foramen cribroethmoidale.[26] The olfactory fila pass through the cribriform plate, along with small dural and arachnoid extensions and branches of the posterior and anterior ethmoid arteries; the largest nasal branch of the anterior ethmoid artery and the anterior ethmoidal nerve leave the cranial cavity through the cribro-ethmoid foramen. In some of our preparations we also found a vein that was connected with an inferior vein of the forebrain passing through the lamina cribrosa.

Not uncommonly, meningo-orbital foramina may be present in the orbital roof; branches of the ophthalmic artery or the middle meningeal artery may pass through these foramina. The planum sphenoidale is located behind the lamina cribrosa. In adults it was 14.19 mm (mean) in front of the tuberculum sellae, while the distance between the foramen cecum and the tuberculum sellae was 42.57 mm (range 28–50 mm). For further details (postnatal growth of these structures, the prechiasmal sulcus, the crista galli, and the lamina cribrosa), see Figure 6. An important landmark on the lateral side of the skull is the frontotemporal point. This most medial part of the superior temporal line in our specimens was situated 17.8 mm (range 11–26 mm) above the frontozygomatic suture and 43.7 mm (range 36–49 mm) above the Frankfort plane. Behind this point is situated the impression of the inferior frontal gyrus and the lateral endofrontal fovea. This part of the anterior skull base is 11.3 mm (range 4–17 mm) below the frontotemporal point. Our measurements of the width of the anterior cranial fossa between this point and the

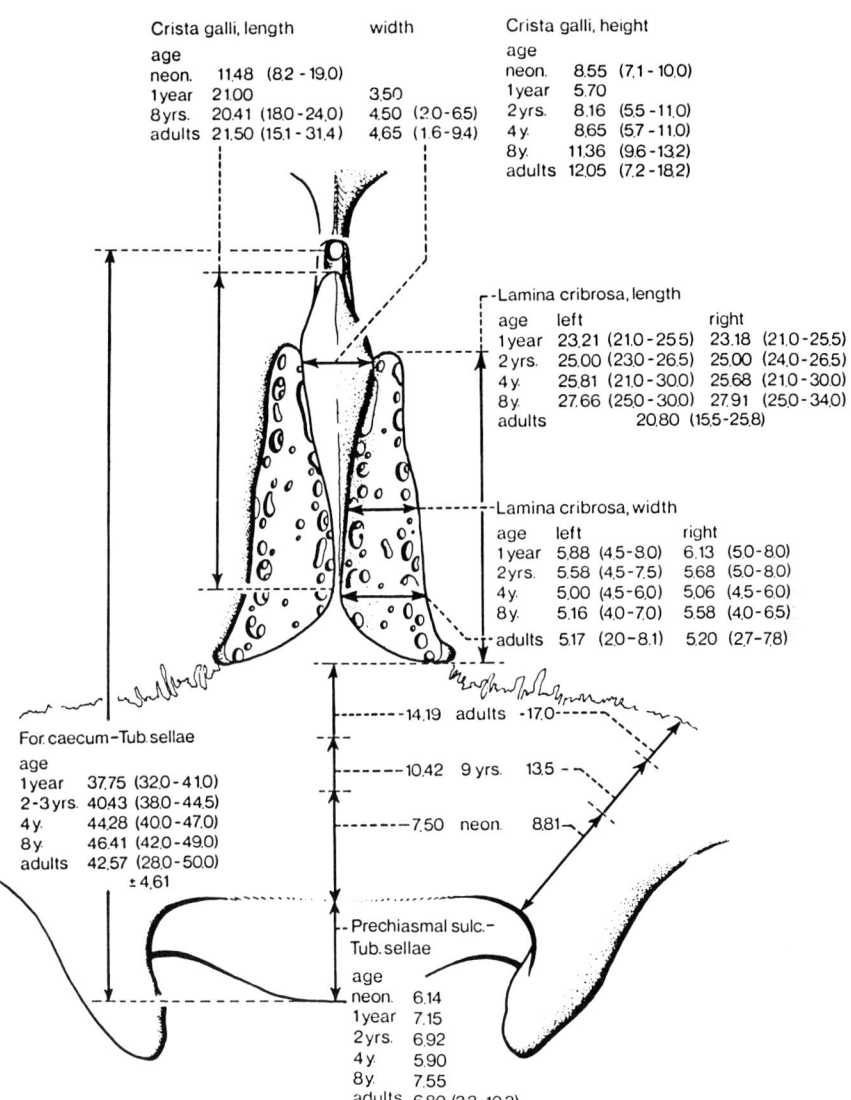

Figure 6: Postnatal changes in dimensions of the middle part of the floor of the anterior cranial fossa. The tuberculum sellae, foramen cecum, crista galli, planum sphenoidale, and optic canal-frontosphenoid suture distance increases with increasing age, while the prechiasmal sulcus and lamina cribrosa do not.

distance between the lateral endofrontal fovea and the optic canal (and their postnatal development) are shown in Figure 7.[13]

The anteroposterior length of the anterior cranial fossa, between the rounded transition zone to the anterior wall and the border of the optic canal, was measured in adults to be about 45 mm (range 36–54 mm). When the midsagittal posterior border of the anterior cranial fossa was used, we estimated the length to be 35 mm (range 28–43 mm) in adults (Fig. 8). Figure 8 shows the distances between the medial borders of the optic canals in adults, postnatal increases in the distance between the optic canal and the lateral border of the lesser wing of the sphenoid bone, the medial and the lateral length of the optic nerve, the width of the optic chiasm, and the distance from the anterior clinoid process to the midsagittal plane.

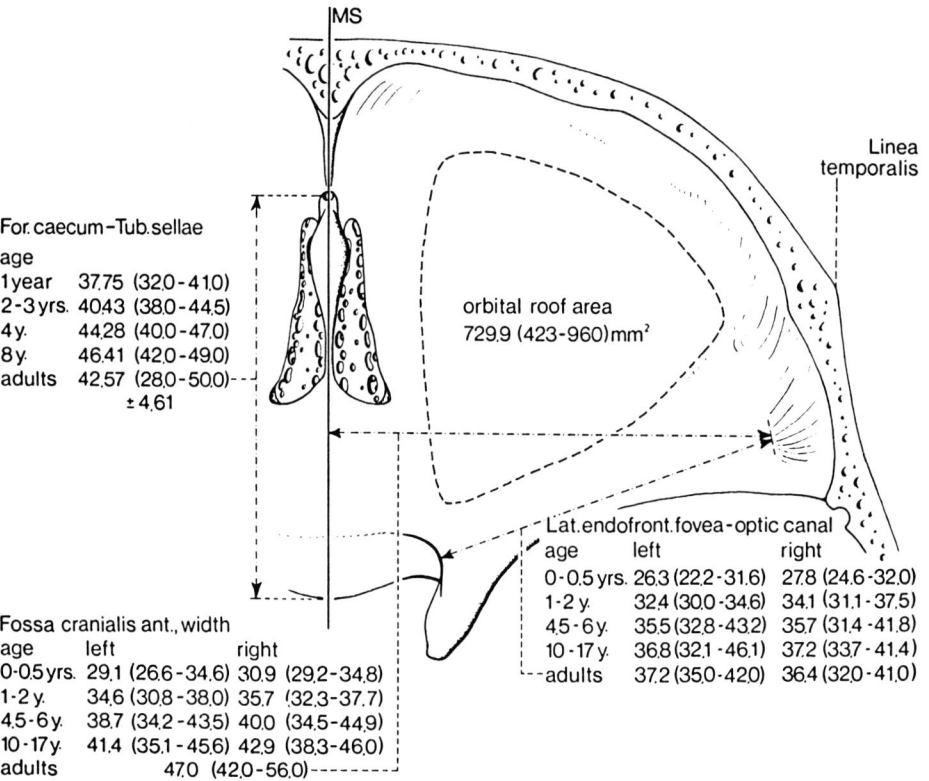

Figure 7: Anterior cranial fossa, showing its width and the postnatal increase in the distance between the lateral endofrontal fovea and the optic canal. The area of the orbital roof is also shown.

Also shown are our measurements of the distance between the intracranial opening of the optic canal and the sphenofrontal suture in the axis of the optic canal.

The anterior cranial base is deeper medially than laterally. The distances from the Frankfurt horizontal plane to the cribriform plate, the medial endofrontal fovea, and endofrontal eminence, and the lateral endofrontal fovea at different stages of postnatal development are shown in Figure 9.

Dura Mater

The dura mater of the anterior cranial fossa consists of collagen fiber systems that are oriented in different directions. Thick zones were seen above the planum sphenoidale and behind the lesser wing of the sphenoid bone. In the latter area we measured the dural thickness to be 2.0 mm (range 1.5–3 mm).[10] In the area of the olfactory fossa we found the dura mater to be relatively thin. The average length of the dura in the olfactory fossa was less than the osseous cribriform plate. We measured the former length to be 15.82 mm (range 11.0–20.0 mm) on the right and 15.92 mm (range 11.0–24.0 mm) on the left. The distance from the olfactory fossa to the anterior rim of the inner skull was 9.62 mm (range 0–21 mm), and the distance from the posterior border of the olfactory fossa to the anterior border of the intracranial aperture of the optic canal was measured to be 18 mm (range 9–26 mm) (Fig. 10). It should be noted that the anterior and posterior borders of the olfactory fossa are covered by small dural folds which we termed olfactory tentoria. The anterior one has an average length of 3.3 mm (range 1.0–5 mm), and the posterior

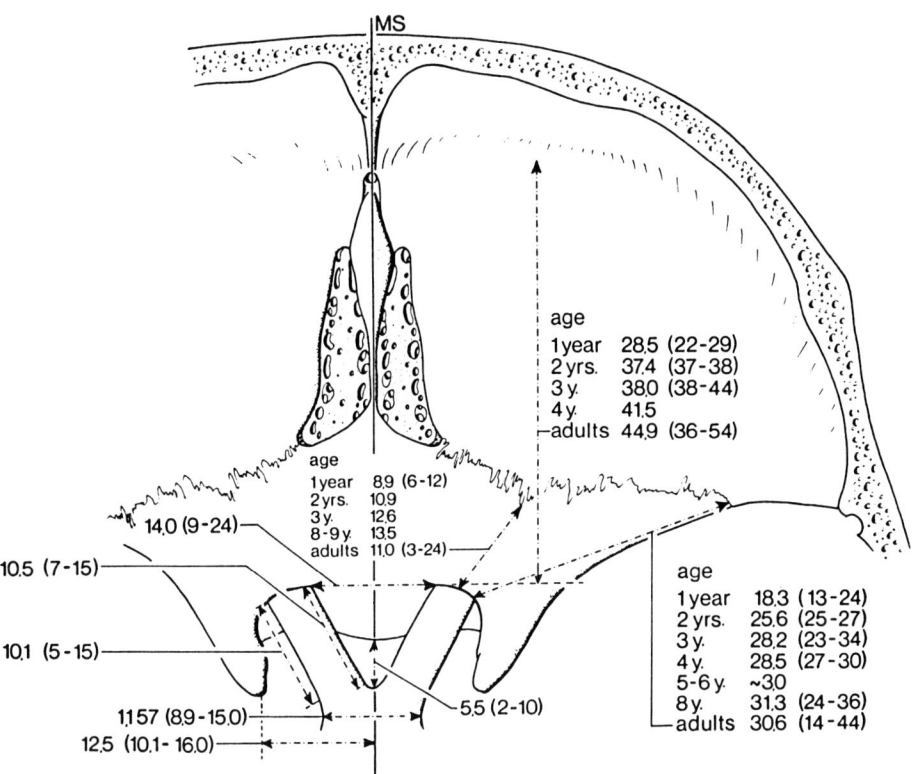

Figure 8: Measurements in adults of the distance from the anterior clinoid process to the midsagittal plane, the width of the optic chiasm, the lateral and medial length of the optic nerve, the distance between the medial borders of the optic canal, and the distance between the tuberculum sellae and the anterior border of the chiasm. Postnatal increases in the distance between the optic canal and the frontosphenoid suture (in the axis of the optic canal), the medial length of the anterior cranial fossa, and the length between the optic canal and top of the lesser wing of the sphenoid bone are also shown.

one a length of 2.6 mm (range 1.5–6.0 mm).

The dura mater and the floor of the anterior cranial fossa are supplied by the ethmoidal arteries, the frontal branch of the middle meningeal artery, and the internal carotid artery. Twigs of the ethmoidal arteries pierce the lamina cribrosa to reach the medial and lateral walls of the nasal cavity. One of the branches that is normally large and well developed is the anterior falx artery, which supplies the falx cerebri. The frontal branch of the middle meningeal artery supplies the lateral area of the floor of the anterior cranial fossa and reaches the orbit through meningo-orbital foramina in most cases (Fig. 11).

Brain and Blood Vessels in the Floor of the Anterior Cranial Fossa

The orbital portion of the frontal lobe has a variable pattern of sulci and gyri, but one feature that remains constant is the olfactory sulcus. The olfactory tract is located near the posterior portion of the olfactory sulcus, in a small olfactory cistern. Medial parts of the orbital surface and the olfactory bulb and tract are supplied by the medial frontobasal artery, which is a twig of the anterior cerebral artery, and in most cases also by branches of the long central artery (recurrent artery of Heubner). The lateral part of the brain in this area is supplied by the lateral frontobasal artery, which is a twig of the middle cere-

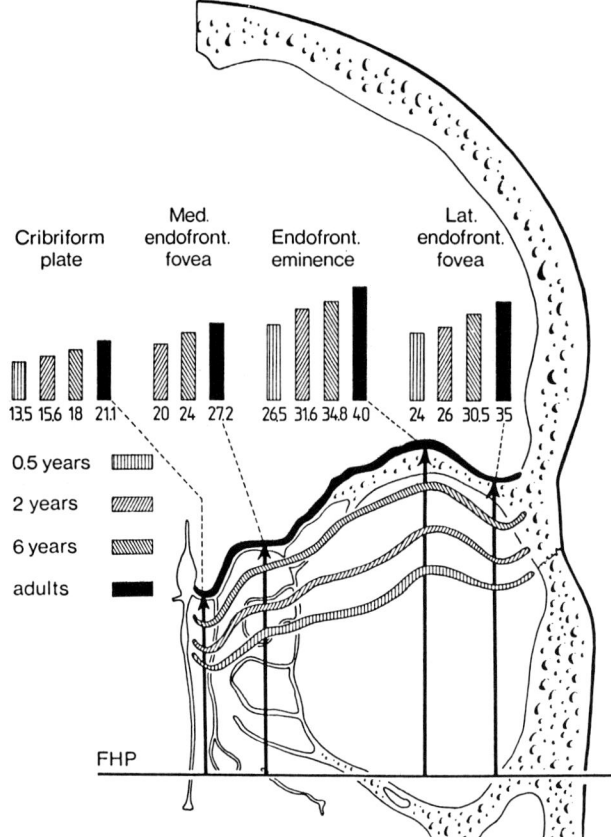

Figure 9: Mean distances in millimeters between the Frankfort horizontal plane (FHP) and (from left = medially to right) structures of the anterior cranial fossa.

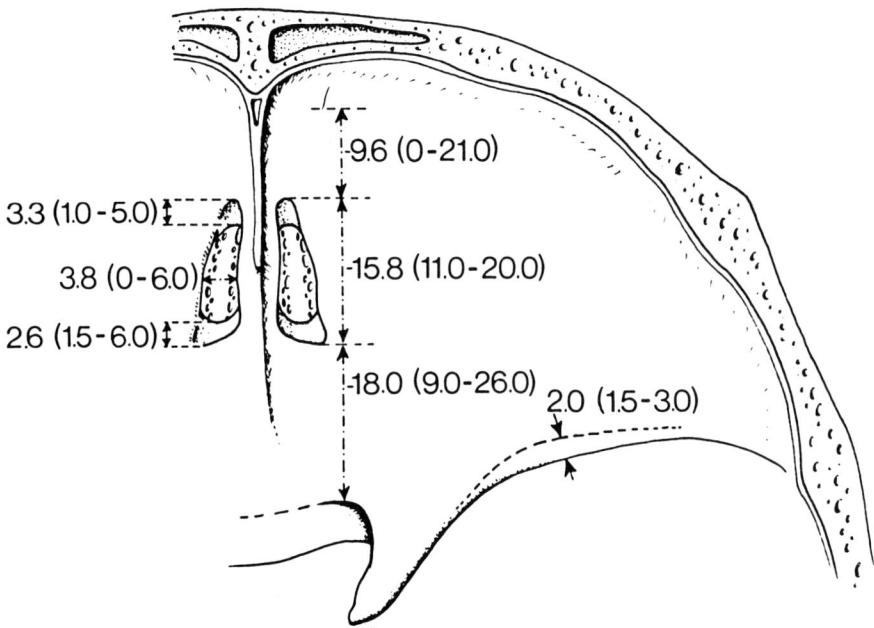

Figure 10: Olfactory fossa dura, measurements and distances to landmarks in adults.

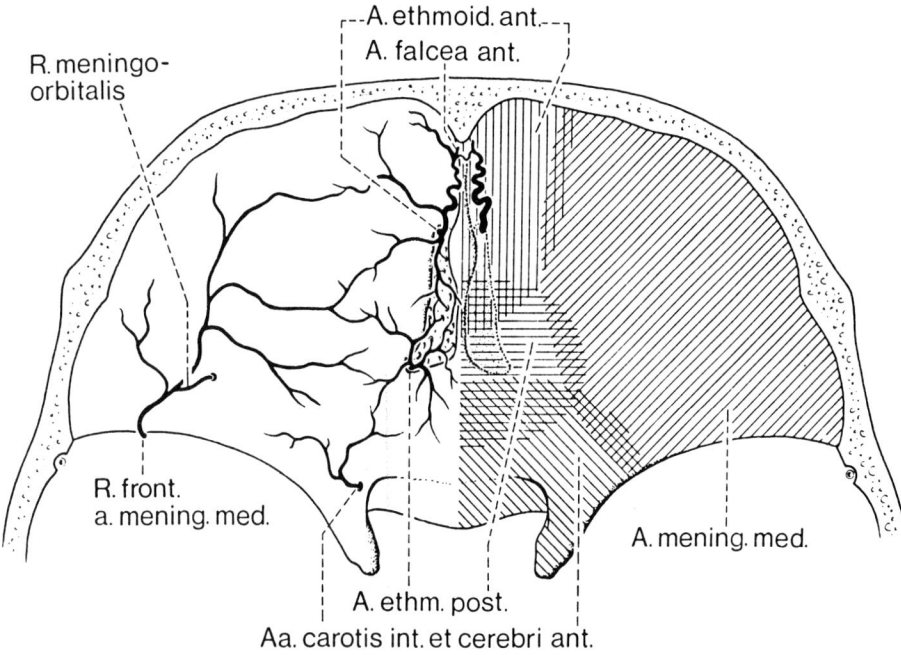

Figure 11: Arterial blood supply to the dura mater and bony parts of the anterior cranial fossa. The branch from the internal carotid artery is very variable.

bral artery. The areas supplied by the anterior cerebral artery and the middle cerebral artery are variable in extent (Fig. 12).

In our specimens, venous drainage of the posteromedial areas of the orbital surface was via the medial orbital vein (well developed in 55% of specimens), the vein of the olfactory gyrus (developed in 80% of our specimens), and the anterior cerebral veins (developed in 88% of specimens). These veins drain the blood to the basal vein of Rosenthal.[13] From the anterior parts of the orbital surface, some veins drain to the superior sagittal sinus and to the inferior sagittal sinus. The lengths of the olfactory bulb, the olfactory tract, the optic nerve, and the optic chiasm are shown in Figure 13, which also shows the distances between the anterior border of the olfactory bulb and the anterior wall of the anterior fossa and the length of the third cranial nerve.[18]

Anterior Cranial Base and Paranasal Sinuses

The paranasal sinuses develop postnatally in the floor of the anterior cranial fossa. The roof of the orbit may be almost doubled in thickness by the addition of the frontal sinus or the anterior superior ethmoid cells. The middle and the posterior superior ethmoid cells can also extend into the floor of the anterior cranial fossa and the anterior clinoid process (Fig. 14). The planum sphenoidale and the anterior clinoid process may also be pneumatized by the sphenoid sinus.[7,10]

Orbit and Optic Canal, Contents

For intracranial approaches to the orbit, the anatomy of the orbital roof is important. This region is shown in Figure 7.[19]

Orbital Walls

The lateral wall of the orbit is formed by the greater wing of the sphenoid bone, the zygomatic bone, and the lateral aspect of the frontal bone. The superior orbital fissure and the inferior orbital fissure are situated in the posterior part of the orbit, between the roof and the floor. The strong

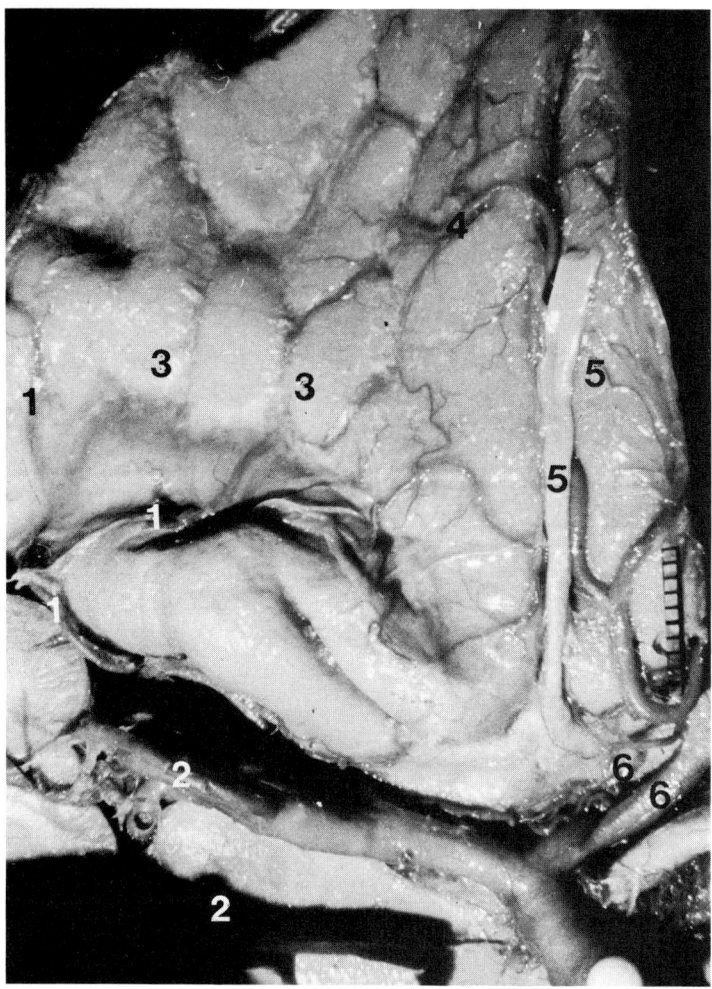

Figure 12: The brain in the floor of the anterior cranial fossa and its arterial blood supply. 1. Lateral frontobasal branch of the middle cerebral artery. 2. Middle cerebral artery, temporal pole, dissected. 3. Orbital gyri of the forebrain. 4. Medial orbitofrontal branch of anterior cerebral artery (A_2 segments). 5. Olfactory tract and gyrus rectus. 6. Anterior recurrent artery and A_1 segment.

zygomatic bone also forms the lateral orbital margin, which is superiorly bordered by the frontal bone. The length of the lateral wall of the orbit in our newborn specimens was measured to be 29.8 mm and in adult specimens to be 47.15 (mean values). In adults we measured the angle between the lateral wall of the orbit and the midsagittal plane and found it to be 35° (range 25.5–52°) on the right and 33.9° (range 23–45.5°) on the left.[19] In this area, the distance between the lateral orbital margin and the lateral border of the superior orbital fissure was estimated to be 34.3 mm (range 25–40 mm) on the right and 34 mm (range 27–40 mm) on the left. The greatest length of the superior orbital fissure we found to be 19.8 mm and the distance from its lateral end to the midsagittal plane was 26.3 mm on the right and 26.9 mm on the left.[21] This length is the shortest distance between the frontozygomatic suture and the dura-covered superior orbital fissure, and therefore also the shortest distance to the anterior border of the middle cranial fossa. These mea-

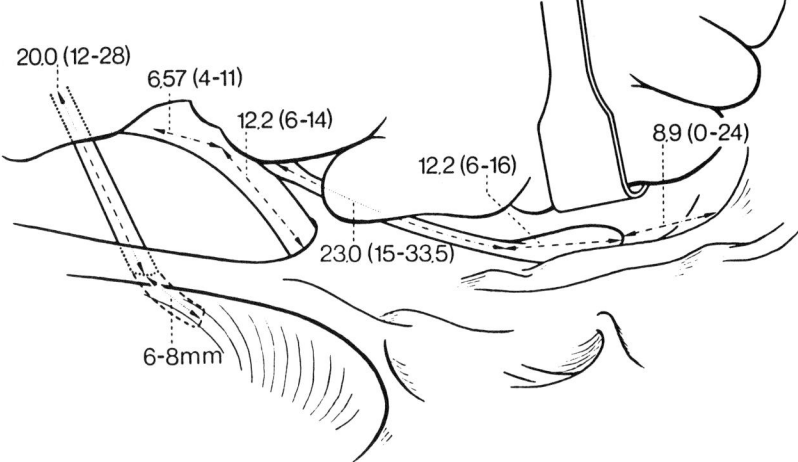

Figure 13: Length of the olfactory bulb and tract, the optic nerve and chiasm, and the third cranial nerve. Also shown is the distance between the anterior border of the olfactory bulb and the anterior border of the anterior cranial fossa. Measurements are given in millimeters (range).

surements are important when the lateral approach to the orbit is utilized.[3] It should be noted that the superior portion of the lateral orbital wall is scalloped to accommodate the lacrimal gland. We estimated the depth of this lacrimal gland fossa to be 4.51 mm (range 0–7.5 mm). The angle of the lateral wall of the orbit between the most lateral point of the orbital margin and the midsagittal plane (through the medial border of the superior orbital fissure) was found to be 46.02° (range 35–56°) on the right and on the left to be 45.1° (mean value).[19]

In the vicinity of the lateral wall of the orbit is the lateral rectus muscle. In

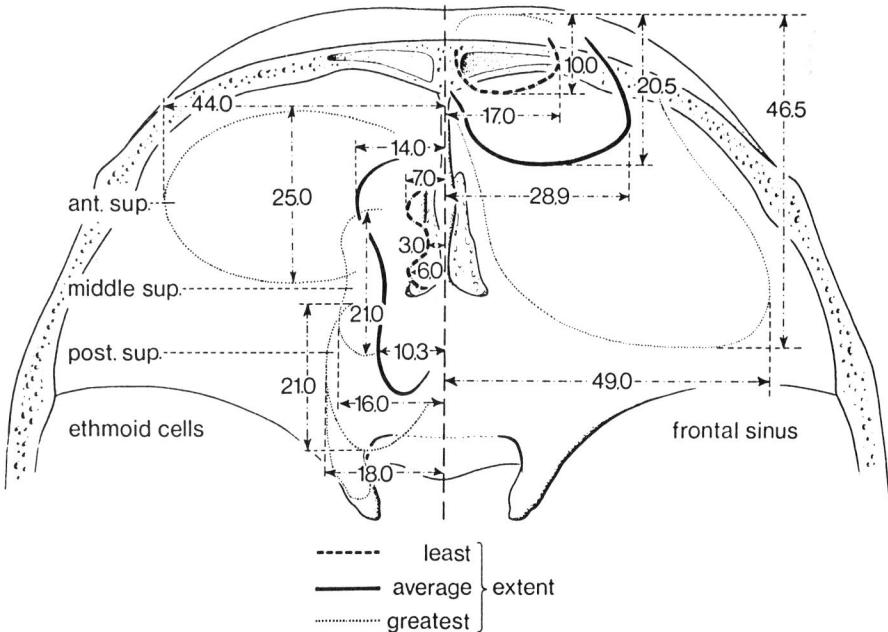

Figure 14: Mean dimensions (in millimeters) of paranasal sinuses in the floor of the anterior cranial fossa.

our specimens the muscle–tendon length was 43.0 mm (range 31.0–50.5 mm) on the right and 44.2 mm (range 33.5–50.0) on the left. The tendons alone measured 7.2 mm long on the right and, on the left, 7.8 mm long.[12] Between this muscle and the orbital wall lies a small amount of fatty tissue and the periorbita. Figure 15 shows the abducens nerve, fibers to the lateral rectus muscle, and distances from the muscle to different landmarks.[18] Figure 16 shows the distance between the lateral orbital margin and the ciliary ganglion, the distance between the cornea and the lateral orbital margin (including skin and orbicularis oculi muscles), and side to side differences.[20] Also shown are the relationship of the courses of the ophthalmic artery and the optic nerve and the length of the lower wall of the optic canal (mean 4.8 mm, range 3–8 mm).[15,18]

Medial to the lateral rectus muscle and behind the ocular bulb lie retrobulbar fatty tissue and the optic nerve, and next to the ciliary ganglion lie the long and short ciliary nerves and branches of the ophthalmic artery and ophthalmic vein. The intraorbital length of the optic nerve and its dural sheath was measured to be about 23 mm in its normal position and 26.8 mm when it was stretched. The dural and arachnoid sheaths of the optic nerve widen in most cases behind the optic bulb, possibly as a result of a rise in intracranial pressure. The measurements of the vertical diameter and also the axis of the optic canal are shown in Figure 17.[18] The medial orbital wall has a mean length in neonates of 29 mm and in adults of 46.2 mm (range 38–52 mm). Its rounded transition zone to the orbital roof is formed by the frontal bone; the posterior portion belongs to the sphenoid bone, middle portion the orbital plate of the ethmoid bone, and the anterior portion is part of the lacrimal bone, which forms the posterior lacrimal crest and the medial wall of the lacrimal sac. The more rounded anterior lacrimal crest is a part of the frontal process of the maxilla. Sometimes the orbital process of the palatine bone has an extension to the medial wall. Important landmarks of the medial wall include the ethmoidal foramina through which pass the anterior and posterior ethmoidal nerves and vessels to the upper parts of the medial orbital wall; from there they pass through the ethmoid cells to reach

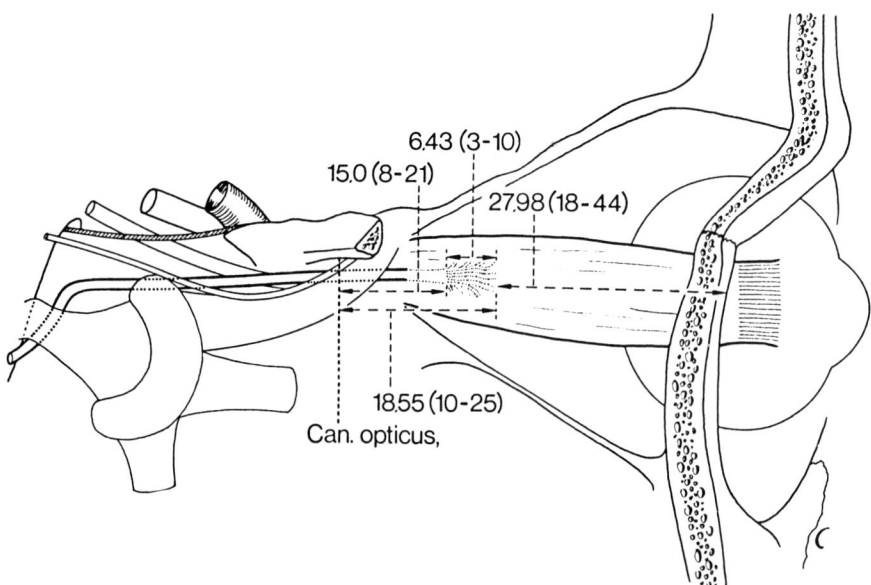

Figure 15: Measurements in millimeters (range) of abducens nerve and lateral rectus muscle. Distances from the lower border of the intraorbital opening of the optic canal and from the lateral orbital wall to the nerve fiber bundles of the sixth cranial nerve are also shown.

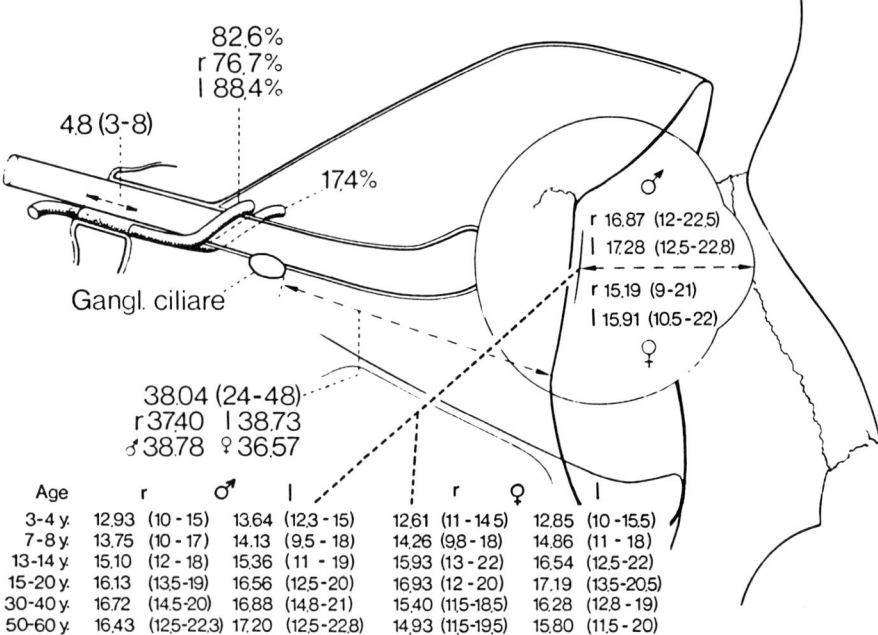

Figure 16: Inferior wall of the optic canal, course of the ophthalmic artery to the optic nerve, and the distance between the lateral rim of the orbit and the ganglion ciliare in adults. The distance between the most anterior point on the cornea and the lateral orbital rim (covered with skin and subcutaneous tissue), postnatal changes, bilateral differences, and sex differences are also shown.

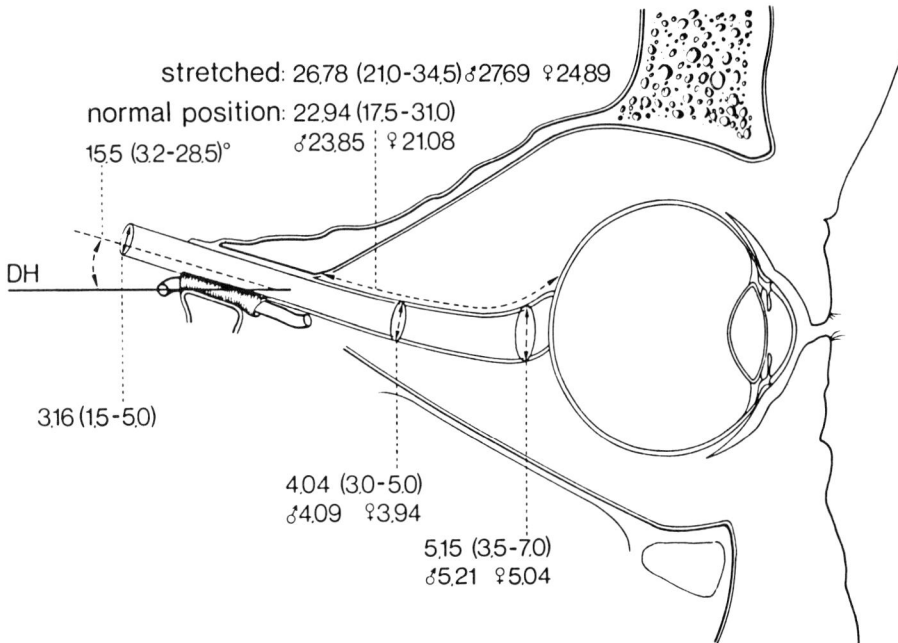

Figure 17: Intraorbital length and height of the optic nerve (with its sheaths) in millimeters (range), with sex differences.[18] The axis of the optic canal with relation to the Frankfort horizontal plane in adults was measured by Lang and Oehmann.[15] Values are given in degrees (range). Also shown is the intracranial height of the optic nerve in adults.

the anterior cranial fossa. The anterior ethmoid foramen has a diameter of 1.5 to 2.5 mm, and is most often situated in the fronto-ethmoid suture. In about 40% of instances it is in the frontal bone above the suture. The distance from the ethmoid foramen to the nasomaxillofrontal point on our specimens was 23.41 mm (range 19–28 mm). The posterior ethmoid foramen is usually smaller but also lies in the vicinity of the fronto-ethmoid suture. Its distance from the nasomaxillofrontal point was found to be 36.4 mm (range 28–42 mm). More important, however, is its distance from the orbital aperture of the optic canal, which we found to be 5.0 mm (range 2.0–11.0 mm). It should be noted that a single orbit may have from one to four ethmoid foramina. Histological preparations have shown that the veins in the end of the anterior ethmoid canal toward the anterior cranial fossa are usually greater in diameter than those near the orbit.[7,10]

On the medial orbital wall are situated the medial rectus and the superior oblique muscles. The total length of the medial rectus muscle on the right we measured to be 40.7 mm (range 35.0–48.5), and of that on the left 41.5 mm (range 36.0–47 mm).[7,12]

Figures 18A and B show the relations of the optic nerve to the orbital walls and muscles.

Floor of the Orbit

The lateral parts of the orbital floor are formed by the zygomatic bone, while the medial portion is composed of maxillary bone and posteriorly the orbital floor is formed by the palatine bone in most cases. The infraorbital nerve and artery enter the orbit through the infraorbital fissure and the orbital foramen. Inside the orbit, these structures are separated from the orbital contents by the periorbita.[5] The

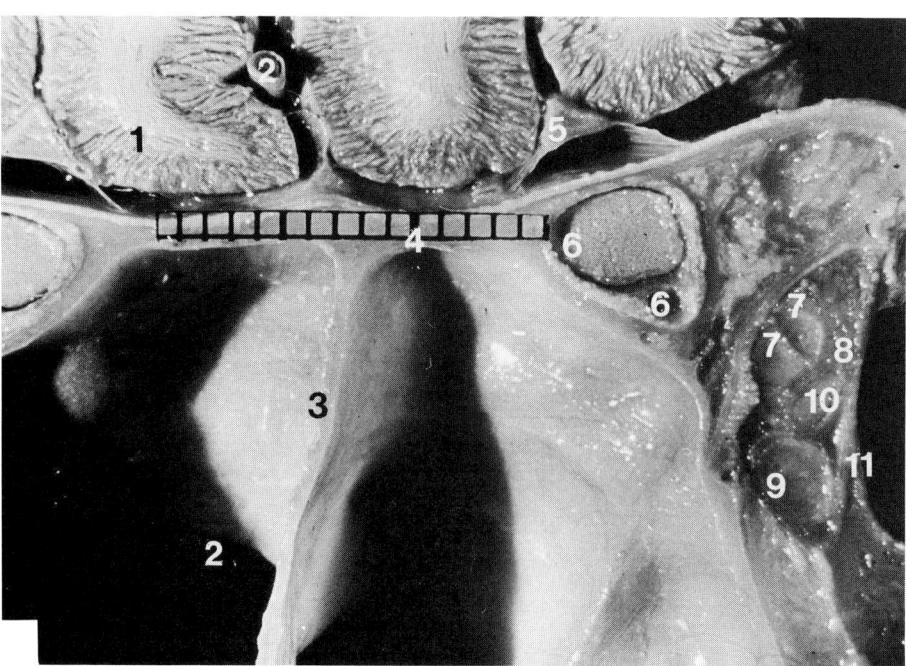

Figure 18A: Coronal section through the optic canal and surrounding structures, viewed from anterior to posterior. 1. Gyrus rectus. 2. Anterior cerebral artery (A_2 segment). 3. Septum of sphenoid sinus. 4. Planum sphenoidale and millimeter scale 5. Olfactory tract, displaced upward. 6. Optic nerve and ophthalmic artery in the optic tract. 7. Trochlear and oculomotor nerves. 8. Ophthalmic nerve. 9. Fatty tissue. 10. Abducens nerve. 11. Lateral walls of the cavernous sinus.

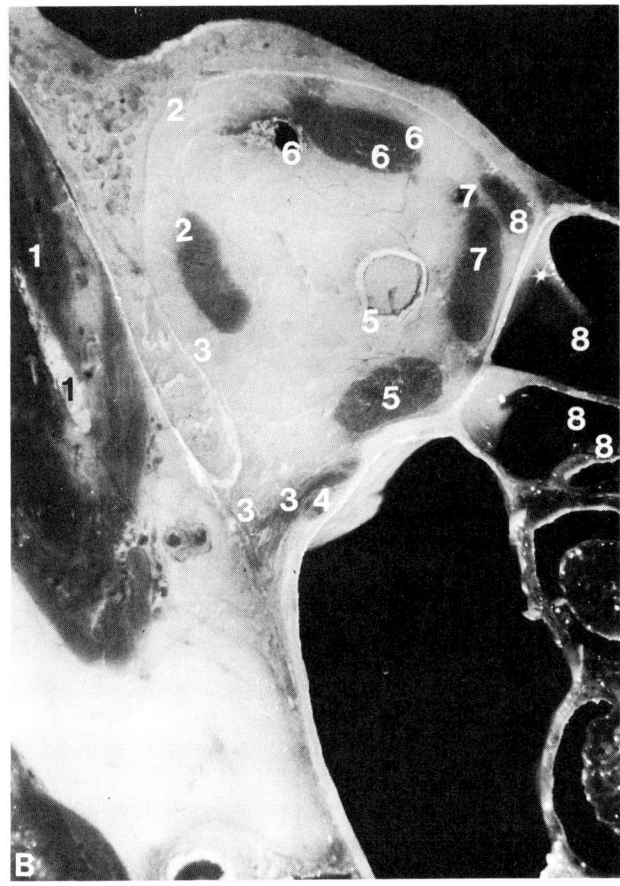

Figure 18B: Coronal section through the anterior border of the planum sphenoidale. 1. Temporal muscle and tendon. 2. Lacrimal nerve and lateral rectus muscle. 3. Orbital fat and m. orbitalis. 4. Infraorbital nerve and artery. 5. Optic nerve with sheaths, inferior rectus muscle, and maxillary sinus. 6. Levator palpebrae, superior rectus muscles, and ophthalmic vein. 7. Supraorbital artery and medial rectus muscle. 8. Superior oblique muscle, ethmoid cells, and millimeter scale.

infraorbital groove becomes roofed for varying lengths and is known as the infraorbital canal. The total length of the inferior orbital groove and canal, from the fissure to the foramen, is 26.5 mm on the right and 27.0 mm on the left (range 21–34 mm). The infraorbital artery usually runs medial to the nerve, and, rarely, lateral to it or within the nerve fascicles. Within the canal the artery was found in most cases below the nerve, less often medial to it, and most rarely lateral to it. The artery gives off an orbital branch, which pierces the orbital floor and the periorbita and anastomoses with twigs of the supraorbital and lacrimal arteries.

The orbital floor is the roof of the maxillary sinus, and surprisingly thin. We measured the thickness medial to the infraorbital groove and canal to be 0.38 mm (range 0.07–1.2 mm), and laterally to be 0.495 mm (range 0.01–1.1 mm).[16] Near the orbital rim, we estimated the bone to have a thickness of more than 1 mm (Fig. 19). It should be noted that we found the lower wall of the infraorbital sulcus or roof to be devoid of a bony covering in 12.0 to 15.4% of cases. The length of the defect was found to be between 2.95 and 11.2 mm.

Blow-out fractures of the orbital floor are the result of trauma transmitted through the orbit contents to the orbit floor. This results in compression of the orbit contents, in particular the inferior rectus muscle or its sheath but rarely the inferior oblique muscle as well.

Optic Canal

The optic canal has a narrower zone in its middle portion, which we called the isthmus of the canal.[15] This zone has a width of 4.63 mm (range 4.0–5.1 mm).

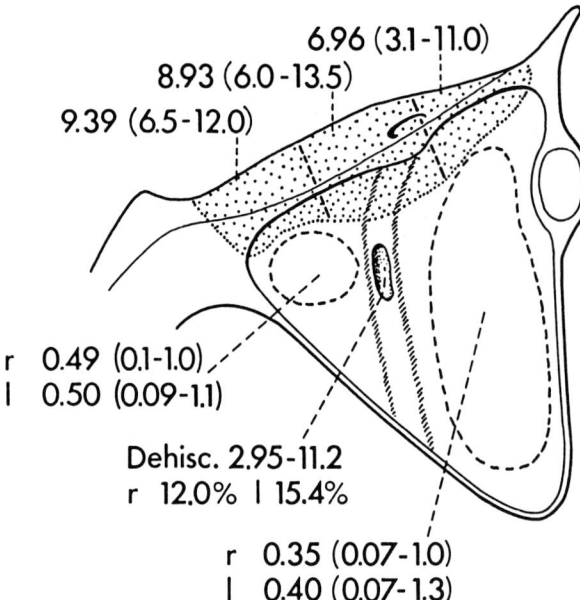

Figure 19: Roof of the maxillary sinus, seen from below. Measurements of the thickness medially and laterally, dehiscences of the infraorbital groove and canal, and the length of the lower orbital rim, which is thicker than 1 mm, are shown.

The length of the floor of the canal was measured to be 4.3 mm (range 3.0–9.3 mm); the roof has a length of 9.8 mm (range 7.3–12 mm), and becomes thin and less dense over its intracranial aperture in older people. In such cases the optic canal is roofed by a dural fold, which has a length of 2.58 mm (range 0.5–8.0 mm).[6,15] The height of the optic canal was measured to be 5.1 mm (range 4.1–6.2 mm) in adults. The thickness of the medial wall of the optic canal was measured by Maniscalco and Habal to be 0.21 mm (range 0.1–0.31 mm).[24] The axis of the optic canal with respect to the midsagittal plane we found in adults to be 39.1° (range 33.0–44.5°). According to van Alyea, the sphenoid sinus reaches to the optic canal and surrounds its upper and lower wall in about 40% of cases.[1] In some 10% of cases, an upper posterior ethmoid cell may be found in the median wall of the optic canal, which also may surround its upper surface. Below the optic nerve, the ophthalmic artery runs together with its dural, pial, and arachnoid sheaths. This artery is usually 1.25 mm wide, and runs into the orbit. At the intracranial opening of the canal, we found the artery to be in 40% of specimens medial to the optic nerve, in the middle of the canal and below the nerve in 55%, and inferolateral to the nerve in 25%.[4] After a short distance within the canal, the artery lies between the dura and the periosteal layer of the canal. Inside the orbit we found the artery lateral to the nerve in about 85% of cases and in 15% of cases medial to it. For further details see Figure 16.

The topography of the muscles, nerves, and vessels of the orbital apex is shown in Figure 20. These relationships should be understood by surgeons operating on gliomas of the optic nerve, which sometimes have intraorbital and intracranial extensions. The superior orbital fissure is an important structure, transmitting the third and fourth cranial nerves, the ophthalmic branch of the fifth cranial nerve, and the abducens nerve. In most cases we found that the ophthalmic nerve divided posterior to the superior orbital fissure into frontal, lacrimal, and nasociliary branches. Division of the third cranial nerve into an upper and lower branch was also found to occur behind the superior orbital fissure.[7] The pathways of these nerves and of the ophthalmic vein are complicated by the fact that in the medial part of the superior orbital fissure lie the zones of origin of the tendons of the lateral, inferior, superior, and medial rec-

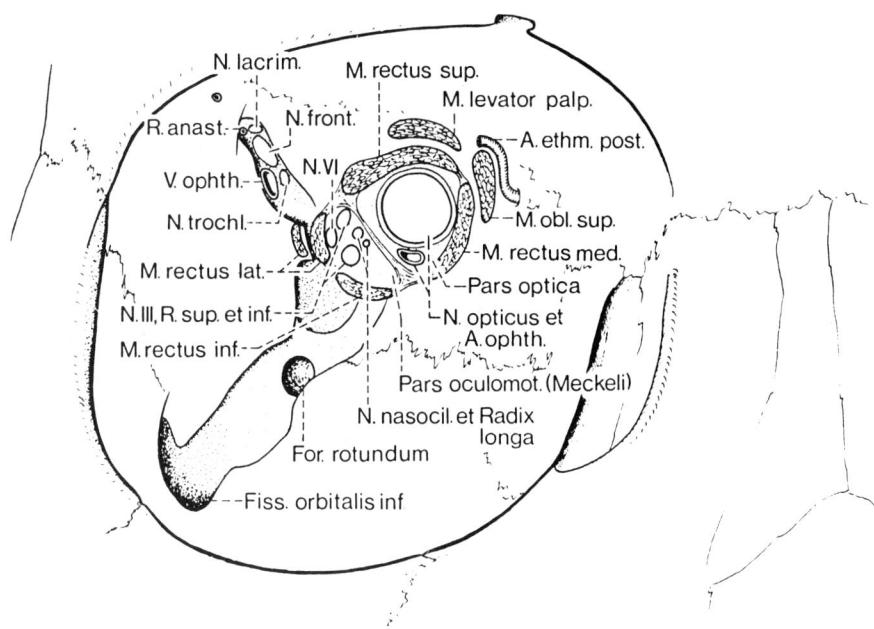

Figure 20: The nerves, vessels, and origins of orbital muscles, viewed from anterolaterally. The zone of origin of the muscles is called the annulus of Zinn. An oblique fibrous structure divides the annulus into optic and oculomotor parts. Also shown are the nerves and vessels that pass through the lateral part of the superior orbital fissure.

tus muscles (annulus of Zinn). An oblique band, with its upper part more lateral than its lower, separates the branches of the third cranial nerve, the nasociliary nerve, and the abducens nerve from the optic nerve and the ophthalmic artery. Lateral and superior to the common tendinous ring, the trochlear nerve, the frontal nerve, and the lacrimal nerve, the anastomotic branch between the middle meningeal artery, and the ophthalmic artery and the ophthalmic vein are situated; only in rare cases did we find the ophthalmic vein running through the common tendinous ring or inferior to the ring.

References

1. Alyea OE Van: Sphenoid sinus anatomic study with consideration of the clinical significance of the structural characteristics of the sphenoid sinus. *Arch Otolaryngol* 34:225-253, 1941.
2. Bergerhoff W, Stilz R: Die Beugung der Schädelbasis im Röntgenbild. *RÖFO (Stuttgart)* 80:618-622, 1954.
3. Berke RN: A modified Kronlein operation. *Trans Am Ophthal Soc* 51:193-231, 1953.
4. Engel A: Ursprungs—und Verlaufsvariationen der ersten Ophthalmica-Strecke. *Med Diss*, Wurzburg, 1975.
5. Lang J: Über die Vascularisation der Periorbita. *Gegenbaurs Morphol Jahrb* 121:174-191, 1975.
6. Lang J: Optic nerve topographic anatomy. In Samii M, Jannetta PJ (eds) *The Cranial Nerves*, New York, Springer-Verlag, 1981, pp 77-84.
7. Lang J: *Clinical Anatomy of the Head. Neurocranium—Orbit—Craniocervical Regions*, translated by Wilson RR and Winstanley DP. Berlin, Heidelberg, New York, Springer-Verlag, 1983.
8. Lang J, Brückner B: Über dicke und dünne Zonen des Neurocranium, Impressiones gyrorum und Foramina parietalia bei Kindern und Erwachsenen. *Anat Anz* 149:11-50, 1981.
9. Lang J, Götzfried HP: Über praktisch-arztlich wichtige Masse an der Fossa cranialis media. *Anat Anz* 151:433-454, 1982.
10. Lang J, Haas R: Neue Befunde zur Bodenregion der Fossa cranialis anterior. *Verh Anat Ges* 73:77-86, 1979.

11. Lang J, Hofmann S, Maier R, et al: Über postnatale Wachstumsveranderungen im Bereich der Fossa cranialis posterior. I. Facies posterior partis petrosae (Porus et Meatus acusticus internus, Fossa subarcuata, Apertura externa aqueductus vestibuli, Apertura externa canaliculi cochleae). *Gegenbaurs Morphol Jahrb* 127:305-342, 1981.
12. Lang J, Horn TH, Eichen U: Über die ausseren Augenmuskeln und ihre Ansatzzonen. *Gegenbaurs Morphol Jahrb* 126:817-840, 1980.
13. Lang J, Koth R, Reiss G: Über die Bildung, die Zuflusse und den Verlauf der V. basalis und der V. cerebri interna. *Anat Anz* 150:385-423, 1981 b.
14. Lang J, Kräussel W: Über das Wachstum der Basis cranii (Abstrands-messungen von aussen und Asymmetrieprobleme). *Anat Anz* 150:455-470, 1981.
15. Lang J, Oehmann G: Formentwicklung des Canalis opticus, seine Masse und Einstellung zu den Schadelebenen. *Verh Anat Ges* 70:567-574, 1976.
16. Lang J, Papke J: Über anatomische Grundlagen der blow-out-fractures der Orbita. 2. *Arb Anat Ges*, Wurzburg, 1980.
17. Lang J, Reiter U: Über den Verlauf des N. abducens vor der Austrittszone aus dem zentralnervosen Organ bis zum M. rectus lateralis. *Neurochirurgia* (Stuttg) 28:1-5, 1985.
18. Lang J, Reiter W: Über praktisch-ärztlich wichtige Masse des N. opticus, des Chiasma opticum und des Tractus opticus. *Gegenbaurs Morphol Jahrb* 131:777-795, 1985.
19. Lang J, Roth CH: Über die Flache des Bodens der vorderen Schadelgrube und des Augenhohlendaches. *Anat Anz* 156:1-19, 1984.
20. Lang J, Schäfer WD, Grafen W, et al: Über Seitenuntershiede der Lage des Hornhautscheitelpunktes zum lateralen Orbitalarand (Messungen mit dem Exophthalmometer nach Hertel). *Klin Monatsbl Augenheilk* 187:521-524, 1985.
21. Lang J, Schlehahn FA: Über die postnatale Entwicklung der Fissurae orbitales. *Gegenbaurs Morphol Jahrb* 127:849-859, 1981.
22. Lang J, Schlehahn FA, Schaefer K: Ueber den Inhalt der Canales ethmoidales. *Verh Anat Ges* 73:87-94, 1979.
23. Lang W: Injuries and diseases of the orbita. *Trans Ophthalmol Soc* 9:41-45, 1889.
24. Maniscalco JE, Habal MB: Microanatomy of the optic canal. *J Neurosurg* 48:402-406, 1978.
25. Schmidt H-M: Über Masse und Niveaudifferenzen der Medianstrukturen der vorderen Schadelgrube des Menschen. *Gegenbaurs Morphol Jahrb* 120:538-559, 1974.
26. Whitaker SR, Sprinkle PM, Chou SM: Nasal glioma. *Arch Otolaryngol* 107:550-554, 1981.

16

Anterior Craniofacial Resection

Victor L. Schramm, Jr., M.D.

Introduction

In the past, the prognosis for patients with neoplasms involving the skull base was extremely poor. Even patients with benign disease originating from the intracranial space but extending into the nose or paranasal sinuses inevitably suffered local recurrence after incomplete transcranial resection, and those with malignancies arising within the nose or paranasal sinuses and extending through the thin, superior bony boundaries were treated incompletely by transfacial resection of the lesion. Radiation therapy was infrequently effective in eliminating persistent local disease. Now, however, the techniques of craniofacial resection offer surgical cure for most patients presenting with disease involving the junction of the cranium and face.

A type of anterior craniofacial resection was first described by Dandy,[1] who in 1941 reported on a technique for resection of orbital tumors by a transcranial approach. Tumors of the frontal and ethmoid sinuses were treated surgically by Smith et al.[10] and Malecki[6] in the 1950s, and in the 1960s Ketcham and van Buren[3-5,11] reported their experiences using a combined surgical approach to manage carcinoma of the paranasal sinuses. However, while the benefits of using this procedure to effect complete tumor resection were considerable, the incidence of complications was high—up to 80% of the patients suffered some type of complication, and 7% died.[4] Then, in 1976, Sisson et al.[9] reported on techniques of management and suggested measures to decrease the incidence of complications following craniofacial surgery to manage sinus tumors. Schramm et al.[8] further modified the surgical approach and introduced a reconstructive technique using a galeal pericranial flap that resulted in much lower morbidity and mortality. Johns et al.[2] also reported on the use of a pericranial flap to protect dural closure after anterior fossa craniofacial resection. These developments have made the anterior craniofacial resection the best tolerated and least complicated of all currently used techniques of skull base surgery.

Indications for Craniofacial Resection

Almost all diseases involving the anterior skull base may be successfully and safely resected by a craniofacial approach. These include benign tumors of the

From: Sekhar LN, Schramm VL Jr, eds: *Tumors of the Cranial Base: Diagnosis and Treatment.* Mount Kisco, New York, Futura Publishing Co, Inc, © 1987.

meninges or skull base, such as meningiomas, fibro-osseous lesions, and tumors of bone or cartilaginous origin that extend through the anterior skull base. In addition, the low subfrontal exposure provided by the technique is ideal for resection of certain suprasellar lesions, and for complete removal of orbital tumors, such as lacrimal adenocystic carcinomas. Tumors of the nasal cavity, including esthesioneuroblastomas, carcinomas, chondrosarcomas of the nasal septum, and mucosal melanomas, may be removed en bloc with intracranial and transfacial resection, and applied tumors of the superior aspect of the paranasal sinuses can also be completely excised by craniofacial techniques. Further, tumors originating from facial skin, even when bone is extensively involved, may be removed satisfactorily by this type of approach.

Nevertheless, tumor location and biological behavior impose some limitations on anterior craniofacial resection. For instance, the resection of tumors that extend to the nasopharynx, cavernous sinus, or middle cranial fossa requires the combination of several surgical approaches, such as transfrontal, transfacial, and infratemporal fossa, although by combining various operative exposures there is virtually no area of tumor extension that cannot be encompassed. The behavior of certain tumors, however, makes their surgical excision ultimately less rewarding. For example, undifferentiated carcinomas or adenocystic carcinomas that extend to involve the brain or optic chiasm, or that have metastasized to cervical lymph nodes, have usually metastasized systemically, limiting the effectiveness of craniofacial resection. For this reason, when patients present with undifferentiated tumors, computerized tomographic scanning of the chest and abdomen is indicated; patients with systemic metastasis are not considered candidates for craniofacial resection at present.

Surgical Anatomy

Anterior cranial exposure is most frequently achieved through a high bicoronal incision, the lateral extent of which is carried to the area above the auricle so that the anterior branches of both temporal arteries are preserved. The galea aponeurotica and the cranial periosteum are supplied by separate supratrochlear and supraorbital vessels, as well as by lateral temporal vessels, and these two layers are separated by loose areolar tissue that is penetrated by numerous fine interconnecting vessels. Thus, an inferiorly based galeal pericranial flap usually has a good blood supply although separate flaps of periosteum and galea may be used when necessary.

Because the frontal bone above the frontal sinus, the temporal squama, and the parietal bone are diploic, they are relatively less resistant to infection than the thin, membrane-like bone of the anterior plate of the frontal sinus. When the frontal sinus is undeveloped, the bone at and above the glabella is generally thick so that a beveled saw cut through this bone permits removal of the anterior table and provides the same low exposure as a transfrontal sinus approach.

The dura is thinnest over the jugum and planum sphenoidale and is closely adherent to the frontal bone, particularly over the midline frontal crest and suture line, making it particularly susceptible to tearing in these areas during extradural elevation. Where superior sagittal sinus begins anteriorly at the foramen cecum through which it receives a vein from the nasal cavity, it is covered only by a thin outer layer of dura at the midline. The dura is penetrated by the olfactory nerves lateral and posterior to the crista galli, which protrudes into a sulcus in the dura posterior to the frontal crest, and transection of these nerves almost invariably produces cerebrospinal fluid leakage.

In the orbit, the anterior and posterior ethmoid arteries penetrate the skull base between the ethmoid and frontal bones and mark the roof of the ethmoid. The optic nerve lies 3 to 7 mm posterior to the posterior ethmoid vessel—with the optic chiasm at the posterior surgical limit of anterior fossa dissection and just superior and medial to the carotid arteries and cavernous sinuses. The cribriform plate lies at a level caudal to the roof of the ethmoid sinus which predisposes it to injury when this area is approached laterally from the ethmoid. Within the sphenoid sinus, the carotid artery may protrude to within 3 or 4 mm of the midline and be dehiscent of bone; when it is thus covered only by dura and sinus mucoperiosteum, it is vulnerable to injury. The ophthalmic artery is also very susceptible to injury, for example, by a bipolar cautery or by the pressure of nasal packing following resection, where it enters the orbit through the optic canal and within the dural sheath of the optic nerve. Blindness will result if the artery is injured or even temporarily compressed.

Patient Evaluation

The resectability of a given lesion is determined by its location and extent, as evidenced by computerized tomography performed with and without contrast medium in the axial and coronal planes. Magnetic resonance imaging is useful for delineation of the intracranial extent and the relationship of the tumor to the petrous and the cavernous carotid artery, while an arteriogram may be helpful in delineating the extent of a vascular lesion, such as a meningioma or angiofibroma, and is often used to determine the best method of managing the carotid artery. Angiographic embolization of vascular tumors is not utilized because of the local inflammatory reaction produced and because current surgical technique circumvents rather than transgresses the tumor, minimizing operative blood loss.

A histological tissue diagnosis is preferred whenever possible. For nasal and paranasal sinus tumors this may be done by intranasal or transnasal biopsy; external facial incisions should be avoided if at all possible to preclude contamination of incisions by tumor and possible difficulties in planning subsequent skin incisions. Certain tumors such as meningioma and fibro-osseous lesions have characteristic radiographic appearances and biopsy is not necessary for their diagnosis.

Once the tumor type and location have been determined, the involved specialists, including the anesthesia team, plan the tumor resection and skull base reconstruction.

Operative Technique

Preparation of the Patient

The tumor bed or nasal cavity should be cultured 24 to 48 hours preoperatively, and prophylactic intravenous antibiotic therapy begun 2 to 6 hours prior to surgery. High doses of penicillin and chloramphenicol have been used most frequently for patients undergoing anterior craniofacial resection, and when this prophylaxis has been utilized, no patient has developed postoperative wound infection or meningitis. Tracheostomy has not been necessary for patients undergoing anterior craniofacial surgery, but securing the oral endotracheal tube by wiring it to the mandibular teeth or by circum-mandibular wiring allows for safe administration of the anesthesia and adequate preparation of the entire scalp and face. A lumbar subarachnoid drain is always placed for fluid drainage of cerebrospinal fluid (CSF).

The patient is placed supine for surgery with the head held on a horseshoe or donut head-holder. The anterior scalp may be shaved; however, we have found it sufficient to shampoo the hair with soap, rinse it with alcohol, and part the hair along the line of the bicoronal incision. No patient who underwent the procedure with the unshaven scalp has developed a complication and all have appreciated the cosmetic results. The operative field is prepared so that anesthesia personnel are located near the foot of the table allowing the surgeon access to both sides of the face as well as to the top of the head.

Intracranial Portion of Procedure

The bicoronal scalp incision should begin laterally just above the midportion of the pinnae, and meet in the frontal area at least 10 cm above the glabella (Figs. 1A, B). The incision area is infiltrated with a combination of 0.5% idocaiane and 1:200,000 epinephrine, and the skin incision is made with a scalpel and extended to a level below the hair follicles. To minimize blood loss, electrocautery can be used to cut the galea and pericranium. Raney clips may be applied to the incised skin edges, but immediate hemostasis with bipolar cautery or ligatures is preferred.

The periosteum is elevated with the coronal flap, generally dividing it along the temporal line laterally. As the supraorbital area is approached, care should be exercised not to injure the neurovascular pedicle at the superior orbital rim. A template of the frontal sinus made from a Caldwell view X-ray, taken at a 6 foot tube-to-patient distance, is used to outline the superior and lateral extent of the frontal sinus (Fig. 2). Then a beveled saw cut is made around the margin of the sinus and the anterior table of the frontal sinus is removed as a free bone flap, after cutting with the saw just above the orbital rims and across the glabella. Next mucosa is removed from the posterior portion of the bone, and the bone is eburnated with a cutting burr, the remaining mucosa is elevated from within the frontal sinus and removed and any remnants are excised with a cutting burr.

A drill with a cutting burr is used to thin the posterior table of the frontal sinus. Dura is initially exposed lateral to the midline, and as dura is elevated, the bone is removed from the entire posterior frontal sinus with a rongeur (Fig. 3). The bone overlying the sagittal sinus in the

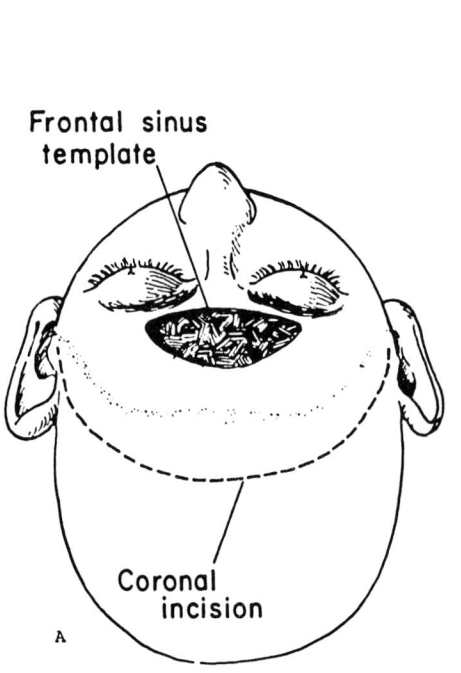
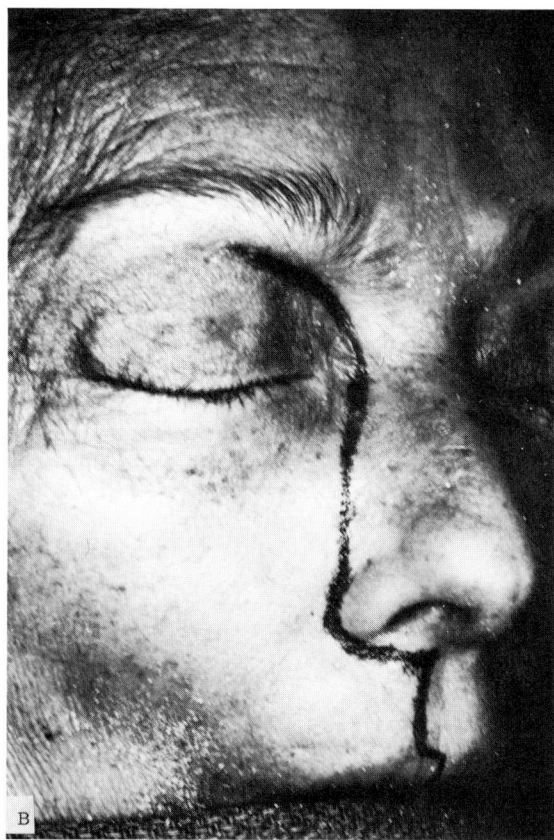

Figure 1: A: Left lateral rhinotomy incision; right bicoronal incision 10 cm above glabella (diagrammatic representation). **B:** Lateral rhinotomy incision marked on a cadaver specimen.

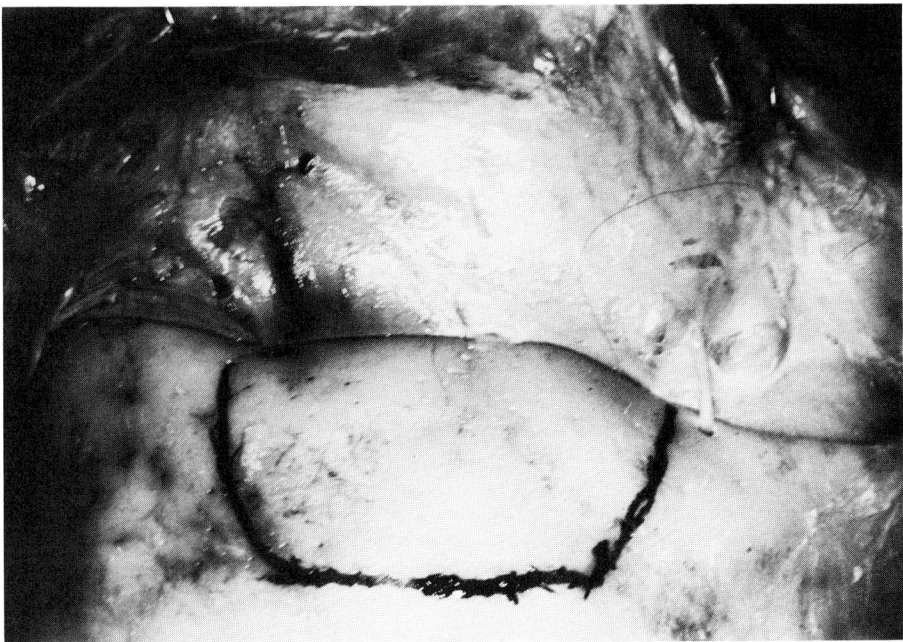

Figure 2: Coronal flap and pericranium elevated to supraorbital rims and outline of frontal sinus.

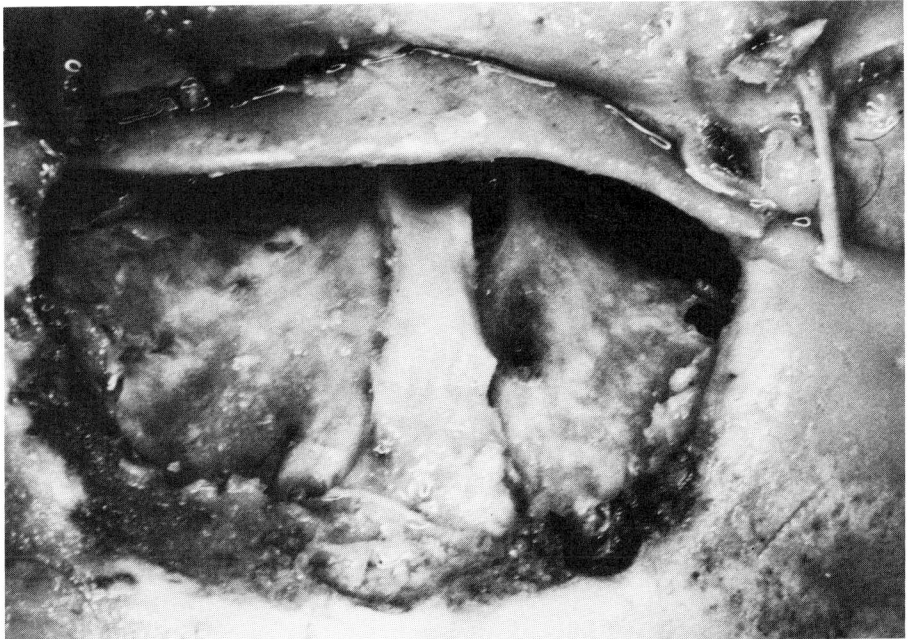

Figure 3: Anterior table of frontal sinus and sinus mucosa removed. Posterior table removed except midline over dural sinus.

midline is removed last after the dura overlying it is elevated from beneath.

As dura is being exposed, CSF is removed through the lumbar subarachnoid drain. Initially only 25 to 30 cc of spinal fluid is removed with further drainage, up to a total of 50 to 70 cc, being done as further dural relaxation is required. Occasionally mannitol, 0.5 to 1 gm/kg bodyweight, is infused intravenously to improve frontal lobe relaxation.

During the intracranial portion of the surgical procedure, the patient is hyperventilated to maintain a low PCO_2. Steroids are occasionally administered, but are usually unnecessary for anterior craniofacial surgery. Anesthetic agents must be given with care to prevent intraoperative hypertension and, in particular, marked swings from hyper- to hypotension.

Even if the frontal sinus is nonexistent, an approach similar to that just outlined is still preferred. A crescent-shaped area of bone 5 to 7 cm in lateral dimension and extending 4 to 6 cm above the glabella may be outlined. Then, utilizing the oscillating saw, the surgeon makes a beveled cut into the cancellous portion of the frontal bone and removes the anterior table. A drill is then used to thin the posterior table, just as for the removal of the posterior table of the frontal sinus, providing similar exposure and subsequent reconstruction to that just described. This approach avoids the necessity for placing burr holes in the forehead which leave postoperative defects and also leaves bone available for reconstruction similar to the membrane-like anterior table.

The next step is to elevate laterally over the roof of the orbit. If the dura has been involved by disease, an intradural dissection may be done so that dura is left in place over the roof of the nose and ethmoid sinuses. As dissection is continued posteriorly in the area of the crista galli, transection of the olfactory nerves nearly always leads to CSF leakage (Fig. 4). Unless intradural dissection is necessary, the crista galli is removed with a needle-nosed rongeur and dural elevation is continued posteriorly to the planum sphenoidale, where care should be taken to preserve dura for subsequent suturing of dural grafts. The dissection is then con-

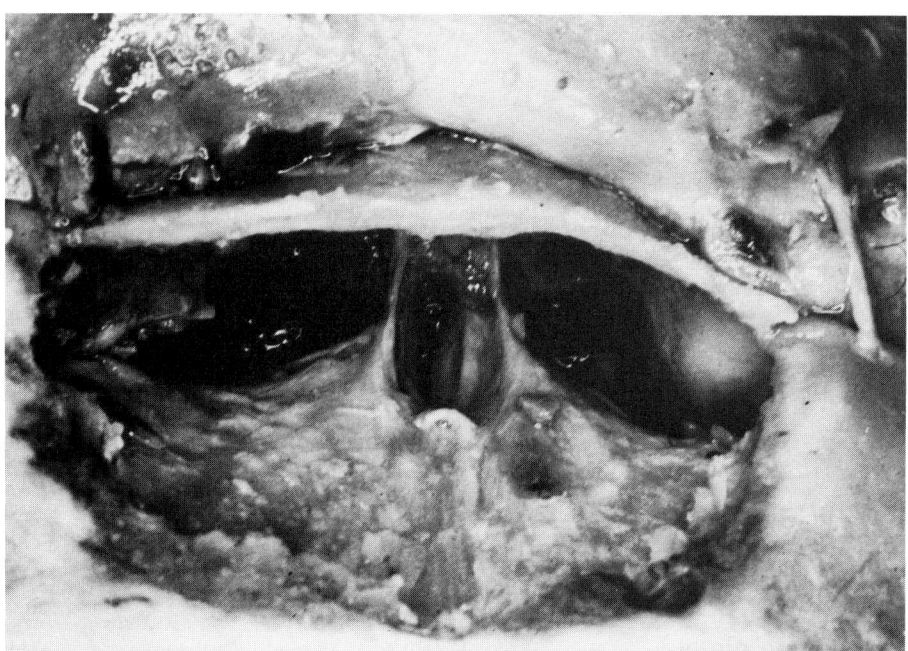

Figure 4: Midline bone and crista removed prior to transection of olfactory nerves.

tinued laterally until it is possible to visualize the intracranial portion of the optic nerves, which must be identified to be preserved prior to total resection of the orbit. During the intracranial portion of the dissection, it is unnecessary to retract the frontal lobe when dural relaxation has been achieved and the exposure is via the low frontal approach.

After the intracranial portion of dissection has been completed, small dural lacerations should be sutured, and if resection of a large portion of dura has been necessary, the dura should be grafted before facial resection is begun. Dural grafting may be done with pericranium obtained from the area posterior to the coronal incision, from temporalis fascia, or fascia lata. The dura is then covered with cottonoids and the bicoronal flap returned to its anatomic position before the facial portion of the resection is undertaken.

Facial Resection

Facial resection is usually approached through a lateral rhinotomy incision.[7] This incision begins just below the medial end of the eyebrow on the side of greatest tumor involvement, extends halfway between the dorsum of the nose and medial canthus, and then along the nasomaxillary groove to the ala before turning around the base of the ala and across the base of the nose, but leaving a rim of the nasal vestibule intact (Fig. 5). If palatal excision is unnecessary, the lip need not be split, although in some cases wider exposure of the maxillary area is

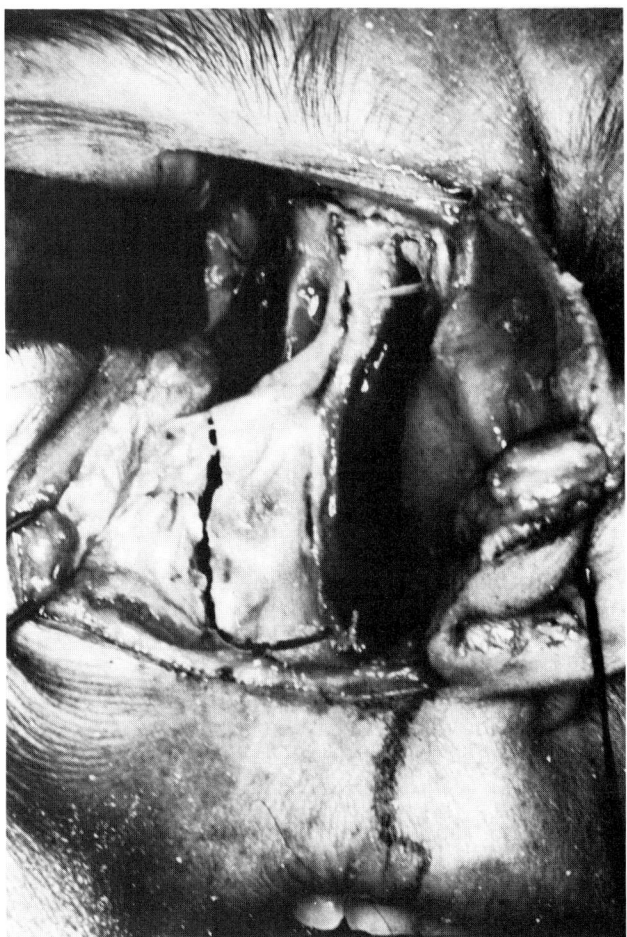

Figure 5: Lateral rhinotomy incision completed, orbital contents retracted and medial maxillectomy bone cuts made.

desirable. This may be accomplished by dividing the lip along the philtrum. A bipolar cautery is a convenient means of controlling bleeding in the area of the angular nasal vessels.

The periosteum is then cut directly beneath the incision, but is not elevated over the nasal bone so that the attachment of the nasal bone and blood supply to the bone are not compromised. Periosteum of the superior and medial orbit is then elevated and the lacrimal sac is transected. The need for further facial exposure depends on the location and extent of the tumor, and may include orbital exenteration, total orbital resection, maxillectomy, rhinectomy, or excision of facial skin.

A nasal osteotomy is done next with a reciprocating saw. A small transverse nasal osteotomy is performed to permit rotation of the nasal bone and exposure of the nasal cavity. Then a contralateral external ethmoid incision is made, and the periorbita elevated across the superior and medial aspects of the orbit, followed by coagulation of the anterior and posterior ethmoid vessels by bipolar cautery. These vessels are then divided, with the stump of the vessel left to mark the roof of the ethmoid. The lacrimal sac may be elevated from its fossa but need not be transected. In most cases it is necessary to resect the entire ethmoid, including the upper nasal septum and medial maxilla on the side of the lateral rhinotomy or total maxillectomy. Following facial resection, the bicoronal flap is turned down and the intracranial area is exposed. Next the frontal lobe is retracted, using a wide malleable retractor, and the rest of the procedure is performed under direct visualization through the orbit as well as intracranially.

Craniofacial Resection

Through the external ethmoid incision, the bone cut in the superior orbit is completed with a reciprocating saw, beginning near the optic canal and extending from posterior or anterior, lateral to the ethmoid sinus. An inferior bone cut at the junction of the maxillary antrum and ethmoid is then made, and extended superiorly at the level of the lacrimal fossa to include excision of the entire ethmoid complex. Bone cuts are then made for medial or total maxillectomy, with the superior bone cut in the orbit being made with simultaneous transfacial and intracranial visualization. The upper septum is divided, but left attached to the cribriform plate. Next a posterior cut into the sphenoid sinus, between the optic nerves, is made transcranially: a small cutting burr is used to make a groove between the optic nerves, and then a curved chisel is used to divide the planum sphenoidale and connect the anterior face of the sphenoid with the specimen. Finally, soft tissue attachments are transected with a heavy curved scissors, with bipolar cautery and suture ligating of the internal maxillary artery being used to achieve hemostasis in the maxillary area and bone edges are smoothed with a double-edged rongeur. If only medial maxillectomy is done, the mucosa is removed completely from the sphenoid and maxillary sinuses to preclude subsequent hypertrophy and difficulty with cavity care.

Intraoperative Repair

Frontal dural repair is most easily accomplished by a combination of transcranial and transfacial suturing; if the dura has been resected posteriorly near the planum sphenoidale, this is done most efficiently through the lateral rhinotomy exposure (Fig. 6). Watertight dural closure is essential, and this can be checked by infusing artificial CSF to re-expand CSF volume and observing for fluid leakage.

We have not found it necessary to graft bone or cartilage to cover the anterior skull base defect, which avoids the problems associated with free graft extrusion. The anterior fossa dura is, however, separated from the nasal and sinus cavities with a galeal pericranial flap. This flap is outlined on the bicoronal flap, beginning lateral to the anterior table bone cut and curving laterally to increase the width of the flap at its midportion (Fig. 7). This dissection should extend to within a centimeter of the bicoronal flap margin. The

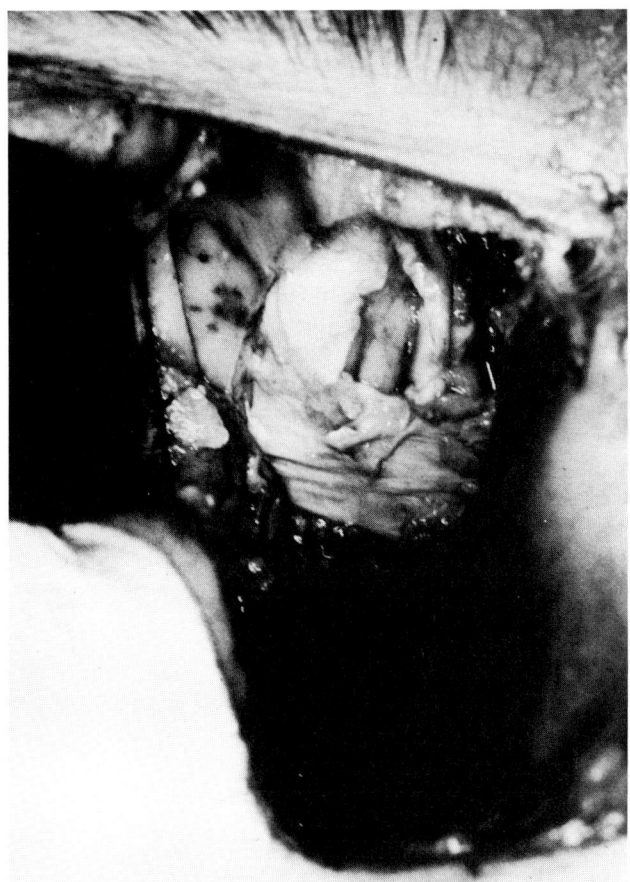

Figure 6: Facial exposure following resection showing dural defect and exposed olfactory bulb.

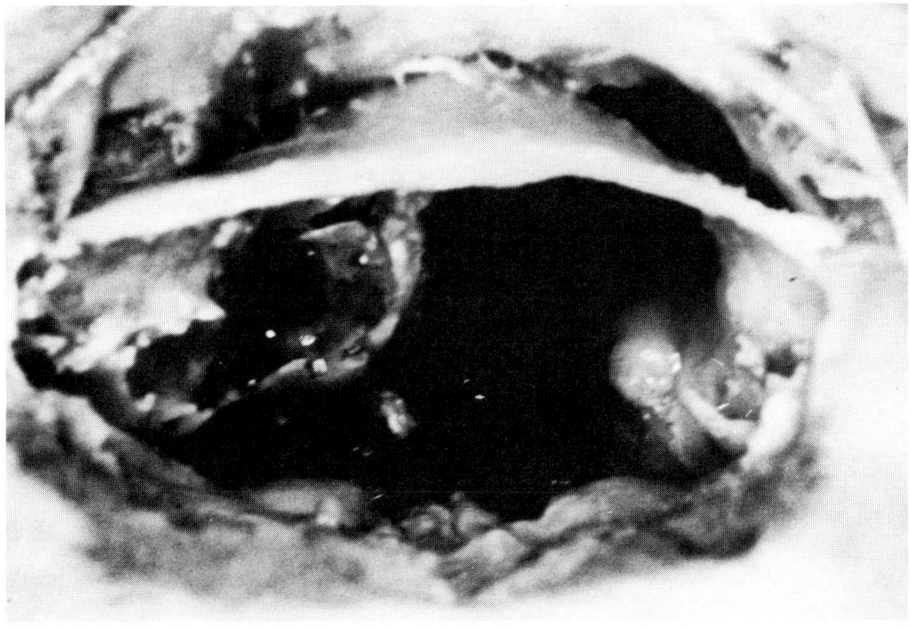

Figure 7: Cranial exposure of nasal cavity and orbital contents following resection.

galea and pericranium are dissected free of subcutaneous tissue, beginning in the area of the incision and continuing toward the supraorbital rim. When the frontalis muscle is encountered, it is split in such a way that a portion is left on the galeal pericranial flap to help ensure preservation of the supraorbital vascular supply (Fig. 8).

After the flap has been dissected to its full length, it is turned over the strut of bone at the glabella and directed posteriorly over the dura at the planum sphenoidale (Fig. 9), then tucked beneath the bone overlying the sphenoid and secured to dura by suturing through the lateral rhinotomy exposure. The flap is continued so that it lies above the superior orbital bone, and a redundant portion is left to cover the posterior aspect of the glabellar strut and fill the potential space between the anterior table of the frontal sinus and dura. The position of the galeal pericranial flap is checked visually, and antibacterial gauze packing is placed transnasally, over the flap.

When a total maxillectomy has been done, a split-thickness skin graft is applied over the galea, in addition to the facial flap. However, a skin graft is not recommended if the cavity resulting from surgical resection is accessible only through the nares, because such skin grafting tends to crust and foster secondary infection and odor in the relatively closed cavity.

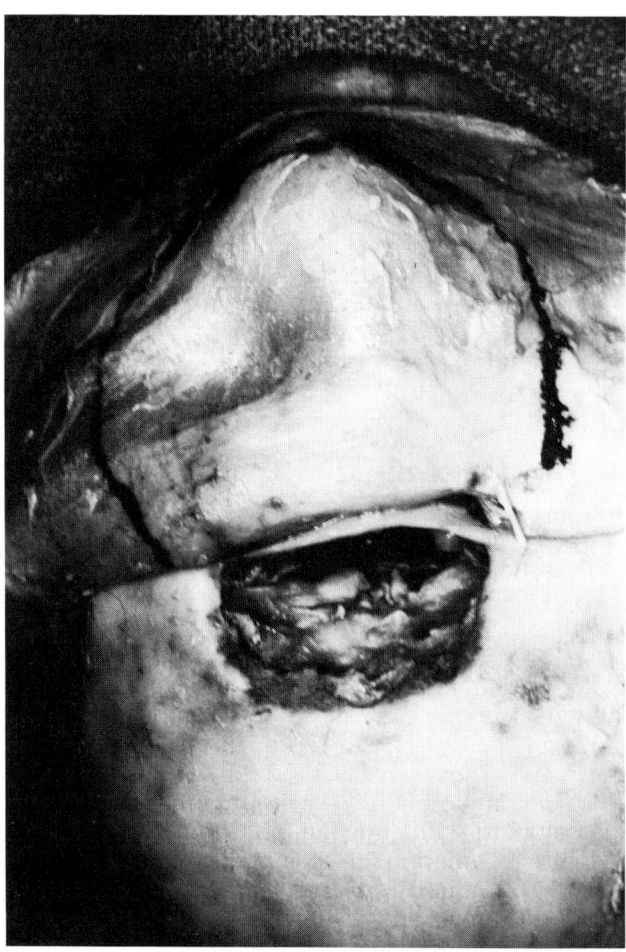

Figure 8: Galeal-pericranial flap outlined on bicoronal flap.

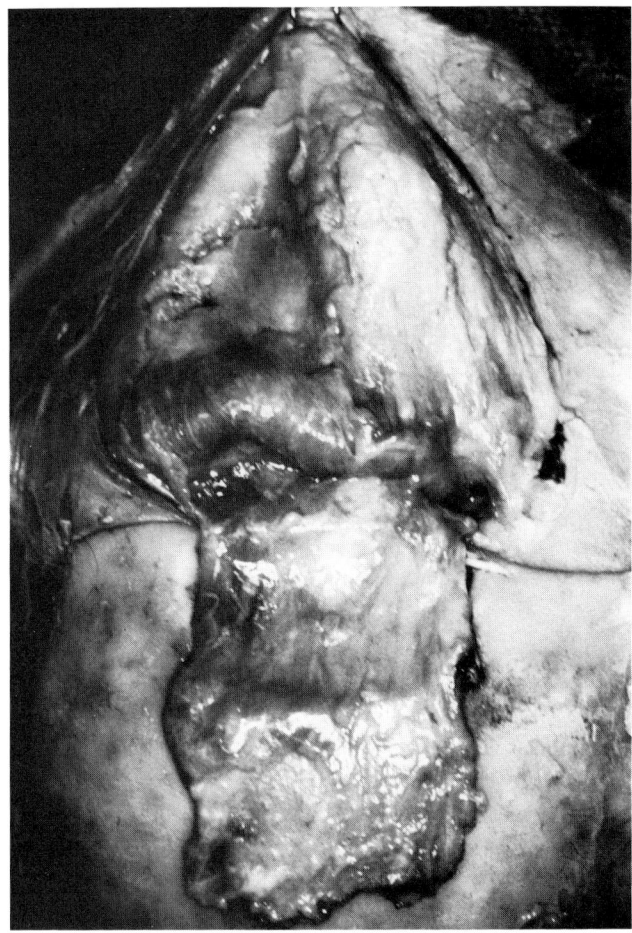

Figure 9: Galeal-pericranial flap elevated to glabella.

Closure

Drill holes are placed along the margin of the frontal bone incision and permanent dural tack-up sutures are placed to bring the dura up against the undersurface of the frontal bone so that epidural hematoma is prevented. Corresponding drill holes are also placed in the frontal bone flap, so that the flap can be secured to the superior margin of the bone incision with permanent, nonmetallic sutures. These sutures should hold the flap superiorly in such a way as to leave space above the galeal pericranial flap (Figs. 10A, B). Metallic sutures are avoided because they have been found to interfere with magnetic resonance imaging, and also may produce local osteoradionecrosis from electron scatter if postoperative radiation therapy is administered.

Closure of the facial approach includes marsupialization of the lacrimal sac and intubation of the superior and inferior canaliculi with Silastic tubing which should be left in place for at least 6 weeks. A permanent suture is placed in the medial canthal ligament and secured through a drill hole in the bone, as far posteriorly and superiorly as possible; such slight overcorrection of the position of the medial canthal ligament is necessary because the ligament will relax postoperatively, leading to drooping of the medial canthus. After subcutaneous tissues and skin have been closed, sterile paper tape is placed over the nose; following closure of the coronal incision, a plas-

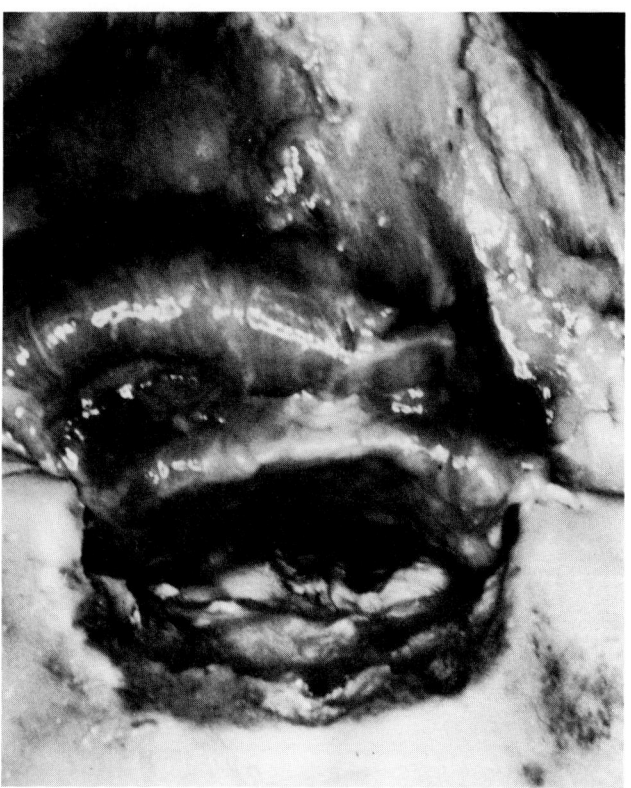

Figure 10A: Flap interposed between repaired dura and nasal cavity.

ter splint is applied to hold the nasal bone in an anatomic position. Scalp closure is completed by closing the periosteum and galea (skin staples are convenient for skin approximation), and bulky pressure dressing is applied. We do not place drains in the frontal area because they may promote leakage of CSF and draw nasal secretions into the wound.

Postoperative Care

Patients should remain intubated until they are fully awake. During the early post-anesthesia recovery phase, patients should be reminded not to cough or try to blow their noses, as such maneuvers cause increased pressure on the dural closure. In addition, it is desirable to keep the dura expanded against the galeal pericranial flap, which may be accomplished by leaving the open lumbar subarachnoid drain in place so that near-normal spinal fluid pressure can be maintained. This drain is generally left open, with the drainage bag in place for 24 to 48 hours following surgery. It should be cultured upon its removal.

Antibiotics should be continued intravenously until the nasal cavity packing is removed, which should be done relatively early when no skin graft has been placed to decrease the likelihood of cavity contamination. Prior to their discharge, which is usually 7 to 10 days following surgery, patients should be instructed in care of the cavity including irrigation. When no skin graft has been placed, the cavity re-epithelializes in 3 to 4 weeks, and if radiation therapy is to be administered postoperatively, it should be delayed until 4 to 6 weeks after surgery to allow for this epithelialization, and for adequate healing of the frontal bone flap.

Results

Sequelae and Complications

Thirty-two patients underwent craniofacial resection in this series (Table I). As a result of the surgical exposure,

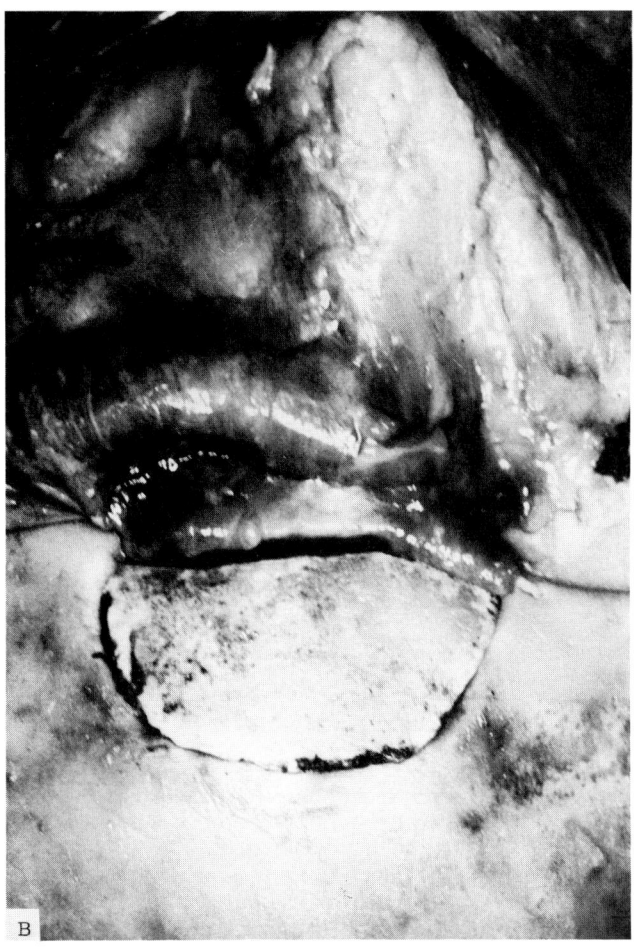

Figure 10B: Anterior frontal sinus table replaced and secured superiorly to provide space for transposed galeal-pericranial flap.

**Table I
Patient Outcome**

Disease	Number	Local Recurrence	Death
Squamous carcinoma	7	0	0
Esthesioneuroblastoma	5	0	0
Chondrosarcoma	3	0	0
Basal cell carcinoma	3	0	0
Undifferentiated carcinoma	3	1	2
Adenoid cystic carcinoma	3	1	2
Melanoma	3	0	2
Clivus chordoma	1	1*	0
Meningioma	4	0	0
	32	3	6

*Anterior craniofacial resection inadequate to excise total tumor.

all patients have become anosmic, although only a few complain of the loss of smell. There is frequently some temporary or permanent alteration in sensation in the forehead area, particularly in the scalp above the coronal incision, and some crusting in the nasal and sinus cavities is inevitable. However, if surgery has resulted in an open cavity, or if no skin graft was placed in a closed cavity, daily irrigations and cleansing are generally adequate for good hygiene.

Cerebrospinal fluid rhinorrhea, meningitis, encephalitis, and neurological sequelae from brain retraction are all potential complications of this type of surgery, but our rate of complication has been remarkably low. Only one patient in our series, the first one who underwent combined resection, developed meningitis.[8] This was the result of inadequate dural reconstruction after resection of a recurrent meningioma, which led to necrosis of the skin graft, pneumocephalus, and subsequent meningitis and cerebritis. Fortunately the patient recovered with no permanent sequelae after the dural defect had been regrafted and protected with a galeal pericranial flap.

Two patients in our series have sustained unilateral visual loss, presumably due to manipulation and compression of the ophthalmic artery, and one patient experienced pain in the lumbar area, presumably related to arachnoiditis from the lumbar subarachnoid drain. All patients undergoing anterior craniofacial resection have survived, and the complication rate utilizing the techniques described has been less than 10%.

Prognosis

Because a variety of tumors may be managed by anterior craniofacial resection, it is not possible to make more than general comments regarding their prognosis. However, of the 28 patients who underwent anterior craniofacial resection for malignancy, most are disease-free. Indeed, as noted by others,[3-5,9,11] the prognosis for patients with differentiated squamous cell carcinoma of the paranasal sinuses is quite good when they are treated by craniofacial resection. Other locally aggressive benign and malignant conditions have also been well managed by craniofacial resection, with patients who have died of the disease most often experiencing distant metastases rather than local recurrence. The techniques described have proven effective in managing disease of the anterior skull base in patients aged 32 months to 82 years.

References

1. Dandy WE: *Orbital Tumor-Results Following the Transcranial Operative Attack.* New York, Oskar Piest, 1941.
2. Johns ME, Winn HR, McLean WC, Cantrell RW: Pericranial flap for the closure of defects of craniofacial resections. *Laryngoscope* 91:952-959, 1981.
3. Ketcham AS, Chretien PM, Van Buren JM, et al: The ethmoid sinuses: A re-evaluation of surgical resection. *Am J Surg* 126:469-476, 1976.
4. Ketcham AS, Moye RC, Van Buren JM, et al: Complications of intracranial facial resection for tumors of the paranasal sinuses. *Am J Surg* 112:591-596, 1966.
5. Ketcham AS, Wilkins RH, Van Buren JM, et al: A combined intracranial facial approach to the paranasal sinuses. *Am J Surg* 106:698-703, 1963.
6. Malecki J: New trends in frontal sinus surgery. *Acta Otolaryngology* 50:137-140, 1959.
7. Schramm VL, Myers EN: How I Do It: Head and Neck. A targeted problem and its solution. Lateral rhinotomy. *Laryngoscope* 88(6):1042-1045, 1978.
8. Schramm VL, Myers EN, Maroon JC: Anterior skull base surgery for benign and malignant disease. *Laryngoscope* 89:1077-1091, 1979.
9. Sisson GA, Bytell DE, Becker SP, Ruge D: Carcinoma of the paranasal sinuses and craniofacial resection. *J Laryngol Otol* 90:59-68, 1976.
10. Smith RR, Klopp CT, Williams JM: Surgical treatment of cancer of the frontal sinus and adjacent areas. *Cancer* 7:991-994, 1954.
11. Van Buren JM, Ommaya AK, Ketcham AS: Ten years experience with radical combined craniofacial resection of malignant tumors of the paranasal sinuses. *J Neurosurg* 28:341-350, 1968.

17

Meningiomas of the Anterior Cranial Base

Robert G. Ojemann, M.D.
Karl W. Swann, M.D.

Introduction

In Cushing's classic two-volume publication on meningiomas, two chapters are devoted to tumors of the anterior cranial base: XII, Suprasellar Meningiomas–The Chiasmal Syndrome–Twenty-Eight Cases, and XIII, The Olfactory Groove meningiomas–With Primary Anosmia–Twenty-Nine Cases.[4] Anterior cranial base meningiomas also include those tumors arising from the orbital roof.[13-15] These locations account for 10% to 14% of all meningiomas.[15,20]

This chapter is based on personal experience with 36 consecutive meningiomas of the anterior cranial base treated with microsurgical techniques from 1968–1985. The location of the tumors was as follows: olfactory groove, 11; suprasellar, 23; and orbital roof, 2. The overall operative mortality was zero. Some of these patients have been included in previous publications.[13-15] In addition, appropriate references are summarized.

General Aspects of Management

Most meningiomas are benign and the majority are potentially curable. It is generally held that the completeness of surgical removal of the tumor is the single most important determinant to the likelihood of recurrence.[4,10,11,17] The objective, therefore, of operation is total removal of the meningioma including the involved dura and bone if at all possible. However, this goal must always be tempered by surgical judgment that holds as first priority the preservation and improvement of neurologic function. In some patients where total removal carries a significant risk of morbidity, it is often best to leave some tumor and plan to follow the patient with regular clinical evaluation and CT scan, considering reoperation at a later time or radiation therapy as indicated.

The use of the operating microscope has greatly reduced mortality due to vascular and hypothalamic injury.[21] In recent

---

From: Sekhar LN, Schramm VS Jr, eds: *Tumors of the Cranial Base: Diagnosis and Treatment*. Mount Kisco, New York, Futura Publishing Co, Inc, © 1987.

Portions of this chapter are reproduced with permission from Ojemann RG: Meningiomas of the basal para-pituitary region; technical considerations. Clin Neurosurg 27:233-262, 1980, and Ojemann RG: Clinical features and surgical management of meningiomas. In Wilkins RH, Rengachary SS (eds): *Neurosurgery*. New York, McGraw-Hill Book Co, 1985, Vol 1, pp 635-654.

series, postoperative medical complications such as pulmonary embolism, pneumonia and gastrointestinal hemorrhage are usually the most frequent causes of mortality.[1,21]

Radiographic Studies

Computerized tomography (CT) is the mainstay of diagnosis for evaluation of tumors of the anterior cranial base. Intravenous infusion of a contrast agent typically discloses a homogenously enhancing mass characteristic of a meningioma.[12] Coronal views of the parasellar region are particularly useful in defining the relationship of the tumor to the skull base.[6] Cerebral angiography is imperative to define arterial and venous relationships to the tumor and to identify the tumor blood supply.

Preoperative Preparation

The patient is given steroids for at least 48 hours before surgery and longer if there is considerable edema in the adjacent brain tissue. This is important in helping prevent the problems caused by cerebral edema that may follow removal of a meningioma.

Preoperative embolization may be indicated in some meningiomas where there is extensive vascularity from external carotid artery branches which might prove difficult to control early in the course of the operation (see Chapter 5). We have not had occasion to use this procedure in our patients with anterior cranial base meningiomas and Al-Mefty et al. could not find any reports of its use in suprasellar meningiomas.[1]

Preparation at the Time of Surgery

The neurosurgeon should have available an anesthesiologist who is knowledgeable in the field of neurosurgery. The operating room should be prepared for neurosurgery including the availability of trained personnel, operating microscope, bipolar coagulation, Cavitron, and laser. The recovery room and intensive care unit should be staffed with individuals familiar with neurosurgical problems.

When the patient arrives in the operating room, a radial artery catheter is inserted for continuous monitoring of blood pressure and blood gases. The arterial pCO_2 is kept near 30 torr during the operation.

A smooth induction of anesthesia without the patient straining or coughing and careful control of blood pressure are important factors in getting the surgery off to a good start. After the insertion of an indwelling Foley catheter, the patient is given 10–20 mg of Lasix. During the preparation and exposure, a 20% solution of mannitol is given in a dosage of 1–1.5 g/kg over 20–30 minutes. Prior to making the skin incision, an antibiotic, usually a cephalosporin, is administered intravenously and continued for 24 hours after surgery.

After careful positioning, the patient's head is held with the three-point skeletal fixation head rest. Care is taken to try and keep the head above the heart level and to avoid compression of the jugular veins in the neck. The position must take into account the effects of gravity, the need to minimize brain retraction, and the avoidance of compression of brain against the edge of the dura.

General Principles of Operation

The entire operation is done using some type of magnification (either loupes or the operating microscope). The skin incision must allow for full exposure of the tumor. Adequate blood supply to the scalp is assured by using a flap that has a wide enough base. Consideration should be given to the cosmetic result of the scar and bone flap.

Use of a free bone flap will allow a wide, expeditious exposure of tumor and can be easily enlarged if needed. The pericranial tissue is kept intact so it can be used for dural graft if necessary. At the end of the operation, the bone flap is wired solidly in place with several #28 stainless steel wires. If burr holes or bone defects will leave a cosmetic deformity, a cranioplasty is done by placing a #28 wire across the opening through holes drilled on each side, and then filling the area with acrylic.

One should always attempt to expose as little normal brain as possible, especially when the brain is full because of the presence of a large tumor mass. Care is taken to avoid excessive retraction. Gentle pressure is placed against the capsule of the tumor or on the dural attachment to help define the plane with adjacent brain tissue. Brain tissue is gently separated from the capsule of the tumor using fine dissectors and bipolar coagulation. As blood vessels between capsule and brain tissue are encountered, they are coagulated with bipolar coagulation and cut with microscissors. In some patients it is best to do an extensive internal decompression of the tumor prior to trying to dissect the capsule. The decompression is facilitated by use of the ultrasonic aspirator (Cavitron) which fragments and aspirates tissue at the tip of the instrument, or the carbon dioxide (CO_2) laser which vaporizes tissue. The use of the CO_2 laser in the operative management of intracranial meningioma has been described in detail.[19] Bleeding from within the tumor will often cease spontaneously but in some cases bipolar coagulation or Surgicel may be needed.

Postoperative Care

Steroids are continued for several days and then gradually tapered. Anticonvulsants are usually given for at least 6 months. Serum electrolytes and urine volume and specific gravity are monitored to detect diabetes insipidus.

Olfactory Groove Meningiomas

Clinical Features

These tumors arise from the midline of the anterior fossa in the region of the cribriform plate and adjacent floor of the anterior fossa extending back onto the planum (jugum) sphenoidale. In Bakay's series of 36 patients, the complaints that led to evaluation were: failing vision, 12; dementia, 8; dementia and failing vision, 5; seizures, 4; seizures and dementia, 3; headache, 3; and urinary incontinence, 1.[2] All patients except one had anosmia on examination but in none was it the presenting symptom. Loss of a sense of smell was recorded "as possibly" the primary symptom in only three of 28 patients in Cushing's series, and he questioned the reliability of this finding.[4] In our series, the most common presenting symptom was a subtle change in mental function or headache alone or in combination, but a disturbance in vision or seizure disorder was also the initial manifestation. None complained of impairment of the sense of smell although it was found on examination.

The tumor may attain a large size before causing symptoms (Fig. 1). Bakay reported that 10 of his patients had meningiomas that were 5–9 cm in diameter.[2] The CT scan and angiographic features are characteristic for the tumor and are illustrated (Figs. 1, 2).

Surgical Management

In planning the operation, it is important to remember that the blood supply comes into the tumor through the bone in the midline of the anterior fossa from branches of the ethmoidal, middle meningeal, and ophthalmic arteries; the posterior capsule may be attached to the optic nerves, chiasm, and anterior cerebral arteries.

A bifrontal craniotomy for removal of these tumors is our usual approach. This leads to the least amount of retraction on the frontal lobes and gives direct access to both sides and posterior surface of the tumor. MacCarty prefers the bifrontal exposure.[9] Kempe describes a unilateral right subfrontal aproach.[7] Logue and Symon use either exposure and also resect part of the frontal lobe.[8,20] Solero et al. use a right frontal craniotomy with frontal lobe resection.[18]

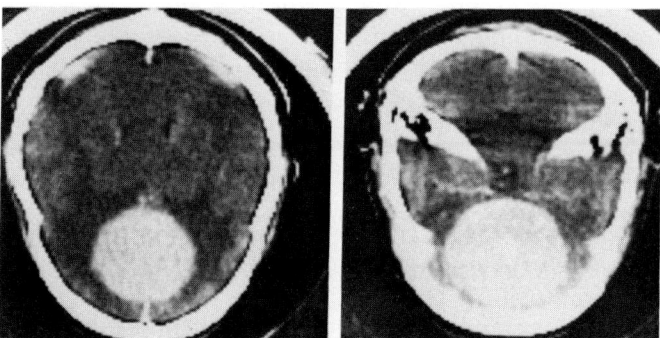

Figure 1: Olfactory groove meningioma. CT scan shows a large, round, midline enhancing mass extending from the floor of the anterior fossa into both frontal lobes with adjacent edema.

The patient is carefully placed in the supine position with the head elevated and slightly extended. Using a coronal incision, skin flap and underlying tissue, including pericranial tissue, are turned down together. Burr holes are placed just below the end of the anterior temporal line and on each side of the sagittal sinus at the level of the skin incision (Fig. 3A).

The high speed craniotome is used to create the bone flap. The frontal sinuses are almost always entered. The mucosa is removed and the sinuses are packed with bacitracin soaked Gelfoam. A flap of pericranial tissue from the back of the skin flap is turned down over the sinuses and sewn to the adjacent dura (Fig. 3B).

The dural incision is made over each

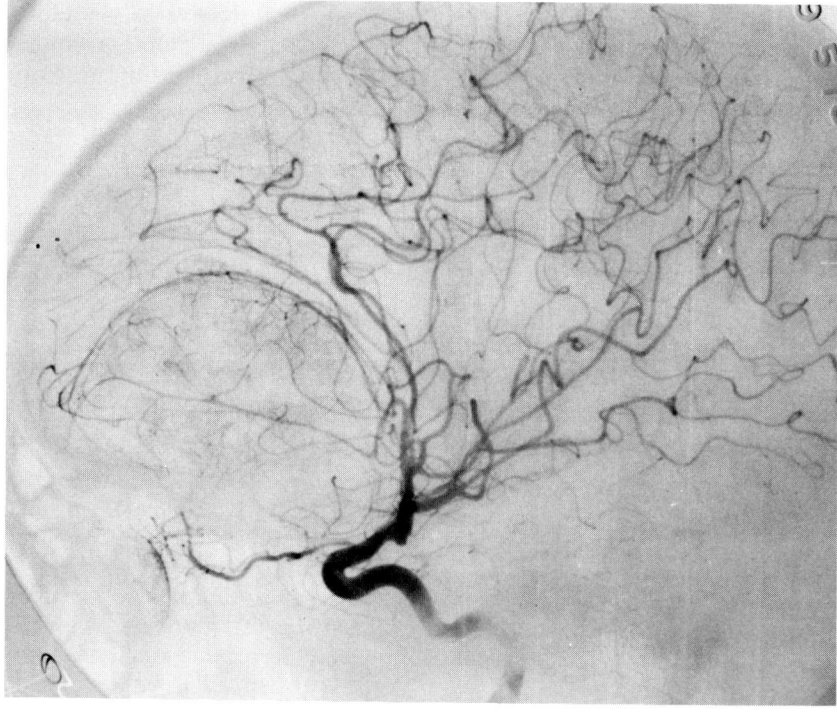

Figure 2: Olfactory groove meningioma. Lateral angiogram showing the typical stretching and elevation of branches of the anterior cerebral artery over the superior surface of the tumor. The main blood supply is coming into the base of the tumor from the branches of the ethmoidal, meningeal, and ophthalmic arteries.

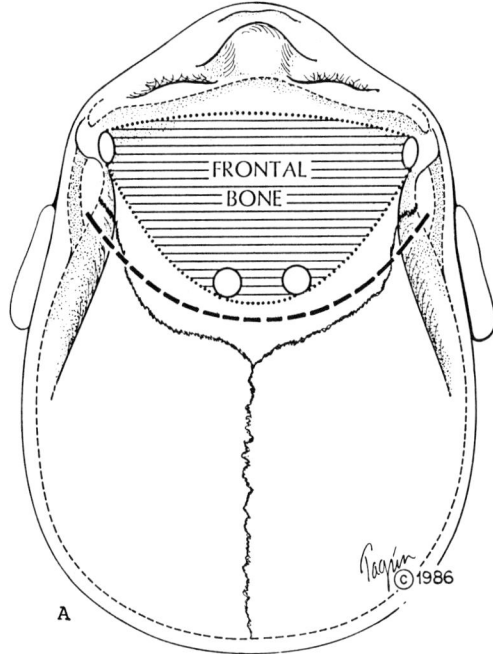

Figure 3: Olfactory groove meningioma. **A:** The skin incision (dashed line) and free bone flap (dotted line) are outlined.

and slightly posteriorly. The tumor will come into view in the midline and at times grows into the region of the crista galli and falx. The anterior capsule of the tumor is exposed and then an extensive internal decompression is done. The base of the tumor in the midline is gradually separated from the underlying bone, interrupting the blood supply which travels through numerous openings in the bone (Fig. 3D). These feeding arteries are occluded with coagulation and bone wax. The capsule can now be reflected into the area of the decompression without undue pressure on the frontal lobes. Great care is taken during the dissection of the posterior portion of the capsule, reflecting it anteriorly, being careful to look for the pericallosal branch of the anterior cerebral artery complex which may be embedded in the tumor. The frontalpolar branch will often be adherent to the tumor and may need to be divided (Fig. 3E). It is usually possible to follow the capsule back to the sphenoid wing and then, working medially, to identify the anterior clinoid processes and the optic nerves. At times it may be difficult to see the nerves because of thickened arachnoid and posterior and inferior displacement by tumor. However, under magnification, the tumor can be reflected off the optic nerves (Fig. 3F).

medial inferior frontal lobe just above the edge of the craniotomy opening. Carefully retracting the frontal lobes, the sagittal sinus is divided between two silk sutures and the falx is cut (Fig. 3C). The frontal lobes are then carefully retracted laterally

Once the bulk of the tumor is re-

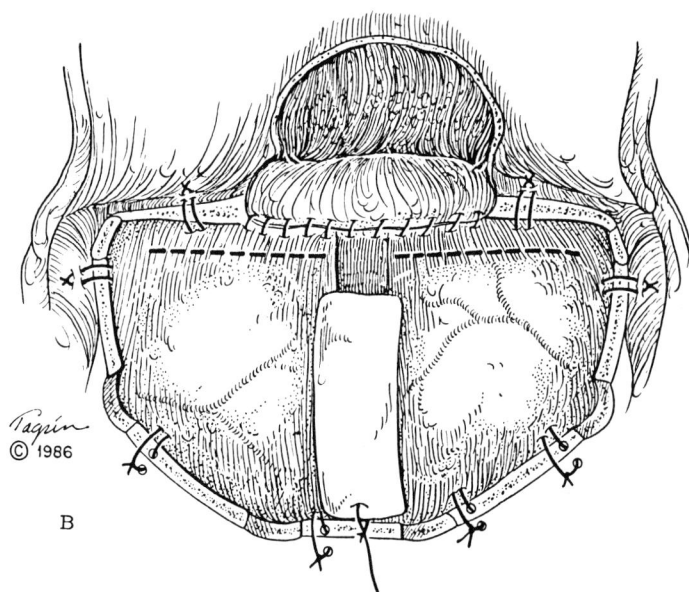

Figure 3B: Frontal sinuses are almost always entered. the mucosa is removed and the sinuses packed with Bacitracin-soaked Gelfoam. The opening is covered with a flap of pericranial tissue sutured to the dura with a continuous stitch.

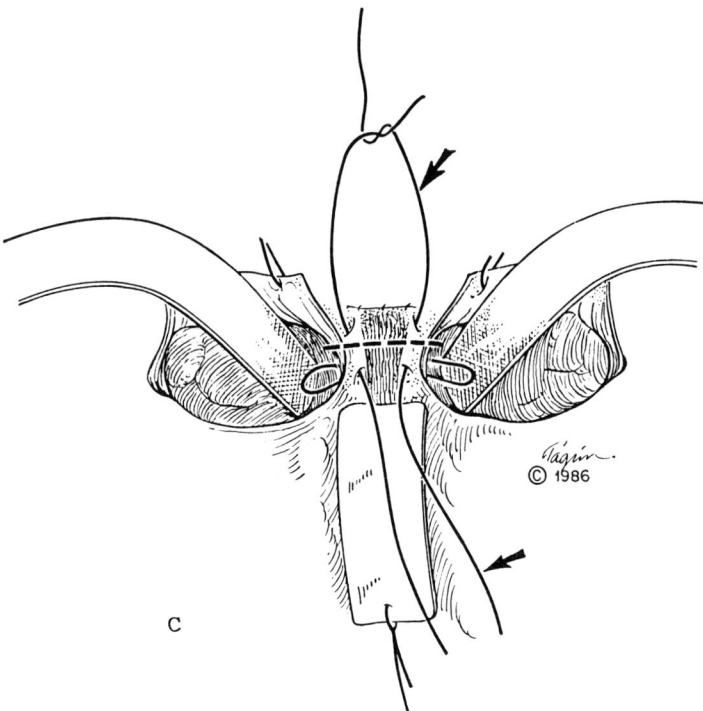

Figure 3C: The anterior sagittal sinus is ligated.

moved, the dural attachment is totally excised and any bone hyperostosis removed (Fig. 3G). The region of the cribriform plate is covered with a graft of pericranial tissue and Gelfoam to prevent a CSF leak. Symon reports that the recurrence rate of these tumors is so low that there is no need to excessively treat the bone and one should avoid entering the ethmoid air cells if possible.[20]

Results

In this series, all 11 tumors were totally removed with restoration of normal mental function and full activity in 10 pa-

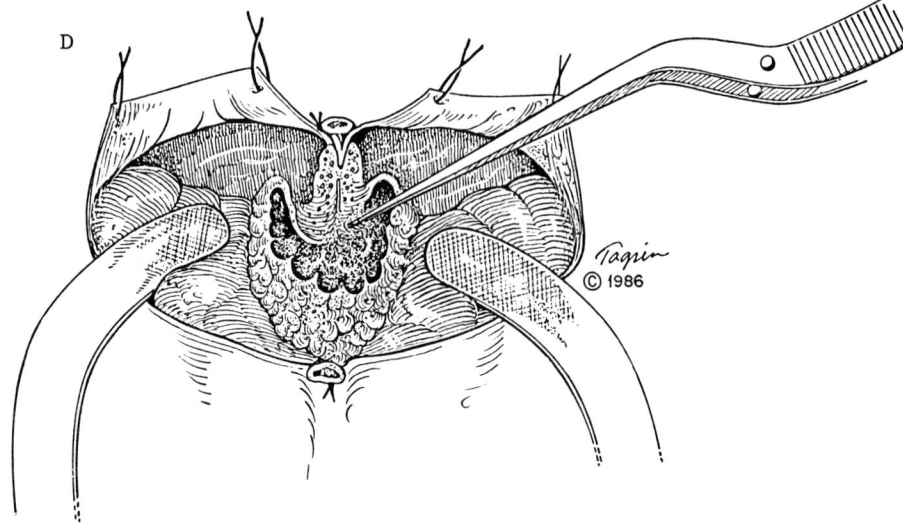

Figure 3D: Internal decompression of the tumor has been accomplished and the blood supply coming through the midline of the frontal fossa is being occluded.

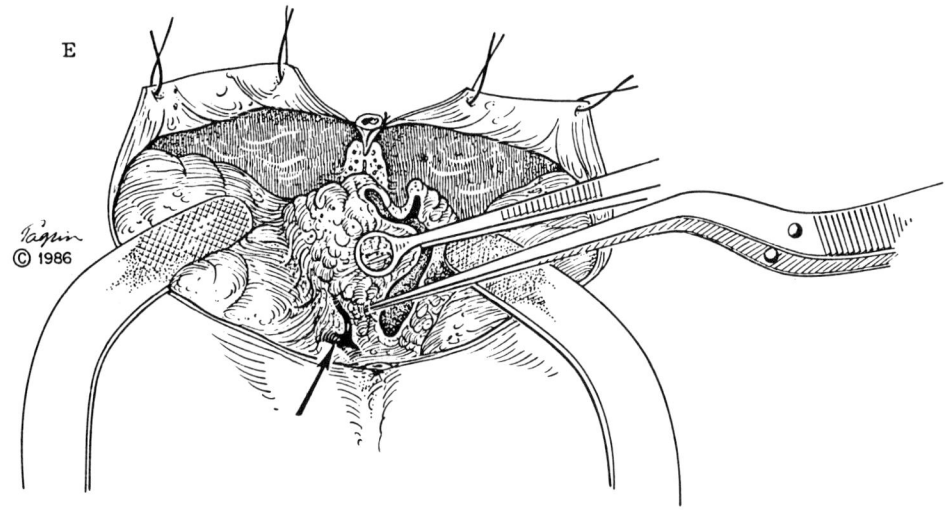

Figure 3E: The posterior capsule is being separated from the frontal lobe. The frontopolar artery is adherent to the tumor capsule and can be divided.

tients. The postoperative course in one patient was complicated by a subdural hydroma that required a subdural-peritoneal shunt. Another had a postoperative wound infection and a third had a CSF leak through the ethmoid sinus that required transethmoid repair. Bakay reported one death in his last 11 patients and MacCarty et al. report a very low mortality rate in their most recent series of meningiomas.[2,9]

Suprasellar Meningiomas

Clinical Features

Suprasellar meningiomas usually arise in the midline from the region of both the tuberculum sellae and planum sphenoidale but they may arise from the diaphragm sellae or be located primarily to one side arising from the anterior

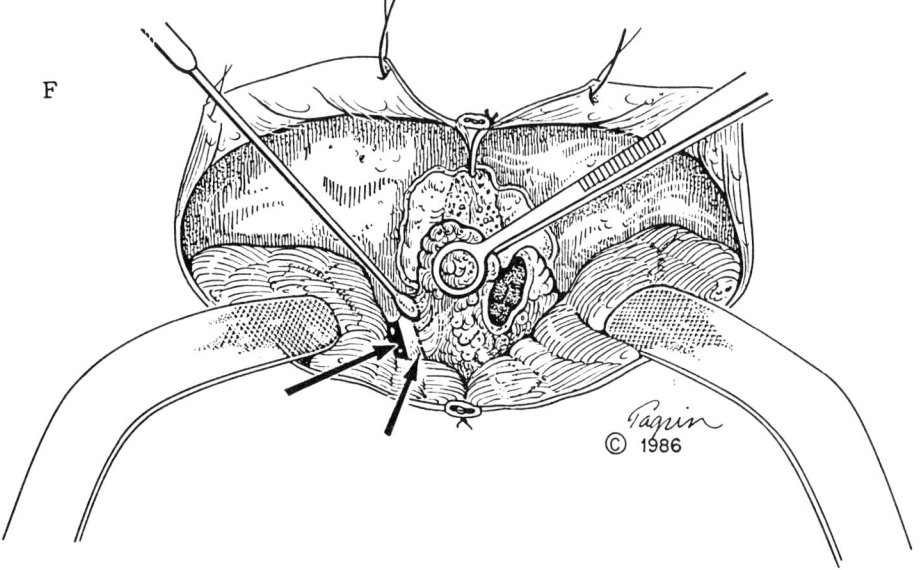

Figure 3F: The left optic nerve and carotid artery (arrows) have been exposed. Tumor is being separated from the arachnoid over the nerve.

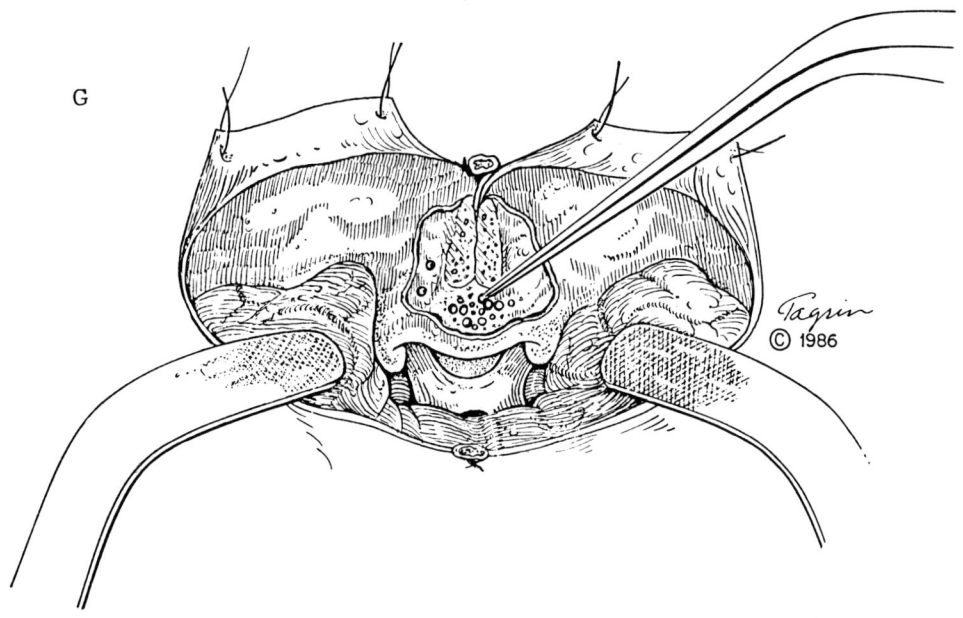

Figure 3G: The tumor has been removed and the dural attachment has been excised. This area will be covered with Gelfoam and a graft of pericranial tissue.

clinoid and adjacent dura.[13,20] In this series, 18 were midline, two extended more to one side, and three arose from the anterior clinoid region.

In our experience the most common symptom is an asymmetrical visual loss starting with a unilateral decrease in central visual acuity or blurring in the visual field, followed by progression to bilateral involvement. The pattern of visual loss may be acute, gradual, or fluctuating.[6] In Symon and Rosenstein's series of 101 patients with meningiomas in this region, symptoms recorded on admission were visual loss in 99%, headache in 45%, and mental changes in 10%. Other symptoms included hyposomia, seizures, diplopia, eye pain, and endocrine dysfunction.[21]

On examination there is almost always a reduction of visual acuity in at least one eye and many patients have bilateral field defects.[6,16] Incongruity and asymmetry of the field defect is the common finding while a symmetrical bitemporal field loss is the exception. Optic atrophy is frequently found and correlates better with the visual acuity loss than with the peripheral field impairment.[5]

Symon and Rosenstein found a visual field defect in all patients and a loss of visual acuity in all but one.[21]

The typical CT scan shows a densely enhancing round mass in the midline above the sella extending anteriorly and laterally (Fig. 4). or in the region of the anterior clinoid processes (Fig. 5). Angiography may show displacement of the distal internal carotid artery and elevation of the A1 segments of the anterior cerebral arteries (Fig. 6).

Surgical Management

The operative approach we prefer in most patients is a right frontal–temporal craniotomy with a lateral subfrontal exposure just in front of the sphenoid wing. In many patients at least one olfactory nerve can be saved and there is minimal trauma to the frontal lobes. Occasionally in large tumors, a bifrontal exposure is indicated. A catheter is often placed in the lumbar subarachnoid space to drain cerebrospinal fluid to help reduce brain tension since drainage from the basal cisterns may not be adequate.

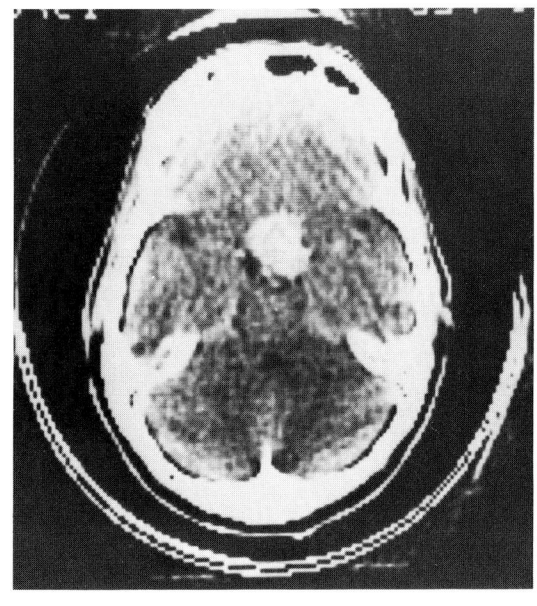

Figure 4: Suprasellar meningioma. CT scan shows the enhancing midline mass just above the sella and extending over the region of the tuberculum and onto the planum sphenoidale.

Kempe also approaches tuberculum sella meningiomas from a right lateral subfrontal exposure.[7] MacCarty et al. use the subfrontal approach from the side of greatest visual loss; they also use a bifrontal craniotomy if the tumor is very large as does Al-Mefty et al.[1,9] Logue and Symon use a unilateral right subfrontal exposure but approach the tumor along the midline.[8,20] In large tumors, Symon resects a portion of the frontal lobe.

The patient is carefully placed in the supine position with the head elevated and held with the three-point skeletal fixation headrest. Most operations have been done with the head rotated 60° to the left so that the anterior zygoma is uppermost (Fig. 7A), but in some the head is kept vertical and a unilateral or bilateral frontal-temporal exposure is done (Fig. 7B). For very large tumors, a bifrontal approach similar to that described for olfactory groove meningiomas is used.

An incision is made beginning just above the zygoma a few millimeters anterior to the ear and then, staying behind the hairline, it extends medially to end in the midline of the forehead. The skin, underlying temporalis muscle, and pericranial tissue are turned down together, exposing the inferior lateral frontal and anterior temporal bone. The most impor-

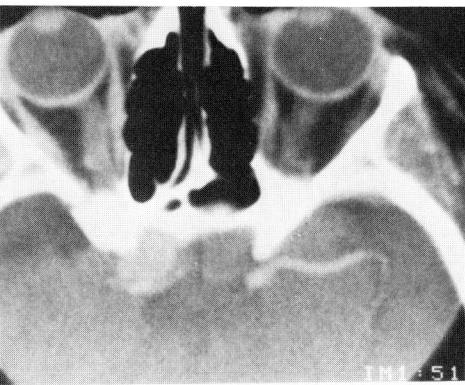 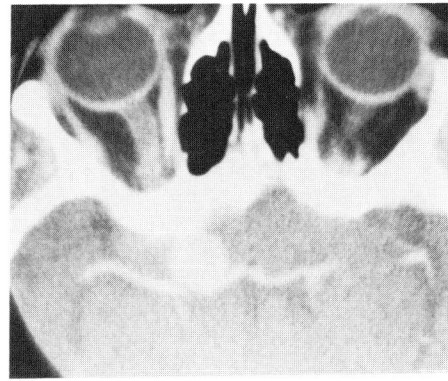

Figure 5: Suprasellar meningioma. This tumor is arising from the region of the left anterior clinoid process.

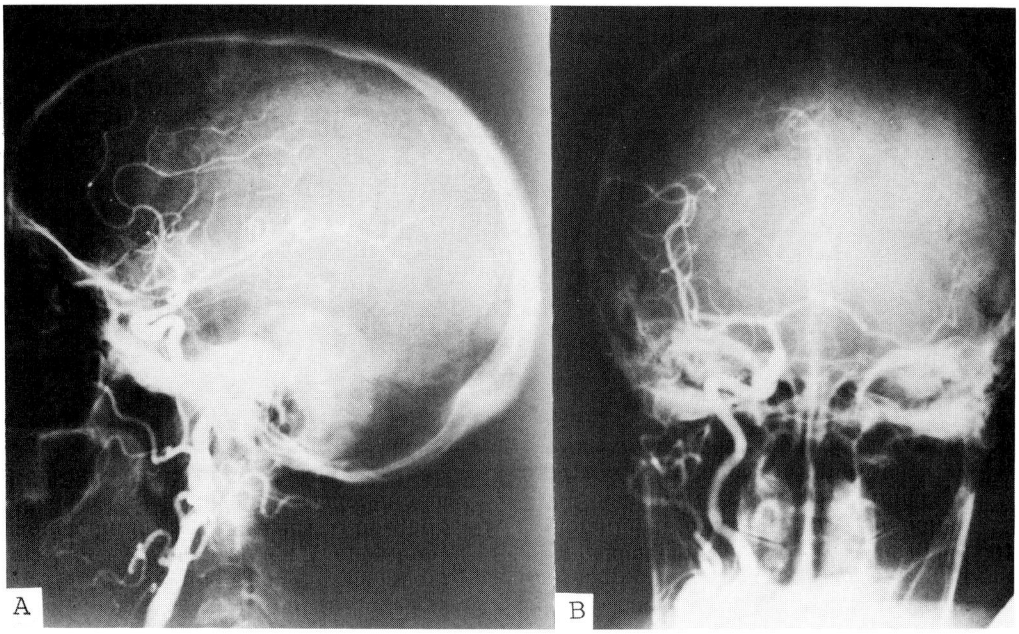

288 • TUMORS OF THE CRANIAL BASE: DIAGNOSIS AND TREATMENT

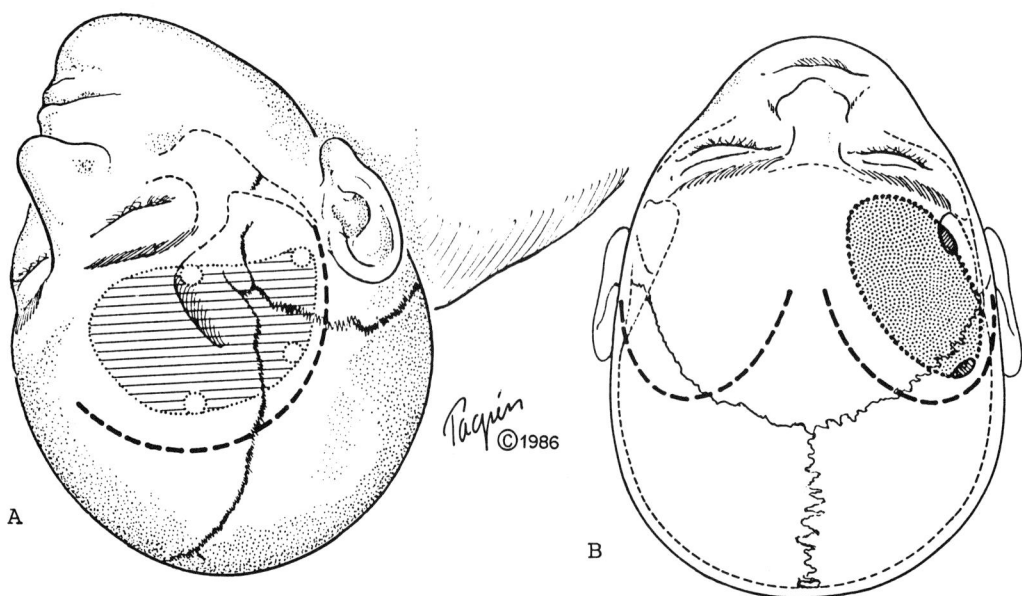

Figure 6: Suprasellar meningioma. **A:** Lateral angiogram showing slight compression of the distal internal carotid artery with displacement both inferiorly and posteriorly. **B:** AP angiogram showing elevation of the A1 segments of the anterior cerebral arteries.

Figure 7: Suprasellar meningioma. **A:** Position, skin incision and bone flap for a right frontal temporal craniotomy preparation for a subfrontal exposure. **B:** Head in vertical position showing bilateral incisions if needed, but usually only the right subfrontal exposure is required.

tant burr hole is the one placed just below the anterior end of the superior temporal line at the level just behind the zygomatic process of the frontal bone. It is important that this hole be properly placed so that the exposure will be on the floor of the anterior fossa. Two or three other burr holes are placed as shown and the bone flap is cut.

The lateral portion of the sphenoid wing is removed, as is bone over the anterior superior temporal region. The dura is opened over the inferior frontal and anterior temporal region. Draining veins from the anterior temporal lobe along the sphenoid wing are divided. The frontal lobe is carefully elevated along the sphenoid wing which reveals the posterior part of the olfactory tract. This normally will lead the surgeon to the optic nerve unless there is significant displacement.

The dura anterior to the optic nerve may be reddish and have increased vascularity. Slightly more exposure reveals the anterior clinoid process, the carotid artery, and a varying portion of the right optic nerve depending on the size of the tumor. In patients with smaller tumors, the arachnoid over the lateral optic nerve and internal carotid artery is opened, and CSF is aspirated to give further decompression. In some patients with larger tumors, tumor may (1) surround both optic nerves; (2) grow beneath the optic nerves to involve the medial wall of the internal carotid artery and its branches; (3) lift the A1 segment of the anterior cerebral arteries off the chiasm and may be adherent to the A2 segments of these arteries (Fig. 8).

The frontal lobe tissue is carefully freed from the surface of the tumor and self-retaining retractors are placed (Fig. 9A). The tumor capsule is opened. Attachments of the tumor along the planum and tuberculum are divided to interrupt the blood supply as it comes into this area. Internal decompression of the tumor is done using bipolar coagulation, Cavitron,

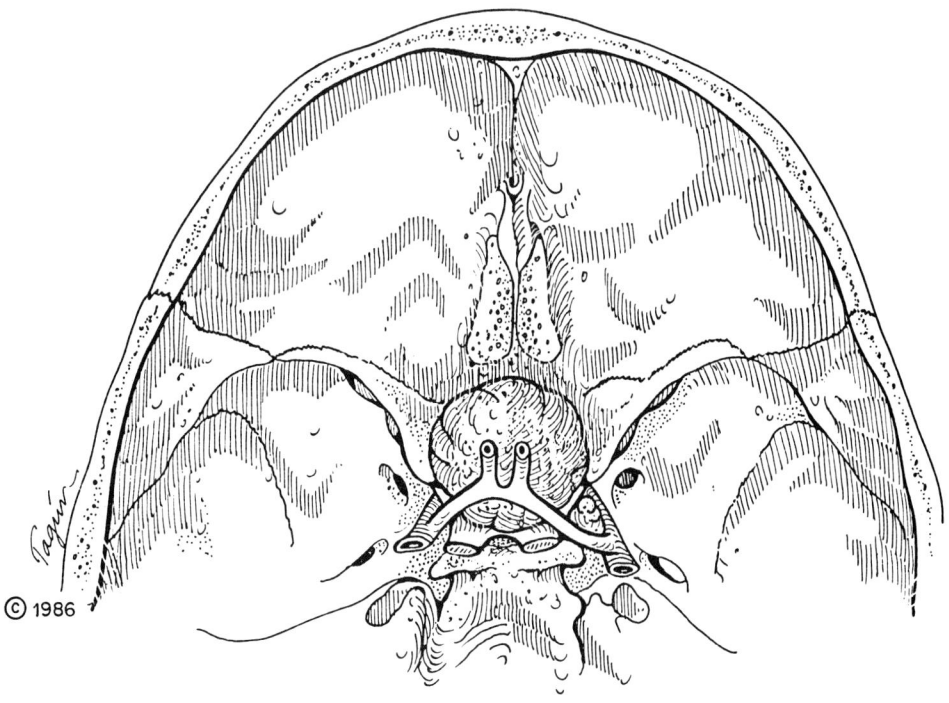

Figure 8: Suprasellar meningioma. Large tumor has displaced the anterior cerebral artery complex away from the optic chiasm. It is growing beneath the right optic nerve to displace the internal carotid artery laterally.

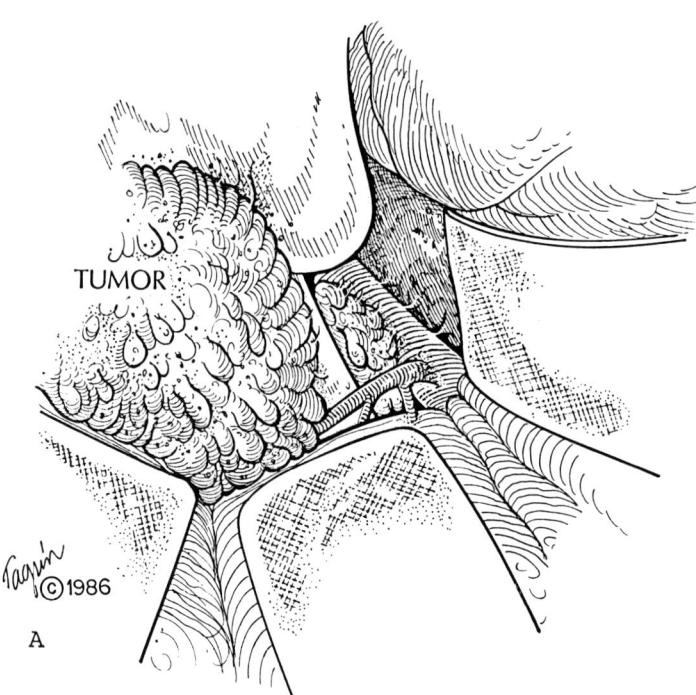

Figure 9: Suprasellar meningioma. **A:** Tumor surrounds a portion of the right optic nerve and right anterior cerebral artery and displaces the right internal carotid artery laterally.

or laser. This is essential before trying to dissect the tumor from the brain, optic nerves, chiasm, and the internal carotid and anterior cerebral arteries.

When a large tumor projects beneath or surrounds a portion of the right optic nerve, it will usually be possible to free the tumor from the nerve, to remove it from its loose attachment to the carotid artery, and to roll it out from beneath the right optic nerve and carotid artery (Fig. 9B). In smaller tumors, the left optic nerve may be seen as the anterior capsule is depressed into the area of decompression. In large tumors, it is sometimes best to identify the chiasm and the left optic nerve by dissection of the posterior capsule, taking great care to visualize directly any attachment to the anterior cerebral vessel or to approach the tumor from a bilateral exposure so that each optic nerve can be seen.

The A1 segment of the anterior cerebral artery and the anterior communicating artery complex may be surrounded by tumor. Usually tumor can be removed from these arteries (Fig. 9C). In some of these patients a small portion of the tumor will need to be left if it is densely adherent. Infrequently, some arterial supply to the tumor will come off the A1 or A2 segments of the anterior cerebral artery and great care must be taken to coagulate and divide this attachment and not avulse it from the artery.

As the tumor is removed from between the optic nerves and in front of the chiasm, arachnoid is encountered which may be thickened. Just beneath this is the pituitary stalk which may have been displaced by the tumor. This structure can usually be preserved.

After tumor removal is completed, the dura over the tuberculum and adjacent area is excised. Usually, this is all that is required, but on occasion there may be hyperostosis which needs to be removed with a diamond burr. In some patients the tumor may grow into the optic foramen and/or involve the dura under the optic nerve and may need to be left in this area.

Results

There was no operative mortality in the patients in this series and Symon and Rosenthal had only one death, due to as-

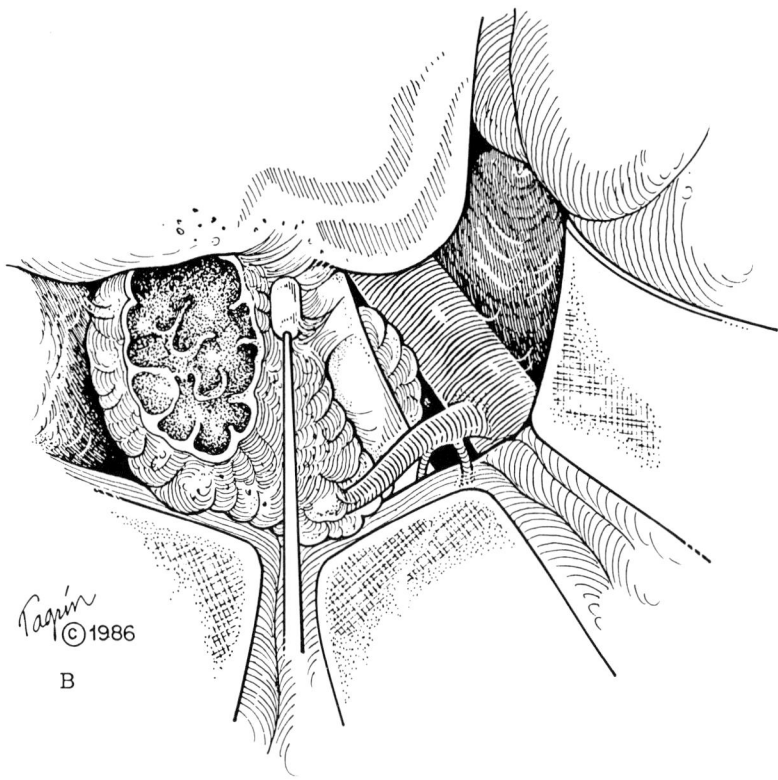

Figure 9B: Internal decompression of the tumor has been accomplished. The attachments to the right optic nerve are being separated as are those from the medial wall of the right internal carotid artery.

piration, in the patients operated with microsurgical technique.[21] These authors also outlined the complications that may be associated with this operation and we have previously discussed the morbidity in these patients.[13,14] The most important morbidity outside the visual system has been the small incidence of permanent frontal lobe syndrome, postoperative seizures, and diabetes insipidus. However, in our series and in Symons', the patients operated on using microsurgical techniques had a very high percentage of good or excellent results usually returning to their normal way of life.

In many of our patients, vision improved but some with extensive growth, particularly recurrent tumors, could not be helped and were occasionally made worse.[13-15] Gregorius et al. found that a long history of decreased visual acuity or a severe visual field defect did not preclude postoperative recovery of vision.[5] They noted that improvement occurred most frequently within the first several weeks after surgery and that further return of vision did not occur after a year. Rosenstein and Symon found that 74% of patients with preoperative visual symptoms for 2 years or less were improved postoperatively compared to only a 43% improvement rate in patients with symptoms for more than 2 years.[16] Furthermore, there was a higher incidence of postoperative visual deterioration in patients with longer duration of symptoms (43% vs. 15%). Other factors that favorably influenced the prognosis for visual function were tumor size less than 3 cm and the presence of normal optic discs.

Residual tumor was left in some patients because of adherence to the visual pathways or vascular structures. This is

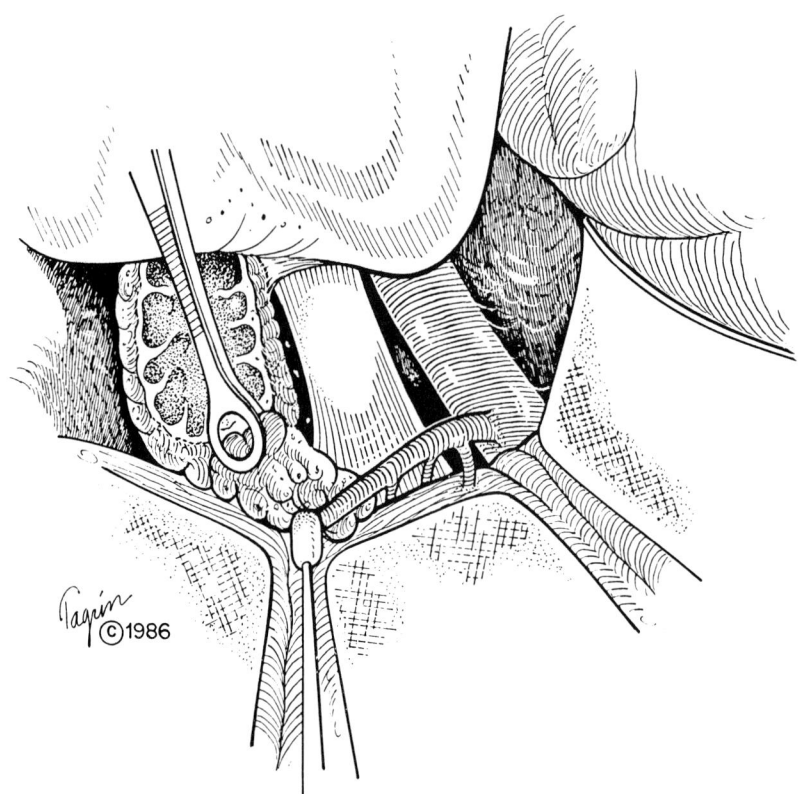

Figure 9C: Tumor surrounding the right anterior cerebral artery is being carefully separated.

almost always true when the patient has had previous surgery. Some of these patients have received radiation therapy, with apparent arrest of tumor growth. This is usually done when the CT scan shows evidence of recurrence and further surgery is considered inadvisable. Benefits of radiation in this group of patients has also been reported by others.[3]

From our experience it is best to do as complete a removal of tumor as possible at the initial operation. The patient should then be carefully followed with regular CT scanning and visual field examination and reoperation or radiation therapy considered if there is evidence of recurrence.

Orbital Roof Meningiomas

Clinical Features and Surgical Management

Meningiomas arising from the floor of the anterior cranial fossa are rare. Cushing operated on one in his series.[4] We have encountered two patients with this type of meningioma: one presenting with seizures and the other with headache. The CT scan shows the homogenously enhancing mass arising from the right orbital roof (Fig. 10). Blood supply comes from the branches of the ethmoidal and meningeal arteries. Surgery is done via a unilateral frontal craniotomy using the same principles discussed for the olfactory groove and suprasellar meningiomas.

References

1. Al-Mefty O, Holoubi A, Rifai A, Fox JL: Microsurgical removal of suprasellar meningiomas. Neurosurgery 16:364-372, 1985.
2. Bakay L: Olfactory meningiomas. The missed diagnosis. JAMA 251 (1):53-55, 1984.

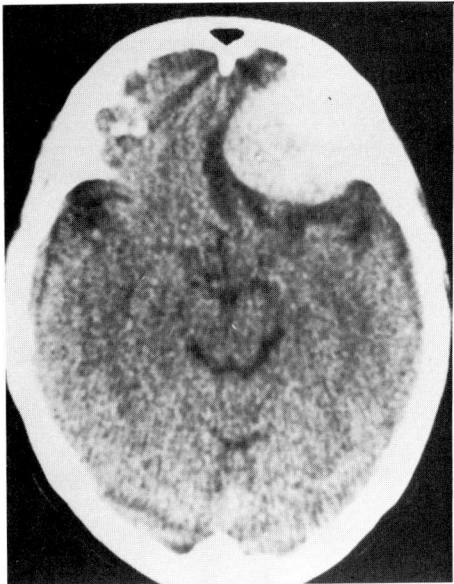 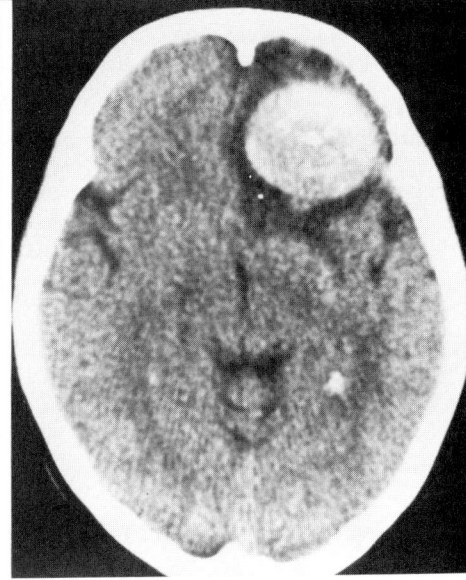

Figure 10: Orbital roof meningioma. CT scan showing the dense enhancing mass arising from the orbital roof projecting directly up into the frontal lobe.

3. Carella RJ, Ransohoff J, Newall J: Role of radiation therapy in the management of meningiomas. Neurosurgery 10:332-339, 1982.
4. Cushing H, Eisenhardt I: *Meningiomas: Their Classification, Regional Behaviour, Life History and Surgical End Results*, Springfield, IL, Charles C. Thomas, 1938.
5. Gregorius FK, Hepler RS, Stern WE: Loss and recovery of vision with suprasellar meningiomas. J Neurosurg 42:69-75, 1975.
6. Kadis GN, Mount LA, Ganti SR: The importance of early diagnosis and treatment of the meningiomas of the planum sphenoidale and tuberculum sellae: A retrospective study of 105 cases. Surg Neurol 12:367-371, 1979.
7. Kempe LG: *Operative Neurosurgery*. Vol 1, New York, Springer-Verlag, 1968.
8. Logue V: Surgery of Meningiomas in Symon L (ed): *Operative Surgery: Neurosurgery*, London, Butterworths, 1979, pp 128-173.
9. MacCarty CS, Piepgras DG, Ebersold NJ: Meningeal Tumors of the Brain in Youmans J (ed): *Neurological Surgery* (2nd ed), Philadelphia, WB Saunders Co, 1982, pp 2936-2966.
10. Maxwell RE, Chou SN: Preoperated evaluation and management of meningiomas. In Schmidek HH, Sweet WH (eds): *Operative Neurosurgical Techniques*, New York, Grune and Stratton, 1982, pp 482-489.
11. Miramanoff R, Dosoretz DE, Linggood RM, Ojemann RG, Martuza RL: Meningioma: Analysis of recurrence and progression following neurosurgical resection. J Neurosurg 62:18-24, 1985.
12. New PFJ, Aronow S, Hesselink JR: National Cancer Institute study: Evaluation of computed tomography in diagnosis of intracranial neoplasms. IV: Meningiomas. Radiology 136:665-675, 1980.
13. Ojemann RG: Meningiomas of the basal parapituitary region: Technical considerations. Clin Neurosurg 27:233-262, 1980.
14. Ojemann RG: Surgical management of meningiomas of the tuberculum sellae, olfactory groove, medial sphenoid wing, and floor of the anterior fossa. In Schmidek HH, Sweet WH (eds): *Operative Neurosurgical Techniques*, New York, Grune and Stratton, 1982, pp. 535-560.
15. Ojemann RG: Clinical features and surgical management of meningiomas. In Wilkins RH, Rengachary SS (eds): *Neurosurgery*. New York, McGraw-Hill Book Co, 1985, Vol 1, pp 635-654.
16. Rosenstein J, Symon L: Surgical management of suprasellar meningioma. Part 2: Prognosis for visual function following craniotomy. J Neurosurg 61:642-648, 1984.
17. Simpson D: The recurrence of intracranial meningiomas after surgical treatment. J Neurol Neurosurg Psychiat 20:22-39, 1957.

18. Solero CL, Giombini S, Morello G: Suprasellar and olfactory meningiomas: Report on a series of 153 personal cases. *Acta Neurochir* (WIEN) 67:181-194, 1983.
19. Strait TA, Robertson JH, Clark WC: Use of the carbon dioxide laser in the operative management of intracranial meningiomas: A report of twenty cases. *Neurosurgery* 10:464-467, 1982.
20. Symon L: Olfactory groove and suprasellar meningiomas. In Krayenbuhl H (ed): *Advances and Technical Standards in Neurosurgery.* Vol 4. Wien, Springer-Verlag, 1977, pp 67-91.
21. Symon L, Rosenstein J: Surgical management of suprasellar meningioma. Part 1: The influence of tumor size, duration of symptoms and microsurgery on surgical outcome in 101 consecutive cases. *J Neurosurg* 61:633-641, 1984.

18

Bony Lesions of the Anterior and Middle Cranial Fossa

P.J. Derome, M.D.
A. Visot, M.D.

Introduction

Many types of bony lesions may involve the anterior cranial base. Primary bone lesions include fibrous dysplasia and tumors such as osteomas, osteoblastomas, ossifying fibromas, chondromas, and chordomas. However, the base of the skull may be involved secondarily by tumors invading superiorly, such as meningiomas, or inferiorly, such as carcinomas and olfactory neuroblastomas. In some cases the bone is destroyed, rather than invaded, by slowly growing lesions such as nasopharyngeal fibromas or large trigeminal schwannomas. Despite the variety of these lesions, the technical problems encountered by the neurosurgeon in their management are the same; thus, all such tumors, with the exception of those malignant lesions that are usually managed primarily by otolaryngological or maxillofacial surgeons, will be discussed in this chapter.

Surgical techniques for managing lesions at the base of the skull have become well established; in particular, the "transbasal" approach has been described extensively.[3,4,6] Such surgery is fairly simple to perform, and is associated with few risks to the patient when indications for operation are clear and the surgeon uses meticulous operative technique. In managing 190 bony lesions of the anterior and middle cranial fossa between 1970 and 1985 (102 of which were resected through a transbasal route), we have identified five elements that we believe are most important to the successful management of such tumors: (1) preoperative evaluation of the feasibility of removal of the lesion; (2) choice of the operative approach; (3) managing technical problems related to pathological involvement of the dura; (4) repair of bone; and (5) evaluating indications for surgery relative to the type of bony lesion in each case.

Tumor Operability and Goals of Surgery

Bony lesions in the anterior or middle cranial fossa often produce few neurological symptoms, except for those due to compression of the cranial nerves exiting

---

From: Sekhar LN, Schramm VL Jr, eds: *Tumors of the Cranial Base: Diagnosis and Treatment.* Mount Kisco, New York, Futura Publishing Co, Inc, © 1987.

the base of the skull: anosmia is found with lesions of the ethmoid area, while oculomotor palsies may occur as a consequence of extradural compression in the supraorbital fissure. On the other hand, compression of the optic nerves in the optic canal is frequent, and visual disturbances are the most frequently seen initial symptoms (they are also the most unpredictable in regard to postoperative improvement). Symptoms of trigeminal compression from middle fossa tumors occur rarely except when an intrinsic lesion of the nerve, such as a schwannoma, is present.

Decompressing the cranial nerves, particularly the optic nerves, is the first goal of surgery (Figs. 1 and 5). This goal is usually easily achieved when the tumor is limited to the bone, and the dura is uninvolved: removal of the greater sphenoid wing will free the inferior edge of the supraorbital fissure and will allow decompression of the foramen rotundum and the foramen ovale; removal of the lesser sphenoid wing and the anterior clinoid process frees the upper aspect of the supraorbital fissure and the lateral and upper boundaries of the optic canal. However, because it is important to free the optic nerves as far centrally as possible, it may be desirable to remove the middle aspect of the sphenoid process to expose the medial (and, if necessary, the lower) edge of the optic canal so that the medial edge of the supraorbital fissure and the root of the pterygoid process can be exposed.[3-5]

Total or near-total excision of the tumor is the second goal of surgery. However, excision may be limited by extensive involvement of bone at the limits of the surgical approach (foramen magnum, basiocciput, pterygoid processes, petrous apex), or because the tumor involves the dura in areas inaccessible to the

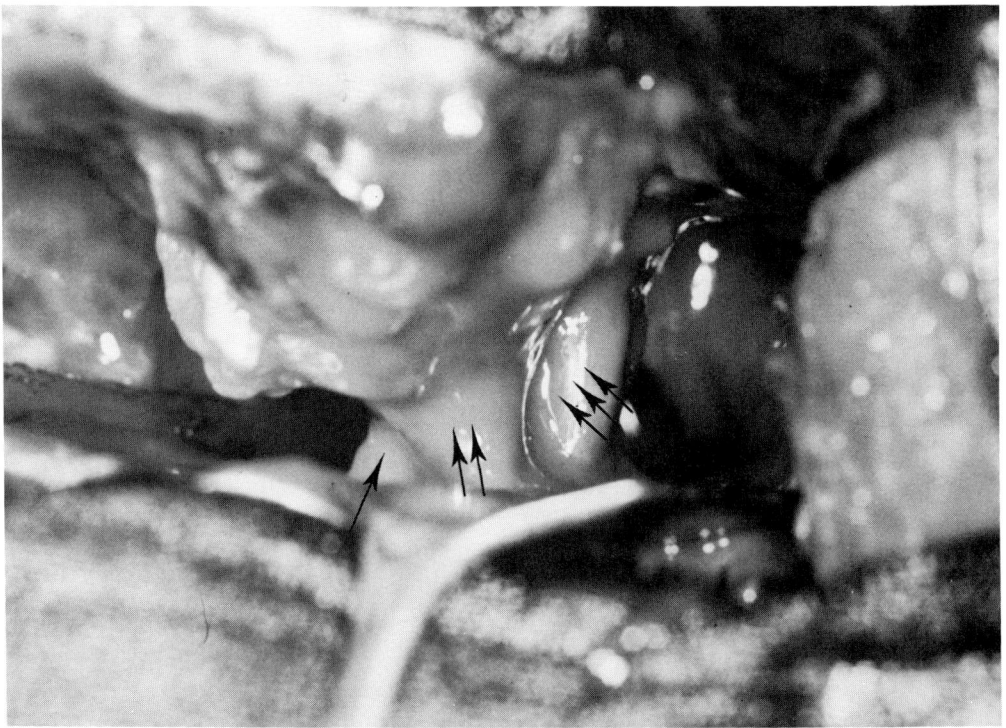

Figure 1: Chordoma. After total resection of the sphenoid body, lesser and greater sphenoid wings, one can see, between the soft tissues of the orbit and the frontal lobe (retracted): the optic nerve (arrow), dura of the supraorbital fissure (double arrows), and second branch of the fifth cranial nerve (triple arrows).

neurosurgeon such as the supraorbital fissure or the cavernous sinus.

Avoiding complications and anatomic reconstruction are the last goals of surgery at the base of the skull. Complications to be avoided include new neurological deficits (except anosmia when the lesion is midline) and infection due to opening of septic facial cavities, while reconstruction may include the correction of large, surgically created craniofacial deformities.

Surgical excision of bony lesions at the base of the skull is technically difficult, and the neurosurgeon may be tempted to try a risky operative procedure to remove such a lesion. However, some of these bony lesions evolve slowly, or even, as with fibrous dysplasias, cease to grow after some time. Thus, it is important to evaluate the nature of the lesion as well as the technical aspects of operative removal before deciding on their surgical management.

Factors that will aid in making this decision include the extent of the tumor, as seen on bone tomography, computed tomography, magnetic resonance imaging, and angiography if necessary; the pathology of the lesion as determined by biopsy of the lesion when this is not otherwise evident; and the possibilities for arresting or improving neurological deficits caused by the lesion. All of these factors must be evaluated before management decisions can be made. The final decision may be to perform radical surgery, subtotal removal, mere surveillance, or, when the lesion is an invasive meningioma, for instance, radiotherapy or embolization.

Choice of the Operative Approach

The choice of operative approach depends upon the location of the tumor.

Involvement of the *middle anterior fossa* (ethmosphenoid area) requires a bilateral frontal approach. The skin incision for this approach is bicoronal, followed by bifrontal elevation of a free bone flap. The surgeon should not hesitate to open the frontal sinuses if they are extensive, as it is important to develop a large anterior pericranial flap, which may be useful for closure of the cranial base (see Chapter 14). Without a bifrontal approach, it is impossible to reach the tuberculum sellae and the most medial limits of the anterior fossa extradurally, and to decompress the optic nerves medially. The patient must be advised preoperatively that the surgery will result in total anosmia.

A unilateral frontal or frontotemporal (pterional) approach may be used for bony tumors located in the *lateral part of the anterior fossa* and the *middle fossa*. Bony lesions restricted to the floor of the middle fossa occur extremely rarely, and usually involve the greater or the lesser sphenoid wing, requiring enlargement of the approach toward the frontal and orbital area. Through such an approach, it is possible to free the contents of the supraorbital fissure and to reach the optic nerve after resection of the anterior clinoid process. However, it is not possible to decompress the optic nerve medially through this approach, as the surgical limits of the pterional approach include the medial edge of the optic canal and the medial orbital wall.

Other approaches are necessary when the tumor overlaps the ethmosphenoid and orbital areas. Posterior and medial extensions of sphenoid tumors that reach the posterior fossa, invade the dorsum sellae, and destroy the clivus are reached through a rhinoseptal approach, which may be combined with the transbasal approach in the same surgical procedures[4,6] (Fig. 2).

Infracranial extensions of tumors may be easily removed through the transbasal approach when they are lobulated, well circumscribed, and soft or pseudogelatinous in consistency (e.g., some meningiomas, chordomas). However, involvement of the facial bones, dense tissue attachments, or a fibrous consistency require the use of another approach: for intramaxillary, infraorbital, or pterygoid extensions, an extended lateral rhinotomy approach is probably the most useful. It may be performed as a separate surgical procedure (as in the case of osteoblas-

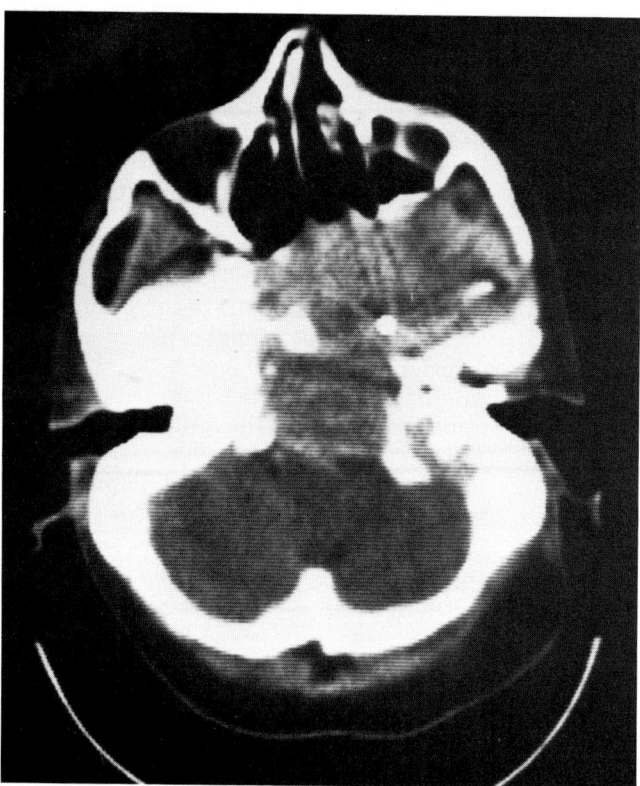

Figure 2: Combined rhinoseptal and transbasal approach is advisable for some cases of chordoma extension.

tomas, Figs. 8A, B), or combined with the transbasal approach in one procedure to attain the extensive surgical exposure necessary to remove very large nasopharyngeal fibromas. Laterally, a transzygomatic, infratemporal approach with sectioning of the mandible may be necessary to remove a large tumor involving the pterygomaxillary fossa. Except for the rhinoseptal approach, which is usually performed by the neurosurgeon, the combined approaches just discussed require the addition of an otolaryngological or maxillofacial surgeon to the surgical team.

Dural Involvement

Pathological involvement of the dura is characteristic of all meningeal tumors, the most frequent bony lesions of the skull base; however, the dura may also be involved with other bony tumors such as ossifying fibromas, chordomas, or olfactory placode tumors. Most instances of incomplete tumor removal are the result of dural involvement of the walls of the cavernous sinus or the supraorbital fissure, with such dural involvement leading in turn to increased risk of cerebrospinal fluid (CSF) leakage and meningitis. These are the most significant postoperative complications of surgery at the base of the skull, and may also result from involvement of the dura adjacent to the air-filled cavities of the face.

The difficulty of repairing the dura intraoperatively is different for bony tumors located laterally (middle fossa, greater or lesser sphenoid wing, orbital roof) and for lesions involving the medial and parasagittal aspect of the anterior fossa. When the tumor is placed laterally, the dura may be exposed widely and the involved area easily removed (except for inoperable extensions) without risk of complication. With midline tumors, however, the risk of CSF leakage is significant unless the dural defect is closed with particular care, as removal of tumor involving the bone will expose the nasal fossae, the frontal sinuses, the ethmoid cells, or the sphenoid sinuses. The boundary between lateral and midline location of a lesion depends upon the extent of basal pneumatization, and usually lies along the axis of the optic nerves.

It is necessary to close the dura in a watertight fashion as soon as possible after resecting a lesion at the base of the skull. The materials most often used are lyophilized dura and fascia lata, with the choice made on the basis of the dural defect to be repaired. Rather than use a foreign material or an aponeurotic graft, we prefer to close the defect with pericranium because of its capacity to form adhesions and to revascularize more quickly. A pericranial graft may be readily obtained from the parietal area, immediately dorsal to the posterior edge of the bone flap.[3,4,6,7] Parietal pericranium is thicker than frontal periosteum, which is reserved for basal reconstruction.

Even when the dura is not involved by tumor (as in fibrous dysplasia), the subfrontal dura is frequently torn during extradural dissection of the anterior cranial fossa, particularly when the olfactory grooves are separated from the cribriform plates. Each dural tear must be closed carefully, and we use a pericranial graft to strengthen the subfrontal dura in the midline.

When a tumor extends intracranially and extranially in the sphenoethmoid area, resection begins with removal of the subfrontal mass. If it is possible to close the dura immediately, a pericranial graft may be stitched to adjacent normal dura, widely overlapping the edges of the defect. With other tumors, especially tuberculum sellae meningiomas, the dura often cannot be sealed after resection because the dural defect extends to the suprasellar cistern and even a very large graft cannot be sutured posteriorly. In these cases, the graft is placed with its posterior edge folded back to overlie the base of the skull by approximately 1 cm; the graft is then stitched anteriorly and laterally to normal dura. After this meningeal reconstruction, the wound is closed. Three to four months later, when watertight closure of the dura has occurred, the second-stage operation is performed: in this procedure, the basal or facial portion of the tumor is approached extradurally, and air-filled cavities are opened with no risk of CSF leakage or infection.

Such staged management of basal tumors requires that several conditions be met. First, if the patient presents with visual disturbances, the optic nerves must be decompressed intra- and extradurally during the first procedure (Fig. 3A), to avoid any worsening of symptoms during the waiting period before the second procedure. Second, in such cases the dural repair should be separated from the tumor by a sheet of foreign material such as Silastic (Figs. 3B, C) so that the graft is not compromised by tumor involvement during the interim between procedures. Interposition of this sheet of Silastic, which will be removed at reoperation, will make dissection and the extradural approach easier.

Bony Reconstruction

Indications for Bony Reconstruction

Bone repair is definitely indicated when removal of a tumor mass produces cosmetic deformities. These may occur whenever the lesion involves not only the skull base but also the frontal vault or orbital rim, as happens frequently with fibrous dysplasia. This condition is often signaled by abnormal bulging in the frontal or supraorbital area, and displacement of the orbital globe.

In contrast, we have found that bony repair is not necessary when a bony lesion is located laterally, involving the greater and/or lesser sphenoid wings and the adjacent floor of the middle fossa. In such cases, the temporal muscle is carefully sutured to the bone flap with nonresorbable sutures to avoid an unattractive depression of the temporal region postoperatively.

Bone repair is optional after removal of the orbital roof. Lack of a supraorbital wall may be responsible for pulsing of the

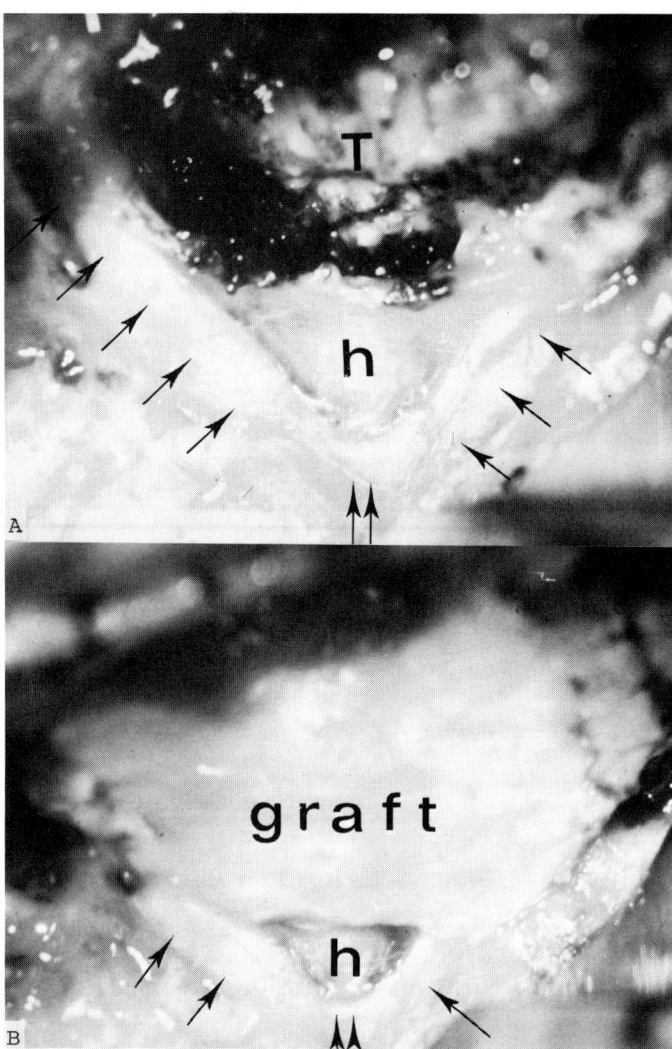

Figures 3A–C: Dural repair of an invasive meningioma of the medial anterior fossa (first operative step after removal of intracranial postion). Arrows = optic nerves; double arrow = optic chiasm; h = pituitary gland, lifted up by involvement of the sphenoid by tumor; T = basal portion of tumor. **A:** optic tract is totally free along its intradural and extradural aspects. **B:** subfrontal dural defect is repaired by placing a pericranial graft so that it covers the extradural portions of the optic nerves. *Continued.*

globe and mild enophthalmos (when several orbital walls have been resected), but these complications are usually not significant unless they lead to difficulties with further attempts at dissection and separation of the periorbita from the subfrontal dura should reoperation be necessary. In our series of patients, we repaired the roof of the orbit only after extensive resection of several orbital walls or after simultaneous resection of the supraorbital rim.

Except for a few cases in which one or two temporal muscles were dissected, rotated, and used for basal closure, we have always reconstructed the sphenoid and ethmoid areas after middle anterior fossa procedures. Such bone reconstruction is additional protection against postoperative leakage of CSF, protects the dura and the brain during any later nasal or facial operations, and eliminates dead space that may be a significant source of secondary hematomas and extradural pneumatocele, with attendant secondary infection or meningoencephalocele (as we observed in one patient who had a large ethmosphenoid dysplastic lesion). Thus, we prefer to repair the skull base with bone in any case where removal of tumor has widely opened the nasal fossae and/or the sphenoid sinuses between the orbits and the optic nerves.

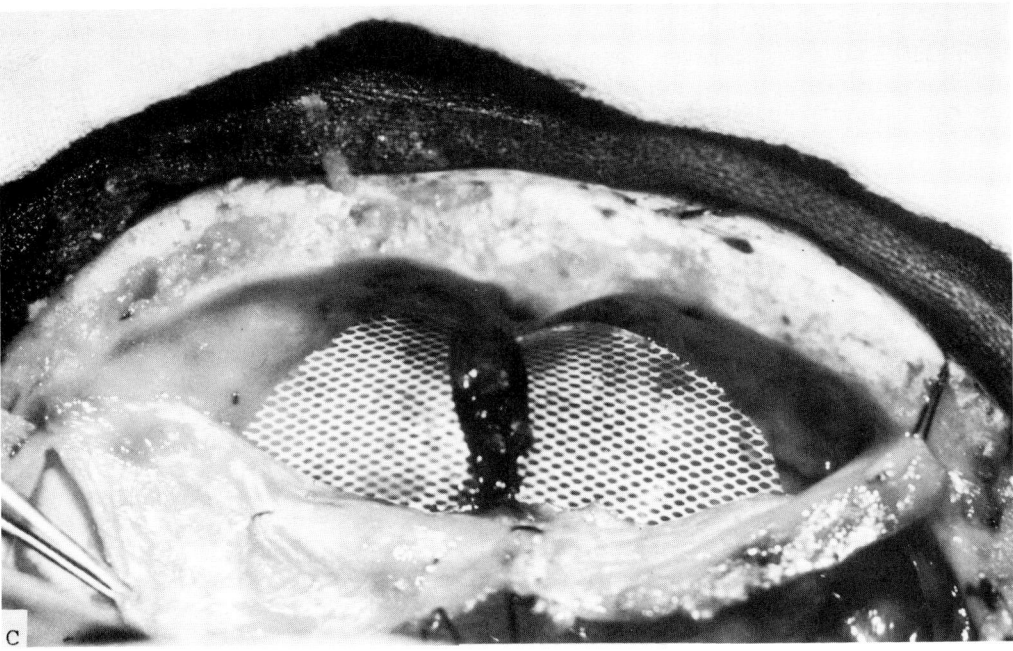

Figure 3C: Sheet of Silastic introduced extradurally, between the pericranial graft and basal meningioma.

Reconstruction Materials

Because any air-filled cavity of the face must be considered to be septic, autogenous bone grafts are recommended for basal reconstruction; we do not recommend that foreign materials such as polymerizable cement be used for reconstruction of the anterior skull base. Further, we believe that cancellous bone grafts are more useful than cortical grafts, as the former are malleable and have better resistance to infection.

Bone from the iliac crest is the best for such reconstruction in patients older than 10 to 12 years, while in children, one can use split-rib grafts or grafts extracted from the parietal cranial vault, behind the bifrontal free flap. Parietal and frontal flaps can be split, with one part being used for the basal reconstruction and the other for closing the vault defect. Bone dust may also be used to complete the repair at the base of the skull, and to close some small cavities (provided that one uses small shavings of bone and not true dust).

In some cases, particularly children, or those with extensive involvement of the frontal vault, it is impossible to obtain a sufficient amount of autogenous bone for grafting. In these patients, autogenous material should be used for repair at the base of the skull and the defect in the vault reconstructed with bone homografts (grafts extracted from cadavers and irradiated with gamma rays). This may be done at the same time, or with polymerizable cement a few months after the basal reconstruction to avoid infectious complications.

Surgery

When bone grafts are used to close an empty cavity, they must be supplied with blood vessels. These vessels may be brought from the dura above or the underlying mucosa; however, frequently the dura itself is devascularized, and the vascularity of the underlying tissues must be assured to avoid necrosis of the graft.

In the sphenoid area the nasopharyngeal mucosa lying just below the sphenoid body is usually easy to locate and provides adequate vascularization. It is difficult to preserve underlying mucosa in the ethmoid area, however, because of the anatomical complexity of the cells. If a few cells are opened, they may be closed readily with grafts of cancellous bone, while when the defect is larger, it may be possible to use septal mucosa for closure of the anterior portion of the nasal fossae.

However, extremely large tumors that involve the nasal fossae and sphenoid sinuses have usually destroyed the mucosal layer. If such a basal defect is anticipated at the beginning of the operation, before trephination, a large anterior pericranial flap should be raised (Fig. 4). As has been described,[3-6] the pericranium should be incised along the temporal crests, as far as possible, 1 or 2 cm behind the coronal sutures. This pericranial flap should be dissected free laterally and posteriorly, leaving the anterior vascular supply intact, and reflected anteriorly during the procedure. After the tumor has been resected, the flap should be brought down over the nasal fossae, between the orbits, and sutured to the subfrontal dura (or the pericranial graft repairing the dura) at the farthest limits of the subfrontal dura in the anterior fossa. This forms a new "mucosal plane," and the autogenous bone grafts will be inserted between this plane and the subfrontal dura (or the free pericranial graft repairing the dural defect).

When cancellous bone grafts are used, they are usually "shingled" over the sphenoethmoid defect and covered with a large cortical graft fitted between the cribriform plates (or the root of the nose) and the posterior wall of the sphenoid sinus (or the clivus) below the sellar floor;[3,4] one must be particularly careful not to compress the optic nerves. From the sphenoethmoid area, reconstruction may be extended to the orbital roofs or orbital rims, with bone dust being used to fill in any dead space.

Bony Lesions

Meningiomas are the bony lesions most frequently encountered at the base of the skull, followed by fibrous dysplasias and chordomas, and then, much less frequently, by various other benign tumors.

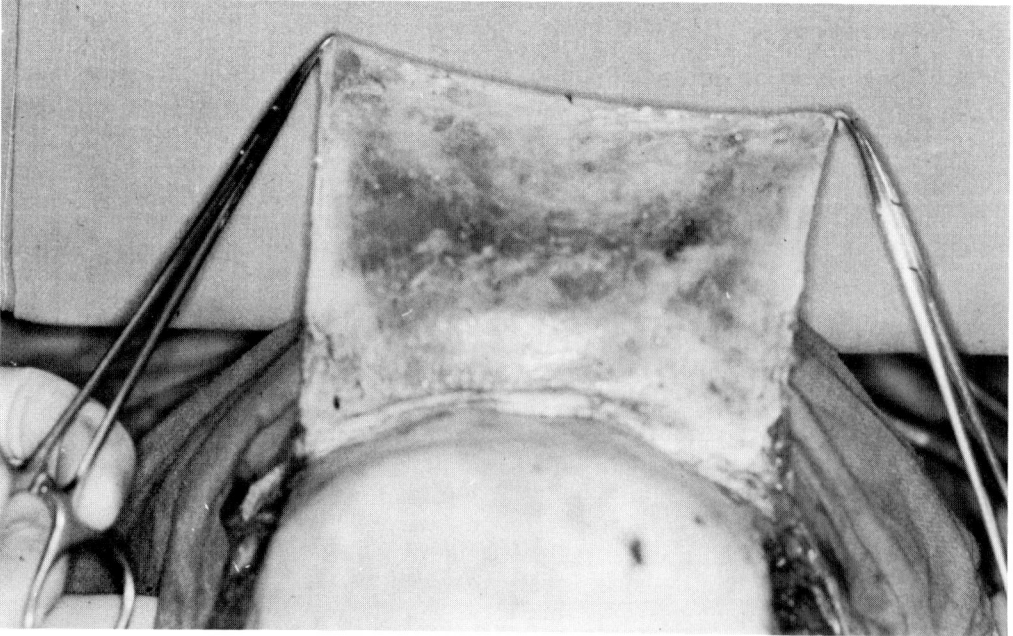

Figure 4: A large anterior pericranial flap is raised at the beginning of a surgical procedure expected to result in a large basal defect and insufficient mucosa.

However, we have found an unusually large proportion of fibrous dysplasias in our study population, perhaps due to our particular interest in this type of tumor.

Meningiomas

A meningioma[2,5,9] becomes a bony lesion (invasive meningioma) when it involves the bone and/or when it extends toward the facial cavities, regardless of whether the dura is involved. In the anterior and middle fossa, two kinds of invasive meningiomas may be seen, differentiated by their locations, anatomical appearances, and growth patterns. Transitional forms have been described, but conceptually these lesions can be divided into hyperostosing meningiomas (en plaques) and true invasive meningiomas (en masse).

Hyperostosing Meningiomas

Hyperostosing meningiomas en plaques[11] are tumors of the greater and lesser sphenoid wings. In our series of patients they were usually located laterally (in 78 cases of 79 operated upon; in the other case, the lesion was found in the middle anterior fossa), sinuses and nasal cavities were spared, there was minimal risk of postoperative leakage of CSF, and basal reconstruction was unnecessary after resection.

For many years neurosurgeons did not resect hyperostosing meningiomas, perhaps because their location at the base of the skull involved approaches most often used by other surgical specialists, and because these lesions grow so slowly. The initial signs of a hyperostosing meningioma are relatively benign: mild exophthalmos, mild bulging of the temporal fossa, no visual disturbances, and rarely retro-orbital headaches. These symptoms worsen slowly, but as the tumor continues to grow, cranial nerves, particularly the optic nerves, may be compressed, and in some cases late invasion of the lateral anterior fossa, middle fossa, and the orbit may cause dramatic proptosis, partial or total oculomotor palsy, unilateral blindness, and extension toward the face. When the lesion has reached this size, cure is not possible, and the prognosis for improvement in clinical symptoms is often poor.

It is for this reason that hyperostosing meningiomas must be resected early. Hyperostosis is not merely a reaction of the bone to pathological involvement of the dura: such en plaque meningiomas do invade the bone, and meningiomatous cells may be found in the bone and Haversian canals. Hyperostosis is responsible for exophthalmos and compression of the optic nerve in the optic foramen, and for invasion of the dura or similar structures such as the periorbita.

A meningiomatous plaque is always found on the cranial side of the hyperostosis, usually in the temporal area around the external portion of the supraorbital fissure; externally the dura appears only thickened and hypervascularized, but examination of the internal aspect of the dura will reveal the meningioma. Similarly, when hyperostosis is found intradurally near the orbit, a periorbital plaque will be seen growing inside the orbit. Sometimes such meningiomatous invasion may be seen in the deeper aspect of the temporal muscle, with infiltration of the aponeurosis and muscle fibers; from these primary plaques, the meningioma will extend and involve progressively the sphenoid fissure, the cavernous sinus, the orbit, and the sheath of the optic nerve.

Surgical management of these meningiomas requires not only total removal of the hyperostosis (since the bone is pathologic), but also the removal of all meningiomatous plaques. The temporal dural defect should be closed with a pericranial graft, and if the periorbital defect left after removing an orbital plaque is large, it should be repaired with the same material.

Invasive Meningiomas of the Midline

These tumors are unusual in that the tumor always grows intracranially and the mass lesion may become extremely large. Initially these tumors are intracranial, originating from the cribriform plates, the planum sphenoidale, or the tuberculum sellae—all skull base areas where the bone is thin. From dural attachment, the bone is progressively involved and/or destroyed, and a path opened for tumor extension toward the sphenoid sinuses, the ethmoid cells, and the nasal fossae.

When an "invasive" meningioma of the midline is resected, contrary to removal of a hyperostosing meningioma en plaque, there is significant risk of CSF leakage and infection postoperatively; for this reason, careful dural and basal reconstruction are necessary after resection of an invasive meningioma. The bony meningiomatous involvement must be totally removed, as any residual tumor may lead to late recurrences, sometimes more than 10 years after removal of an olfactory or planum meningioma. In a few cases, the recurrence has been known to involve the skull base only, with extradural compression of the optic nerves into the optic foramina; more often, however, the recurrence grows intracranially, in the skull base, and into adjacent cavities. Problems encountered during surgery to remove such recurrences are much the same as those of the primary procedure, and the solutions are also the same: watertight closure of the dura, which may require surgery to be performed in more than one step. We removed 28 such tumors through a transbasal approach.

However, under two sets of conditions, a different approach may be used. Sometimes the basal abnormalities appear to be mere bony reactions, without true involvement of the bone, close to the attachment of the meningioma: the lesion appears as a small osteoma, without apparent bony involvement. In such cases, basal surgery is not necessary, but the patient must be followed closely for many years.

In other cases, total removal of an invasive meningioma is impossible because of bony and dural involvement of the sellar and parasellar area. In these cases, tumor embolization and/or radiotherapy may be considered.

Fibrous Dysplasia

Fibrous dysplasia of the skull (Fig. 5)[1-7] is a disease of unknown etiology marked by the presence of intraosseous proliferating connective tissue that causes extreme thickening of the bone in the affected areas. Endocrine disorders such as hyperthyroidism, acromegaly, Cushing's disease, gynecomastia, acceleration of skeletal growth, and McCune-Albright's syndrome are sometimes associated with fibrous dysplasia. There are three main radiologic manifestations of this disorder: a sclerotic ("compact") form, found in 50% of our 58 cases, in which there is homogeneous opacification and thickening of the bone; a "lytic" form (found in 15% of our cases), called *soufflante* because the lesion did not destroy the bony structures; and the "pseudo-Pagetoid" or mixed form, marked by alternating sclerotic and radiolucent areas, found in 35% of our cases.

The most common presenting symptoms of this disorder are progressive orbitocranial swelling (which may reach enormous proportions and lead to major craniofacial deformity) and exophthalmos. The patient usually complains only of the cosmetic deformity, but the main risk of fibrous dysplasia is compression of the cranial nerves in the foramina of the skull base, particularly of the optic nerves. Notable visual symptomatology was present in 35% of our patients: of 12 patients with unilaterally impaired vision, seven were completely blind in one eye, and of eight patients with bilateral visual impairments seven were blind in one eye. The occurrence of visual symptoms is quite unpredictable, and may be due to one or more of several mechanisms: external compression of the optic nerve in a stenosed optic canal, external compression by a cystic dysplastic lesion, stretching of the optic nerve by a very large medial craniofacial dysplasia, or ischemia due to compression of the ophthalmic artery.

Fibrous dysplasia is not a true tumor. We have reviewed the literature and our own experiences to evaluate the evolution of this curious disease, and found that it

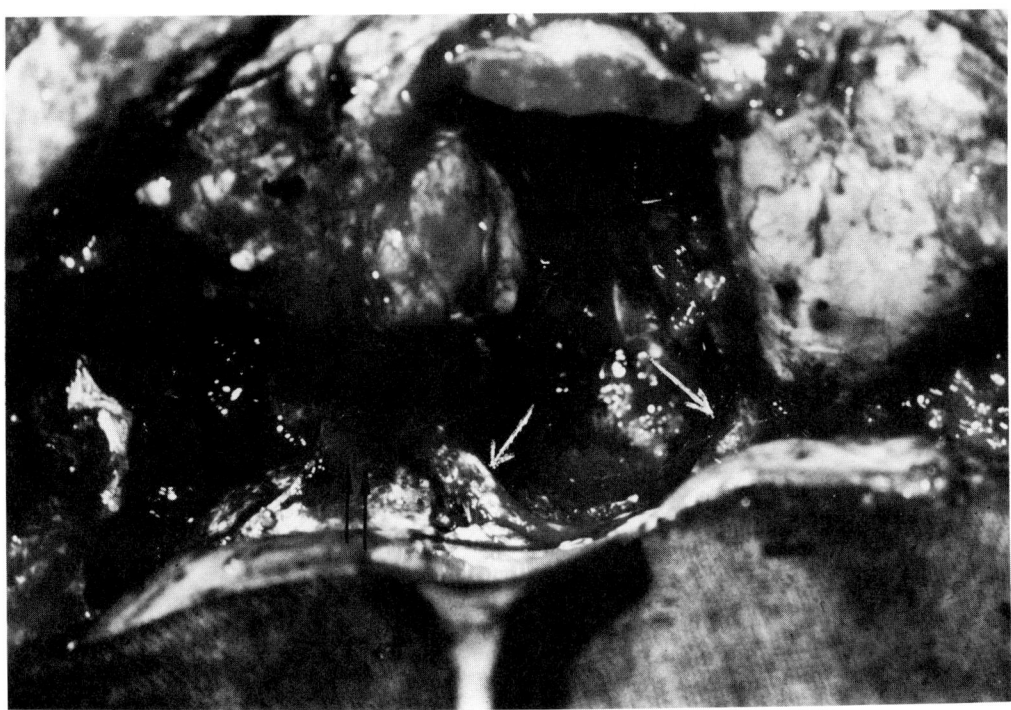

Figure 5: Total resection of a very large basal fibrous dysplasia. The optic nerves (white arrows) and supraorbital fissure (double black arrows) are totally free and, between the soft orbital tissues, the cavum mucosa is visible in the midline.

occurs mainly in younger patients, stabilizing after 25 or 30 years of age in all but a few cases. It is possible to identify two growth periods: the first during the first decade of life, and the second between 12 and 22 years. Cystic forms are more dangerous than sclerotic forms, particularly in terms of visual complications. Puberty does not stop the disease, and does not play a role in its stabilization; we have seen many complications in patients beyond puberty. The risk of malignant transformation of fibrous dysplasia varies between 0.4 and 4% and seems to be more significant in monostotic locations, particularly the maxilla and mandible. In 44% of irradiated patients, degeneration increased with radiotherapy, which is ineffective and carries great risks, and thus is not recommended.

Treatment for fibrous dysplasia is surgical, but because of the particular evolution of this disease, the indications for surgery depend upon patient symptomatology and the location and morphology of the lesion. The neurosurgeon must be aware that the major complication is visual impairment, including blindness, and that such complications occur unpredictably. We consider visual disturbance an absolute indication for operation, while preventive operation might be considered in patients younger than 25 years if the optic canals are involved and if the lesion is heterogenous or cystic in form; in adults without progressive symptomatology it seems logical to follow the patient on a regular basis, since in many cases the disease will stabilize. Indications for cosmetic surgery must be evaluated carefully, taking into account the degree of the deformity; mild cranio-orbitofacial deformity may be corrected by remodeling using resected bone.

In our series of patients, 42 individuals with basal dysplasia underwent surgery. Forty-two percent of those who had visual impairment preoperatively had improved vision postoperatively, often quite dramatic, and all of the young pa-

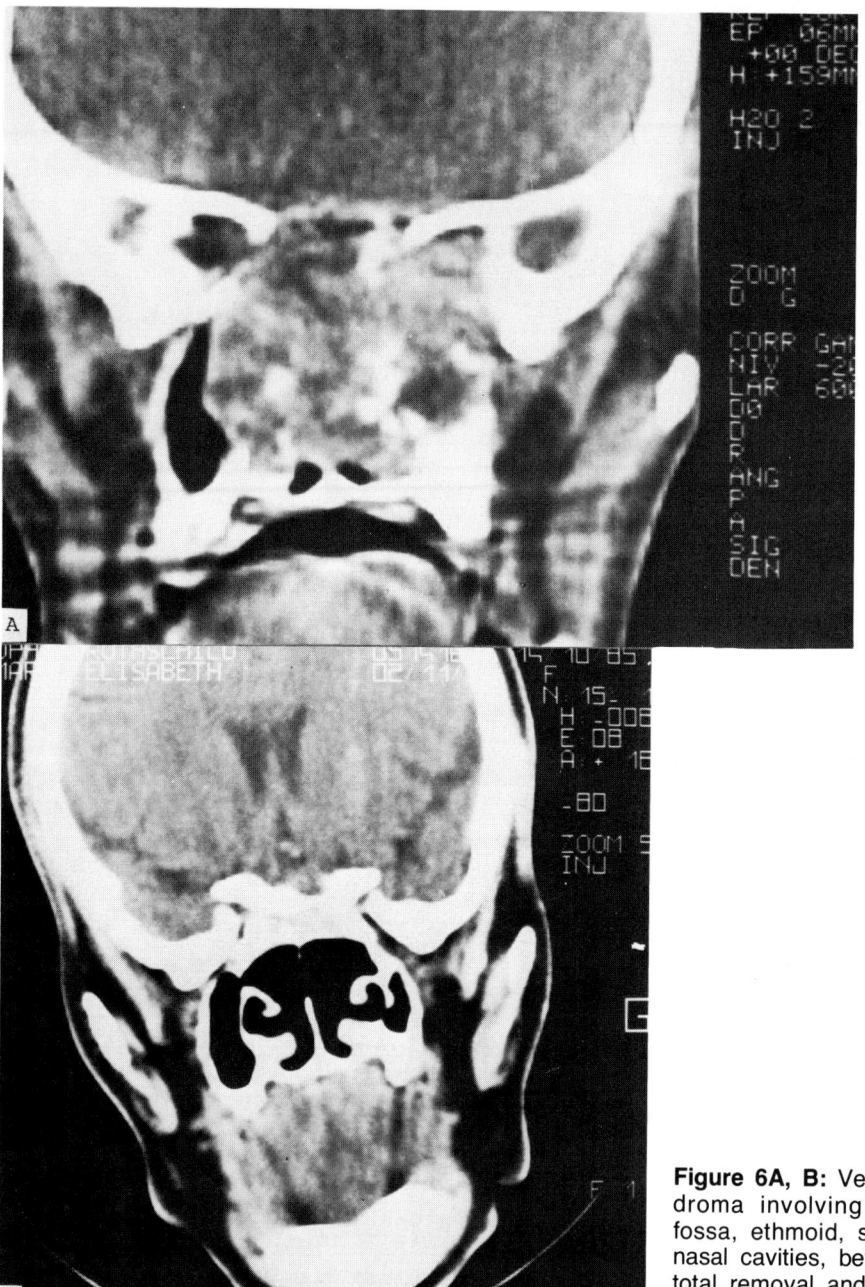

Figure 6A, B: Very large chondroma involving the anterior fossa, ethmoid, sphenoid, and nasal cavities, before and after total removal and basal reconstruction.

tients in whom the basal dysplasia involved the optic canal uni- or bilaterally underwent preventive surgery with no worsening of vision postoperatively. When surgery was performed on patients with very large craniofacial defects, maxillofacial surgeons assisted to correct facial deformity or hypertelorism.

While obtaining dural closure may be a major problem following resection of a basal meningioma, the dura is never involved in fibrous dysplasia and dural closure is easily performed after resection of such a lesion. However, technical problems may occur with basal reconstruction following the latter operation. Because mucosa may be lacking when a very large medial dysplasia is removed, an anterior pericranial flap may be particularly useful for closure, while removal of a dysplasia that extends toward the frontal vault may leave a defect too large to be filled by bone autografts. In this case another material such as irradiated homografts may be used. The technical aspects of surgery to manage fibrous dysplasia have been described previously.[7]

Chordomas

Chordomas are discussed in the chapter "Management of Cranial Chordomas."

Other Basal Tumors

Chondromas are usually localized in the sellar and parasellar areas,[10] and are often extensive, calcified, and grow intracranially. Total removal may be associated with high risk, or be impossible, because of involvement of the carotid arteries, optic tract, and cranial nerves.

However, in the anterior fossa, chondromas are more often destructive lesions that do not involve the dura, and they may be removed totally despite extensive basal involvement (Figs. 6A, B); the prognosis for cure depends upon the amount of posterior extension toward the parasellar area (cavernous sinuses, petrous apex). Of the five patients with lesions of this type in our series (followed for up to 17 years in one case), two have been operated upon for recurrences and one patient died after three subtotal resections and radiotherapy. Because of malignant degeneration in the patient that died following radiotherapy, we believe that radiation therapy is inadvisable except when a primary chondrosarcoma is present.

Olfactory placode tumors are usually removed in two surgical steps because their removal creates large dural defects. The resection is similar to that for invasive meningiomas localized to the midline, and total removal is usually possible (Figs. 7A, B). However, the patient's

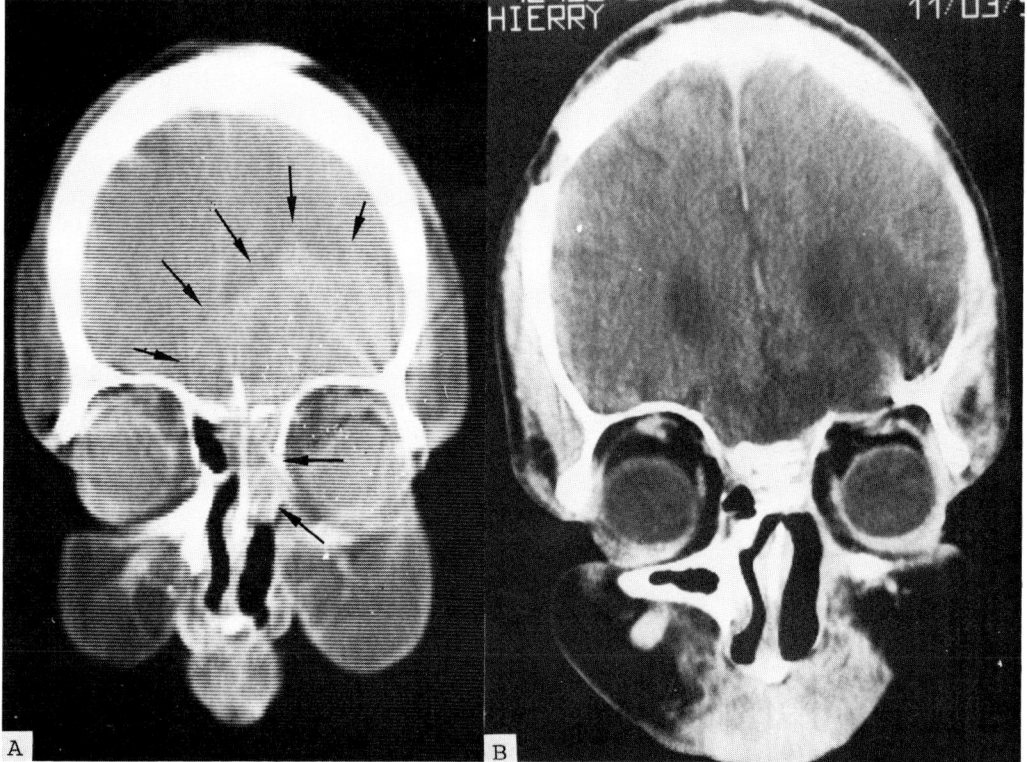

Figure 7A, B: Esthesioneurocytoma before and after a two-stage resection. Note bone autografts used to repair the ethmosphenoid area **B**.

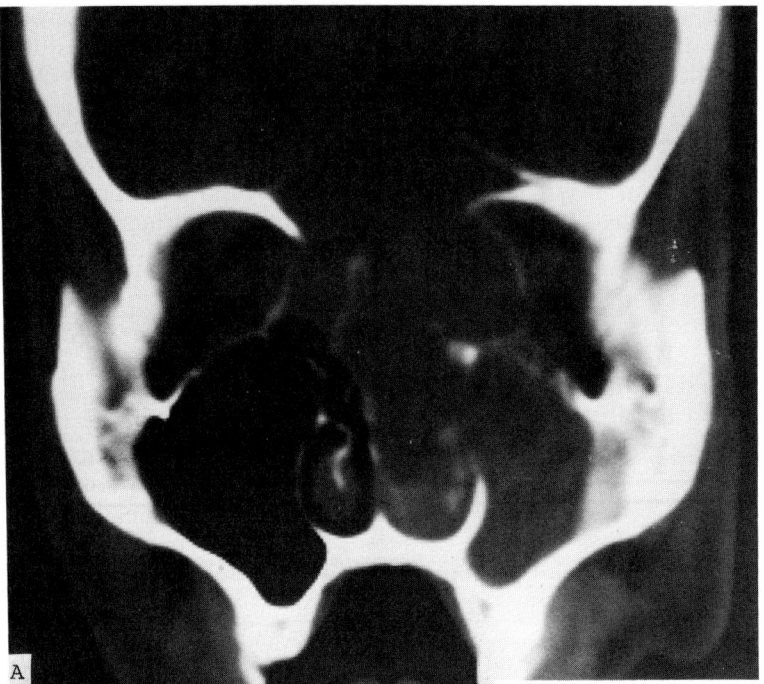

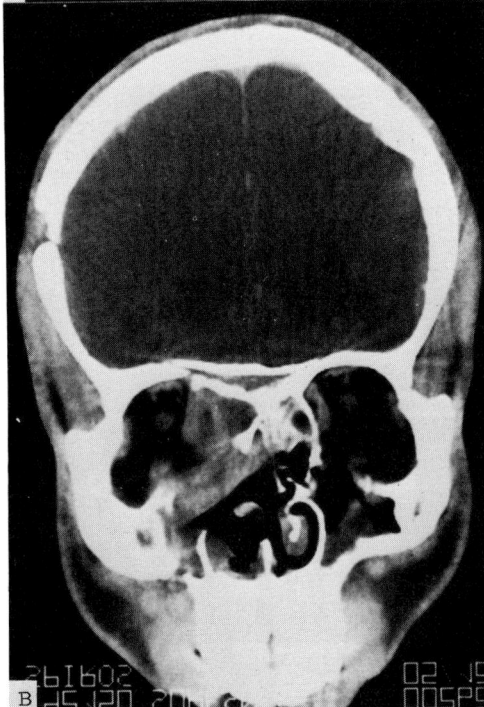

Figure 8A, B: Osteoblastoma involving the anterior cranial base, nasal fossae, and left maxillary sinus. **A:** Before surgery; **B:** (figure reversed) after transbasal and paralateral nasal approaches to resect the lesion.

prognosis depends upon the tumor type: it is good if the lesion is an esthesioneurocytoma, but poor with esthesioneuroblastomas, despite postoperative radiotherapy. Three of our six patients with olfactory placode tumors had malignant lesions, and died following local craniofacial invasion and metastasis.

Ossifying fibromas are totally benign tumors. In the three cases we have managed, they were very extensive intracranial lesions that involved the skull base (similar to invasive meningiomas en masse of the midline), except in one case in which the lesion resembled ethmosphenoid fibrous dysplasia.

Osteoblastomas are also benign lesions. They usually appear sclerotic on neuroradiological studies, and have a very firm consistency. One of the four patients we treated for such a lesion was unusual in that the osteoblastoma simulated a lytic fibrous dysplasia involving the nasal cavities (Figs. 8A, B). In this case, two surgical approaches, transbasal and lateral rhinotomy, were necessary for tumor removal.

Pure osteomas occur rarely, although

we have treated two patients with such lesions. They grow from ethmoid cells, or frontal or sphenoid sinuses, and particular care must be taken during their removal to preclude postoperative extradural pneumatoceles.

In our series of patients, two *dermoid cysts* and one *bony angioma* occurred in the greater sphenoid wing. Hypervascularized lesions such as angiomas (or nasopharyngeal fibromas) must be embolized preoperatively. Another bony tumor that may be found at the base of the skull, although exceptionally rarely, is the giant cell tumor; these lesions occur within the sphenoid bone, with parasellar and intradural involvement in some cases, which is the most frequent cause of incomplete removal.[8] However, radiotherapy may lead to long survival, as happened in the only individual with such a lesion that we followed in our series of patients with basal tumors.

References

1. Akerman M, Oddou B, Visot A, Derome P: Dynamic bone scintigraphy in craniofacial dysplasia. Eur J Nucl Med 8:A-22, 1983.
2. Castellano F, Guidetti B, Olivecrona H: Pterional meningiomas 'en plaque.' J Neurosurg 9:188-196, 1952.
3. Derome P, et al: Les tumeurs sphenoethmoidales. Possibilities d'exerese et de reparation chirurgicales. Neurochirurgie 18(Suppl 1), 1972.
4. Derome PJ: the transbasal approach to tumors invading the base of the skull. In Schmidek HH, Sweet WH (eds): Current Technics in Operative Neurosurgery. New York, Grune & Stratton, Inc, 1977, pp 223-245.
5. Derome P, Guiot G: Bone problems in meningiomas invading the base of the skull. Clin Neurosurg 25:435-451, 1978.
6. Derome PJ, Guiot G, et al: Surgical approaches to the sphenoidal and clival areas. Adv Tech Stand Neurosurg 6:101-136, 1979.
7. Derome PJ, Visot A, et al: Fibrous dysplasia of the skull. Neurochirurgie 29 (Suppl 1), 1983.
8. Geissinger JD, Siqueira EB, Ross ER: Giant cell tumors of the sphenoid bone. J Neurosurg 32:665-670, 1970.
9. Guiot G, Derome P: A propos des meningiomes en plaque du pterion. Le traitement chirurgical des meningiomes osseux hyperostosants. Ann Chir 20:C1109-C1127, 1966.
10. Krayenbuhl H, Yasargil MG: Chondromas. Progr Neurol Surg 6:435-463, 1975.
11. Pompili A, Derome PJ, Visot A, Guiot G: Hyperostosing meningiomas of the sphenoid ridge. Clinical features, surgical therapy and long-term observations: Review of 49 cases. Surg Neurol 17:411-416, 1982.

VII

Middle Cranial Base

19

Middle Cranial Base Anatomy

Johannes Lang, M.D.

Introduction

The middle cranial base comprises the bony floor of the middle cranial fossa and the sella turcica region. The bony floor of the middle cranial fossa is bounded anteriorly by the posterior border of the lesser wing of the sphenoid bone and its lateral extension, the crista alaris (Sylvii). The frontal bone, the parietal bone, the squama of the temporal bone, and the greater wing of the sphenoid bone meet here, in most cases in an H-shaped suture zone called the pterion. However, sometimes we found only the temporal squama connected to the frontal bone, or the greater wing of the sphenoid bone connected by a suture to the parietal bone.[16]

In this normally thick bony area, we found, on the right and left sides in about 35% of cases, a bony canal for the frontal branch of the middle meningeal artery, or a meningeal sinus.[3] A little bit below the crista alaris we found (in 21% of cases) canals between the middle cranial fossa and the orbit called the posterior meningo-orbital foramina. Through these canals run vessels which anastomose with the middle meningeal artery and branches of the ophthalmic artery, most commonly the lacrimal artery. The greater wing of the sphenoid bone forms the major part of the floor and a part of the lateral wall of the middle cranial fossa. In its medial part, the greater wing extends further dorsally than in its lateral part. Laterally the greater wing of the sphenoid bone connects to the squamous portion of the temporal bone, which also constitutes the lateral bony floor of the middle cranial fossa. Medially and posteriorly the greater wing abuts the petrous part of the temporal bone and the bony carotid canal (Fig. 1).

Figure 2 shows the mean values of the lateral-medial dimension of the middle cranial fossa, measured between the crista alaris and the superior margin of the petrous temporal bone.

Rostral to the petrous part of the temporal bone in each case we determined the thickest and thinnest bone structures of the middle cranial fossa.[17] In 80% of cases the thickest bone was found in the area of the mandibular eminence rostral to the fossa mandibularis. The mandibular fossa was the thinnest area of the floor of the middle cranial fossa in 67% of cases. In 20% of cases we found a tubercle in the area of the greater wing of the sphenoid bone, which was the thickest area of the floor, and found a gyral impression behind and lateral to the foramen rotundum (Fig. 3).

From: Sekhar LN, Schramm VL Jr, eds: *Tumors of the Cranial Base: Diagnosis and Treatment*. Mount Kisco, New York, Futura Publishing Co, Inc, © 1987.

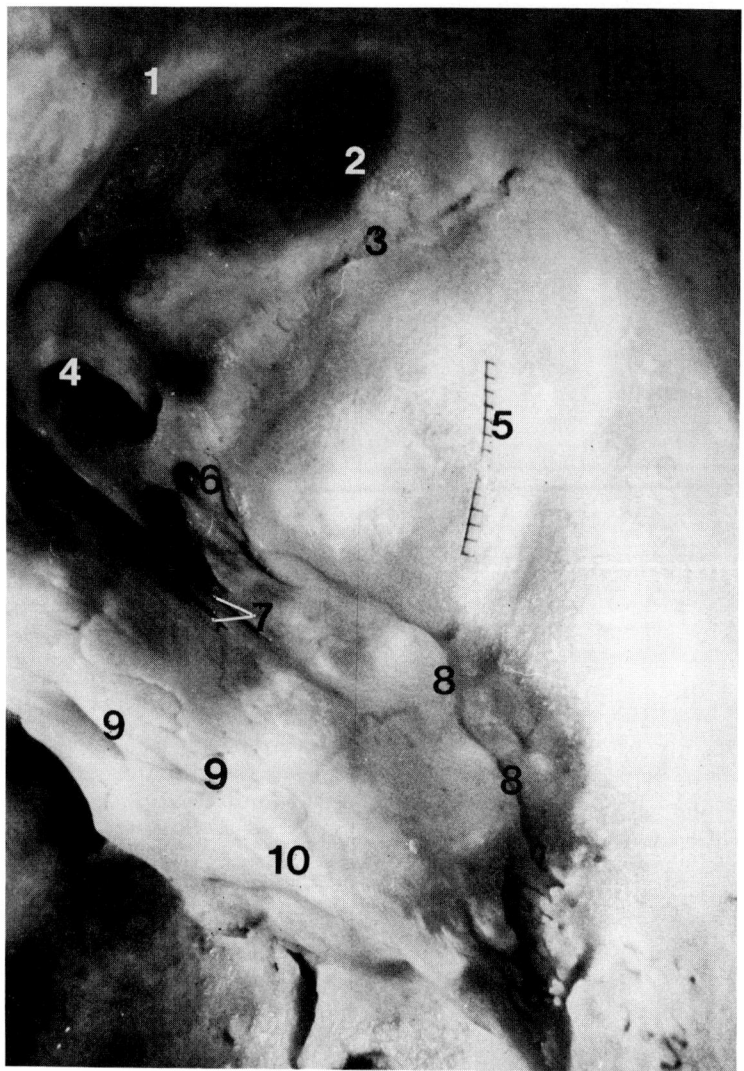

Figure 1: Middle cranial base (4-year-old child). 1. Lesser wing of sphenoid bone. 2. Greater wing of sphenoid bone. 3. Sphenosquamosal suture. 4. Foramen ovale. 5. Squamous part of temporal bone. 6. Foramen spinosum. 7. Crus for the lesser and greater petrosal nerves. 8. Petrosquamosal suture. 9. Internal auditory meatus and subarcuate fossa. 10. Sulcus sinus petrosi superioris.

We measured the depth of the middle cranial fossa between the anterior petroclinoid fold (at the level of the diaphragmatic foramen) and the deepest area of the middle cranial fossa. This dimension was 20.55 mm (range 17.0–23.0 mm) on the right and 18.0 mm (range 14.2–22.6 mm) on the left. The average difference in depth between the two sides was 2.54 mm (Fig. 4).[4] The deepest area of the middle cranial fossa is the area of the upper border of the zygomatic process of the temporal bone, in the vicinity of its articular tubercle. The deepest point is on the average 0.9 mm below this landmark, with extreme variations being found 6 mm above to 9 mm below the upper border of the zygomatic process. In adults the deepest point is 6.4 mm (range 0–15 mm) behind this landmark[18] (Fig. 5).

Middle Cranial Base Anatomy • 315

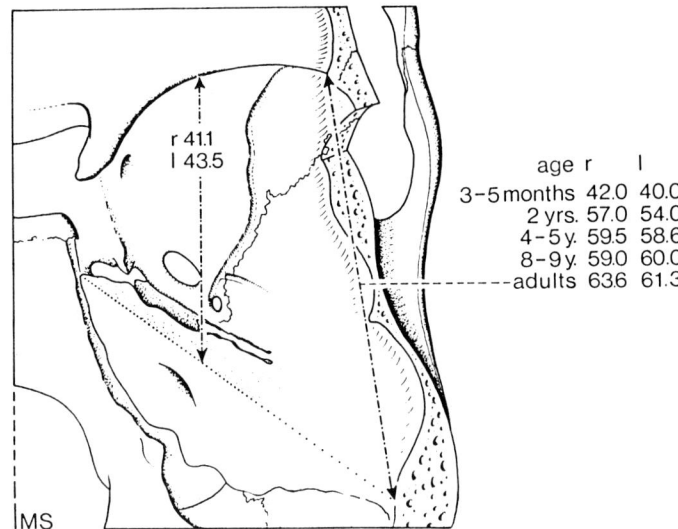

Figure 2: Length of the middle cranial fossa in the lateral area, with postnatal increases in the medial part given as mean values in millimeters for right (r) and left (l) sides separately. MS, Midsagittal line.

Middle Cranial Fossa Orifices

Superior Orbital Fissure

The medial part of the superior orbital fissure is wide; its lateral extent narrows and turns upward and forward. Its upper border is formed by the lower surface of the lesser wing, and its medial boundary by the inferior root of the lesser wing and by a part of the body of the sphenoid bone. The inferior border of the superior orbital fissure is the upper margin of the greater wing of the sphenoid bone. The length of the fissure from the

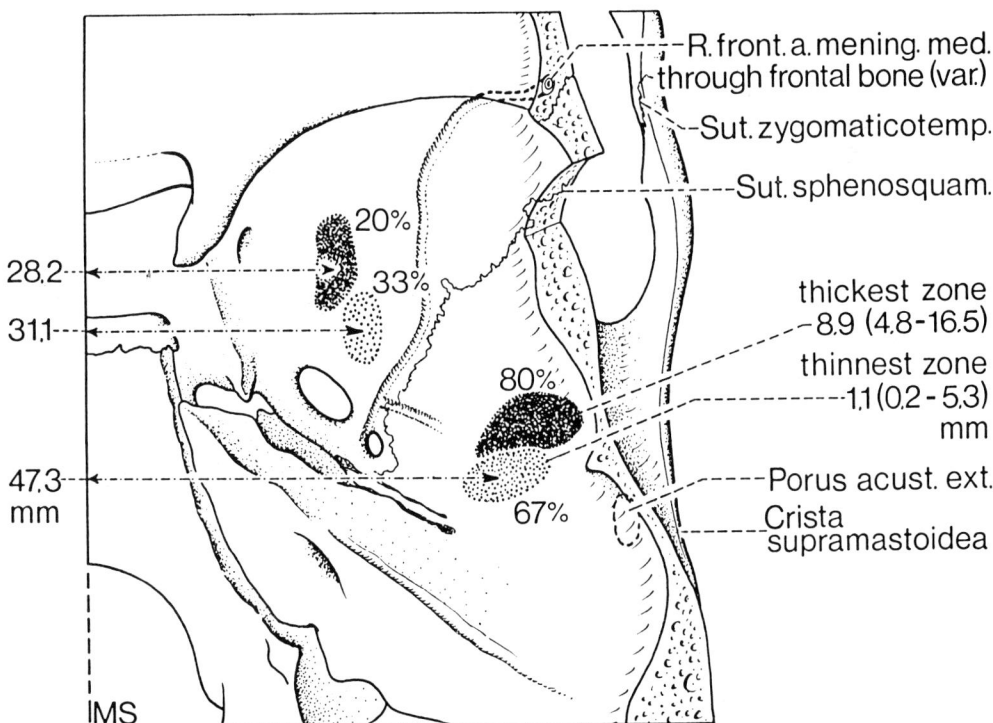

Figure 3: Thin and thick areas of the floor of the middle cranial fossa (excluding the thickness of the petrous part).

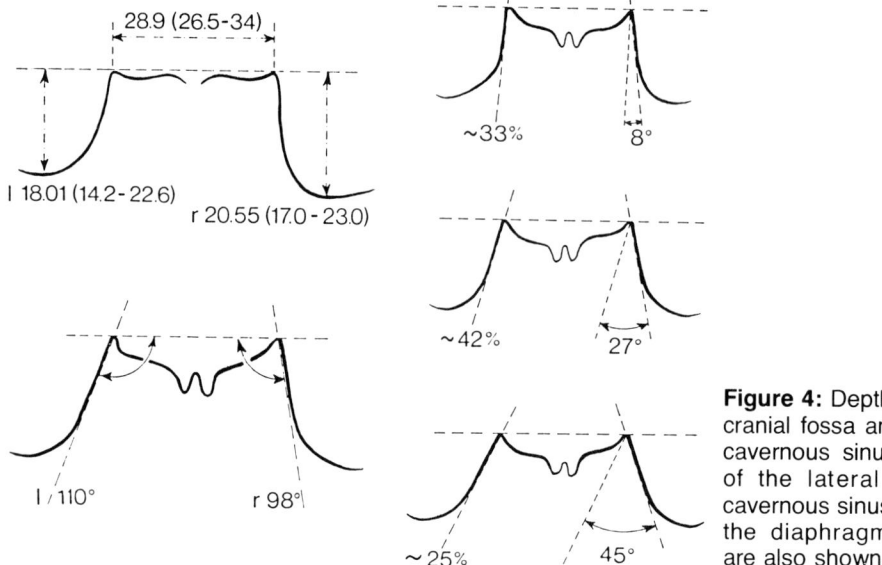

Figure 4: Depth of the middle cranial fossa and width of the cavernous sinus. The angles of the lateral walls of the cavernous sinus in the area of the diaphragmatic foramen are also shown.

lateral end to the medial end on the right side in our specimens averaged 19.91 mm (range 12–26 mm). On the left side, the length of the fissure averaged 19.62 mm (range 12–26 mm).

The superior orbital fissure is always widest medial to the spine for the lateral rectus muscle; its width was 6.46 mm (range 3.8–11.0 mm) on the right and 6.39 mm (range 3.4–11.5 mm) on the left.[36] The superior orbital fissure was narrowest about 5 mm medial to its lateral end, and the width here was estimated to be 2.22 mm on the right and 2.11 mm on the left

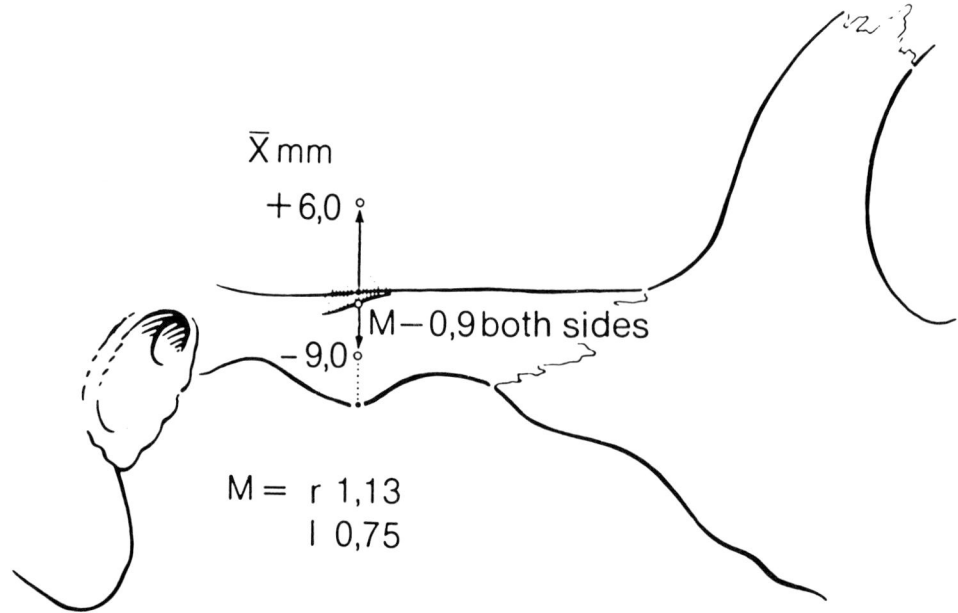

Figure 5: The deepest point of the middle cranial fossa is in the area of the upper border of the zygomatic arch. The extremes and means for right and left are also shown.

side. The extremes were 0.3 and 5.3 mm.

The lateral end of the superior orbital fissure was situated 26.27 mm (range 13.2–34.2 mm) from the sagittal plane on the right side, and on the left, 26.86 mm (range 13.8–34.2 mm).

Angle of the Superior Orbital Fissure with Transverse Horizontal Axis

In our specimens we found the longitudinal axis of the superior orbital fissure on the right side to be at an angle 44.66° (range 31–61°) and on the left to be 42.86° (range 28–61°) to the horizontal axis (Fig. 6).

Foramen Rotundum

In adults, the foramen rotundum is a canal about 4 mm in length. Its internal aperture is situated below the inferior medial border of the superior orbital fissure at a distance of 3.61 mm (range 0.7–7.8 mm) and 3.57 mm (range 1.3–6.6 mm) on the left. The width of the canalis rotundus on the intracranial aperture was found in adults to be 3.34 mm (range 2.2–4.9 mm) on the right and 3.52 mm (range 2.1–5.2 mm) on the left. Its height was found to be 2.7 mm (range 1.4–3.8 mm) on the right and 2.76 mm (range 1.6–5.5 mm) on the left side.

Canalis Rotundus, Axis

We found that in the first year of life, the axis of the canalis rotundus is oriented 13° (range 7°–17°) inferior to the Frankfort horizontal plane. This downward projection of the axis was found in most skulls of children less than 1 year old, while in older children and adults we found the axis to be tilted up to 36° downward and up to 24° forward and upward. In newborns, the short canal in most cases is directed forward and medially a maximum of 7°. Between the second and fourth years of life, the canal becomes more anteriorly oriented, and in adults it is located for-

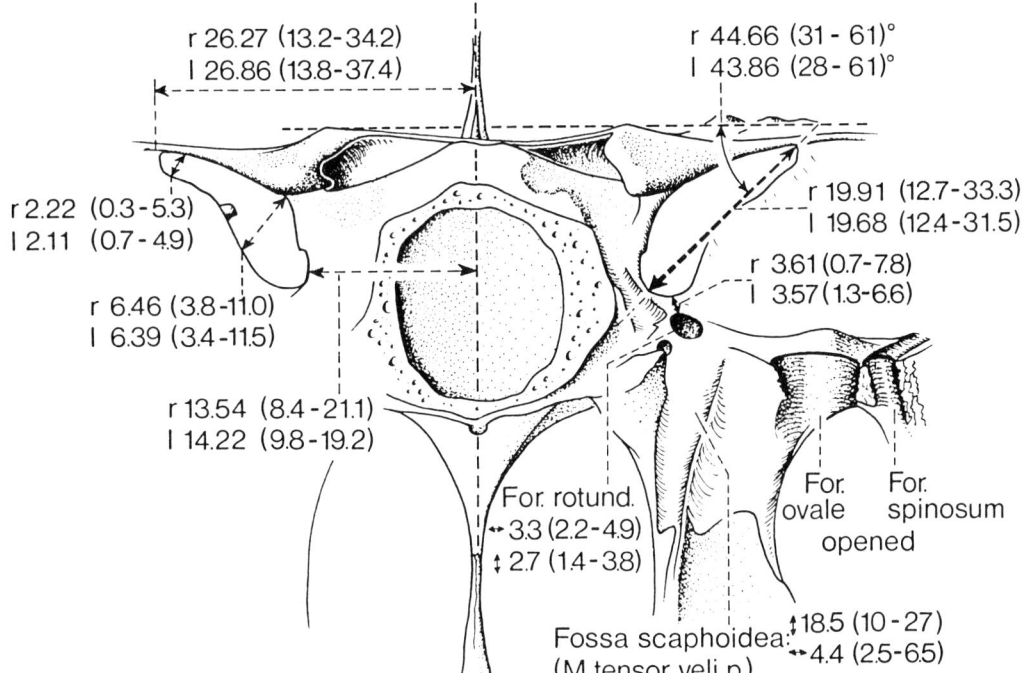

Figure 6: Superior orbital fissure (viewed from posterior to anterior), postnatal enlargement. Also given are the distance to the foramen rotundum, our measurements of the latter, and right and left differences. Measurements are in millimeters (range).

ward and laterally at an angle up to 15° from the longitudinal axis of the head. Postnatal enlargement of the foramina rotundum, ovale, and spinosum and their topographical changes have been described previously.[20]

Postnatal shifting of the foramen rotundum (and the foramina ovale and spinosum) is shown in Figure 7. The maxillary nerve runs through the middle cranial fossa to the pterygopalatine fossa. Its intracranial length between the trigeminal ganglion and the foramen rotundum were measured in our specimens to be 10.34 mm (range 4.5–15.1 mm) on the right and 10.33 mm (range 5.5–16.0 mm) on the left. The cross-sectional area of the nerve ranges from 4.6 to 15.3 mm². Within the foramen rotundum the nerve contains an average of 14 fascicles, each with an average thickness of 173 µm; there are also two arteries with lumina of average diameter 135 µm. Occasionally we found only one fascicle within the foramen, but in other instances, up to 30 fascicles have been counted.[19] In one case with agenesis of the internal carotid artery, a large branch of the maxillary artery that was found to be piercing the foramen rotundum, and another one that coursed through the foramen ovale, united rostal to the trigeminal ganglion.[6] The branches supplied one hemisphere of the brain. Sondheimer found, in about 10% of cases studied, veins in the foramen rotundum with diameters between 1 and 3 mm; these veins were on the medial circumference of the foramen rotundum and were seen to be coming from the pterygoid process of the sphenoid bone.[33] In our specimens, we found these veins arising in the fovea granularis medial to the foramen rotundum.

Foramen Ovale

In adults, the average length of the foramen ovale is 7.26 mm (range 4.2–9.9 mm) on the right and 7.15 mm (range 3.2–9.7 mm) on the left side. Its width was

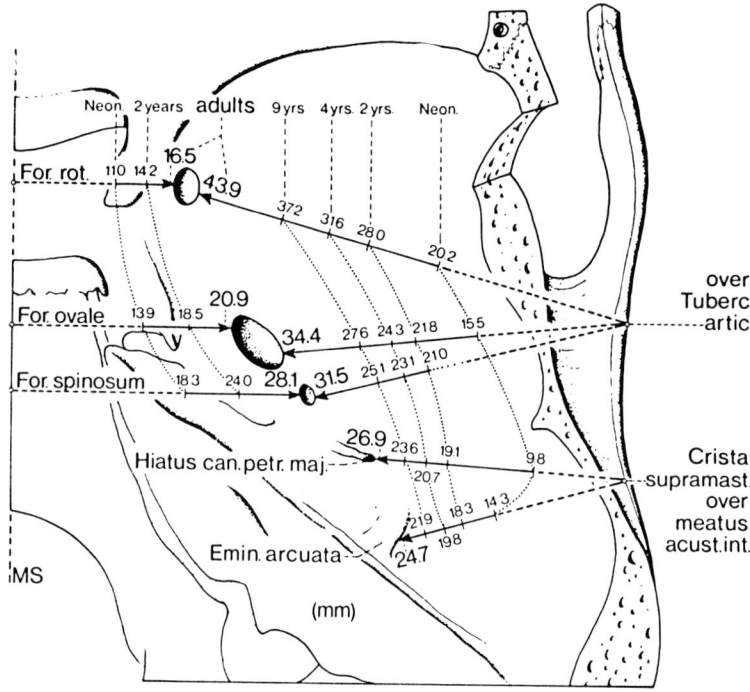

Figure 7: Postnatal shift of the foramina rotundum, ovale, and spinosum, from the midsagittal plane (MS) and the zygomatic arch over the articular tubercle. Also given are the distances between the supramastoid crest (over the external auditory meatus) and the exit zone of the superior petrosal nerve and the arcuate eminence. Measurements are in millimeters.

found to be 3.65 mm (2.2–6.7 mm) on the right and 3.77 mm (1.7–5.9 mm) on the left. During development of the skull, the posterior border of the foramen ovale (and the foramen spinosum) closes at a relatively late stage. According to Wood-Jones (1931), the posterior border is absent to a greater or lesser extent in 8% of cases; the defect was found bilaterally in 3% and unilaterally in 5% of cases.[15,38] The postnatal displacement of the foramen ovale is shown in Figure 7.

Through the foramen ovale, the mandibular nerve leaves the middle cranial fossa. Its intracranial length between the trigeminal ganglion and the foramen ovale was measured to be 6.6 mm (range 2.9–11.5 mm) on the right side and 6.63 mm (range 2.8–9.8 mm) on the left side.[34] In our specimens, its cross-sectional area varied between 7.8 and 14.5 mm^2 on the right and between 10.4 and 16.2 mm^2 on the left.[35] Besides the mandibular nerve, the foramen ovale occasionally carries the accessory meningeal branch from the middle meningeal artery and the meningeal branch of the mandibular nerve. Also within the foramen ovale is a large-caliber venous plexus that connects the foramen ovale to the cavernous sinus and usually to the middle meningeal vein, though less commonly to a paracavernous sinus. The plexus extends upward as far as the region of the trigeminal ganglion in 68% of cases, and always reaches the proximal part of the maxillary nerve and the anterior upper half of the intracranial part of the mandibular nerve.[32] Below the skull, this plexus is connected with the pterygoid venous plexus.

Foramen Spinosum

In most cases (about 98%), the foramen spinosum is located behind and lateral to the foramen ovale.[3] The distance between the foramen ovale and the anterior border of the foramen spinosum in our specimens was an average of 2.61 mm (range 0.3–5.6 mm) on the right side and 2.59 mm (range 0.6–5.8 mm) on the left. Its length was found to be 2.57 mm (range 1.2–4.3 mm) on the right and 2.6 mm (range 1.0–4.7 mm) on the left. The width of the foramen was estimated on the right side in adults to be 2.05 mm (range 1.1–3.8 mm), and on the left to be 2.10 mm (range 1.2–3.7 mm).[20]

The foramen spinosum is, like the foramen rotundum, a short bony canal. Measured along the lateral side in our specimens, the length of the canal was estimated to be 7.4 mm (range 2–15 mm) on the right and 7.3 mm (range 3–13 mm) on the left side. As a rule, the canal is shortest on the medial side: 5.6 mm (range 2–11 mm) long on the right and 5.5 mm (range 2–10 mm) long on the left. Between the perinatal period and adult life, the length of the canal approximately doubles.[7]

Duplicate foramina spinosa have been found in dried skulls and in roentgenographs.[26] According to Sondheimer, the duplication of the foramen spinosum is not associated with early bifurcation of the middle meningeal artery outside the skull.[33] According to Lindblom, the foramen spinosum is absent in 0.4% of cases and the middle meningeal artery arises from the ophthalmic artery instead of entering the skull through the foramen spinosum.[26] This vessel is surrounded by the middle meningeal veins, which are really sinuses.

Foramina Rotundum, Ovale, and Spinosum, Right–Left Differences

On the right side, we found these foramina situated more medially than on the left, while on the left side, the foramina are situated slightly more rostrally than on the left.[24]

Foramen Venosum of Vesalius

This foramen transmits the basal emissary vein from the cavernous sinus and was present in our specimens on the right side in 49% and on the left in 36%. It is situated dorsal to (more frequently mediodorsal to and less frequently laterodorsal to) the foramen rotundum. A small nerve may also pass through the foramen venosum into the cavernous sinus (nervulus sphenoidalis lateralis). In our specimens the foramen had an average diameter of 1.14 mm and an average length of 2.04 mm on the right and smaller dimensions on the left side. The average distance of the foramen venosum from the median plane was 15.78 mm (range 12.6–24.9 mm) on the right and 17.62 mm (range 13.3–26.2 mm) on the left. In rare cases we also found the foramen venosum (Vesalii) incomplete dorsally.[15]

Anterior Surface of the Petrous Bone

The anterior surface of the petrous part of the temporal bone has an impression, called the trigeminal impression. On the superior crest of the petrous bone, the trigeminal incisura is visible in this area. The impression is usually found on the lateral margin of the trigeminal incisura, in most cases extending deeper laterally than medially. The impression extends downward and forward to the foramen lacerum internum and the sulcus of the greater superficial petrosal nerve (GSPN). In cases with large foramina lacera interna, the trigeminal impression is small, about 3 mm, while when the foramen lacerum internum is small, the impression could be up to 13 mm in diameter.[39] In most cases an upper, a dorsal, a medial, and an anterior lower and lateral part of this impression can be identified; they touch one another in the area of the sphenoid lingula. In the area of the upper medial part the pars triangularis of the trigeminal nerve is situated while in the lower lateral portion lies a part of the trigeminal ganglion. The upper side of the impression is the trigeminal incisura, while the medial border is directed parallel to the midsagittal plane, between the medial end of the incisura and the apex of the sphenoid lingula. This part is between 6 and 11 mm long. The lateral border of the trigeminal impression is directed upward and anteriorly toward the outer border of the trigeminal incisura, then downward and laterally; it is between 4 and 6 mm long. The anterior and lower sides are curved and its convexity is oriented downward and laterally. The medial end of the impression reaches the apex of the lingula sphenoidalis.

In about 50% of cases, a small ridge forms the border of the lower end of the trigeminal impression. The triangular part of the trigeminal nerve is situated above the dura mater, which covers the trigeminal impression, and a depression for the trigeminal ganglion is situated lateral to the impression for the pars triangularis of the trigeminal nerve. In addition, in cases in which the carotid canals on the anterior side were entirely closed (4% of our cases) (Fig. 8), the depression for the trigeminal ganglion developed below the trigeminal impression. In about 1% of our cases, the impression for the trigeminal ganglion was found in the dorsal part of the greater wing of the sphenoid bone.

Below the impression for the triangular part of the trigeminal nerve runs the canal for the internal carotid artery. Its upper anterior surface was dehiscent in 96% of our cases. This dehiscence, which was closed by connective tissue and which we called the inferior petrosphenoid ligament, varied in size and shape (Fig. 8). Lateral to the trigeminal impression the openings for the greater and lesser petrosal nerves may be identified.

The canal of the facial nerve was covered by a bony lamella, but was uncovered by bone in about 15% of cases. When the canal was exposed, the ganglion lay directly below the dura mater of the middle cranial fossa. The opening for the lesser petrosal nerve lies slightly inferior, on the anterior surface of the petrous portion. Distal to their openings, the two nerves are 2.19 mm (range 1.27–3.1 mm) apart on the right and 2.59 mm (range 1.82–3.36 mm) apart on the left side.[23] The distance between the opening of the canal for the greater petrosal nerve and the supramastoid crest above the external auditory meatus was found to be 26.96 mm (range 21–34 mm) on the right and 26.84 mm (range 21–38 mm) on the left in adults (see Fig. 7). The groove for the greater petrosal nerve was on the average 1.54 mm wide (range 0.4–3.8 mm), and lay at an angle of

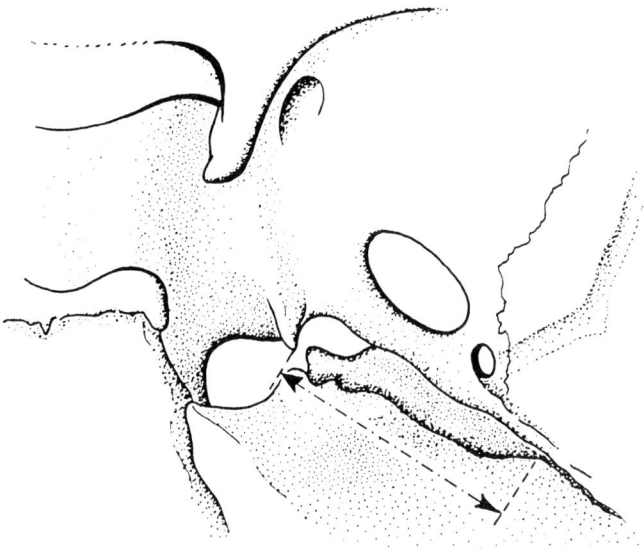

Carotid canal,
dehiscence of its upper wall

age	left	right
0 - 0.5 yrs.	7.7 (3.8 - 11.0)	8.2 (3.9 - 11.9)
2.5 - 4 y.	8.8 (5.9 - 11.9)	8.5 (6.2 - 12.1)
10 - 17 y.	12.6 (8.0 - 15.6)	11.8 (7.1 - 19.1)
adults	12.5 (6.0 - 13.8)	

missing in 4%

Figure 8: In 96% of our cases the upper wall of the carotid canal had dehiscences. Shown are the length of the dehiscence, its postnatal change, and right and left differences. Measurements are in millimeters (range).

28° to 68° to the midsagittal plane. (The average angle was 45.89° on the right and 49.36° on the left.)

The average width of the groove for the lesser petrosal nerve in our specimens was 0.9 mm (range 0.3–1.8 mm), and its angle to the midsagittal plane averaged 46.94° on the right side and 50.91° on the left.[36] The greater and lesser petrosal nerves run forward, medially, and downward, embedded in dura mater close to the bone. Below the trigeminal ganglion, the GSPN then pierces the transverse part of the inferior sphenopetrosal ligament and is joined by sympathetic fibers (deep petrosal nerve). Together with these fibers, it then enters the pterygoid canal, where it forms the nerve of the pterygoid canal. This nerve runs forward to the pterygopalatine ganglion in the pterygopalatine fossa. The lesser petrosal nerve passes into the middle cranial fossa somewhat lower down and more rostrally. It is embedded in the external layer of dura mater and pierces the transverse part of the inferior sphenopetrosal ligament to end in the otic ganglion. In about 15% of cases, however, the lesser petrosal nerve pierces the greater wing (usually lateral and dorsal to the foramen spinosum) to reach the lower surface of the skull (Arnold's canal).

The GSPN is accompanied by an arterial branch from the middle meningeal artery (less frequently from one of the caroticocavernous branches): the petrosal branch. This twig runs to the geniculate ganglion and to parts of the labyrinthine and tympanic segments of the facial nerve. The lesser petrosal nerve is also accompanied by a twig of the middle meningeal artery: the superior tympanic artery. This branch supplies the tensor tympani muscle and the mucosa of the tympanic cavity.

The arcuate eminences of newborns and young children are always visible. In later childhood, bony tubercles sometimes develop in this area, and the eminence is clearly visible in only 50% of adults. In 26% of our specimens, the eminence was not visible on the right nor on the left, while in the remainder of the specimens, it was more often seen on the left than on the right.[20] This landmark is important for the subtemporal approach to the internal auditory meatus, as described by House.[9] Below the area of the arcuate eminence is found the anterior semicircular canal and its "blue line" (after drilling away the superficial part of the petrous bone in this area). The distances from the arcuate eminence to landmarks on the skull are shown in Figure 2.

The upper border of the petrous temporal bone forms a variable angle with the midsagittal plane. In adults the angle averages 128.7° on the right and 127.0° on the left. Lateral to the arcuate eminence, the often very thin tegmen tympani is located. Slightly inferior and lateral to the tegmen is found the internal petrosquamosal suture. This suture is visible in most skulls of young children and sometimes in those of adults. In frontal sections of the temporal bone, this suture is found above the lateral part of the tympanic cavity and overlaps the squamous part of the temporal bone laterally (Fig. 9).

In newborns, a fissure is visible in this area; it is filled with connective tissue and connects the dura mater and the tympanic cavity. After the fifth month of postnatal life, the inferior process of the tegmen tympani grows inferiorly to the lateral skull base, where it forms the anterior border of the petrotympanic fissure (Glaseri). This process extends also to the cleft between the annulus tympanicus and the squama. Thus, between these two bony structures, the fissura tympanosquamosa anterior (Gruber) is formed, and is completely separated from and lateral to the tympanic cavity. Because in young children the inferior process of the tegmen tympani has not lengthened fully, both fissures on the outer skull base are united. Inside the skull, in the roof of the tympanic cavity, there is also a transitional zone between the dura mater of the middle cranial fossa and the tympanic cavity and the mastoid process. Through this suture, small twigs of the middle meningeal artery reach the tegmen tympani area[30,37] (Figs. 1, 9). The superior petrosal sinus is found along the upper rim of the petrous bone, embedded in dura mater forming the tentorium cerebelli posteriorly.

Dura Mater of the Middle Cranial Fossa, Blood Supply

The arteries supplying the floor of the middle cranial fossa are mainly twigs of the middle meningeal artery, while in the medial parts of the middle cranial fossa numerous anastomoses with twigs of the caroticocavernous branches are found (Fig. 10). The parts of the brain that are situated in the floor of the middle cranial fossa are shown in Figure 11.

Pituitary Region

Osteology

That the bone surrounding the pituitary may vary greatly is partly the result of the complicated embryology of the sphenoid. In 10% of skulls of neonates and young children, the median craniopharyngeal canal is visible. This canal runs through the body of the sphenoid to the base of the skull, or it may lead into the sphenoid sinus. Arey found an open craniopharyngeal canal in 0.42% of adults, with a diameter of 1 to 1.5 mm and a length of 15 to 16 mm.[1] In our specimens (newborns and adults), we found arterial and venous branches piercing the bottom of the hypophyseal fossa (see Fig. 144 in Lang,[15]). It has been suggested that canals of this kind represent relics of the path taken by Rathke's pouch.

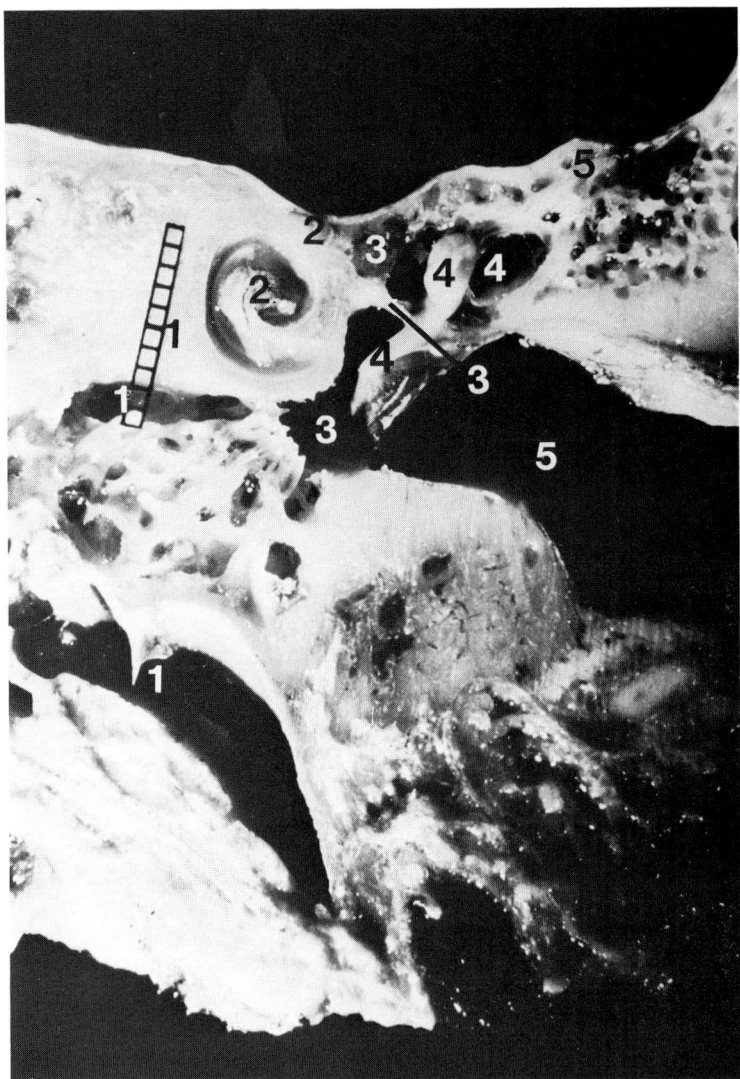

Figure 9: Vertical section through temporal bone, viewed posterior to anterior. 1. Scale in 1 mm blocks, inframeatal cells, and internal jugular vein. 2. N. facialis and cochlea. 3. Pars tympanica of the facial nerve and tendo m. tensoris tympani and cavum tympani. 4. Epitympanic recess, head of malleus, and manubrium mallei. 5. Petrosquamosal suture and external auditory meatus.

In about 5 to 6% of cases, sella bridges, intraclinoid taeniae, and caroticoclinoid foramina may be seen, the latter located at different angles to the Frankfort plane, horizontal plane, the midsagittal plane, and the vertical plane.[14,15]

The sellar spine was first described on a skull of a 23-year-old Caucasian man.[14] The osseous spine was 4.35 mm long and protruded from the dorsal side of the pituitary fossa into the fossa itself. The tip of the spine was 1.25 mm long. Dietemann et al. noted that in five cases examined anatomically and radiologically, the spine protruded into the pituitary fossa.[5] Further, we have not uncommonly found in adults dehiscences in the dorsum sellae, through which were running twigs of the caroticocavernous branches and veins between hypophyseal and clival arterial and venous networks.

The postnatal enlargement of the

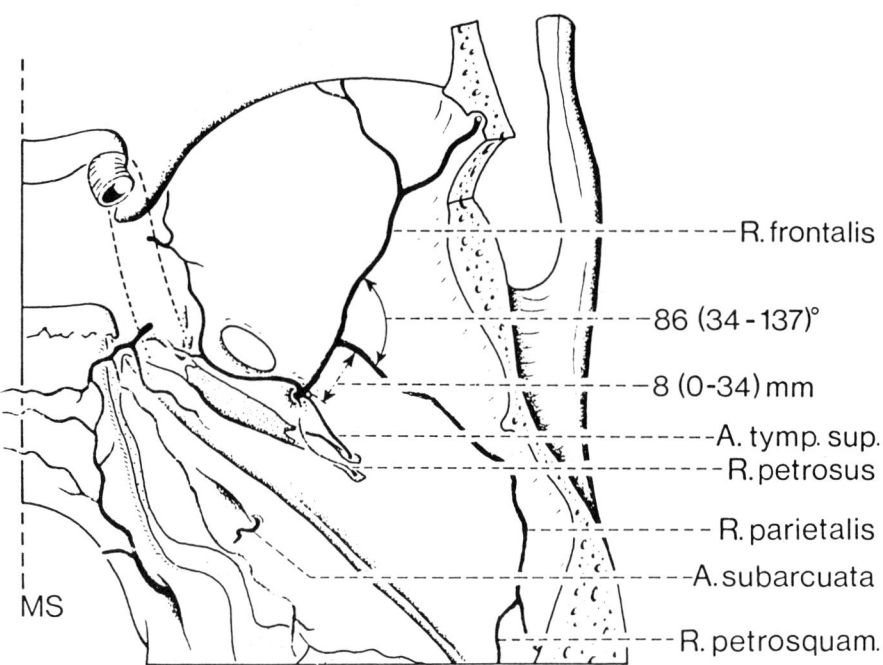

Figure 10: Arterial supply of middle cranial base. The main artery is the middle meningeal artery with its branches. Medial parts are supplied by twigs of the caroticocavernous trunks and have anastomoses with twigs of the middle meningeal artery.

hypophyseal area is shown in Figure 12. It should be noted that we found no increase in the length between the anterior border of the prechiasmic sulcus and the tuberculum sellae, but great variations of the distances between the anterior clinoid and the posterior clinoid processes during postnatal development. The width of the sella floor was measured by Renn and Rhoton to be 14.0 mm (range 10–16 mm).[31] We found that it is widest (3–7.5 mm) dorsal to the tuberculum sellae and that the right margin of the pituitary fossa is less often lower in relation to the Frankfort horizontal plane than the left.[25] Only in 50% of our casts of 71 skulls could we see a hypophyseal fossa; in 15.5% the bottom of the sella was a horizontal plateau, in about 20% we found a plateau and a small impression, and in 6% a plateau and a convexity, while in each of 4.23% of cases we found a concavity, a convexity or a concavity, or a plateau and a convexity on the sella floor. The lateral wall of the sphenoid bone in the hypophyseal area is more vertical on the right side than on the left side (as are the lateral walls of the cavernous sinus, see Fig. 4). Further, we found that impressions of the internal carotid artery in dorsal parts of the sphenoid bone were more pronounced on the left side than on the right. In the anterior area (below the anterior clinoid process), we found such impressions in 53.3% of cases.

Distances between the anterior and posterior clinoid processes, the tuberculum sellae, and the dorsum sellae and the prechiasmal sulcus are given in Figure 12. In our specimens the average distance (oblique line) from the middle of the anterior clinoid process to the middle of the posterior clinoid process was 12.23 mm (range 8–17 mm) on the right and 12.58 mm (range 9–16 mm) on the left.[8] Differences of up to 3 mm in this dimension were found between the right and left sides of some skulls. In 60 subjects (20 women and 40 men) aged between 30 and 93 years, there was no evidence of any correlation between this distance and cranial length, cranial width, or cranial in-

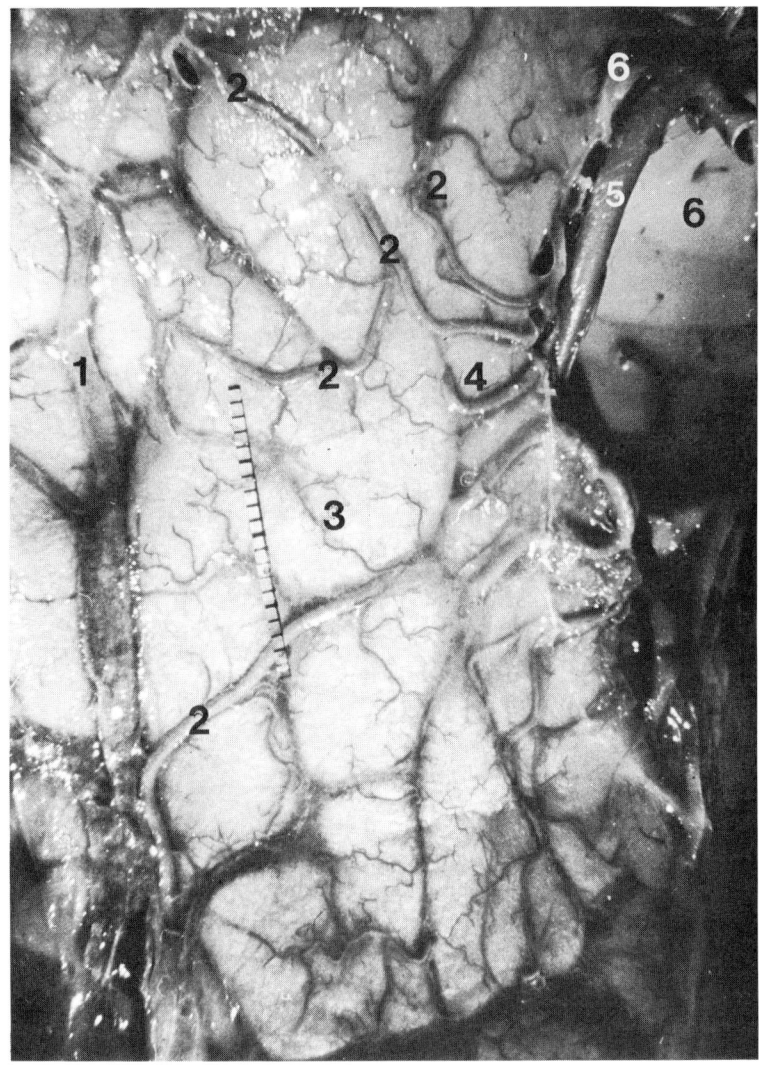

Figure 11: Portions of the brain and its arteries in relation to the floor of the middle cranial fossa. 1. Inferior anastomotic vein, runs on the lower surface of the inferior temporal gyrus (var.). 2. Inferior temporal rami of the posterior cerebral artery; scale in millimeters. 3. Occipital temporal gyrus. 4. Parahippocampal gyrus. 5. Posterior cerebral artery. 6. Uncal notch and midbrain, cut.

dex. Measurements of the hypophysis are given in Figure 13.[27,28] Especially for the transsphenoidal approach, it is important to know the distance between the two internal carotid arteries. Figure 13 shows the dural plate on the intracranial opening of the optic canal. In cases in which the arteries are elongated, or the optic nerves are compressed from below, we found grooves on the upper side of the optic nerve that had been cut from the posterior border of the lamella.

We also measured the angle between the two petroclinoid folds. The posterior petroclinoid fold extends from the apex of the petrous ridge to dorsum sellae in its upper lateral zone. Its fibers consist mainly of contributions from the anterior fibers of the tentorium cerebelli, including fibers of the anterior petroclinoid fold, which extends to the anterior clinoid process. The angle between the two petroclinoid folds was measured to be 38° (range 25–50°) on the right and 37° (range

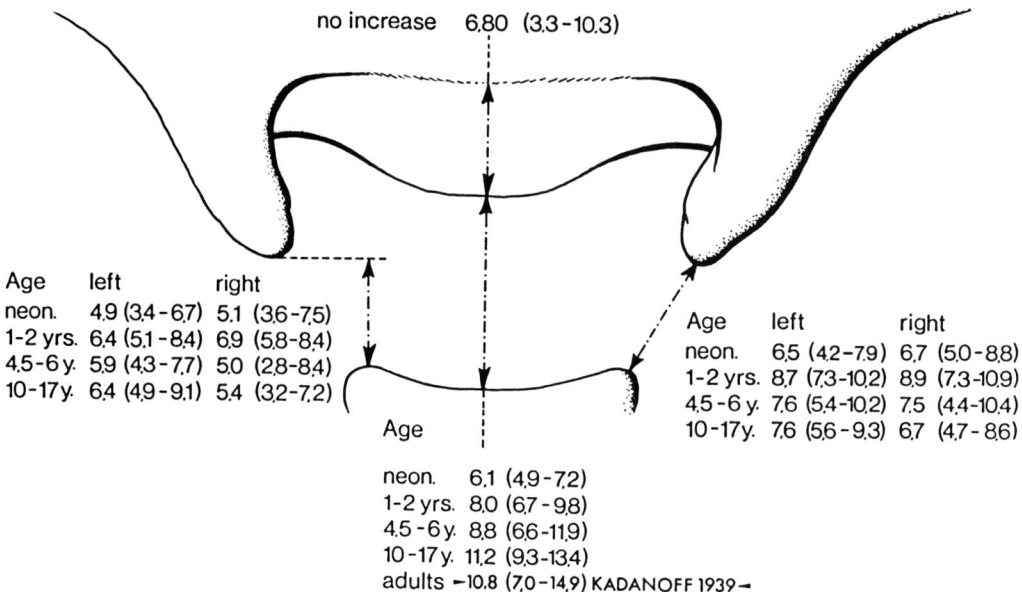

Figure 12: Distances between bony portions of the hypophyseal area at different postnatal ages. Right and left measurements are given in millimeters (range).

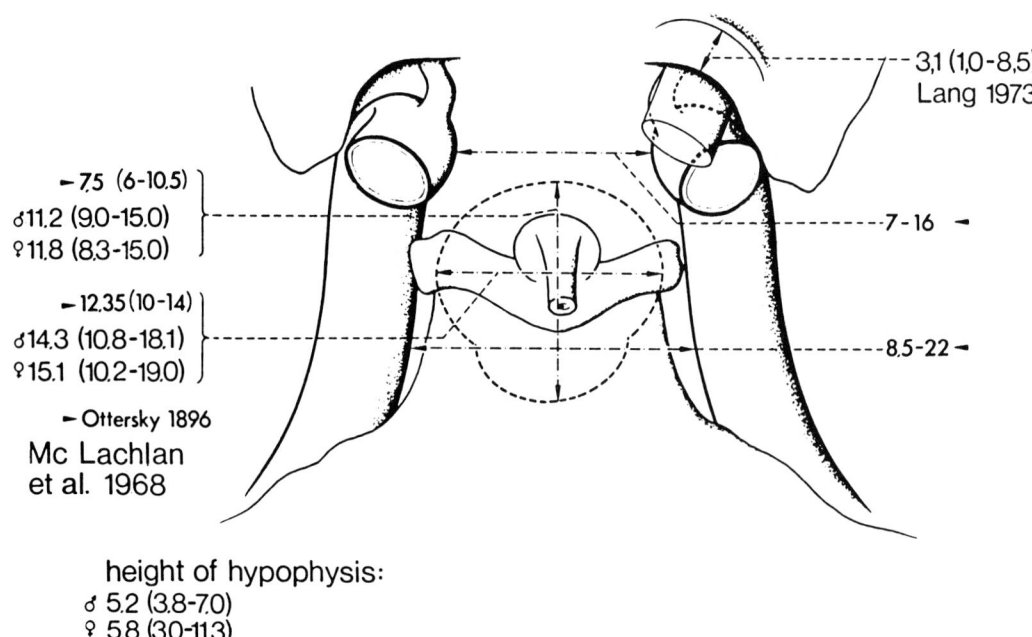

Figure 13: Hypophyseal area as seen from above, showing measurements of the length and width of the hypophysis and the distances between the posterior and anterior medial borders of the internal carotid arteries. Also given is the length of the dural roof of the optic canal. All measurements are given in millimeters (range) and by sex.

20–55°) on the left. Most values for the angle were between 30° and 50°. The anterior petroclinoid fold lies against part of the parahippocampal gyrus and produces the uncal notch in the latter, but when the fold is rounded, this notch may not be present. In space-occupying lesions, the oculomotor nerve may be compressed against the posterior petroclinoid fold.

The diaphragma sellae extends from the origin of the tuberculum sellae to the upper border of the area of the dorsum sellae and the posterior clinoid processes. Its average length was measured by Renn and Rhoton (1975) to be 8 mm (range 5–13 mm), and its width to be 11 mm (range 6–15 mm). In the middle area of the diaphragma lies the foramen diaphragmatis, which is round in 54% of cases and transverse oval in 46% of cases.[31] It has a diameter of 5 mm or more.[2] The diaphragma sellae is attached anteriorly to the tuberculum sellae and posteriorly to the anterior part of the posterior clinoid processes and the dorsum sellae. Medial to the anterior clinoid process, the internal carotid artery traverses the diaphragma sellae; below this area this vessel curves convexly forward and medially, then passes through the dural portal of the diaphragma sellae which is rounded in outline and sometimes situated exactly in the transverse plane. More frequently, its anterior border is somewhat higher than its posterior. Through the diaphragma courses an extension of the arachnoid membrane and subarachnoid space that is known as the pituitary cisterna. In the Würzburg specimens, the pituitary cisterna was clearly demonstrated in corrosion casts. Bergland et al. could identify the cistern inside the sella turcica in roughly 20% of cases studied by roentgenographic methods (Fig. 14).[2]

Hypophyseal Vessels

The superior hypophyseal arteries, usually two (range one to four) in number, branch off mostly from the medial and upper surface of the subarachnoid part of the internal carotid artery shortly after it passes through the diaphragma sellae. In some cases we found the origin of these arteries below the diaphragma and inside the cavernous sinus. Then the arteries run upward and backward toward the infundibulum, reaching it at various levels. Some twigs of this artery supply the lower surface of the optic chiasm and nerve, the infundibulum, and the tuber cinereum. At the pituitary stalk the arteries usually form an arterial circle round the infundibulum, and then descend on the anterior or lateral circumference of the pituitary stalk in the direction of the foramen diaphragmatis. As they run inferiorly, they often give off several fine arterioles on the anterior and posterior surfaces of the pituitary stalk. Inside the stalk they form glomeruli hemocapillares— spatial vessels—with a narrow afferent and a wide efferent capillary loop. These vessels have an unusual wall structure, which makes them easily permeable to certain substances. The wide efferent capillary loops run to the portal vein system of the hypophysis, which reaches the anterior loop and supplies its cell groups with blood. Besides the superior hypophyseal artery, we also found accessory hypophyseal arteries, small branches of the posterior communicating arteries, which run to the tuber cinereum and contribute to the supply of the infundibulum and anastomose with the superior hypophyseal artery (Fig. 15).[22]

In the material we studied, we found two to six small arteries arising from the cavernous part of the internal carotid artery. In most instances there were two main trunks, which we labeled the posterior and lateral caroticocavernous trunks. The posterior caroticocavernous trunk branches off in the vicinity of the posterior sinus curve of the internal carotid artery. This branch runs at first dorsally for 2 to 7 mm inside the cavernous sinus, then divides into two or three branches which partly supply the dorsum sellae, the clivus, and the dura mater portions of the petrous apex region. The latter branches anastomose with the ascending pharyngeal artery and with branches of the vertebral artery. The main branch to

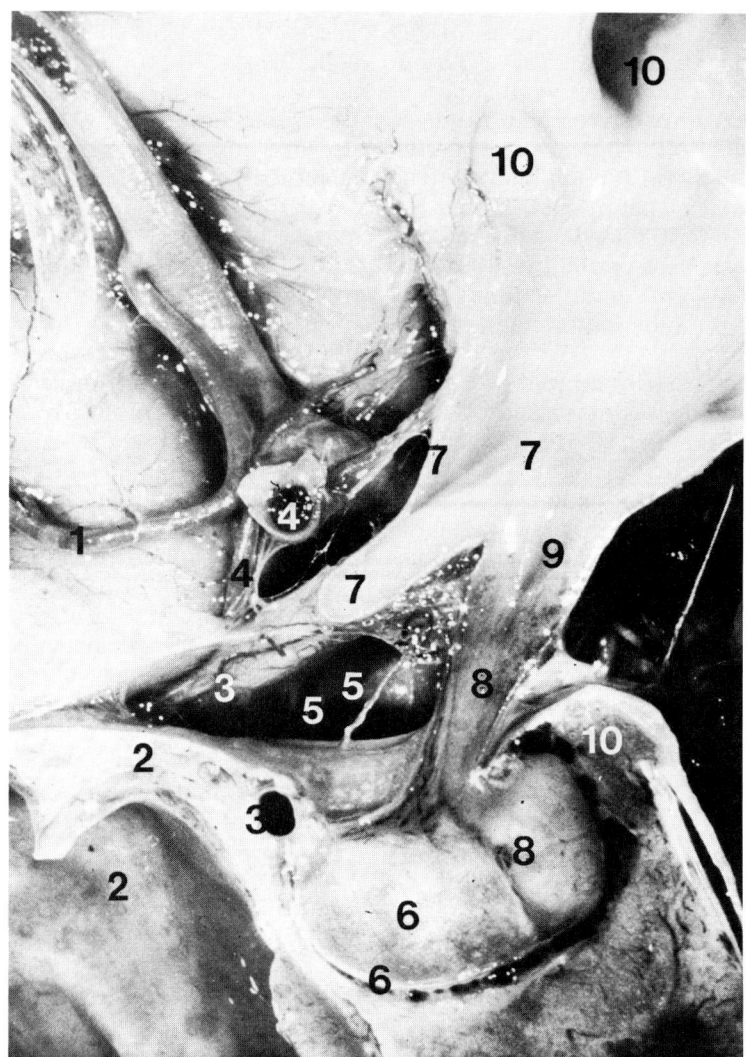

Figure 14: Hypophyseal area seen in midsagittal section, viewed from medial to lateral. 1. R. frontopolaris. 2. Planum sphenoidale and sinus sphenoidalis. 3. N. opticus with vessels and intercavernous anterior sinus. 4. A. communicans ant. and r. orbitofrontalis med. 5. A. carotis int. and ophthalmic artery, origin. 6. Adenohypophysis and capsule. 7. Lamina terminalis and chiasm. 8. Infundibulum and neurohypophysis. 9. Recessus infundibuli. 10. Comm. rostralis (ant.) and foramen interventriculare.

the hypophyseal area is the inferior hypophyseal artery, which divides into two branches that embrace the posterior lobe of the hypophysis. The ramus superior runs on the upper posterior part of the adenohypophysis and the ramus inferior on the lower area of its posterior lobe. Some of the twigs of the lower artery supply the floor of the pituitary fossa, penetrate the capsule of the hypophysis from below, and contribute to the blood supply of the pituitary. Left–right anastomoses between the pituitary arteries are common.

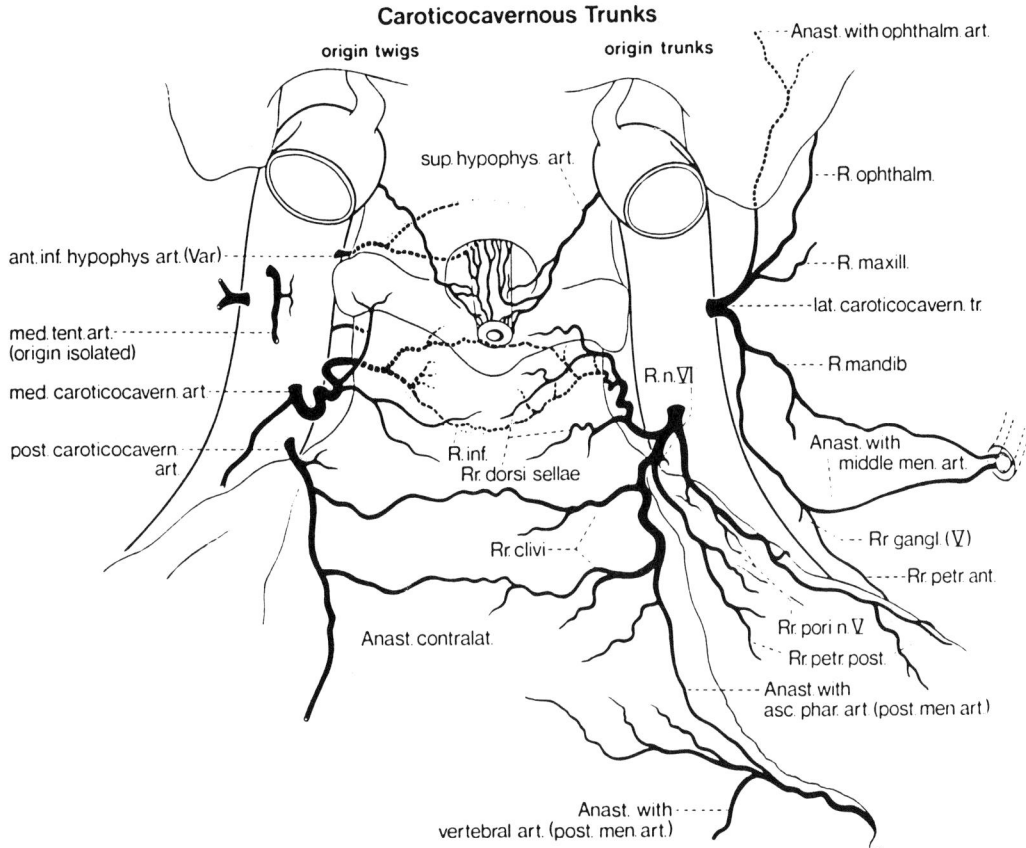

Figure 15: Caroticocavernous trunks and their twigs to the hypophysis and surrounding structures. Also visible are the superior hypophyseal arteries and anastomoses. On the right side the most common zones of origin are shown; on the left some variations are visible.

Cavernous Sinus

The cavernous sinus, which surrounds the hypophysis, contains the internal carotid artery and the abducens nerve and its venous blood space, which is connected with the opposite cavernous sinus through the anterior, inferior, and posterior intracavernous sinuses. These in turn are very variable in presentation. The upper wall of the cavernous sinus is composed of dura mater, which we call the transverse plate. In our specimens it has a width in the area of the diaphragmatic foramen of 38.9 mm (range 26.5–34.0 mm). In most cases the lateral edge is the anterior petroclinoid fold, which is placed 20.55 mm (range 17.0–23.0 mm) above the dural floor of the middle cranial fossa on the right and 18.01 mm (range 14.2–22.6 mm) on the left (see Fig. 4). The distance between this area and the greatest cranial width on the right side was 53.75 mm (range 45–61 mm) and on the left was 51.46 mm (range 45–57 mm). In the upper surface of the dura, the third and fourth cranial nerves course to the lateral wall of the cavernous sinus (Figs. 16A, B). It should be noted that these two nerves (and the abducens nerve) are enclosed for a certain distance in dural and arachnoidal sheaths inside the cavernous sinus (Fig. 17).[12,13,15] Parkinson introduced a surgical approach to the cavernous sinus portion of the internal carotid artery through a triangle formed by the course of

330 • TUMORS OF THE CRANIAL BASE: DIAGNOSIS AND TREATMENT

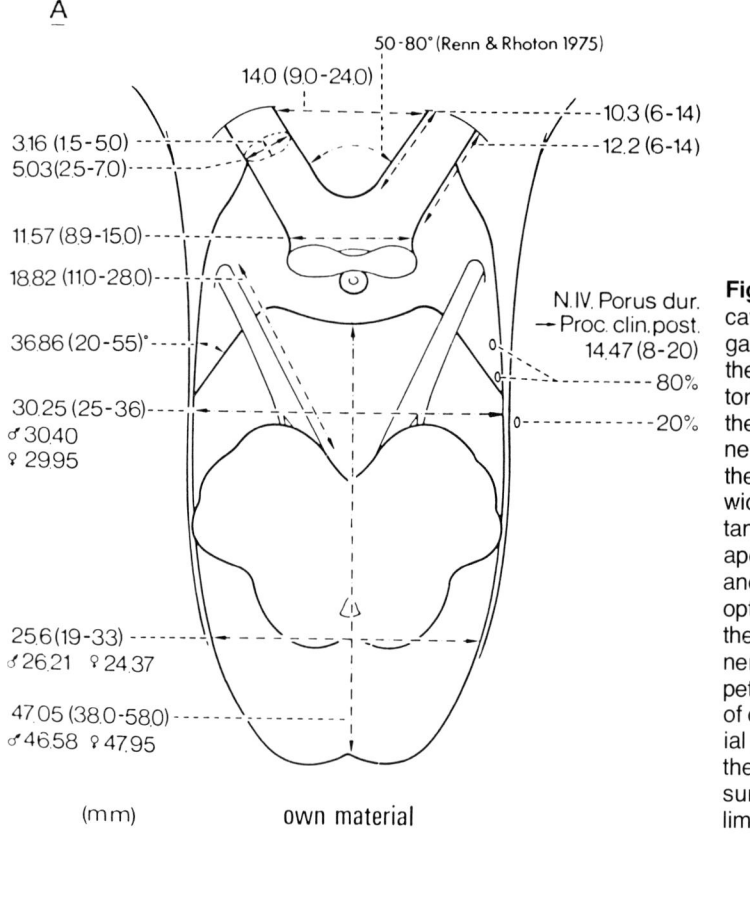

Figure 16A: Upper wall of the cavernous sinus and tentorial gap. The width and height of the cavernous sinus and tentorial gap are shown, as are the medial length of the optic nerve and the lateral length of the nerve to the chiasm, the width of the chiasm, the distance between the intracranial apertures of the optic canal, and the angle between the two optic nerves. Also shown are the length of the third cranial nerve, the angle between the petroclinoid folds, the results of our measurements of tentorial gap, and the dural pores for the fourth cranial nerve. Measurements are given in millimeters (range).

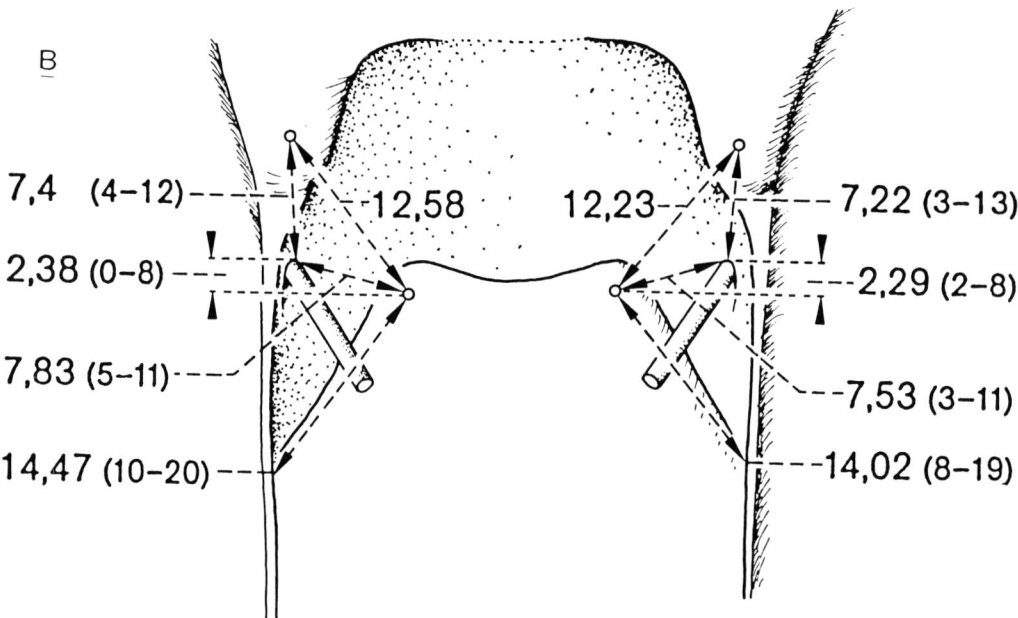

Figure 16B: Distances from the anterior border of the dural pore of the third cranial nerve to some landmarks.

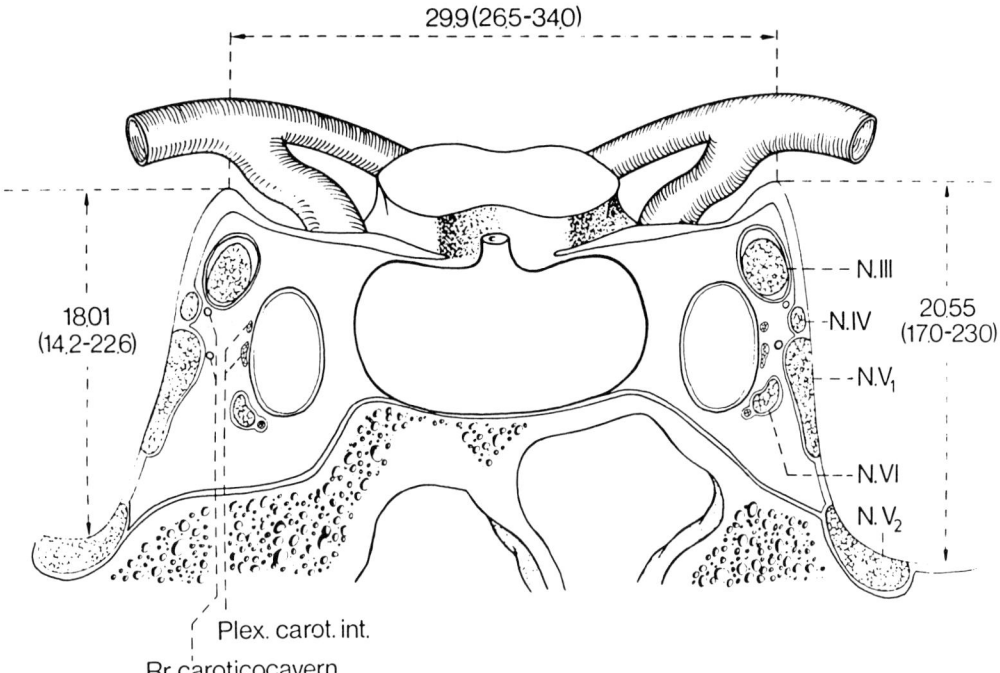

Figure 17: Frontal section through the cavernous sinus, showing the course of the cranial nerves inside the sinus and in its lateral wall. Measurements are given in millimeters (range).

the trochlear nerve, the posterior petroclinoid fold, and a line along the upper border of the ophthalmic nerve.[29] This triangle was measured in our specimens as well (Fig. 18).[21] We noted that in most cases the lower border of the triangle (on the ophthalmic nerve) projected through the upper corner of the trigeminal ganglion backward to the clivus. In the area of the posterior curve of the internal carotid artery inside the cavernous sinus, we found the distance between the ophthal-

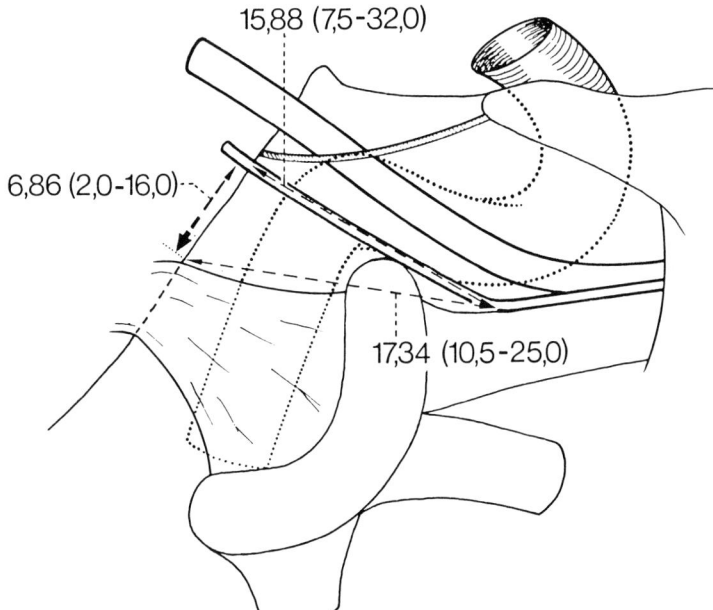

Figure 18: Measurements (in millimeters) of Parkinson's triangle on 89 heads split in half.

mic and trochlear nerves to be 2.51 mm (range 0.0–6.5 mm), and we found distances of 4 mm or more in about 30% of cases (more often on the right than on the left side). The course of the trochlear nerve inside the lateral wall of the cavernous sinus is quite variable.[12,15] The variations that we found in the last preparations studied are shown in Figure 19.[21]

The abducens nerve runs in the posterior segment of the cavernous sinus around the lateral wall of the internal carotid artery and is separated from the trigeminal ganglion by the medial wall of the cavum trigeminale. In our specimens the nerve ran below the upper border of the trigeminal ganglion in about 80%, about 1.5 mm (range 0–6 mm) from the upper edge of the ganglion. When the nerve ran upward from the upper edge of the trigeminal ganglion area (in about 20% of cases), the distance to the ganglion was approximately 1.23 mm (range 0.3–3.0 mm).[15] Where the abducens nerve runs in the cavernous sinus, it usually makes a lateral deviation around the internal carotid artery before running either parallel to the midsagittal plane or rostrolaterally toward the superior orbital fissure.

Below the triangular part of the trigeminal nerve and ganglion and medial to it the inferior sphenopetrosal ligament separates the trigeminal cave from the internal carotid artery. We divided this ligament, which extends between the sphenoid lingula and the petrous bone, into both a sagittal part and a transverse part. The sagittal part separates the ganglion bed from the cavernous part of the internal carotid artery, while the transverse separates it from the transverse

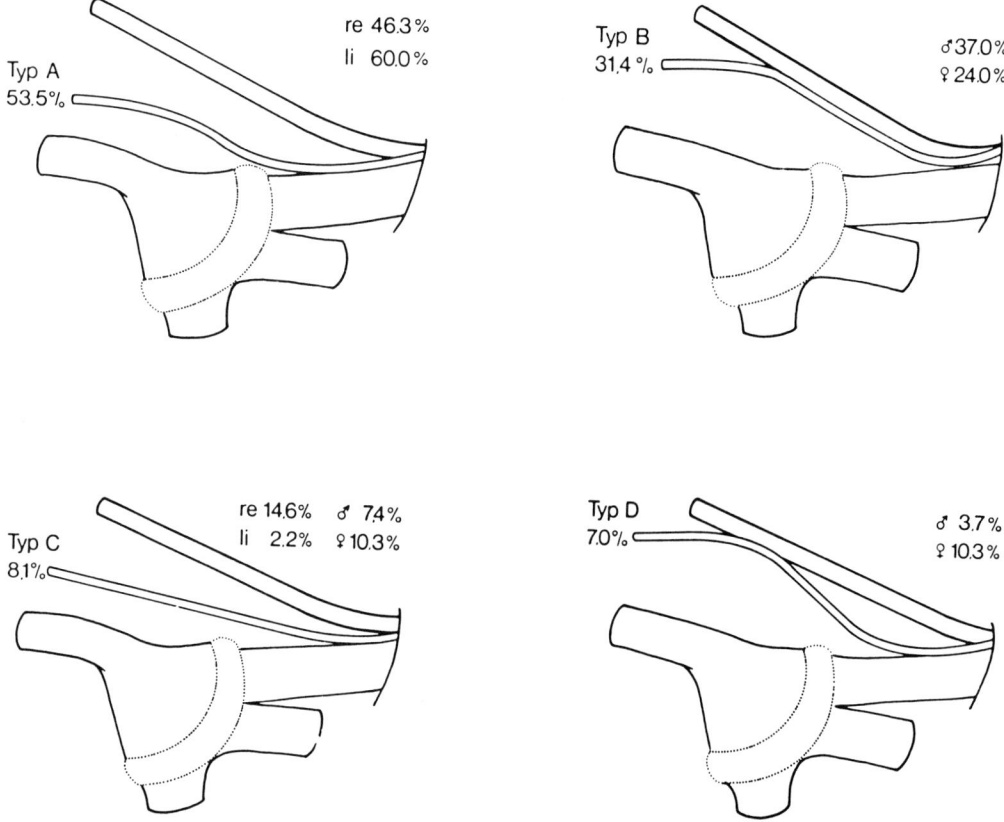

Figure 19: Different courses of the trochlear nerve in the lateral wall of the cavernous sinus. Percentages are given for right (re) and left (li) sides by sex.

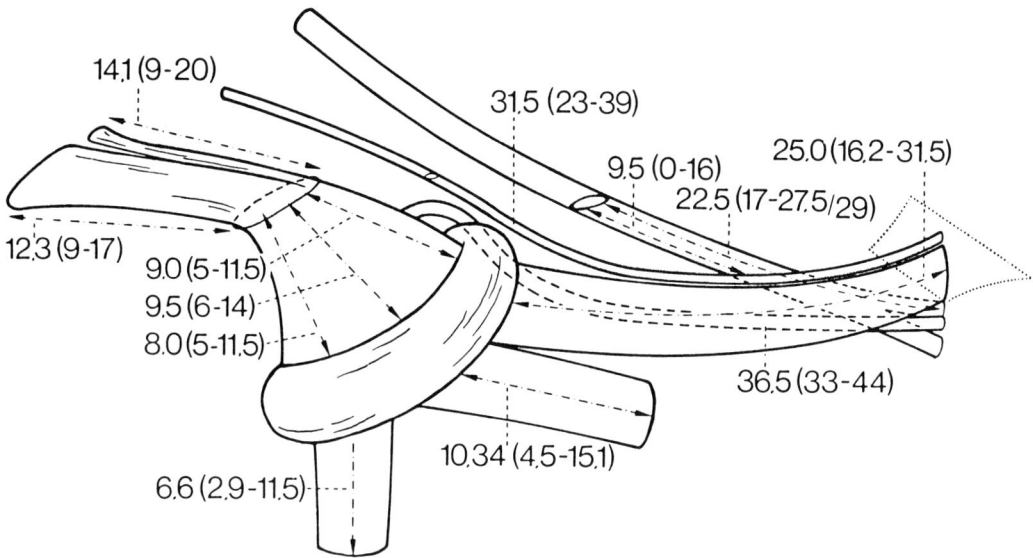

Figure 20: Lengths of the third and fourth cranial nerves and the ophthalmic nerve between their dural portals and the anterior border of the trigeminal ganglion and the inferior border of the intraorbital aperture of the optic canal. The maxillary and mandibular nerves are measured between the inner borders of the foramina rotundum and ovale to the trigeminal ganglion. Lengths of the triangular and compact parts of the trigeminal nerve in the middle and posterior cranial fossae are also given. All measurements are given in millimeters (range).

petrous part of the internal carotid artery.[15] Measurements of the trigeminal nerve and ganglion area are shown in Figure 20.

References

1. Arey LB: The craniopharyngeal canal reviewed and reinterpreted. *Anat Rec* 106:1-16, 1950.
2. Bergland R, Ray B, Torack R: Anatomical variations in the pituitary gland and adjacent structures in 225 human autopsy cases. *J Neurosurg* 28:93-99, 1968.
3. Chandler SB, Derezinski CF: The variations of the middle meningeal artery within the middle cranial fossa. *Anat Rec* 62:309-319, 1935.
4. Dausacker J: Praktisch-anatomische Befunde an der mittleren und hinteren Schädelgrube. *Med Diss Würzburg,* 1974.
5. Dietemann JL, Lang J, Francke JP, Bonneville JF, Clarisse J, Wachenhein A: Anatomy and radiology of the sellar spine. *Neuroradiology* 21:5-7, 1981.
6. Fisher AG: Case of complete absence of both internal carotid arteries with a preliminary note on development of stapedial artery. *J Anat Physiol* 48:37-46, 1914.
7. Hassmann H: Form, Masseund Verläufe der Schädelkanäle: des Canalis infraorbitalis, Canalis incisivus, Canalis palatinus major, Foramen spinosum und Meatus acusticus internus. *Med Diss Würzburg* 1975.
8. Horn W: Variationen am Sinus cavernosus und benachbarter Regionen. *Med Diss Würzburg* 1978.
9. House WP: Early and late complications of stapes surgery. *Arch Otolaryngol* 78:606-613, 1963.
10. Kadanoff D: Über die Beziehung zwischen der Schädelbasiskrümmung und dem Ganzprofilwinkel. *Anat Anz* 87:321-368, 1939.
11. Lang J: Zur Vascularisation der Dura mater cerebri. II Vascularisierte Durazotten am Eingang in den Canalis opticus. *Z Anat Entwickl Gesch* 141:223-236, 1973.
12. Lang J: Eintritt und Verlauf der Hirnnerven (III, IV, VI) "im" Sinus cavernous. *Z Anat Entwickl Gesch* 145:87-99, 1974.
13. Lang J: Über die Pori durales der Nn. III, IV und VI. *Verh Anat Ges* 69:785-791, 1975.
14. Lang J: Structures and postnatal organization of heretofore uninvestigated and in-

frequent ossifications of the sella turcica region. *Acta Anat* (Basel) 99:121-139, 1977.
15. Lang J: *Clinical Anatomy of the Head. Neurocranium—Orbit—Craniocervical Regions.* Translated by Wilson RR and Winstanley DP. New York, Springer Verlag, 1983a.
16. Lang J: Über die Pteriongegend und deren klinisch wichtigem Abstand zum Nervus opticus. 1 Pteriongegend. *Neurochirurgia* 26:161-163, 1983b.
17. Lang J, Brückner B: Über dicke und dunne Zonen des Neurocranium, Impressiones gyrorum und Foramina parietalia bei Kindern und Erwachsenen. *Anat Anz* 149:11-50, 1981.
18. Lang J: Götzfried HP: Über praktisch-arztlich wichtige Masse an der Fossa cranialis media. *Anat Anz* 151:433-453, 1982.
19. Lang J, Keller H: Über die hintere Pfortenregion der Fossa pterygopalatina und die Lage des Ganglion pterygopalatinum. *Gegenbaurs Morphol Jahrb* 124:207-214, 1978.
20. Lang J, Maier R, Schafhauser O: On the postnatal magnification of the foramina rotundum, ovale et spinosum and their topographical changes. *Anat Anz* 156:351-387, 1984.
21. Lang J, Reiter U: Ober den Verlauf der Hirnnerven in der Seitenwand des Sinus cavernosus. *Neurochirurgia* 27:93-97, 1984.
22. Lang J, Schäffer K: Über Urpsrung und Versorgungsgebiete der intracavernoesen Strecke der A. carotis interna. *Gegenbaurs Morphol Jahrb* 122:182-202, 1976.
23. Lang J, Strobel F: Über de Einbau des Ganglion trigeminale. *Verh Anat Ges* 72:437-439, 1978.
24. Lang J, Tisch-Rottensteiner K: Lage und Form der Foramina der Fossa cranii media. *Verh Anat Ges* 70:557-565, 1976.
25. Lang J, Tisch-Rottensteiner K: Über Form und Formvarianten der Sella turcica. *Verh Anat Ges* 71:1279-1282, 1977.
26. Lindblom K: A roentgenographic study of the vascular channels of the skull. *Acta Radiol* (Suppl) 30:146, 1936.
27. McLachlan MSF, Williams ED, Doyle FH: Applied anatomy of the pituitary gland and fossa. *Br J Radiol* 41:782-788, 1968.
28. Ottersky E: Untersuchungen Über Weichteile und Knochen der mittleren Schädelgrube insbesondere uber die Lage des Chiasma opticum. Inauguraldissertation, Königsberg (i Pr) 1896.
29. Parkinson D: A surgical approach to the cavernous portion of the carotid artery. *J Neurosurg* 23:474-483, 1965.
30. Proctor B, Nielsen E, Proctor C: Petrosquamosal suture and lamina. *Otolaryngol Head Neck Surg* 89:482-495, 1981.
31. Renn WH, Rhoton AL Jr: Microsurgical anatomy of the sellar region. *J Neurosurg* 43:288-298, 1975.
32. Simoes S: Relacoes Anatomicas do seio Emissario do forame ovale suas implicacoes clinico-cirurgicas. *Arq Neurosiquiatr* 31:1-9, 1973.
33. Sondheimer FK: In Newton TH, Potts TG (eds): *Radiology of the Skull and Brain*, Vol. 1, The Skull, St. Louis, CV Mosby Co., 1971.
34. Strobel FJ: über Lagebeziehungen des Ganglion trigeminale. *Med Diss Würzburg* 1980.
35. Thorsteinsdottir K: über Faserzahlen des N. oculomotorius, N. trochlearis, N. abducens, N. ophthalmicus, N. maxillaris und N. mandibularis sowie die Faszikelanzahl des N. maxillaris. *Med Diss Würzburg* 1982.
36. Tisch-Rottensteiner K: Öffnungen und Varietaten der mittleren Schädelgrube. *Med Diss Würzburg* 1975.
37. Wagenhäuser GJ: Beiträge zur Anatomie des kindlichen Schlaefenbeines. Über die Fossa subarcuata. *Arch Ohrenheilk* 19:95-126, 1882.
38. Wood-Jones F: The non-metrical morphological characters of the skull as criteria for racial diagnosis. Part II. *J Anat* (Lond) 65:368-378, 1930/31.
39. Zander R: Über die Impressio trigemini der Felsenbeinpyramide des menschlichen Schaedels. *Anat Anz* 9:681-686, 1894.

20

Large Tumors of the Pituitary Gland

Paul B. Nelson, M.D.

Introduction

Large pituitary tumors remain a common problem for the neurosurgeon.[4,7,31-34,36,42-44,46,47,49] They are usually nonhormonal-secreting tumors, but there has been increased awareness of prolactin-secreting tumors that have reached a large size.[12,14,15,24,25,28,32,35,37,44,50,53] Large pituitary tumors are more commonly seen in males than in females, and the average age for presentation is much later than in patients with microadenomas. Whereas microadenomas most commonly present in the second and third decades, large pituitary tumors are more common in the fourth and fifth decades. The description of large pituitary tumors remains controversial. The terminology varies from author to author and the definitions are often not precise.

Macroadenomas are defined as tumors that are greater than 1–2 cm (Fig. 1).[7,8] Giant pituitary tumors are defined as tumors that are greater than 4 cm above the planum sphenoidale, less than 6 mm from the foramen of Monroe, and tumors with multidirectional spread.[47,48] Although the usual direction of expansion of large pituitary tumors is into the suprasellar area, occasionally the tumors may extend into the anterior, middle, or posterior fossa (Fig. 2).

Invasive adenomas have been defined as tumors that extend beyond the pituitary capsule and invade surrounding tissue.[24,32] The cavernous sinus is a common site of extension of invasive tumors.[33,44] The plain skull x-ray and CT scan may show destruction of the sellar floor and skull base (Fig. 3). The term invasive adenoma as commonly used is imprecise in that only block pathological examination can truly reveal invasion. Destruction of the floor of the sella and skull base as seen on radiographic studies may merely be secondary to chronic pressure from an encapsulated tumor rather than due to true invasion. Laws et al. recently described dural invasion in 87% of macroadenomas and 97% of tumors with suprasellar extension.[27] In general, the term invasive adenoma should probably be limited to the pathologist who has histological proof of actual tumor invasion. Examples of a block section of a normal pituitary gland as well as two tumors of increasing size show progressive lateral extension into the cavernous sinus (Fig. 4).

Malignant or carcinomatous pituitary tumors are even more difficult to define.[3,13,40] Jefferson originally defined malignant tumors as tumors that invaded surrounding tissue with or without metastases and with anaplastic changes.[20,21]

From: Sekhar LN, Schramm VL Jr, eds: *Tumors of the Cranial Base: Diagnosis and Treatment.* Mount Kisco, New York, Futura Publishing Co, Inc. © 1987.

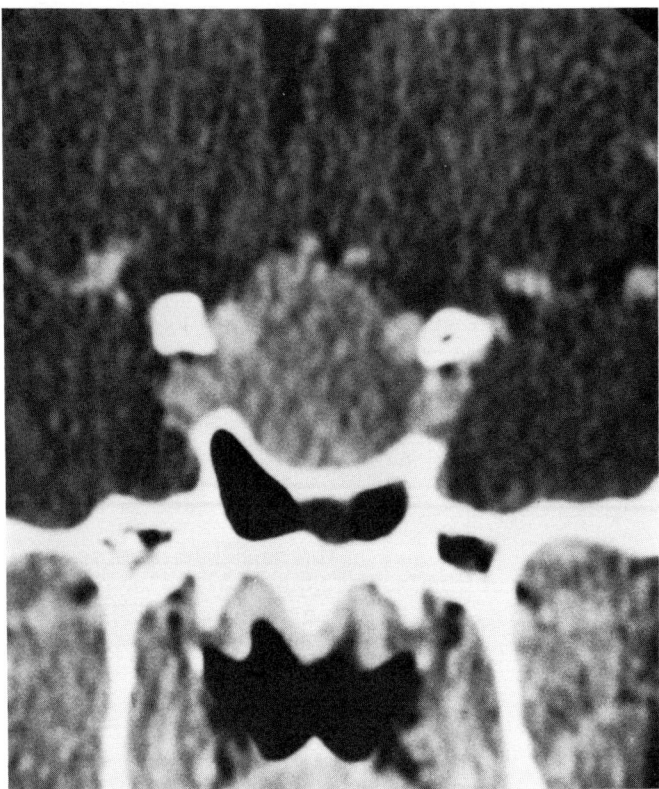

Figure 1: An example of a macroadenoma with typical sellar and suprasellar extension.

Others have defined malignant tumors as those with local invasion and/or metastases.[5,19,41] The strictest definition of malignant tumors is that there are proven metastases outside the central nervous system.[22,35] The metastatic tumor may, however, appear benign histologically.[49] The most common site of metastases from pituitary tumors has been the liver.[49]

It has been generally accepted that the biological activity rather than the histology determine the degree of invasiveness or malignancy.[23,35] Tumors may be grossly malignant but histologically benign, they may be grossly and histologically benign but metastasize, or they may be grossly and histologically malignant with or without metastases.[35]

A classification of pituitary tumors that would be most useful for the practicing physician is one based upon the radiological studies that are obtained for evaluation of pituitary tumors. Wilson has recently described classification of pituitary adenomas that is a modification of Hardy's original classification:[52]

Grade I – less than 10 mm, sella normal or focally expanded.
Grade II – greater than 10 mm, sella enlarged.
Grade III – focal perforation of the sellar floor.
Grade IV – diffuse perforation of sellar floor.
Grade V – spread of the tumor by CSF or hematogenous pathways.
Stage 0 – no suprasellar extension.
Stage A – suprasellar extension without deformation of the third ventricle.
Stage B – suprasellar extension with obliteration of the anterior recess of the third ventricle.
Stage C – suprasellar extension with elevation of the floor of the third ventricle.
Stage D – intracranial extension into the
   1. anterior fossa
   2. middle fossa
   3. posterior fossa.
Stage E – invasion of cavernous sinus.

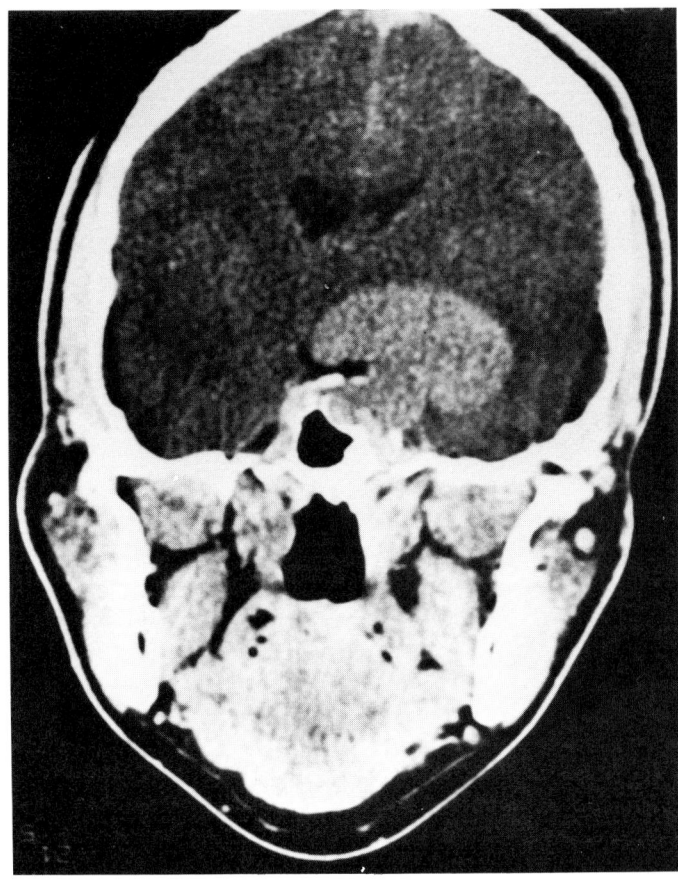

Figure 2: Coronal CT scan showing extension of a large pituitary tumor into the middle fossa.

Clinical Presentation

The most common presentation is one of visual deterioration and loss of pituitary function.[1,26,29,38,39] The visual loss is usually a bitemporal visual field abnormality. Superior temporal cuts from infrachiasmal compression are present early and are seen long before the patient develops complete temporal cuts. Impaired visual acuity and complete blindness are a late finding. Extraocular muscle palsies from lateral extension are seen less frequently.

Loss of pituitary function from extension of large pituitary tumors usually occurs in a progressive fashion. Loss of gonadotropin function and decreased response of a growth hormone to arginine and insulin stimulation are the earliest abnormalities. Decreased thyroid function generally occurs next, and loss of adrenal function is generally the last hormonal deficit to appear. Diabetes insipidus in a patient with a pituitary mass should make one suspicious of a metastases to the pituitary gland rather than a primary pituitary tumor.[5,19,22]

Large pituitary tumors that are prolactin-secreting usually produce serum prolactin values of greater than 1000 ng/ml. Patients with large pituitary tumors that have only modest prolactin elevations (50–90 ng/ml) have prolactin elevations secondary to hypothalamic compression and inhibition of prolactin inhibitory factor and not generally because of prolactin secretion by the tumor.

Less common modes of presentation of large pituitary tumors include pituitary apoplexy, hydrocephalus, and pituitary abscess.[40] Apoplexy develops secondary to hemorrhage or infarction within the pituitary tumor and the patient may present with acute visual loss, headache, depressed level of consciousness, and ad-

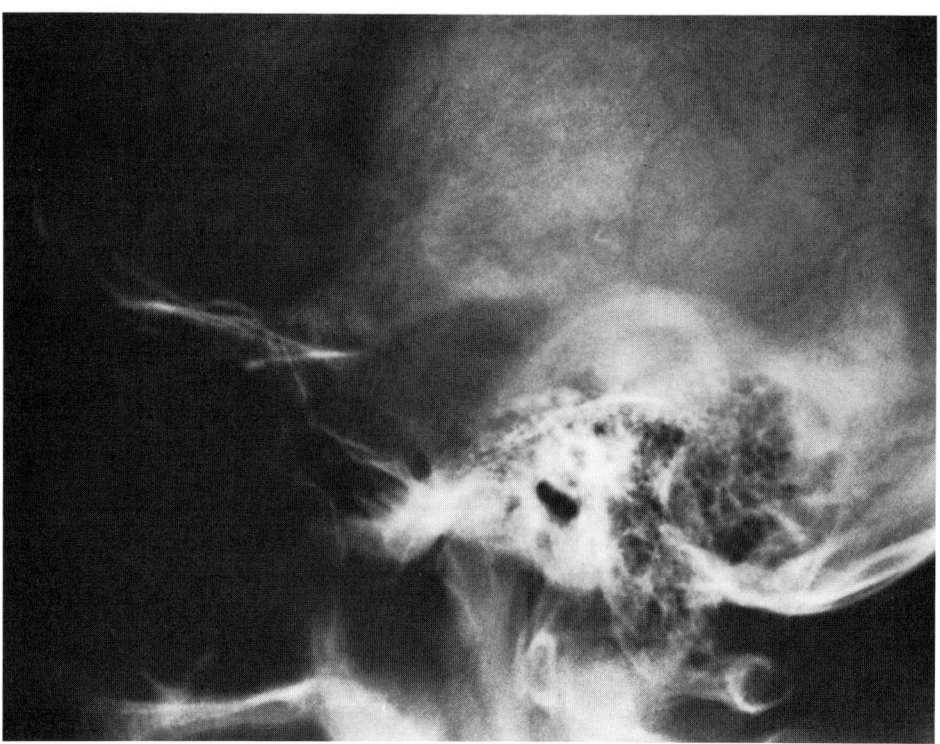

Figure 3A: Skull x-ray of a patient with an "invasive adenoma" showing almost complete destruction of the sellae turcica. Continued.

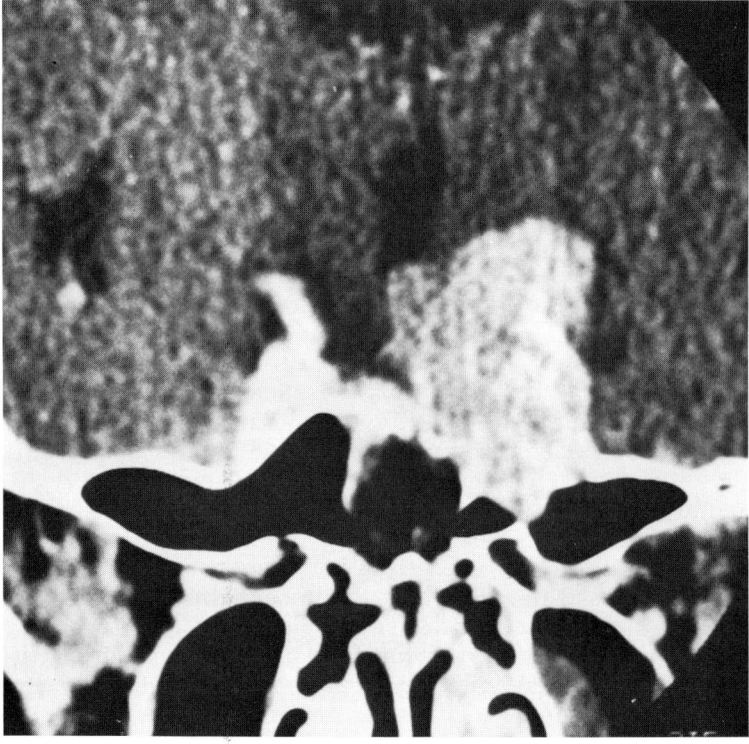

Figure 3B: Coronal CT scan showing parasellar extension with destruction of the skull base.

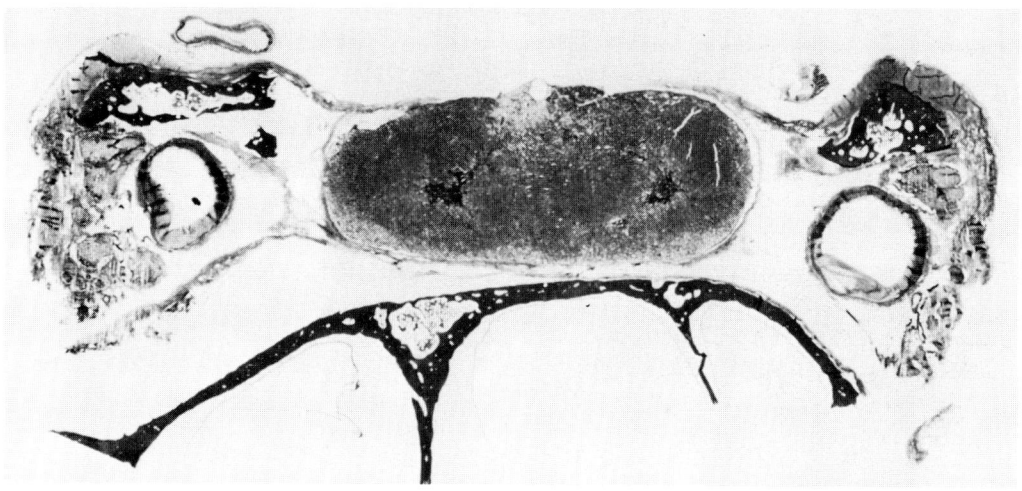

Figure 4A: Cross-section of a normal pituitary gland showing the usual relationship of the pituitary gland and the adjacent cavernous sinus. Continued.

renal insufficiency. Acute hydrocephalus may occur with suprasellar extension which occludes the foramen of Monroe. Abscesses have occasionally been reported in tumors that have invaded the paranasal sinuses and become secondarily infected with nasal flora. These patients may have headache, fever, and a parameningeal response in their spinal fluid. The spinal fluid culture is usually negative.

Diagnostic Evaluation

There is still a place for plain skull x-rays in the evaluation of large sellar-parasellar masses. If the tumor originates in the sella, the pituitary fossa is usually enlarged and ballooned with thinning of the floor of the sella and erosion and posterior displacement of the dorsum sella. The anterior clinoids may be undercut.

A tuberculum sellae meningioma

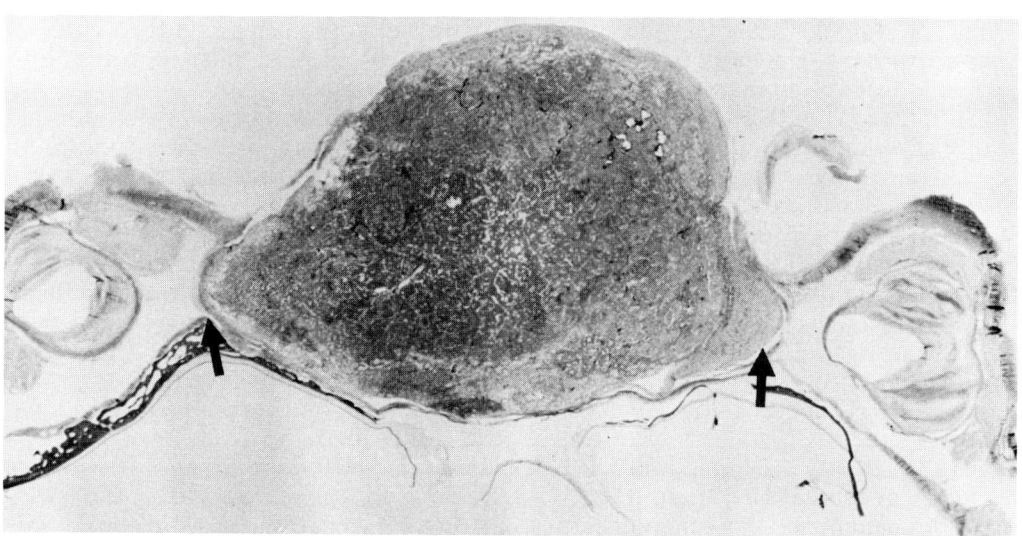

Figure 4B: Cross-section of a macroadenoma that is beginning to protrude into the cavernous sinus (arrows). Continued.

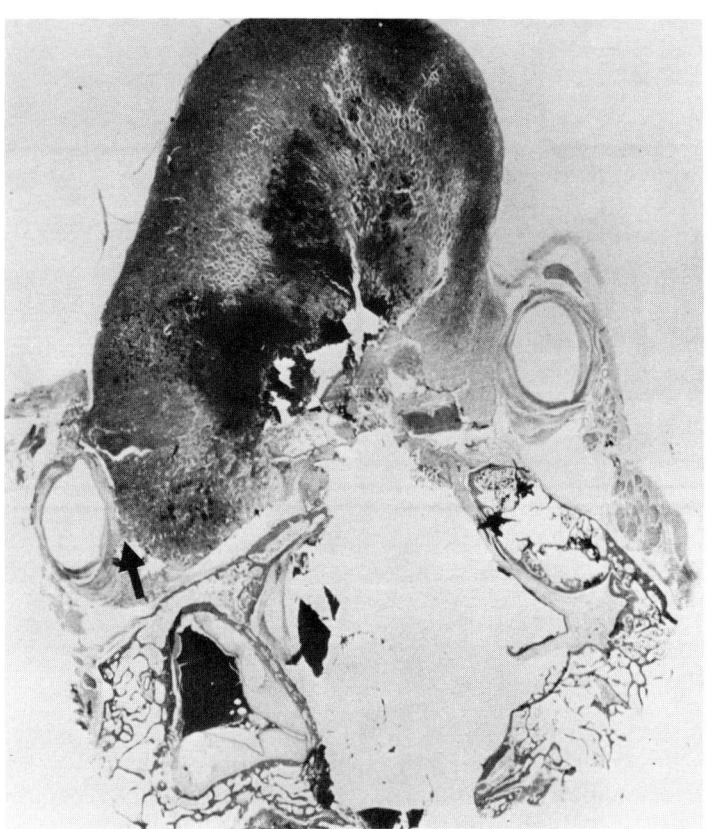

Figure 4C: Cross-section of a large pituitary tumor that has invaded the cavernous sinus on the right side (arrow). The patient has had a previous transsphenoidal operation.

may resemble a pituitary tumor on computed tomography (CT), but the skull x-ray will usually show an intact sellar floor. The dorsum sella may be eroded from above but the sella is not markedly enlarged. Reactive bone formation or blistering in the area of the tuberculum sellae is an inconstant finding.

The best way to evaluate large pituitary tumors is with contrast-enhanced coronal CT scanning, using 3 mm slices. Third-generation CT scanners are capable of showing good anatomical delineation of the sphenoid sinus and the pituitary tumor. The relationship of the tumor to the internal carotid artery and anterior cerebral artery can usually be defined with this study. CT metrizamide cisternography is seldom needed in the preoperative evaluation.

The anatomy of the sphenoid sinus varies considerably from patient to patient. The transsphenoidal surgeon must have a good understanding of the sphenoid sinus anatomy. If the CT scan leaves any question concerning the sphenoid sinus anatomy, one may elect to obtain anteroposterior hypocycloidal tomography of the sella turcica and sphenoid sinus.

Angiography may also be used in patients with large pituitary tumors to further define the anatomy of the carotid artery in the skull base and sphenoid sinus, and to be sure that there is not an associated aneurysm or that the sellar–suprasellar mass is not an aneurysm itself. If available, anteroposterior digital subtraction angiography is probably all that is needed to obtain this information.

The role of magnetic resonance imaging (MRI) in the evaluation of pituitary tumors is yet to be defined. MRI studies will probably be more useful in the evaluation of large tumors than small microadenomas. The relationship of the tumor to the internal carotid artery and the anterior cerebral arteries can be well defined. MRI may be better able to define cavernous sinus extension and may also be a good study to differentiate between pituitary tumor and giant aneurysm. The bony anatomy of the sphenoid sinus, however, may not be as well visualized as compared to CT scanning and bone tomography.

Endocrine evaluation of patients with nonhormonal-secreting large pituitary tumors is directed towards looking for evidence of pituitary hypofunction. It is important to test pituitary function in the basal state and after stimulation. A patient may have normal basal levels but an abnormal response to stimulation. Luteinizing hormone (LH) and follicle-stimulating hormone (FSH) are measured both before and after GNRH administration. Growth hormone and cortisol levels are evaluated both before and after insulin hypoglycemia, and thyroid stimulating hormone (TSH) and prolactin are determined both before and after TRH administration.

Preoperative visual evaluation should include visual acuity testing, color vision, funduscopic evaluation, swimming flashlight testing, formal visual fields, and extraocular muscle function.

Treatment

The most common method of treatment of nonhormone-secreting large pituitary adenomas with midline suprasellar extension is transsphenoidal decompression and radiation therapy.[6,7,16,17,51,52] Cushing initially advocated a transsphenoidal approach for large pituitary tumors, but abandoned this approach because of poor lighting, CSF leaks, and inability to remove adequate amounts of the tumor.[18] The majority of pituitary tumors reported by Cushing were operated by a right frontal approach. With the refinement of the transsphenoidal technique and the use of the microscope, there has been a return to using primarily the transsphenoidal approach. Wilson's contraindications to the transsphenoidal approach are dumbbell-shaped adenomas, tumors with lateral extensions, massive suprasellar extension, and tumors that are associated with an incompletely pneumatized sella.[51,52] Some authors feel that if there is extensive destruction of the base of the skull, these tumors should be merely biopsied and radiated because of the increased risk of CSF leaks and meningitis.[24] Symon has also suggested biopsy and radiation as the treatment of choice for tumors with massive suprasellar extensions.[47]

Several authors have suggested a more aggressive surgical approach to the pituitary adenomas with extrasellar extension.[31,33] Mackay and Hosobuchi recommended a transcranial approach to intracavernous extensions.[33] They recommended preoperative venography and angiography to evaluate the anatomy of the cavernous sinus and also test occluded the carotid in case the carotid had to be sacrificed during the surgical procedure. A frontotemporal craniotomy was used to expose the tumor and the floor of the middle fossa. They described an incision of the lateral wall of the cavernous sinus in the Parkinson's triangle between the trochlear and ophthalmic nerves (Fig. 5). Electromyographic activity of the extraocular and temporalis muscles was monitored in an attempt to preserve cranial nerve function.

Loyo et al. described a combined suprasellar and intrasellar approach for very large pituitary tumor, hourglass tumors, or tumors with extension into the middle or posterior fossa.[31] They recommended two neurosurgical teams. The transsphenoidal decompression was done first. The tumor is then dissected from the carotid and visual apparatus from above and pushed down into the sella for further removal by the transsphenoidal surgeons.

Most patients with nonhormone-secreting tumors should undergo radiation therapy following tumor removal. Cushing found that he could significantly decrease his recurrence rate with postoperative radiation therapy.[18] There was about a 20% recurrence rate if there was no radiation therapy given to large pituitary tumors as compared to about a 10% recurrence rate with radiation therapy.[7] A common dosage given is 4500 rads in 5 weeks at 180 rads per fraction.[9]

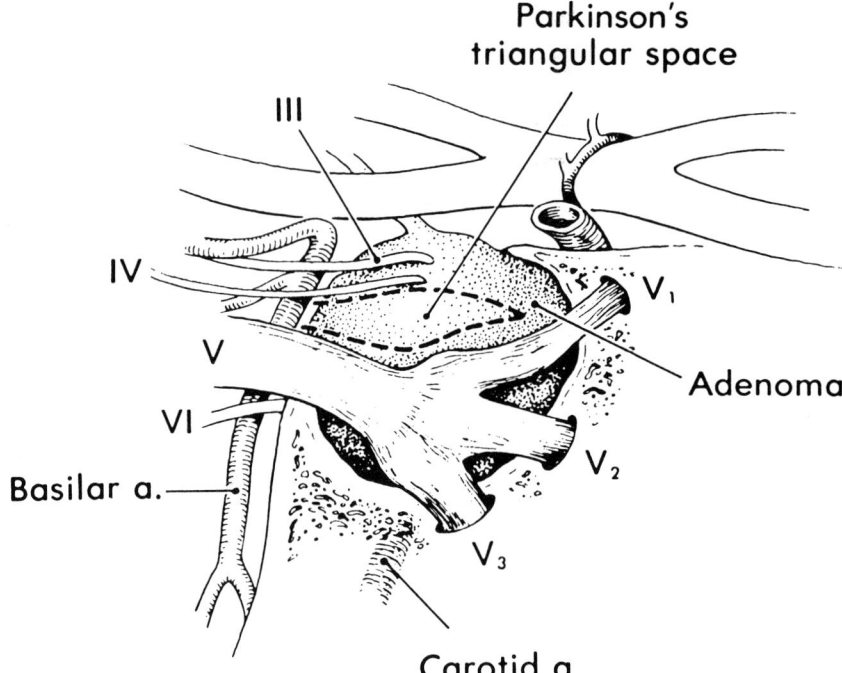

Figure 5: Structures of the right cavernous sinus when intrasellar tumor has bowed the sinus laterally and expanded Parkinson's "triangular space." (From Mackay H, Hosobuchi Y.[33])

The treatment of large pituitary tumors that are prolactin-secreting tumors is somewhat different than the nonhormone-secreting tumors.[12,14,15,24,25,28,30,32,35,37,44,45,50,53] Weiss has shown that preoperative treatment with bromocriptine in large pituitary tumors may improve the postoperative results.[50] Landolt has suggested that preoperative treatment with bromocriptine in prolactin-secreting microadenomas may actually adversely affect the postoperative outcome, but did not note this adverse effect in larger secreting adenomas.[25] Extremely high prolactin levels may be secondary to cavernous sinus invasion.[44] It is common to reduce the prolactin level but uncommon to reduce the prolactin level to a normal range following transsphenoidal surgery in large prolactin-secreting tumors. If the prolactin remains elevated following decompressive surgery, bromocriptine may be used either alone or in conjunction with radiation therapy.

Mortality and Morbidity

Cushing had a 5.3% mortality rate from transsphenoidal surgery.[18] Subsequent series of large pituitary tumors operated upon from a transsphenoidal approach report a mortality rate of 1–2%.[7,28,51,52] The incidence of early CSF leaks has been reported to be approximately 3–7%. Delayed-onset CSF leaks, however, have been reported in patients receiving radiation therapy and bromocriptine for prolactin-secreting tumors that involve the skull base.[24] The visual and endocrine morbidity will be summarized in the subsequent reviews of the visual and endocrine outcome.

Visual Outcome

Approximately 80% of patients with preoperative visual field defects will improve after transsphenoidal decompression of their tumors.[11,26,29] Approximately 5% of patients will, however, show a delayed worsening of vision without radiological evidence of tumor recurrence.[7] This may be due to scarring or may be a post-irradiation effect. The incidence of early worsening of the visual field or extraocular muscle palsy following transsphenoidal surgery is 1–2%.[51] The visual outcome from transcranial pituitary procedures has also been good. However, there have been occasional reports of blindness after transcranial procedures.[42,47]

Endocrine Outcome

The endocrine outcome in patients with large pituitary tumors in general is not as good as the visual outcome.[1,2,38,39] Approximately 70–90% of the patients will have no change in their preoperative endocrine status. Larger series have reported approximately 10% incidence of improvement in function after decompression. The incidence of worsening in endocrine function immediately after operative decompression is approximately 10%. If the patients are followed long enough after radiation therapy, however, pituitary function may worsen in another 20% of the patients. Delayed worsening may in part be a post-irradiation effect. All patients who have had operative decompression and radiation therapy for large pituitary tumors should have at least yearly evaluation of their endocrine function.

CT Outcome

A CT scan obtained soon after transsphenoidal decompression of large pituitary tumors will show persistent sellar and suprasellar mass effect in approximately 50% of the patients.[7] With surgical decompression and radiation therapy, at 1 years, only 20–25% of the patients will have persistent suprasellar mass effect. As long as the visual deficits are stable or improved, the persistent mass effect seen on early postoperative CT scan can be followed with serial CT scans and visual field determinations. If mass effect is seen after operative decompression and the visual fields worsen, one should begin corticosteroids and consider a transcranial operative decompression.

Summary of Author's Series

Thirty-one patients who underwent operative decompression for large sellar and suprasellar tumors by the author from 1980 until 1984 were studied prospectively. There were 22 males and 9 females. The mean age of patients was 49 ± 2.5 years. The mean follow-up was 21.3 ± 2.9 months. Thirty patients had transsphenoidal operations. One patient had a transcranial operation.

Twenty-seven of the patients had hormonally inactive tumors, and four of the patients had prolactin-secreting pituitary adenomas. All of the patients who had hormonally inactive tumors had postoperative radiation therapy. Two patients with prolactin-secreting tumors had postoperative radiation and bromocriptine therapy, and two patients with prolactin-secreting tumors had bromocriptine therapy alone.

Eighty-six percent of the patients had improvement in their preoperative visual field defects. In the early postoperative period, 83% of the patients had no change in their endocrine status and 13% had worsening in their pituitary function. Twenty-three percent of the patients developed delayed worsening of their pituitary function without evidence of tumor recurrence 1 to 2 years following surgery. Fifty-five percent of the patients had persistent suprasellar mass effect in the early postoperative period. Persistent suprasellar mass effect decreased to 20% of the patients on serial CT scanning done over a 12 to 18 month period.

Conclusion

Large pituitary tumors are still a common problem for the practicing neurosurgeon. Patients are older and predominantly male. Most of these tumors are nonhormone-secreting tumors; however, there has been an increased number of these tumors that have been found to be prolactin-secreting. The most common method of treatment is transsphenoidal decompression followed by radiation therapy for the nonhormone-secreting tumors and bromocriptine treatment for the prolactin-secreting tumors with persistent prolactin elevations. Vision will usually be improved following operative decompression but a few patients will have developed visual deterioration. Endocrine function is usually unchanged following surgery but there is a 20% incidence of delayed worsening in pituitary function, perhaps as a result of the radiation therapy. Patients with persistent suprasellar mass effect on the early postoperative scan may be followed by serial CT scans if vision is improved or stable, since many of these patients will have progressive resolution of the mass effect in approximately 1 year.

References

1. Abboud CF, Laws R Jr: Clinical endocrinological approach to hypothalamic-pituitary disease. *J Neurosurg* 51:271-291, 1979.
2. Arafah BM, Brodkey JS, Manni A, et al: Recovery of pituitary function following surgical removal of large nonfunctioning pituitary adenomas. *Clin Endocrinol* 17:212-222, 1982.
3. Bailey OT, Cutler EC: Malignant adenomas of the chromophobe cells of the pituitary body. *Arch Pathol* 29:368-399, 1940.
4. Bakay L: The results of 300 pituitary adenoma operations (Prof. Herbert Olivecrona's series). *J Neurosurg* 7:240-255, 1950.
5. Buonaguidi R, Ferdeghini M, Faggionato F, et al: Intrasellar metastasis mimicking a pituitary adenoma. *Surg Neurol* 20:373-378, 1983.
6. Ciric IS, Tarkington J: Transsphenoidal microsurgery. *Surg Neurol* 2:207-212, 1984.
7. Ciric IS, Mikhael M, Stafford T, et al: Transsphenoidal microsurgery of pituitary macroadenomas with long-term follow-up results. *J Neurosurg* 59:395-401, 1983.
8. Cohen HR, Cooper PR, Kupensmith MJ, et al: Visual recovery after transsphenoidal removal of pituitary adenomas. *Neurosurgery* 17:446-452, 1985.
9. Coulter C: In Berholz PE (ed): *Principles of Pituitary Irradiation in Management of Pituitary Disease*, NY, John Wiley & Sons, 1985.
10. Eastman R, Gorden P, Roth J: Conventional supervoltage irradiation is an effective treatment for acromegaly. *J Clin Endocrinol Metab* 48#6:931-940, 1979.
11. Fager CA, Poppen JL, Saltzman FA, et al: Long-term results of the treatment of pituitary adenomas. *Lahey Clin Found Bull* 28:53-63, 1976.
12. Faria MA Jr, Tindall GT: Transsphenoidal microsurgery for prolactin secreting pituitary adenomas: Results in 100 women with the amenorrhea-galactorrhea syndrome. *J Neurosurg* 56:33-43, 1982.
13. Feiring EH, Davidoff LM, Zimmerman HM: Primary carcinoma of the pituitary. *J Neuropathol Exp Neurol* 12:205-223, 1953.
14. Goodman LA, Chang R: Pregnancy after bromocriptine-induced reduction of an extrasellar prolactin-secreting pituitary macroadenoma. *Obstet Gynecol* 63#3: (Supplement) 25-75, 1984.
15. Grossman A, Cohen BL, Charlesworth M, et al: Treatment of prolactinomas with megavoltage radiotherapy. *Br Med J* 288:1105-1109, 1984.
16. Hardy J: Transsphenoidal microsurgery of the normal and pathological pituitary. *Clin Neurosurg* 16:185-217, 1969.
17. Hardy J: Transsphenoidal surgery of hypersecreting pituitary tumors. In Kohlor PO, Ross GT (eds): *Pituitary Tumors: Diagnosis and Treatment*, Amsterdam, Excerpta Medica, pp 179-194, 1973.
18. Henderson WR: The pituitary adenomato: A follow-up study of the surgical results in 338 cases (Dr. Harvey Cushing's series). *Br J Surg* 26:811-921, 1939.
19. Hoi SU, Johnson C: Metastatic prolactin-secreting pituitary adenoma. *Human Pathol* 15:94-94, 1984.
20. Jefferson G: Extrasellar extensions of pituitary adenomas. *Proc Royal Soc Med* 33:433-458, 1940.

21. Jefferson G: The invasive adenomas of the anterior pituitary. The Sherrington Lectures, Vol 3, Liverpool, Univ. Liverpool Press, 1955.
22. Kistler, M, Pibram HW: Metastatic disease of the sella turcica. Am J Roentgenol 123:13-21, 1985.
23. Landolt AM: Ultrastructure of human sellae tumor. Acta Neurochir 22:94-103, 1975.
24. Landolt AM: Cerebrospinal fluid rhinorrhea. A complication of therapy for invasive prolactinomas. Neurosurgery 11#3:395-400, 1982.
25. Landolt AM, Keller PJ, Froesch ER, et al: Bromocriptine: Does it jeopardise the result of later surgery for prolactinomas: Lancet 2:657-658, 1982.
26. Laws ER Jr, Trauman JC, Hollenhorst RW Jr: Transsphenoidal decompression of the optic nerve and chiasm: Visual results in 62 patients. J Neurosurg 46:717-722, 1977.
27. Laws ER Jr, Scheithauer BW, Selman WA: Invasion of the dura in pituitary adenomas. Presented at the Neurosurgical Society of America, Charleston, South Carolina, May 20, 1985.
28. Laws ER Jr, Ebersold MJ, Piepgras DG: The results of transsphenoidal surgery in specific clinical entities. In Laws ER Jr, Randall RV, Kern EB (eds): Management of Pituitary Adenomas and Related Lesions with Emphasis on Transsphenoidal Microsurgery, New York, Appleton-Century-Crofts, 1982, pp 277-306.
29. Lennerstrand G: Visual recovery after treatment for pituitary adenoma. Acta Ophthalmol 61:1104-1117, 1983.
30. Liuzzi A, Dallabonzana D, Giuseppe O, et al: Low doses of dopamine agonists in the long-term treatment of macroprolactinomas. New Engl J Med 313:656-659, 1985.
31. Loyo M, Kleriga E, Mateos H, et al: Combined supra-infrasellar approach for large pituitary tumors. Neurosurgery 14:485-488, 1984.
32. Lundberg PO, Drettner B, Hemmingsson A, et al: The invasive pituitary adenoma: A prolactin-producing tumor. Arch Neurol 34:742-749, 1977.
33. Mackay A, Hosobuchi Y: Treatment of intracavernous extensions of pituitary adenoma. Surg Neurol 10:377-383, 1978.
34. Maeda T, Ushiroyama T, Okuda K, et al: Effective bromocriptine treatment of a pituitary macroadenoma during pregnancy. Obstet Gynecol 61#1:117-121, 1983.
35. Martin NA, Hales M, Wilson CB: Cerebellar metastasis from a prolactinoma during treatment with bromocriptine. J Neurosurg 55:615-619, 1981.
36. Martins Captain AN, Hayes Colonel GJ, Kempe Lt Colonel LG: Invasive pituitary adenomas. J Neurosurg 22:268-276, 1965.
37. McGregor AM, Scanlon MF, Hall K, et al: Reduction in size of a pituitary tumor by bromocriptine therapy. New Engl J Med 291-293, 1979.
38. McLanahan CS, Christy JH, Tindall GT: Anterior pituitary function before and after transsphenoidal microsurgical resection of pituitary tumors. Neurosurgery 3#2:142-145, 1978.
39. Nelson AT Jr, Tucker H, St. George Jr, et al: Residual anterior pituitary function following transsphenoidal resection of pituitary macroadenomas. J Neurosurg 61:577-580, 1984.
40. Nelson PB, Haverkos H, Robinson AG: Abscess formation within pituitary tumors. Neurosurgery 12#3, 1983.
41. Oglivy KM, Jakubowski J: Intracranial dissemination of pituitary adenomas. J Neurol Neurosurg Psych 36:199-205, 1973.
42. Sanchis J, Bordes M: Immediate visual deterioration after attempts at radical excision of pituitary adenomas. Acta Neurochir 38:251-258, 1977.
43. Serri O, Rasio E, Beauregard H, et al: Recurrence of hyperprolactinemia after selective transsphenoidal adenomectomy in women with prolactinoma. New Engl J Med 309#5:280-283, 1983.
44. Schucart WA: Implication of very high prolactin levels associated with pituitary tumors. J Neurosurg 52:226-228, 1980.
45. Spark RF, Baker R, Bienfang DC: Bromocriptine reduces pituitary tumor size and hypersecretion: Requiem for pituitary surgery? JAMA 247:311-316, 1982.
46. Srivastava VK, Marayanaswamy KS, Rao T: Giant pituitary adenoma. Surg Neurol 20:379-382, 1983.
47. Symons L, Jakubowski J, Kendall B: Surgical treatment of giant pituitary adenomas. J Neurol Neurosurg Psych 42:973-982, 1979.
48. Teasdale G: Surgical management of pituitary adenoma. Clin Endocrinol Metab 12#3:789-823, 1983.
49. Virapongse C, Bhimani S, Sarwar M, et al: Prolactin-secreting pituitary adenomas: CT appearance in diffuse invasion. Radiology 152:447-451, 1984.
50. Weiss MH, Wycoff RR, Yadley R, et al: Bromocriptine treatment of prolactin-

secreting tumors: Surgical implications. *Neurosurgery* 12#6:640-642, 1983.
51. Wilson CB, Dempsey LC: Transsphenoidal microsurgical removal of 250 pituitary adenomas. *J Neurosurg* 48:13-22, 1978.
52. Wilson CB: A decade of pituitary microsurgery. The Herbert-Olivecrona lecture. *J Neurosurg* 61:814-833, 1984.
53. Zervas NT, Martin JB: Current concepts in cancer management of hormone-secreting pituitary adenomas. *New Engl J Med* 210-214, 1980.

21

Craniopharyngiomas: Diagnosis and Treatment

Edward R. Laws, Jr., M.D.

Introduction

Craniopharyngiomas continue to be one of the most difficult therapeutic problems for the neurosurgeon. Although numerous technical advances have occurred, the long-term results of surgical therapy are less than totally satisfactory for many patients, and the challenge of improving the outlook for these patients continues.

Historical Aspects

In 1857, Zenker reported a postmortem study of a patient with a cystic suprasellar lesion that contained cholesterol crystals and squamous epithelium. Luschka, in 1860, described the presence of squamous cell nests in the infundibular area, and noted the similarity of these cells to the epithelium of the oral cavity. In 1899, Mott and Barrett postulated that cystic tumors might arise from the hypophyseal duct. Erdheim discussed the embryology of the pituitary, the relationship of cystic suprasellar tumors to Rathke's pouch, and the etiology of congenital cysts and tumors in this area. Kiyono and, later, Carmichael also described epithelial cell nests extending from the hypothalamus and tuber cinereum along the pituitary stalk to the gland within the sella (Fig. 1). The term craniopharyngioma was coined by Frazier in 1931 and was adopted by Cushing in 1932. Other terms utilized for this tumor were adamantinoma and ameloblastoma (because of the similarity of the solid portion of the tumor to the epithelial structures which give rise to erupting teeth), Rathke's pouch tumor, Rathke cleft cyst or tumor, hypophyseal duct tumor, and epithelioma.

Babinski and Erdheim both described the clinical picture of sexual infantilism and adiposity which characterized specific patients with cystic lesions of the sella and suprasellar space.

The first surgical removal of a craniopharyngioma was probably performed by A.E. Halstead of Chicago in 1908. He used a transsphenoidal approach with an incision below the nose, and described a cystic tumor. The patient survived surgery, but ultimately died of

From: Sekhar LN, Schramm VL Jr, eds: *Tumors of the Cranial Base: Diagnosis and Treatment*. Mount Kisco, New York, Futura Publishing Co, Inc. © 1987.

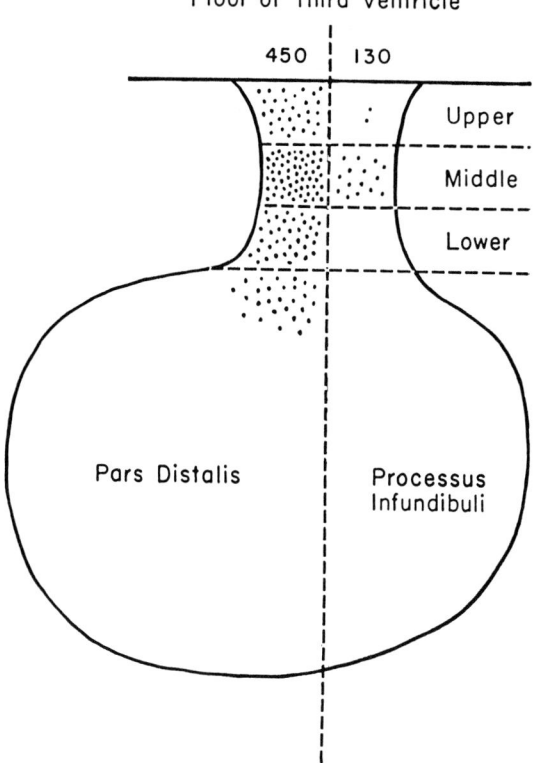

Figure 1: Location of epithelial nests in autopsy specimens of normal pituitary glands, reproduced with permission from the Journal of Neurosurgery (Svien, 1965).

complications. In 1910, Dean Lewis successfully performed a craniotomy for a cystic suprasellar tumor in a patient with delayed sexual maturation and dystrophic adiposity. Cushing encountered 92 craniopharyngiomas between 1908 and 1927 and operated on 13 using the transsphenoidal approach.

Cushing and Frazier both had pioneered the transcranial approach for this tumor. Later, Love, Kahn, and Ingraham were successful in operating on significant series of craniopharyngiomas prior to the introduction of steroids, and their results improved once this advance had been made. Matson, working in the post-steroid era, made a vigorous case for the concept of total removal of these tumors in children. This approach has been moderated somewhat by Shillito, but is still espoused by Sweet, Hoffman, Patterson, and Carmel, among others, in North America and by other surgeons in Europe and Japan.

With the exception of a few proponents, the transsphenoidal approach lay relatively dormant until revived by Guiot who utilized it both alone and in combination with craniotomy for the management of craniopharyngioma. In 1962, Hardy described the transsphenoidal removal of a giant craniopharyngioma, and some additional isolated case reports were published. Laws presented a series of craniopharyngiomas treated by transsphenoidal surgery, and described the indications for and limitations of the approach.

A recent conceptual advance has been presented by Ciric. He describes the relationship of craniopharyngiomas to the pia-arachnoid, and makes the point that, depending on the site of origin of the tumor, it may be extra-arachnoid, subarachnoid extra-pial, or intra-pial. This concept explains many aspects of the spectrum of pathology seen in the craniopharyngiomas.

Pathology and Pathologic Anatomy

In the United States, craniopharyngiomas represent approximately 3% of intracranial tumors. They are more frequent in children than in adults, comprising some 9% of childhood brain tumors. There is an incidence peak in childhood (ages 5–10) and then the frequency for the third through seventh decades is relatively constant, though there is a tendency towards a second smaller peak at 50–60 years of age. Sex distribution is nearly equal with a slight male predominance.

These tumors can be considered as part of a spectrum with regard to a number of characteristics: size (microscopic to "giant"); constitution (cystic to solid to calcified with varying combinations); nature of histology (cuboidal to columnar to respiratory to squamous epithelium); contents (clear fluid to yellow-brown, to "purulent" to viscid, with cholesterol crystals, flakes, calcific, and keritinized debris); invasiveness (well circumscribed to invasive of surrounding brain); and anatomic location (third ventricle to hypothalamus to tuber cinereum to infundibulum to pars intermedia to neurohypophysis to "pharyngeal," intraventricular to interpeduncular to retroclival to suprasellar to intrasellar to intrasphenoidal). These various aspects of the tumors make it impossible to generalize with regard to any single mode of management, and make evident the fact that each patient suffering from a craniopharyngioma must be considered individually.

Because these tumors are usually related to the pituitary stalk, their blood supply normally arises from small branches of the internal carotid, anterior cerebral, or posterior communicating arteries. This is true even in intraventricular or retroclival lesions which rarely if ever have blood supplied by the basilar bifurcation or posterior cerebral arteries.

When craniopharyngiomas enlarge, particularly the cystic lesions, they may extend along cisternal pathways and protrude into the posterior or middle fossae, as well as superiorly to involve the third ventricle and frontal lobes. They may also extend along and be adherent to major blood vessels.

Hardy has maintained that enlargement of the sella turcica in cases of craniopharyngioma reflects an origin of the tumor within the sella and below the diaphragm. Subsequent suprasellar extension may occur, but these tumors with sellar enlargement are almost invariably extra-arachnoid. The incidence of such sellar enlargement varies from 25% to 67% of various series of craniopharyngiomas studied.

Because of the age spectrum and the histologic continuum from simple to squamous epithelium, debate continues as to whether these tumors are strictly congenital or developmental in origin or whether epithelial cell nests undergo squamous metaplasia over time. There is evidence to suggest that both mechanisms are valid in the pathogenesis of these lesions.

Clinical Presentation

The signs and symptoms of craniopharyngioma relate to the age of the patient and the size and location of the tumor. Symptom categories include endocrine, visual, mental, and those related to increased intracranial pressure.

Endocrine symptoms are most prominent in children who usually present with retardation of growth and sexual development. Primary amenorrhea occurs in girls. Diabetes insipidus may occur as well, either in conjunction with or, less frequently, independent of impairment of growth and development. Endocrine symptoms in adults are usually related to hypopituitarism. Fatigue and impotence may occur as well as diabetes insipidus. Young adult women may present with a pseudoprolactinoma syndrome of amenorrhea and galactorrhea, with infertility and hyperprolactinemia, usually of modest degree. These effects presumably result from involvement of the pituitary stalk and interference with the effect of hypothalamic prolactin-inhibiting factor (PIF) on pituitary lactotrophs.

Visual symptoms are most often related to chiasmal compression, although optic nerve and optic tract type visual field defects may also occur. Obviously, visual symptoms may be difficult to detect and to characterize in young children. Mental symptoms, particularly memory loss and dementia, are more common in adults, especially those with large tumors. A Korsakoff-like syndrome has been reported, and other, more generalized symptoms may be present.

Increased intracranial pressure may occur when craniopharyngiomas obstruct the normal pathway of CSF circulation. The usual symptoms are headache, nausea, vomiting, and ataxia. Rarely, cranial nerve palsies may occur either by direct or secondary effects of pressure. Diagnostic findings of increased intracranial pressure include Macewen's sign in young children and papilledema. Increased intracranial pressure, growth retardation, visual loss, and diabetes incipidus are a symptom complex characteristic of craniopharyngioma in childhood.

Diagnosis

Important features of physical diagnosis document the symptoms and signs previously discussed. In children, the height, weight, and growth curve should be plotted as carefully as possible over time. Secondary sexual characteristics are documented and staged both by examination and by history. In women, menstrual history (menarche, regularity), breast development, and presence of galactorrhea are all noted. Similar physical and historical features of sexual function are sought in men. Radiologic bone age should be determined in children and adolescents. Appropriate endocrine laboratory tests are obtained including growth hormone, somatomedin-C, morning and evening blood corticosteroid levels, serum thyroxine and TSH, prolactin, FSH, LH and testosterone, and additional tests (blood and urine osmolality, urinary steroids, dynamic endocrine tests) as necessary.

Visual assessment includes funduscopic examination, determination of the visual fields with tangent screen and perimeter, and tests of visual acuity. Mental functioning can be tested when indicated with psychometric assessment of intellect and memory.

The rapid advances that have occurred in diagnostic imaging have revolutionized the diagnosis and, to some extent, the therapy of craniopharyngioma. The plain skull radiograph, particularly the lateral projection, continues to be useful (Figs. 2, 3). The size and shape of the

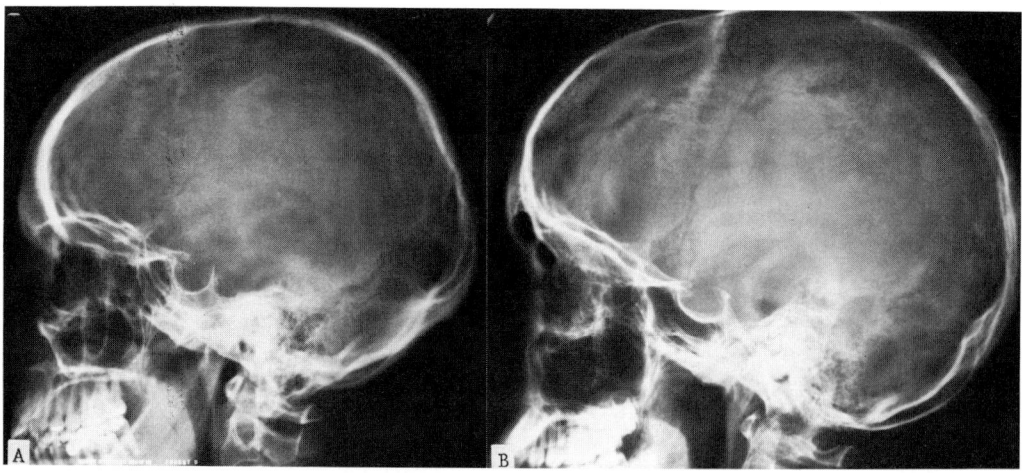

Figure 2A, B: Lateral skull films showing sellar enlargement in cases of craniopharyngioma.

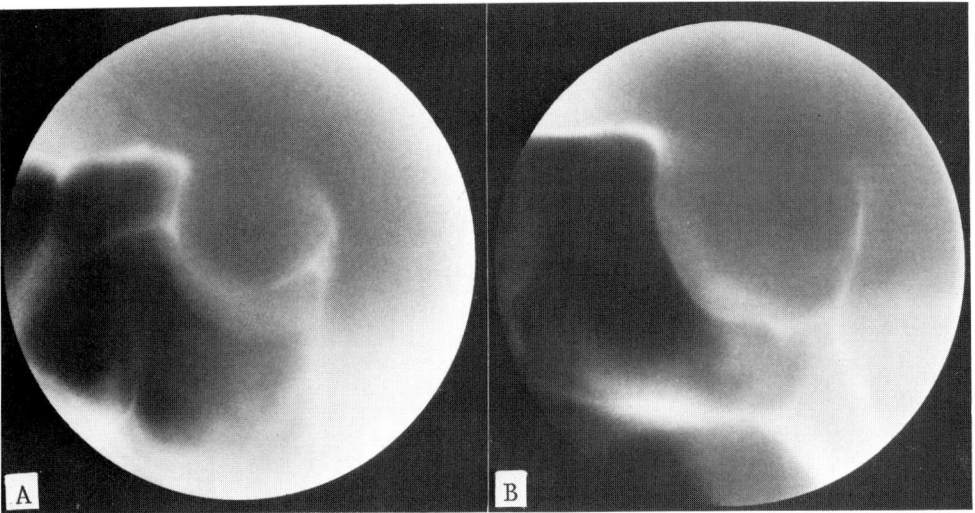

Figure 3A, B: Lateral sellar polytomograms showing sellar enlargement in cases of craniopharyngioma.

sella are of paramount importance, and the presence of sellar or suprasellar calcification may be detected. An enlarged sella suggests that the tumor originated below the diaphragm. Erosion or amputation of the posterior clinoid processes signifies a posteriorly located suprasellar lesion. In children with increased intracranial pressure, spreading of the sutures may be present. The size and pneumatization of the sinuses may influence the choice of surgical approach.

The primary modality for imaging and anatomic diagnosis of craniopharyngiomas currently is the CT scan with contrast enhancement (Figs. 4, 5). Magnetic resonance imaging (MRI) may become equally or even more important as it develops (Fig. 6), but it is likely that the two studies will remain complementary. CT is capable of showing the epicenter and the extent of the lesion. It usually can distinguish readily between cystic and solid components, and will detect calcification when present. With contrast enhancement, relationships to major blood vessels can often be determined. Hydrocephalus, when present, is obvious as are other secondary effects on normal brain such as compression and reactive edema. Angiography is generally recommended when craniotomy is planned, primarily to document the relationship of vessels to the tumor rather than to search for vessels actually feeding the tumor. In most cases bilateral carotid and vertebrobasilar angiograms should be obtained, with the latter being particularly important in posteriorly situated and retroclival tumors.

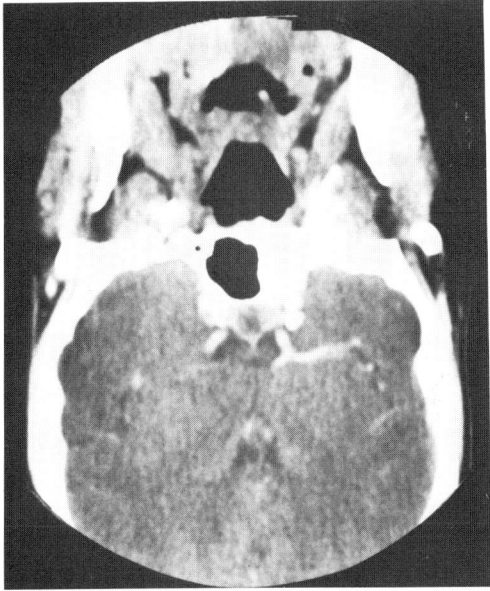

Figure 4: CT scan showing craniopharyngioma, primarily intrasellar.

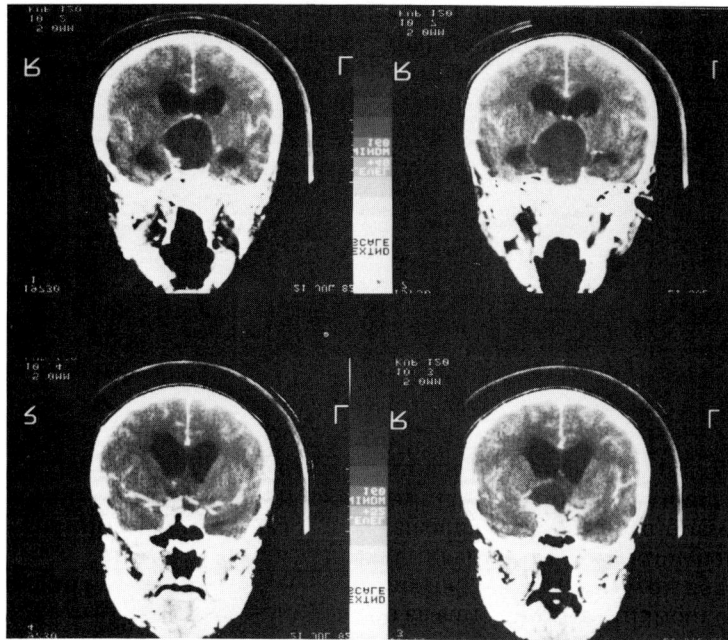

Figure 5: CT scan showing intra- and suprasellar craniopharyngioma approached both transsphenoidally and by subsequent craniotomy for gross total removal.

Polytomography, radionuclide brain scanning, and pneumoencephalography, although useful in the past, have been effectively supplanted by CT imaging and currently are not generally employed in the diagnosis of craniopharyngioma.

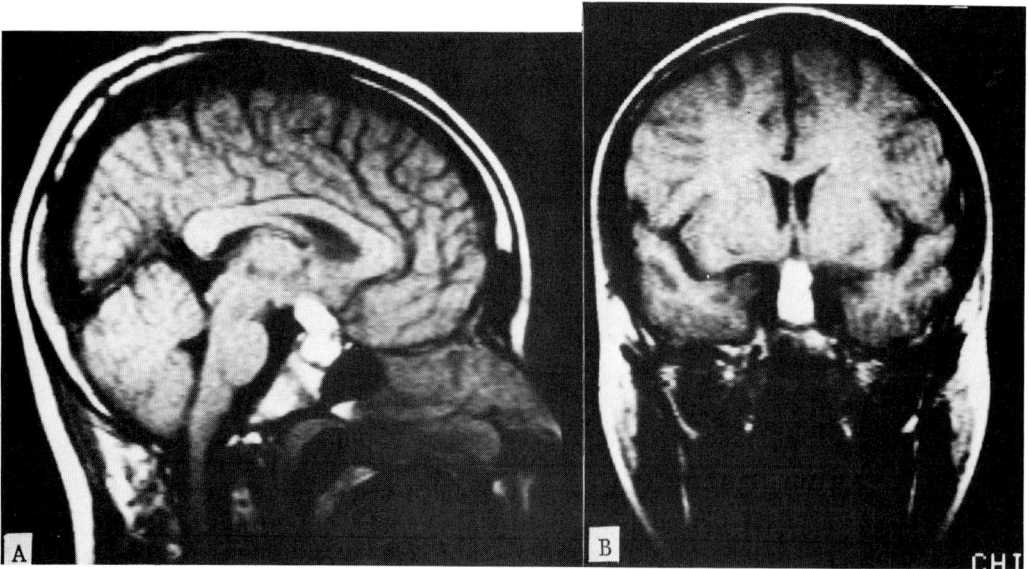

Figure 6A, B: MR scan of intra and suprasellar craniopharyngioma—gross total removal transsphenoidally.

Differential Diagnosis

The differential diagnosis of craniopharyngioma theoretically includes a rather large variety of sellar and suprasellar lesions. In fact, when laboratory evaluation and imaging studies are complete, the correct diagnosis is usually evident. Pituitary adenomas, particularly those with cystic change or calcification, can mimic craniopharyngioma. As mentioned previously, craniopharyngioma can produce all the symptoms and signs of a pituitary prolactinoma. Other lesions to be considered are aneurysms of the anterior circle of Willis, arachnoid cyst, germinoma, dermoid or epidermoid cyst, optic nerve, chiasmal or hypothalamic glioma, colloid cyst of the third ventricle, histiocytosis X, and hamartoma or teratoma in the sellar-suprasellar region.

Therapeutic Approaches

Major factors to be considered in choosing a therapeutic approach include the following:

1. Is this the initial attempt at treatment or has there been prior therapy with recurrence or persistence of the tumor?
2. Is the lesion primarily cystic, solid, or a combination; is there a major degree of calcification?
3. Is hypopituitarism present (anterior and/or posterior)?
4. Is the sella enlarged or normal in size?
5. What is the nature and degree of visual loss?
6. In what anatomic location does the tumor arise and in what directions does it extend?

With these factors and others considered, the surgeon must then decide upon the goal of therapy. The goal can range from total excision which is desirable if it can be accomplished with reasonable risk of mortality and morbidity, to palliation which may be more prudent, particularly in recurrent tumors. Subtotal excision and cyst aspiration have been advocated because of the technical difficulty and attendant morbidity associated with some tumors. In cases where tumor is incompletely excised, radiotherapy has been demonstrated to be effective, and can provide long-term control in many cases. Other methods of palliation include reservoir drainage, transsphenoidal drainage, intra-cystic instillation of radioactive isotopes, and CSF shunting procedures when associated hydrocephalus is present.

Craniotomy

A large number of craniotomy approaches for craniopharyngioma have been developed and utilized. Historically, the unilateral subfrontal approach has been the most common. Most surgeons recommend fashioning the bone flap on the side of worse vision. Bifrontal craniotomy with subfrontal or interhemispheric approach has also been advocated. Heuer and Dandy advocated a unilateral approach along the sphenoid wing for tumors of the hypophyseal region. This approach has matured into the pterional craniotomy which has become favored by many surgeons using microsurgical techniques (Fig. 7). Poppen suggested a temporal approach and this has been sophisticated and adapted to microtechniques by Symon. Transventricular and transcallosal approaches have been advocated for tumors lying primarily within the third ventricle.

A variant of transfrontal craniotomy has been proposed by Patterson—a transcranial, transsphenoidal approach wherein the tuberculum sellae is drilled away and the sphenoid sinus is entered, giving access to the anterior wall of the sella.

The choice of craniotomy approach depends on the nature and the anatomy of the tumor. Once the brain is exposed, access to the tumor may be obtained by several routes. Some lesions may be removed from between the optic nerves. In many patients, particularly children, the optic chiasm is prefixed, limiting access between the nerves. Further dissection along the dorsal surface of the optic

354 • TUMORS OF THE CRANIAL BASE: DIAGNOSIS AND TREATMENT

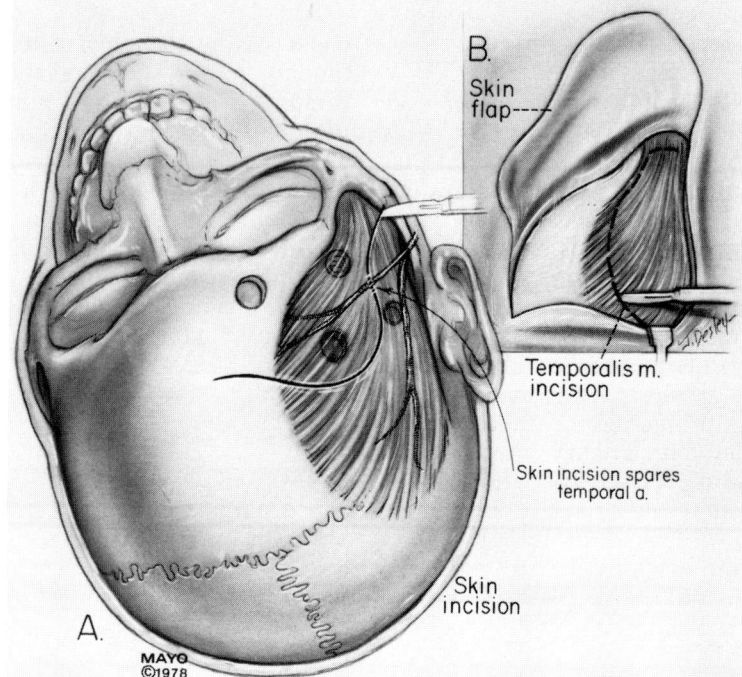

Figure 7A-C: Pterional approach utilized in some cases of craniopharyngioma.

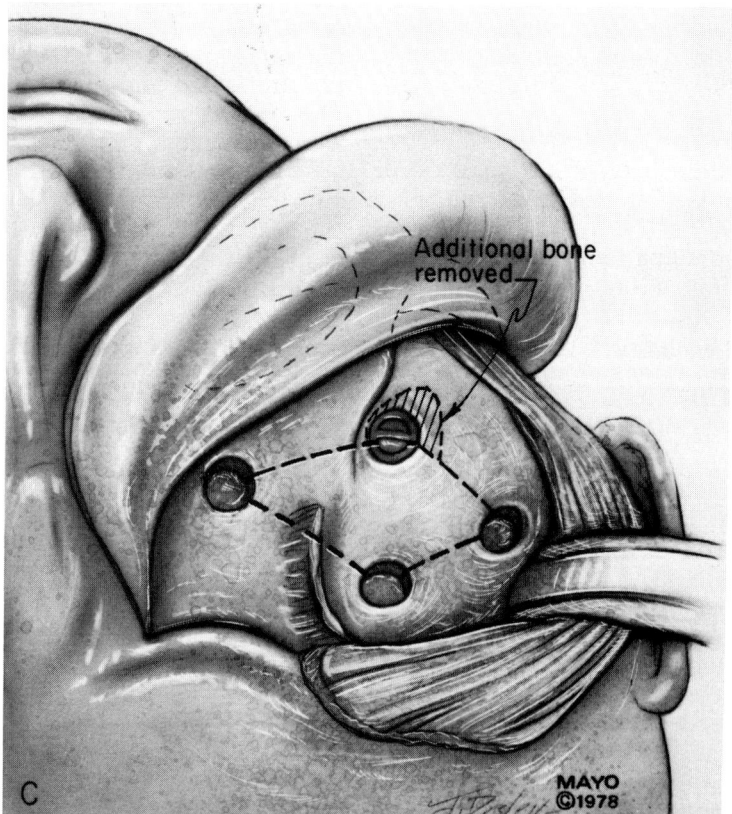

Figure 7C.

chiasm allows an approach through the lamina terminalis. This has the advantage of midline exposure, but may limit visualization of the lateral extents of the tumor. An approach between the optic nerve and the carotid artery allows good exposure of the lateral aspect of the tumor, but may be limited by the optic tract posteriorly and by other aspects of the anatomy of the supraclinoid carotid and the optic apparatus. The temporal approach requires either surgical removal or extensive mobilization and retraction of the anterior temporal lobe. This provides good access to the lateral and posterior aspects of the tumor, but is limited again by the anatomic relationships of the optic nerve and tract, the carotid artery and its branches, and the third cranial nerve. Combinations of these approaches, along with the transcranial, transsphenoidal exposure mentioned earlier, may be required to remove particularly difficult tumors.

Stereotactic approaches to craniopharyngiomas have been utilized for biopsy, aspiration of cystic contents, and instillation of radioactive isotopes.

Transsphenoidal Approaches

Craniopharyngioma patients with enlarged sellas may in general be presumed to harbor tumors that have started below the diaphragm and have subsequently expanded. These tumors are almost invariably extra-pial and extra-arachnoid. They are usually well circumscribed and the tumor will expand the sella, displacing and flattening normal gland anteriorly in most cases. The dorsal capsule of the tumor fuses with the diaphragm of the sella, and both may expand intracranially. The enlarged sella gives the transsphenoidal surgeon the room and maneuverability necessary to deal with the tumor.

Transsphenoidal approaches, like transcranial ones, can be used either for definitive removal of tumor or for palliative subtotal removals or drainage procedures. The latter are favored in patients who have had prior surgery and are suffering from persistent or recurrent tumor.

Surgical techniques are similar to those used for the transsphenoidal management of pituitary adenomas. Patients with large tumors having suprasellar extensions have a lumbar needle inserted so that air may be injected or CSF withdrawn during the operative procedure. The sella is carefully and widely exposed. In children with poorly pneumatized sphenoid sinuses, it is usually possible to create a sellar floor by removing first the cortical bone and then the medullary bone of the sphenoid. The posterior cortical surface then becomes the floor of the sella. This may be done with a drill or with a combination of fine chisel and curette.

The floor of the sella is then removed as widely as possible so as to create the greatest possible working area. Lateral exposure should extend from one cavernous sinus to the other, and vertical exposure from the floor of the sella to the junction of the face of the sella with the anterior fossa. The dura should be opened with caution so that the capsule of the tumor is not violated. If pituitary gland tissue is present, it usually lies just behind the dura and may be displaced laterally and preserved. Once a plane of cleavage has been established, the cystic component of the tumor may be aspirated. Further vigorous dissection may be necessary to detach the capsule of the craniopharyngioma from the dural walls of the sella. When the intrasellar portion of the tumor has been fully mobilized, it is then necessary to incise the diaphragm, usually at its anterolateral margin. This creates a sizable CSF leak. Further dissection will mobilize the anterior attachment of the diaphragm which is fused with the dorsal aspect of the tumor capsule. As the tumor is depressed into the sella, the pituitary stalk is usually visualized. Careful bipolar cauterization and sharp dissection allow detachment of the tumor from the stalk with minimal trauma. Further intracranial dissection is performed under direct microscopic visual and fluoroscopic control, and the majority of tumors associated with enlarged sellas can be completely removed (Figs. 8A, B).

The resection of the diaphragm makes effective closure a major portion of the operative procedure. Occlusive packing of the sella with homograft or autograft muscle or fat is preferred. This is done under fluoroscopic control. Once packed, the sella is carefully reconstructed. The floor is replaced with a plate of nasal cartilage or bone designed to apply broad pressure to the graft. Epidural placement of the bone is preferred when feasible. If septal bone and cartilage are not available, bank bone or methacrylate fashioned to form a plate may be used. In most cases, the sphenoid sinus is also packed with muscle or fat. The use of biologic glue or postoperative spinal drainage has not been necessary.

Steroid support is given before and after surgery until accurate baseline blood corticosteroid determinations can be made. Diabetes insipidus is controlled with DDAVP parenterally until the nasal formulation can be used (ordinarily the fourth postoperative day).

In a number of cases, planned transsphenoidal and craniotomy approaches have been used in the same patient (Fig. 5). This has occurred in urgent situations where temporizing transsphenoidal decompression was subsequently followed by definitive transcranial surgery and also when a solid tumor has both intracranial and intrasellar extensions.

The transsphenoidal route has been used for palliative partial resections and also for attempts at prolonged drainage of cystic lesions. If the subarachnoid space is not entered, it may be possible to insert a silastic drain from the tumor cavity to the posterior nasal space. Although such drainage tubes tend to become obstructed and are eventually extruded, they have functioned well as long as 5 years in some patients.

Other Surgical Procedures

Other palliative means of dealing with craniopharyngiomas have been utilized. The insertion of the tube of an Ommaya reservoir into a cystic lesion may permit repeated aspirations. Tumors that obstruct the foramen of Monro or other CSF pathways either directly or secondary to an inflammatory response may produce hydrocephalus. Ventricular CSF shunting procedures may then be indicated, and often must be performed bilaterally.

Recent Surgical Experience at the Mayo Clinic

The most recently treated 100 cases of craniopharyngioma (1973–1986) have reflected the interest in the transsphenoidal approach and its indications and limitations. For that reason, 59 cases were treated with initial transsphenoidal operations. Subsequent craniotomy was performed in four of these patients. There was one patient who had an exploratory craniotomy and a subsequent transsphenoidal removal of her tumor.

Patients generally were divided into primary (virgin) cases, previously operated cases, and "salvage" cases (Figs. 8A–E). The goal with the primary cases was total removal whenever possible. In previously operated cases, the goal usually was radical subtotal removal. In "salvage" cases, palliation was the goal for patients with tumors that had escaped control.

Among the craniotomy cases were two bifrontal approaches, two temporal approaches (modification of Symon's technique without brain resection), two large frontotemporal craniotomies with transventricular or transcallosal approaches, 18 frontotemporal approaches, and 17 pterional approaches. Among the 32 craniotomy cases where total removal was thought to have been accomplished, there has been one recurrence to date.

Among the transsphenoidal cases, total removal was thought to have been accomplished in 27 cases and there have been four recurrences to date in this group. Palliation of visual loss was accomplished in 25 of 27 patients. The difficult nature of those patients with residual tumor is emphasized by the fact that 13 of these patients required subsequent surgical procedures. Radiation therapy has been used only sparingly in

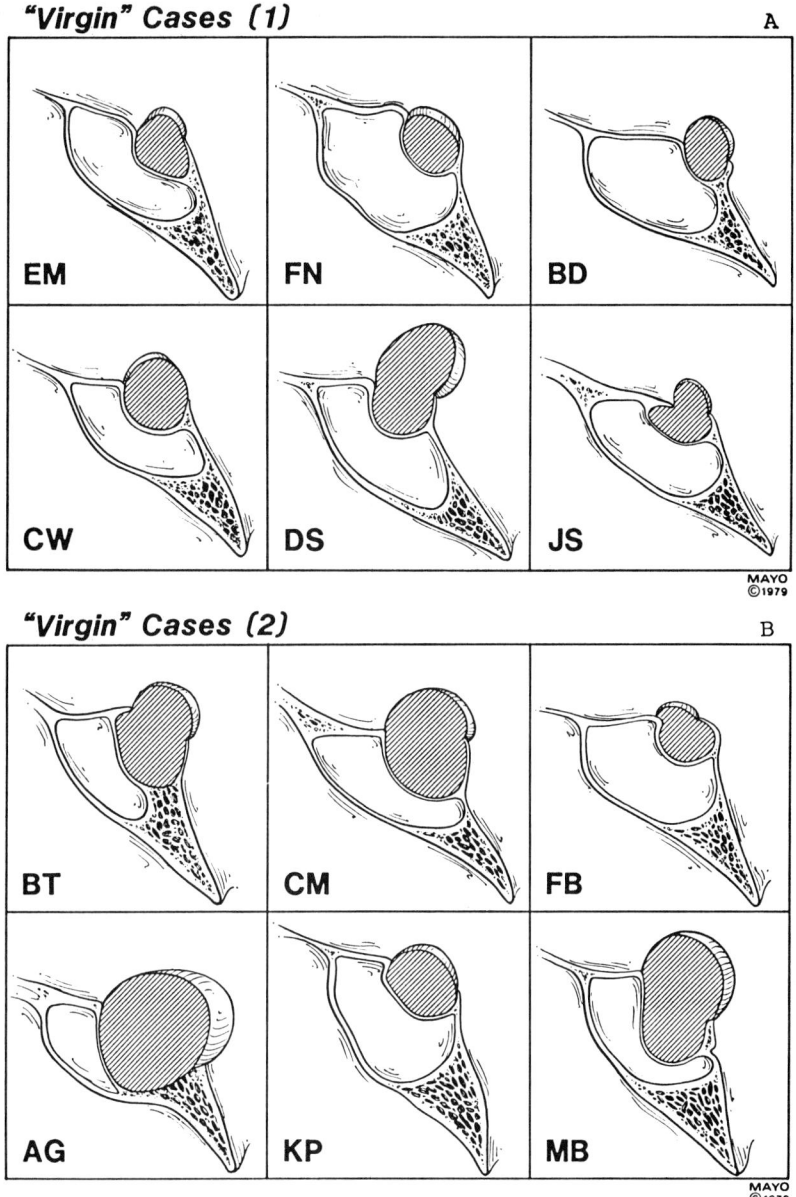

Figure 8 A-E: Diagrammatic representations of craniopharyngiomas treated by transsphenoidal surgery.

this group of patients, and insufficient time has passed to allow for any comment on its effectiveness.

Operative mortality for the series as a whole has been low (2%). One patient with a calcified intrasellar tumor (Fig. 9) died after developing carotid thrombosis, presumably from transsphenoidal intrasellar dissection of the tumor, causing spasm and occlusion of both cavernous carotid arteries.

Radiation Therapy

Lesions of the pituitary region have been treated by various forms of radiation therapy since 1909. Such therapy has

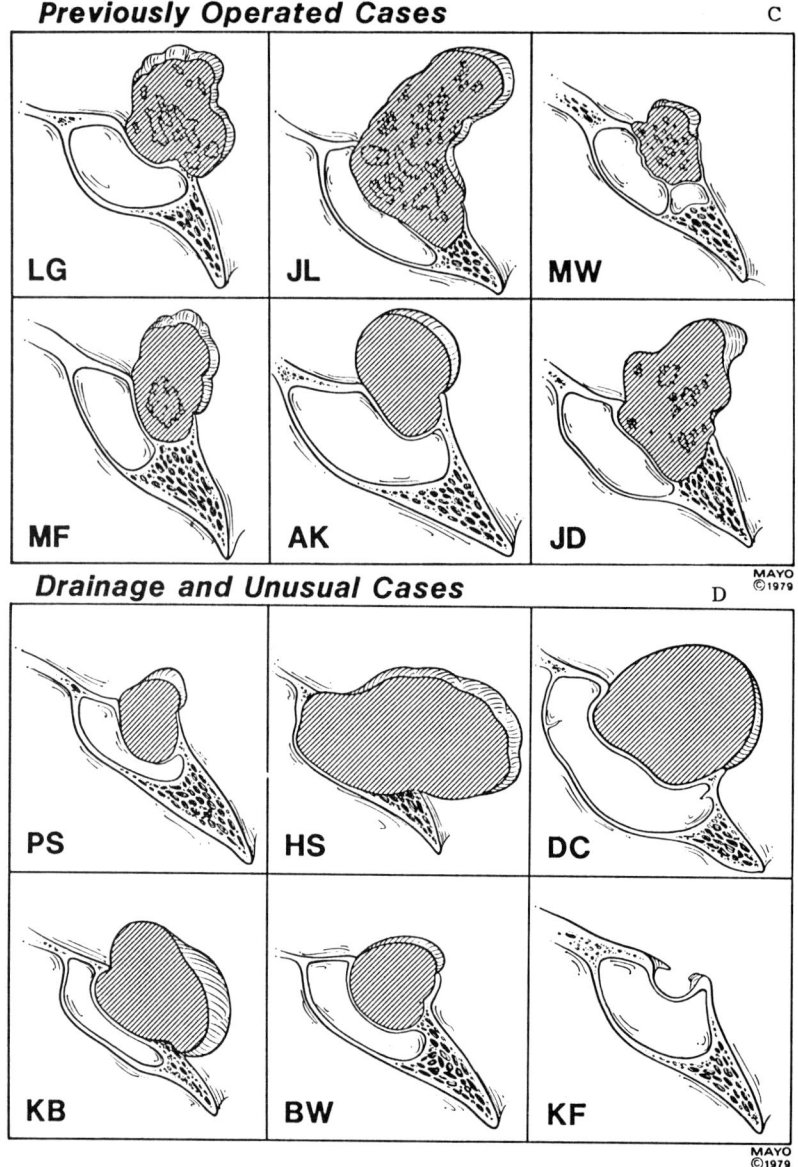

Figure 8C, D.

evolved along several different lines and still remains a matter of investigation and, occasionally, controversy. Conventional teletherapy with gamma radiation from ^{60}Co or a linear accelerator has been demonstrated to be of benefit in patients with craniopharyngioma. Total tumor dose ranges of 4500–5500 rads have been recommended, and careful attention to technique (multiple ports with shielding of the eyes) and fractionation (no more than 180 rads/day) is mandatory. Other radiotherapeutic approaches have included the use of high energy particles—protons, alpha particles, or neutrons generated by cyclotrons and deposited in the area of the tumor using the Bragg peak effect. Some patients have been treated with stereotactically applied external gamma irradiation from multiple sources accurately aimed at the tumor as a focal point.

"Salvage" Cases

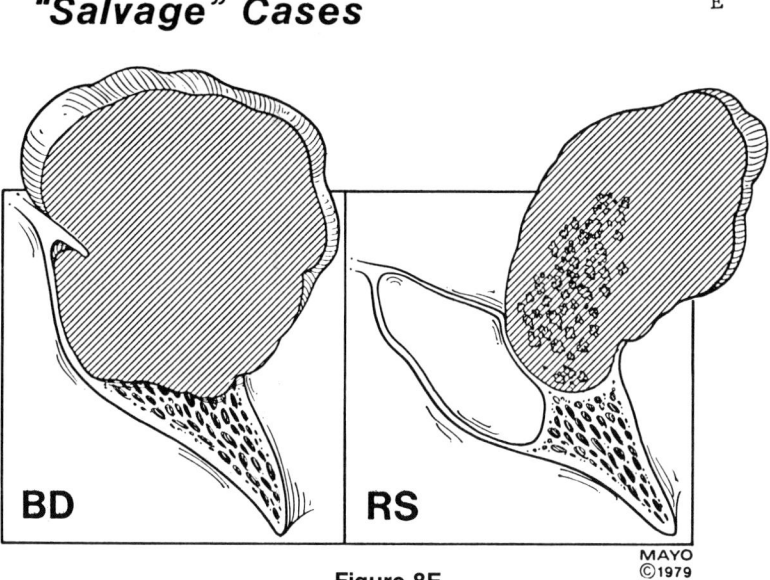

Figure 8E.

Cystic tumors have been treated by the injection of radioactive solutions containing beta emitters such as ^{32}P, ^{90}Y, ^{198}Au, or ^{186}Rh. Stereotactic implantation of beta-emitting seeds into solid portions of the tumor has also been performed.

All of the radiotherapeutic approaches share the risk of damage to normal structures—the pituitary gland, the optic nerves and chiasm, the hypothalamus, and the vasculature in the region of the sella. These effects continue after cessation of treatment and are difficult to predict or to treat. In infants and children, radiation therapy has been implicated in the mental retardation, growth, and development abnormalities, and psychological disorders so common in youngsters with craniopharyngioma. Patients of all ages are subject to the small risk of radiation necrosis of the brain and radiation-induced malignancies which have occasionally been reported.

Selection of Therapeutic Approach

Because each craniopharyngioma is different, it is important to individualize the plan of management to the patient and to what is known about the anatomy and biology of the tumor. In previously untreated patients, several issues should be addressed. Total removal remains a reasonable goal in many tumors, especially those with enlargement of the sella and no major involvement of or attachment to the hypothalamus or the optic apparatus. In infants and children who are growing normally, it is occasionally prudent to delay therapy until growth is complete. In

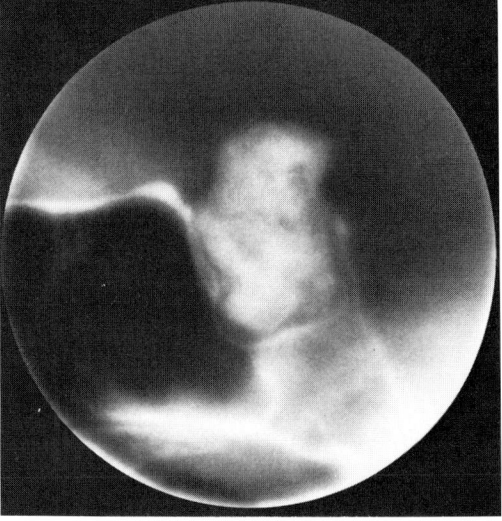

Figure 9: Calcified intrasellar craniopharyngioma. Transsphenoidal removal of this lesion resulted in carotid thrombosis and death.

adults, the question of growth and sexual development is less important. For many patients, satisfactory results can follow subtotal tumor removal and subsequent radiation therapy. The effects of radiation, particularly on the immature brain and neuroendocrine system, must be carefully considered.

In patients who have persistent or recurrent craniopharyngioma, the goals of therapy must also be thoroughly analyzed. Although in some cases total removal may be accomplished, in most instances palliation is the desired result. Relief of pressure on the optic apparatus, decompression of a cystic portion of the tumor or relief of hydrocephalus all may be necessary components of an overall plan of therapy.

The goal of treatment, a neurologically intact patient living as normal a life as possible, is accomplished by using a judicious combination of careful surgery, meticulous medical and endocrine management, and appropriate radiation therapy. Improvements in diagnosis and in the technical and conceptual aspects of medical, surgical, and radiotherapeutic management should lead to continuing improvement in the outlook for patients with craniopharyngioma.

General Bibliography

1. Agnetti V, Carreras M, Roccas A, et al: Epithelial cysts related to the Rathke's cleft. *J Neurosurg Sci* 18:65-69, 1974.
2. Aiba T, Sueyoshi S, Kumagai N, et al: Microsurgical resection of craniopharyngioma preserving the pituitary stalk. Excerpta Medica, International Congress Series, Third International Congress of Neurological Surgery, No. 418, p. 91, 1977.
3. Aiba T, Yamada S: Surgery of craniopharyngiomas in adults. *Neurol Med Chir* (Tokyo), 20:439-451, 1980.
4. Alpers BJ: The cerebral epidermoids (cholesteatomas). *Am J Surg* 43:55-65, 1939.
5. Alvord EC: Growth rates of epidermoid tumors. *Ann Neurol* 2:367-370, 1977.
6. Amacher AL: Craniopharyngioma: the controversy regarding radiotherapy. *Childs Brain* 6:57-64, 1980.
7. Antunes JL, Muraszko K. Quest DO, Carmel PW: Surgical strategies in the management of tumours of the anterior third ventricle. In Brock M (ed): *Modern Neurosurgery*. Berlin, Springer-Verlag, 1982, pp 215-224.
8. Arendt AA: Evaluation of surgical management of craniopharyngiomas. In Opukholi gipofiza i kraniofaringiomy (Tumors of the hypophysis and craniopharyngiomas). Moscow, pp 81-84, 1962. (in Russian)
9. Arutyunov AI, Rostotskaya VI, Mareyeva TG: Surgical treatment of craniopharyngiomas in children. In Materialy nauchnoi konferentsii neirokhirurgov USSR (Proceedings of Scientific Conference of Ukrainian Neurosurgeons), Zaporozhye, pp 187-189, 1972. (in Russian)
10. Arutyunov AI, Rostotskaya VI, Krasnova TS: Principles of treating craniopharyngiomas. In Opukholi golovnogo mozga (Tumors of the Brain). Moscow, pp 114-121, 1975. (in Russian)
11. Atwell WJ: The development of the hypophysis cerebri in man with special reference to the pars tuberalis. *Am J Anat* 37:159-193, 1926.
12. Avioli LV, Earley LE, Kashima HK: Chronic and sustained hypernatremia, absence of thirst, diabetes insipidus and adrenocorticotrophin insufficiency resulting from widespread destruction of the hypothalamus. *Ann Intern Med* 56:131-140, 1962.
13. Azar-Kia B, Kreshnan UR, Schecter MM: Neonatal craniopharyngioma: Case report. *J Neurosurg* 42:91-93, 1975.
14. Babinski MJ: Tumeur du corps pituitare sans acromegalie et avec arret de developpement des organes genitaux. *Rev Neurol* (Paris) 8:531-533, 1900.
15. Backlund EO: Studies on craniopharyngiomas. I. Treatment: past and present. *Acta Chir Scand* 138:743, 1972.
16. Backlund EO: Studies on craniopharyngiomas. III. Stereotaxic treatment with intracystic yttrium-90. *Acta Chir Scand* 139:237-247, 1973.
17. Backlund EO: Studies on craniopharyngiomas. IV. Stereotaxic treatment with radiosurgery. *Acta Chir Scand* 139:344-351, 1973.
18. Backlund EO, Johansson L, Sarby B: Studies on craniopharyngiomas. II. Treatment by stereotaxis and radiosurgery. *Acta Chir Scand* 138:749-759, 1972.

19. Bailey P: Note concerning keratin and keratohyalin in tumors of the hypophyseal duct. Ann Surg 74:501-505, 1921.
20. Banna M: Craniopharyngioma in adults. Surg Neurol 1:202-204, 1973.
21. Banna M: Craniopharyngioma: based on 160 cases. Br J Radiol 49:206-223, 1976.
22. Banna M, Hoare RD, Stanley P, Till K: Craniopharyngioma in children. J Pediatr 83:781-785, 1973.
23. Barnett DJ: Radiologic aspects of craniopharyngiomas. Radiology 72:14-18, 1959.
24. Bartlett JR: Craniopharyngiomas. An analysis of some aspects of symptomatology, radiology and histology. Brain 94:725-732, 1971.
25. Bartlett JR: Craniopharyngiomas: a summary of 85 cases. J Neurol Neurosurg Psychiat 34:37-41, 1971.
26. Bayoumi ML: Rathke's cleft and its cysts. Edinburgh Med J 55:745-749, 1948.
27. Beckmann JW, Kubie LS: A clinical study of twenty-one cases of tumour of the hypophyseal stalk. Brain 52:127-170, 1929.
28. Belza J: Double midline intracranial tumors of vestigial origin: contiguous intrasellar chordoma and suprasellar craniopharyngioma. Case report. J Neurosurg 25:199-204, 1966.
29. Benes V: Results of surgical treatment of craniopharyngiomas. Excerpta Medica, International Congress Series No. 60, Second European Congress of Neurological Surgeons, Rome, 1961, pp 60-61, Abstract No. 35.
30. Bergland R, Ray BS: The arterial supply of the human optic chiasm. J Neurosurg 31:327-334, 1969.
31. Berry RG, Schlezinger NS: Rathke-cleft cysts. Arch Neurol (Chicago) 1:48-58, 1959.
32. Bhagwati SN, Vuckovich DM: Craniopharyngioma presenting with acute blindness: case report. Arch Neurol 8:101, 1963.
33. Bingas B, Wolter M: Das Kraniopharyngeom. Fortschr Neurol Psychiat 3:117-195, 1968.
34. Block MA, Goree JA, Jiminez JP: Craniopharyngioma with optic canal enlargement simulating a glioma of the optic chiasm: case report. J Neurosurg 39:523-527, 1973.
35. Bloom HJG: Combined modality therapy for intracranial tumors. Cancer 35:111-120, 1975.
36. Bloom HJG: The role of radiotherapy in the management of chiasmal compression. Proc R Soc Med 70:319-326, 1977.
37. Bloom HJG: Recent concepts in the conservative treatment of intracranial tumours in children. Acta Neurochir 50:103-116, 1979.
38. Bloom HJG, Harmer CL: Craniopharyngiomas. Br. Med J 2:288-289, 1972.
39. Bloom HJG, Harmer CL: Craniopharyngiomas: general aspects and treatment. In Di Tumori Infantili, Bucalossi P, Veronesi U, Emanueli H, et al (eds). Editerce Ambrosiana, Milan, pp 119-128, 1976.
40. Bode U, Oliff A, Bercu BB, et al: Absence of CT brain scan and endocrine abnormalities with less intensive CNS prophylaxis. Am J Pediatr Hematol Oncol 2:21-24, 1980.
41. Bollati A, Giunta F, Lenzi A, et al: Third ventricle intrinsic craniopharyngioma: Case report. J Neurosurg Sci 18:216-219, 1974.
42. Bouche J, Rougerie J, Freche Ch, Derome P, Chaiz G: L'abord des craniopharyngiomes par la voie trans-sphenoidale basse. Ann Otolaryngol (Paris), 84:655-658, 1967.
43. Braun IF, Pinto RS, Epstein F: Cystic craniopharyngiomas. AJNR 3:139-141, 1982.
44. Bruce DA: Craniopharyngioma. In Long DM (ed): Current Therapy in Neurological Surgery. Philadelphia, B.C. Decker, 1985, pp 36-37.
45. Burns EC, Tanner JM, Preece MA, et al: Growth hormone treatment in children with craniopharyngioma: Final growth status. Clin Endocrinol 14:587-595, 1981.
46. Cabezudo JM, Vaquero J, Areitio E, Martinez R, de Sola RG, Bravo G: Craniopharyngiomas: a critical approach to treatment. J Neurosurg 55:371-375, 1981.
47. Cabezudo JM, Vaquero J, Garcia-de-Sola R, Leunda G, Nombela L, Bravo G: Computed tomography with craniopharyngiomas: a review. Surg Neurol 15:422-427, 1981.
48. Calvet J, Claux J: Les craniopharyngiomas —le traitement par voie basse. Rev Otoneuroopht 27:121-128, 1955.
49. Campbell JB, Hudson FM: Craniobuccal origin, signs, and treatment of craniopharyngiomas. Surg Gynecol Obstet 111:183-191, 1960.
50. Carmel PW: Surgical syndromes of the hypothalamus. Clin Neurosurg 27:133-159, 1979.
51. Carmel PW: Craniopharyngiomas. In Wilkins RH, Rengachary SS (eds):

Neurosurgery. New York, McGraw-Hill Book Company, 1985, pp 905-916.
52. Carmel PW, Antunes JL, Chang CH: Craniopharyngiomas in children. Neurosurgery 11:382-389, 1982.
53. Carmichael H: Squamous epithelial rests in the hypophysis cerebri. Arch Neurol Psych 26:966-975, 1931.
54. Carpenter RC, Chamberlin GW, Frazier CH: The treatment of hypophyseal stalk tumors by evacuation and irradiation. Am J Roentgenol 38:162-177, 1937.
55. Carrea R, Mora H: Microneurosurgical intracranial radical removal of craniopharyngiomas. In Handa H (ed): Microneurosurgery. Baltimore, Maryland, University Park Press, 1975, pp 161-172.
56. Carrea R, Mora H, Leston J, Girado JM, Schuster G: Cirugia radical de los craniofaringiomas. Acta Neurol Latinoamer 11:109-136, 1965.
57. Carrea R, Mora H, Lanari E: Radical surgery and radioactive chromic phosphate in the treatment of craniopharyngiomas. Excerpta Medica Int Congress Series No. 193, p 29, 1969.
58. Cashion EL, Young JM: Craniopharyngioma in the third ventricle. J Tenn Med Assoc 55:156-160, 1962.
59. Cashion EL, Young JM: Intraventricular craniopharyngioma—report of two cases. J Neurosurg 34:84-87, 1971.
60. Cavazzuti V, Fischer EG, Welch K, et al: Neurological and psychophysiological sequelae following different treatments of craniopharyngioma in children. J Neurosurg 59:409-417, 1983.
61. Chadduck WM, Roberts M: Long term survival with craniopharyngioma: report of a patient in 29th year after treatment, seen for a second intracranial tumor. J Neurosurg 25:312-314, 1966.
62. Cheetham HHD: Experimental squamous metaplasia and squamous epthelioma formation in the pituitary of the rat. Br J Cancer 17:657-662, 1963.
63. Choux M, Lena G: Bases of surgical management of craniopharyngioma in children. Acta Neurochir (Suppl) 28:348, 1979.
64. Ciric I: Neuroepithelial cysts. J Neurosurg 44:134, 1976.
65. Ciric I: On the origin and nature of the pituitary gland capsule. J Neurosurg 45:596-600, 1977.
66. Ciric IS, Cozzens JW: Craniopharyngiomas: transsphenoidal methods of approach—for the virtuoso only? Clin Neurosurg 27:169-187, 1980.
67. Clopper RR, Meyer WJ III, Udvarhelyi GB, et al: Postsurgical IQ and behavioral data on twenty patients with a history of childhood craniopharyngioma. Psychoneuroendocrinology 2:365-372, 1977.
68. Cobb CA, Youmans JR: Brain tumors of disordered embryogenesis in adults. In Youmans JR (ed): Neurological Surgery, 2d ed. Philadelphia, Saunders, 1982, pp 2899-2935.
69. Cobb JP, Wright JC: Studies on a craniopharyngioma in tissue culture. I. Growth characteristics and alterations produced following exposure to two radiomimetic agents. J Neuropath Exp Neurol 18:563-568, 1959.
70. Cooper PR, Ransohoff J: Craniopharyngioma originating in the sphenoid bone: case report. J Neurosurg 36:102-106, 1972.
71. Costin G, Kogut MD, Phillips LS, Daughaday WH: Craniopharyngiomas: The role of insulin in promoting postoperative growth. JCE + M 42:370-379, 1976.
72. Craig WM: Tumors of hypophyseal region. In Bancroft FW, Pilcher C (eds): Surgical Treatment of the Nervous System. Philadelphia, Lippincott, 1946, pp 176-203.
73. Critchley M, Ironside RN: The pituitary adamantinomata. Brain 49:596-600, 1977.
74. Crompton MR, Layton DD: Delayed radionecrosis of the brain following therapeutic X-radiation of the pituitary. Brain 84:85-101, 1961.
75. Cushing H: The craniopharyngiomas. In Intracranial Tumors. Notes upon a series of two thousand verified cases with surgical mortality percentages pertaining thereto. Springfield, IL, Charles C. Thomas, 1932, pp 93-98.
76. Dandy WE: Hypophyseal duct tumors. In Lewis DD (ed): Practice of Surgery. Hagerstown, W.F. Prior Co, 12:598-605, 1932.
77. Danoff BF, Cowchock S, Kramer S: Childhood craniopharyngioma: survival, local control, endocrine and neurologic function following radiotherapy (meeting abstract). Int J Radiat Oncol Biol Phys 7:1238, 1981.
78. Decker RE, Malis LI: Surgical approaches to midline lesions at the base of the skull: a review. Mt Sinai J Med (NY), 37:84-102, 1970.
79. Deery GM: Syndromes of tumors in the chiasmal region; a review of 170 cases re-

ceiving a transfrontal operation. *J Nerv Ment Dis* 71:383-396, 1930.
80. Di Lorenzo N, Nolletti A, Palma L: Late cerebral radionecrosis. *Surg Neurol* 10:281-290, 1978.
81. Djordjevic M, Djordjevic Z, Janicijevic M, et al: Surgical treatment of craniopharyngiomas in children. *Acta Neurochir Suppl* 28:344-348, 1979.
82. Dobos EI, Freed CG, Ashe SMP: An intrinsic tumor of third ventricle. *J Neuropath Exp Neurol* 12:232-243, 1953.
83. Douglas FS, Smith FG: Return of normal growth following removal of a craniopharyngioma. *Am J Dis Child* 116:311-314, 1968.
84. Drachman DA: See-saw nystagmus. *J Neurol Neurosurg Psychiatr* 29:356-361, 1966.
85. Drummond WAC: Intrasellar adamantinoma. *Proc Roy Soc Med* 32:200-207, 1939.
86. Duff TA, Levine R: Intrachiasmatic craniopharyngioma: Case report. *J Neurosurg* 59:176-178, 1983.
87. Duffy WC: Hypophyseal duct tumors. *Ann Surg* 72:537-555, 1920.
88. Erdheim J: Zur normalen und pathologischen histologie der glandula thyreoidea, parathyreoidea und hypophysis. *Beitr Path Anat* 33:158-236, 1903.
89. Erdheim J: Uber hypophysengangsgeschwulste und hirncholesteatome. *Sitzungsb d Kais Akad Wissench Math Naturw Klin* 113:537-726, 1904.
90. Erdheim J: Uber einen neuen fall von hypophysengangsgeschwulst Zentralblatt fur Allg. *Pathol Pathol Anat* 17:209-215, 1906.
91. Erdheim J: Uber einen hypophysentumor von ungewohnlichen sitz. *Beitr Path Anat Allg Path* 46:223, 1909.
92. Fager C, Carter H: Intrasellar epithelial cysts. *J Neurosurg* 24:77, 1966.
93. Fairburn B, Larkin IM: A cyst of Rathke's cleft. *J Neurosurg* 21:223-225, 1964.
94. Fischer EG, Welch K, Belli JA, Wallman J, Shillito JJ Jr, Winston KR, Cassady R: Treatment of craniopharyngiomas in children: 1972-1981. *J Neurosurg* 62:496-501, 1985.
95. Fitz CR, Wortzman G, Harwood-Nash DC, Holgate RC, Barry JF, Boldt DW: Computed tomography in craniopharyngiomas. *Radiology* 127:687-691, 1978.
96. Frazier CH: A review—clinical and pathological—of parahypophyseal lesions. *Surg Gynecol Obstet* 62:1-33, 1936.
97. Frazier CH: Alpers BJ: Adamantinoma of the craniopharyngeal duct. *Arch Neurol Psych* 26:905-965, 1931.
98. Frazier HC, Alpers BJ: Tumors of Rathke's cleft. *Arch Neurol Psych* 32:973-984, 1934.
99. Fujii K, Chambers SM, Rhoton AL Jr: Neurovascular relationships of the sphenoid sinus: A microsurgical study. *J Neurosurg* 50:31-39, 1979.
100. Fulstow M: An epithelial cyst of the hypophysis. *Am J Pathol* 4:87-90, 1928.
101. Galatzer A, Nofar E, Beit-Halachmi N, et al: Intellectual and psychosocial functions of children, adolescents and young adults before and after operation for craniopharyngioma. *Child Care Health Dev* 7:307-316, 1981.
102. Gamblin GT, James LP, Thomas J, Six E, Eil C: Simulation of a prolactin-secreting adenoma by an intrasellar craniopharyngioma. *Neurosurgery* 16:689-692, 1985.
103. Garcia-Uria J: Surgical experience with craniopharyngioma in adults. *Surg Neurol* 9:11-14, 1978.
104. Gass HH: Large calcified craniopharyngioma and bilateral subdural hematomata present at birth: survey of neonatal brain tumors. *J Neurosurg* 3:514, 1956.
105. Ghatak NR, Hirano SA, Zimmerman HM: Ultrastructure of a craniopharyngioma. *Cancer* 27:1465-1475, 1971.
106. Ghatak NR, White BE: Delayed radiation necrosis of the hypothalamus: report of a case simulating recurrent craniopharyngioma. *Arch Neurol* 21:425-430, 1969.
107. Gillman T: The incidence of ciliated epithelium and mucous cells in the normal Bantu pituitary. *S Afr J Med Sci* 5:30-40, 1940.
108. Goldberg GM, Eshbaugh DE: Squamous cell nests of the pituitary gland as related to the origin of craniopharyngiomas. *Arch Pathol* 70:293-299, 1960.
109. Gordy PD, Peet MM, Kahn EA: The surgery of the craniopharyngiomas. *J Neurosurg* 6:503-517, 1949.
110. Grant DB, Lyen K: Hypopituitarism after surgery for craniopharyngioma. *Child's Brain* 9:201-204, 1982.
111. Grekhov VV: Morphology of craniopharyngiomas. In Opukholi gipofiza i kraniofaringiomy (Tumors of the hypophysis and craniopharyngiomas). Moscow, pp 104-108, 1962. (in Russian)
112. Grisoli F, Vincentelli F, Farnarier P, Gondim-Oliveira J, Vigouroux RP: Transsphenoidal microsurgery in the management of non-pituitary tumours of the

sella turcica. In Brock M (ed): *Modern Neurosurgery*. Berlin, Springer-Verlag, 1982, pp 193-204.
113. Grover WD, Rorke LB: Invasive craniopharyngioma. *J Neurol Neurosurg Psychiat* 31:580-582, 1968.
114. Guidetti B, Fraioli B: Craniopharyngiomas. Results of surgical treatment. *Acta neurochir* (Wien) (Suppl) 28:349-351, 1979.
115. Guiot G: Par ou faut-il aborder l'hypophyse? *Presse Med* 78:209-210, 1970.
116. Gutin PH, Klemme WM, Lagger RL, et al: Management of the unresectable cystic craniopharyngioma by aspiration through an Ommaya reservoir drainage system. *J Neurosurg* 52:36-40, 1980.
117. Halstead AE: Remarks on the operative treatment of tumors of the hypophysis. *Surg Gynecol Obstet* 10:494-502, 1910.
118. Hamberger CA, Hammer G, Norlen G, Sjogren B: Surgical treatment of craniopharyngioma; radical removal by the transantrosphenoidal approach. *Acta Otolaryngol* (Stockh) 52:285-292, 1960.
119. Hamer J: Removal of craniopharyngiomas by sub-nasal trans-sphenoidal operation. *Neuropediatrie* 9:312-319, 1978.
120. Hamlin H: Discussion of Leksell L, Backlund EO: The treatment of craniopharyngiomas (summary of paper.) *Acta Neurol Scand* 43:240, 1967.
121. Hardy J: Transsphenoidal hypophysectomy. *J Neurosurg* 34:581-594, 1971.
122. Hardy J, LaLonde J: L exerese par voie trans-sphenoidale d'un craniopharyngiome geant. *Un Med Canada* 92:1124-1129, 1963.
123. Hardy J, Vezina JL: Transsphenoidal neurosurgery of intracranial neoplasms. In Thompson RA, Green JR (eds): *Advances in Neurology*. New York, Raven Press, 15:261-274, 1976.
124. Harris JR, Levene MB: Visual complications following irradiation for pituitary adenomas and craniopharyngiomas. *Radiology* 120:167-171, 1976.
125. Harris FS, Rhoton AL Jr: Anatomy of the cavernous sinus: A microsurgical study. *J Neurosurg* 45:169-180, 1976.
126. Hirano A, Ghatak NR, Zimmerman HM: Fenestrated blood vessels in craniopharyngioma. *Acta Neuropath* (Berlin) 26:171-177, 1973.
127. Hoff JT, Patterson RH Jr: Craniopharyngiomas in children and adults. *J Neurosurg* 36:299-302, 1972.
128. Hoffman HJ: Supratentorial tumors in childhood. In Youmans J (ed): *Neurological Surgery*. Philadelphia, WB Saunders, 1982, pp 2702-2732.
129. Hoffman HJ: Craniopharyngiomas. In *Pediatric Neurosurgery*. New York, Grune and Stratton, 1982, pp 501-511.
130. Hoffman HJ, Hendrick EB, Humphreys RP, Buncic JR, Armstrong DL, Jenkin RDT: Management of craniopharyngioma in children. *J Neurosurg* 47:218-227, 1977.
131. Holbach KH, Gullotta F: Zur formalgenese intrasellarer und intraventrikularer zysten. *Neurochirurgia* (Stuttgart) 20:186-188, 1977.
132. Hoogenhout J, Otten BJ, Kazem I, Stoelinga GB, Walder AH: Surgery and radiation therapy in the management of craniopharyngiomas. *Int J Radiat Oncol Biol Phys* 10(12):2293-2297, 1984.
133. Horwitz NH, Rizzoli HV: *Postoperative Complications in Neurosurgical Practice*. Baltimore, Williams and Wilkins, 1967, pp 59-63.
134. Humphreys RP, Hoffman HJ, Hendrick EB: A long-term postoperative follow-up in craniopharyngioma. *Childs Brain* 5:530-539, 1979.
135. Hunter AJ: Squamous metaplasia of cells of the anterior pituitary gland. *J Pathol Bact* 69:141-145, 1955.
136. Illum P, Elbrond O, Nehen AM: Surgical treatment of nasopharyngeal craniopharyngioma: Radical removal by the transpalatal approach. *J Laryngol Otolaryngol* 91:227-233, 1977.
137. Ingraham FD, Matson DD, McLaurin RL: Cortisone and ACTH as an adjunct to the surgery of craniopharyngiomas. *N Engl J Med* 246:568-571, 1952.
138. Ingraham FD, Matson DD: *Neurosurgery of Infancy and Childhood*, Springfield, IL, Charles C. Thomas, 1954, p 292.
139. Ingraham FD, Scott HW: Craniopharyngiomas in children. *J Pediatr* 29:95-116, 1946.
140. Iyer CGS: Case report of an adamantinomata present at birth. *J Neurosurg* 9:221-228, 1957.
141. Jackson H: Craniopharyngeal duct tumors. *JAMA* 66:1082, 1916.
142. James AE Jr, DeLand FH: Hodges FJ, Wagner HN: Radionuclide imaging in the detection and differential diagnosis of craniopharyngiomas. *Am J Roentgenol* 109:692-700, 1970.
143. Job JC, Lambertz J, Sizonenko PC, Rossier A: La croissance des enfants atteints de craniopharyngiome. *Arch Franc Pediat* 27:341:353, 1970.

144. Johnson NE: Craniopharyngioma—review with a discussion of transpalatal approach. *Laryngoscope* 72:1731-1749, 1962.
145. Kahn EA: Some physiologic implications of craniopharyngioma. *Neurology* 9:82-90, 1959.
146. Kahn EA, Gosch HH, Seeger JF, Hicks SP: Forty-five years experience with craniopharyngiomas. *Surg Neurol* 1:5-12, 1973.
147. Kapcala LP et al: Galactorrhea, oligo/amenorrhea and hyperprolactinoma in patients with craniopharyngiomas. *J Clin Endocrinol Metab* 51:798-800, 1980.
148. Katz EL: Late results of radical excision of craniopharyngiomas in children. *J Neurosurg* 42:86-90, 1975.
149. Kempe LG: Craniopharyngioma. In Kempe LG (ed): *Operative Neurosurgery, Vol. 1, Cranial, Cerebral and Intracranial Vascular Disease.* New York, Springer-Verlag, 1968, p 90.
150. Kennedy HB, Smith RJS: Eye signs in craniopharyngioma. *Br J Ophthalmol* 59:689-695, 1975.
151. Kenny FM, Iturzaeta NF, Mintz D, Drash A, Garces LY, Susen A, Askari HA: Iatrogenic hypopituitarism in craniopharyngioma: unexplained catch up growth in three children. *J Pediatr* 72:766-775, 1968.
152. Kepes JJ: Transitional cell tumor of the pituitary gland developing from Rathke's cleft cyst. *Cancer* 41:337-343, 1978.
153. Kernohan JW: Tumors of congenital origin. In Minckler J (ed): *Pathology of the Nervous System.* New York, McGraw Hill, 1971, pp 1927-1937.
154. Kernohan JW, Sayre JP: *Tumors of the Central Nervous System: Atlas of Tumor Pathology.* Fascicle 35. Washington Armed Forces Institute of Pathology, 1952.
155. Kerr AS: Craniopharyngiomata—Proc Soc Brit Neurol Surgeons. *J Neurol Neurosurg Psychiat* 31:646-650.
156. Killeffer FA, Stern WE: Chronic effects of hypothalamic injury: report of a case of near total hypothalamic destruction resulting from removal of a craniopharyngioma. *Arch Neurol* (Chicago) 22:419-429, 1970.
157. King TT: Removal of intraventricular craniopharyngiomas through the lamina terminalis. *Acta Neurochir* (Wien) 45:277-286, 1979.
158. Kiyono H: Uber das vorkommen von plattenepithelherden in der hypophyse. (Zugleich ein Beitnag zur Kenntnis der Hypophysenganggewachse). *Virchow's Arch f Path Anat* 252:118-145, 1924.
159. Kjellberg RN: Craniopharyngiomas. In Tindall GT, Collins WF (eds): *Clinical Management of Pituitary Disorders.* New York, Raven Press, 1979, pp 373-388.
160. Kobayashi T: Recent progress in the treatment of craniopharyngioma. Proc of Japanese Congress of Neurological Surgeons, Tokyo, 1983, pp 101-112.
161. Kobayashi T, Kageyama N, Ohara K: Internal irradiation for cystic craniopharyngioma. *J Neurosurg* 55:896-903, 1981.
162. Kobayashi T, Kageyama N, Yoshida J, et al: Pathological and clinical basis of the indications for treatment of craniopharyngiomas. *Neurologia Medico-Chirurgica*, 21:39-47, 1981.
163. Kodama T, Matsukado Y, Uemura S: Intracapsular irradiation therapy of craniopharyngiomas with radioactive gold: Indication and follow-up results. *Neurol Med Chir* (Tokyo) 21:49-58, 1981.
164. Konovalov AN: Operative management of craniopharyngiomas. In Krayenbuhl H (ed): *Advances and Technical Standards in Neurosurgery,* Vol. 8. Wien, Austria, Springer-Verlag, 1981, pp 281-318.
165. Konovalov AN: Microsurgery of craniopharyngiomas. In Rand RW (ed): *Microneurosurgery.* St. Louis, CV Mosby, 1985, pp 196-213.
166. Koos WT, Bock FW, Salah S: Experiences in the microsurgery of craniopharyngiomas. In Handa H (ed): *Microneurosurgery,* Baltimore, MD, University Park Press, 1975, pp 151-160.
167. Koos WT, Miller MH: *Intracranial Tumors of Infants and Children.* Stuttgart, George Thieme Verlag, 1971.
168. Korsgaard O, Lindholm J, Rasmussen P: Endocrine function in patients with suprasellar and hypothalamic tumours. *Acta Endocr* (Kobenhavn) 83:1-8, 1976.
169. Kramer S: Radiation therapy in the management of craniopharyngiomas. In Deeley TJ (ed): *Central Nervous System Tumours.* London, Butterworths, 1974, pp 204-223.
170. Kramer S, McKissock W, Concannon JP: Craniopharyngiomas. Treatment by combined surgery and radiation therapy. *J Neurosurg* 18:217-226, 1961.
171. Kramer S, Southard M, Mansfield CM: Radiotherapy in the management of craniopharyngiomas: Further experiences and late results. *AJR* 103:44-52, 1968.

172. Krayenbuhl H: Hypophyseal adenomas and craniopharyngiomas. Excerpta Medica, International Congress Series No. 36, Second International Congress of Neurological Surgery, Washington, DC, 1961, Abstract No. S7.
173. Krayenbuhl H, Prader A: Traitement endocrinien des troubles de la croissance chez des malades operes d'un craniopharyngiome. Neurochirurgie 8:223-233, 1962.
174. Kunicki A, Lechowski S, Madroszkiewicz E, Szwagrzyk E: Guzy kieszonki Rathkego wieku dzieciecego w materiale kliniki neurochirurgii AMW Krakowie. Neurochir Pol 5:715-720, 1971.
175. Kunicki A, Lechowski S, Madroszkiewicz E, Szwagrzyk E: Rathke's pouch tumors of childhood in the material of the Department of Neurosurgery. Medical Academy in Cracow. Pol Med J 11:985-990, 1972.
176. Kurze T: Microtechniques in neurological surgery. Clin Neurosurg 11:128-134, 1964.
177. Landolt AM: Die ultrastruktur des kraniopharyngeoms. Schwez. Arch Neurol Neurochir Psychiat 111:313-329, 1972.
178. Lascelles PT, Lews PD: Hypodipsia and hypernatremia associated with hypothalamic and suprasellar lesions. Brain 95:249-264, 1972.
179. Laws ER Jr: Transsphenoidal microsurgery in the management of craniopharyngioma. J Neurosurg 52:661-666, 1980.
180. Laws ER Jr: Transsphenoidal approach to lesions in and about the sella turcica. In Schmidek HH, Sweet WH (eds): Operative Neurosurgical Techniques. New York, Grune and Stratton, 1982, pp 327-341.
181. Laws ER Jr, Kern EB: Complications of transsphenoidal surgery. Clin Neurosurg 23:401-416, 1976.
182. Laws ER Jr, Randall RV, Kern EB, Abboud CF (eds): Management of Pituitary Adenomas and Related Lesions. New York, Appleton-Century-Crofts, 1982, pp 376.
183. Laws ER Jr, Randall RV, Abboud CF, Hayles AB: Craniopharyngioma—The transsphenoidal microsurgical approach. In Givens JR (ed): The Hypothalamus, Chicago, Year Book Medical Publishers, 1984, pp 335-347.
184. LeGros Clarke WE, Beattie J, Riddoch G, Dott NM: Oliver and Boyd (ed): The Hypothalamus, 1938.
185. Leksell L: Stereotaxis and Radiosurgery: An Operative System. Springfield, IL, Charles C. Thomas, 1971.
186. Leksell L, Backlund EO, Johansson L: Treatment of craniopharyngiomas. Acta Chir Scand 133:345-350, 1967.
187. Leksell L, Liden K: A therapeutic trial with radioative isotopes in cystic brain tumour. In Oxford HM: Radioisotope Techniques, Stationery Office, 1951, pp 76-78.
188. Lewis DD: Contribution to the subject of tumors of the hypophysis. JAMA 55:1002-1008, 1910.
189. Lichter AS, Wara WW, Sheline GE, et al: The treatment of craniopharyngiomas. Int J Radiat Oncol Biol Phys 2-675-683, 1977.
190. Lindgren E, Di Chiro G: Suprasellar tumors with calcification. Acta Radiol 36:173-195, 1951.
191. Liszczak T, Richardson EP, Phillips JP, Jacobson S, Kornblith PL: Morphological, biochemical, ultrastructural, tissue culture and clinical observations of typical and aggressive craniopharyngiomas. Acta Neuropathol (Berlin) 43:191-203, 1978.
192. Liwnicz BH, Berger TS, Liwnicz RG, Aron BS: Radiation-associated gliomas: a report of four cases and analysis of postradiation tumors of the central nervous system. Neurosurgery 17:436-445, 1985.
193. Long DM, Chou SN: Transcallosal removal of craniopharyngioma within the third ventricle. J Neurosurg 39:563-567, 1973.
194. Love JG, Marshall TM: Craniopharyngiomas. Surg Gynec Obstet 90:591-601, 1950.
195. Love JG, Sheldon CH, Kernohan JW: Tumor of the hypophyseal duct (Rathke's cysts). Arch Surg 39:28-56, 1939.
196. Lucas G, Benderitter T, Choux M: L'exploration endocrinienne pre- et postoperatoire des craniopharyngiomes de l'enfant. Arch Fr Pediatr 39:303-307, 1982.
197. Lundberg PO, Osterman PO, Wide L: Serum prolactin in patients with hypothalamus and pituitary disorders. J Neurosurg 55:194-199, 1981.
198. Luschka H: Der Hirnanhand und die Steissdruese des Menschen. Berlin, Von Georg, Reimer, 1860.
199. Luse SA, Kernohan JW: Squamous cell rests of the pituitary gland. Cancer 8:623–628, 1955.
200. Lyen KR, Grant DB: Endocrine function, morbidity, and mortality after surgery for

craniopharyngioma. *Arch Dis Child* 57:837-841, 1982.
201. Maira G, DiRocco C, Anile C, Roselli R: Hyperprolactinemia as the first symptom of craniopharyngioma. *Child's Brain* 9:205-210, 1982.
202. Majlessi H, Shariat AS, Katirai A: Nasopharyngeal craniopharyngioma. Case report. *J Neurosurg* 49:119-120, 1978.
203. Manaka S, Teramoto A, Takakura K: The efficacy of radiotherapy for craniopharyngioma. *J Neurosurg* 62:648-656, 1985.
204. Martin AM, Johnson JS, Henry JM, Stoffel TJ, DiChiro G: Delayed radiation necrosis of brain. *J Neurosurg* 47:336-345, 1977.
205. Matson DD: Craniopharyngioma. *Clin Neurosurg* 10:116-129, 1964.
206. Matson DD: Craniopharyngioma. In Matson DD (ed): *Neurosurgery of Infancy and Childhood*. Springfield, IL, Charles C. Thomas, 1969, pp 544-574.
207. Matson DD, Crigler JF Jr: Radical treatment of craniopharyngioma. *Am Surgery* 152:699-704, 1960.
208. Matson DD, Crigler JF Jr: Management of craniopharyngioma in childhood. *J Neurosurg* 30:377-390, 1969.
209. McKenzie KG, Sosman MC: The roentgenological diagnosis of craniopharyngeal pouch tumors. *Am J Roentgenol* 11:171-176, 1924.
210. McKissock W, Ford RK: Results of treatment of the craniopharyngiomas. *J Neurol Neurosurg Psychiat* 29:475, 1966 (abstract).
211. McLean AJ: Die craniopharyngealtaschentumoren (Embryologie, Histologie, Diagnose und Therapie). *Ztschr f d ges Neurol u Psychiat* 126:639-682, 1930.
212. McLone DG, Raimondi AJ, Naidich TP: Craniopharyngiomas. *Child's Brain* 9:188-200, 1982.
213. McMurry FG, Hardy RW Jr, Dohn DF, Sadar E, Gardner WJ: Long-term results in the management of craniopharyngioma. *Neurosurgery* 1:238-241, 1977.
214. Meadows AT, Gordon J, Massari DJ, et al: Decline in IQ scores and cognitive dysfunction in children with acute lymphoblastic leukaemia treated with cranial radiation. *Lancet* 2:1015-1018, 1981.
215. Michelsen WJ, Mount LA, Renaudin J: Craniopharyngioma: a thirty-nine year survey. *Acta Neurol Latinoam* 18:100-106, 1972.
216. Mihalkovics VV: Wirbesaite und hirnanhang. *Arch Mikrosc Anat* 11:389-439, 1875.
217. Mikhael MA: Radiation necrosis of the brain: correlation between patterns on computed tomography and dose of radiation. *J Comput Assist Tomogr* 3:241-249, 1979.
218. Mori K, Handa H, Murata T, et al: Results of treatment for craniopharyngioma. *Childs Brain* 6:303-312, 1980.
219. Moss HA, Nannis ED, Poplack DG: The effects of prophylactic treatment of the central nervous system on the intellectual functioning of children with acute lymphocytic leukemia. *Am J Med* 71:47-52, 1981.
220. Mott FW, Barrett JOW: Three cases of tumor of the third ventricle. *Arch Neurol (Lond)* 1:417-440, 1899.
221. Muller PJ, Russell NA, Morley TP: Craniopharyngioma: results of surgical treatment without radiotherapy. In Morley TP (ed): *Current Controversies in Neurosurgery*. Toronto, WB Saunders Co, 1976, pp 344-350.
222. Muller R, Wohlfart G: Craniopharyngiomas. *Acta Med Scand*, 138:121-138, 1950.
223. Mundinger F: The treatment of brain tumors with radioisotopes. *Progr Neurol Surg* 1:202-257, 1966.
224. Naidich TP, Pinto RS, Kushner MJ, et al: Evaluation of sellar and parasellar masses by computed tomography. *Radiology* 120:91-99, 1976.
225. Nakagawa Y, Tsuru M: Studies on postoperative course of craniopharyngioma. *No To Shinkei* 23:993-1002, 1971.
226. Nakayama T, Kodama T, Matsukado Y: Treatment of inoperable craniopharyngioma with radioactive gold. *No To Shinkei* 23:509-513, 1971.
227. Northfield DWC: Rathke-pouch tumors. *Brain* 80:293-312, 1957.
228. Northfield DWC: *The Surgery of the Central Nervous System: A Textbook for Postgraduate Students*. Oxford, Blackwell Scientific, 1973, pp 314-327.
229. Obrador S, Blazquez MG: Pituitary abscess in craniopharyngioma: case report. *J Neurosurg* 36:785-789, 1972.
230. Olivecrona H: On suprasellar cholesteatomas. *Brain* 55-122-134, 1932.
231. Olivecrona H: Experiences with 107 cases of craniopharyngiomas. Excerpta Medica, International Congress Series No. 60, Second European Congress of Neurological Surgeons, Rome, 1961, pp 66-67, Abstract No. 40.
232. Olivecrona H: The craniopharyngiomas. In Olivecrona H, Tonnis W (eds): *Handbuch der Neurochirurgie*, Vol. IV/4.

233. Onoyama Y, Ono K, Yabumoto E, et al: Radiation therapy of craniopharyngioma. *Radiology* 125:799-803, 1977.
234. Patrick BS, Smith RR, Bailey TO: Aseptic meningitis due to spontaneous rupture of craniopharyngioma cyst: case report. *J Neurosurg* 41:387-390, 1974.
235. Pecker J, Guy G, Scarabin J: Third ventricle tumors. In *Handbook of Clinical Neurology*, Vol 12 part II. Amsterdam, pp 440-473, 1974.
236. Peet MM: Pituitary adamantinomas. *Arch Surg* 15:829-854, 1927.
237. Pennybacker J, Russell D: Necrosis of the brain due to radiation therapy: clinical and pathological observations. *J Neurol Neurosurg Psychiat* 11:183-198, 1948.
238. Pertuiset B: Craniopharyngiomas. In *Handbook of Clinical Neurology*, Vol. 18, part III. Amsterdam-New York, pp 531-572, 1975.
239. Petitto CK, Degirolami U, Earle MK: Craniopharyngiomas, a clinical pathologic review. *Cancer* 37:1944-1952, 1976.
240. Podochin L, Rolan L, Altman MM, Peyser E: 'Pharyngeal' craniopharyngioma. *J Laryngol Otol* 84:93-99, 1970.
241. Poletti CE, Ojemann RG: Stereo Atlas of Operative Neurosurgery. St. Louis, CV Mosby Co., 1985, pp 78-90.
242. Poppen JL: *An Atlas of Neurosurgical Techniques.* Philadelphia, W.B. Saunders Co., 1960, pp 122-125.
243. Post KD, Kasdon DL: Sellar and parasellar lesions mimicking adenoma. In Post KD, Jackson I, Reichlin S (eds): *The Pituitary Adenoma.* New York, Plenum, 1980, pp 159-216.
244. Prasad U, Kwi NK: Nasopharyngeal craniopharyngioma. *J Laryngol Otolaryngol* 89:445-452, 1975.
245. Raimondi AJ: *Pediatric Neuroradiology.* Philadelphia, W.B. Saunders, 1972, pp 571-590.
246. Rand RW: Transfrontal transsphenoidal craniotomy in pituitary and related tumors. In Rand RW (ed): *Microneurosurgery*, St. Louis, CV Mosby, 1978, pp 93-104.
247. Rand RW, Jannetta PJ: Microneurosurgery: application of the binocular surgical microscope in brain tumors, intracranial aneurysms, spinal cord disease, and nerve reconstruction. *Clin Neurosurg*, 15:319-342, 1968.
248. Rand RW, Konovalov AN: Craniopharyngiomas. In Rand RW (ed): *Microneurosurgery.* CV Mosby, St. Louis, 1985, pp 187-195.
249. Randall RV, Clark EC, Dodge HW Jr, Love JG: Polyuria after operation for tumors in the region of the hypophysis and hypothalamus. *J Clin Endocrinol* 20:1614-1621, 1960.
250. Randall RV, Laws ER Jr, Abboud CF: Clinical presentation of craniopharyngioma: A brief review of 300 cases. In Givens JR (ed): *The Hypothalmus.* Chicago, Year Book Medical Publishers, 1984, pp 335-347.
251. Randall RV, Scheithauer BW, Laws ER Jr, Abboud CF: Pseudoprolactinomas. *Trans Am Clin Climatolog Assoc* 94:114-121, 1982.
252. Raskind R, Brown HA, Mathis J: Recurrent cyst of the pituitary: 26 year follow-up from first decompression. Case report. *J Neurosurg* 28:595-599, 1968.
253. Rathke H: Ueber die entstchung der glandula pituitaria. *Arch Anat Physiol Wissensch Med* 5:482-486, 1838.
254. Ray BS: Surgery of recurrent intracranial tumors. *Clin Neurosurg* 10:1-30, 1964.
255. Ray BS: Intracranial operations on the pituitary (Audio Visual Education in Neurosurgery). The Society of Neurological Surgeons, Research Foundation, Inc., 1972.
256. Renn WH, Rhoton AL Jr: Microsurgical anatomy of the sellar region. *J Neurosurg* 43:288-298, 1975.
257. Rhoton AL Jr, Hardy DG, Chambers SM: Microsurgical anatomy and dissection of the sphenoid bone, cavernous sinus and sellar region. *Surg Neurol* 12:63-104, 1979.
258. Rhoton AL Jr, Harris FS, Renn WH: Microsurgical anatomy of the sellar region and cavernous sinus. *Clin Neurosurg* 24:54-85, 1977.
259. Rhoton AL Jr, Maniscalco J: Microsurgery of the sellar region. In Glaser JS (ed): *Neuro-ophthalmology*, Vol. IX. St. Louis, CV Mosby, 1977, pp 106-127.
260. Rhoton AL Jr, Yamamoto I, Peace DA: Microsurgery of the third ventricle: Part 2. Operative approaches. *Neurosurgery* 8:357-373, 1981.
261. Riccio A: Su di un caso di craniofaringioma del clivus. *Minerva Neurochir* 13:13-15, 1969.
262. Richmond IL, Wilson CB: Parasellar tumors in children. II. Surgical management, radiation therapy, and follow-up. *Childs Brain* 7:85-94, 1980.

263. Richmond IL, Wara WM, Wilson CB: Role of radiation therapy in the management of craniopharyngiomas in children. Neurosurgery 6:513-517, 1980.
264. Ringel SP, Bailey OT: Rathke's cleft cyst. J Neurol Neurosurg Psychiat 35:693-697, 1972.
265. Rosenberg D, David L, Bertrand J, Ruitton-Ugliego A, Lapras C, Picot C, Monnet P: Craniopharyngiome. Reprise de croissance apres l'intervention malgre deficit en hormone somatotrope. Arch Franc Pediat 27:355-369, 1970.
266. Ross Russell RW, Pennybacker JB: Craniopharyngioma in the elderly. J Neurol Neurosurg Psychiat 24:1-13, 1961.
267. Ross HS, Rosenberg S, Friedman AH: Delayed radiation necrosis of the optic nerve. Am J Ophthalmol 76:683-686, 1973.
268. Rostotskaya VI, Mareyeva TG, Nersesyants SI, Artaryan AA: Basic principles of surgical treatment of chiasmal-sellar-diencephalic tumors in children. Vopr Neirokhirurg 2:9-13, 1971. (in Russian)
269. Rougerie J: What can be expected from the surgical treatment of craniopharyngiomas in children. Report of 92 cases. Childs Brain 5:433-449, 1979.
270. Rougerie J, Fardeau M: Les Craniopharyngiomes. Masson et Cie, Paris, 1962.
271. Rougerie J, Raimondi AJ: Craniopharyngiomas. In Amador LV (ed): Brain Tumors in the Young. Springfield, IL, Charles C. Thomas, 1983, pp 599-621.
272. Rowbotham GF, Clarke PRR: Colloid cyst of the pituitary gland causing chiasmal compression. Br J Surg 44:107-108, 1956.
273. Rubinstein LJ: Tumors of the Central Nervous System: Atlas of Tumor Pathology, Series 2, Fascicle 6. Washington, DC, Armed Forces Institute of Pathology, 1972, p 293.
274. Rush JL, Kusske JA, deFeo DR, Pribram HW: Intraventricular craniopharyngioma. Neurology (Minn) 25:1094-1096, 1975.
275. Russell DS, Rubinstein LJ: Pathology of Tumors of the Nervous System, 4th edition. Baltimore, Williams & Wilkins, 1977.
276. Samaan NA, Bakdash MM, Cadero JB, Cangir A, Jesse RH, Balantyne AJ: Hypopituitarism after external irradiation—evidence for both hypothalamic and pituitary origin. Ann Intern Med 83:771-777, 1975.
277. Scarff JE: A new method for treatment of cystic craniopharyngioma by intraventricular drainage. Arch Neurol Psychiat (Chicago) 46:843-867, 1941.
278. Schachter T: A light and electron microscope study of Rathke's pouch in fetal rabbits. Gen Comp Endocrinol 14:53-67, 1970.
279. Seemayer TA, Blundell JS, Wigglesworth FW: Pituitary craniopharyngioma with tooth formation. Cancer 29:423-430, 1972.
280. Servo A, Puranen M: Moyamoya syndrome as a complication of radiation therapy. Case report. J Neurosurg 48:1026-1029, 1978.
281. Shalet SM, Beardwell CG: Endocrine consequences of treatment of malignant disease in childhood: A review. J Royal Soc Med 72:39-41, 1979.
282. Shanklin WH: On the presence of cysts in the human pituitary. Anat Rec 104:379-399, 1949.
283. Shanklin WM: The incidence and distribution of cilia in the human pituitary with a description of micro-follicular cysts derived from Rathke's cleft. Acta Anat 11:361-382, 1951.
284. Shanklin WH: The histogenesis and histology of an integumentary type of epithelium in the human hypophysis. Anat Rec 109:217-231, 1951.
285. Shapiro K, Till K, Grant DN: Craniopharyngiomas in childhood. A rational approach to treatment. J Neurosurg 50:617-623, 1979.
286. Sharma V, Tandon PN, Saxena KK, et al: Craniopharyngiomas treated by a combination of surgery and radiotherapy. Clin Radiol 25:13-17, 1974.
287. Shealy CN: Craniopharyngioma diagnosed after head trauma. Arch Neurol 13:217-218, 1965.
288. Shillito J Jr: The treatment of craniopharyngiomas of childhood. In Morley TP (ed): Current Controversies in Neurosurgery. Philadelphia, WB Saunders, 1976, pp 332-335.
289. Shillito J Jr: Craniopharyngiomas: the subfrontal approach, or none at all? Clin Neurosurg 27:188-205, 1980.
290. Shillito J Jr, Matson DD: Craniopharyngioma. In Shillito J, Matson DD (eds): An Atlas of Pediatric Neurosurgical Operations. Philadelphia, WB Saunders Co., 1982, pp 295-303.
291. Shuangshoti S, Netsky MG, Nashold BS: Epithelial cysts related to sella turcica: proposed origin from neuroepithelium. Arch Pathol Lab Med 90:444-450, 1970.

292. Shucart WA, Jackson I: Management of diabetes insipidus in neurosurgical patients. Neurosurgery 44:65-71, 1976.
293. Slooff ACJ, Slooff JL: Supratentorial tumours in children. In Vinken PJ, Bruyn GW (eds): *Handbook of Clinical Neurology*, Vol. 18. Amsterdam, North-Holland Publishing Co., 1975, pp 305-386.
294. Smith RA, Bucy PC: Pituitary cyst: Lined with a single layer of columnar epithelium. J Neurosurg 10:540-543, 1953.
295. Soffer D, Pittaluga S, Feiner M, et al: Intracranial meningiomas following low-dose irradiation to the head. J Neurosurg 59:1048-1053, 1983.
296. Sogg RL, Donaldson SS, Yorke CH: Malignant astrocytoma following radiotherapy of a craniopharyngioma. Case report. J Neurosurg 48:622-627, 1978.
297. Streja D, Teichner F, Marliss E: Fifty year survival after surgery for craniopharyngioma. JAMA 234:510-511, 1975.
298. Sung DI, Chang CH, Harisiadia L, Carmel PW: Treatment results of craniopharyngiomas. Cancer 47:847-852, 1981.
299. Susman W: Embryonic epithelial rests in the pituitary. Br J Surg 19:571-576, 1932.
300. Svien HJ: Experiences with craniopharyngiomas. J Neurosurg 23:148-155, 1965.
301. Svolos DG: Craniopharyngiomas. A study based on 108 verified cases. Acta Chir Scand (Suppl) 403:1-44, 1969.
302. Sweet WH: Radical surgical treatment of craniopharyngioma. Clin Neurosurg 23:52-79, 1976.
303. Sweet WH: Recurrent craniopharyngiomas: therapeutic alternatives. Clin Neurosurg 27:206-229, 1980.
304. Sweet WH: Craniopharyngiomas, with a note on Rathke's cleft or epithelial cysts and on suprasellar cysts. In Schmidek HH, Sweet WH (eds): *Operative Neurosurgical Techniques*. New York, Grune and Stratton, 1982, pp 291-325.
305. Symon L: The temporal approach for resection of craniopharyngioma. In Symon L (ed): *Operative Surgery: Neurosurgery*. London, Butterworth, 1979, pp 185-186.
306. Symon L: Operative surgery in craniopharyngiomas. In Edwards JMR (ed): *Topical Reviews in Neurosurgery*. Wright-PSG, Bristol/London/Boston, Vol. 1, 1982, pp 134-160.
307. Symon L, Logue V, Jakubowski J: The surgical treatment of craniopharyngioma. In Brock M (ed): *Modern Neurosurgery*. Berlin, Springer-Verlag, 1982, pp 187-192.
308. Symon L, Sprich W: Radical excision of craniopharyngioma. J Neurosurg 62:174-181, 1985.
309. Tabaddor K, Shulman K, Dal Canto MC: Neonatal craniopharyngioma. Am J Dis Child 128:381-383, 1974.
310. Takeda F, Tsunoda T, Sasaki R, Aiba T, Kawafuchi J: Hypothalamo-pituitary dysfunctions and their management in craniopharyngioma, chromophobe adenoma and suprasellar meningioma. Neurol Med Chir 12:155-158, 1972.
311. Taylor JC: Craniopharyngioma: a radiological technique for outlining the anatomy of large cysts. J Neurol Neurosurg Psychiat 34:105, 1971.
312. Thomsett MJ, Conte FA, Kaplan SL, et al: Endocrine and neurologic outcome in childhood craniopharyngioma: review of effect of treatment in 42 patients. J Pediatr 97:728-735, 1980.
313. Tiberin P, Goldberg GM, Schwartz A: Craniopharyngiomas in the aged. Neurology 8:51-54, 1958.
314. Till K: Craniopharyngiomas. Child's Brain 9:179-187, 1982.
315. Tinley F: The glands of the brain with special reference to the pituitary gland. Res Pub Assoc Nerv Ment Dis 17:1-12, 1938.
316. Toglia JU, Netsky MG, Alexander E: Epithelial (epidermoid) tumors of the cranium, their common nature and pathogenesis. J Neurosurg 23:384-393, 1965.
317. Torkildsen A: Should extirpation be attempted in cases of neoplasm in or near the third ventricle of the brain? Experiences with a palliative method. J Neurosurg 5:249-275, 1948.
318. Trippi AC, Garner JT, Kassabian JT, Shelden CH: A new approach to inoperable craniopharyngiomas. Am J Surg 118:307-310, 1969.
319. Trokoudes KM, Walfish PG, Holgate RC, Pritzker KPH, Schwartz ML, Kovacs K: Sellar enlargement with hyperprolactinemia and a Rathke's pouch cyst. JAMA 240:471-473, 1978.
320. Turkington RW: Secretion of prolactin by patients with pituitary and hypothalamic tumors. J Clin Endocrinol Metab 34:159-164, 1972.
321. Tytus JS, Seltzen HS, Kahn EA: Cortisone as aid in the surgical treatment of craniopharyngiomas. J Neurosurg 12:555-564, 1955.
322. Urdaneta N, Chessin H, Fischer JJ: Pituitary adenomas and craniopharyngiomas:

analysis of 99 cases treated with radiation therapy. *Int J Radiat Oncol Biol Phys* 1:895-902, 1976.
323. Van den Bergh R, Brucher JM: L'abord transventriculaire dans les craniopharyngiomes du troisieme ventricule. Aspects neuro-chirurgieaux et neuropathologiques. *Neuro-chirurgie* (Paris) 16:51-65, 1970.
324. Van Gilder JC, Inukai J: Growth characteristics of experimental intracerebrally transplanted oral epithelium. *J Neurosurg* 38:608-615, 1973.
325. Vladykova J: Kraniofaryngeom z hlediska oftalmologa. *Cesk Oftal* 29:109-116, 1973.
326. Waga S, Handa H: Radiation-induced meningioma: With review of literature. *Surg Neurol* 5:215-219, 1976.
327. Waltz TA, Bronwell B: Sarcoma: A possible late result of effective radiation therapy for pituitary adenoma. *J Neuosurg* 24:901-907, 1966.
328. Weiss SR, Raskind R: Non-neoplastic intrasellar cysts. *Int Surg* 51:282-288, 1969.
329. Wertheimer P, Corradi M: Les craniopharyngiomes apres 40 ans. Etude anatomo-clinique et resultats operatoires. (A propos de 18 observations). *Neurochirurgie* 3:3-21, 1957.
330. Wise BL, Brown HA, Naffziger HC, Boldrey EB: Pituitary adenomas, carcinomas, and craniopharyngiomas. *Surg Gynecol Obstet* 101:185-193, 1955.
331. Witt JA, MacCarty CS, Keating FR Jr: Craniopharyngioma (pituitary adamantinoma) in patients more than 60 years of age. *J Neurosurg* 12:354-360, 1955.
332. Wycis HT, Robbins R, Spiegel-Adolf M, Meszaros J, Spiegel EA: Studies in stereoencephalotomy. III. Treatment of a cystic craniopharyngioma by injection of radioactive P^{32}. *Confin Neurol* 14:193-202, 1954.
333. Yasargil MG: *Microsurgery*. Thieme, Stuttgart, 1969, pp 151-152.
334. Yoshida J, Kobayashi T, Kageyama N, Kanzaki M: Symptomatic Rathke's cleft cyst: Morphological study with light and electron microscopy and tissue culture. *J Neurosurg* 47:451-458, 1977.
335. Zenker FA: Enorme Cystenbildung im Gehirn, vom Hirnanhang ausgehend. *Virch Arch Path Anat Physiol und Klin Med* 12:454-466, 1857.
336. Zozulya AG, Patsko YaV, Shamayev MI: Topographic prerequisites for radical surgery for craniopharyngiomas. *Vopr Neirokhirug* 2:3-9, 1978. (in Russian)
337. Zulch KJ: *Brain Tumors: Their Biology and Pathology*, 2nd Amer Ed. New York, Springer-Verlag, 1965.

22

Meningiomas of the Sphenoid Wings

Joël Pierre Bonnal, M.D.
Jacques Brotchi, M.D.
Jacques Born, M.D.

Introduction

The sphenoid ridge is the second most common location for intracranial meningiomas.[36] Cushing and Eisenhardt[15] classified these meningiomas into three groups: tumors of the deep or clinoidal third, the middle ridge tumors, and the pterional tumors, again divided into two groups: "en plaque" or hyperostosing lesions of ala magna, and "global" or sylvian point tumors. Each of these locations have their anatomical connections and pathological extensions producing typical clinical signs and surgical problems. To get a better clinical and preoperative surgical assessment of these meningiomas, we should emphasize three remarks:

1. Clovis Vincent, and David and Mahoudeau showed that deep or clinoidal meningiomas usually involved the cavernous sinus.[16] They called them sphenocavernous meningiomas.

2. Grant classified basilar meningiomas into those with a narrow dural attachment, and those with a broad dural attachment. The former can be easily removed with minimal morbidity. Attempted total removal of the diffuse variety with the dura is very difficult and will usually result in crippling neurologic sequelae for the patient.[26]

3. In preceding publications, we have emphasized the great tendency of a meningioma "en masse" or "en plaque" of the sphenoid ridge which has a broad dural attachment, to be closely related to the internal carotid artery and cranial nerves, to invade the hyperostotic bone and the base of the skull, to spread into the dura of the anterior, middle, and posterior fossae, and finally to invade the craniofacial cavities.[5-7]

Fifteen microscopic pathological examinations of hyperostotic bone were performed: in 13 cases, the greater sphenoidal wings and the anterior clinoid process were invaded by the tumor. This has great surgical significance: "hyperostosing meningiomas" are truly *invading meningiomas* (Fig. 1).

Progress made in diagnosis and operative techniques enables us to approach these invading meningiomas in a more hopeful frame of mind from that of Grant or Castellano et al.[10,26] One of the contributions of Derome and Guiot was the description of a technique for a very

From: Sekhar LN, Schramm VL Jr, eds: *Tumors of the Cranial Base: Diagnosis and Treatment.* Mount Kisco, New York, Futura Publishing Co, Inc. © 1987.

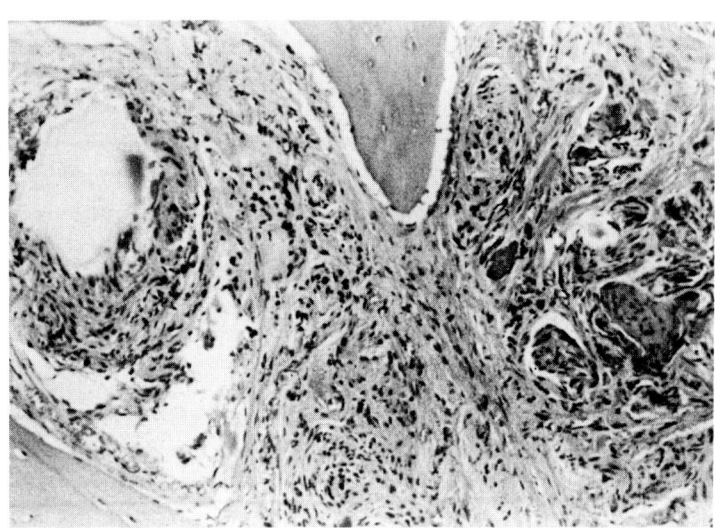

Figure 1: Histological study of the hyperostotic ala magna, showing meningiomatous cells in the bone.

wide removal of these lesions.[8,17,18,27,45] Various opinions have been expressed by different authors[6,11,12,20,24,28,36,44,47,55,57,62] showing that there is not yet agreement about the classification and treatment of these meningiomas. We will first describe three groups of invading meningiomas of the sphenoid ridge (Fig. 2): clinoidal or sphenocavernous meningiomas (group A, 15 cases), invading meningiomas of sphenoid wings en plaque (group B, 11 cases), and invading meningiomas of sphenoid wings en masse (group C, 11 cases). We will then describe two classic groups: middle ridge meningiomas (group D, 5 cases), and pterional global meningiomas or sylvian point tumors (group E, 10 cases). There are many technical problems in the first three groups (invading meningiomas) (37 cases), and fewer difficulties in the latter two groups.

Group A: Deep or Clinoidal or Sphenocavernous Meningiomas "En Masse"

These tumors extend upward into the cranial cavity from the dura of the cavernous sinus, the dura, the anterior clinoid process, or from the dura of the inner aspect of the sphenoidal wings. They are in close contact with the internal carotid artery and its branches (which are shifted, stretched, or embedded) and with the optic nerve and tract.[2] The total removal of this meningioma is difficult even with the help of magnification and ultrasonic aspiration. Bone is not involved except for the anterior clinoid process, nor are the craniofacial cavities involved. These meningiomas can spread intracranially to the midline, invading the dura of the tuberculum sellae and the dura of the clivus. We have sometimes observed meningiomas with a variable lateral extension from the dura of the cavernous sinus. These tumors compress the temporal lobe rather than the frontal lobe. The first category of Ojemann's sphenoid wing meningioma is the same as our group A. The second category is similar to our group B.[42]

Group B: Invading Meningioma "En Plaque" of the Sphenoid Wings

We prefer this term to "pterional tumors en plaque," or to "hyperostosing lesion of the ala magna" for two reasons: the meningiomatous cells invade the hyperostosing bone, and the meningioma spreads "en plaque" into the dura of the sphenoid wings and into the cavernous sinus. Very rarely the plaque can be limited to the dura of the anterior clinoid process. The internal carotid artery and its branches, the optic nerve, and the optic

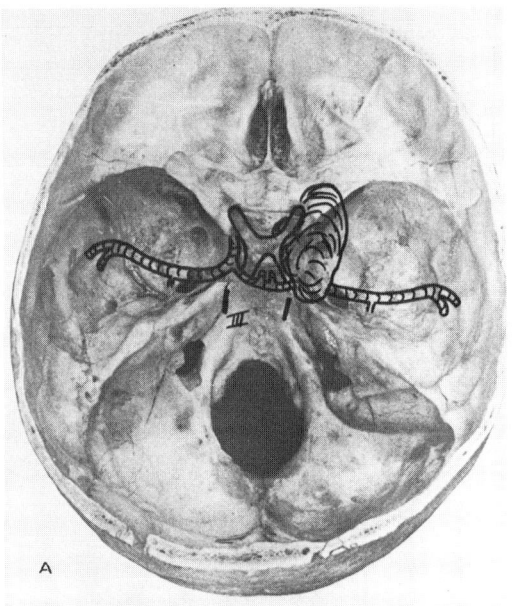 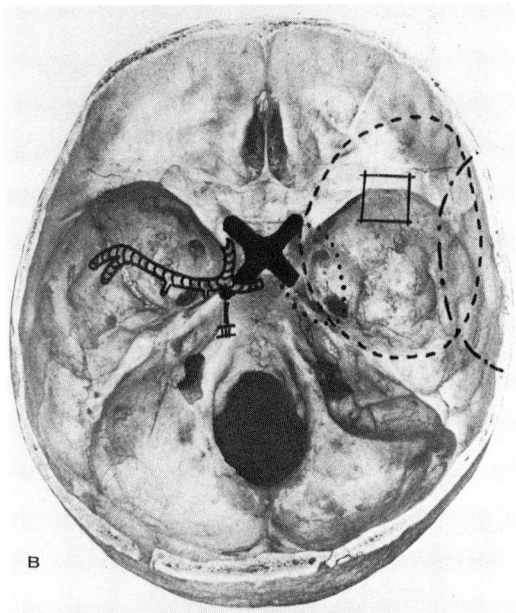

Figure 2A: Site of sphenocavernous meningioma group A and relationship with optic nerve and tract and internal carotid artery and its branches. **B:** Dural attachments of group A dotted line, of groups B and C dashed line, of group D solid line, group E dotted-dash line.

tract are not involved intracranially but in some cases the optic nerve is compressed within the optic canal. These tumors extend downward through the base of the skull. They penetrate into the craniofacial cavities, especially the orbit, and often the infratemporal fossa, pterygomaxillary fossa, parapharyngeal space, Eustachian tube, nasoethmoidal cavities, and the sphenoidal, frontal, and maxillary sinuses.[34] The extent of the invasion of the dura, bone, and craniofacial cavities limits the surgical possibilites.

Group C: Invading Meningiomas of Sphenoid Wings "En Masse"

This group combines the features of the two preceding groups.

Group D: Middle Ridge Tumors

These are not invasive meningiomas. Cushing described them as "meningiomas straddling the mid-sphenoidal ridge involving in varying degrees both frontal and temporal lobes; they have a surprisingly good surgical prognosis." These meningiomas can be readily removed because their dural attachment is small. In some instances, the dural attachment is situated deeper but remains small without close connections to the internal carotid artery and optic system. Then the surgical procedure remains easy.

Group E: Pterional Global Tumors or Sylvian Point Tumors

These meningiomas are attached to the external part of the sphenoid wings (pterion) at the level where the base of the skull ends and the vault begins, and the dural attachment is limited. These tumors compress the frontal and temporal lobes. They invade the bone minimally, more at the vault rather than the base. They can be totally removed without much difficulty.

Clinical Features

The different location of the meningiomas in each group explains the differences in clinical features.

Group A

These patients exhibited optic nerve or optic tract involvement with unilateral loss of vision, optic atrophy, and often hemianopsia. Oculomotor palsy was observed if the cavernous sinus was involved. Furthermore, frontal and temporal lobe compression caused seizures, especially temporal lobe epilepsy, and hemiparesis, aphasia, and intracranial hypertension.

Groups B and C

In these patients, the thickening of the sphenoid wings explained the early occurrence of unilateral exophthalmos, and sometimes a fullness of the temporal fossa. Later, we observed unilateral loss of vision with optic atrophy. Group C patients also presented with seizures, hemiparesis, aphasia, and intracranial hypertension. In these two groups, epistaxis indicated an invasion of frontal sinus or ethmoid cells by the tumor. A unilateral deafness might be due to compression of the Eustachian tube.

Group D

Only the signs of temporal and frontal lobe compression were present in this group. Epilepsy and intracranial hypertension were the first clinical features.

Group E

In addition to the signs of group D, these patients presented with fullness of the frontotemporal areas, sometimes with prolonged and localized pain.

Early diagnosis of all groups may lead to improved outcome.[30]

Radiologic Findings

At present, computed tomography (CT) with and without contrast injection enables us not only to diagnose the presence of meningiomas but also to determine their extension within or beyond the skull. In particular, one has to look for the extension of "en plaque" and "en masse" meningiomas into the orbit and the extracranial fossae. The increase in volume of the cavernous sinus should point towards its invasion especially if an oculomotor deficit exists. However, it is only during the surgical procedure that this suspicion can be confirmed. CT scanning also reveals the presence of peritumoral edema.[51] According to Fine et al.,[23] the occurrence of the edema appears to be related in part to the location of tumor in the middle cranial fossa and its proximity to the major venous pathways of this area.[23] Finally, CT scanning, plain skull films, and tomography reveal the presence of hyperostosis of the sphenoid wings. They pinpoint the limits of tumoral extension to the anterior clinoidal process, lateral portion of sphenoid body, sphenoid fissure, and orbital roof. Opacification of the sphenoid sinus or of ethmoid cells is a probable sign of their invasion. Internal carotid angiography is essential to determine the relationship between the tumor and the carotid-sylvian axis. This investigation shows stretching, displacement, narrowing, or even an occlusion of the artery (Fig. 3). It remains difficult to predict with certainty the relationships between meningiomas and vessels. However, when one of these angiographic appearances is associated with an ipsilateral loss of vision or optic atrophy, one is probably dealing with a deeply situated meningioma which surrounds the arteries.[13,19] Intracranial occlusion of the internal carotid artery has been observed by several authors.[33,41,52,53] An occlusion of the middle cerebral artery was observed in two of our cases (Fig. 4). External carotid angiography often reveals the precise blood supply of the tumor and enables us to consider if preoperative embolization is necessary.

Diagnosis of Extension

The clinical signs and the neuroradiological findings greatly increase our

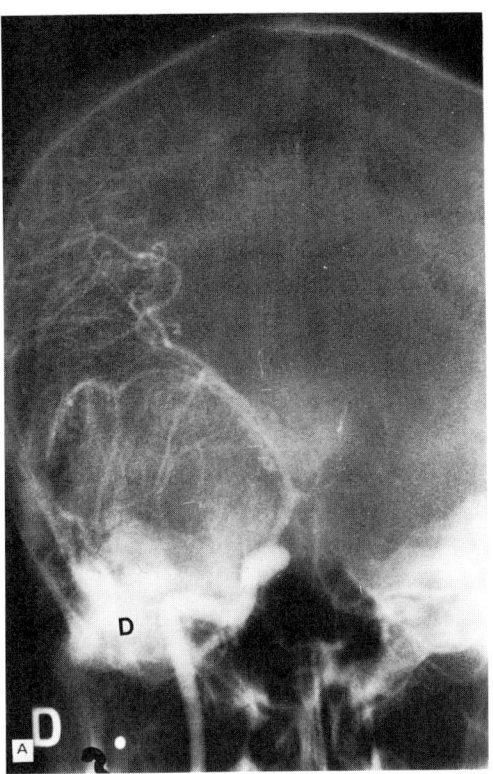

Figure 3: Carotid angiography AP view **(A)** and lateral view **(B)**. Sphenocavernous meningioma group A. Internal carotid and middle cerebral arteries were stretched, shifted and narrowed. The microsurgical dissection was difficult, the arteries were almost surrounded.

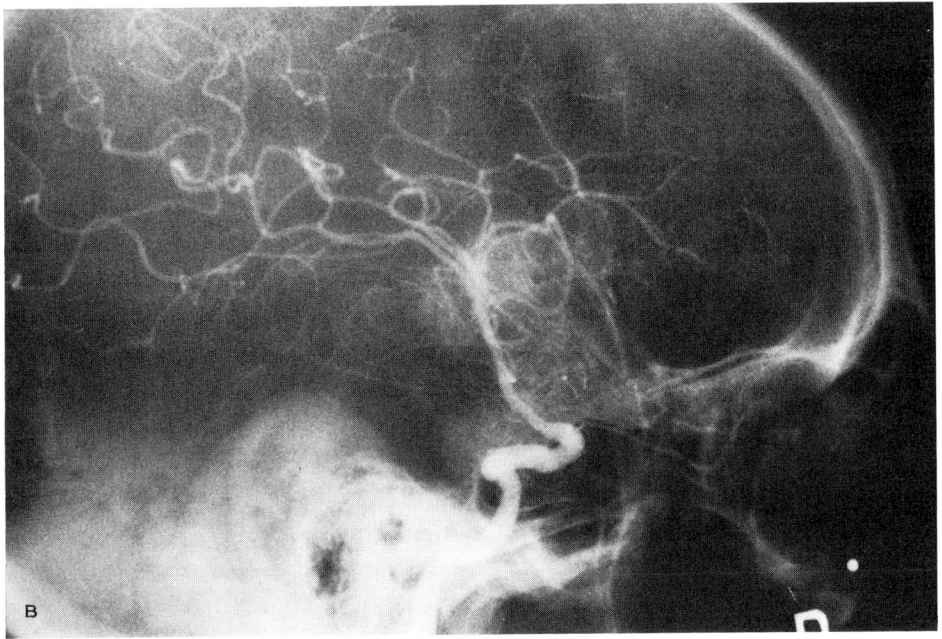

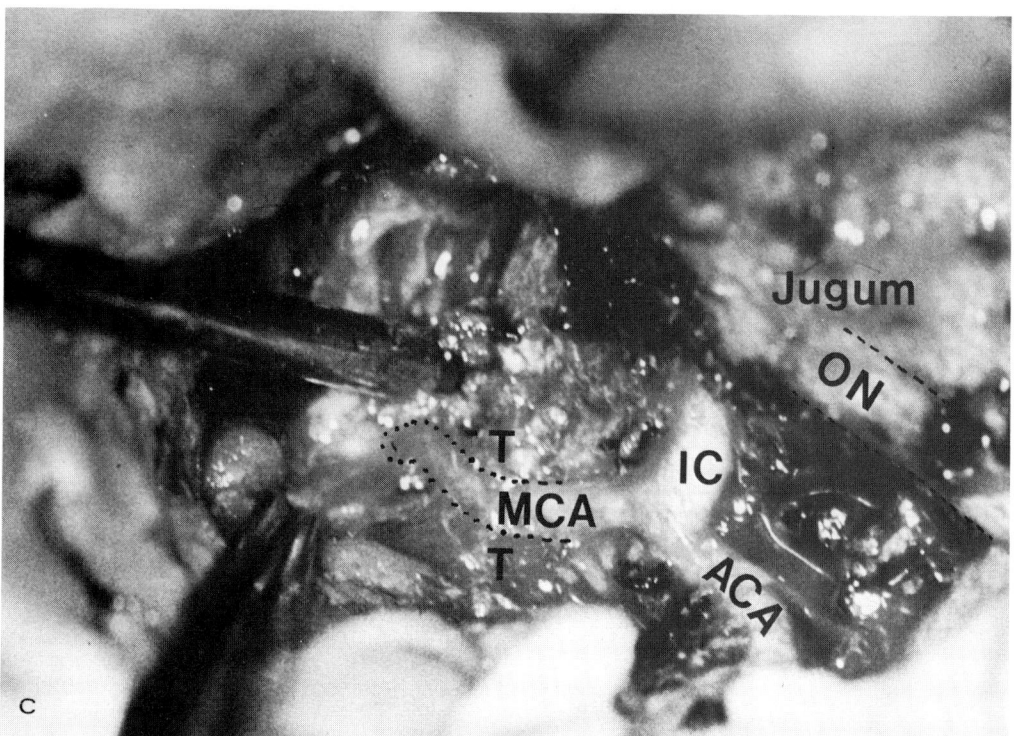

Figure 3C: Operative view shows the internal carotid (IC) and the middle cerebral (MCA) arteries in the meningioma. Anterior cerebral artery (ACA); optic nerve, (ON); tumor (T); jugum sphenoidale (Jugum).

knowledge of the tumor's arterial and neural relationships and the extent of their spread into the dura, the skull base, and the extracranial cavities. This knowledge is necessary to plan the best surgical technique and to be in a position to perform the most complete removal of the tumor. However, the surgical findings and the postoperative follow-up examinations are the best means of judging the extent of these invading meningiomas and our surgical efficiency. Tables I, II, III, and IV give our personal experience of these extensions.

Surgical Technique

Surgical Approach

We used a frontotemporal pterional approach similar to but more extensive than the one described by Yasargil for intracranial aneurysms.[35,48] The patient is placed in the supine position with the head raised and rotated about 45° to the opposite side. The vertex is lowered a little to permit a better approach to the base of the skull. The skin incision extends behind the normal hair line, beginning beyond the midline of the head and ending in front of the ear at the level of the zygoma. The frontotemporal craniotomy has to be as basal as possible to allow a direct view to the floor of the frontal and temporal intracranial fossae so that the orbit can be easily opened. In group A, the craniotomy extends more frontally near the midline. In groups B, C, and E, the external pterional bone can be very thick and the craniotomy more difficult, with more bleeding. First we remove the external part of the invaded bone until a communication between the orbit and the frontal and temporal fossae is achieved.

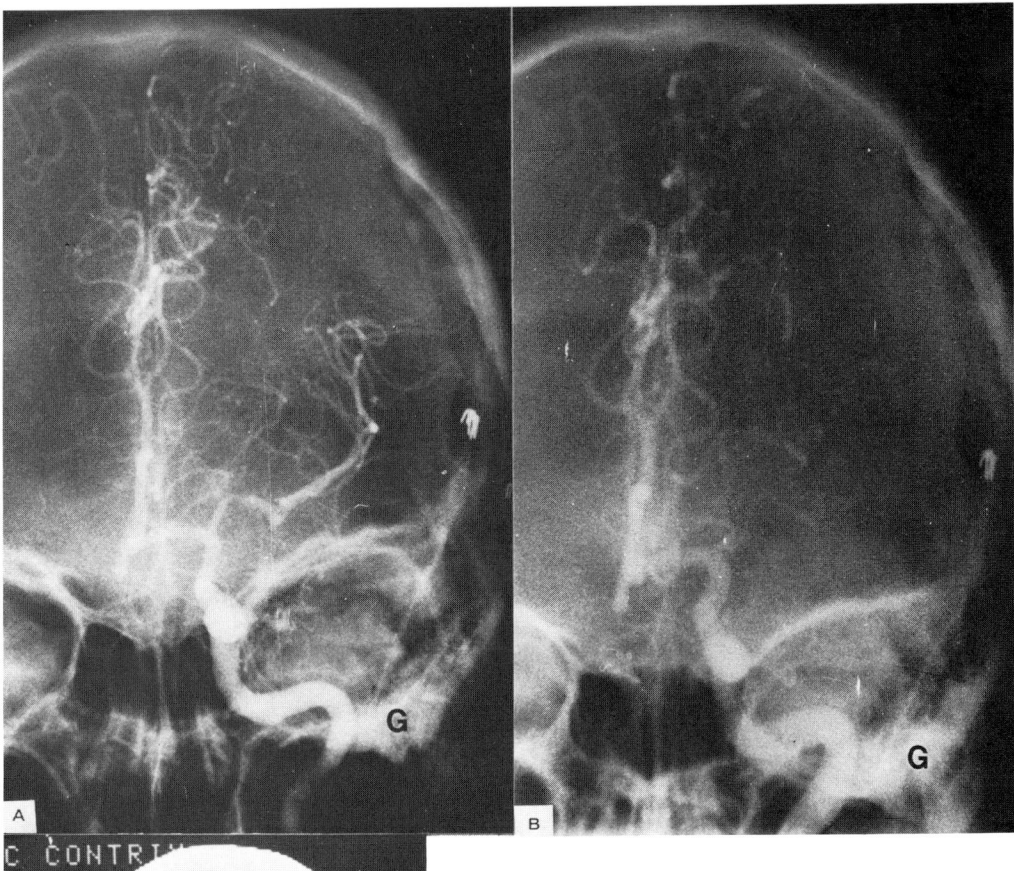

Figure 4: In 1974, carotid angiography **(A)** showed a narrowing of middle cerebral artery. In 1977, carotid angiography **(B)** showed the occlusion of middle cerebral artery by a sphenocavernous deep or clinoidal meningioma **(C)**.

The Tumor and its Arterial Relationships

In groups A and C, the only way to remove these tumors without fear of arterial injury is to begin the intradural surgical procedure by dissecting the distal part of the middle cerebral artery in the sylvian fissure under the surgical microscope. The middle cerebral artery is followed medially to the internal carotid artery, removing the tumor piecemeal, and dissecting the tumor away from the arteries. The dural attachment of the tumor should

Table I
Arterial Involvement by Meningioma in this Series

Involvement	ICA	MCA	ACA
stretched, compressed, or half surrounded	12	17	6
embedded	12	4	4
obstructed or invaded	0	2	0
total			
Groups A & C (26 cases)	24	23	10
Group B (11 cases)	0	0	0

ICA = internal carotid artery; MCA = middle cerebral artery; ACA = anterior cerebral artery.

Table II
Invasion of Basilar Dura by Meningiomas in This Series*

Feature Involved	Group A ($n=15$)	Group B ($n=11$)	Group C ($n=11$)
cavernous sinus	13	6	7
sella turcica dura	6	1	4
anterior fossa dura beyond midline	7	2	2
clivus	4	0	1

*For a description of patient groups, see text.

Table III
Invasion of Skull by Meningiomas in This Series*

Area of Skull Invaded	Group A	Group B	Group C
anterior clinoid process	8	8	9
optic foramen	0	6	6
ala magna	0	11	11
lateral portion of sphenoid body	0	4	6
sphenoid fissure	0	7	7
orbital roof	0	10	9
ethmoid bone	0	1	4
pterional bone	0	6	4
malar bone	0	1	1

*For a description of patient groups, see text.

not be exposed before having first dissected the internal carotid artery. During microsurgical dissection, we can distinguish the cases in which arteries are entirely embedded in tumor from those in which arteries are only shifted, stretched and compressed or partially surrounded. In the last case, the tumor remains separate from the artery in the arachnoidal plane. Arterial microdissection enables us to coagulate and cut close to the main arterial trunk without traction of the small arterial branches feeding the tumor. It is necessary to preserve the perforating vessels, the lenticulostriate arteries, and the anterior choroidal artery, but not always the posterior communicating artery. The Cavitron Ultrasonic Aspirator (CUSA)* is a useful tool to dissect the tumor away from these arteries. In two of our cases, preoperative angiography showed that the middle cerebral trunk was obstructed. In one case in which the meningioma invaded the wall and lumen of the middle

*Cooper Laser Services, Inc., Stamford, Conn.

Table IV
Invasion of Intra- and Extracranial Fossae by Meningiomas in This Series*

Fossae	Group A (n=15)	Group B (n=11)	Group C (n=11)	Group D (n=5)	Group E (n=10)
Intracranial fossae					
anterior	12	9	11	4	5
middle	13	11	11	4	8
posterior	7	0	3	0	0
Extracranial fossae					
orbit	0	7	7	0	0
Zinn's annulus	0	4	3	0	0
extratemporal region	0	7	4	0	0
infratemporal region	0	4	3	0	0
Eustachian tube	0	1	0	0	0
frontal sinus	0	1	3	0	0
ethmoid cells	0	1	2	0	0

*For description of patient groups, see text.

cerebral artery, the vessel was clipped without postoperative hemiplegia. In another case, we injured an embedded carotid artery at the origin of a branch, but gentle pressure with Surgicel and cottonoids permitted us to obtain a good hemostasis without any postoperative problems. In all the other cases, the arterial dissection ended without injury, but was limited by the basilar dura. The arterial dissection was never carried into the cavernous sinus. The removal of the tumor proceeds piecemeal with the help of electrical cautery or the CUSA. We protect the cerebral cortex and its vessels as much as possible. This is accomplished by grasping the arachnoid membranes on the tumor's surface with forceps, and detaching the tumor from the brain, coagulating and dividing several bridging vessels.

Optic Nerve and Tract

During the dissection of the internal carotid artery and the anterior cerebral artery, the ipsilateral optic nerve and tract were seen and easily separated from the meningioma. The optic nerve and tract were shifted and compressed but rarely embedded in the tumor. In two cases where dura of the tuberculum and the diaphragma sellae was invaded, the ipsilateral optic nerve was embedded in the meningioma.

Invasion of the Basilar Dura (Fig. 5)

It is quite easy to remove "en masse," mobile, noninvasive meningiomas with a narrow dural attachment. They should be distinguished from meningiomas with a large dural extension and with invasion of hyperostotic bone. Most of this invaded dura must be resected but we have never attempted to excise the portion invading the cavernous sinus and the dura of the sella turcica. There was frequent involvement of the cavernous sinus. In three cases, the sinus was swollen, had lost its normal shape, and was totally invaded. We believe that opening the sinus to remove the meningioma is not only insufficient to obtain a complete removal but also leads to oculomotor palsy and even carotid injury. Fortunately, in many cases, only the sinus walls seemed to be involved and we carefully coagulated them. The invasion of the dura of the sella turcica and clivus is best handled by very cautious coagulation avoiding injury to the optic chiasm and the pituitary stalk. In 10 cases, a large bud of meningioma extended into the posterior fossa through the tentorial notch. It was always easily removed.

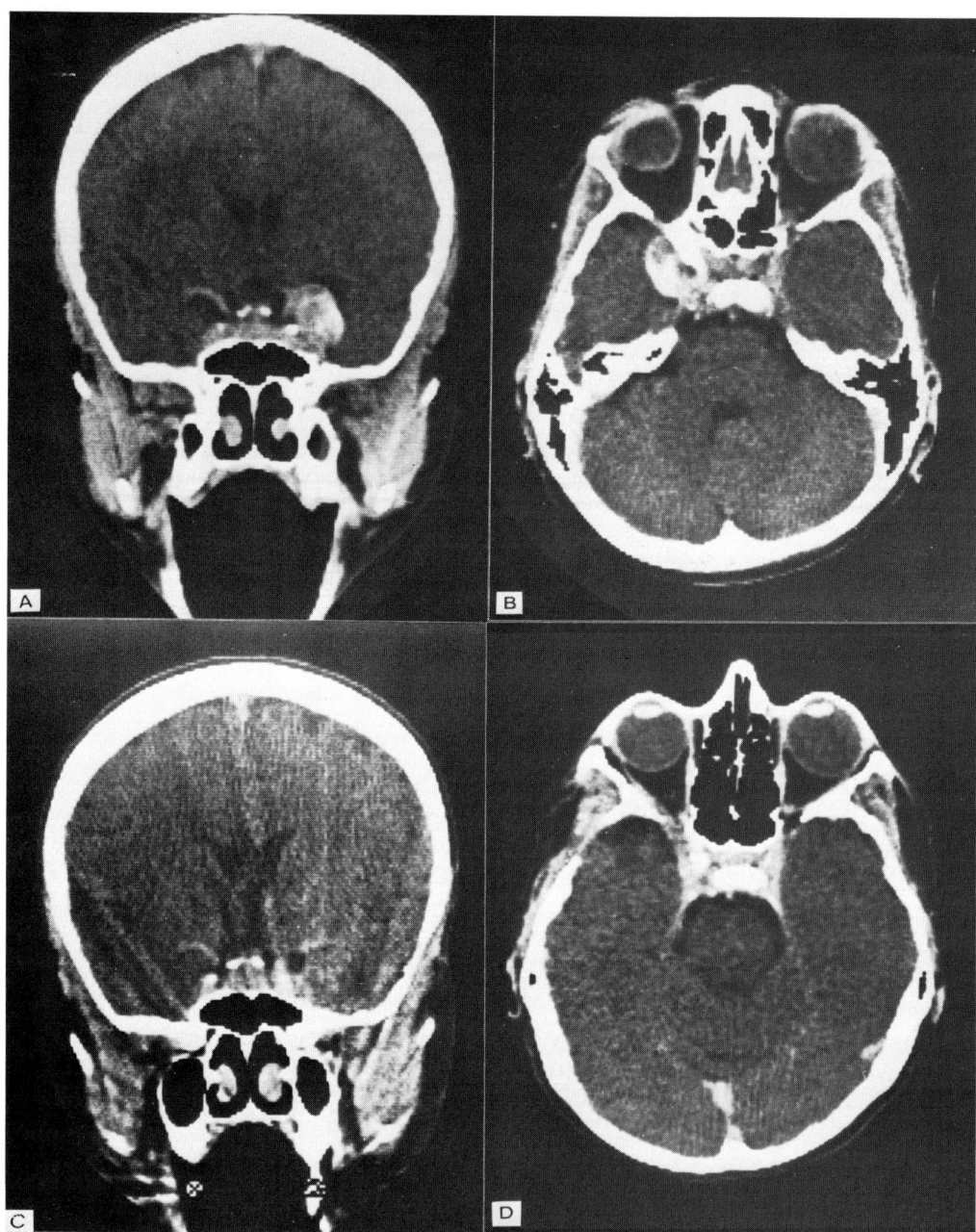

Figure 5: Sphenocavernous meningioma with hyperostotic anterior clinoid process. **A,B:** preoperative CT scans. **C,D:** postoperative CT scans. All CT scans were performed with contrast.

Invasion of the Base of the Skull (Figs. 6–10)

In groups B and C, the greater sphenoidal wing was always involved often from the pterion to the sphenoid body. We removed it in 16 cases, opening the foramen rotundum, the foramen ovale, and the sphenoid fissure, but we could not remove the glenoid cavity of the temporomandibular joint and the lateral part of the sphenoid body medial to the fora-

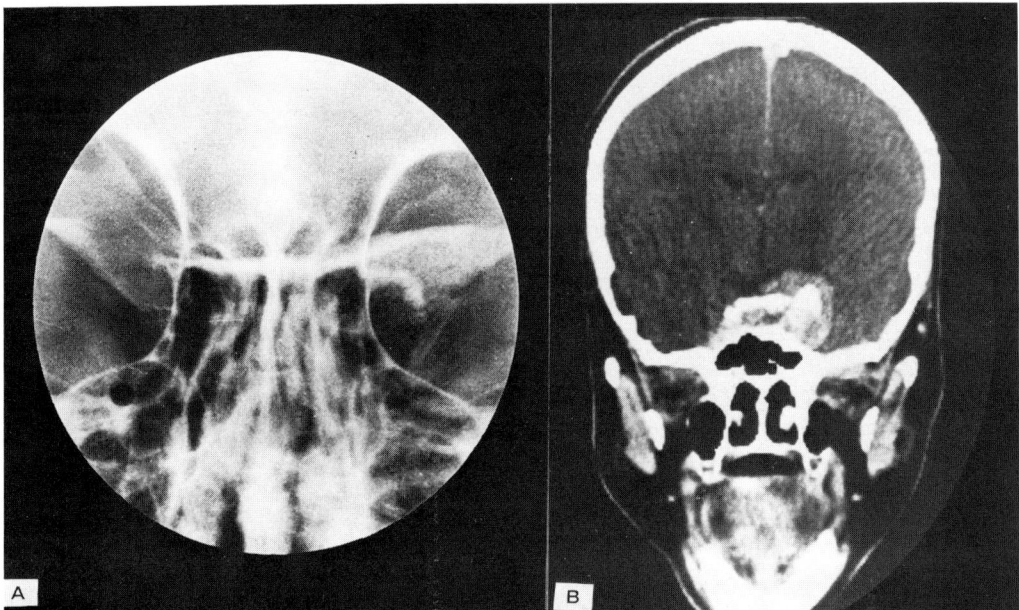

Figure 6: Sphenocavernous meningioma with hyperostotic anterior clinoid process. **A:** Plain radiograph. **B:** coronal CT scan with contrast.

men ovale and the foramen rotundum. The roof of the orbit was most often invaded, sometimes as far as the optic foramen and the frontal sinus. The anterior clinoid process involved in 17 cases had to be removed with the help of a high speed drill so as to open the optic foramen and to remove its bony walls thus completely forcing the optic nerve. Special problems were due to the invasion of the planum ethmoidale and the tuberculum sellae. In contrast, the invasion of the supraorbital arch was observed only exceptionally during surgery and it was seldom necessary to remove it, an important fact from a cosmetic point of view. The maxillary and the zygomatic bones were seldom involved except in pterional global meningiomas.

Invasion of Craniofacial Cavities

The presence of meningiomas "en plaque" or "en masse" on each side of a thickened bone was proof of the invasion of this bone. Broad removal of the invaded sphenoid wings and of the orbital roof afforded a wide approach to the orbit (which was invaded in 14 cases in groups B and C), and to the infratemporal and zygomatic fossae. Operating with the help of the microscope, we carefully removed the tumor in the orbit, often totally, without injuring the ocular muscles and nerves. The adhesion of the meningioma to Zinn's common tendinous ring is a limiting factor to surgery. The removal of this ring destroys the motility and the stability of the eye. Enucleation was not indicated unless vision was totally lost. Mass extensions into the infratemporal, pterygomaxillary, and zygomatic fossae can be seen on preoperative CT scans and on external carotid angiograms. Their partial removal was carried out, following the course of the mandibular and the maxillary nerves, to avoid injuring them. The temporal muscle and the pterygoid muscle were involved. In one case, the extracranial meningioma spread to the Eustachian tube, but this extension was not removed. In this case, embolization of the branches of the external carotid artery feeding the meningioma yielded a good result without loss of blood during surgery. In three

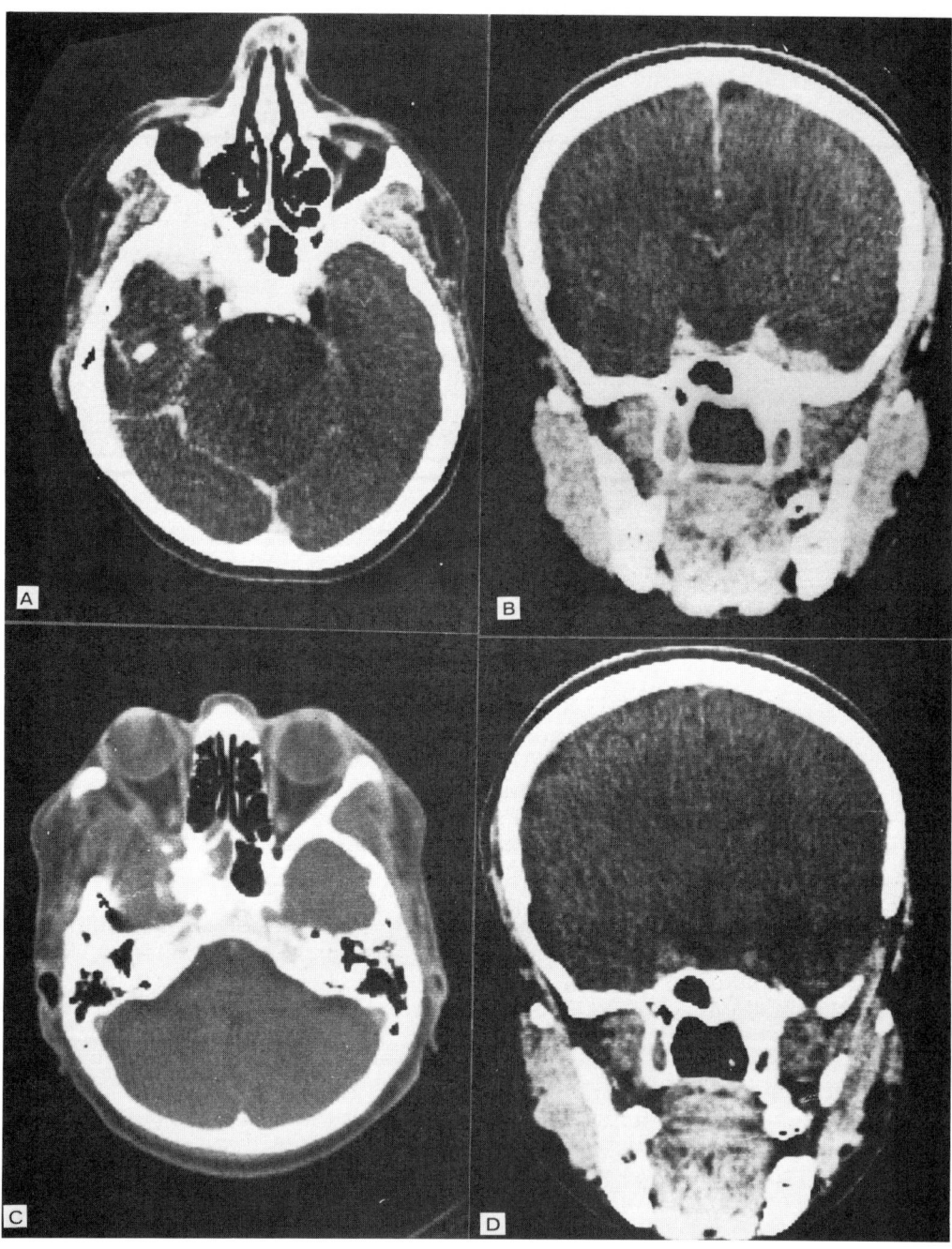

cases, a bud of the meningioma was removed in the frontal sinus. If the wall of this sinus seemed invaded on the X-ray films or on the CT scan, we always opened the sinus and found the meningioma within. In two cases, the tuberculum sellae, nasoethmoidal cells, and sphenoid body were seen to be invaded in the preoperative neuroradiological studies, so we performed a second surgical procedure using the Derome and Giuot's technique with a combined bifrontal and transnasal approach.[18] When the meningioma spread into the lower part of the orbit and into pterygomaxillary fossa, Basso et al. used, in addition to the pteri-

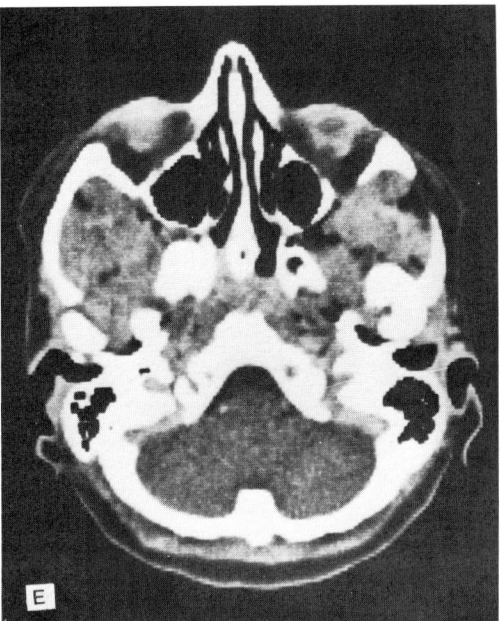

Figure 7: Invading meningioma en plaque group B. Preoperative **(A,B)** and postoperative **(C,D,E)** CT scans show the limits of operability and the hyperostotic lateral part of the sphenoid body **(A,C)** and the hyperostotic base of pterygoid process **(B,D,E)**.

onal approach, a temporary resection of malar bone, while Pellerin et al. used an orbito-fronto-malar approach with removal of the superior orbital edge.[4,43] In these cases, reconstruction of the orbital walls is necessary to obtain a good cosmetic result.

Dural and Bone Reconstruction

A dural graft is always necessary after removal of such invading meningiomas. We used fascia lata rather than pericranial tissue or lyophilized dura for the reconstruction. Bone reconstruction is not always necessary, if only the sphenoid wings are resected. We observed few poor cosmetic results when the orbital arch was conserved, as is usually possible. However, if bone resection was very large, reconstruction was done with iliac bone. Postoperative infections were rare in our experience. These are frequent with lengthier operative procedures and with the opening of craniofacial cavities.

Adjunctive Techniques

Preoperative embolization can be useful because sphenoid wing meningiomas are tumors in which many feeding vessels can be reached only after removal of the tumor.[46] In fact, any large convexity or sphenoid wing meningioma may benefit from external carotid embolization[29,39] and it is particularly helpful in patients who are high anesthetic risks or whose meningioma has invaded bone and soft tissue.[58] Fukui et al. recommended preoperative radiation for highly vascular meningiomas.[25] When nerves or vessels are stretched or embedded, the laser or CUSA may be useful.[56] We have no personal experience with the laser but, as stated by Bartal and associates, at sites where bone is infiltrated by the tumor, the beam bares the bone at high power and erodes it to the desired depth.[3] This could be helpful to resect as much bone as possible. On the other hand, to remove the interior of the tumor, the laser doesn't seem superior to ultrasonic aspiration which allows safe removal of the tumor parenchyma with sparing of adjacent vessels. When a bud of meningioma lies between carotid artery and optic tract, there is an obvious advantage to using ultrasonic aspiration, as well as when a vessel is stretched or embedded by the tumor. A limitation to the use of ultrasonic aspiration is the hardness of the tumor. Very rarely, the invading meningioma is so huge that the carotid artery cannot be spared. In that situation, it is convenient to perform an extra-intracranial bypass prior to dissecting the carotid artery, but this procedure does not absolutely protect against hemiplegia as reported by Fardoun et al.[22]

Natural History and Operative Results

Meningiomas are generally benign, well circumscribed, and slow-growing

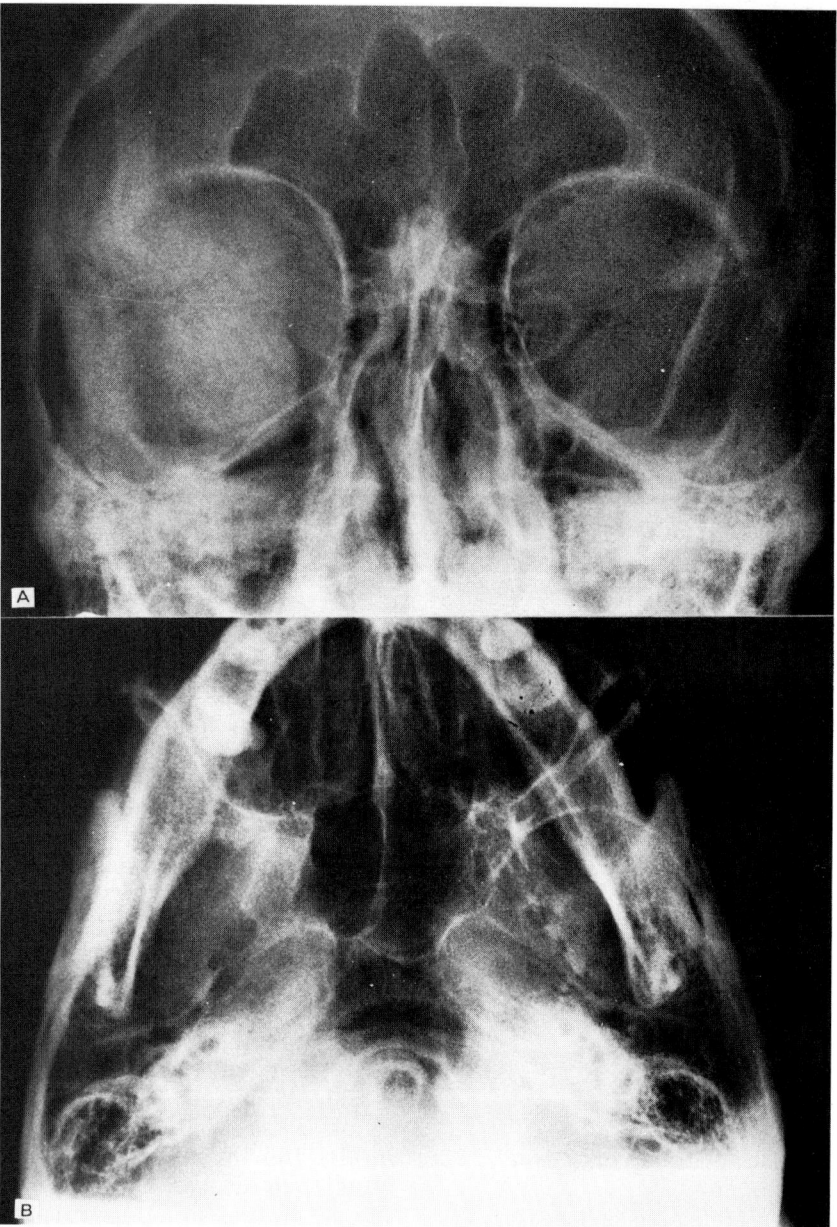

Figure 8: Invading meningioma of sphenoid wing en plaque. Preoperative **(A,B)** and postoperative **(C,D)** x-ray films show the total removal of hyperostotic bone, as in Fig. 10A.

tumors. However, they can be accompanied by extensive hyperostosis, or encasement of major blood vessels or they may grow to massive proportions preventing a total surgical removal. Even in cases where advanced age or the wide extension of the lesion contraindicate surgery, patient survival is very long (5 to 22 years in our five cases). The main disability is loss of one eye on the invaded side by enucleation, blindness, and oculomotor palsy. However, some of these tumors produce intracranial hypertension, neurological deficit, or seizures which oblige the neurosurgeon to have a more aggressive attitude, especially when the patient is a

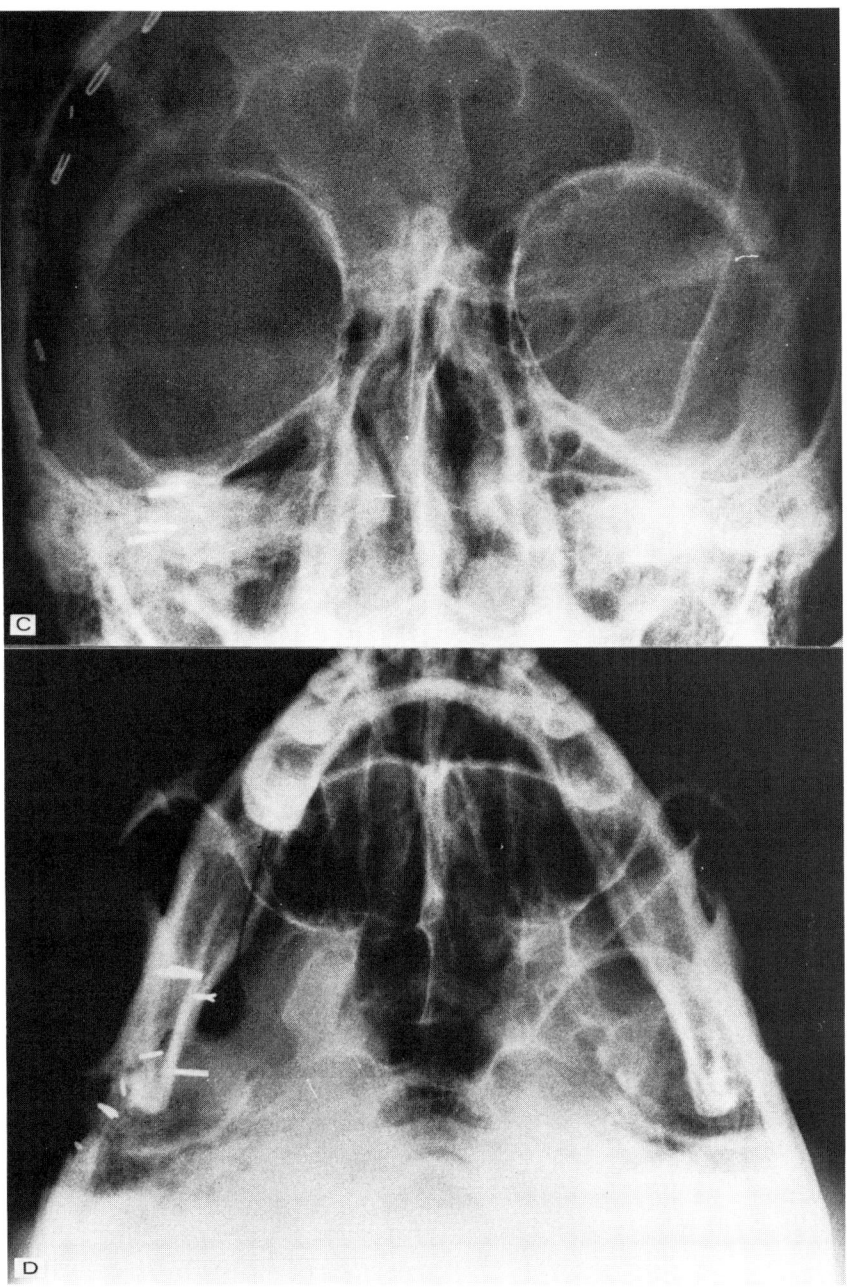

young adult. Postoperative mortality is low in our series (7.7%) and was observed only in group A. Our aim has been to demonstrate that a total or at least a wide removal with conservation of ocular function gave better results than partial resection. On the other hand, partial excisions do not obviate a continuing evolution of the disease, and afford no additional benefit for the patients as compared to the avoidance of surgery. Five to ten years after a total or near-total removal of meningiomas, follow-up CT scans showed three cases with recurrence, and

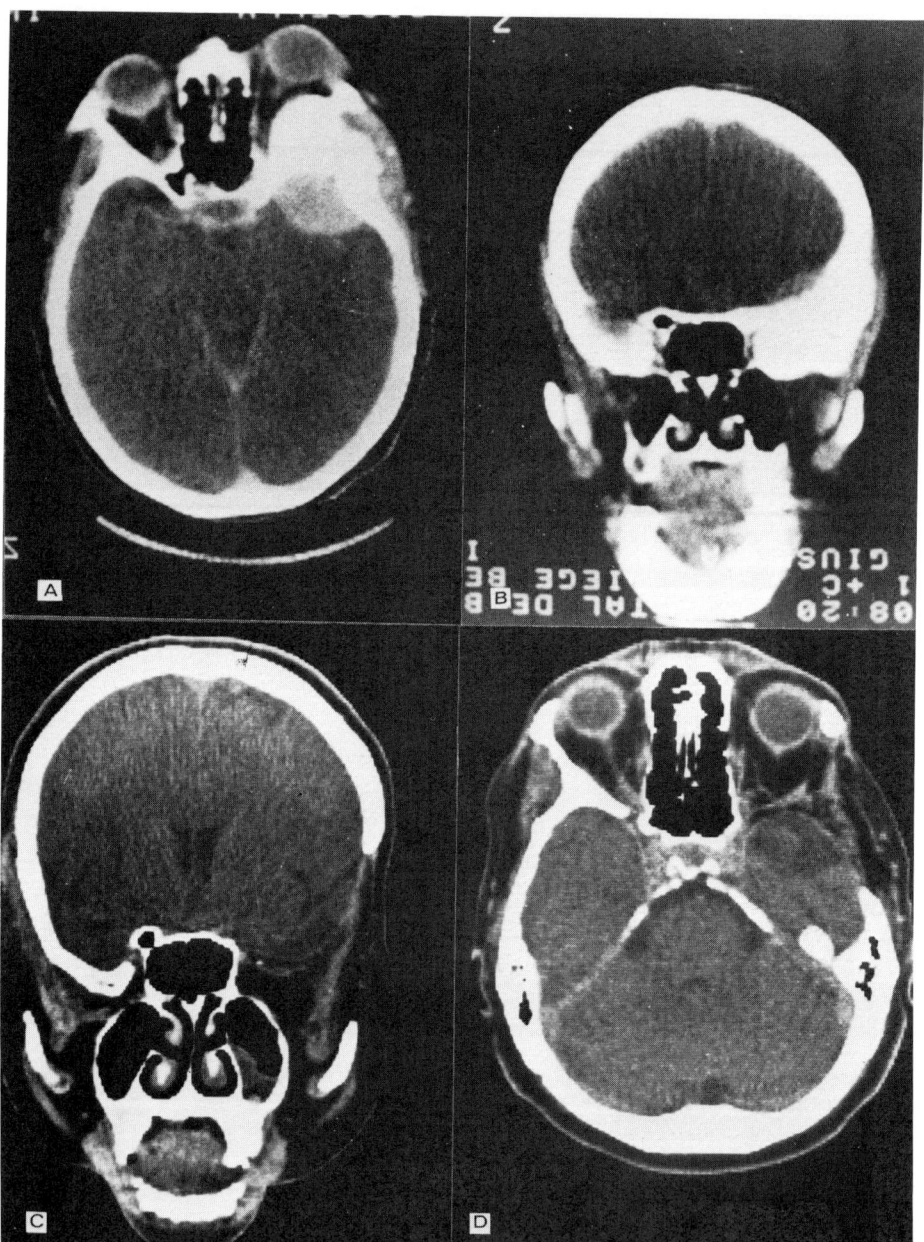

Figure 9: Invading meningioma of sphenoid wing en masse. Preoperative **(A,B)** and postoperative **(C,D)** CT scans show the total removal of the meningioma and the hyperostotic bone.

eight cases without any evidence of recurrence and any evidence of evolution of the hyperostotic lateral part of the sphenoid body. Nevertheless, we observed two cases with multiple meningiomas and von Recklinghausen's disease. Even in these cases, repeated wide excision gave us long survival without serious sequelae. With improvements of our surgical technique and with postoperative radiotherapy, we can hope for better results.

The Problem of Recurrence: Radiotherapy?

First of all, it is necessary to distinguish a recurrence from a residual tumor.

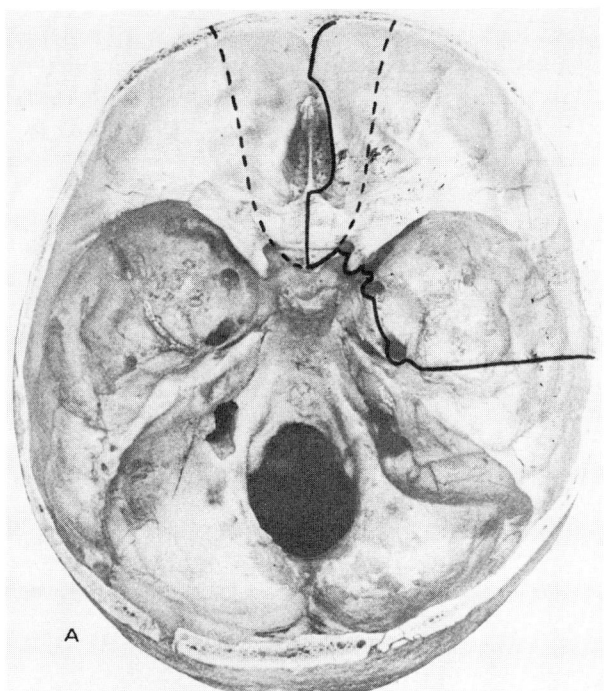

Figure 10A: The portion of the skull base delimited by the solid line is removed through basilar pterional frontotemporal craniotomy. The midline part of the skull base delimited by the broken line is removed with Derome and Guiot's technique.

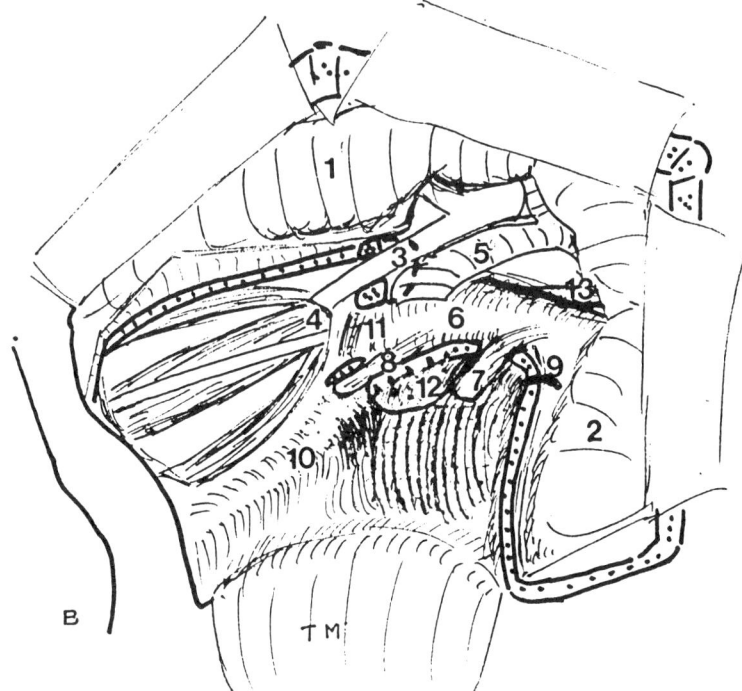

Figure 10B: Surgical sketch after removal of an invading meningioma of the sphenoid ridge (groups B and C); the superior and external walls of the orbit, the anterior clinoid process (3), and the temporal base of the skull have been removed. Optic foramen (3), superior sphenoid fissure (11), inferior sphenoid fissure (10), foramen rotundum (8), foramen ovale (7), and foramen spinosum (9) have been opened. The optic nerve (3), the internal carotid artery (5), the oculomotor nerve (13), the cavernous sinus (6), the V_2 (8) and V_3 (9), the muscles of the orbit, Zinn's common tendinous ring (4), the lateral part of the sphenoid body (12), and the base of the pterygoid process (12) are visible.

Early postoperative CT scanning is very helpful. Following tumor removal, it allows early recognition of tumor recurrence.[38,49,50] Hence, CT scanning is not only important in making an early diagnosis of meningioma prior to the first operation but it is also useful in follow-up assessment and in recognizing early tumor recurrence.[9] It is important to remove as much tumor as possible during the first operation. Tumor removal should be as radical as is safe for the patient.[37] Reoperations are possible, but the dissection of nerves and vessels is more difficult. The anterior clinoidal process has to be resected every time even if normal, in types A, B, and C, because recurrence will start from that point. In their series of 225 patients with meningioma who underwent surgery as the only treatment modality between 1962 and 1980, Mirimanoff et al. stated that among the sphenoid ridge meningiomas (which represent 16% of their series), only 28% were totally resected.[40] These meningiomas have the highest risk of recurrence or progression at 5 and 10 years (34% and 54%). The role of radiation therapy in meningioma treatment is still controversial. It is recommended by some authors following subtotal removal of a benign meningioma.[59,60] On the other hand, King et al.[31] were unable to demonstrate any benefit of radiotherapy in reducing the rate of recurrence. This is not the opinion of Wara et al. who advocated a tumor dose at least 5000 rads for incomplete meningioma resection and certain previously nonirradiated recurrent tumors and also preoperatively in a attempt to improve resectability of certain highly vascular meningiomas.[60] Carella et al. gave an usual dose of 5000–6000 rads. In their experience, radiotherapy is effective in cases of incomplete resection and recurrence, even when histology reveals a malignant meningioma.[9] In spite of the opinion of Yanashita, who stated that radiotherapy for recurrent meningioma is of little value, we believe that it must be added to surgery when it is obviously impossible to perform a total resection without sequelae or when recurrence is invading inoperable sites (cavernous sinus, sella turcica, common tendinous ring of Zinn, pterygomaxillary fossa, lateral part of sphenoid body and pterygoid process). Radiosurgery or proton beam therapy are perhaps interesting tools for the future, according to the experience of Steiner et al. and Kjellberg et al., but at present it is too early to draw any conclusion about the effect of these techniques on the remaining bud of tumor, for example, when cavernous sinus is invaded.[32,54] The problem of recurrence is also linked to the histological types.[49] Crompton and Gautier-Smith suggested that syncytial meningiomas are most likely to recur and fibroblastic meningiomas the least likely, but the results of Adegbite et al. directly contradict that finding.[11,14] High cellularity was found more frequently among recurring tumors as was an increase in mitotic figures.[1,50]

The Future

Newer tools will probably provide a better resection of these invading meningiomas. Newer therapy will help to control growth in those patients with incomplete removal. One can hope that the high concentration of estrogen-receptor protein found in some meningiomas[21] will permit another approach to their treatment. However, at present, one must recognize that complete resection of invading meningiomas of the sphenoid ridge remains a challenge.

ACKNOWLEDGMENT: *The autnors are grateful to Dr. W.F. Collins, Editor of the* Journal of Neurosurgery, *for the permission to reproduce part of the text of the paper "Invading Meningiomas of the Sphenoid Ridge," which appeared in the* Journal of Neurosurgery 53:587-599, 1980.

References

1. Adegbite AB, Khan ML, Paine KW, et al: The recurrence of intracranial meningiomas after surgical treatment. J Neurosurg 58:51-56, 1983.
2. Agnoli A, Otto H, Voit D: Kompressionen von Hirnarterien durch intrakranielle Tumoren. Z Neurol 200:33-44, 1971.

3. Bartal AD, Heilbronn YD, Avram J, et al: Carbon dioxide laser surgery of basal meningiomas. Surg Neurol 17:90-95, 1982.
4. Basso A, Carrizzo A, Kreutel A, et al: La chirurgie des tumeurs spheno-orbitaires. Neurochirurgie 24:71-82, 1978.
5. Bonnal J, Sedan R, Paillas JE: Problemes cliniques, evolutifs et therapeutiques souleves par les meningiomes envahissants de las base du crane. Neurochirurgie 7:108-117, 1961.
6. Bonnal J, Castermans A, Stevenaert A, et al: Les meningiomes des etages anterieurs et moyens de la base du crane. Conduite a tenir vis-a-vis des envahissements osseux et des prolongements dans les cavites de la face. Neurochirurgie 18:441-451, 1972.
7. Bonnal J, Thibaut A, Brotchi J, et al: Invading meningiomas of the sphenoid ridge. J Neurosurg 53:587-599, 1980.
8. Bucy PC: Editorial: Removal of involved bone with meningioma. Surg Neurol 17:416, 1982.
9. Carella RJ, Ransohoff J, Newall J: Role of radiation therapy in the management of meningioma. Neurosurgery 10:332-339, 1982.
10. Castellano F, Guidetti B, Olivecrona H: Pterional meningiomas "en plaque." J Neurosurg 9:188-196, 1952.
11. Cook AW: Total removal of large global meningiomas at the medial aspect of the sphenoid ridge: Technical note. J Neurosurg 34:107-113, 1971.
12. Cophignon J, Lucena J, Clay C, et al: Limits to radical treatment of spheno-orbital meningiomas. Acta Neurochir Suppl 28:375-380, 1979.
13. Cophignon J, Doyon D, Dijndjian R, et al: Les tumeurs du sinus caverneux et de la region; opacification arterielle et veineuse. Neurochirurgie 19:7-27, 1973.
14. Crompton MR, Gautier-Smith PC: The prediction of recurrence in meningiomas. J Neurol Neurosurg Psychiatry 33:80-87, 1970.
15. Cushing H, Eisenhardt L: Meningiomas, Vol. 2. New York, Hafner Publishing Company, 1962, p 733.
16. David M, Mahoudeau D: Les meningiomes de la petite aile du sphenoide. Gazette Medicale de France, pp 111-131, 1935.
17. Derome PJ: Les tumeurs sphenoethmoidales. Neurochirurgie 15 (Suppl) 1:1-164, 1972.
18. Derome PJ, Guiot G: Bone problems in meningiomas invading the base of the skull. Clin Neurosurg 25:435-451, 1978.
19. Dilenge D, Metzger J, Ramee A, et al: L'angiographie des tumeurs de la region du sinus caverneux. J Radiol Electrol Med Nucl 11:615-628, 1966.
20. Dolenc V: Microsurgical removal of large sphenoidal bone meningiomas. Acta Neurochirurgica (Suppl) 28:391-396, 1979.
21. Donnell MS, Meyer GL, Donegan WL, Estrogen-receptor protein in intracranial meningiomas. J Neurosurg 50:499-502, 1979.
22. Fardoun R, Mercier P, Guy G: Limites de l'anastomose extra-intracranienne preventive. A propos d'un meningiome clinoidien stenosant la carotide interne. 28/6:391-394, 1982.
23. Fine M, Brazis P, Palacios E, et al: Computed tomography of sphenoid wing meningiomas: Tumor location. Surg Neurol 13:385-389, 1980.
24. Fischer G, Fischer C, Mansuy L: Pronostic chirurgical des meningiomes de l'arete sphenoidale. Neurochirurgie 19:323-346, 1973.
25. Fukui M: Radiosensitivity of Meningioma: Analysis of five cases of highly vascular meningioma treated by preoperative irradiation. Acta Neurochirurgica 36:47-60, 1977.
26. Grant FC: The surgery of meningiomas at the base of the brain. Clin Neurosurg 5:25-38, 1958.
27. Guiot G, Derome PJ: A propos des meningiomas en plaques du pterion. Ann Chir 20:19-20, 1109-1127, 1966.
28. Guyot JF, Vouyouklakis D, Pertuiset B: Meningiomes de l'arete sphenoidale. A propos de 50 cas. Neurochirurgie 13:571-585, 1967.
29. Hieshima GB, Everhart FR, Mehringer CM, et al: Preoperative embolization of meningiomas. Surg Neurol 14:119-127, 1980.
30. Kadis GN, Mount LA, Ganti SR: The importance of early diagnosis and treatment of the meningiomas of the planum sphenoidale and tuberculum sellae: 105 cases. Surg Neurol 12:367-372, 1979.
31. King DL, Chang CH, Pool JL: Radiotherapy in the management of meningiomas. Acta Radiol (Ther) (Stockholm) 5:26-33, 1966.
32. Kjellberg RN, David KR, Lyons S, et al: Bragg peak proton beam therapy for arteriovenous malformation of the brain. Clin Neurosurg 31:248-290, 1984.
33. Lepoire J, Montaut J, Renard M: Une cause rare de thrombose de la carotide interne supraclinoidienne; un meningiome de la petite aile du sphenoide. Ann Med Nancy 3:1143-1149, 1964.

34. Leroux-Robert J, Guiot G, Paquelin F, et al: La propagation des meningiomes dans le massif maxillo-facial. Ann Otolaryngol 83:617-631, 1966.
35. Logue V: Operative Surgery: Neurosurgery. England, Butterworths, 2nd edition, 1971, p 320.
36. MacCarty CS: Meningiomas of the sphenoidal ridge. J Neursurg 36:114-121, 1972.
37. MacCarty CS, Piepgras DG, Ebersold MJ: Meningeal Tumors of the Brain. In Youmans J (ed): Neurological Surgery, 1982, pp 2936-2966.
38. Melamed S, Sohar A, Beller AS: The recurrence of intracranial meningioma. Neurochirurgia 22:47-54, 1979.
39. Merland JJ, Riche M, Chirars J, et al: Therapeutic angiography in neuroradiology. Classical data: recent advances and perspectives. Neuroradiology 21:111-121, 1981.
40. Mirimanoff RO, Dosoretz DE, Linggood RM, et al: Meningioma analysis of recurrence and progress following neurosurgical resection. J Neurosurg 62:18-24, 1985.
41. Momose KJ, New PFJ: Nonatheromatous stenosis and occlusion of the internal carotid artery and its main branches. Am J Roentgenol Radium Ther Nucl Med 118:550-566, 1973.
42. Ojemann RG: Meningiomas of the basal parapituitary region: Technical considerations. Clin Neurosurg 27:233-262, 1980.
43. Pellerin P, Lesoin F, Dhellemmes P, et al: Usefulness of the orbitfrontomalar approach associated with bone reconstruction for fronto-temporo-sphenoid meningiomas. Neurosurgery 15:715-718, 1984.
44. Pertuiset B, Guillaumat L, Pialoux P, et al: Meningiome cranio-facial (temporo-obrito-jugal) opere en trois temps. La Presse Medicale 66:1863-1865, 1958.
45. Pompili A, Derome PJ, Visot A, et al: Hyperostosing meningiomas of the sphenoid ridge: Clinical features. Surgical therapy and long-term observations. Review of 49 cases. Surg Neurol 17:411-415, 1982.
46. Richter HP, Schachenmayr W: Preoperative embolization of intracranial meningiomas. Neurosurgery 13:261-268, 1983.
47. Sadar ES, Conomy JP, Benjamin SP, et al: Meningiomas of the paranasal sinuses: Benign and malignant. Neurosurgery 4:227-232, 1979.
48. Seeger W: Fronto-temporal operations, anatomical principles. In Special Microsurgical Operative Procedures of the Brain. Part II. Microsurgery of the Brain—Anatomical and Technical Principles 1, NY, Springer-Verlag, 1980.
49. Simpson D: The recurrence of intracranial meningiomas after surgical treatment. J Neurol Neurosurg Psychiatry 20:22-40, 1957.
50. Skullerud K, Loken AC: The prognosis in meningiomas. Acta Neuropathol (Berl) 29:337-344, 1974.
51. Smith HP, Challa VR, Moody DM, et al: Biological features of meningiomas that determine the production of cerebral edema. Neurosurgery 8:428-433, 1981.
52. Sole-Llenas J, Tolosa E, Fuenmayor P: Occlusion des arteres cerebrales en rapport avec des lesions expansives intracraniennes. Acta Radiol (Diagn) (Stockh) 9:487-493, 1969.
53. Spallone A: Occlusion of the internal carotid artery by intracranial tumors. Surg Neurol 15:51-57, 1981.
54. Steiner L, Leksell L, Forster DMC, et al: Stereotactic radiosurgery in intracranial arteriovenous malformations. Acta Neurochir (suppl) 21:195-209, 1977.
55. Stern WE: Meningiomas in the cranio-orbital junction. J Neurosurg 38:428-438, 1973.
56. Strait TA, Robertson JH, Clark WC: Use of the carbon dioxide laser in the operative management of intracranial meningiomas: A report of twenty cases. Neurosurgery 10:464-467, 1982.
57. Stroobandt G, Cornelis G, Thauvoy C, et al: Meningiomes hyperostosants "en plaque" du pterion. Intervention precoce et intervention tardive. Acta Neurologica Belgica 74:64-69, 1974.
58. Teasdale E, Patterson J, McLelland D, et al: Subselective preoperative embolization for meningiomas. A radiological and pathological assessment. J Neurosurg 60:506-511, 1984.
59. Van Effenterre R, Bataini JP, Cabanis EA: High energy radiotherapy in the treatment of meningioma of cavernous sinus. Acta Neurochir (Suppl) 28:464-467, 1979.
60. Wara WM, Sheline GF, Newman H: Radiation therapy of meningioma. AJR 123:453-458, 1975.
61. Yanashita J, Handa H, Twaki K: Recurrence of intracranial meningioma with special reference to radiotherapy. Surg Neurol 14:33-40, 1980.
62. Zozulia YA, Romodanov SA, Patsko YV: Diagnosis and surgical treatment of benign craniobasal tumors involving the cavernous sinus. Acta Neurochir (Suppl) 28:387-390, 1979.

23

Operative Management of Tumors Involving the Cavernous Sinus

Laligam N. Sekhar, M.D.

Introduction

The cavernous sinus (CS) is a small venous space enclosed by leaves of dura and periosteum and located on either side of the sella turcica, medial to the temporal lobes. The cavernous sinus contains very critical neural and vascular structures and its lateral well contains cranial nerves III, IV, V_1, and sometimes V_2.[15,42] The results of injection and corrosion studies favor the view that the cavernous sinus contains a plexus of veins, rather than being a large venous space with multiple trabeculations.[41] These studies are also corroborated by our intraoperative observations after the removal of intracavernous tumors. The internal carotid artery (ICA), the abducens nerve, and the sympathetic nerves also lie within the CS.

Tumors that originate primarily within the cavernous sinus are rare, usually meningiomas and neurilemmomas. However, many tumors may invade the sinus secondarily from adjacent areas, including meningiomas, neurilemmomas, chordomas, chondromas, chondrosarcomas, pituitary adenomas, nasopharyngeal carcinomas, esthesioneuroblastomas, nasopharyngeal angiofibromas, and metastatic lesions. In addition, giant aneurysms of the cavernous carotid artery often present with signs and symptoms resembling a tumor of this space. Fungal infections, particularly mucormycosis and aspergillosis, and noninfectious granuloma (Tolosa-Hunt syndrome) may also present clinically with signs and symptoms resembling an intracavernous neoplasm.

Tumors invading the cavernous sinus have generally been considered inoperable because of the likelihood of bleeding from the cavernous venous plexus, or of injury to the internal carotid artery (ICA) or to the cranial nerves III, IV, and VI. However, during the last 3 years, 16 patients with intracavernous neoplasms have been operated upon by this author with no mortality, no strokes, and minimal cranial nerve morbidity (Tables I and II). This chapter will emphasize our approaches to the preoperative evaluation of these patients, intraoperative monitoring, operative management, and postoperative problems.

Both benign and malignant neoplasms invading the cavernous sinus were

From: Sekhar LN, Schramm VL Jr, eds: *Tumors of the Cranial Base: Diagnosis and Treatment*. Mount Kisco, New York, Futura Publishing Co, Inc, © 1987.

Table I
Neoplasms of the Cavernous Sinus Operated During 1983–1986

Tumor Type	Number	Complete Resection
Meningioma	6	5
Trigeminal neurinoma	2	2
Pituitary adenoma	1	1
Chordoma	1	1
Chondrosarcoma	3	2
Adenoid cystic carcinoma	2	2
Squamous cell carcinoma	1	1
Total	16	14

removed. Indications for tumor removal included recurrence of tumor from a residue left in the region during a previous operation, the appearance of cranial nerve symptoms (ophthalmoplegia or intractable pain), or the prospect of achieving a total cure or long-term control of the lesion with operation alone or with operation and radiation therapy.

Preoperative Evaluation

The preoperative evaluation included a careful physical and neurological examination, axial and coronal computed tomographic (CT) scans, cerebral angiography, and neurophysiological testing of the function of the second, seventh, and eighth cranial nerves. In the more recent cases (14 patients), a balloon occlusion test of the ipsilateral ICA was performed with repeated neurological examinations and the measurement of cerebral blood flow (CBF).[47] One patient in this group developed numbness on the contralateral side of the body 8 minutes after test occlusion, and the balloon was immediately deflated. No blood flow studies were performed in this patient. He was considered to be at high risk for the development of stroke if the carotid artery had to be permanently occluded. The other 13 patients tolerated the test occlusion well clinically with varying degrees of CBF reduction. If the CBF values were diminished to between 15 and 30 ml/100 gm/min during test occlusion, the patient was considered to be at high risk for the development of stroke following permanent occlusion of the artery. Those with reductions of CBF between 30 and 40 ml/100 gm/min were considered to be at moderate risk, with a possibility of developing stroke if there was hypotension or hypovolemia during the intraoperative or postoperative period. Those with CBF values above 40 ml/100 gm/min were considered to be at minimal risk for the development of stroke following permanent occlusion, provided thromboembolism from a stump is avoided.

Table II
Complications of Intracavernous Operations

Death	0
Stroke	0
Carotid pseudoaneurysm (infection)	1
Wound infection	1
Cerebrospinal fluid leak	2
Cranial nerve palsy (permanent)	
II (significant decrease)	1
III (tumor invasion)	1
IV	2
V (V_1, V_2 or V_3, partial loss)	3
VI	1
Improved cranial nerve function	3

Intraoperative Monitoring (See Chapter 7)

Intraoperative monitoring of the third, fourth, and sixth cranial nerves was done by recording the action potentials (EMG) from the extraocular muscles (Fig. 1). The cranial nerves were stimulated with 150 μs rectangular pulses at 5 or 10 per second using a hand-held monopolar electrode (Grass Instruments Co., type 5D9 Stimulator), the return electrode being a 25 gauge metal hypodermic needle placed in the wound. The lateral rectus muscle (N VI) was reached by placing a needle electrode (Grass Instruments Co., type E2 subdermal electrodes) through the skin at the lateral corner of the eye, aimed away from the globe to avoid injury to the conjunctiva. The medial rectus (N III) and the superior oblique muscles (N IV) were reached in a similar way, by inserting

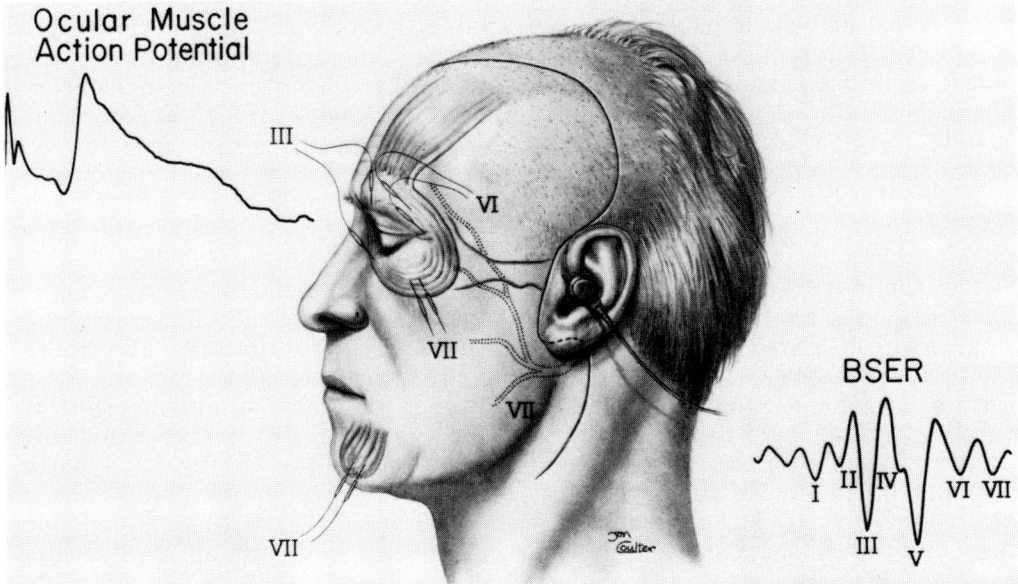

Figure 1: The incision used for operations within the cavernous sinus and the location of monitoring devices are shown. The extension of the incision below the ear facilitates the isolation of the genu and vertical segment of the petrous ICA, and aids in the inferior approach to the cavernous sinus.

needle electrodes through the skin over these muscles. Reference electrodes were placed on the opposite side of the forehead and ground electrodes were placed nearby. Responses from facial muscles were recorded individually from two electrodes, one placed in the mentalis muscle and one in the orbicularis oculi muscle.

The recorded potentials were amplified by four separate amplifiers (Grass Instruments Co., type P511J) with a bandpass of 0.3 to 3 kHz, and displayed on oscilloscopes. The potentials could also be made audible through a loudspeaker one channel at a time and the stimulus artifacts were suppressed by a technique described earlier.[22]

In some patients, the optic nerve was also monitored by recording visual evoked potentials (VEPs) from electrodes placed on the scalp, and directly on the optic nerve. The stimuli used were short light flashes generated by light-emitting diodes that were glued to plastic contact lenses. Scalp VEPs were recorded by placing needle electrodes in the occipital and parietal areas (O_z and C_z), with a ground electrode placed on the opposite side of the head. Direct VEPs were recorded by placing a malleable Teflon-insulated silver wire with a cotton wick sutured to its uninsulated tip directly on the optic nerve (Moller AR, Burgess J, Sekhar LN: unpublished data, 1986). The reference electrode was a 25 gauge all-metal hypodermic needle placed in the wound.

The VEPs recorded from the scalp and directly from the optic nerve were amplified (Grass Instruments Co., type P511J) with a bandpass of 0.3 to 300 Hz and were averaged using a minicomputer (LSI 11/23). The results were displayed on an oscilloscope and stored on disk.

Operative Technique

Anesthesia and Patient Positioning

All patients are operated upon under general endotracheal inhalational anesthesia. Short-acting neuromuscular blocking agents are used during induction. After the conclusion of the major portion of the operation, the anesthesiologist is allowed to paralyze the patient so that the requirements for inhalational agents can be reduced. Furosemide, 40 mg, is administered intravenously at the time of skin incision, and if required, 50 gm of mannitol can also be given intravenously. Cerebrospinal fluid drainage is accomplished by the opening of cisterns at operation, and sometimes by lumbar subarachnoid catheter.

The patient's head is placed in a three-point pin fixation device in the usual fashion for a frontotemporal craniotomy. A "reverse question mark" incision is made starting in the frontal scalp extending backward and then downward in front of the ear, below the earlobe and then forward along a cervical skin crease (Fig. 1). The skin and subcutaneous tissues are dissected and reflected forward, carefully avoiding injury to the frontal and zygomatic branches of the facial nerve. The facial nerve is identified just outside the stylomastoid foramen using the external ear cartilage as a landmark and traced to its bifurcation within the parotid gland. The parotid gland itself is mobilized from the underlying masseteric fascia to enable the dislocation or excision of the mandibular condyle without any stretch of the facial nerve. The cervical ICA is dissected behind the angle of the mandible and a tape is passed around it for control if necessary. The stylomandibular ligament is divided. The zygomatic arch is divided anteriorly and posteriorly and the temporalis muscle is reflected downward and forward. A frontotemporal craniotomy is then made extending anteriorly to about the midpoint of the eyebrow, posteriorly to just above the pinna of the ear. Through a burr hole made low in the temporal area and using brain relaxation achieved by the lumbar subarachnoid catheter, the dura of the middle fossa is separated from the lateral aspect of the floor. The capsule of the temporomandibular joint is then dissected free of the lower articular surface of the temporal bone and the condyle of the mandible is dislocated downward for a distance of 1 cm to 1½ cm. The bone is then cut with a Stryker drill just medial to the articular surface of the temporal bone to include the root of the zygoma and the entire bone flap, and the articular surface of the temporomandibular joint is fractured and removed as a single piece, if possible. Alternatively, the frontal and temporal bone flaps can be removed in two pieces and subsequently reconnected. The bone of the pterion is drilled away and the lateral wall of the orbit is unroofed. The lesser wing of the sphenoid and a portion of the roof of the orbit are removed almost to the anterior clinoid process. Anteroinferiorly, the greater wing of the sphenoid is removed with rongeurs to unroof the superior orbital fissure completely and to unroof and identify the maxillary nerve (V₂) exiting through the foramen rotundum, the mandibular nerve (V₃) exiting through foramen ovale, and the middle meningeal artery exiting through the foramen spinosum.

A self-training retractor is then placed under the temporal dura with minimal or no pressure. Starting at the level of the floor of the middle fossa, immediately deep to the temporomandibular joint, bone is removed with a high speed cutting drill. The tensor tympani muscle and the bony eustachian tube are identified and removed. The genu of the petrous carotid artery lies just deep to the bony eustachian tube, often covered by a thin sliver of bone or no bone at all. It is unroofed with a bone punch or a curette. The vertical segment of the petrous carotid artery can then be unroofed working downward toward the carotid canal with the aid of curettes, bone punches, and the drill. There is often a dense cartilaginous ring surrounding the carotid artery at its entrance to the carotid canal which has to be divided. The periosteal sheath covering the carotid artery is attached to this and must be detached at this level (Figs. 2 and 3). The horizontal segment of the petrous internal carotid artery can then be traced in an anteromedial direction. The greater superficial petrosal nerve often lies superficial and parallel to it. It must be identified and divided to avoid traction on the geniculate ganglion (Fig. 4). The geniculate ganglion of the facial nerve and the cochlea lie posterosuperior to the genu of the petrous carotid artery and drilling

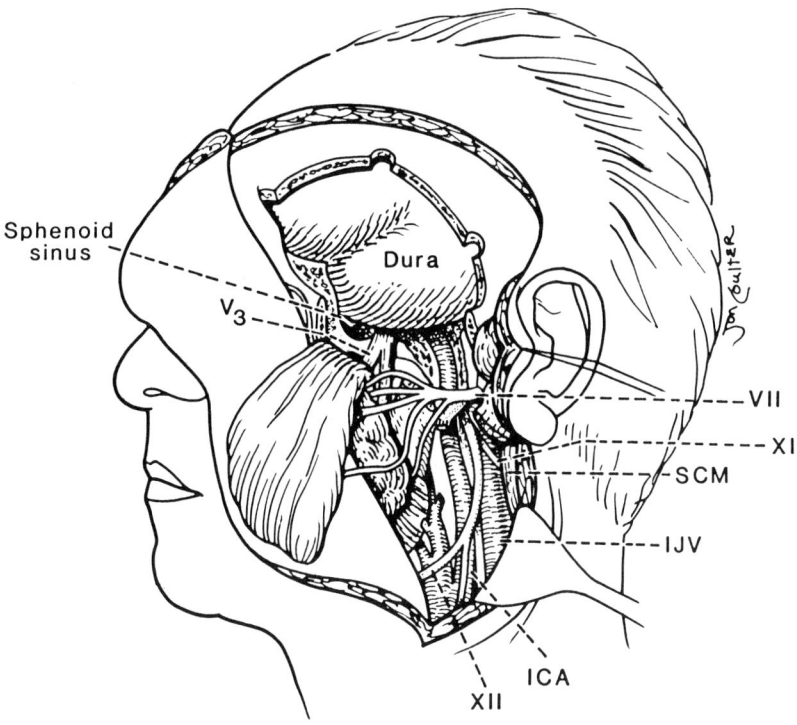

Figure 2: The temporalis muscle has been reflected down and forward after the division of the zygomatic arch. The facial nerve and its branches have been dissected. The mandibular condyle has been dislocated downward. The vertical segment and genu of the petrous ICA has been exposed. The mandibular nerve (V₃) has been unroofed. The location of the sphenoid sinus is shown, but it is preferable not to expose this unless the tumor extends into it.

must be avoided in this area to prevent injury to them. The horizontal segment of the petrous internal carotid artery can then be followed to the point where it is crossed by V₃ (Fig. 5). The entire petrous carotid artery is then mobilized from the carotid canal with the aid of a Rosen microdissector and a vessel loop or a ligature is passed around it in preparation for temporary occlusion if this should become necessary.

The frontotemporal dura is then opened in a curvilinear fashion and tacked forward. Under the microscope, the frontal lobe is elevated and the optic nerve and carotid cisterns are opened. The extent of the tumor is inspected and a decision is made regarding the operative approach to the cavernous sinus to be employed. Tumors such as pituitary adenomas and meningiomas will be found to be both intradural and extradural within the cavernous sinus whereas tumors such as chordomas and neurilemmomas will be predominantly extradural within the cavernous sinus. When the neoplasm has already extended into the middle fossa and elevated or thinned the temporal lobe, one can merely split the sylvian fissure and hold up the temporal tip with a retractor and work here. Alternatively, when the tumor is predominantly within the region of the cavernous sinus, it may be essential to remove the anterior 3 or 4 cm of the temporal tip including the inferior and middle temporal gyrus, sparing the superior temporal gyrus and the uncus, hippocampus, and amygdala. Distal control of the internal carotid artery just beyond the ophthalmic artery can be easily achieved by preparing a segment of the artery for temporary clipping.

The following operative approaches

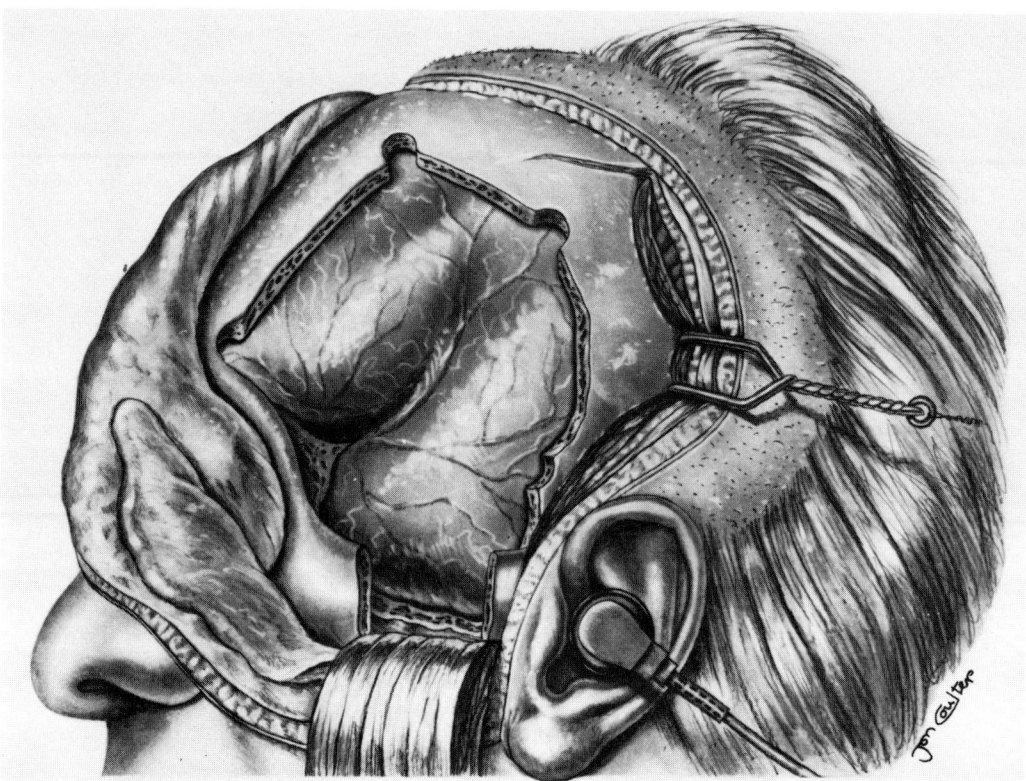

Figure 3: Craniotomy and exposure when it is not necessary to expose the vertical segment of the petrous ICA.

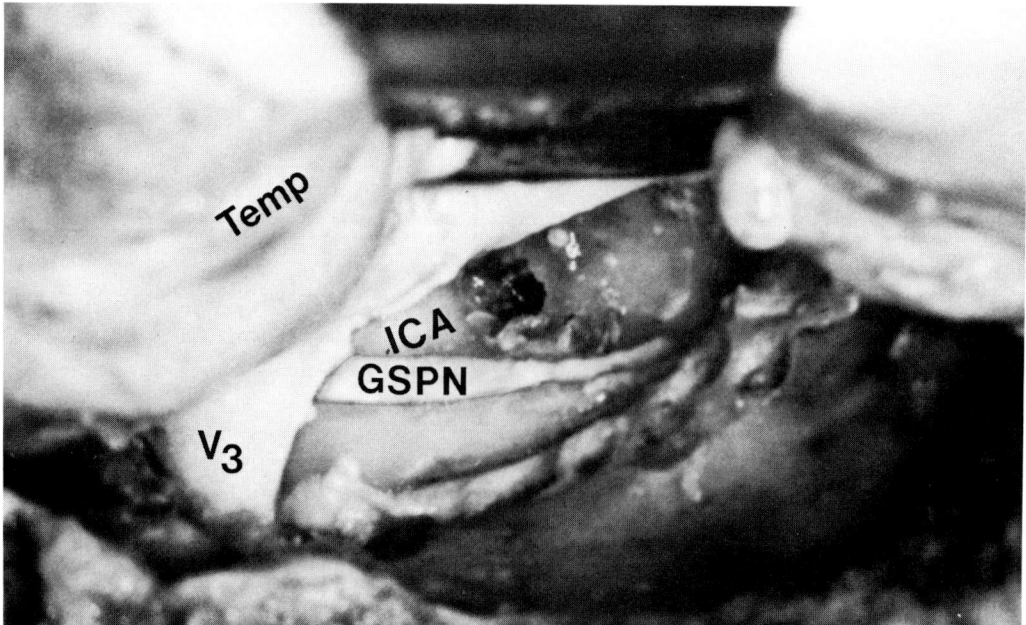

Figure 4: Landmarks in the floor of the middle cranial fossa for the exposure of the horizontal segment of the petrous ICA. Temp = temporal dura; V_3 = mandibular nerve; GSPN = greater superficial petrosal nerve; ICA = internal carotid artery seen through a defect in the bone.

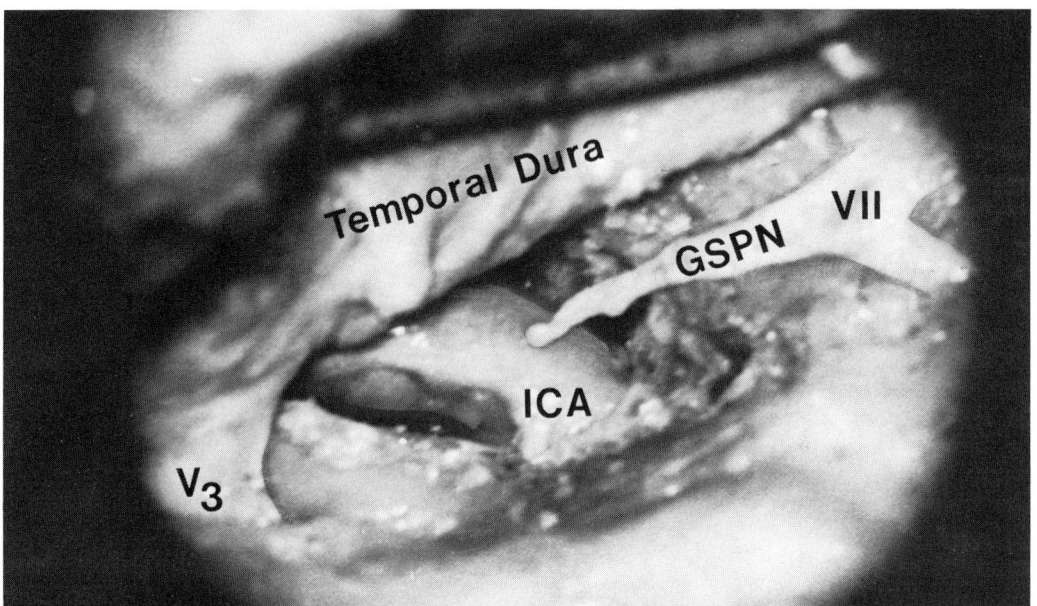

Figure 5: The horizontal segment of the petrous ICA has been exposed by drilling bone away. The geniculate ganglion of the facial nerve (VII) need not be exposed, but its relationship is shown here.

to the cavernous sinus are then employed (Fig. 6).

Lateral Approach

This approach enters the cavernous sinus through its lateral wall between the trochlear and ophthalmic nerves (the extended Parkinson's triangle), or between the ophthalmic and maxillary nerves. The surgeon can usually easily identify the oculomotor nerve prior to its entry into the lateral wall of the CS. However, the precavernous trochlear nerve is often difficult to identify without dividing the tentorium and is best identified by dissection in the lateral wall of the CS. An incision is started along the lateral wall of the CS parallel to the approximate location of V_1 and extending toward the superior orbital fissure. The outer layer of the dura is then peeled from the inner layer and another incision is made in a vertical direction. The outer layer of the dura is then further dissected from either the inner layer or the underlying tumor, carefully identifying the trochlear and oculomotor nerves which lie within the two layers of the dura superiorly, and the ophthalmic and maxillary nerves which usually lie inferiorly. Sutures can be used to hold the dural leaves apart. The tumor is then debulked by means of the bipolar cautery and suction irrigation. The intracavernous ICA is usually identified by its pulsatility before its wall is reached, or one of its branches (usually the meningohypophyseal) may be traced to it. The tumor is then dissected sharply from its wall. The surgeon must be prepared to temporarily clip and repair any tears in the wall should these occur. The location of the oculomotor and the trochlear nerves in the CS is relatively constant whereas the location of the ophthalmic and the abducens nerve is very variable. Intermittent stimulation of the area with observation of the evoked EMG activity from the lateral rectus is useful to identify the abducens nerve.

Inferior Approach

This approach is possible only when the cavernous sinus is aproached from the infratemporal fossa with the exposure of the petrous carotid artery (as described). The horizontal segment of the petrous carotid artery is traced into the cavernous

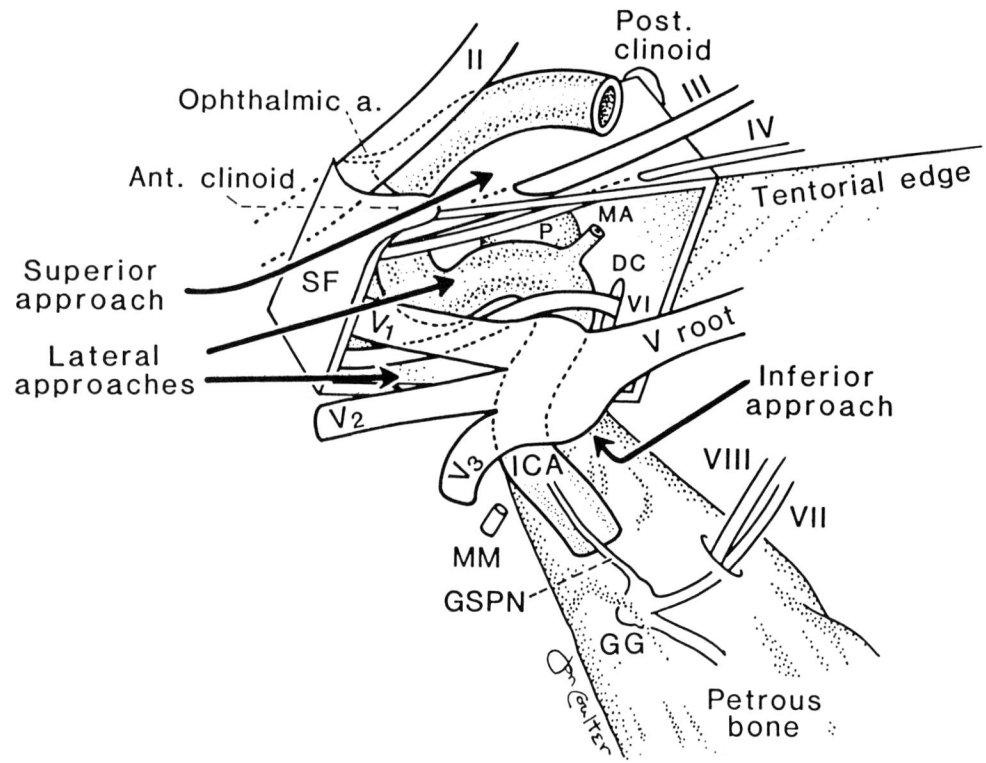

Figure 6: Operative approaches to the cavernous sinus shown schematically. II, III, IV, V_1, V_2, V_3, VI, VII, VIII = cranial nerves; P = pituitary gland; DC = Dorello's canal; MM = middle meningeal artery; GG = geniculate ganglion; MA = meningohypophyseal branch of the cavernous ICA.

sinus. V_3 may have to be temporarily retracted either anteriorly or posteriorly to do so. When this nerve is invaded by tumor, it may be divided. More anteriorly, one can expose the ophthalmic, maxillary, and mandibular nerves between the leaves of the dura and enter the CS between V_1 and V_2 or between V_2 and V_3. One can usually get up to the level of the abducens nerve with this approach but the superior aspect of the CS is not optimally exposed.

Superior Approach

This enters the CS from an anterior and superior direction. The anterior clinoid process is removed with a drill after opening a dura over it. The bony optic canal is unroofed in its superior and lateral aspects and the dural sheath over the optic nerve is opened. In this fashion, the optic nerve is completely mobilized. After removal of the anterior clinoid process, the dura over the superior aspect of the cavernous sinus is normally thin in this region. The ICA is densely attached to the dura where it emerges from the superior wall of the CS just medial to the anterior clinoid process. The superior wall of the CS itself is devoid of any cranial nerves. It can be opened just lateral to the ICA and one can follow the ICA into the CS dissecting it and removing tumor around it. Tumor in the orbital apex area can also be easily removed by this approach, after removing the bone covering the orbital apex superiorly and laterally.

Vascular Management

With the majority of the benign neoplasms invading the cavernous sinus, one can dissect the tumor away from the wall of the ICA. Any lacerations may be sutured with 8-0 or 7-0 nylon after proximal and distal temporary clipping of the ICA. If the artery is irreparably injured, if it is found impossible to dissect the tumor away from the wall of the artery, or if the neoplasm is malignant, one has the following options. (1) The artery may be simply occluded just proximal to the ophthalmic artery with a clip. This can be safely performed if the patient tolerated the balloon occlusion test with blood flow values above 40 ml/100 gm/min.[36] Those with CBF values between 30 and 40 ml/100 gm/min will also probably tolerate permanent ICA occlusion without a stroke if careful attention is given to avoid hypovolemia and hypotension. (2) If the blood flow values were between 15–30 ml/100 gm/min after the balloon occlusion test but the patient did not develop any neurological deficits, the abnormal arterial segment may be excised and replaced by a short saphenous vein graft (5 cm or less). Since such a graft is short in length and carries a high volume of blood flow, the patency rate would be expected to be high. The perioperative use of high dose steroids, aspirin, and dipyridamole, as well as the long-term use of aspirin and dipyridamole, would be expected to improve the patency of the graft. (3) If the patient did not tolerate the balloon occlusion test clinically or if the blood flow values were lower than 15 ml/100 gm/min during the test, tumor must be left behind or the surgeon may perform a long vein graft from the external carotid artery to one of the major branches of the middle cerebral artery and subsequently remove the tumor that has invaded the carotid artery. A superficial temporal to middle cerebral artery anastomosis does not reliably carry enough blood acutely precluding its use for acute ICA occlusion. Long saphenous vein grafts do have a higher rate of complications and this has to be weighed against the risk of leaving tumor behind. With malignant neoplasms, we have increasingly preferred to excise the invaded artery after intraoperative arterial occlusion.

Cranial Nerve Management

The oculomotor and trochlear nerves are relatively easy to preserve during operations of the cavernous sinus because they traverse a very short length of the lateral wall of the cavernous sinus and are usually easy to find. The greatest difficulty occurs with the preservation of the sixth nerve since its position is very variable when displaced by tumors. We have found the intermittent intraoperative stimulation of the nerves to be useful for locating them and for preserving their function. After extensive dissection of the nerves, the patient usually exhibits an ophthalmoplegia postoperatively but makes a complete functional recovery within 12 months. When the sixth nerve is involved by malignant neoplasms, it may be worthwhile to excise it, and then reconstruct with a graft from the posterior fossa to the orbit. For this purpose, the apex of the petrous bone posterosuperior to the horizontal segment of the petrous carotid artery is removed. After occlusion of the superior petrosal sinus with clips or ligature, the dura of the anterior clivus is opened exposing the anterior surface of the pons, the basilar and anterior inferior cerebellar arteries, and the proximal abducens nerve. To expose the distal portion of the abducens nerve, the bone over the orbital apex is unroofed. After the dura is opened, dissection is performed in the fat plane laterally to identify the lateral rectus. The abducens nerve can be identified on the medial surface of the lateral rectus muscle. Although we have performed this kind of grafting only in cadaver specimens to date, a good recovery may be possible in patients after such grafting since the abducens nerve innervates a single muscle and is purely motor (Sekhar LN, Burgess J, Akin O: unpublished data). If the oculomotor nerve is irreparably damaged either by tumor or by operation, reconstruction may be performed either by direct suture or with a graft. The nerve divides into two divisions either shortly before or immediately after passing through the superior orbital fissure. Aberrant regeneration does occur in the oculomotor distribution but does not usually present a functional problem. Recovery of function after the suture of an injured oculomotor nerve has been reported in one patient (Professor Yasargil: personal communication, 1985). We have resutured the oculomotor nerve after removal of an abnormal segment which was found to be encased and invaded by neoplasm, but it is too early to assess the results. In experimental studies in cats, transection of the oculomotor nerve followed by repair with fibrin glue or a silicone sheath was followed by good results in 10/15 and fair results in 5/15. Return of pupillary light reaction, convergence, caloric nystagmus, the ocular electromyographic activity were documented.[29,30] The successful recovery of trochlear nerve function after suture of the trochlear nerve has been reported by Grimson et al.[13] Samii has also reported the reconstruction of the ophthalmic nerve in a small number of patients.[28]

Avoidance of Cerebrospinal Fluid Leakage

The cavernous sinus is bordered medially by the sphenoid sinus. Some tumors may extend into the bone of the sphenoid or into the cavity of the sphenoid itself. Removal of the cavernous sinus tumor along with the lateral wall of the sphenoid sinus exposes the patient to the risk of postoperative CSF leakage and infection since it is usually impossible to repair the dura in a watertight fashion. In these cases, the surgeon must perform the operation in two stages. During the first stage of the operation, the bony wall of the sphenoid sinus and any tumor within it are removed. The sphenoid sinus is then occluded, preferably with vascularized tissue such as a rectus abdominis free flap. When this is not feasible, one may use a devascularized muscle and/or fat. Tumor within the cavernous sinus is then removed at a second stage operation 4 to 6 weeks later.

Management of Venous Bleeding

Bleeding from the venous plexus within the cavernous sinus usually indicates the margin of tumor in the area. Packing with Surgicel and gentle pressure applied over a cotton patty are adequate for control. Further elevation of the head may also be utilized. Unless the intracavernous ICA is injured, the surgeon never encounters torrential bleeding which does not stop with packing.

Case Reports

Patient P.K.: Recurrent Meningioma

A 51-year-old woman was referred for management of a recurrent meningioma, 4 years after an initial operation to remove a middle fossa tumor. On examination, trismus, fullness of the right side of the face and the nasopharynx, and diminished sensation in the trigeminal distribution were present. CT scan revealed a very large tumor involving the petrous bone and clivus, parapharyngeal area, infratemporal fossa, the sphenoid sinus, the middle fossa, the cavernous sinus, and the tentorial notch area on the right side (Figs. 7 and 8). On cerebral angiography, the neoplasm was quite vascular and predominantly supplied by the external carotid artery. A trial balloon occlusion was well tolerated by the patient clinically, but CBF was significantly reduced with mean flow values of 27 ml/100 gm/min.

The neoplasm was resected in two stages. During the first operation, a subtemporal and preauricular infratemporal fossa approach was utilized (see Chapter 34). The neoplasm was totally removed from the infratemporal fossa, including the invaded muscles, the mandibular nerve, and a portion of the nasopharyngeal wall. The petrous ICA was encased by tumor involving the petroclival bone. The vertical segment of the petrous ICA

Operative Management: Cavernous Sinus • 403

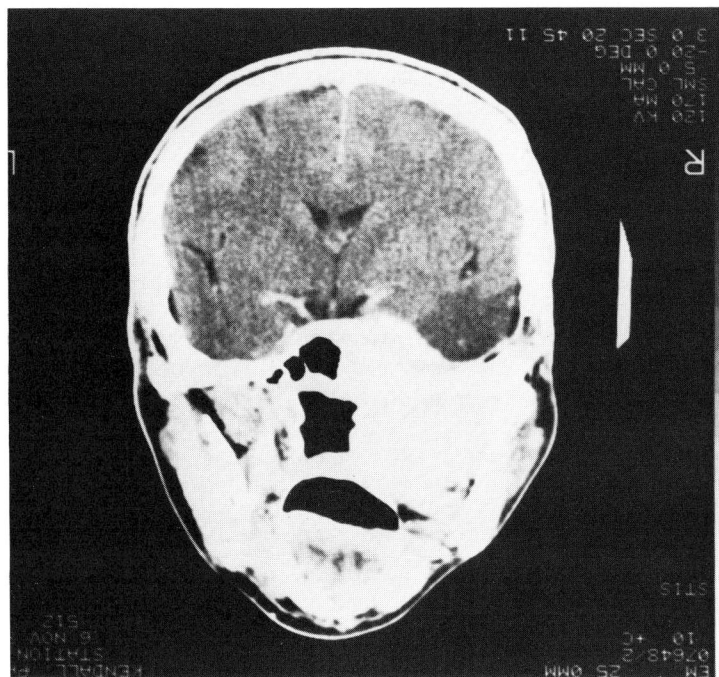

Figure 7: Preoperative coronal enhanced CT scan of patient P.K. showing tumor in the infratemporal fossa, sphenoid sinus, middle fossa, the cavernous sinus, and the petroclival area (see Fig. 8).

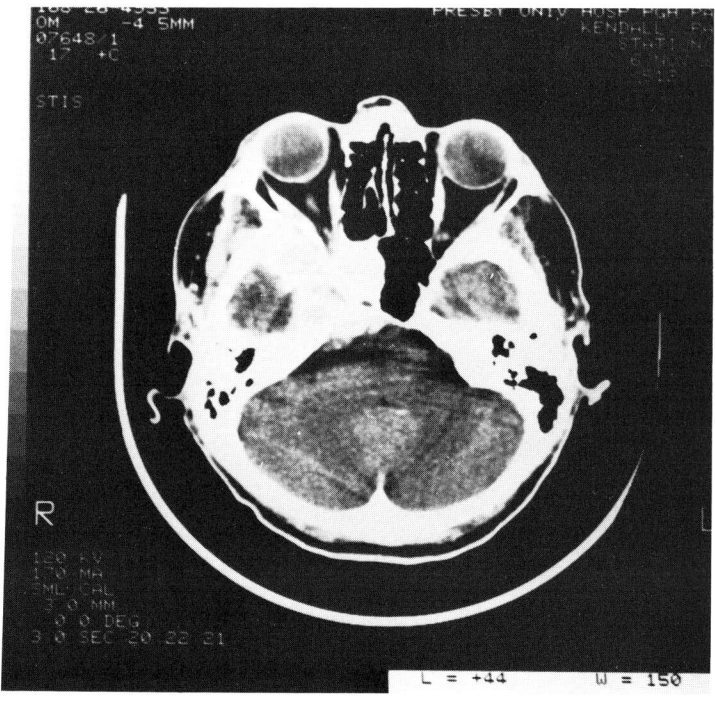

Figure 8: Same patient as in Figure 7, axial view.

was identified, and the entire petrous ICA was dissected free of tumor. Tumor was then removed from the basal cavernous sinus (inferior approach) by dissecting it away from the cavernous ICA and the abducens nerve (Fig. 9). The petroclival bone and the sphenoid sinus were also cleared of tumor. At the end of the operation, a vascularized rectus abdominis flap was used to fill the infratemporal fossa, the sphenoid sinus, and the defect in the nasopharyngeal wall. Postoperatively, the patient had a facial and an abducens nerve palsy.

During the second-stage operation, a frontotemporal approach to the lesion was performed. Residual tumor was found in the upper cavernous sinus area, the dura overlying the trigeminal nerve in the middle fossa, the tentorial notch, and the clival area. Through a lateral and superior approach, the neoplasm was totally removed from the CS. Cranial nerves III, IV, V_1, and V_2 were dissected from the tumor and preserved (Fig. 10). Two lacerations of the cavernous ICA were sutured with 8-0 nylon after temporary clipping of the petrous and supraclinoid ICA. The remaining intracranial tumor was also removed.

The patient had a complete third and fourth cranial nerve paralysis postoperatively, in addition to her previous sixth nerve palsy, but otherwise had an uneventful recovery. A postoperative angiogram revealed the ICA to be patent and normal. Radiation therapy was given to the infratemporal fossa region as an adjunct to tumor resection. On follow-up 1 year later, the patient had completely recovered from the palsies of the cranial nerves III, IV, and VI. However, the facial paralysis did not recover and required graft reconstruction. There is no evidence of tumor recurrence on CT scans obtained 2½ years later (Fig. 11).

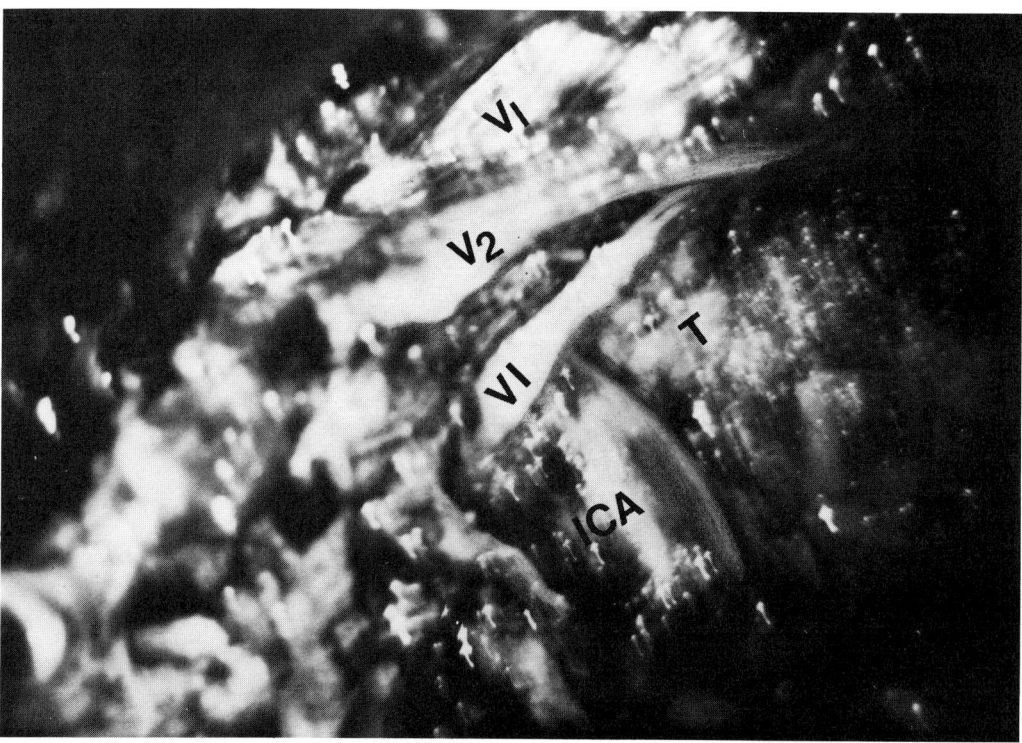

Figure 9: Operative exposure of the tumor in the basal cavernous sinus during the first stage operation. V_1, V_2, VI = cranial nerves; T = tumor.

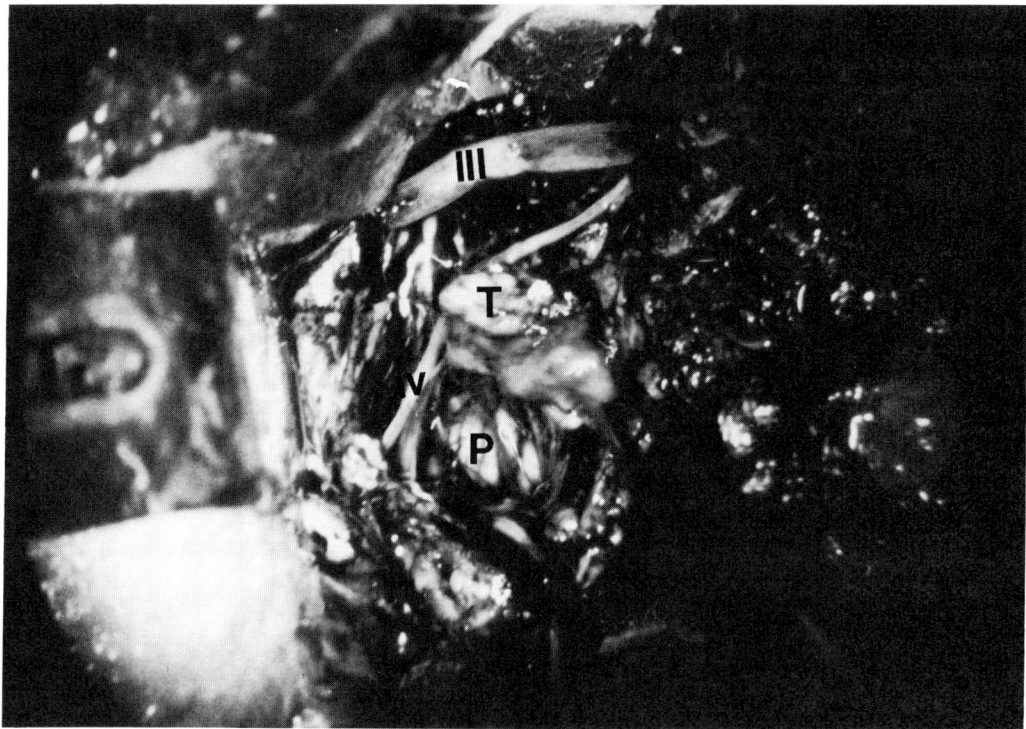

Figure 10: Operative exposure of the tumor during the second stage operation. The oculomotor (III) and trochlear (IV) nerves have been completely dissected in the lateral wall of the cavernous sinus. Tumor (T) is being removed from the cavernous sinus. The pons (P) is visible following the division of the tentorium and the removal of the tumor from the petroclival area.

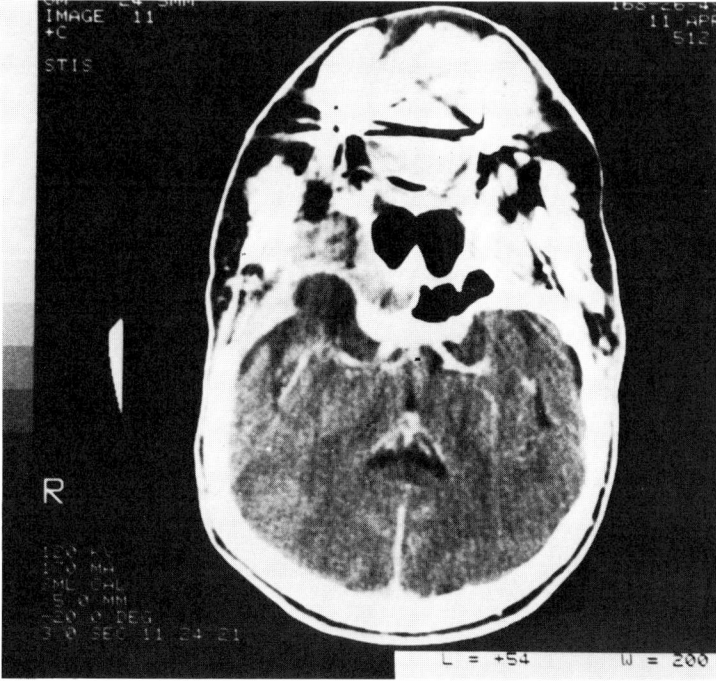

Figure 11: CT scan 1 year after operation. Note the now atrophic muscle filling the sphenoid sinus, and the infratemporal fossa.

Patient D.L.: Chordoma

A 24-year-old man presented with a 4-year history of headaches, tingling around the eyes, and intermittent double vision. He had recently developed an abducens and oculomotor paresis. CT scanning showed a hyperdense lesion involving the left CS, middle fossa, posterior fossa, and infratemporal fossa, which enhanced after contrast administration (Fig. 12). Cerebral angiography revealed a displacement of the petrous and cavernous ICA, but no tumor blush was apparent.

The tumor was approached through a left frontotemporal craniotomy, with monitoring of the third, sixth, and seventh cranial nerves. The temporal lobe was significantly elevated by the tumor, and after splitting the sylvian fissure, it had to be merely held in place with a retractor. The supraclinoid ICA and the third cranial nerve were found to be displaced anteromedially by the tumor, which occupied the CS and basal middle fossa and extended into the clival area medial to Meckel's cave. After an incision in the lateral wall of the CS, the trigeminal nerve and its branches were found to be displaced laterally by the tumor (Fig. 13). A yellowish-red soft tumor was easily removed with suction irrigation and blunt microdissection. The sixth cranial nerve and the cavernous ICA were found to be displaced medially and downward (Fig. 14). The infratemporal fossa was entered through the enlarged foramen ovale and tumor removed from there. After division of the tentorium, the portion of the tumor in the posterior fossa was removed. Tumor in the cavernous sinus and the middle and posterior fossae was thought to have been completely resected.

Postoperatively, the patient has had a permanent V₃ palsy. The pathology of the lesion was chondroid chordoma. Proton beam radiation therapy was administered. On follow-up 9 months later, the abducens and oculomotor paresis had resolved completely. CT scans obtained 2 years later have revealed no evidence of recurrent tumor (Figs. 15 and 16).

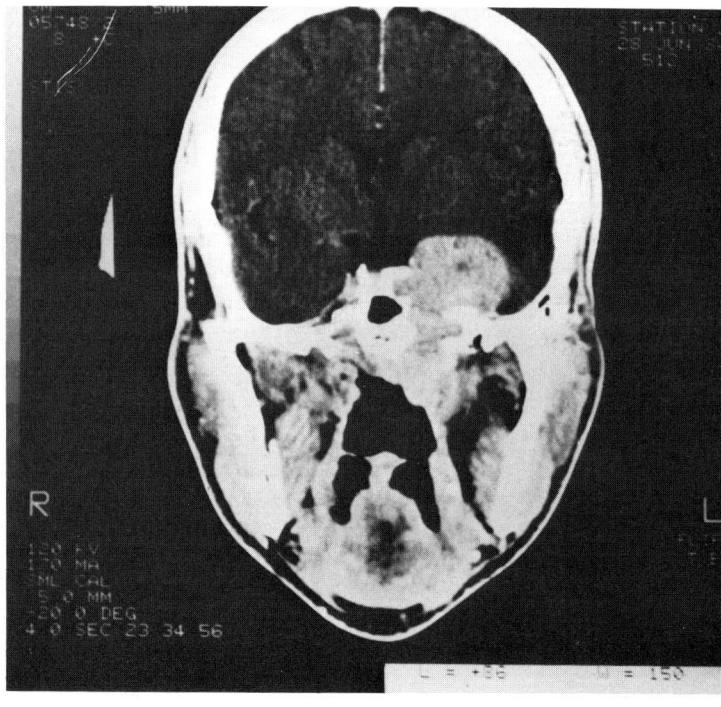

Figure 12: Coronal CT scan of patient D.L. showing tumor in the cavernous sinus and the infratemporal fossa.

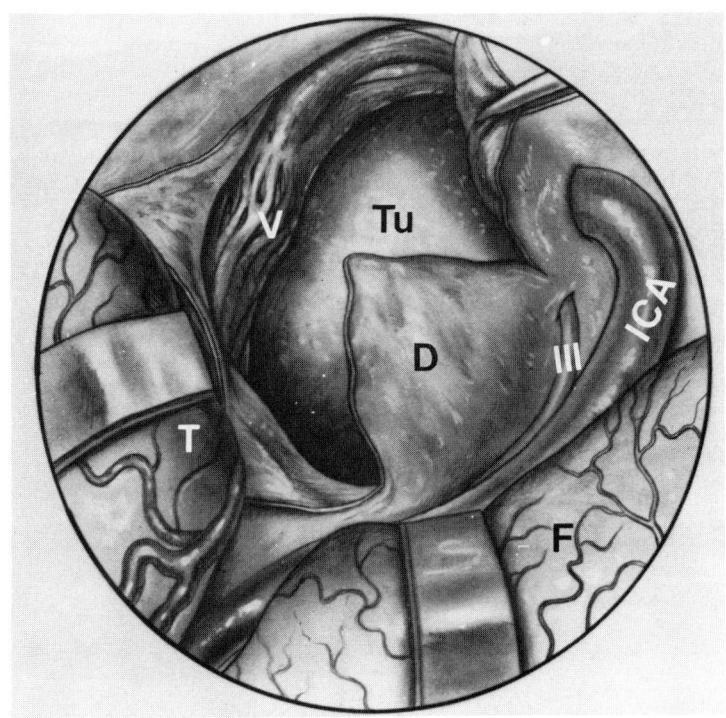

Figure 13: Operative exposure in patient D.L. The dura (D) has been opened in a cruciate fashion over an extradural, intracavernous tumor. The oculomotor, and trigeminal nerves are displaced by the tumor (Tu). T = temporal lobe; F = frontal lobe.

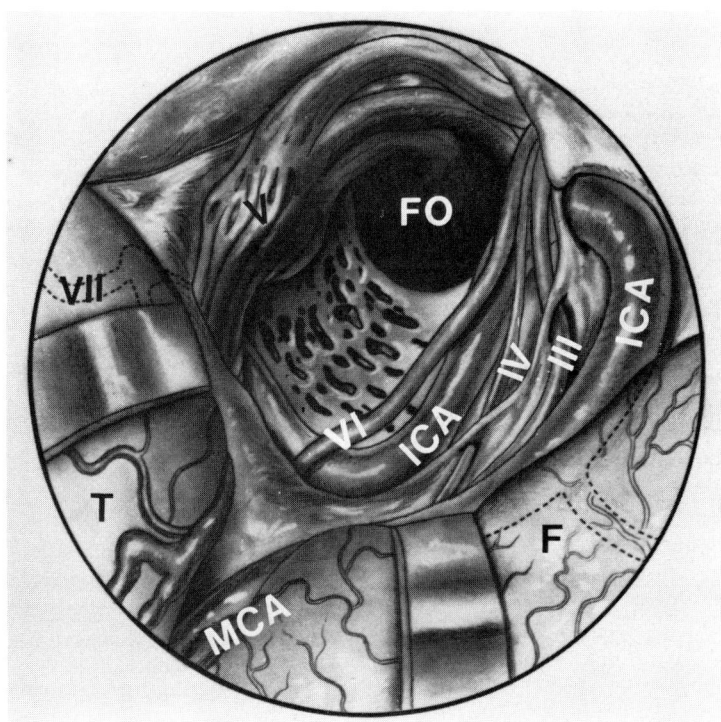

Figure 14: After the removal of the tumor, the abducens (VI) and trochlear (IV) nerves, and the intracavernous carotid artery (ICA) are seen to be markedly displaced by the tumor. The location of the facial nerve (III) and the middle cerebral artery (MCA) are shown.

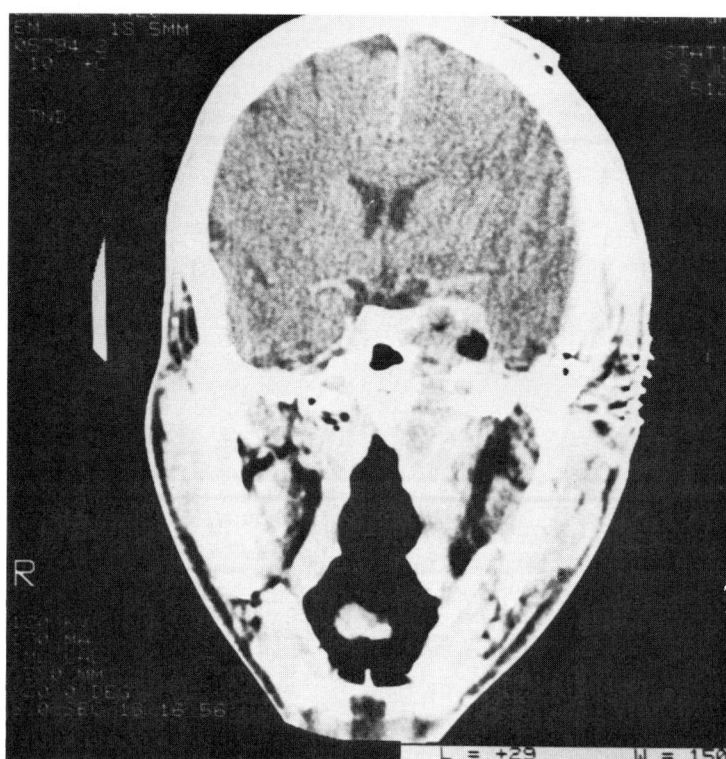

Figure 15: Coronal CT scan in the immediate postoperative period (see Fig. 16).

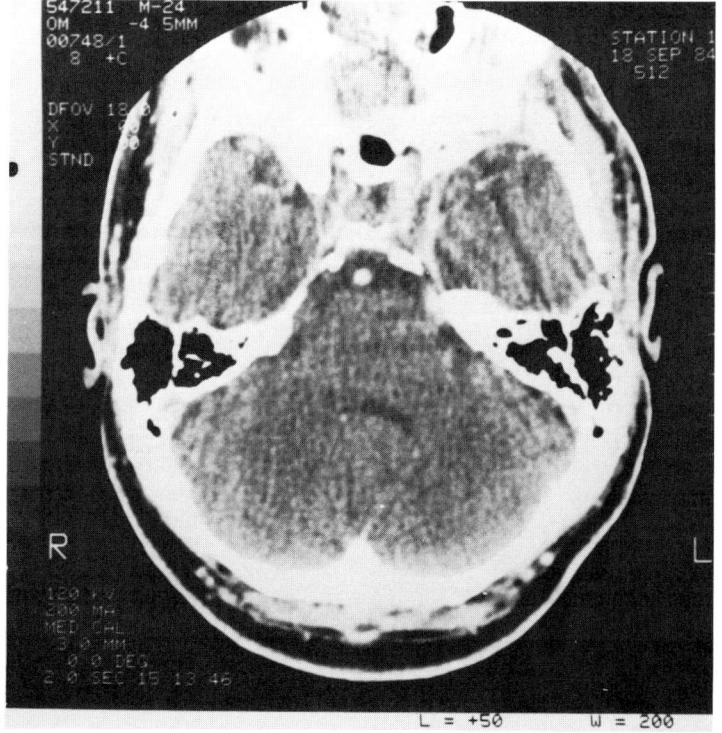

Figure 16: Same patient as in Figure 15—axial CT scan 3 months postoperatively showing no residual tumor.

Patient M.U.: Invasive Pituitary Adenoma

A 76-year-old woman presented with a 4-year history of atypical trigeminal neuralgia in the distribution of cranial nerves V₁, V₂, and V₃ and the recent onset of drooping of the right eyelid. On examination, the visual acuity in the right eye was reduced to finger counting, with a central scotoma. A complete paralysis of cranial nerves III, IV, and VI and diminished sensation in all divisions of the trigeminal nerve was present. CT scan revealed a sphenoid, sellar, suprasellar, and parasellar mass (Fig. 17).

By a transsphenoidal approach, a yellowish and friable tumor was removed from the sphenoid sinus, the sella, and the suprasellar area. The sphenoid sinus was packed with fat and fascia lata. The pathology was nonsecretory chromophobe adenoma. Postoperatively, the patient continued to have persistent facial pain and ophthalmoplegia and her vision was unimproved. It was felt by the neuroophthalmology service that an extradural compression of the optic nerve was responsible for her visual problem. A further neurosurgical procedure was performed to relieve her pain and ophthalmoplegia and to improve the chances of a cure of the tumor.

Ten days after the first operation, the tumor was reapproached through a right frontotemporal craniotomy. The bony and dural canals of the optic nerve were completely unroofed. The tumor was found to be extruding from the superior surface of the cavernous sinus, and the third nerve was humped and splayed over it as it entered the dura (Fig. 18). The lateral wall of the cavernous sinus was opened, and tumor was removed from within. The third nerve was decompressed by opening the dura of the lateral wall along its course. The superior surface of the cavernous sinus was then entered and further tumor resection was accomplished. At the beginning of the operation, there was no response from the respective extraocular muscles upon electrical stimulation of the third and fourth nerves, but after an incision was made in the lateral wall of the cavernous sinus, some spontaneous activity was noticed in

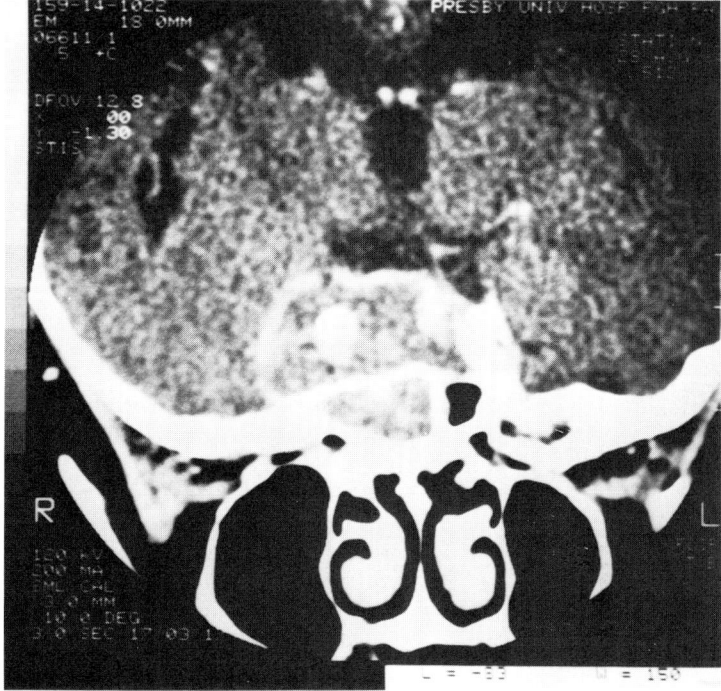

Figure 17: Coronal CT scan of patient M.U. revealing tumor within the sella, the sphenoid sinus, suprasellar area, and the cavernous sinus.

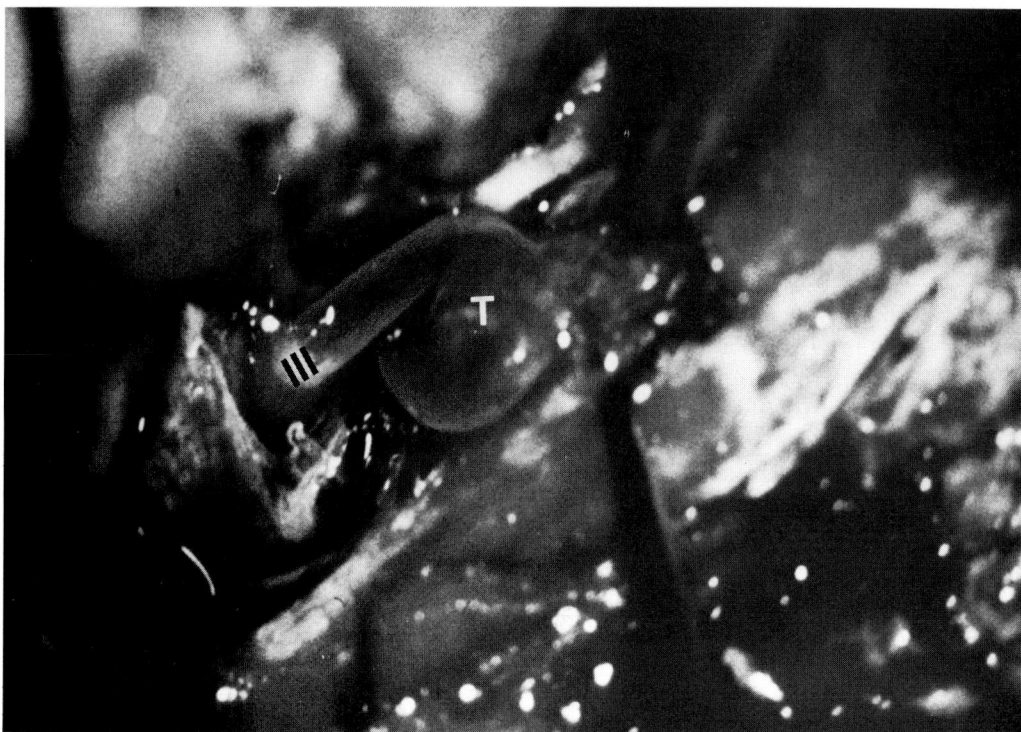

Figure 18: Operative exposure in patient M.U. Note the oculomotor (III) nerve humped and splayed by tumor (T) extruding from the cavernous sinus.

the muscles supplied by the third and fourth cranial nerves (Fig. 19).

This patient received postoperative radiation therapy. On follow-up 6 months later, her visual acuity had improved to 20/70, and the facial pain was considerably reduced, requiring only an occasional analgesic. Except for a mild ptosis, she recovered normal extraocular muscle function. CT scans obtained 8 months after the operation showed no evidence of tumor recurrence (Fig. 20). However, 9 months after the operation, the patient developed septicemia from a urinary tract infection, and died suddenly of a massive myocardial infarction. Permission for an autopsy could not be obtained.

Patient H.L.: Recurrent Meningioma

This 56-year-old woman presented to another neurosurgeon 2 years previously with a history of transient right hemiparesis and dysphasia, increasing dizziness, headaches, and memory loss. A CT scan revealed a tumor arising from the clivus area. The lesion was exposed by a left frontotemporal transsylvian approach, and meningioma arising from the upper clivus was removed. There was extension of the tumor around the exit of the left carotid artery from the left cavernous sinus area which was coagulated. During this operation, the right third nerve was seen to be humped over tumor. The patient had a transient third nerve paresis on the left side postoperatively but recovered from this completely. Follow-up CT scan a year later revealed a recurrent tumor arising from the right cavernous sinus area and occupying the tentorial notch and the upper clivus region on the right side (Fig. 21, 22A and B).

She was then referred to us for further evaluation and treatment (Fig. 23A and B). Her neurological examination upon admission was entirely normal. A balloon occlusion test of the right ICA was well tolerated, without any change in CBF. In

Operative Management: Cavernous Sinus • 411

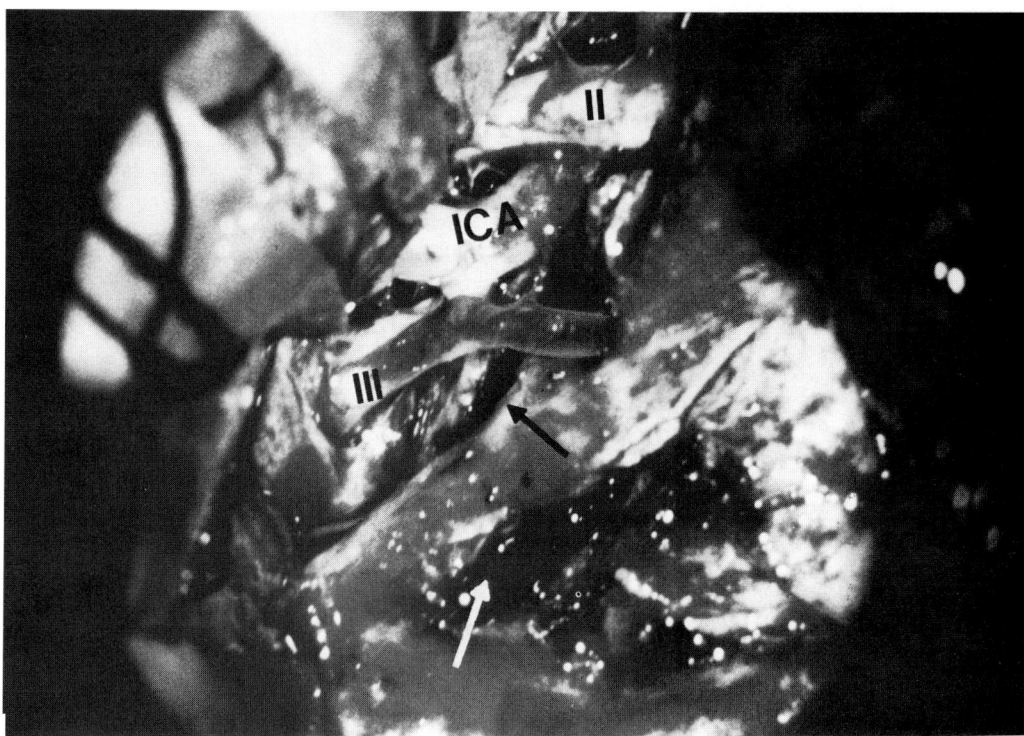

Figure 19: After tumor removal. The oculomotor nerve is now well decompressed. The black arrow indicates entry into the cavernous sinus by the superior approach, and the white arrow the entry by the lateral approach.

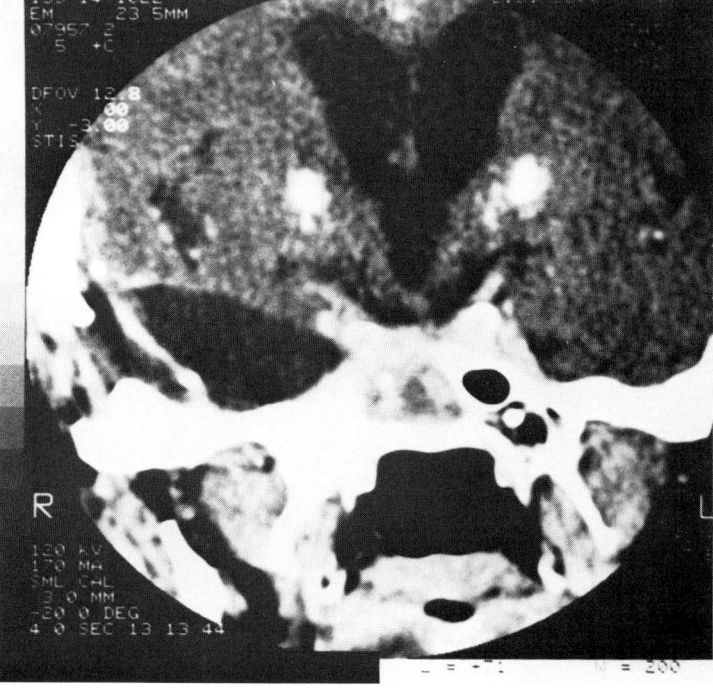

Figure 20: Postoperative CT scan showing the absence of tumor.

412 • TUMORS OF THE CRANIAL BASE: DIAGNOSIS AND TREATMENT

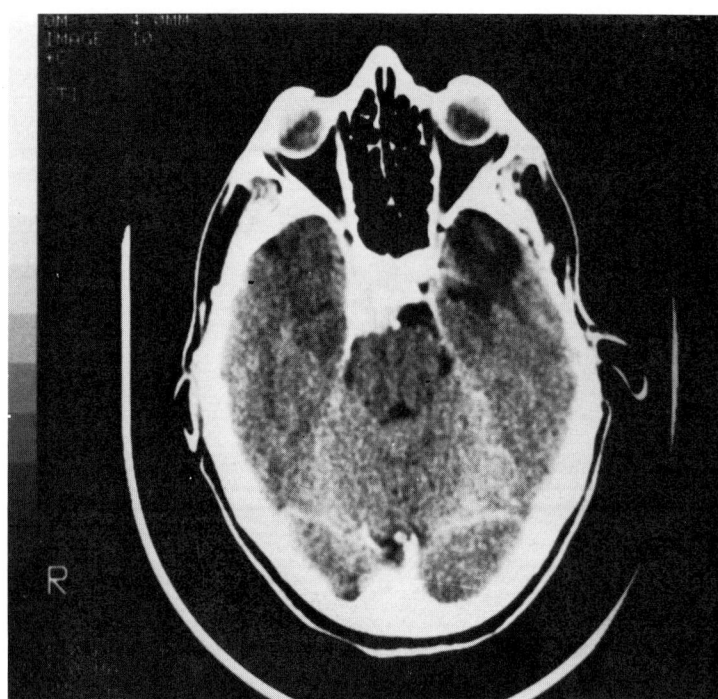

Figure 21: Preoperative axial CT scan of patient H.L. showing tumor in the cavernous sinus and the petroclival area (see Figs. 22A, B).

November 1985, the tumor was reached by us through a combined right frontotemporal and infratemporal fossa approach. The vertical and horizontal segments of the petrous carotid artery were exposed and prepared for temporary clipping. Tumor was noted to be occupying the region of the cavernous sinus, tentorial notch, and the clivus. It was breaking through the dura of the cavernous sinus superiorly, and the third cranial nerve was markedly humped and splayed over the tumor. Through a lateral approach, tumor was totally removed from all the

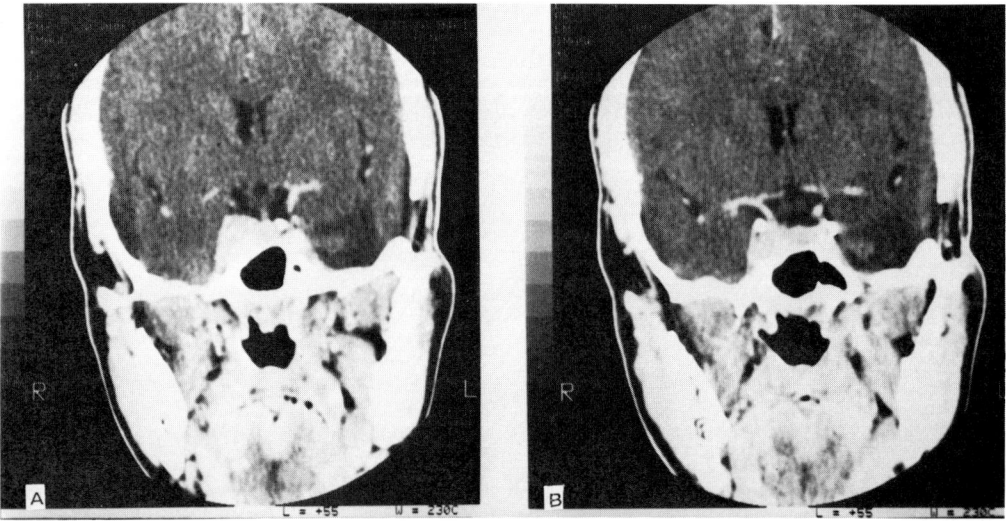

Figure 22A, B: Coronal CT scans of patient H.L. (see Fig. 21).

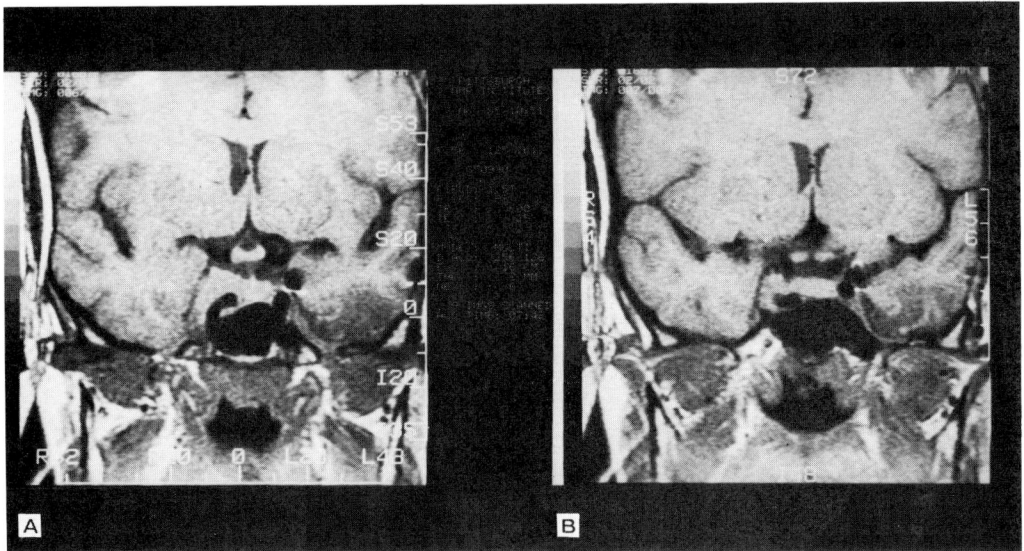

Figure 23A, B: Coronal magnetic resonance images of patient No. 8 showing tumor within the cavernous sinus and its relationship to the internal carotid artery and the pituitary gland.

regions described. The third nerve was widely decompressed to the superior orbital fissure. The meningohypophyseal and the capsular branches of the cavernous ICA artery were enlarged and supplying the tumor and were coagulated.

Postoperatively, the patient was noted to have a paresis of the facial nerve and the abducens nerve and a paralysis of the third and fourth cranial nerves. On the second postoperative day, she developed a delayed deterioration of vision in the right eye to light perception only. Cerebrospinal fluid leakage occurred through an opening in the external ear canal and this resolved with spinal fluid drainage. There was no residual tumor noted on postoperative CT scans (Figs. 24, 25A and B).

On follow-up examination 8 months later, the facial weakness had resolved. The function of the third and sixth nerves had improved considerably and was almost normal. However, visual function did not improve beyond light perception.

Comment: Even though the optic nerve was not unroofed in this particular patient and the superior approach to the cavernous sinus was not used, a delayed deterioration of vision occurred. This may have been due to a delayed occlusion of the ophthalmic artery or due to swelling of the optic nerve and compression within the optic canal.

Summary of Cases and Operative Results

A total of 16 intracavernous neoplasms were operated on which included six meningiomas, one chordoma, three chondrosarcomas, one pituitary adenoma, two trigeminal neurinomas, one squamous cell carcinoma, and two adenoid cystic carcinomas (Table I). The majority of the neoplasms were extensive, and involved other areas besides the CS. Among the meningiomas, four lesions involved the interior of the CS, whereas two involved the lateral wall only. Fourteen of the 16 neoplasms were judged to have been removed totally and two subtotally, on the basis of postoperative CT and MRI scans. Patients with malignant tumors underwent radiation therapy postoperatively. On follow-up ranging from 3 months to 2½ years, there was no evidence of tumor regrowth in any of these patients, but the follow-up period is inadequate to judge this. All the patients are independent for daily living, and 14 have

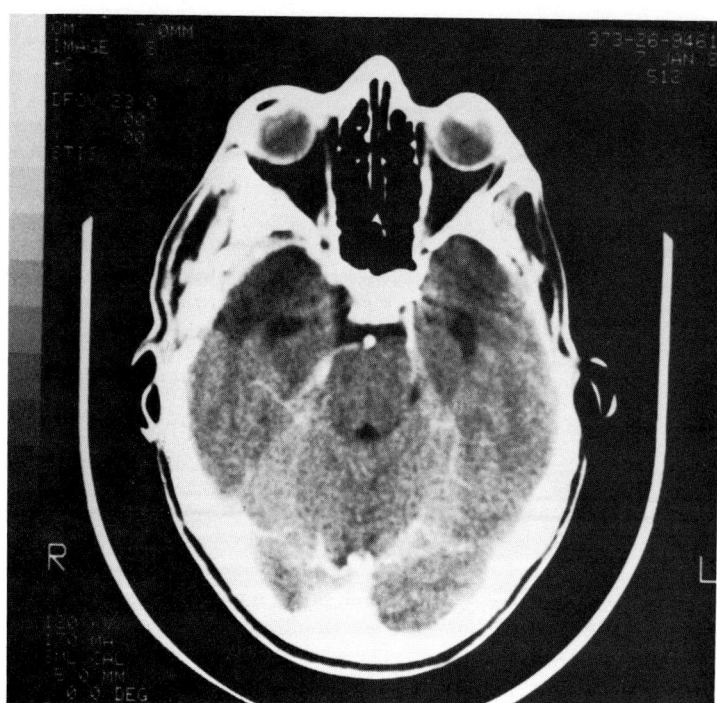

Figure 24: Postoperative axial CT scan obtained after tumor excision (see Figs. 25A, B).

returned to their previous work. Two patients have taken permanent disability from work for economic reasons.

Complications (Table II)

There were no deaths or strokes postoperatively. One patient (J.K.) suffered a postoperative wound infection with gram negative organisms secondary to invasion from a previous maxillectomy cavity which communicated with the wound despite free rectus flap reconstruction. A pseudoaneurysm of the ICA and a sentinel hemorrhage occurred. A permanent balloon occlusion of the ICA, subsequent anticoagulation, removal of the bone flap, and antibiotic therapy have produced an excellent outcome in this patient. The permanent cranial nerve complications are seen in Table II. Although four patients suffered a complete ophthalmoplegia and four others suffered abducens paralysis immediately after the operation, most of these patients recovered function 3 to 9 months later. In one patient with a preoperative subtotal oculomotor palsy, the oculomotor nerve was found to be invaded by tumor at its entrance into the CS. The abnormal segment was excised and the nerve was resutured with 10/0 nylon. It is too early to know whether there will be meaningful functional recovery. In one patient with a malignant tumor, the invaded abducens nerve was excised with the neoplasm. Permanent partial trigeminal nerve deficits occurred in three patients due to tumor invasion. Cranial nerve function also improved postoperatively in three patients. There were two postoperative CSF leaks. One patient required re-exploration and packing of the sphenoid sinus with fat, and the other responded to spinal fluid drainage alone.

Discussion

Previous Reports

Previous reports of operations within the cavernous sinus for aneurysms and neoplasms and our current report are

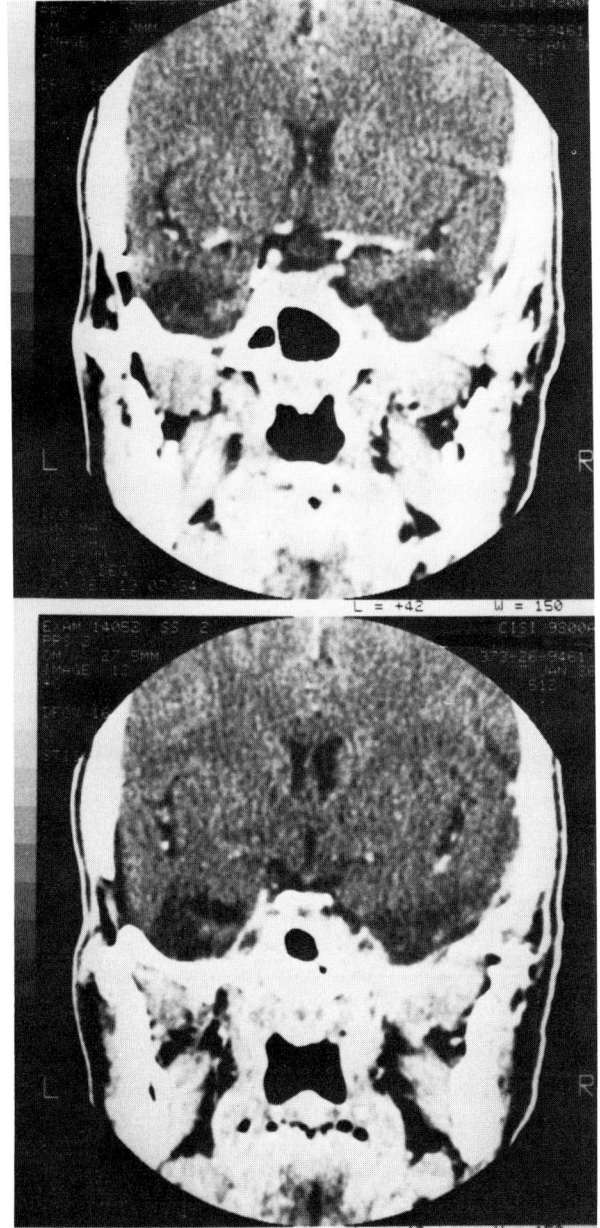

Figure 25A, B: Coronal scans obtained after excision of tumor in same patient as in Figure 24.

listed in Table III. Reports of operations for carotid cavernous fistulae are excluded because the majority of these are best managed at present by intravascular catheter techniques. Parkinson pioneered the operative approach to intracavernous lesions, and reported on 31 lesions.[26,27] A lateral approach to the CS was utilized. Data concerning the completeness of tumor excision, and long-term follow-up were not available. Dolenc reported three cases of giant aneurysms managed by direct clipping or aneurysmorraphy. Although his approach to the CS was lateral, it differed from Parkinson's in that a complete dissection of the cranial nerves in the lateral wall was performed.[9] Hakuba et al. used four approaches during opera-

Table III
Published Reports of Direct Operations For Intracavernous Aneurysms and Neoplasms

Author/Year	Aneurysms (Number)	Neoplasms (Number and Type)	Approaches	Outcome
Gordy 1965[12]	—	1 Trigeminal neuroma	Lateral	Good
Parkinson 1965[26,27]	1	12	Lateral	1 Death; other details unavailable
Nakahara et al. 1975[23]	1	—	Lateral	Good
Mackay et al. 1978[21]	—	2 Pituitary adenomas	Lateral	1 Poor 1 Good
Zozulia et al. 1979[48]	—	Number not known Meningiomas, Pituitary adenomas	Not known	Not known
Johnston 1979[17]	1	—	Lateral	Fair
Unsold et al.[43]	—	1 Metastatic carcinoma (biopsy)	Not known	Fair
Schubiger et al. 1980[31]	—	1 Neurinoma (origin not identified)	Lateral	Good
Kline and Galbraith 1981[18]	—	1 Epidermoid	Lateral	Good
Hakuba et al. 1982[14]	6	4 Meningiomas 1 Neurinoma 1 Teratoma 3 Pituitary adenomas 2 Chordomas	Lateral 3 Anterolateral 6 Anteromedial 2 Posterior 1 Combined 2	1 Death 1 Hemiplegia 13 Good
Dolenc 1983[9]	3	—	Lateral	Good 1 Fair*
Sekhar 1986	—	6 Meningiomas 2 Trigeminal neurinomas 1 Pituitary adenoma 1 Chordoma 3 Chondrosarcomas 2 Adenoid cystic Ca 1 Squamous cell Ca	Lateral 15 Superior 6 Inferior 3 Medial 1	15 Good 1 Fair **

*One patient died 3 months postoperatively as a result of infection after a good initial outcome.
**Died 8 months following the operation as a result of a myocardial infarction.

tions for six aneurysms and 13 neoplasms.[14] The lateral approach was through the Parkinson's triangle. Their anterolateral approach consisted of removing the anterior clinoid and the wall of the optic nerve canal to expose the anterior intracavernous portion of the ICA. The anteromedial approach was through the planum sphenoidale and the sphenoid sinus to reach the opposite CS. Their posterior approach was an exposure of the petrous apex, without entering the CS. The authors did not emphasize the preservation of cranial nerve function. Complications included one death, one stroke, one loss of vision and two other multiple cranial nerve palsies.[14] Laws et al. used a transethmoidal, transsphenoidal approach to occlude a carotid cavernous fistula, with a balloon in the cervical ICA for proximal control.[20] We do not recommend transsphenoidal approaches to the CS because of inadequate exposure, poor proximal and distal control of the ICA, and the danger of CSF leakage.

Philosophy of Management of Tumors of Cavernous Sinus

The current options for managing a neoplasms of the cavernous sinus include doing nothing, operative removal, and radiation therapy with or without operation. Until more data become available concerning the response to different therapeutic modalities, the decision should be individualized according to the patient's age and physiological condition, the pathology of the neoplasm, and its biological behavior. With regard to basal meningiomas, involvement of the CS has been the limitation for radical tumor resection, and the cause of recurrence, in a number of series.[1,2,7,32,35,46] However, the biological behavior of meningiomas is variable. Recurrence may occur very quickly in some patients, while in others it may be delayed for years. Radiation therapy of intracavernous meningiomas has been shown to improve the symptoms, but to cause no apparent change on CT.[34,44] Thus younger patients and those with recurrent meningiomas must be considered for a radical tumor resection, with or without radiation therapy. Pituitary adenomas have been treated successfully in many cases by subtotal tumor resection and radiation However, it has been pointed out by Mackay and Hosobuchi[21] and others[25,38] that a major cause of recurrence of pituitary tumors is the intracavernous and extradural portions of the tumor. A radical operation in which intracavernous portions of the tumor are removed may therefore be indicated in those with recurrent pituitary tumors.

In patients with chordomas and chondrosarcomas of the cranial base, many reports have established that the combination of a radical operative resection and postoperative radiation therapy gives the best long-term results.[4,5,8,11,39,45] When these tumors involve the CS, removal of tumor from within the CS permits more complete resection. Reports on series of esthesioneuroblastomas and juvenile angiofibromas include evidence that involvement of the cavernous sinus is a limitation for radical tumor excision and impairs the eventual outcome.[3,10,16,19,33,37] The majority of adenoid cystic, acinar cell, and squamous cell carcinomas involving the cranial base and the CS are currently managed by biopsy, radiation, and chemotherapy and have a poor outcome. Removal of the CS portion of the tumor may facilitate the total resection of the cranial base neoplasm, and in combination with radiation therapy, may improve the patient survival.

A question that remains to be answered is whether treatment of CS tumors by radical operation with or without radiation therapy is better than radiation therapy alone. Since radiation can induce sarcomas, cause temporal lobe necrosis, and produce cranial nerve palsies, and its effects on benign tumors are variable, it should be avoided for benign tumors that can be excised totally. For malignant tumors, radiation is more likely to be effective when the tumor cell mass is considerably reduced. Long-term follow-up of a number of patients is required to answer this question.

References

1. Adegbite AB, Khan MI, Paine KW, et al: The recurrence of intracranial meningiomas after surgical treatment. J Neurosurg 58:51-56, 1983.
2. Bonnal J, Thibaut A, Brotchi J, et al: Invading meningiomas of the sphenoid ridge. J Neurosurg 53:587-599, 1980.
3. Chapman P, Carter RL, Clifford P: The diagnosis and surgical management of olfactory neuroblastoma: the role of craniofacial resection. J Laryngol Otol 95:785-799, 1981.
4. Chetiyawardana AD: Chordoma: results of treatment. Clin Radiol 35:159-161, 1984.
5. Cianfriglia F, Pompili A, Occhipinti E: Intracranial malignant cartilaginous tumors: Report of two cases and review of literature. Acta Neurochir (Wien) 45:163-75, 1978.
6. Ciric I, Mikhael M, Stafford T, et al: Transsphenoidal microsurgery of pituitary macroadenomas with long term follow up results. J Neurosurg 59:395-401, 1983.
7. Cophignon J, Lucena J, Clay C, et al: Limits to radical treatment of sphenoorbital meningiomas. Acta Neurochir (Suppl) 28:375-380, 1979.
8. Cummings BJ, Hodson OI, Bush RS: Chordoma: The results of megavoltage radiation therapy. Int J Radiol Oncol Biol Phys 9:633-42, 1983.
9. Dolenc V: Direct microsurgical repair of intracavernous vascular lesions. J Neurosurg 58:824-831, 1983.

10. Fisch U: The infratemporal fossa approach for nasopharyngeal tumors. *Laryngoscope* 93:36-44, 1979.
11. Gay I, Elidan J, Kopolovic J: Chondrosarcoma at the skull base. *Ann Otol Rhinol Laryngol* 90:53-5, 1981.
12. Gordy PD: Neurinoma of the gasserian ganglion. Report of a case and review of the literature. *J Neurosurg* 22:90-94, 1965.
13. Grimson BS, Ross MJ, Tyson G: Return of function after intracranial suture of the trochlear nerve. *J Neurosurg* 61:191-192, 1984.
14. Hakuba A, Nishimura S, Tsukamoto M: Surgical approaches to the cavernous sinus. Report of 19 cases. *Neurol Med Chir (Tokyo)* 22:295-308, 1982.
15. Harris FS, Rhoton AL: Anatomy of the cavernous sinus: A microsurgical study. *J Neurosurg* 45:169-180, 1976.
16. Jafek BW, Krekorian EA, Kirsch WM, et al: Juvenile nasopharyngeal angiofibroma. Management of intracranial extension. *Head Neck Surg* 2:119-128, 1979.
17. Johnston I: Direct surgical treatment of bilateral intracavernous ICA aneurysms. *J Neurosurg* 51:98-102, 1979.
18. Kline LB, Galbraith JG: Parasellar epidermoid tumor presenting as painful ophthalmoplegia. *J Neurosurg* 54:113-117, 1981.
19. Krekorian EA, Kato RH: Surgical management of nasopharyngeal angiofibroma with intracranial extension. *Laryngoscope* 87:154-164, 1977.
20. Laws E Jr, Onofrio BM, Pearson BW, et al: Successful management of bilateral carotid-cavernous fistulae with a transsphenoidal approach. *Neurosurgery* 4:162-167, 1979.
21. Mackay A, Hosobuchi Y: Treatment of intracavernous extensions of pituitary adenomas. *Surg Neurol* 10:377-383, 1978.
22. Moller AR, Jannetta PJ: Preservation of facial function during removal of acoustic neuromas: Use of monopolar constant-voltage stimulation and EMG. *J Neurosurg* 61:757-760, 1984.
23. Nakahara A, Asakura T, Kawabatake H, et al: A giant aneurysm of the internal carotid artery treated by intracranial direct surgery. *No Shinke: Geka* 3:783-789, 1975.
24. Nelson PB: Large tumors of the pituitary gland. In Sekhar LN, Schramm VL (eds): *Tumors of the Cranial Base: Diagnosis and Treatment.* Mt. Kisco, NY, Futura Publishing Co. (in press).
25. Northfield DWC: *The Surgery of the Central Nervous System.* Oxford, Blackwell, 1973, p 285.
26. Parkinson D: A surgical approach to the cavernous portion of the carotid artery: Anatomical studies and case report. *J Neurosurg* 23:474-483, 1965.
27. Parkinson D, West M: Lesions of the cavernous sinus region. In Youmans JR (ed): *Neurological Surgery,* Vol 5, Second Ed. Philadelphia, WB Saunders, 1982, pp 3004-3023.
28. Samii M: Reconstruction of the trigeminal nerve. In Samii M, Jannetta PJ (eds): *The Cranial Nerves.* New York, Springer-Verlag, pp 352-358, 1981.
29. Sandvoss G, Cervos-navar OJ, Yasargil MG: Intracranial suture of oculomotor nerve in cats. *Neurochirugia* (in press).
30. Sandvoss G, Smith RD, Yasargil MG: Experimentelle, Microchirurgische freilegung der hirnerver III, IV, und VI bei der Katze. *Neurochirurgia* 27:129-132, 1984.
31. Schubiger O, Valavanis A, Hayek J, et al: Neuroma of the cavernous sinus. *Surg Neurol* 13:313-316, 1980.
32. Sekhar LN, Jannetta PJ: Cerebellopontine angle meningiomas. Microsurgical excision and follow up results. *J Neurosurg* 60:500-505, 1984.
33. Shah JP, Fehgali J: Esthesioneuroblastoma. *Am J Surg* 142:456-458, 1981.
34. Sheline GE: Radiation therapy of brain tumors. *Cancer* 39:873:881, 1977.
35. Simpson D: The recurrence of intracranial meningiomas after surgical treatment. *J Neurol Neurosurg Psychiatr* 20:22-39, 1957.
36. Spetzler RF, Carter PL: Revascularization and aneurysm surgery: Current status. *Neurosurgery* 16:111-116, 1985.
37. Standefer J, Holt GR, Brown WE, et al: Combined intracranial and extracranial excision of nasopharyngeal angiofibroma. *Laryngoscope* 93:772-779, 1983.
38. Stern WE, Batzdorf U: Intracranial removal of pituitary adenomas. An evaluation of varying degrees of excision from partial to total. *J Neurosurg* 33:564-573, 1970.
39. Suit HD, Goitein M, Munzenrider J, et al: Definitive radiation therapy for chordoma and chondrosarcoma of base of skull and cervical spine. *J Neurosurg* 56:377-85, 1982.
40. Symon L, Jakuboski J, Kendall B: Surgical treatment of giant pituitary adenomas. *J Neurol Neurosurg Psychiatr* 42:973-982, 1979.
41. Taptas JN: The so-called cavernous sinus:

A review of the controversy and its implications for neurosurgeons. *Neurosurgery* 11:712-717, 1982.
42. Umansky F, Nathan H: The lateral wall of the cavernous sinus: With special reference to the nerves related to it. *J Neurosurg* 56:228-234, 1982.
43. Unsold R, Sajran AB, Sagran E, et al: Metastatic infiltration of nerves in the CS. *Arch Neurol* 37:59-61, 1980.
44. Van Effenterre R, Bataini JP, Cabanis EA, et al: High energy radiotherapy in the treatment of meningiomas of the cavernous sinus. *Acta Neurochir* (Suppl) 28:464-467, 1979.
45. Wold LE, Laws ER Jr: Cranial chordomas in children and young adults. *J Neurosurg* 59:1043-7, 1983.
46. Yasargil MG, Mortara RW, Curcic M: Meningiomas of the basal posterior cranial fossa. In Krayenbuhl H (ed): *Advances and Technical Standards in Neurosurgery*, Vol. 7. Wien, Springer-Verlag, 1980, pp 3-115.
47. Yonas H, Wolfson SK, Gur D, et al: Clinical experience with the use of Xenon-enhanced CT blood flow mapping in cerebral vascular disease. *Stroke* 15:443-450, 1984.
48. Zozulia YA, Romodanov SA, Patskio YV: Diagnosis and surgical treatment of benign craniobasal tumors involving the cavernous sinus. *Acta Neurochir* (Suppl) 28:387-390, 1979.

24

Infratemporal Fossa Surgery

Victor L. Schramm, Jr., M.D.

Introduction

The application of skull base surgery has expanded rapidly in recent years with the advent of improved diagnostic techniques to map tumor location and with the cooperative efforts of the head and neck surgeon, neurosurgeon, and the microvascular reconstructive surgeon. Surgical exposure of the infratemporal fossa is a pivotal procedure that provides access for excision of a variety of neoplasms as well as other diseases such as carotid aneurysms. These diseases approach or involve the parapharyngeal space, petroclival area, or cavernous sinus from both intracranial and extracranial origins. This chapter will describe the evolution of infratemporal fossa surgery, the indications for such surgery, as well as anesthesia considerations, specific surgical anatomy, surgical technique and the sequela and complications of this surgery. The results of this approach when applied for the care of 63 patients will also be documented.

Evolution of Infratemporal Fossa Surgery

Surgical approaches and exposure in the infratemporal fossa initially stemmed from the need to control the anterior extension of benign tumors arising from the temporal bone such as glomus tumors into the area of the petrous carotid artery. In 1976, House[1] described a transcochlear approach to the infratemporal fossa and Fisch[2] in 1977 independently published a report of his posterolateral infratemporal fossa approach. These techniques were expanded to allow surgical resection of tumors arising primarily in the infratemporal fossa and clivus as well as tumors that had parasellar or sphenoid extension, either for intracranial lesions or tumors arising in the nasopharynx. The surgical innovations of Fisch[3-5] have provided the primary impetus for surgical treatment of lesions involving the temporal bone and base of skull. Sequelae of the postauricular transtemporal approach to the infratemporal fossa included a conductive or complete sensory neural hearing loss as well as varying degrees of facial nerve dysfunction. Problems of cerebrospinal fluid leakage, meningitis, and limited anterior visualization were common problems involved with this approach. The technique as described by Fisch has improved the postoperative functional mandibular result.

Terez[6] has applied a craniofacial approach for resection of tumors invading the pterygoid fossa but described unsatisfactory outcomes because of residual

From: Sekhar LN, Schramm VL Jr, eds: *Tumors of the Cranial Base: Diagnosis and Treatment.* Mount Kisco, New York, Futura Publishing Co, Inc, © 1987.

tumor due to inadequate surgical removal in the area of the petrous carotid artery and nasopharynx. In an attempt to improve this outcome, Friedman[7] described a stylohamular dissection for tumors involving the infratemporal fossa. He also had difficulty controlling the cervical and petrous carotid artery and reported a 25% cerebrovascular accident rate. In addition, the technique of stylohamular dissection required resection of the ascending ramus of the mandible as well as the condyle and coronoid process to gain access. This produces unnecessary disability in patients who have benign tumors. The experience of Fisch in caring for squamous cell and nonkeratinizing carcinoma of the nasopharynx produced encouraging results for stage I and stage II disease, but when tumor had extended to the foramen ovale or involved the petrous carotid artery, early death was reported and the technique was not advised. Many of the problems involved in resection of nasopharyngeal carcinoma including carotid artery management and reconstruction of the skull base to isolate the cerebrospinal fluid from the pharynx and paranasal sinuses have been solved with techniques described elsewhere in this book.

Indications for Infratemporal Fossa Surgery

Tumors that are located anterior to the tympanic cavity and internal auditory canal may be treated by a preauricular infratemporal fossa dissection. Primary tumors of the parapharyngeal space including neurogenic tumors, rhabdomyosarcomas, and tumors that extend into the parapharyngeal space such as deep lobe parotid tumors, synovial tumors of the temporomandibular joint and extensive glomus vagale and carotid body tumors may be treated by infratemporal dissection alone. A further approach may be used for nasopharyngeal tumors such as teratomas, angiofibromas, and carcinomas as well as clivus chordomas or chondrosarcoma or tumors of the petrous apex such as primary epidermoid. The preauricular infratemporal fossa approach may also be used as a part of a combined approach for tumors extending into the area including meningioma and craniopharyngioma. Maxillary sinus tumors or tumors of the ethmoid which extend to the sphenoid may also be treated with a transfacial as well as an infratemporal fossa approach. Oral cavity and oral pharyngeal carcinoma may be resected when tumors extend into the pterygomaxillary space or infratemporal fossa and tumors of the anterior cranial fossa which extend into the cavernous sinus are best approached through a combined anterior cranial and lateral infratemporal fossa approach.

A postauricular transtemporal approach is reserved for tumors that involve the mastoid as well as the infratemporal fossa. These include extensive benign tumors of the temporal bone as well as lateral malignancy such as basal cell carcinoma or squamous cell carcinoma of the ear canal. Malignancy involving the mastoid and eustachian tube require total temporal bone resection and this procedure is described in another chapter.

Contraindications for extensive infratemporal fossa surgery are few. Tumors may be dissected from around the petrous carotid artery or the carotid artery may be replaced. Even tumors extending into the cavernous sinus may be dissected with only the expected sequelae of limitation of extraocular movement. A consideration against infratemporal fossa surgery need be given only for patients with aggressive undifferentiated malignancy and for those with distant metastases. This surgery, however, should be done only in centers with the surgical and medical expertise and support required for the care of these patients.

Special Anesthesia Considerations

When oral endotracheal intubation is used, the endotracheal tube should be wired in place to mandibular dentition and prepped into the field. The oral cavity and endotracheal tube may be covered with an adherent plastic drape but should be visible during the procedure when head movement and prolonged surgical time may alter the endotracheal tube position. Nasotracheal intubation has not been found necessary to improve the ability to displace the mandible, and actually makes the surgical preparation of the face more difficult. Tracheostomy should be considered when airway compromise may be produced by the surgical manipulation or postoperative swelling and may be preferable in patients who may require vigorous postoperative pulmonary therapy or ventilatory assistance. Physiologic monitoring of facial nerve function and extraocular muscle function is often desirable and anesthesia producing muscle paralysis should be avoided. In addition to lumbar subarachnoid drainage which is routine for patients having temporal craniotomy, means for monitoring of arterial and central venous pressure, particularly in elderly patients, should be provided. A Swan-Ganz catheter is now used routinely in these situations.

Surgical Anatomy

The cervicofacial skin flap utilized in the preauricular infratemporal fossa dissection has an abundant blood supply. Even though this flap is elevated to the level of the lateral orbital rim and anterior border of the masseter muscle, the blood supply from the facial artery, infraorbital artery, and collateral from the opposite temporal artery are preserved. However, if the skin flap is folded acutely rather than over a moist gauze sponge and if prolonged pressure and dessication are allowed, marginal skin necrosis can occur. When a postauricular approach is utilized, the external ear is denervated and is also partially devascularized so that pressure intraoperatively or postoperatively can produce necrosis of the external ear skin and cartilage.

One of the primary considerations in infratemporal fossa surgery is the preservation of facial nerve function. Anteriorly, as the branches of the facial nerve exit the parotid gland, they lie beneath the platysma and facial musculature and elevation of the cervicofacial flap generally does not disturb or injure the facial nerve. The upper division, however, frequently sustains prolonged retraction and sequelae may be minimized by preserving its surrounding fibrofatty envelop by dissecting superficially in the subcutaneous tissue below the zygomatic arch and superiorly just above the level of the temporalis fascia. When the temporomandibular joint is dislocated and the mandible retracted anteriorly and inferiorly, the facial nerve is stretched at the stylomastoid foramen area, even if a superficial parotidectomy has been completed. Only by mobilizing the parotid away from the masseter fascia can the mandible be transposed without producing excessive nerve trauma. Displacement of the mandible may also be done without skeletonizing the facial nerve between the stylomastoid foramen and the mandible, and some additional support to the nerve is afforded if a cuff of soft tissue is left surrounding the centimeter of nerve between the stylomastoid foramen and mandible. The nasopharynx or petroclival area can be reached without transposing the facial nerve out of the fallopian canal. However, when the facial nerve needs to be transposed within the temporal bone, the blood supply, particularly in the area of the vertical segment, is severely compromised and results in the inevitable loss of facial function which occurs at least temporarily.

The vascular supply to the temporalis muscle comes primarily from the external carotid system through the temporal vessel superficially and the internal maxillary artery medially. Additional blood supply is provided by vessels coming through the foramen ovale as well as from communications through the squamous portion of the temporal bone. The internal maxillary artery contribution may be preserved if the temporal artery is dissected beneath the parotid to half the distance from the angle of the mandible to the zygomatic arch. If the temporalis muscle is divided inferiorly and retracted superiorly, the blood supply from the internal maxillary artery and foramen ovale areas is disrupted and the transtemporal blood supply is inadequate for muscle survival. Transposition of the temporalis muscle for skull base reconstruction is facilitated by dividing the attachment to the coronoid process of the mandible and subsequent mandibular function is not significantly compromised.

To mobilize the mandible, the ligamentous attachments from the styloid to the posterior ascending ramus of the mandible must be divided as must the sphenomandibular ligament and a portion of the adjacent pterygoid musculature. Mobilization of the temporomandibular joint capsule requires transection of the attachments at the various sutures and the vascular supply coming through the sutures can produce enough bleeding to obscure visualization unless they are coagulated prior to division. The pterygoid plexus and middle meningeal artery lie just medial and anterior to the medial aspect of the mandibular condyle. As the skull base is approached, a venous communication is present between the infratemporal fossa and the medial cavernous sinus, surrounding the lower division of the trigeminal nerve. The motor division of V_3 is most lateral with the inferior alveolar nerve being more medial. Mobilization of the lateral pterygoid muscle and its fascial attachment to the mandible exposes the pharyngobasilar fascia and the mucosa of the nasopharynx. The mucosa with its firm attachment to the medial pterygoid and skull base may be easily torn in this area. The petrosphenoid and petroclival articulations are filled with fibrocartilage, forming a synchondrosis which may be mistaken for tumor.

The bone overlying the posterior maxillary sinus, the lower lateral orbit, the inferior lateral sphenoid sinus, and the intercranial lateral orbital plate adjacent to the superior orbital fissure is thin and may be easily transgressed in the dissection. Exposure of cerebrospinal fluid to sinus secretions, injury to the lateral rectus muscle, or nerve and vessel injury in the superior orbital fissure may result.

Cranial nerves IX through XII are frequently injured in the area of the jugular foramen, particularly during dissection for extensive glomus jugulare tumors. Identification of these nerves during the cervical portion of the dissection may be done simultaneously with the isolation of the internal and external carotid arteries and jugular vein. To preserve cranial nerve function, the nerves may be followed through the skull base by dividing the jugular vein at the jugular foramen and dissecting it along with the jugular bulb in a retrograde fashion, keeping the nerves in view as they traverse the temporal bone.

The transverse process of the atlas may be exposed by removing the attachments of the sternocleidomastoid muscle, the trapezius, and longus capitus muscles, however, the position of the vertebral artery which lies just posterior, must be taken into consideration.

Preauricular Infratemporal Fossa Technique

The patient is placed in the supine position on the operating table with horseshoe or pin head fixation. The operating table is flexed 10° to improve peripheral venous return and minimize the possibility of stasis and venous thrombosis with postoperative pulmonary embolism. The head is shaved or alternatively, for aesthetic reasons, the hair may be parted for the surgical incision if no intradural dissection is planned. The scalp, face, and neck are surgically prepped and if carotid exposure and intradural dissection are contemplated in association with nasopharynx or sinus exposure, further preparation includes the abdomen as well as the groin and leg as donor sites for a free rectus muscle flap, saphenous vein graft, or small vein grafts for microvascular anastomosis. Antibiotic prophylaxis is begun preoperatively with considerations for nasal and nasopharyngeal flora as well as *Pseudomonas aeruginosa* if infected ear tumors are to be resected.

The surgical incision begins above the hairline, 8 cm above the mid-brow, extends above the temporal line, curving to the level of the posterior helix, and then into a preauricular skin crease. The incision is further extended around the lobule of the ear, over the mastoid, to the posterior border of the sternocleidomastoid and then anteriorly in an upper cervical skin crease, 3 or 4 cm below the angle of the mandible (Fig. 1). If a simultaneous neck dissection is to be completed, the upper cervical incision can be continued across the midline and a McFee incision made above the clavicle. At the level of the zygomatic arch, the dissection halts temporarily, to be continued in the preauricular area. The incision here is carried to the parotid fascia and then anteriorly in a subcutaneous plane extending anterior to the parotid gland. The fibrofatty soft tissue over the zygomatic arch is left to be developed as a soft tissue envelope around the upper division of the facial nerve (Figs. 2, 3). This soft tissue envelope needs to be mobilized so that exposure can be obtained to the level of the lateral orbital rim. The cervical portion of the flap is elevated initially superficial to the platysma muscle and then the platysma muscle is divided and retracted to protect the mandibular division of the facial nerve. The anterior border of the sternocleidomastoid muscle is then dissected and the muscle retracted posteriorly to expose the jugular

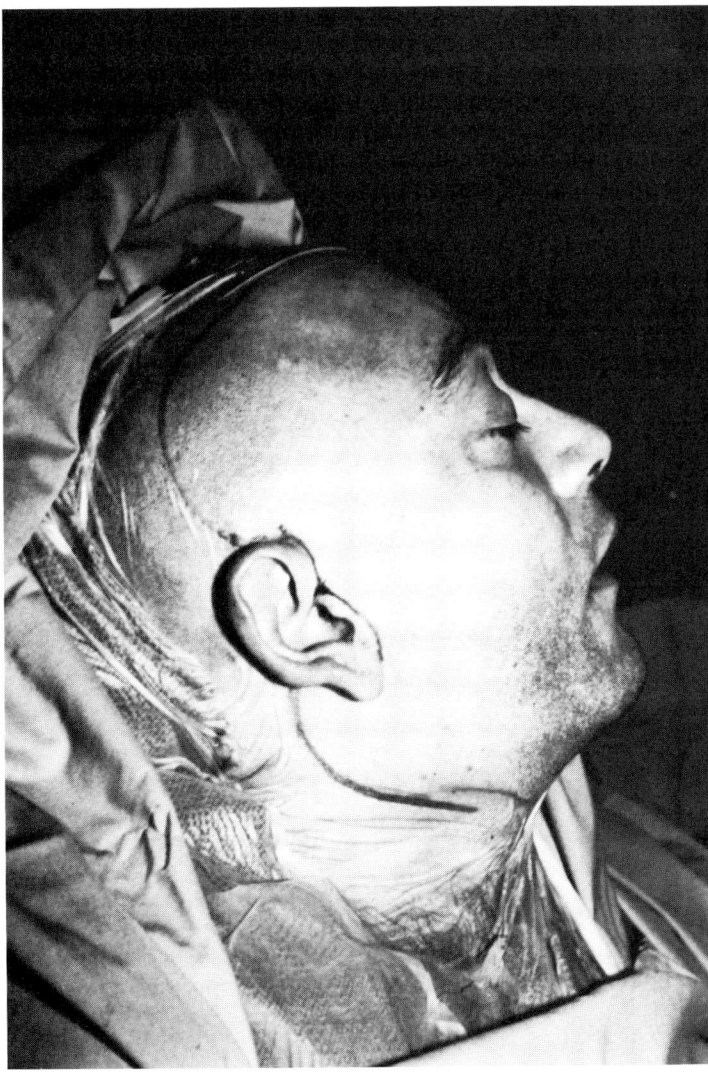

Figure 1: Incision for preauricular infratemporal fossa dissection.

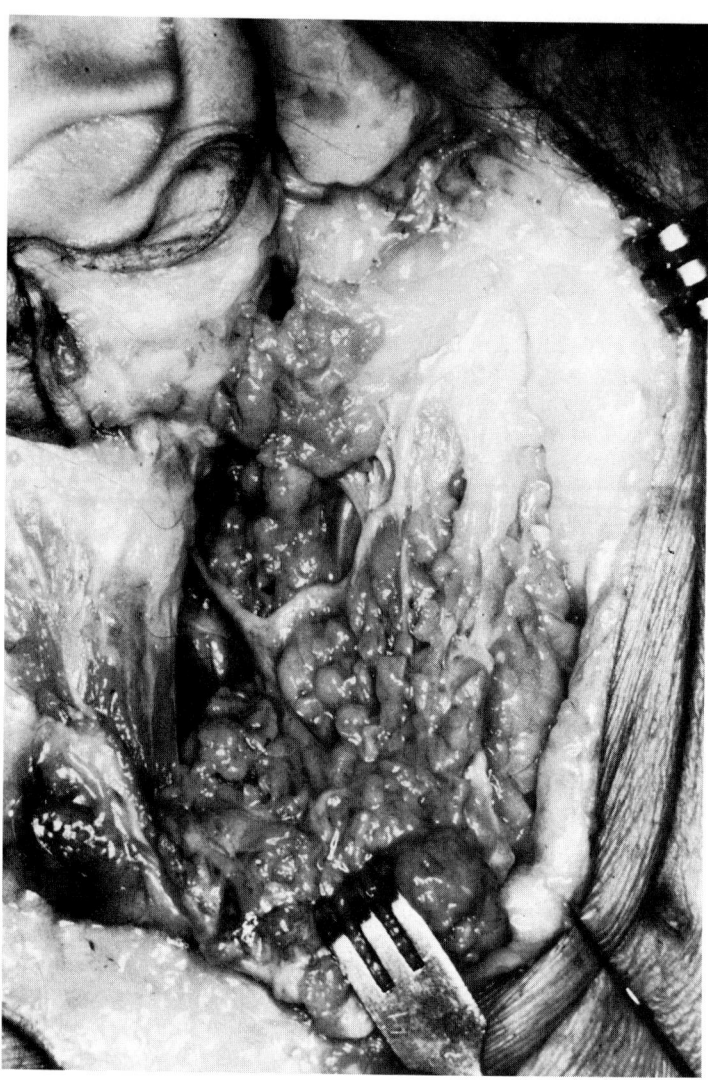

Figure 2: Facial nerve exposure between stylomastoid foramen and parotid gland. Extratemporal facial nerve trunk and upper division are dissected from surrounding soft tissue for demonstration but are not exposed during surgical dissection.

vein, the internal and external carotid arteries, and cranial nerves IX through XII. These structures are dissected superiorly to the skull base with retraction or division of the posterior belly of the digastric muscle. The styloid process is then identified medial to the mandible and the facial nerve. The stylomandibular ligament is divided with either an elevator or a scissors, leaving soft tissue remaining around the trunk of the facial nerve between the stylomastoid foramen and the mandible. The temporal artery and vein should then be dissected into and deep to the parotid gland and ligated beneath the parotid. These vessels must be treated carefully, particularly if a microvascular free muscle flap is to be used in reconstruction as they provide the most suitable donor vessels. The parotid is further mobilized over the masseter muscle with blunt dissection to the level of the zygomatic arch.

Exposure of the infratemporal fossa begins by dividing the pericranium just above the temporal line and mobilizing the temporal muscle from the underlying temporal squama. Hemostasis is facilitated during elevation of the muscle by electrocautery dissection and bone wax occlusion of the arterial and venous anastomoses through the temporal squama.

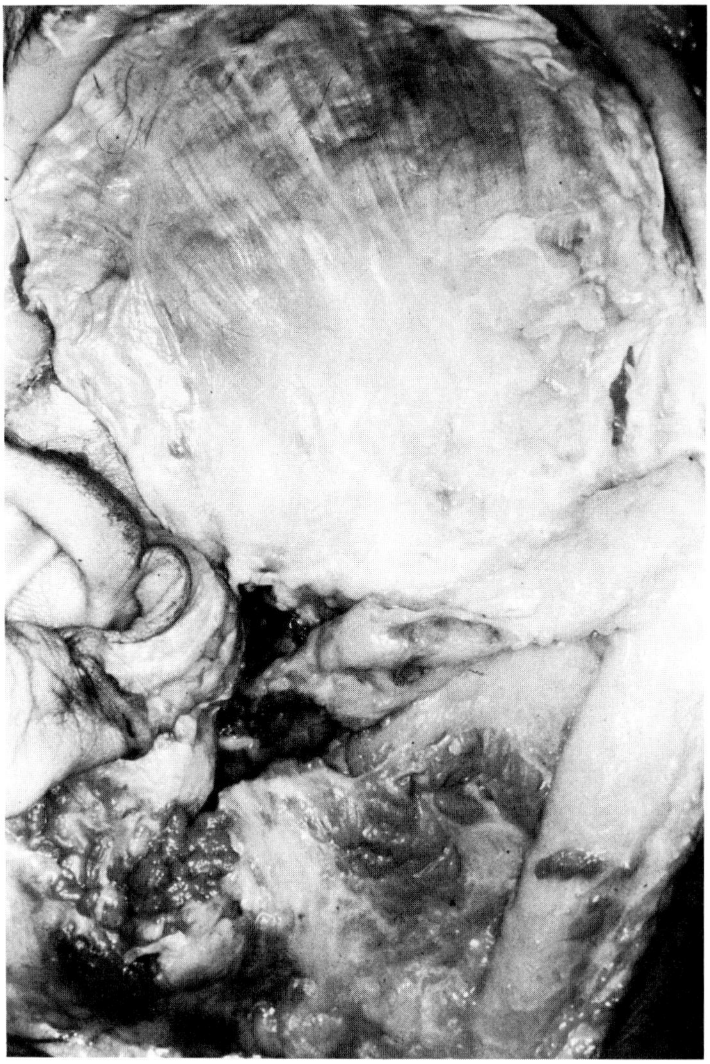

Figure 3: Periosteum incised around temporalis muscle for elevation of muscle from temporal squama.

The temporalis muscle is mobilized along the upper and lateral border of the orbital rim as well as along the posterior root of the zygoma.

Further exposure of the infratemporal fossa is limited by the presence of the zygomatic arch. The arch may be mobilized and left attached to the temporalis muscle or may be divided posteriorly and anteriorly and removed (Fig. 4). When a more anterior exposure is desirable for visualization of the clivus and petrous apex it is preferable to remove the zygomatic arch along with the lateral orbital rim and lateral orbital wall. If the arch and lateral orbital rim are to be removed, the overlying fascia and periosteum are incised at the upper border of the zygomatic arch, and a subperiosteal dissection completed both lateral and medial to the arch. Retraction of the overlying soft tissue containing the upper division of the facial nerve should be done in a lateral rather than an inferior fashion, in order to avoid subsequent facial nerve paralysis (Fig. 5). Drill holes are placed on either side of the proposed bone incision and the bone cuts are most conveniently done with a reciprocating saw. If the zygomatic arch is to be transposed with the temporal muscle, the fascial attachments are left intact except anteriorly and posteriorly. The posterior

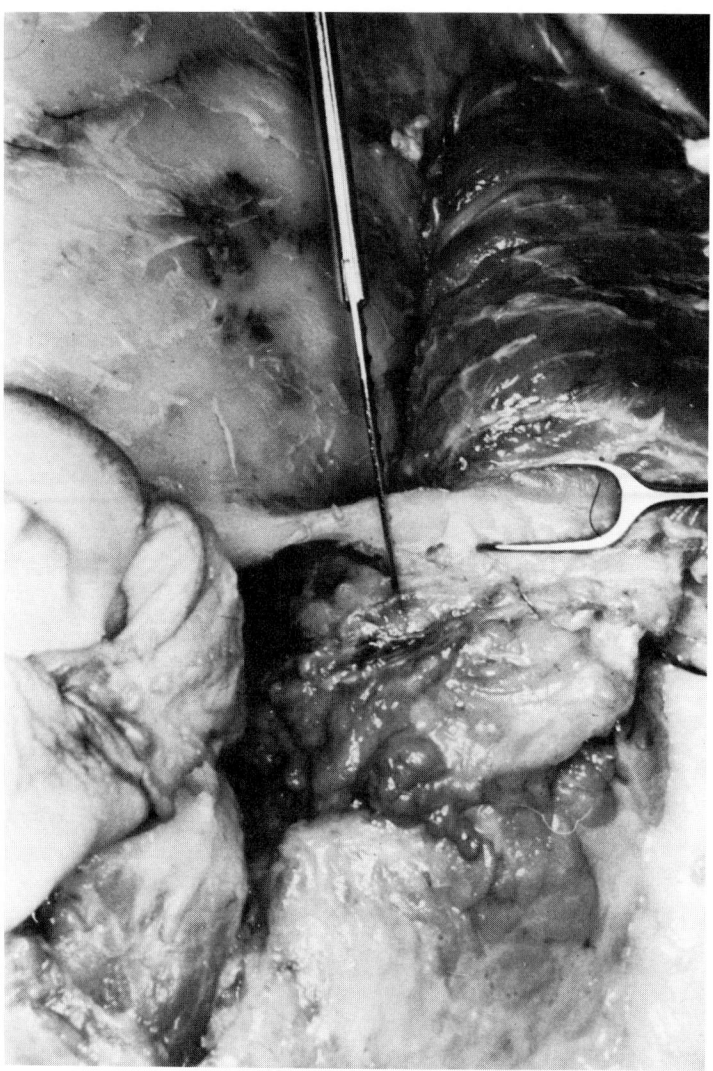

Figure 4: Posterior zygomatic arch divided with reciprocating saw after initial mobilization of temporomandibular joint capsule.

saw cut is placed above and tangential to the capsule of the temporomandibular joint.

After mobilization or removal of the zygomatic arch, further dissection deep to the facial nerve and surrounding tissue is possible over the mandibular condyle and neck as well as ascending ramus of the mandible, to complete the parotid mobilization. Mobilization of the mandibular condyle and surrounding temporomandibular joint capsule is most easily accomplished with an Adson neurosurgical elevator and with bipolar cautery assisted by suction dissection (Fig. 6). During soft tissue elevation anterior to the mandibular joint capsule, bipolar cautery is necessary to obtain hemostasis and to facilitate exposure of the middle meningeal artery. The middle meningeal artery may be coagulated by bipolar cautery and the venous plexus in the area also needs to be cauterized prior to division of the sphenomandibular ligament and pterygoid attachment from anterior and medial to the mandible. Convenient and relatively atraumatic retraction of the cervical-facial flap as well as the temporalis muscle may be obtained by suturing rubber bands to these structures and attaching the rubber bands to surrounding drapes. After mobilization of the mandibular condyle, it

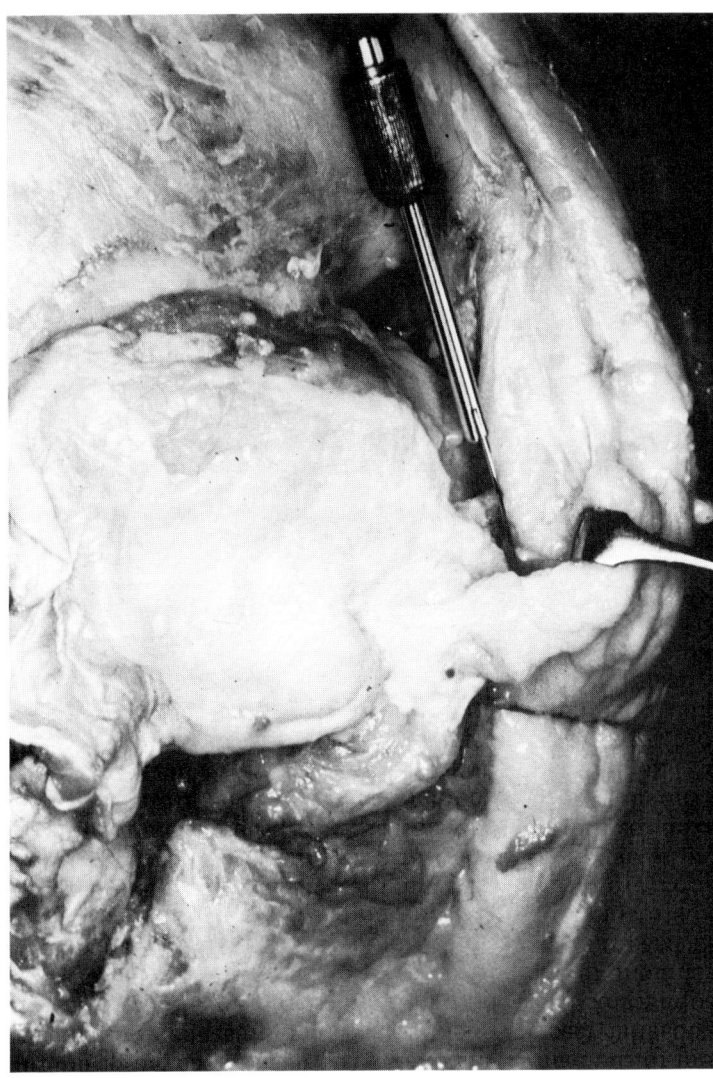

Figure 5: Soft tissue around upper division of facial nerve retracted laterally for transection of anterior zygomatic arch at lateral orbital rim.

can be held in an anterior and inferior position by a Fisch retractor or alternatively by a Green thyroid retractor, again attached to rubber band traction.

The subsequent infratemporal fossa dissection depends on the tumor location and biology. A subperiosteal dissection is continued to the level of the foramen ovale and bleeding again controlled with bipolar cautery. Anterior dissection over the lateral orbit and maxilla allows identification of the lateral pterygoid muscle and the pterygomaxillary fissure (Fig. 7). If extracranial dissection is adequate for tumor removal, the infratemporal bone may be thinned with a cutting burr and drill as the dissection proceeds. If total or partial mobilization of the carotid artery or if intracranial dissection are necessary, a low temporal craniotomy is completed. The craniotomy extends anteriorly to the anterior extent of the middle fossa and posteriorly includes the glenoid fossa. An incision anterior to the ear canal with a fine cutting burr allows later replacement and normal function of the glenoid fossa.

A decision must next be made as to the management of the third division of the trigeminal nerve in the foramen ovale. If the nerve is intimately involved with a malignant tumor, it should be sacrificed;

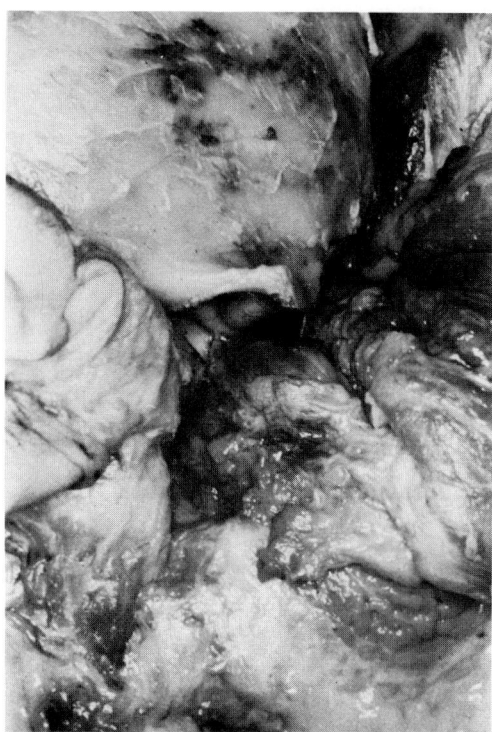

Figure 6: Mobilization of mandible from glenoid fossa prior to division of middle meningeal artery and sphenomandibular ligament.

however, it may be mobilized and dissected from a benign tumor, particularly if an intracranial dissection is included. Anterior dissection and removal of the lateral pterygoid plate or division of the posterior wall of the maxillary sinus allows exposure of the lateral wall of the nasopharynx. If extracranial dissection is adequate for the medial extent of the infratemporal dissection, the dissection may be continued superiorly along the pterygomaxillary fissure to the lateral orbit and then medial to the level of the medial pterygoid plate. Nasopharyngeal exposure may be obtained anteriorly at the maxilla, inferiorly at the level of the soft palate, and superiorly, either via the lateral wall of the sphenoid sinus or vault of the nasopharynx. The posterior dissection may include the clivus. Further surgical exposure of the sphenoid sinus may be obtained through a contralateral external ethmoid-sphenoid approach. For oral cavity and oropharyngeal carcinoma, standard techniques may be combined with the infratemporal fossa dissection. Simultaneous transfrontal sinus craniotomy and anterior fossa dissection over the orbit to the anterior cavernous sinus is also relatively easily accomplished.

Postauricular Infratemporal Fossa Dissection

For the postauricular transtemporal infratemporal fossa dissection, the same temporal and cervical incisions are made, but they are connected behind the ear, approximately 3 cm behind the concha. When tumor does not necessitate removal of the mastoid periosteum, this layer should be included with the flap elevation. The entire ear canal is elevated at the level of the bony canal, and the dissection is then continued forward as for the preauricular approach. The ear canal is closed by dissecting the cartilage from the lateral canal skin and then everting the skin with a subcutaneous closure. A sec-

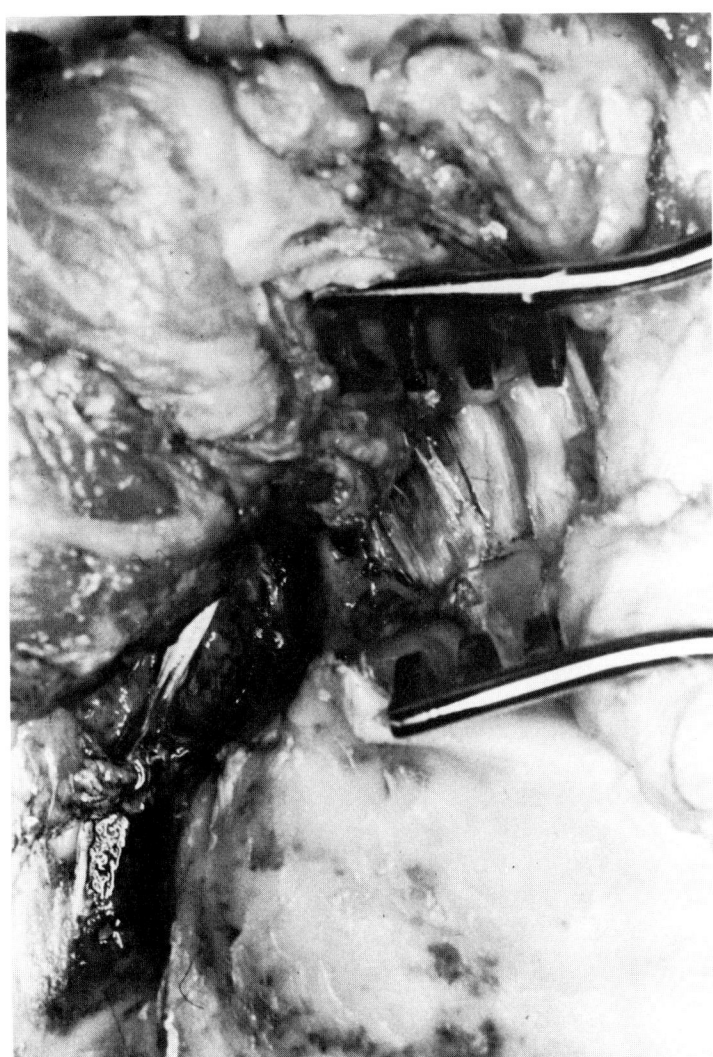

Figure 7: Retraction of mandible after division of V_3 at foramen ovale and partial dissection of pterygoid muscle from skull base.

ond layer closure over the ear canal is obtained by mobilizing the mastoid periosteum from the postauricular flap and advancing and closing it over the skin closure. Management of the cervical dissection, mobilization of the temporalis muscle and zygomatic arch, and dissection of the mandibular condyle are completed in a fashion identical to that described for the preauricular infratemporal fossa approach. The ear canal skin and tympanic membrane are removed, and the incudostapedial joint disarticulated. A complete mastoidectomy is then accomplished with dissection continuing superiorly and posteriorly to the tumor, exposing dura above the mastoid and posterior to the sigmoid sinus. The entire bone ear canal is removed to communicate the mastoid dissection with the glenoid fossa. With removal of the styloid process, bone removal can be continued along the medial aspect of the glenoid fossa to expose the carotid artery (Figs. 8, 9). Further dissection depends on the type and location of the tumor to be removed.

For extensive benign disease of the mastoid extending into the infratemporal fossa, particularly for glomus jugulare tumors, the initial dissection is designed to surround the tumor. The facial nerve may be identified at the stylomastoid

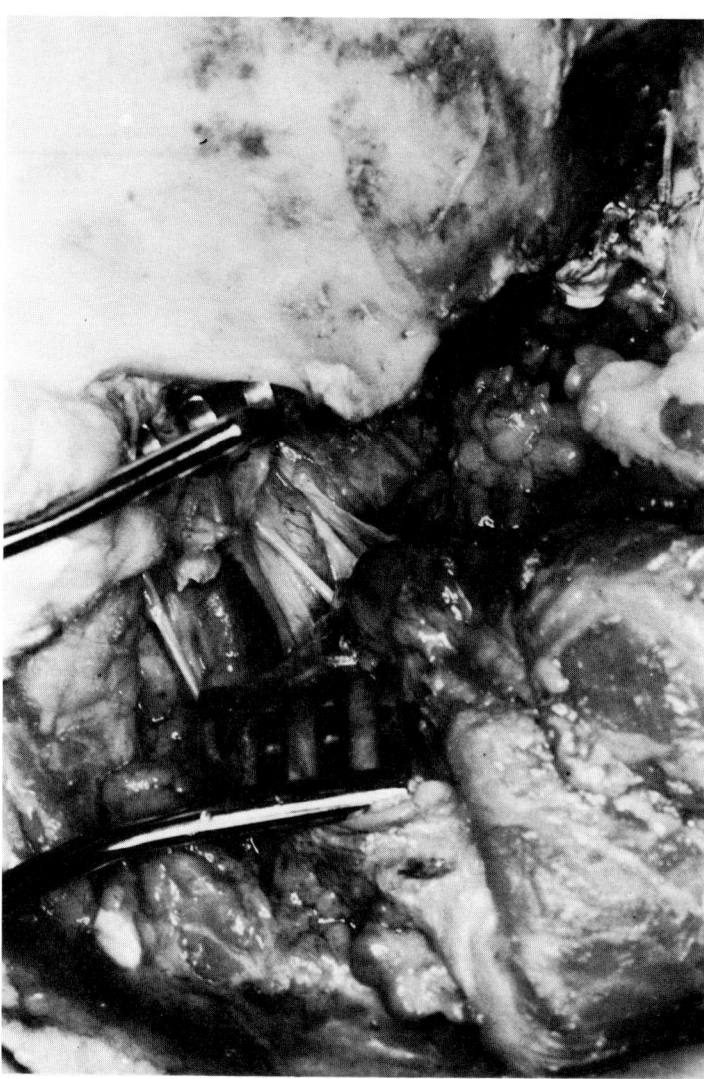

Figure 8: Exposure of cranial nerves IX–XII, internal carotid artery and jugular vein after removal of styloid process.

foramen and the surrounding fibrous attachments removed. After removing the tip of the mastoid, the decompression of the facial nerve is continued superiorly with final dissection around the facial nerve accomplished with a diamond drill and suction irrigation. Mobilization of the facial nerve from the Fallopian canal needs to be done to the level of the geniculate ganglion (Fig. 10). A trough in bone can then be made from the labyrinthine segment toward the parotid. Prior to tumor removal, the main feeding arteries, particularly the ascending pharyngeal artery, may be temporarily or permanently ligated, even if embolization of a vascular tumor has been accomplished preoperatively. The jugular vein is then divided below the jugular foramen and bone from around the foramen removed with a cutting drill and rongeurs. The sigmoid sinus above the level of the tumor must be ligated. This may be accomplished by incising dura anterior and posterior to it, and passing a ligature with a ligature carrier or aneurysm needle. Alternatively, the dura may be split, and the sigmoid sinus occluded with vascular clips. The jugular

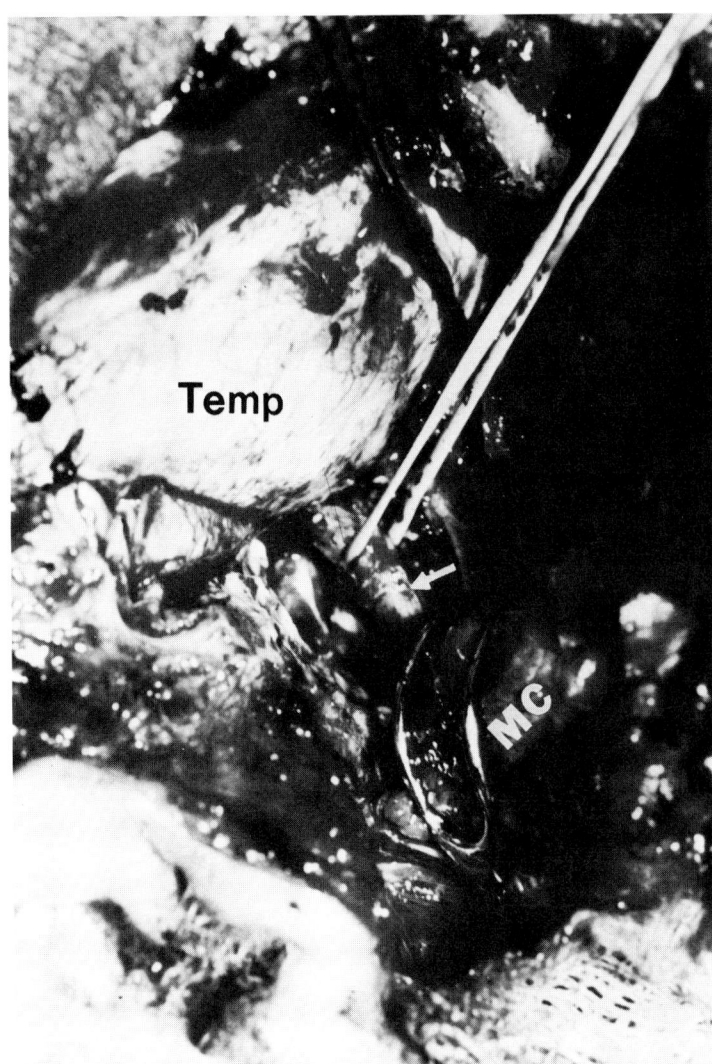

Figure 9: Petrous carotid artery dissection following displacement of mandibular condyle (MC) and low temporal craniotomy (temp). Carotid retracted with vascular tape (arrow).

vein is then dissected retrograde into the mastoid, with dissection and preservation of the cranial nerves exiting in the area of the jugular foramen. The tumor is dissected from posterior to anterior over the posterior fossa dura. If intracranial extension of the glomus tumor or other tumor is present, a retrosigmoid intradural dissection is carried out simultaneously. An infralabyrinthine dissection is accomplished if inner ear function has not been lost, or alternatively, a translabyrinthine dissection may be utilized for complete tumor clearance. The anterior dissection may extend medial to the petrous carotid artery to the level of the petroclival synostosis without displacing the carotid artery.

Surgical Reconstruction

A watertight dural closure may be obtained by direct suturing or by dural graft using pericranium or temporalis fascia. The application of surgical glue or placement of free fat grafts has not been satisfactory for reconstruction and frequently

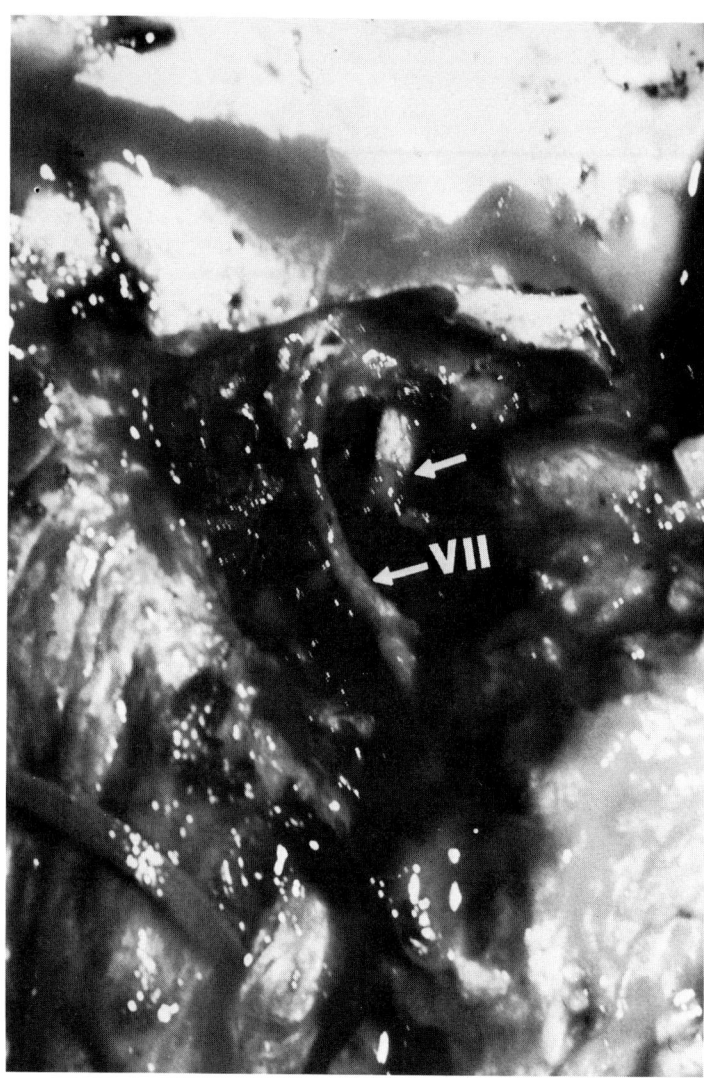

Figure 10: Intratemporal facial nerve (VII) completely decompressed and carotid artery (arrow) exposed anterior to tympanic cavity.

leads to postoperative cerebrospinal fluid leak. When the defect left by surgical resection is relatively small, and when the temporalis muscle is viable, the mastoid and surgical defects may be filled by splitting the temporalis muscle and rotating the posterior half of the muscle into the defect. If there has been extensive dural resection, and carotid exposure and nasopharyngeal or sinus exposure, consideration should be given to transposition of a pectoralis or myocutaneous flap. Alternatively, a free muscle transfer, such as rectus muscle free flap, should be considered in situations where there is tenuous dural closure.

If a temporal craniotomy has been completed, the temporal bone flap is replaced and burr holes filled with bone dust. Tack-up sutures from dura to the bone flap should be placed to ensure that an epidural hematoma does not accumulate. The zygomatic arch segment is secured with 00 monofilament nylon or titanium wire. These materials are chosen so that subsequent radiographic or magnetic resonance scanning may be done without artifact. The temporal muscle is secured to surrounding periosteum. Suction drains are positioned so that direct exposure to dura or to pharyngeal closure is avoided. If the nasopharynx has been exposed, a transnasal nasopharyngeal pack is positioned and unless postoperative Doppler monitoring of microvascular anastomosis is necessary, a bulky external dressing is applied.

Postoperative Management

Perioperative intravenous antibiotic therapy is continued for 24 hours or until nasopharyngeal packing has been removed. The lumbar subarachnoid drain is left in place for 24 hours with the drainage collection bag left at ear level. Hemovac drains are routinely connected to wall suction and usually left in place for 2–3 days postoperatively. When tracheotomy has been utilized, the tracheostomy tube is left in place for 24 to 48 hours or until the patient demonstrates a satisfactory upper airway. If vocal cord paralysis has been produced by the dissection, vocal cord injection with Gelfoam paste or Teflon is done under local anesthesia prior to the removal of the tracheostomy tube. Patients undergoing prolonged operative procedures should have a nasogastric tube placed for early postoperative gastric decompression and for subsequent feeding if vocal cord paralysis is present. Oral feeding is begun after nasopharyngeal packing has been removed and after the patient demonstrates glottic competence.

Outcome of Infratemporal Fossa Dissection

A variety of benign and malignant tumors have been treated by infratemporal fossa dissection alone, or simultaneously with other surgical approaches. The type of dissection and disease is outlined in Table I. Of the 63 patients included in the series, 18 have been treated for benign disease and 45 for various types of malignancy. Though the length of patient follow-up varies from less than 1 year to more than 10 years, the overall outcome has been encouraging. Of the patients with benign disease, 17 are currently alive and free of disease and one patient has persisting meningioma with no current symptoms. Twenty-seven of the 45 patients treated for malignant tumor are currently alive and free of disease (Table II). Six patients who have been treated for malignant tumors survived but later died of causes other than their malignancy, and six patients have succumbed to their malignant tumors. Five patients are currently living with disease, though only two of those patiients have local persistence following infratemporal fossa dissection.

There have been a variety of expected sequelae from the infratemporal fossa surgery. All patients have had a conductive hearing loss when a postauricular infratemporal fossa procedure had been done, but the patients who have had preauricular dissection have normal conductive hearing, though many require placement of tympanostomy tubes. Pa-

Table I
Type of Dissection and Disease

Dissection	Benign	Malignant	Total
ITF	11	15	26
ITF & Ant	3	14	17
ITF & Post	4	13	17
ITF & Ant & Post	0	3	3
	18	45	63

ITF = Infratemporal fossa dissection.
Ant = Combined with anterior fossa or facial dissection.
Post = Combined with posterior fossa dissection.
Ant & Post = Combined with anterior and posterior fossa dissection.

Table II
Disease Outcome—Infratemporal Fossa Dissection

Tumor	NED	AWD	DOD	DOC	No
Benign	17	1*	0	0	18
Malignant	27	5**	6	6	45
	44	6	6	6	63

*Persistent meningioma after second resection asymptomatic.
**Three patients with systemic metastasis and two with local persistence.
NED = no evident disease, AWD = alive with disease; DOD = dead of disease; DOC = dead other causes.

tients undergoing transposition of the facial nerve from the Fallopian canal have had prolonged postoperative facial paralysis and most often incomplete return of function with persisting synkinesis. Patients undergoing a preauricular dissection, where the parotid has been mobilized and the upper divisions of the facial nerve protected, have had excellent return of facial function (Fig. 11).

Despite displacement of the mandibular condyle, only one of 40 patients required a temporary guide plane to reestablish normal occlusion. There has been some limitation of mandibular movement which often requires persisting mandibular exercise. Patients undergoing condylar resection for disease or to allow placement of a microvascular free flap have had centric occlusion postoperatively, though a persisting mandibular shift with jaw opening is routinely present.

Cranial nerve dysfunction is frequent, but depends on the extent of dissection and type of disease treated. Patients who have had the third division of the trigeminal nerve dissected, but not transected, have had return of muscle function and frequently return of facial and oral sensation. Vocal cord paralysis with glottic incompetence has required vocal cord injection in 12 patients. No patients have required permanent tracheostomy and aspiration has been eliminated by vocal cord injection and swallowing therapy, so that all patients have been able to continue a normal oral diet.

As might be expected, such extensive skull base surgery is not without complication (Table III). Complications related to carotid artery dissection or resection have occurred in four patients. Postoperatively, two patients have had carotid artery rupture, one requiring angiographic occlusion and the other, resection of the ruptured area and reanastomosis. The latter patient ultimately died of ensuing further

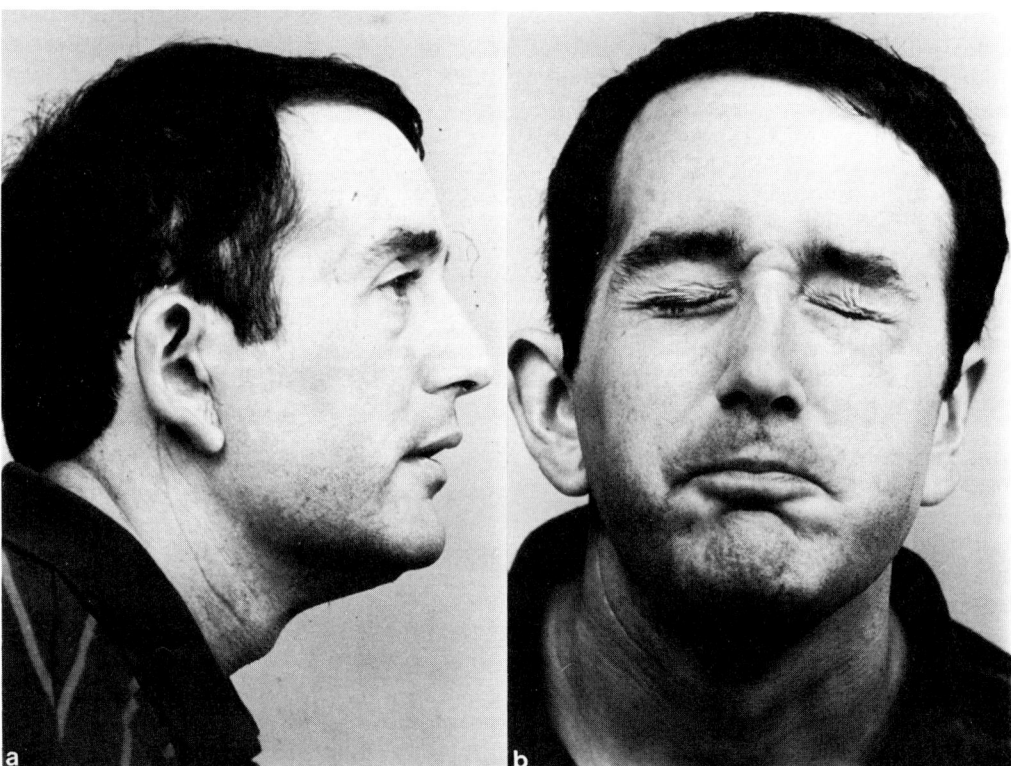

Figure 11: Lateral appearance **(A)** and facial nerve function **(B)** 3 months following preauricular transtemporal infratemporal resection of postradiation persistent nasopharyngeal carcinoma.

Table III
Complications of 63 Infratemporal Fossa Dissections

Massive intraoperative bleeding	6
Postoperative hematoma	4
Postoperative CSF leak	4
Meningitis	2
Temporalis muscle necrosis	3
Carotid rupture	2
Postoperative death	1*

*Delayed following carotid rupture.

complications and is the only fatality in the series. One patient sustained a carotid graft thrombosis, with the graft being removed, but no further sequelae. One patient had a postoperative cerebrovascular accident which cleared incompletely. Cerebrospinal fluid leakage occurred in four patients, with two requiring a secondary procedure for closure. Two patients have been treated for meningitis with intravenous antibiotic therapy and sustained no further sequelae. Massive intraoperative bleeding, presumably due to fibrinolysis or clotting factor deficiency, occurred in six patients. This experience has led to the routine use of platelet replacement and fresh frozen plasma for every four units of blood transfused. Postoperative wound hematoma has occurred in four patients, two of whom required urgent tracheostomy for airway obstruction. The hematoma complication was related to incomplete factor replacement in two patients, and to aspirin anticoagulation in two patients who had undergone a free flap with microvascular anastomosis.

There are also several factors which cannot be quantified that have been important for the surgeons performing and for the patients undergoing extensive infratemporal fossa surgery. A majority of the patients treated have been previously considered in a hopeless situation or have had persisting disease despite prior radiation therapy or surgical resection. For these patients, the hope of survival and the pain relief provided by the surgery have more than compensated for the rigors that they have undergone, even when their disease has ultimately persisted. Several patients, after lengthy discussion, have chosen surgery as an alternative to suicide for alleviation of pain, and have survived free of narcotic addiction for months to years following their surgery. Because of the lack of long-term disability, the patients have returned to a lifestyle that has been productive and enjoyable.

References

1. House WF, Hitselberger WE: The transcochlear approach to the skull base. *Arch Otolaryngol* 102:334-342, 1976.
2. Fisch U: Infratemporal fossa approach for extensive tumors of the temporal bone and base of skull. In Silverstein H, Norell N (eds): *Neurological Surgery of the Ear*, Birmingham, Aesculepius Publishers Inc, 1977, pp. 35-53.
3. Fisch U, Pilsbury HC: Infratemporal fossa approach to lesions in the temporal bone and base of skull. *Arch Otolaryngol* 105:9, 1979.
4. Fisch U, Fagan P, Valvanis A: The infratemporal fossa approach for the lateral skull base. *Otolaryngol Clin North Am* 17:513-552, 1984.
5. Fisch U: The infratemporal fossa approach for nasopharyngeal tumors. *Laryngoscope* 93:36-44, 1983.
6. Terez JJ, Alksne FJ, Lawrence W: Craniofacial resection for tumors invading the pterygoid fossa. *Am J Surg* 118:732-740, 1969.
7. Friedman WH, Katsantonis GP, Cooper MH, Lee JM, Strelzow VV: Stylohamular dissection: A new method of en bloc resection of malignancies of the infratemporal fossa. *Laryngoscope* 91:1869-1879, 1981.

VIII

Posterior Cranial Base

25

Posterior Cranial Base Anatomy

J. Lang, M.D.

Posterior Cranial Fossa, Bony Parts

The clivus is located in the middle area of the posterior cranial fossa. Its upper portion develops from the sphenoid bone, while its lower portion is the basilar part of the occipital bone. Normally, the spheno-occipital synchondrosis closes between 13.5 and 18.5 years starting at the intracranial end and progressing to the outer skull base area. The total length of the clivus in our specimens was measured to be 45.0 mm (range 37–52 mm) (Lang et al., unpublished data). Holsten and Herrmann estimated the normal length of the basilar part of the clivus to be 32 mm, a value which compares well with our measurements of this structure during postnatal development.[11] A shortened pars basilaris of the occipital bone has also been described and called occipital hypoplasia; this structure was approximately 24 mm in length.[31] The pars lateralis of the occipital bone in childhood is bordered anteriorly by the anterior intra-occipital synchondrosis and posteriorly by the posterior intra-occipital synchondrosis. The posterior synchondrosis closes earlier than the anterior one, which is situated in the area of the anterior border of the hypoglossal canal. Behind the pars lateralis of the occipital bone, the squama occipitalis forms the posterior border of the foramen magnum and a large part of the floor of the posterior cranial fossa. Anteriorly and laterally, the petrous part of the temporal bone is connected to the squama of the occipital bone.

Between the basilar part of the occipital bone and the petrous bone is situated the synchondrosis petro-occipitalis. In this area, cartilage is also found in the skulls of children and young adults; in specimens from older individuals we noted synostoses between the two bone parts. This area also includes the inferior petrosal sinus, which also extends to the jugular foramen area. In anatomical terms, this is called the sulcus sinus petrosi inferioris of the occipital bone; there is also a sulcus sinus petrosi inferioris of the temporal bone. Occasionally the petrous temporal bones in our specimens had such a sulcus only in the upper area (sometimes it was absent) and the whole sulcus was grooved in the basilar part of the occipital bone. In the lower part, the suture between the occipital and petrous bones is situated in most cases near the petrous bone. The posterior part of the posterior skull base is usually thickened

From: Sekhar LN, Schramm VL Jr, eds: *Tumors of the Cranial Base: Diagnosis and Treatment.* Mount Kisco, New York, Futura Publishing Co, Inc, © 1987.

by the internal occipital crest, and above this crest by the internal occipital protuberance. Near the foramen magnum a flattened or hollowed area (Vermian impression or triangle) can be seen in most cases. Laterally are the cerebellar fossae, on which lie the lower surfaces of the cerebellar hemispheres, separated from the bone by dura and subarachnoid space. Other important landmarks are the grooves for the lateral and sigmoid sinuses. In approximately 3% of our specimens, the occipital sinus (normally embedded in the falx cerebelli) had two limbs arranged in a V-shaped pattern around the foramen magnum and running toward the jugular foramen. This arrangement was found more often in children then in adults.[14] Landmarks of the posterior fossa are shown in Figure 1.

The thickest and thinnest zones of the posterior part of the posterior cranial base, its sutures in adults, the mastoid emissary vein, and some measurements are given in Figure 2. It should be noted that the thickest portion of the floor (except for the clivus and the petrous bone) is found in the area of the jugular tubercle and the anterior part of the occipital condyle. The thinnest area, as measured in our specimens, was near the posterior margin of the foramen magnum.[16] Figure 2 shows the sutures of the posterior fossa floor. The thickness of the posterior border of the foramen magnum was 5.4 mm (range 1.7–9 mm). The condylar canal was absent in our specimens on both sides in 22%, on only the right side in 14%, and on only the left in 10%.

The foramen magnum in our new-

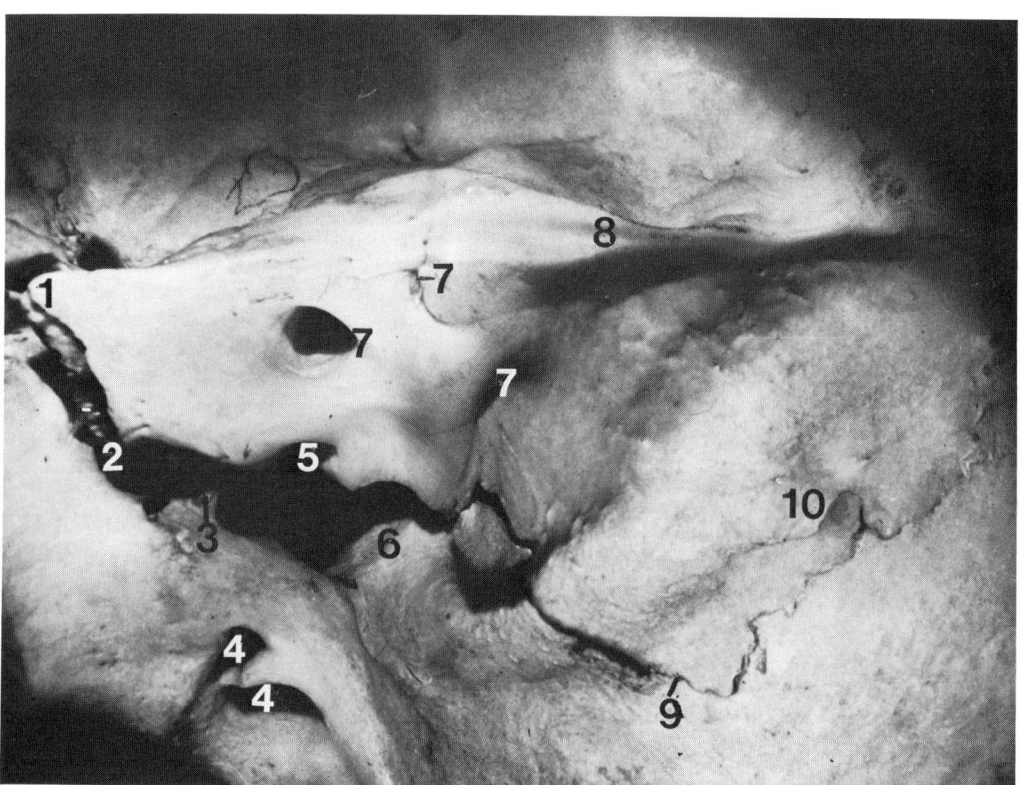

Figure 1: Posterior surface of petrous bone. 1. Petrosus apex. 2. Sulcus sinus petr. inferioris. 3. Proc. hamatus. 4. Two pori of the hypoglossal canal. 5. Apertura externa canaliculi cochleae. 6. Margo terminalis sigmoidea. 7. Internal auditory meatus, lateral lip, fossa subarcuata, rima sacci endolymphatici. 8. Sulcus sin. petrosi sup. 9. Sutura occipitomastoidea. 10. Sulcus sin. sigmoidei, area.

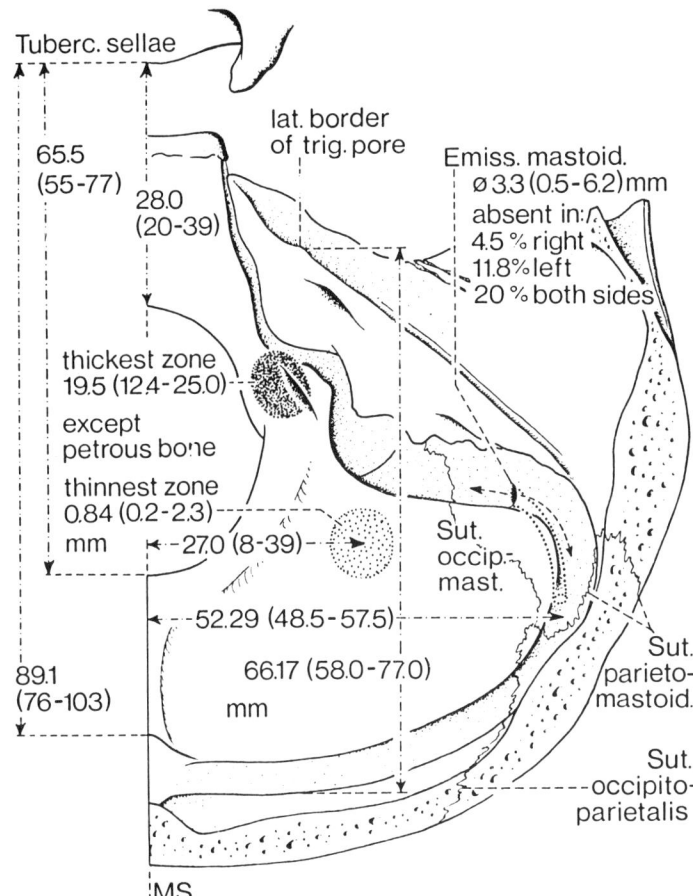

Figure 2: Lengths were measured on skulls in the Frankfurt horizontal plane. The thickest zone (except the petrous part) is situated between the jugular tubercule and the occipital condyle.

born specimens was 20.85 mm long (range 14–25 mm), in 1-year-old children it was 28.71 mm long (range 26–31 mm), and in 4-year-old children it was 32.5 mm (range 29–36 mm). In 9- to 11-year-old children the length was 33.14 mm (range 31–35 mm), and in adults the length was 35.33 mm (range 30–41.4 mm). The width of the foramen magnum was estimated to be 15.3 mm (range 13–18 mm) in newborns, 22.79 mm (range 19–28 mm) in 1-year-olds, 26.5 mm (range 24–30.5 mm) in 4-year-old children, 28.14 mm (range 26–30 mm) in 9- to 11-year-old children, and 29.67 mm (range 21.4–37.6 mm) in adults. In adults, we found the foramen magnum in most cases to be shaped like two half circles of different radii.[20] For further details see Figure 3. It is well known that in cases of long-standing pressure which accompanies syringomyelia and intra- or extramedullary tumors, the foramen magnum becomes widened. It may be focally eroded by neoplasms such as chordoma or metastases. Meningiomas are also occasionally found in this region.[29]

Jugular Foramen

In most cases the foramen jugulare on the right side is wider than that on the left, and it is usually triangular. Its posterior border is part of the occipital bone. The anterior margin of the jugular foramen is formed by the posterior inferior border of the petrous bone and is called the incisura jugularis; in most cases this appears as a processus intrajugularis. Medial to this processus is the opening of the cochlear aqueduct. We measured the upper and

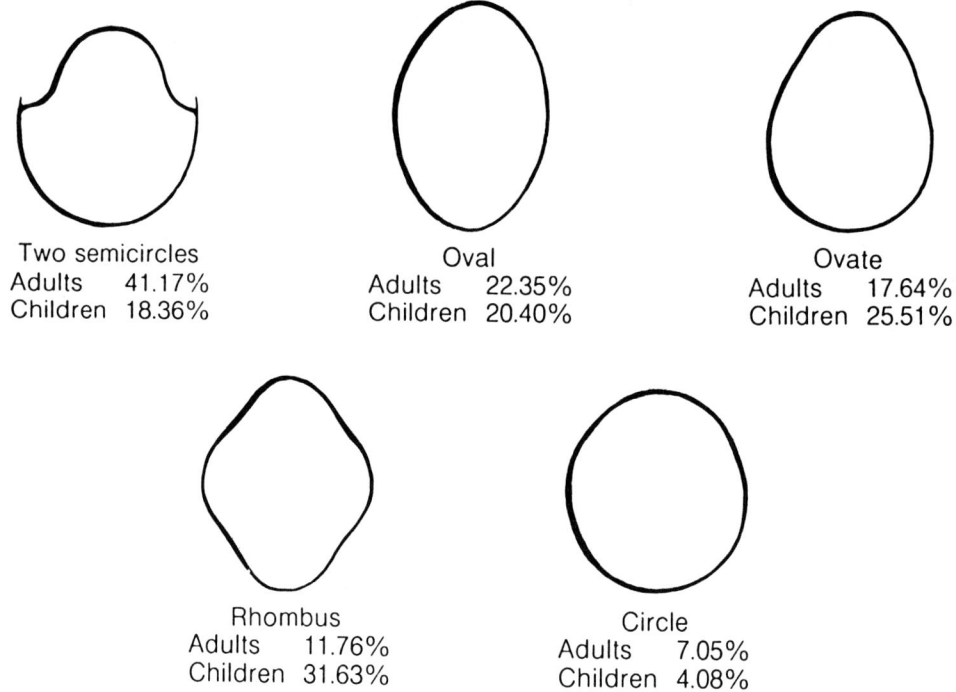

Figure 3: Shape of the foramen magnum in children and adults.

lower length and the width of the foramen jugulare at various stages in postnatal development and found that the width, in particular, increases with increasing age. Figure 4 shows the distance between the medial border of the jugular foramen and the midsagittal plane. The border between the sigmoid sinus and the jugular foramen has been called the terminal sigmoid border. Occasionally this ridge is duplicated. From this point the blood from the sigmoid sinus flows forward and laterally into the bulb of the internal jugular vein. It should be noted that in 14.6% of our adult specimens, and in 11.6% of skulls of infants, the jugular foramen was divided.[21] DiChiro et al. found divided foramina unilaterally in 13.2% of skulls and bilaterally in 4.7%.[7] It should be noted that the bridges in the jugular foramen were found in different directions and levels. A canal medial to the jugular foramen was present on one side of the skull in 6% of our specimens.[4] In about 50%, this foramen transmitted the inferior petrosal sinus, and in the other half carried the glossopharyngeal nerve.[22] In cases with chondrodysplasia, the jugular foramen is narrow.

We measured the hypoglossal canal in newborns to be 4–6 mm long, in specimens from individuals in the second year of life it was 5–9 mm long, and in adults it was 6.4–14.1 mm long.[20] In most corrosion casts the canal is S-shaped, although sometimes we found a right-angled canal with the apex upward. In about 20% of specimens, the intracranial opening of the hypoglossal canal is duplicated.[30] The width of the intracranial pore in newborns was measured to be 2.5–4.0 mm and in adults to be 5.6 mm (range 3–10 mm). The angle of the hypoglossal canal to the midsagittal plane was found to be 33.17° (range 30–36.0°) in newborns and 45° (range 16–60°) in adults.[20,32] The postnatal changes in the angle of the hypoglossal canal are shown in Figure 5.

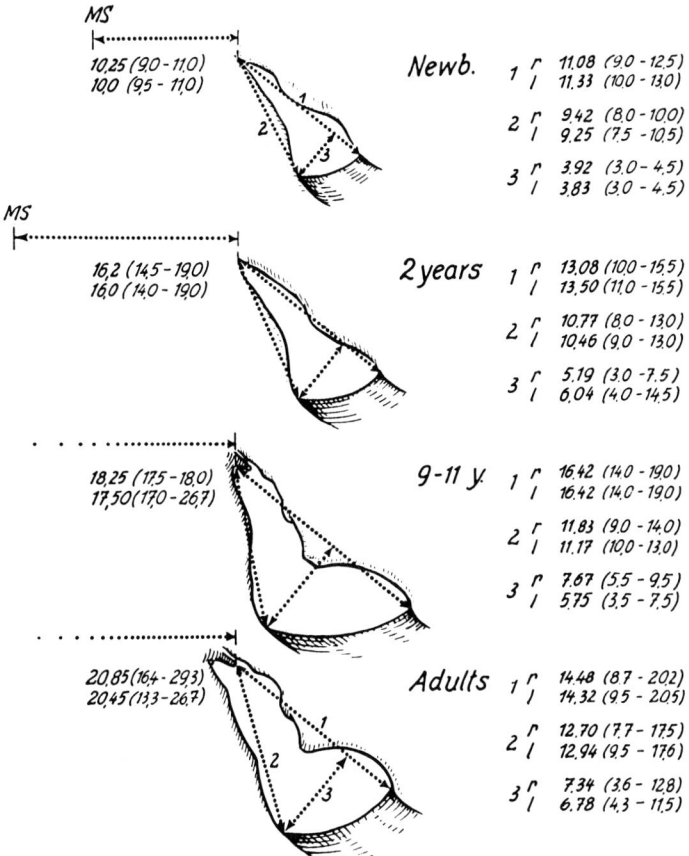

Figure 4: Jugular foramen, postnatal shift and enlargement. *MS*, midsagittal plane.

Posterior Cranial Fossa, Dura Mater

In the floor of the posterior cranial fossa, a depression was located in the clivus area. In one-third of the cases, the depression had a radius of 65–74 mm and in two-thirds, a radius of 17–42 mm.[6]

An oblique dural plica was found in approximately 60% of our specimens between the posterior part of the foramen magnum area, directed anteriorly and laterally to the area of the internal auditory meatus. The venous sinuses were described by Lang.[13]

The arterial supply of the posterior cranial base and the dura mater in the floor of the fossa are shown in Figure 6. Rarely, we found anastomoses between the meningeal arteries of the posterior cranial fossa and arteries of the brain (for example, the posterior inferior cerebellar artery).[19] Near all orifices of the posterior cranial fossa (as in the anterior and middle cranial fossae), the dura mater extends around the nerves or veins through these portals to the outer skull base. In the area of the jugular foramen, a connective tissue septum develops between the dura mater and the connective tissue on the outer skull base. This septum usually transmits cranial nerves IX, X, and XI, and sometimes it transmits the blood from the inferior petrosal sinus. In most cases (48%), this sinus passes to the jugular bulb between the ninth and tenth cranial nerves. However, in 30% of cases, the sinus runs anterior to the ninth cranial nerve, and in

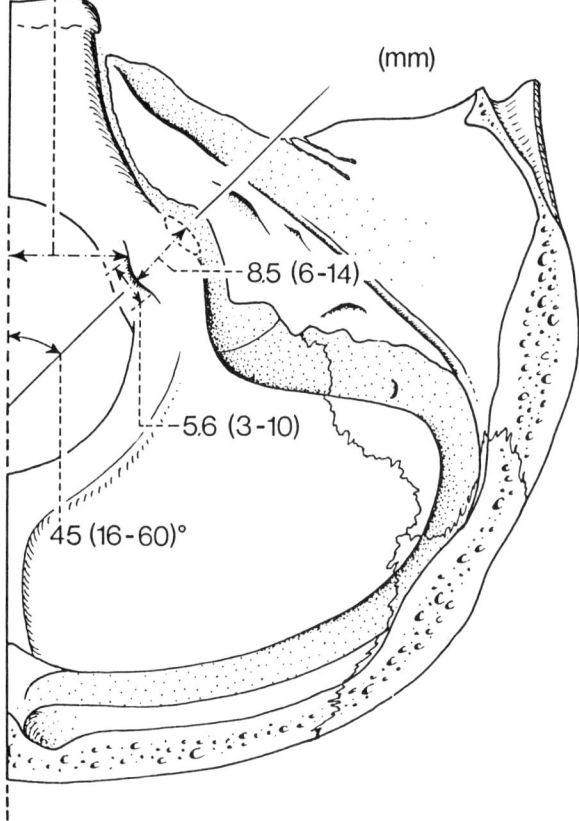

age	left		right	
neon.	7.00	(6.5 - 7.5)	7.10	(6.5 - 7.5)
1 year	10.67	(9.5 - 11.5)	11.00	(10.0 - 12.0)
2 yrs.	10.75	(10.0 - 12.0)	11.42	(10.0 - 13.5)
5 yrs.	11.89	(10.5 - 15.0)	12.00	(11.0 - 14.0)
adults	14.24	(11.0 - 17.0)	14.69	(11.0 - 17.0)

Figure 5: Angle of the hypoglossal canal to the midsagittal plane and lateral shift of the internal pore of the canal. Also shown are our measurements of the width of the internal pore and the length of this canal in adults. Measurements are in millimeters (range).

16%, two holes are present in the septum, one anterior to and the other posterior to the tenth cranial nerve. In about 6% of specimens, the sinus runs between the tenth and eleventh cranial nerves. We also found differences in the height of this sinus: in 23% of specimens, the inferior petrosal sinus runs into the middle of the jugular bulb, and in 33% it runs into the lower portion of the bulb. The sinus terminates extracranially in the internal jugular vein in 21% of cases, and in the jugular bulb in 17.3%. In approximately 7% of the cases, the inferior petrosal sinus entered the internal jugular vein well below the jugular foramen.

In about 4% of cases, Fiegler identified a median basilar canal in the clivus area which carries an emissary vein running between the basilar venous plexus and the veins outside the cranium. According to Fiegler, the length of this canal is 5–17 mm and its width 1–3 mm. In most cases the opening on the external cranial base was found anterior to the pharyngeal tubercle, in a small groove.[8,10]

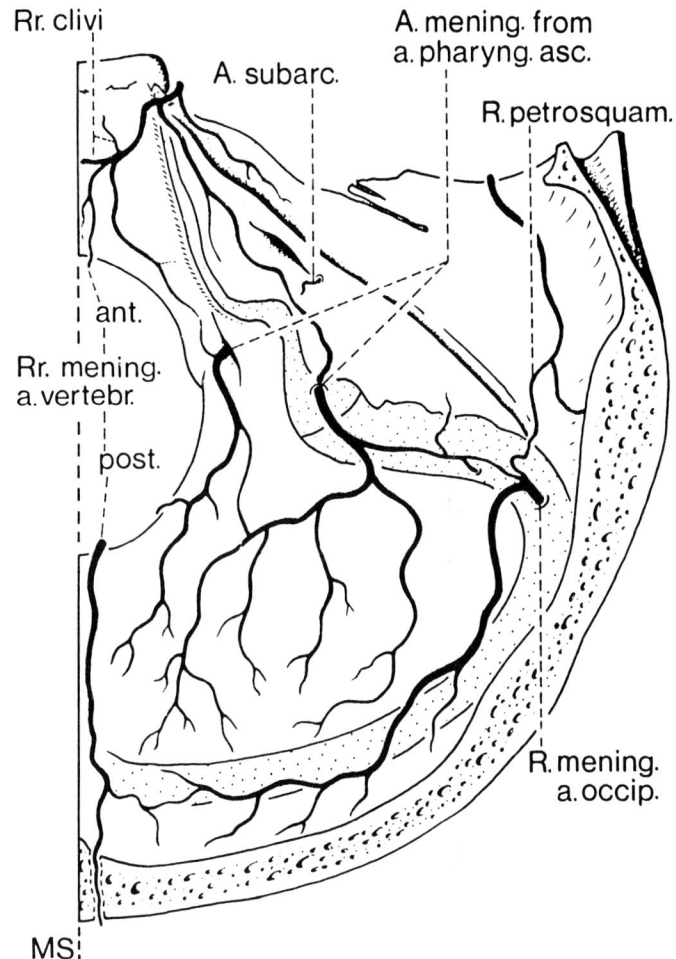

Figure 6: Arteries supplying the floor of the posterior cranial fossa. In many cases the arteries are found inside the sinuses.

Brain Stem and Cranial Nerves in the Floor of the Posterior Cranial Fossa

Figure 7 shows the portions of the brain lying in the midline, with our measurements of the lengths of the central segments of the lower cranial nerves on the left side of the figure (the right side of the brain). On the right side of the figure (left side of the brain), our measurements of intracisternal length are shown. Figure 8 shows the lower cranial nerves and their intracisternal courses in the posterior fossa as seen through a retrosigmoid approach, along with the lengths of the central segments of the nerves.[13] The nerve-vessel relations in the area of the internal auditory meatus as measured by Sunderland and Mazzoni are shown in Figure 9.[25,35] The anterior inferior cerebellar artery, or other arteries in the posterior cranial fossa, veins, or tumors, may compress the central segments of these nerves and cause trigeminal neuralgia, hemifacial spasm, or glossopharyngeal neuralgia. These conditions may be treated by neurovascular decompression.[12]

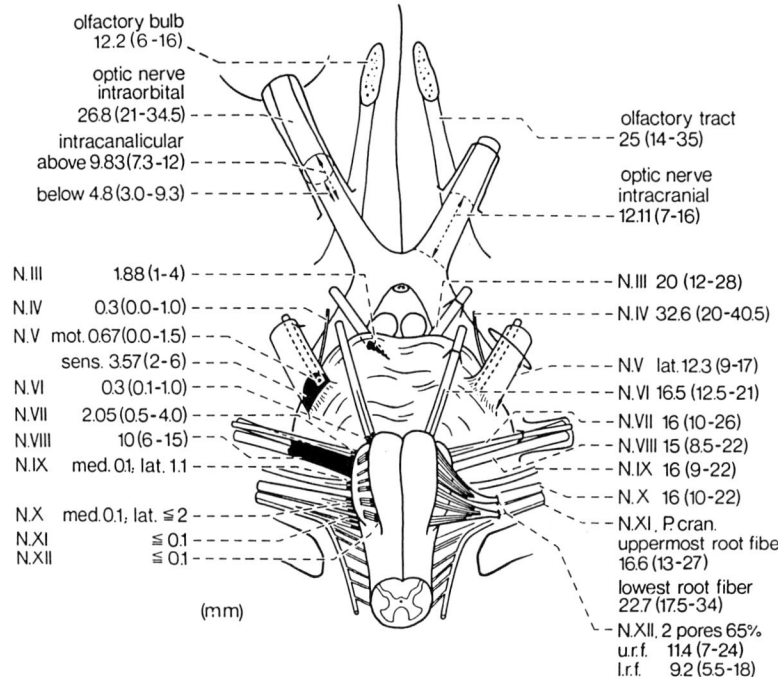

Figure 7: On the left side of the figure (right side of the brain) are given our measurements of the lengths of different nerves and their central segments (black). On the right side of the figure (left side of the brain) the intracisternal lengths of the cranial nerves and the lengths of the root fibers of cranial nerves XI and XII are shown. Values are given in millimeters (range).

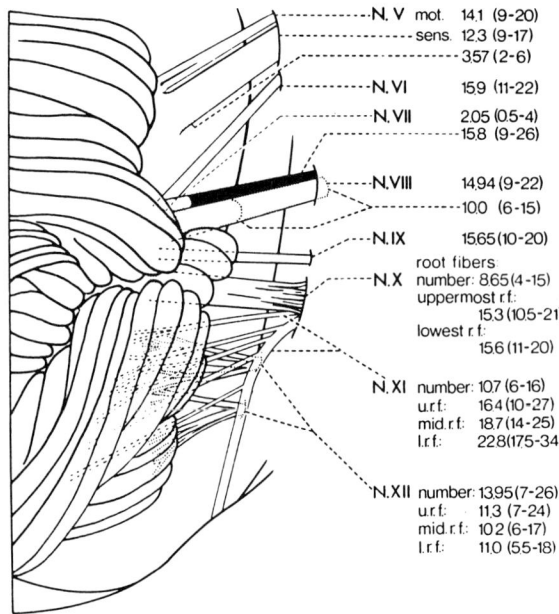

Figure 8: Lengths of the intracisternal courses of the lower cranial nerves, viewed as through a retrosigmoid approach. Also shown are the lengths of the central segments of the nerves. Measurements are given in millimeters (range). The seventh cranial nerve, peripheral segment, is shown in black.

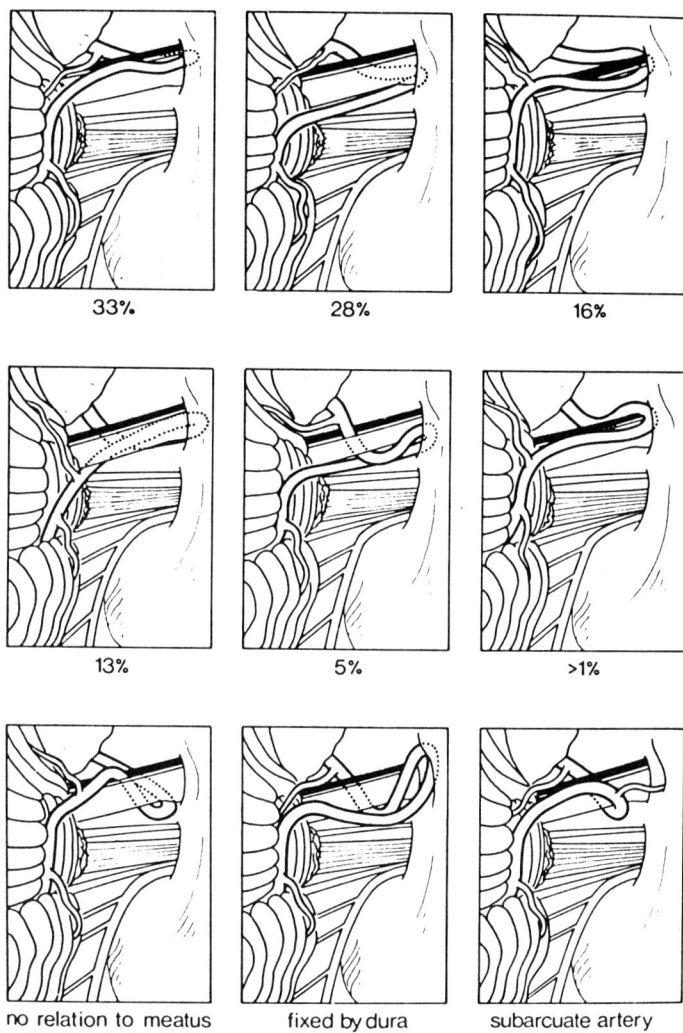

Figure 9: Nerve–vessel relations (AICA) on the porus or in the internal auditory meatus according to Sunderland (1945) and Mazzoni (1969). The facial nerve is shown in black.

Cerebellopontine Angle and Internal Acoustic Meatus

The cerebellopontine angle is bordered anteriorly by the dura mater, which covers the posterior surface of the petrous bone, posteriorly by the anterior surface of the inferior part of the pons and the middle cerebellar peduncle, inferiorly by the biventral lobule, and inferomedially by the medullary olives (see Fig. 7). In this angular area, the exit zones of the seventh and eighth cranial nerves are located more cranially and those for cranial nerves IX, X, and XI more caudally. Two important structures in this area are the flocculus and the lateral aperture of the fourth ventricle (see Fig. 8). For operations on the cerebellopontine angle, structures on the posterior surface of the petrous portion are important landmarks. In Figures 10 A–C, measurements of important landmarks on the posterior surface of the right petrous part of the temporal bone are shown.[15,17,33]

Tumors of the eighth cranial nerve arise in most cases in the peripheral segment of the vestibular part or from the

450 • TUMORS OF THE CRANIAL BASE: DIAGNOSIS AND TREATMENT

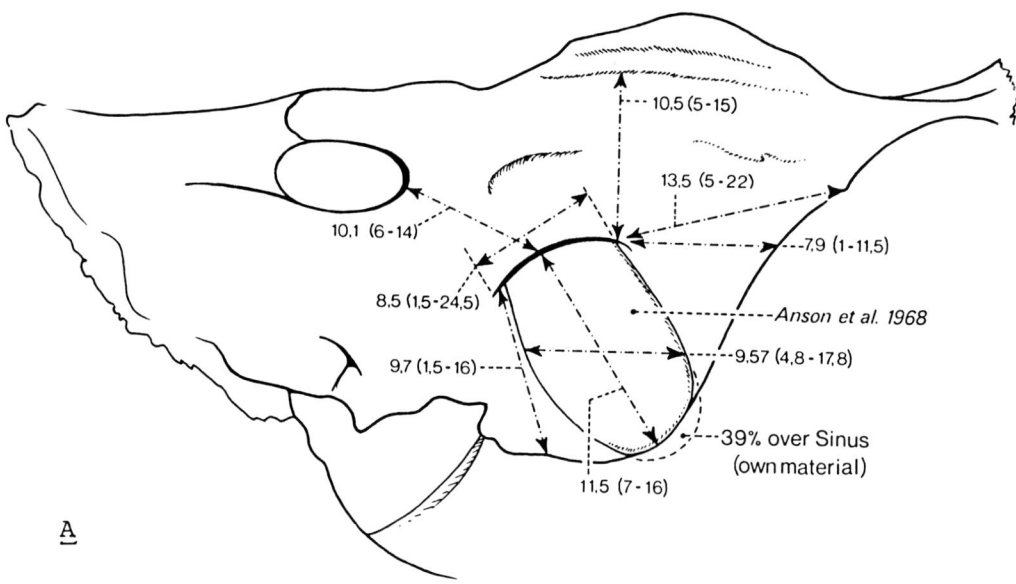

Figure 10A: Distances from the rim of the endolymphatic sac to different landmarks and dimensions of the endolymphatic sac itself according to Anson et al. (1968).

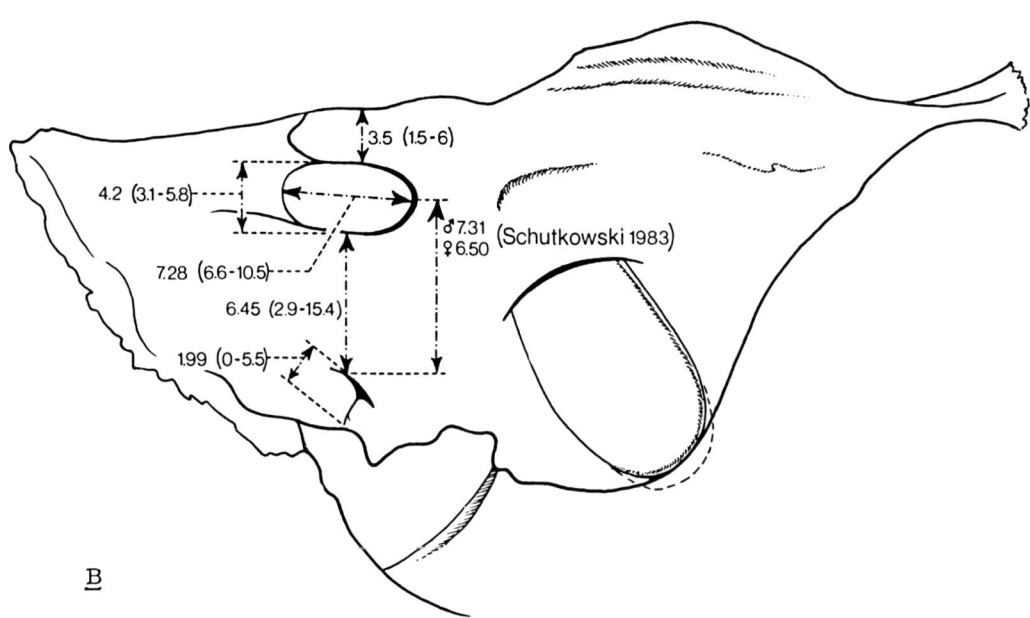

Figure 10B: Dimensions of the internal auditory meatus and distances from its upper border to the lower surface of the tentorium and from its lower border to the janua arcuata, which covers the perilymphatic duct. Also shown are some measurements of Schutkowski (1983) (sex-differences). Measurements are given in millimeters (range).

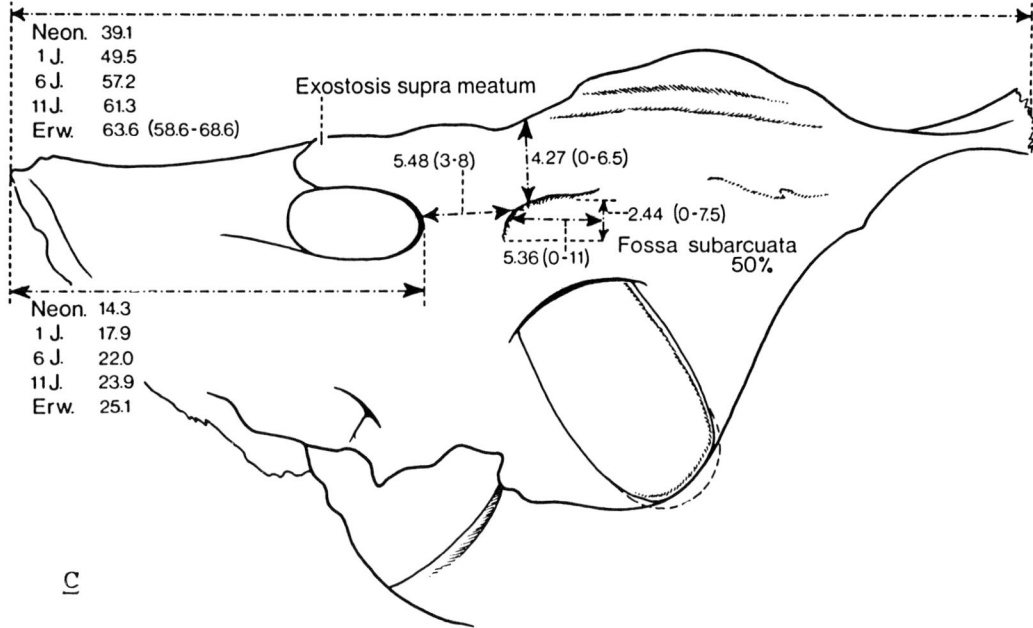

Figure 10C: Orientation of the lateral rim of the internal auditory meatus relative to the subarcuate fossa, which is developed in 50% of adults. Also shown is the distance of the latter to the upper border of the petrous bone, its width and height in adults. Values are given in millimeters (range).

Obersteiner-Redlich zone. The latter is located in the posterior fossa, near the internal acoustic meatus (IAC), or inside the internal acoustic meatus. When the tumor is in such a location, the posterior lip of the IAC must be drilled off. Figure 11 shows the results of measuring a temporal bone cut transversely through the

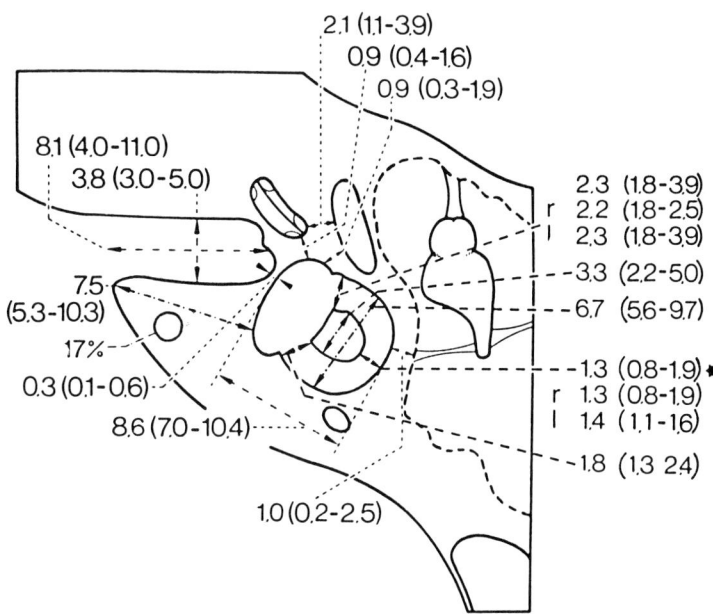

Figure 11: Transverse section through the temporal bone along the axis of the internal auditory canal. Dimensions of various canals in the inner ear and distances from these canals to landmarks in the internal auditory meatus are shown. Air cells were present in the lateral pore in 17% of cases. Values are given in millimeters (range) and some bilateral variations are noted.

axis of the internal auditory canal.[17] We found air cells in the posterior wall of the IAC in 17% of specimens and behind the sigmoid sinus in 42%. Figure 11 also shows the relationships of the medial wall of the vestibule to the internal auditory meatus, dimensions of the lateral semicircular canal, and distances between the cochlea and the facial nerve canal and the vestibule and the facial nerve canal.

In Figure 12, the double-headed arrows at the top show the relationships of the posterior semicircular canal to the posterior tip of the IAC. Also shown are distances between the anterior crus of the anterior semicircular canal and the area of the geniculate ganglion, between the lateral crus of the posterior semicircular canal and the posterior surface of the petrous bone, and between the lateral crus and the sigmoid sinus.

By studying coronal sections cut along the axis of the internal auditory canal, we found that the meatus is 4.37 mm high (range 1.5–7.4 mm) (Fig. 13). The length of the canal, including the distance behind the transverse crest, was found to be 12.33 mm (range 5.8–18.2 mm) on the upper side and 11.29 mm (range 7.3–24.3 mm) on the lower side. Figure 13 also shows measurements of the upper and lower fundus, with suprameatal and inframeatal air cells. The axis of the internal auditory canal in our specimens turned laterally, away from the midcoronal plane, about 15° (range 5–35°).

When surgeons use a translabyrinthine or retrolabyrinthine approach to the internal auditory meatus in the jugular foramen region, it is important to know the locations of the facial nerve canal, the sigmoid sinus, and other structures in the temporal bone. Figures 14 A and B show the relationships of these canals and nerves in the petrous bone. The length of the transverse part of the internal carotid canal, its angle to the midsagittal plane, and distances between landmarks on the outer skull base are given in Figure 15.[20,21] As is well known, aneurysms may arise in this part of the internal carotid artery.

After parts of the temporal and occipital bone have been removed, the course of the cranial nerves IX to XI in the area of the jugular foramen and below the skull base may be seen (Fig. 16). The internal

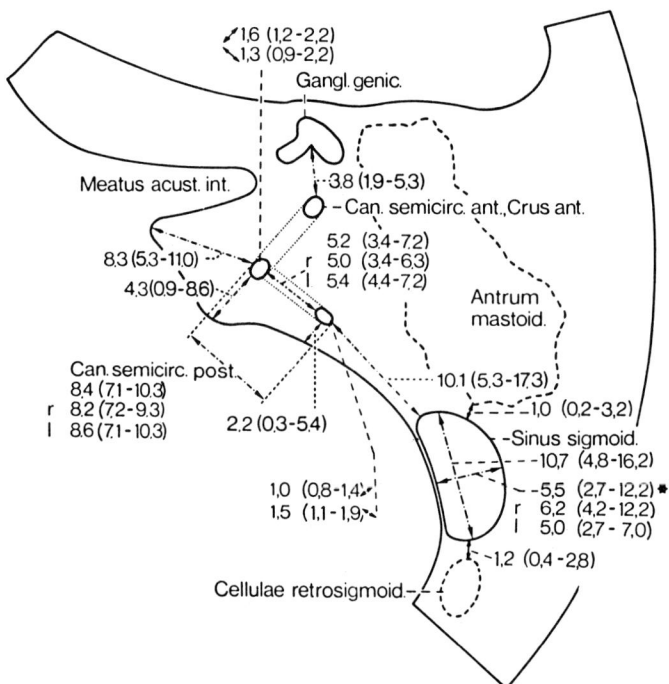

Figure 12: Transverse section through the upper part of the internal auditory canal. Measurements from the canals to different landmarks in the upper part of the internal auditory meatus are shown. Retrosigmoid cells were found in 42% of cases. Values are given in millimeters (range).

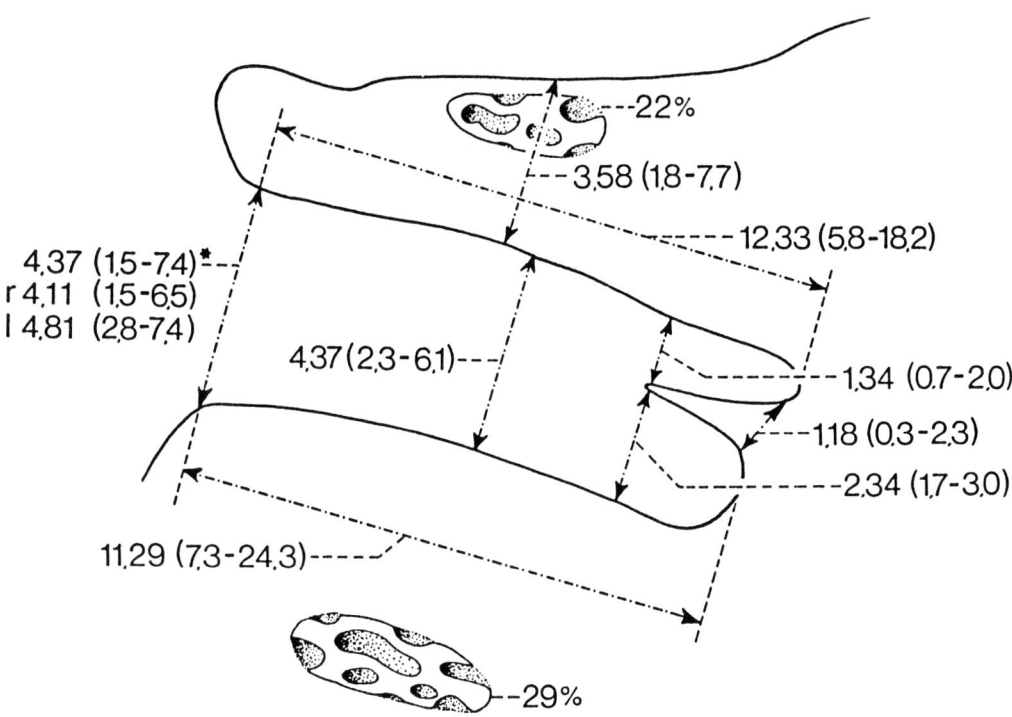

Figure 13: Dimensions of the internal auditory canal as measured on coronal sections. Measurements of the transverse crest and the distance to the upper border of the petrous bone are also shown as is the development of supra- and inframeatal air cells. All measurements are given in millimeters (range).

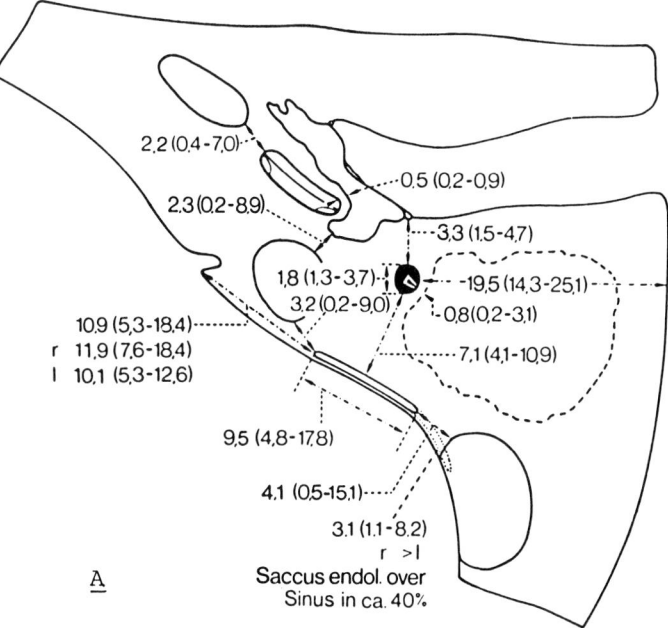

Figure 14A: Transverse section through the temporal bone showing the internal auditory canal and basal turn of the cochlea. Distances from the mastoid portion of the facial canal (black) to the outer surface of the temporal bone, to the fibrous annulus, to the antrum, and to the endolymphatic sac area are shown in millimeters (range).

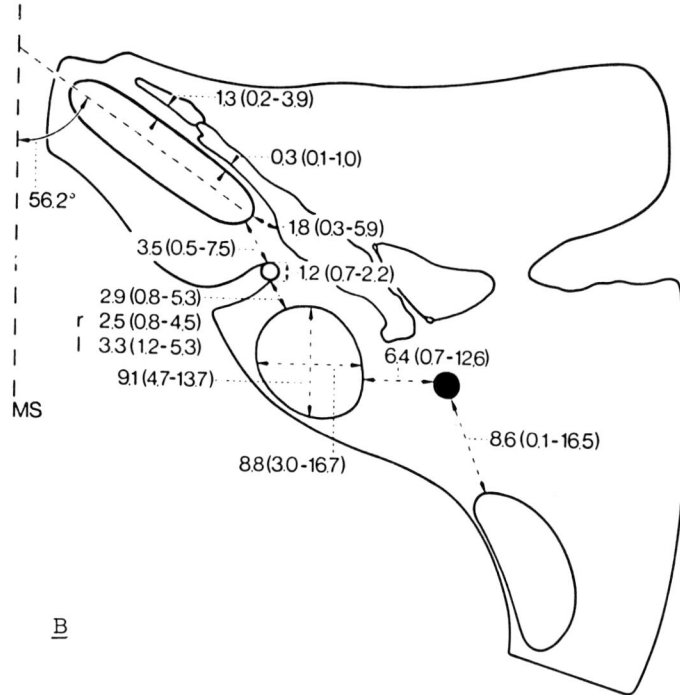

Figure 14B: Transverse section through the temporal bone near the petrous portion of the carotid canal. Distances to the auditory tubercle and to the ninth and seventh cranial nerves, the width of the jugular bulb, and the distances from the mastoid portion of the facial canal to the jugular bulb and to the sigmoid sinus are shown. Measurements are given in millimeters (range) with bilateral variations.

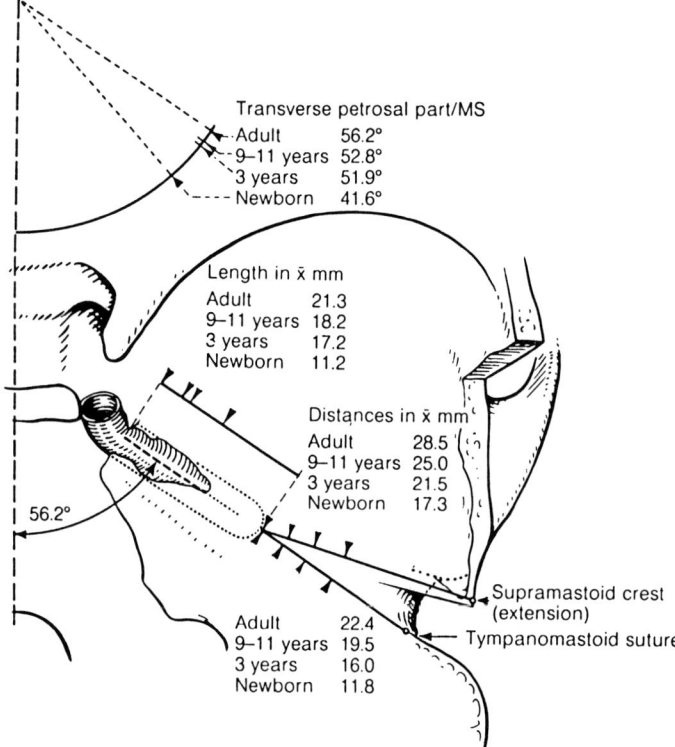

Figure 15: Transverse part of the internal carotid canal, its angle to the midsagittal plane, its length, and its distance from landmarks on the outer skull base. Mean values are given in degrees and in millimeters.

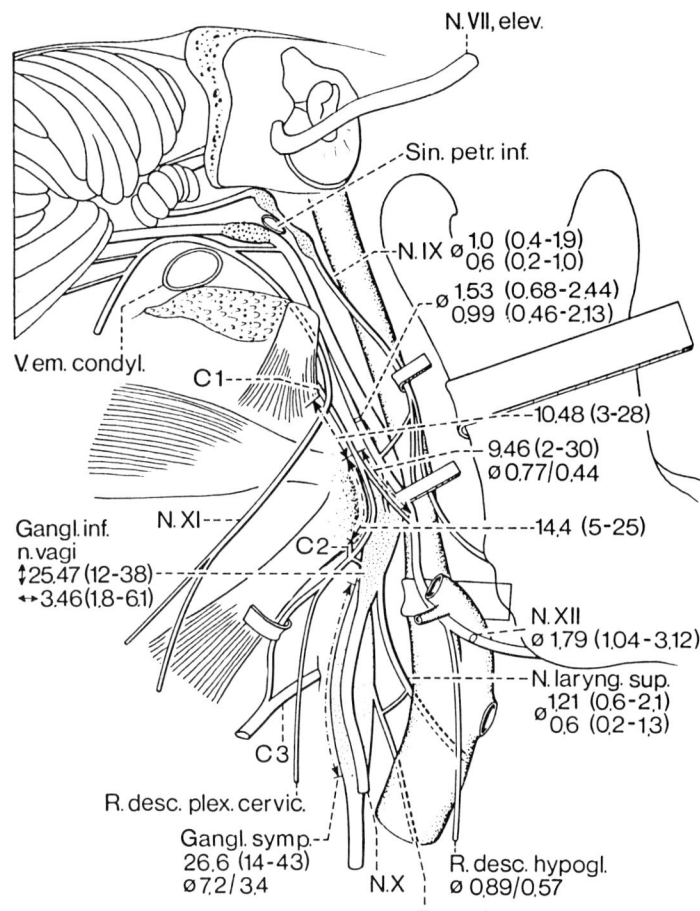

Figure 16: Courses of cranial nerves IX–XI through the jugular foramen region and below the skull base, viewed from lateral to medial. Also given are the thicknesses and lengths of nerves, anastomoses, and ganglia. Measurements are given in millimeters (range).

jugular vein in this preparation was removed, as was the external carotid artery at its origin. The diameters of the nerves, the length of the inferior ganglion of the tenth cranial nerve, and the superior ganglion of the sympathetic trunk were measured, as were various distances between structures. Figure 17 shows the location of the glomeruli in the courses of the tympanic nerve and the auricular branch of the vagus nerve. In most cases, glomus tumors are found in the tympanic cavity, but they may also be found in the area of the jugular fossa or elsewhere in the petrous bone. They are supplied by many vessels, the principal of which is the ascending pharyngeal artery and its twigs.[18]

Clivus Region

The petrous apex is also part of the clivus region. Epidermoids of this apex may cause different symptoms, i.e., if the fifth and sixth cranial nerves are involved, diplopia may be present; involvement of the cochlear portion of the auditory canal may lead to other symptoms.[26] Other tumors originating in the petrous apex area are chondromyosarcomas, neurofibromas, or other lesions that may have formed from the matrix of the fibrocartilago basalis.[9] Finally, chordomas or chondromas may also invade the apex region. Different approaches to this area have been described: subtemporal, transcentral, transapical (apex partis petrosae),

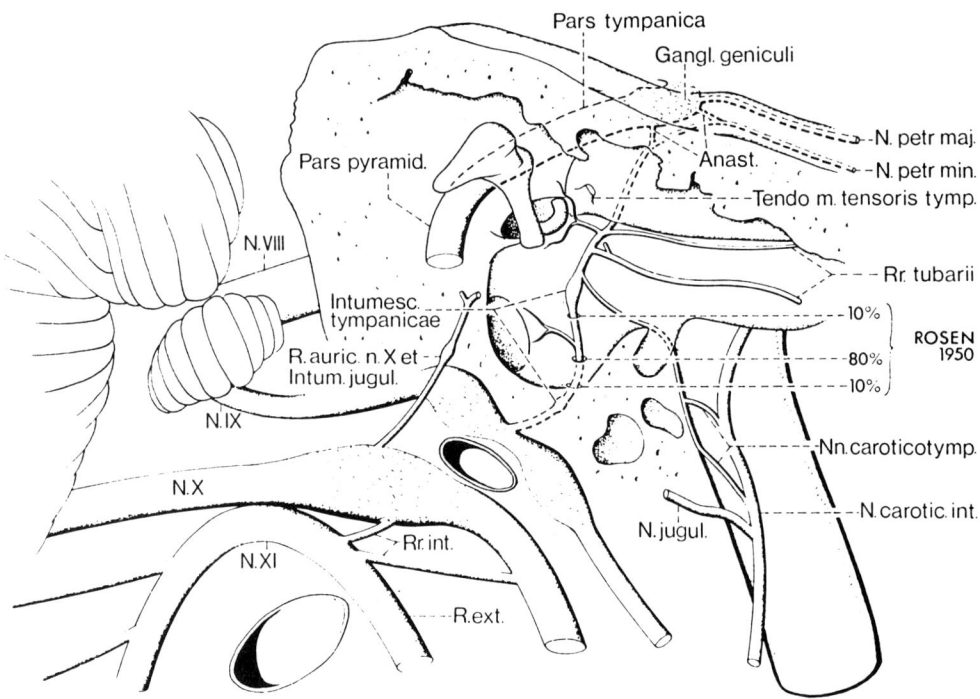

Figure 17: Glomeruli of the tympanic nerve and auricular branch of the vagus nerve.

transoral, subglossal, rhinoseptal, transpalatine, transcervical, and others.[2,34] Chordomas arise from the notochordal remnants, and occupy the clivus, the sphenoid parasellar region, the foramen magnum, and upper cervical areas (Fig. 18).[1,5,23,27-29] Chondromas of the clivus area have been described by many authors, for example Mabrey.[24] Such tumors are sometimes called osteochondromas, and in the clivus area they are found in the neighborhood of the spheno-occipital (Fig. 18). As mentioned before, we measured the length of the clivus in adults on its inner surface to be 45 mm (range 37–52 mm). On its outer surface, we measured the distance between the posterior part of the ala vomeris and the basion (anterior border of the occipital foramen) in adults to be 27.9 mm (range 19–34 mm) (see Fig. 19). Also given are distances from these two landmarks to the pharyngeal tubercle, to the lateral border of the choana, to the apex partis petrosae, and between the outer opening of the hypoglossal canal and the midsagittal plane in adults.

Figure 20 shows the width of the clivus in its anterior region to be 22.5 mm (range 13–28 mm). This small anterior projection of the lower surface of the clivus is about 11 mm (range 8–18 mm) long. The clivus then broadens as it nears the medial border of the jugular foramen to a width of 42.7 mm (range 33–52 mm). Figure 20 also shows distances between the anterior and posterior borders of the hypoglossal canal, outer opening. It should be noted in children that this external aperture of the hypoglossal canal is situated in most cases lateral to the occipital condyles, which in adults, this area is in most cases found superior to the lateral surface of the condyli occipitales. Shown on the left side of Figure 20 are our measurements of the length and width of the foramen lacerum externum, which is closed by the fibrocartilage.

For inferior approaches to the clivus area, the external opening of the internal carotid canal is also an important landmark. The distance between this canal and the midsagittal plane, and the dis-

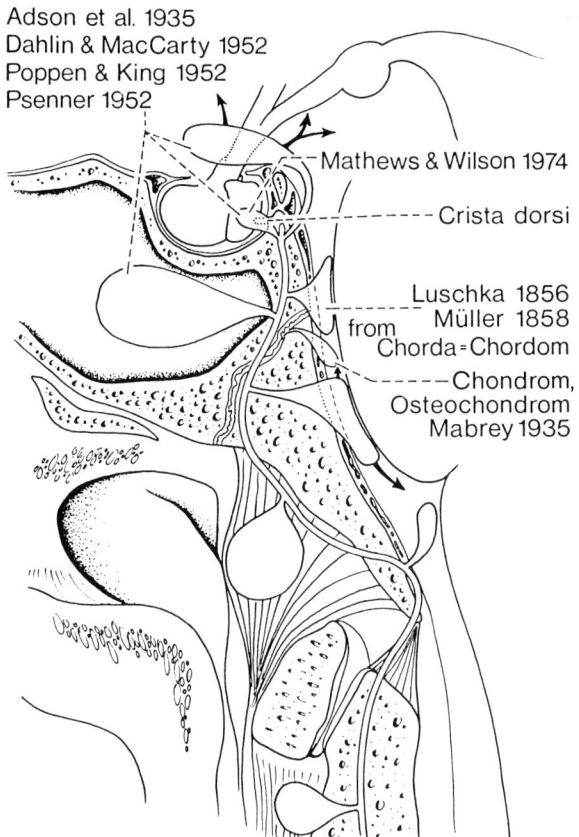

Figure 18: Course of the notochord from which chordomas may develop. Also shown is the petro-occipital synchondrosis, from which, in rare cases, chondromas have been known to develop.

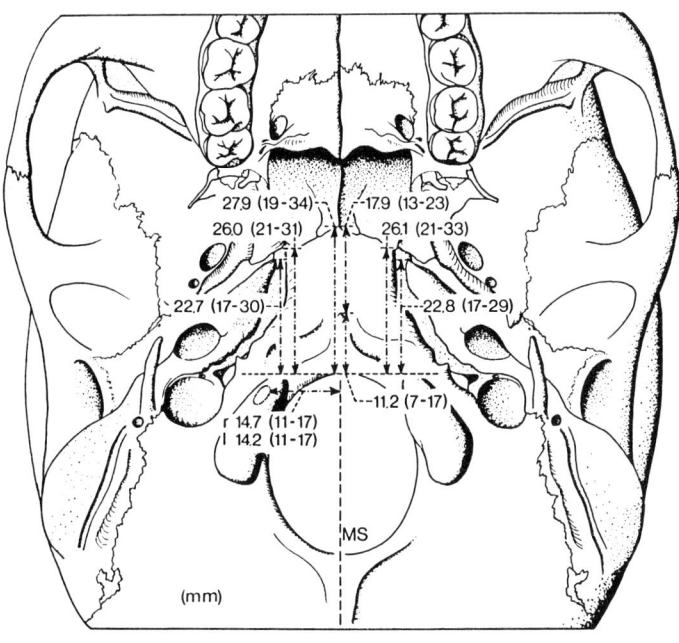

Figure 19: Measurements of clivus length from below, the distances between the posterior border of the vomer and the pharyngeal tubercle and the basion, and distances between the lamina medialis and the basion and the apex of the petrous part and the basion. Also given is the distance between the anterior border of the outer opening of the hypoglossal canal and the midsagittal plane. Values are given in millimeters (range).

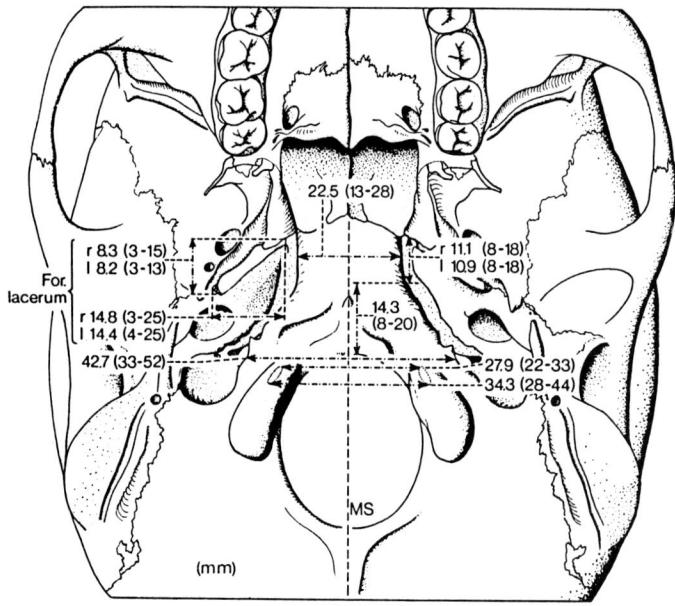

Figure 20: Outer skull base, showing widths and lengths of the small anterior and broad posterior areas of the clivus, and its length. Distances between the anterior and posterior borders of the outer opening of the hypoglossal canal are also shown, as are measurements of the foramen lacerum on the outer skull base. All measurements were made on adult skulls and are given in millimeters (range).

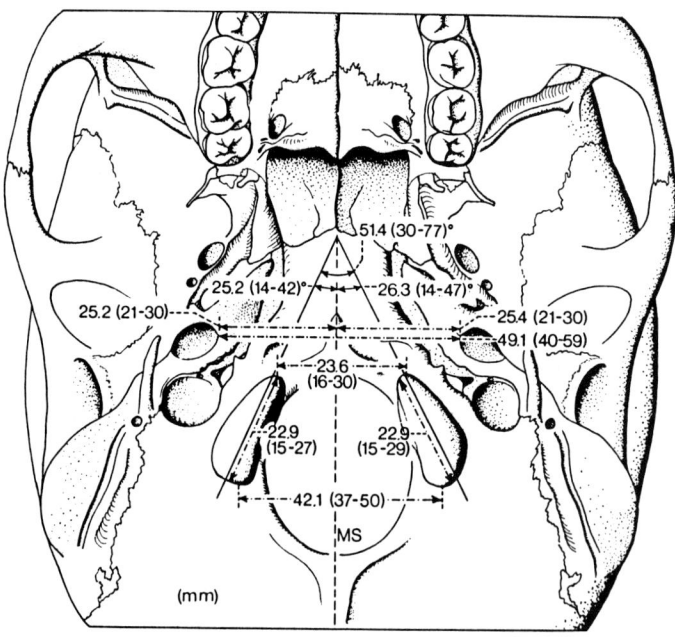

Figure 21: Distance between the external apertures of the internal carotid canal (with bilateral variation) and angles and distances from the apertures to the occipital condyles. Measurements are given in millimeters (range) and degrees (range).

tance between the two internal carotid canal openings, are shown in Figure 21, in which the length of the occipital condyles, the distance between its anterior and posterior borders, its angle to the midsagittal plane, and the angle between the two long axes of the condyles in adults are also shown.

References

1. Adson AW, Kernohan JW, Woltman HW: Cranial and cervical chordomas: A clinical and histologic study. Arch Neurol Psychiat (Chicago) 33:247-261, 1935.
2. Alonso WA, Black P, Connor GH, et al: Transoral transpalatal approach for resection of clival chordoma. Laryngoscope 81:1626-1631, 1971.
3. Anson BJ, Warpeha RL, Rensink MJ: The gross and macroscopic anatomy of the labyrinths. Ann Otol Rhinol Laryngol 77:1-25, 1968.
4. Bonorden B: über die allgemeine und spezielle Morphologie des menschlichen Foramen jugulare. Med Diss Würzburg 1976.
5. Dahlin DC, MacCarty CS: Chordoma: A study of fifty-nine cases. Cancer 5:1170-1178, 1952.
6. Dausacker J: Pratisch anatomische Befunde an der mittleren und hinteren Schädelgrube. Med Diss Würzburg 1974.
7. DiChiro G, Fisher RL, Nelson K: The jugular foramen. J Neurosurg 21:447-460, 1964.
8. Fiegler W: Der Canalis basilaris medianus im Röntgenbild und Computer-tomogramm. Fortschr Röntgenstr 133:416-419, 1980.
9. Gacek RR: Diagnosis and management of primary tumor of the petrous apex. Ann Otol (suppl) 18, 84:1-20, 1975.
10. Gruber W: über den anomalen Canalis basilaris medianus des Os occipitale beim Menschen. Mém Acad Imp Sci, St. Pétersbourg (Sér 7) 27/9, 1880.
11. Holsten RD, Herrmann E: Röntgenbefunde bei okzipitaler Dysplasie. In Trostdorf E, Stender H St (eds): Wirbelsäule und Nerven-system. Stuttgart, Georg Thieme Verlag, 1970.
12. Jannetta PJ: Hemifacial spasm. In Samii M, Jannetta PJ (eds): The Cranial Nerves. New York, Springer Verlag, 1981, pp 484-493.
13. Lang J: über Bau, Länge und Gefässbeziehungen der "zentralen" und "peripheren" Strecken der intrazisternalen Hirnnerven. Ein Beitrag zur vaskularen Hirnnervenschädigung und Dekompressionsbehandlung bei Trigeminusneuralgie, okularer Neuromyotonie, Spasmus hemifacialis, Tinnitus und Vertigo, Glossopharyngeusneuralgie und Caput obstipum spasticum. Zbl Neurochirurgie 43:217-258, 1982.
14. Lang J: Clinical Anatomy of the Head: Neurocranium—Orbit—Craniocervical Regions. Translated by Wilson RR and Winstanley DP. Berlin, Heidelberg, New York, Springer Verlag, 1983.
15. Lang J: Clinical anatomy of the cerebellopontine angle and internal acoustic meatus. Adv Otorhinolaryngol 34:8-24, 1984.
16. Lang J, Brückner B: über dicke und dünne Xonen des Neurocranium, Impressiones gyrorum and Foramina parietalia bei Kindern und Erwachsenen. Anat Anz 149:11-50, 1981.
17. Lang J, Jack CH: über Lage und Lagevariationen der Kanalsysteme im Os temporale. Teil I. Kanäle der Pars petrosa zwischen Margo superior und Meatus acusticus internus. HNO 33:176-179, 1985.
18. Lang J, Heilek E: Anatomisch-klinische Befunde zur A. pharyngea ascendens. Anat Anz 156:177-207, 1984.
19. Lang J, Müller J: über bisher unbekannte topographische Beziehungen von Kleinhirnarterien. Verh Anat Ges 69:823-828, 1975.
20. Lang J, Schafhauser O, Hoffmann S: Contribution to the postnatal development of the cranial base. Canalis caroticus, foramen jugulare, canalis hypoglossalis, canalis condylaris and foramen magnum. Anat Anz 153:315-357, 1983.
21. Lang J, Schreiber TH: über Form und Lage des Foramen jugulare (Fossa Jugularis) des Canalis caroticus und des Foramen stylomastoideum sowie deren postnatale Lageveränderungen. HNO 31:80-87, 1983.
22. Lang J, Weigel M: Nerve-vessel relations in jugular foramen region. Anat Clin 5:1-16, 1983.
23. Luschka H: Die Altersveranderungen der Zwischenwirbelknorpel. Virchow's Arch 13:9-311, 1856.
24. Mabrey RE: Chordoma: A study of 150 cases. Am J Cancer 25:502-517, 1935.
25. Mazzoni A: Internal auditory canal: Arterial relations at the porus acusticus. Ann Otol Rhinol Laryngol 78:797-814, 1969.
26. Montgomery WW: Cystic lesions of the petrous apex: transsphenoidal approach. Ann Otol 86:429-435, 1977.
27. Müller H: über das Vorkommen von Resten der Chorda dorsalis bei Menschen nach der Geburt und uber die Verhältnisse zu den Gallertgeschwülsten. Z Rat Med 2:202-236, 1858.
28. Poppen JL, King AB: Chordoma: Experience with thirteen cases. J Neurosurg 9:139-163, 1952.

29. Psenner L: Beitrag zur Klinik und zur Rontgendiagnostik des Chordoms der Schadelbasis. *Rofo* 77/4:425-433, 1952.
30. Resnikoff S, Cardenas YC: Meningioma at the foramen magnum. *J Neurosurg* (Chicago) 21:301-302, 1964.
31. Schmidt H, Fischer E: *Die okzibpitale Dysplasie*. Stuttgart, Georg Thieme Verlag, 1960.
32. Schmidt TH: Der Canalis hypoglossi, Topographie, Form, Länge, Durchmesser und Volumen. *Med Diss Würzburg* 1975.
33. Schutkowski H: über den diagnostischen Wert der Pars petrosa ossis temporalis für die Geschlechtsbstimmung. *Z Morphol Anthropol* 74:129-144, 1983.
34. Stevenson GC, Stoney RJ, Perkins RK, Adams JE: A trancervical transclival approach to the ventral surface of the brain stem for removal of a clivus chordoma. *J Neurosurg* 24:544-551, 1966.
35. Sunderland S: The arterial relations of the internal auditory meatus. *Brain* 68:23-27, 1945.

26

Inferior Skull Base Anatomy

Johannes Lang, M.D.

Osteology

Inferior Orbital Fissure

The anterior border of this area is the tuber maxillae, which increases in size postnatally, especially between the fifth and eighth years of life. The pterygopalatine fossa is situated behind the medial posterior part of the tuber. The inferior orbital fissure is narrower medially and wider laterally, and is bordered above by the greater wing of the sphenoid bone and below by the tuber maxillae. The anterior lateral border is formed in about 50% of individuals by the zygomatic bone, and in the other 50% by the sphenoid and maxillary bones. In rare cases (mainly in older people), this part of the fissure is thinned and orbital fat may project into the temporal fossa as a "fat hernia" (Fig. 1).[93] Below the inferior orbital fissure are the foramina alveolaria through which the rr. alveolares superiores posteriores are transmitted to the lateral wall of the maxillary sinus.[87] These nerves and the accompanying vessels supply the mucous membrane of the maxillary sinus, the molars of the upper jaw, and parts of the gingiva.

Infratemporal Fossa

Behind the infraorbital fissure is the infratemporal fossa, located mainly below the greater wing of the sphenoid bone. Dorsolaterally the squama of the temporal bone forms the temporomandibular joint. Immediately behind the inferior orbital fissure a groove is present in most cases, and behind this groove is the crista sphenomaxillaris.[53] Behind this crista and in the lateral part of the infratemporal fossa is the infratemporal spine, which is shaped like a pyramid with three sides. This infratemporal spine connects with the sphenomaxillary crest anteriorly and the infratemporal crest laterally and posteriorly.[147]

Pterygoid Process (Fig. 2)

Medial to the infratemporal fossa the lamina lateralis of the pterygoid process projects downward. The whole pterygoid process grows postnatally, as does the maxillary bone, inferiorly.[83] The lateral lamina of the pterygoid process is oriented dorsally and laterally. Between the lamina lateralis of the pterygoid process and the spine of the ala extends the ligamentum

From: Sekhar LN, Schramm VL Jr, eds: *Tumors of the Cranial Base: Diagnosis and Treatment*. Mount Kisco, New York, Futura Publishing Co, Inc., © 1987.

Fissura orbitalis inf. and Foramen rotundum, viewed from below and behind

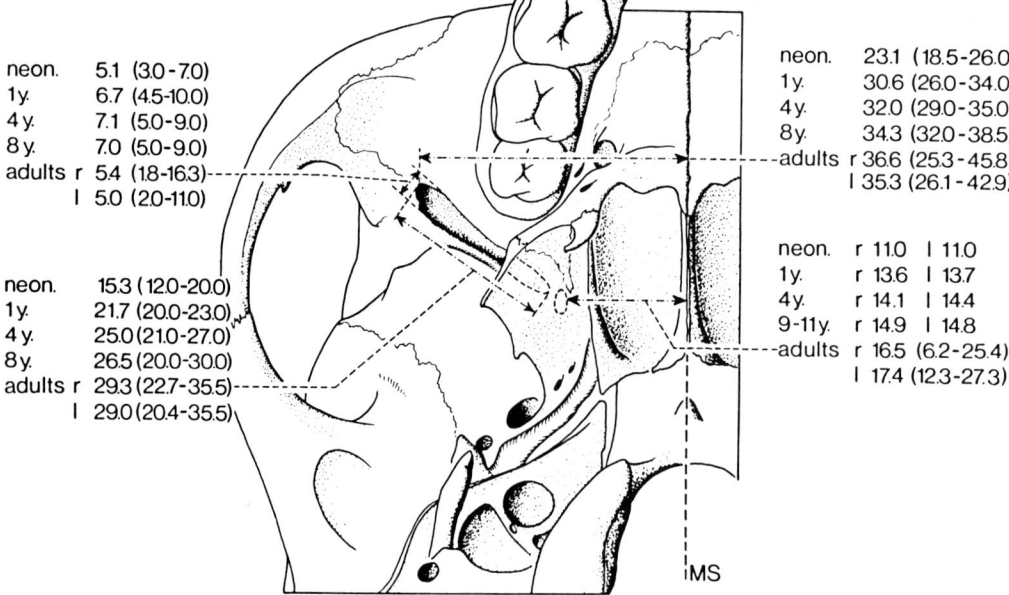

Figure 1: Inferior orbital fissure, showing measurements of width and length and distances from the midsagittal plane at different stages of postnatal development. Measurements from the foramen rotundum to the midsagittal plane are also given.

pterygospinosum. Sometimes this ligament becomes ossified, in both children and adults. These bony bridges are called *laminae pterygospinosae*, and are situated medial to the foramen ovale, below this foramen, or laterally. In the last case, thermocoagulation of the trigeminal ganglion may be difficult or impossible. The so-called spinous processes of the lateral pterygoid lamina have different shapes, are sometimes duplicated, and may lie in the upper or lower part of the lateral lamina.

The lamina medialis of the pterygoid process is shorter than the lamina lateralis. In adults we measured the anteroposterior length of the medial lamina to be 6.78 mm (range 2–12 mm), and of the lamina lateralis to be 14.9 mm (range 9–28 mm).[83] The length of the pterygoid fossa, measured between the uppermost point of the fossa and the most caudal point on the pyramidal process of the palatine bone, averaged 7.38 mm in newborns, 15.7 mm in 4- to 7-year-olds, and 23.4 mm in adults.[83]

Fissura Sphenomaxillaris (Fig. 3)

The superior and anterior part of the pterygoid process is situated slightly posterior to the tuber maxillae. The space between these two bony structures is called the sphenomaxillary fissure, and forms the lateral border of the pterygopalatine fossa. In this fossa are located the pterygopalatine ganglion, the pterygopalatine part of the maxillary artery, veins, and fatty tissue. The sphenomaxillary fissure was 19.87 mm (range 13–29 mm) long and 5.66 mm wide (range 2–12 mm) in adults.

Pterygopalatine Fossa, Walls

The anterior wall of the pterygopalatine fossa is the tuber of the maxilla; the medial wall is composed of the lamina verticalis ossis palatine, and the posterior wall is the pterygoid process. The portals of the pterygopalatine fossa are shown in Table I.

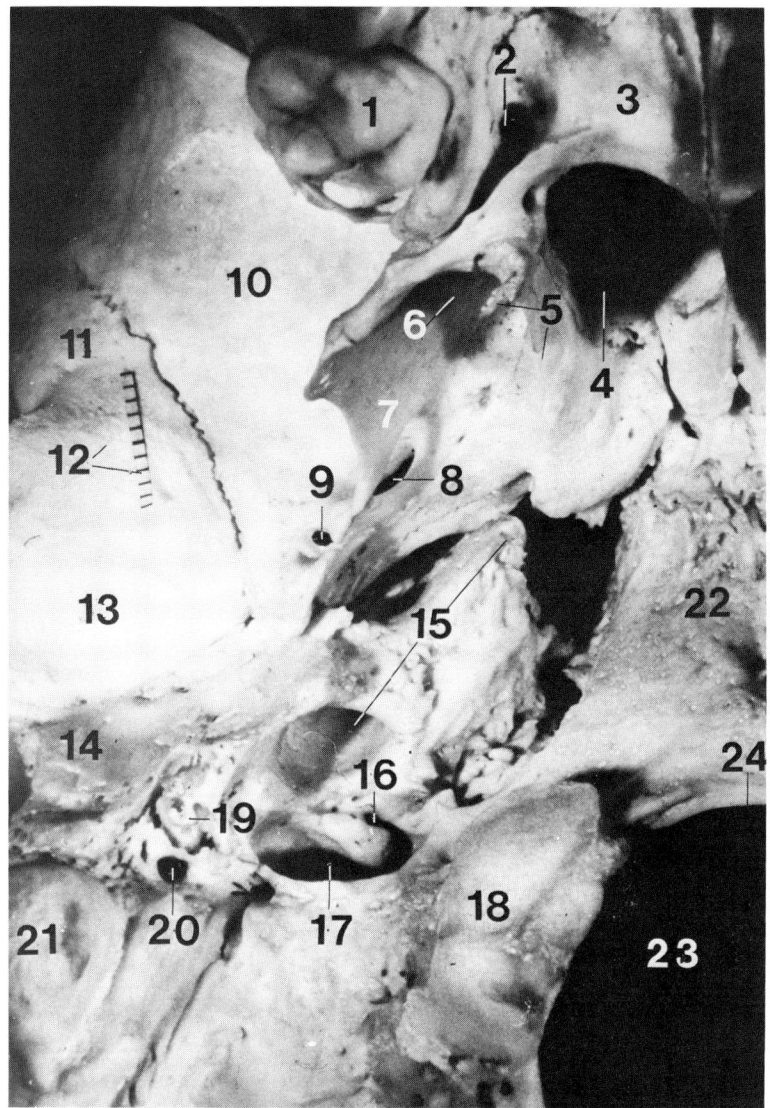

Figure 2: Inferior aspect of the skull base of a 15-year-old child. 1. Second molar tooth. 2. Foramen palatinum majus. 3. Lamina horizontalis ossis palatini. 4. Choana. 5. Lamina media of the pterygoid process and hamulus. 6. Fossa pterygoidea. 7. Lamina lateralis, extending to sphenoid spine (lamina pterygospinosa). 8. Foramen ovale. 9. Foramen spinosum. 10. Greater wing of sphenoid bone. 11. Squama of temporal bone. 12. Eminentia articularis. 13. Fossa articularis. 14. Pars tympanica. 15. Carotid canal and apex of petrous part. 16. Fossula petrosa. 17. Foramen jugulare. 18. Condylus occipitalis. 19. Styloid process (dissected). 20. Stylomastoid foramen. 21. Mastoid process. 22. Clivus. 23. Foramen magnum. 24. Basion.

Mandibular Fossa, Articular Tubercle, and Articular Eminence (Fig. 4)

The posterior and lateral parts of the fossa infratemporalis are bounded by the squamous temporal bone. This part is triangular in shape. Behind the squama the tympanic part of the temporal bone and the inferior process of the tegmen tympani are situated. The lateral ligament of the temporomandibular joint originates in the articular tubercle. Medial to this is the articular fossa; this fossa may be

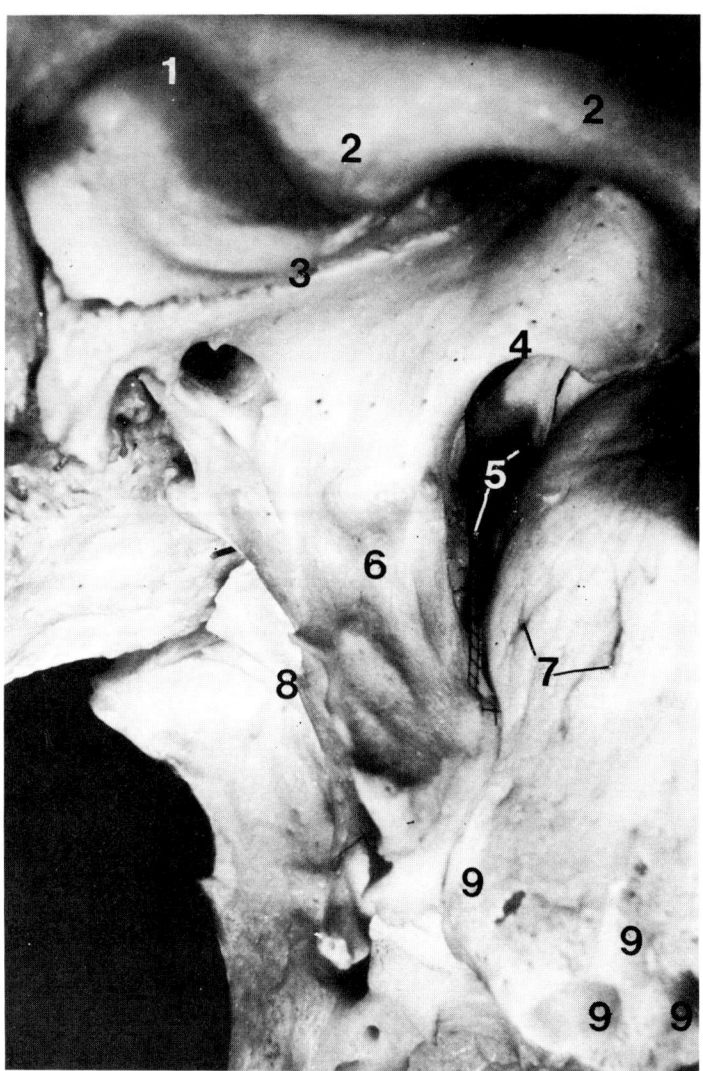

Figure 3: Fissura sphenomaxillaris (adult), viewed from lateral to medial and inferior (and slightly dorsally) to superior. 1. Fossa mandibularis. 2. Tuberculum articulare and processus zygomaticus. 3. Sutura sphenosquamosa. 4. Fissure sphenomaxillaris, upper border. 5. Foramen sphenopalatis (scale in millimeters). 6. Lamina lateralis of pterygoid process. 7. Portals of the superior posterior alveolar nerves and vessels. 8. Vomer, posterior border. 9. Tuberculum postmolare and alveoles of third molar.

transverse or oblique, and fibrous cartilage covers part of the joint between the articulate disc and the squamous part of the temporal bone. Medial to the articular tubercle is the articular eminence. Like the articular fossa, this structure is covered by thin fibrous cartilage. The articular eminence in adults has a height of 6.83 mm on the right and 6.86 mm on the left (mean values).[85]

The largest transverse diameter of the caput mandibulae was measured in our specimens to be 20.91 mm on the right and 20.73 mm on the left (range 16.0–24.7 mm). In most cases the mandibular fossa is the thinnest zone of the middle cranial fossa. It should be remembered that the gonion angle of the mandible, which in our material measured 124° (range 105–139°) in adults, prevents direct transmission of forces from the corpus mandibulae to the ramus. The caput mandibulae lie anterior to a line on the posterior side of the ramus mandibulae, and at an angle to that line of 30.1° (range 4–52.2°)[86,92] Posterior to the articular fossa the retroarticular process is situated, directed inferiorly.[111]

Table I
Fossa Pterygopalatina, Portals

Portals		Contents	and Course
1. lateral portal	Fissura pterygo-maxillaris	A. maxillaris, Aa., Vv., Nn. alveolares sup. post.	Fossa infratemp.
2. dorsal portals	a. Foramen rotundum, above and lat.	N. maxillaris and artery	middle cranial fossa
	b. Canalis pterygoideus, above and med.	N. pterygoideus, A. can.pteryg.	inferior cranial base
	c. Canalis vomerovaginalis, more medially	small arteries and nerves	Fornix pharyngis
	d. Canalis palatovaginalis, medially	Rr. pharyngei of Gangl. pterygo-pal. and artery	Roof of the pharynx
3. medial portal	Foramen sphenopalatinum, above and med.	Rr. nasales post., A. sphenopalat.	nasal cavity
4. ventral portal	Fissura orbitalis inf., above and ventr.	A. and N. infraorbitalis, N. zygomaticus	Orbita
5. inferior portal	Canalis palatinus major	As., Vv., Nn. palatini maj. et min.	Palat. durum et molle, nasal cavity

Fissura Petrotympanica (Fig. 4)

Between the retroarticular process and a small zone medial to it, the tympanic part of the petrous bone connects with the squamous part via the tympanosquamous suture. The petrotympanic fissure is situated more medially. The inferior process of the tegmen tympani grows downward shortly before and after birth, and later, between this process and the tympanic part of the temporal bone, one or two foramina may be found through which run the chorda tympani nerve and the inferior tympanic artery.

Pars Tympanica

Posterior to the tympanosquamous and tympanopetrous suture and fissure lies the tympanic part of the temporal bone. An annulus tympanicus has been identified in newborns, shaped like a horseshoe, situated nearly horizontally. The pars tensa of the tympanic membrane is embedded in this ring-shaped bone. Where the annulus is absent, in the incisura Rivini (named after Augustus Rivinus, 1652–1723), the pars flaccida of the eardrum may be found loosely attached. During childhood, tympanic bone grows laterally, medially, and anteriorly to form the solum tympani and the lower wall of the canalis musculotubalis. Posterior to and against the carotid canal and the jugular fossa, the vagina processus styloidei grows inferiorly.

Processus Styloideus, Processus Mastoideus

The styloid process develops from a portion of the second branchial arch (as do the malleus, the styloid ligament, the lesser horn of the hyoid bone, and the

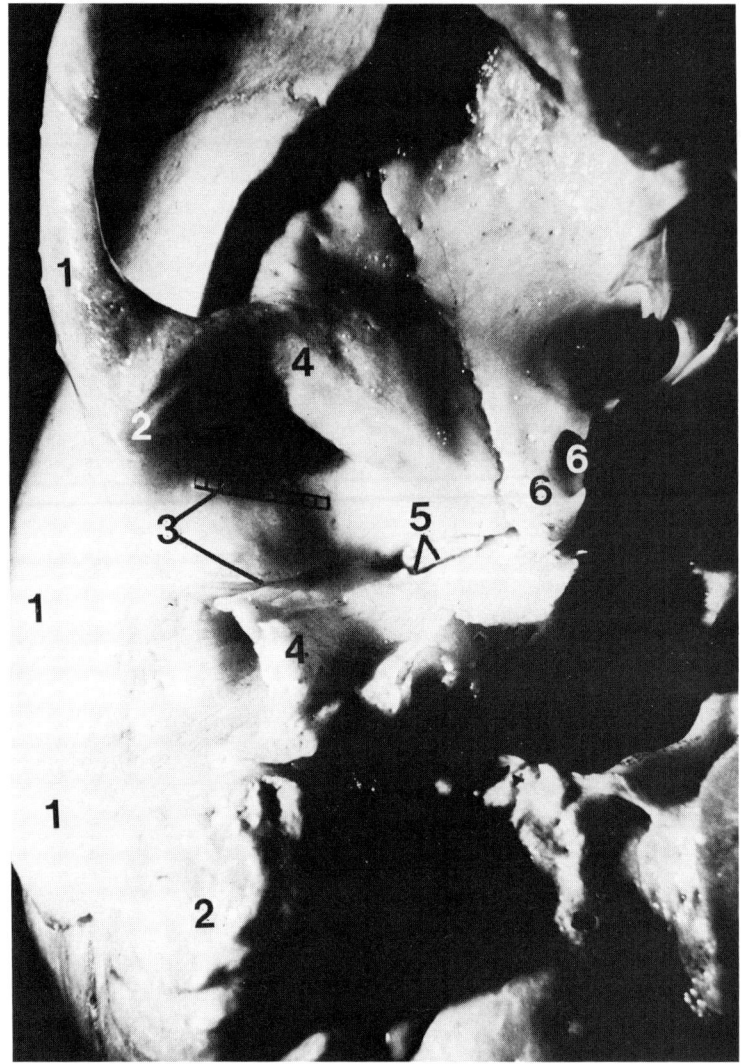

Figure 4: Temporomandibular joint, socket and surrounding structures. 1. Zygomatic process and temporal squama. 2. Tuberculum articulare and mastoid process. 3. Fossa mandibularis, with scale in millimeters and temporosquamosal suture. 4. Eminentia articularis and tympanic part of temporal bone. 5. Processus inferioris tegminis partis petrosae and fissura petrotympanica. 6. Spina ossis sphenoidalis and foramen spinosum.

upper part of the corpus ossis hyoidei). In newborns the styloid process is directed anteriorly and medially, later more vertically. The styloid process is 32.6 mm long (range 16–58 mm) and 4.4 mm thick in men, and 29.7 mm (range 14–55 mm) long and 3.85 mm wide in women.[7,34] Rarely, the styloid process may reach the hyoid bone. Bony and cartilaginous chips are sometimes found in the stylohyoid ligament. In these cases, and when the styloid process reaches the hyoid bone, compression of the blood vessels of the neck and of cranial nerves V, VII, IX, and X, may occur, especially with extension of the head. Attacks of unconsciousness and/or lesions of the recurrent nerve, the phrenic nerve, the glossopharyngeal nerve, and the superior laryngeal nerve have been described in such cases.[99]

Foramen Stylomastoideum (Fig. 5)

Behind and lateral to the styloid process is the opening of the facial canal, the stylomastoid foramen. The foramen in our specimens was 2.05 mm (1.2–3.9 mm) wide on the right and 2.01 mm (range 1.0–2.2 mm) on the left. In 80% of cases studied, the foramen was round and in 20% oval. The distance from the lateral border of the stylomastoid foramen to the tympanomastoid suture was 11.1 mm (range 7.2–19.2 mm) on the right and 11.4 mm (range 6.–17.7 mm) on the left.[94]

Processus Mastoideus

Behind the pars tympanica or the annulus tympanicus, the mastoid process develops postnatally. The mastoid process varies in height and in thickness, depending partly on variations in pneumatization. The intermastoid line (the line between the apices of the two mastoid processes) is situated in most cases in the area of the posterior part of the occipital condyle. Medial to the mastoid process is a groove called the sulcus digastricus. On its medial border a ridge is present, in 93% of specimens, called the paramastoid crest.[24] The posterior belly of the digastric muscle arises in the digastric sulcus and the paramastoid crest. In well-pneumatized mastoid processes this sulcus is visible from inside the mastoid process, and the surgeon may follow it to the mastoid part of the facial canal. In most cases a groove, called the sulcus a. oc-

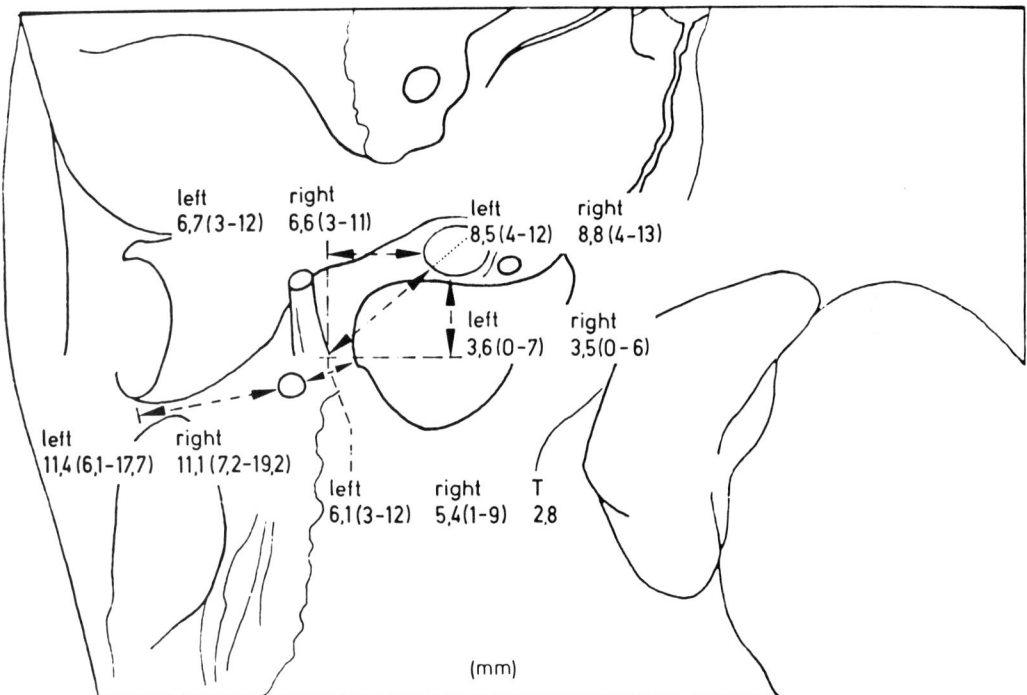

Figure 5: Stylomastoid foramen and inferior opening of the carotid canal are shown, with distances to surrounding structures, between the tympanomastoid fissure (in the middle portion of the external auditory meatus), and the lateral border of the stylomastoid foramen. Also shown are distances between the external opening of the carotid canal and the medial border of the styloid process, measured in the transverse plane; the oblique, sagittal distance between the lateral border of the carotid canal and the anterior border of the stylomastoid process; and the shortest distance of the jugular fossa to the styloid process. The distance between the transverse line along the posterior border of the styloid process and the posterior border of the external opening of the carotid canal are also shown.

468 • TUMORS OF THE CRANIAL BASE: DIAGNOSIS AND TREATMENT

cipitalis, may be found medial to the paramastoid crest, and the occipital artery runs in this groove.

Inferior Cranial Base: Portals for Nerves and Vessels

The maxillary nerve runs through the foramen rotundum into the pterygopalatine fossa. Within the foramen rotundum the nerve contains an average of 14 fascicles (range 1–30), with an average thickness of 173 μm. There are also two arteries, with average diameters of 135 μm.[84]

The mandibular nerve exits through the foramen ovale. The dimensions of the foramen ovale and the other foramina of the outer skull base are shown in Figure 6. A venous plexus surrounds the mandibular nerve and connects veins and sinuses of the inner skull base with veins on the outer skull base. The middle meningeal artery, surrounded by a venous plexus of the middle meningeal veins, runs through the foramen spinosum. In about 30% of specimens we found a foramen Vesalii transmitting a sphenoid emissary vein. This foramen was located on the outer skull base, on the upper border of the pterygoid fossa, lateral to the fossa scaphoidea (origin zone for the tensor veli palatini muscle).

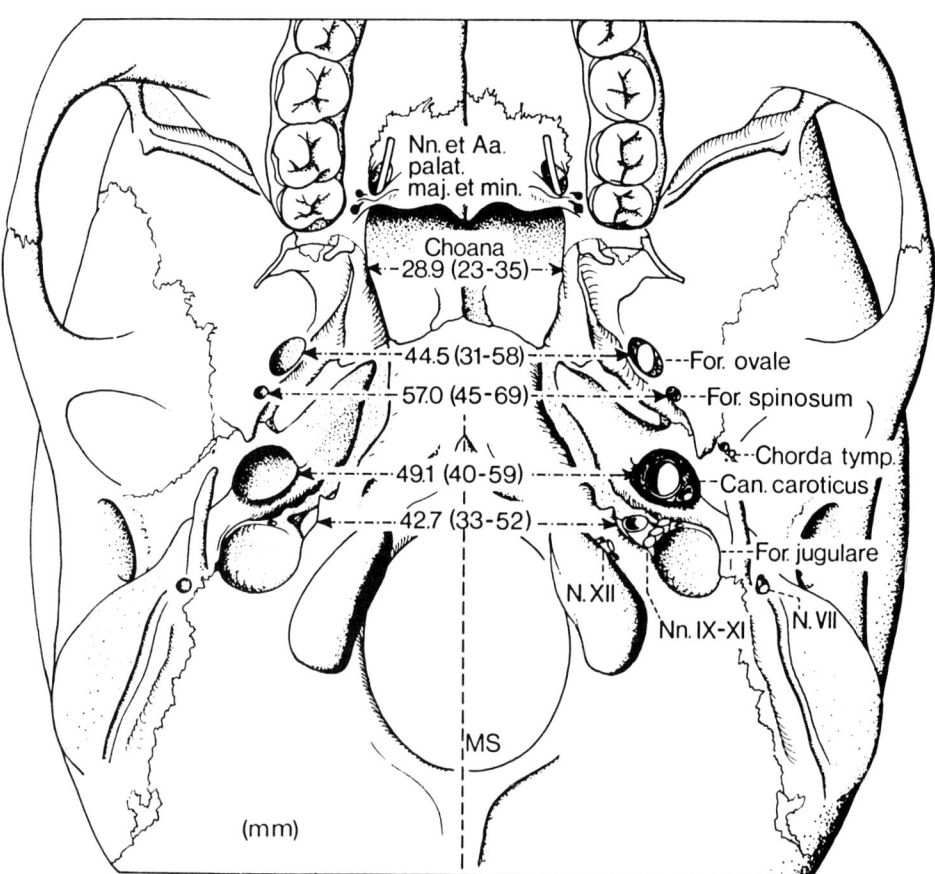

Figure 6: Paramedian distances of foramina on the lower skull base are shown, with measurements of the width of the choana, distances between the foramina ovalia and spinosa bilaterally, dimensions of the outer opening of the carotid canal, and of the most medial portion of the jugular foramen.

Eustachian Tube

Dorsal and medial to the foramen spinosum, the opening of the canalis musculotubalis is found. The pars ossea of the auditory tubercle is the lower part and the groove for the tensor tympani muscle is the upper part of this tube. The two grooves are divided by a bony bridge of variable thickness. The bony part of the Eustachian tube in adults is 11–12 mm long. The angles of the canal (opening anteriorly) to the midsagittal plane are given in Figure 7.

The cartilaginous portion of the Eustachian tube has a length of between 24 and 25 mm. This part runs obliquely from laterally to medially and inferiorly, with an angle to the horizontal plane of the skull of between 30° and 40°. The pharyngeal opening of the Eustachian tube is therefore placed about 15 mm below the tympanic opening. The angle between the osseous and the cartilaginous

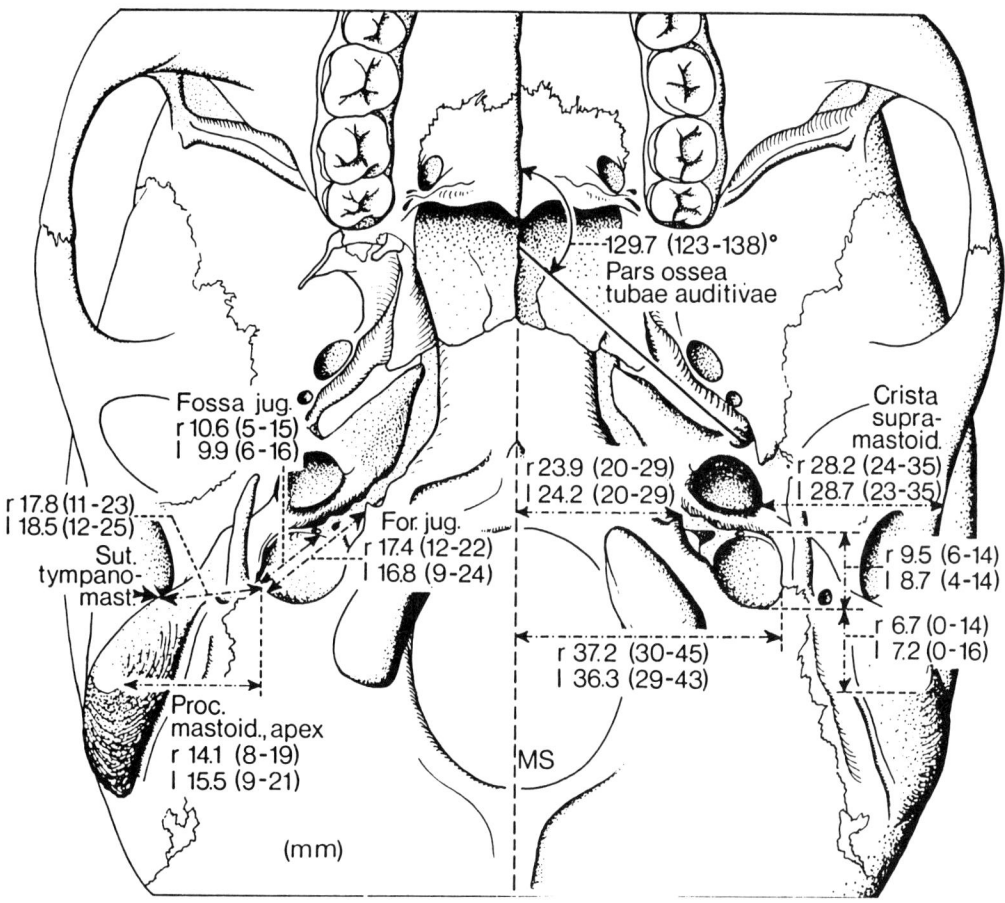

Figure 7: Measurements on the lower skull base are shown, including the angle of the osseous Eustachian tube with the midsagittal plane (right side), length of the jugular foramen and jugular fossa, and distance from the jugular fossa to the tympanomastoid suture and tip of the mastoid process. Also given are distance from the midsagittal plane to the medial and lateral borders of the jugular foramen, posteroanterior length of the foramen, distance to the tip of the mastoid process, and distance from the lateral border of the foramen to the midsagittal plane. The distance from the supramastoid crest to the lateral border of the internal carotid canal on the outer skull base is also shown.

parts of the auditory tube is about 5°, opening ventrocaudally. This narrowed area is called the isthmus of the auditory tube, and is absent in about 48% of cases, spiral-shaped in 30%, and pronounced in 22%.[134] The width of the auditory tube is indicated in Figure 7.

Carotid Canal (Fig. 8)

The outer opening of the carotid canal is oval in most cases, with its long axis oriented mediorostral to laterodorsal. In newborns, the greatest diameter of the carotid canal was 3.5 mm (range 3.0–4.5 mm); in children 2 years old, this opening was 5.6 mm (range 4–8 mm) wide; and in adolescents and adults it was 6.42 mm (range 6–7 mm) wide on the right and 6.8 mm (range 6.0–8.0 mm) wide on the left.[91]

The carotid canal carries the internal carotid artery, the venous plexus and veins around the artery, and the sympathetic nerves. The first part of the canal is directed superiorly and anteriorly, at an angle to the Frankfort horizontal plane of 122° (range 113–135°) in newborns, 121° (range 110–130°) in 5-year-old children, and 99.1° (range 86–110°) in adults.[94] The length of the ascending portion of the canal was 3.8 mm (range 3.5–4.5 mm) in newborns, 5.7 mm in 1-year-old children, 7.3 mm in 3-year-old children, 10.0 mm in 15-year-old children, and in adults 10.13 mm (range 6.5–13.5 mm).

Foramen Jugulare

The dimensions of the jugular foramen measured in our specimens are shown in Figure 8. The distances from the outer border of the jugular foramen to the apex of the mastoid process and the tympanomastoid suture, and from the posterior border of the jugular formen to the tip of the mastoid process are given in Figure 7. It should be noted that we found the jugular foramen to be undivided in about

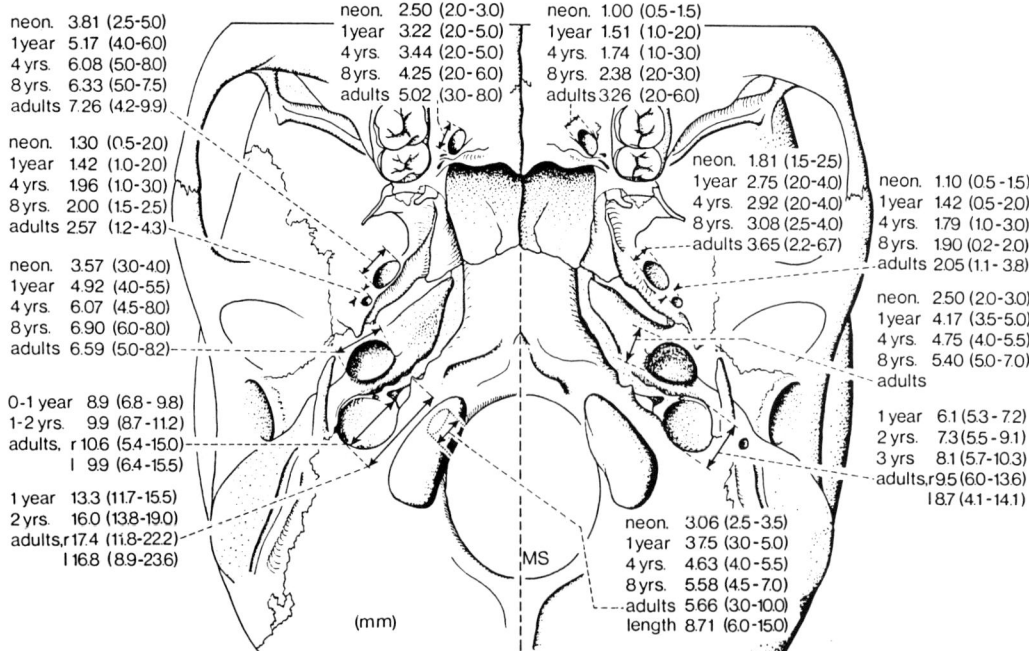

Figure 8: Measurements of the lengths and widths of openings on the lower skull base: foramen palatinum majus, foramen ovale, foramen spinosum, carotid canal, and jugular foramen.

54% of adult specimens and 60% of pediatric specimens. However, an intrajugular process of the petrous bone had developed in all cases, and we found an intrajugular process of the occipital bone in 30% of adult specimens and in 24.3% of pediatric specimens. Completely divided jugular foramina were found in 14.6% of adult specimens and in 11.6% of pediatric specimens. The glossopharyngeal nerve and/or the inferior petrosal sinus may course between divided foramina. In most cases the width of the right foramen jugulare is greater than the left, but not its length. The glossopharyngeal, vagus, and accessory nerves run through the jugular foramen in a connective tissue layer that joins the dura mater intracranially and the pericranium extracranially. This "guide plate" is situated in most cases between the jugular foramen area and the inferior petrosal sinus, and contains an opening for the inferior petrosal sinus, usually between the glossopharyngeal and the vagus nerves. In some cases we found more than one opening for this sinus. The location of the jugular bulb and the drainage of the inferior petrosal sinus are very variable (Fig. 9).

Fossula Petrosa and Canaliculus Tympanicus

A small depression, called the fossula petrosa, is located between the external aperture of the internal carotid canal and the jugular foramen. In this area, the inferior ganglion of the glossopharyngeal nerve is also located. One twig of this nerve is the tympanic nerve, which extends from the fossula area laterally to the cavum tympani. In most cases the channel between the fossula petrosa and the cavum tympani is 3–5 mm long. Two to six glomeruli[42] are embedded in this nerve, from which glomus tumors can develop, either in the channel or in the tympanic cavity. The inferior tympanic artery, a twig of the ascending pharyngeal artery, may run through this channel to the middle ear, or in its own small canal in the neighborhood of the internal carotid canal.

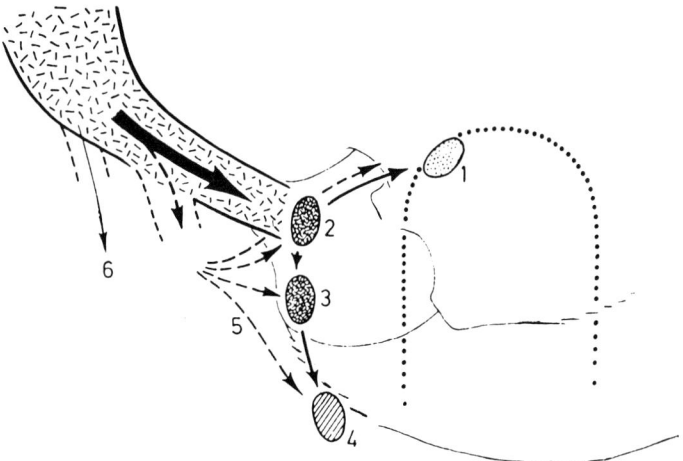

Figure 9: Height of the inferior petrosal sinus in relation to the internal jugular vein (percent of cases for each relationship): 1. Upper level of the bulb (right 11.53%, left 5.76%). 2. Upper level of the jugular foramen (right 9.61%, left 13.46%). 3. Opening in the transitional zone between the bulb of the jugular vein and the vein itself (right 15.38%, left 17.3%). 4. Opening in the sinus below the skull in the internal jugular vein (right 11.53%, left 9.61%). 5. Additional connection with the inferior petrosal sinus through small canals in the cranial base (right 10%, left 7.3%). 6. Inferior petrosal sinus, piercing the skull base (right 1.92%, left 3.84%, in its own canal). In very rare cases, we found two veins immediately below the skull base, the deeper vein draining the inferior petrosal sinus.

Apertura Externa Canaliculi Cochleae

The external aperture of the bony channel for the perilymphatic aqueduct is situated behind the external aperture of the carotid canal and below the internal auditory meatus (Fig. 10). In most cases we also found a second channel anterior to the cochlear canaliculus, through which the labyrinthine vein passed. Inferior and slightly caudad to this opening, the superior ganglion of the glossopharyngeal nerve may be seen, with its upper surface in contact with cerebrospinal fluid and its inferior surface embedded in the channel for the lower cranial nerves.

Canaliculus Mastoideus

In the upper surface of the jugular fossa of many specimens we identified a transverse groove for the auricular branch of the vagus nerve. This groove enters a small channel (canaliculus mastoideus), which is also directed laterally to the mastoid part of the facial nerve canal. The auricular branch of the vagus nerve runs posterior to the facial nerve in this area, although sometimes anterior to the facial nerve and lateral to the channel to the tympanomastoid suture. Some fibers of the auricular branch of the vagus nerve connect to the facial nerve, and glomeruli were identified along its course. The nerve supplies a portion of the outer surface of the tympanic membrane and the posterior wall of the external auditory meatus and the pinna.

Hypoglossal Canal

The internal opening of the hypoglossal channel is located medial and in-

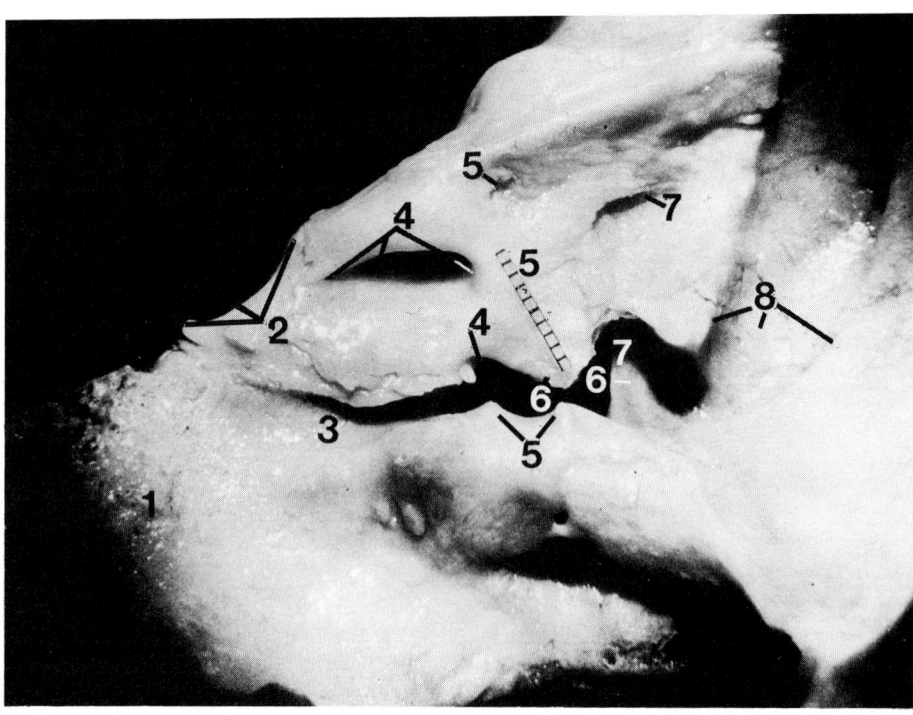

Figure 10: Posterior surface of the petrous bone and jugular bulb: variations, viewed from medial to lateral. 1. Clivus. 2. Incisura trigemini. 3. Sulcus sinus petrosi inferioris. 4. Internal auditory meatus and arcuate janua. 5. Subarcuate fossa, millimeter scale, and groove in the jugular tubercle. 6. Jugular foramen. 7. Rim of the endolymphatic sac and terminal sigmoid crest. 8. Sulcus sinus sigmoidei.

ferior to the jugular foramen. In some adults the intracranial openings of the channel were divided; this was found in 14.8% of specimens on the right and in 27.47% of specimens on the left. Three intracranial openings were found on the right sides of each of two specimens and on the left side in one specimen of the 142 examined. So-called lingulae (bony spurs) were seen in a different area of the internal meatus of the channel in approximately 39% of specimens. Figure 12 shows the results of our measurements of the hypoglossal canal.

Foramen Lacerum

The foramen lacerum externum is an irregular pore on the outer skull base between the sphenoid bone anteriorly, the basilar part of the occipital bone medially, and the apex of the petrous temporal bone laterally and dorsally. We measured the distance of the foramen from the external auditory meatus (Fig. 11), and its width and length (Fig. 12). The foramen lacerum is covered by fibrocartilage externally, and transmits the internal carotid artery internally.

Upper Wall of the Nasal Cavity and Its Channels (Fig. 13)

The upper wall of the nasal cavity is composed most anteriorly by the nasal bone, immediately posteriorly by the superior nasal spine of the frontal bone, and posterior to the latter's bony portion by the lamina cribrosa. Posterior to this

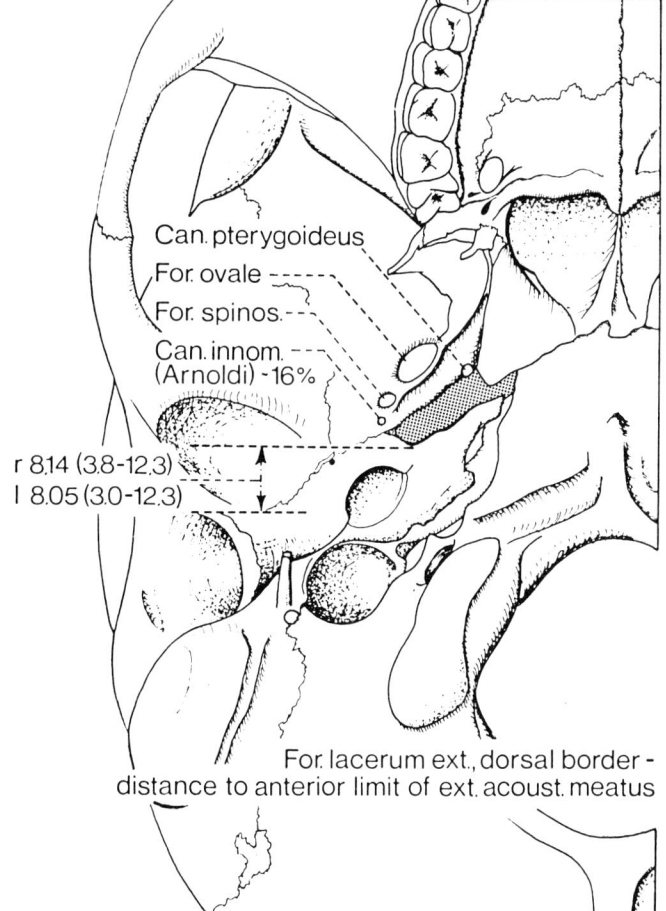

For. lacerum ext., dorsal border - distance to anterior limit of ext. acoust. meatus

Figure 11: Distance in millimeters (range) from the posterior border of the foramen lacerum externum to the anterior border of the external auditory meatus, and to canals anterior to the foramen lacerum.

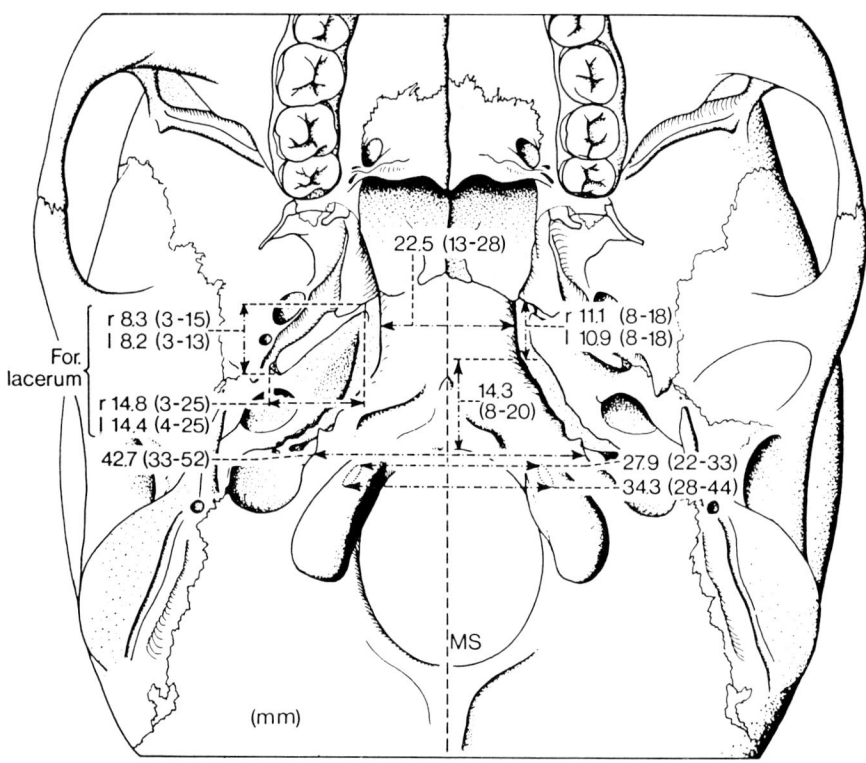

Figure 12: Widths and lengths of the narrow and wide portions of the clivus. The anterior narrow portion is about 11 mm long, the posterior wide portion 14.3 mm (range 8–20 mm). Width and length of the foramen lacerum and distances between the most medial border of the jugular foramen and the anterior and posterior borders of the hypoglossal canal on the outer skull base are also given.

area, the sphenoid bone and the aperture of the sphenoid sinus are located.

Between the ethmoid labyrinth and the sphenoid bone lies a sphenoethmoid recess on each side. Behind and inferior to this recess and the sphenoid bone lies the foramen sphenopalatinum. Its superior border is the sphenoid bone, its anterior border is the processus orbitalis, and its posterior border the processus sphenoidalis of the lamina perpendicularis ossis palatini.

A more or less developed ridge may be noted on the lower medial surface of the sphenoid bone. This ridge is called the rostrum sphenoidale, and it connects to the ala vomeris, the middle part of the roof of the choanae. The processus vaginalis of the sphenoid bone develops laterally in the roof area.

Channels in the Upper Wall of the Nasal Cavity (see Fig. 13)

Canalis Vomerobasilaris

In most cases, a vomerobasilar canal is present between the sphenoid bone and the alae vomeris. Small veins, connective tissue, and, in the posterior part, the pharyngeal hypophysis are located in this canal.

Canalis Palatovaginalis

The superior border of the palatovaginal channel is the inferior surface of the processus vaginalis of the sphenoid bone. Anteriorly, the floor of this short channel is formed by the processus sphenoidalis of

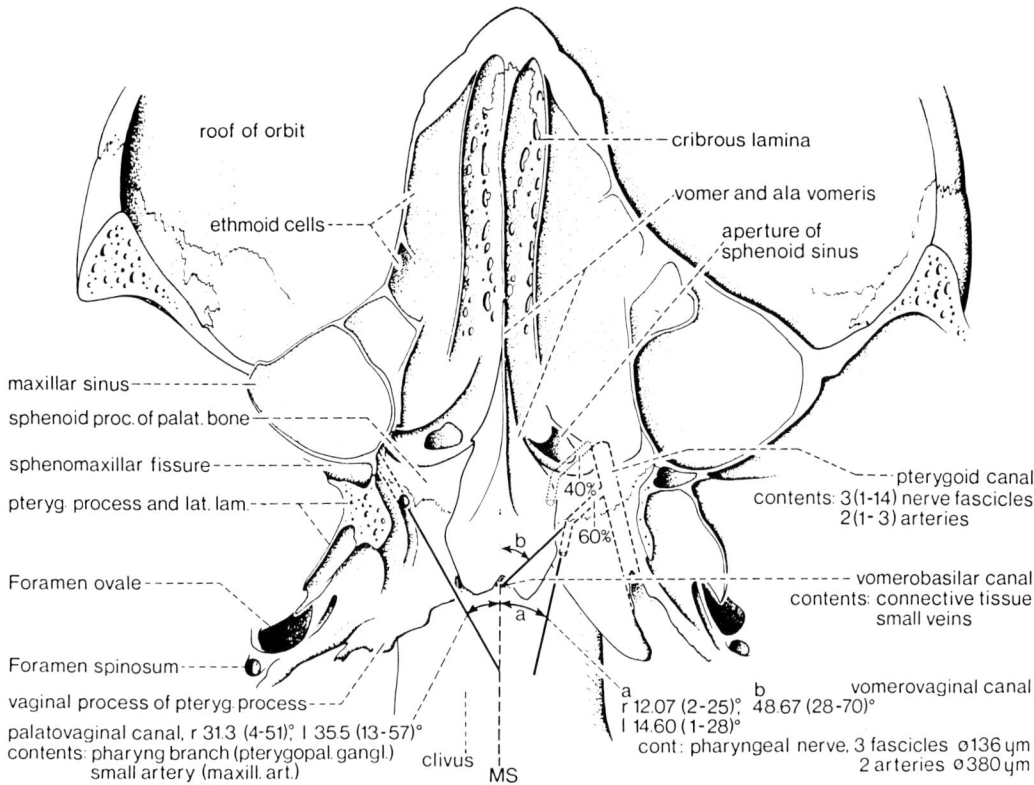

Figure 13: Roof of the nasal cavity and orientation of canals in the upper area of the pharynx, including the pterygoid canal.

the lamina perpendicularis ossis palatini, and the channel opens into the pterygopalatine fossa. Its posterior opening lies on the inferior surface of the processus vaginalis of the sphenoid bone, and in most cases a groove is present on the inferior surface of the process, posterior to the opening. Through this small channel runs a pharyngeal branch of the pterygopalatine ganglion and a small twig of the a. maxillaris to the mucous membrane of the roof of the pharynx, posterior and superior to the pharyngeal opening of the Eustachian tube.

Canalis Vomerovaginalis (see Fig. 13)

The superior wall of the vomerovaginal channel is the inferior surface of the processus vaginalis of the pterygoid process, and sometimes also the lateral border of the ala vomeris. In 60% of our specimens, this channel began in the pterygoid channel, posterior to the anterior aperture of the latter, and in 40% of our specimens the canalis vomerovaginalis began in the pterygopalatine fossa medial to the anterior opening of the pterygoid channel.[84] The channel was seen to contain an average of three (range one to six) nerve fiber bundles, with thicknesses of 136 μm (range 55–370 μm). In addition, the channel also contained one to three arteries, with lumina of 381 μm (range 74–814 μm).

Canalis Craniopharyngealis Medialis

We found this channel in only about 0.5% of our adult specimens. When it was present in fetal and newborn specimens, the channel contained small veins and arteries running between the hypophyseal fossa and the superior surface of the ala vomeris.

Canalis Craniopharyngeus Lateralis

Between the medial border of the superior orbital fissure and the canalis vomerovaginalis, a channel may be identified in specimens from individuals 6 years of age or less. It is thought that this channel may carry a vein, and that the channel forms lateral septae in the sphenoid sinus.

Canalis Pterygoideus (Fig. 14)

The pterygoid channel is located in the body of the sphenoid bone. In our specimens its posterior aperture was located 15.2 mm (range 12–19.2 mm) lateral to the midsagittal plane. It was estimated to be 1.63 mm wide (range 0.7–2.5 mm).[94] The anterior aperture of the channel is located in the posterior wall of the pterygopalatine fossa, 12.3 mm (range 5.5–17.5 mm) from the midsagittal plane.[84] In 44% of our specimens, the channel ran dorsolaterally to anteromedially, forming an angle to the midsagittal plane of 14° (range 5–45°). In 32% of specimens, the course of the channel

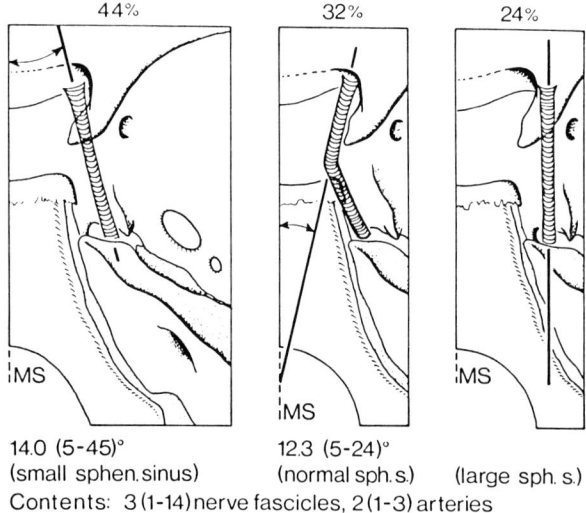

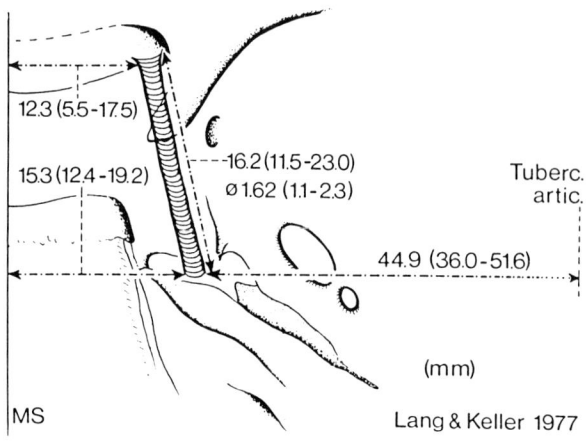

Figure 14: Orientations of the pterygoid canal with respect to the midsagittal plane, in degrees, and percentages. Distances of the posterior and anterior pores of the canal from the midsagittal plane and from the posterior pore to the tuberculum articulare are also shown.

curved medially, and in 24% of specimens, the axis of the canal lay in the sagittal plane. The canal was estimated to be 16.2 mm long (range 11.5–23 mm).

In 18% of specimens the channel appeared on the inferior surface of the sphenoid sinus as a bony ridge, while in 34% of specimens the channel was separated from the sphenoid sinus by very thin bone. The bony roof of the canal was dehiscent in 10% of specimens. Between one and 14 nerve fascicles (mean three) having thicknesses of 407 μm (range 74–1,924 μm) were found in the channel, and one to three (mean two) arteries having lumens of 122 μm (range 54–222 μm).

Fibers of the greater superficial petrosal nerve (GSPN) run in this channel, specifically, pre- and postganglionic sympathetic fibers to the pterygopalatine ganglion. These fibers arise in the superior salivatory nucleus and travel through the nervus intermedius. It is thought that gustatory fibers also travel in this nerve to reach the geniculate ganglion cells.

The deep petrosal nerve carries postganglionic sympathetic fibers from the superior cervical sympathetic ganglion; these fiber bundles pass around the internal carotid artery to unite with the GSPN above the fibrocartilage covering the foramen lacerum externum. The nerve then pierces this connective tissue layer to reach the posterior opening of the pterygoid channel. Chorobsky and Penfield[20] found small accumulations of ganglion cells in the area where the GSPN and the deep petrosal nerve united, and also along the course of the pterygoid canal. The location of this union was identified by Zolotarewa and Strynck[148] as lying 3 to 4 mm behind the posterior aperture of the pterygoid channel. In addition, they described a duplicated pterygoid canal (and nerve) in the posterior course.

Sphenoid Sinus

Development of the Sphenoid Sinus

The sphenoid sinus begins to develop in the third month of fetal life as a mucosal bud arising from the superoposterior region of the nose. This well-vascularized mucosal bud penetrates the presphenoid portion of the sphenoid bone, which is still cartilaginous. Cope[23] states that the bud does not develop further posteriorly until puberty, when it begins to develop dorsally and dorsolaterally. However, incomplete septa often persist at the location of the former intrasphenoid synchondrosis.

The anterior wall of the sphenoid sinus is bounded by the sphenoid concha (conchae sphenoidales, ossicula Bertini), which begins to develop in the fifth month of fetal life. During the first year of postnatal life, the conchae continue to grow, increasing chiefly in height and to a lesser extent in breadth, and covering the developing sphenoid sinus except in the vicinity of the ostium. Between 4 and 9 years of age, the sphenoid sinus increases in width, and the concha region covers its medial and anterior portions. During this time the ostium migrates medially.

The lateral and superior margins of the bony ostium of the sphenoid sinus are derived from the ethmoid bone. The sphenoid conchae fuse with the body of the sphenoid between 9 and 12 years of age.[136] If the conchae remain small, the most posterior ethmoid cell grows further dorsally and forms the medial wall of the optic canal or even comes to underlie the floor of the pituitary fossa. We noted this condition to be present in about 10% of our specimens (Fig. 25).

Rostrum of the Sphenoid Bone

The sphenoid rostrum is the prominent median ridge, wedge-shaped or more or less rounded, that projects from the anterior and inferior surface of the body of the sphenoid. At the boundary between the anterior and posterior segments of the body, there is a funnel-shaped cleft, sometimes extending transversely, that penetrates the body of the sphenoid. This cleft may terminate within the sphenoid, or it may continue as a small channel as far as the pituitary fossa. Between 1 and 3 years of age the rostrum enlarges, usually becoming narrower and more pointed, although it has been noted to become broader and more obtuse in some cases.

Ostium of the Sphenoid Sinus

Lateral to the superior and posterior portions of the septum and behind the posterior nasal concha we found a sphenoethmoid recess in 48.3% of specimens. In this small recess, or, when it is absent, slightly medial to this location, the aperture of the sphenoid sinus is located. In 70% of our specimens,[90] we found the aperture to be less than 3.5 mm in diameter, while in 15% of cases the aperture was pinhead size. Sometimes the aperture is very small. In 28% of our specimens we noted that the aperture was oval, with the longer diameter lying in a nearly vertical plane, sometimes obliquely or transversely oriented. This aperture is notable as the point where the surgeon begins to open the sphenoid sinus for the approach to the hypophysis.

Morphology of the Sphenoid Sinus

Most anatomists classify the sphenoid sinus as conchal, presellar, or sellar. When the sinus is of the conchal type (3% of cases) the surgeon encounters thick bone in the floor of the pituitary fossa when approaching transnasally. The anterior wall of the sella is pneumatized in sinuses of the presellar type (11%), while in sellar sinuses (86%) the entire floor of the sella is occupied by the sphenoid sinus.[45,46]

Septum of the Sphenoid Sinus

As the mucosal buds arising from the nasal cavity grow posteriorly on either side of the midsagittal plane, they create the septum between the two sphenoid sinuses, which is actually formed from the central segment of the sphenoid bone. The septum may be oblique or even transverse. The septum has developed in the vertical midsagittal plane in 25% of cases,[46] while in other cases the septum may be completely absent or the sinuses may be lacking.[12] In the latter case the space is filled with bone resembling the diploë.

Transverse Septa

A transverse septum (called a septum transsphenoidale by Cope[23]) was seen frequently in our specimens.[4] It was usually located in the roof of the sinus, immediately below the tuberculum sellae, also known as the olivary eminence. Transverse septa on the floor of the sphenoid bone are seen less frequently.

Walls of the Sphenoid Sinus

The *superior wall* of the sphenoid sinus varies in length and width. When the sinus is large, it abuts rostrally on the planum sphenoidale, the roof of the lesser wing of the sphenoid, the optic channel, and the floor of the sella. Occasionally it extends into the dorsum sellae and the clivus. The upper wall may be very thin, especially in the vicinity of the optic channel.

The *inferior wall* of the sphenoid sinus may form part of the upper wall of the nasal cavity or may even be situated behind the latter, forming part of the roof of the nasopharynx. It is usually the thickest wall of the sphenoid sinus, except for the posterior wall.

As a rule, the *posterior wall* of the sphenoid sinus is oriented vertically, and is slightly concave anteriorly. Depending upon the development of the sphenoid sinus, it may be situated in the presphenoid or postsphenoid portion of the sphenoid bone, or even occasionally in the clivus portion of the occipital bone.

The *anterior wall* of the sphenoid sinus is also oriented more or less vertically, and its upper part is extremely thin. The bony ostium of the sphenoid sinus, an orifice that is narrowed by reduplication of the mucosa, is situated here, 14.3 mm (range 9–21 mm)[70] from the sella floor.

The *lateral wall* of the sphenoid sinus is formed by the body of the sphenoid.

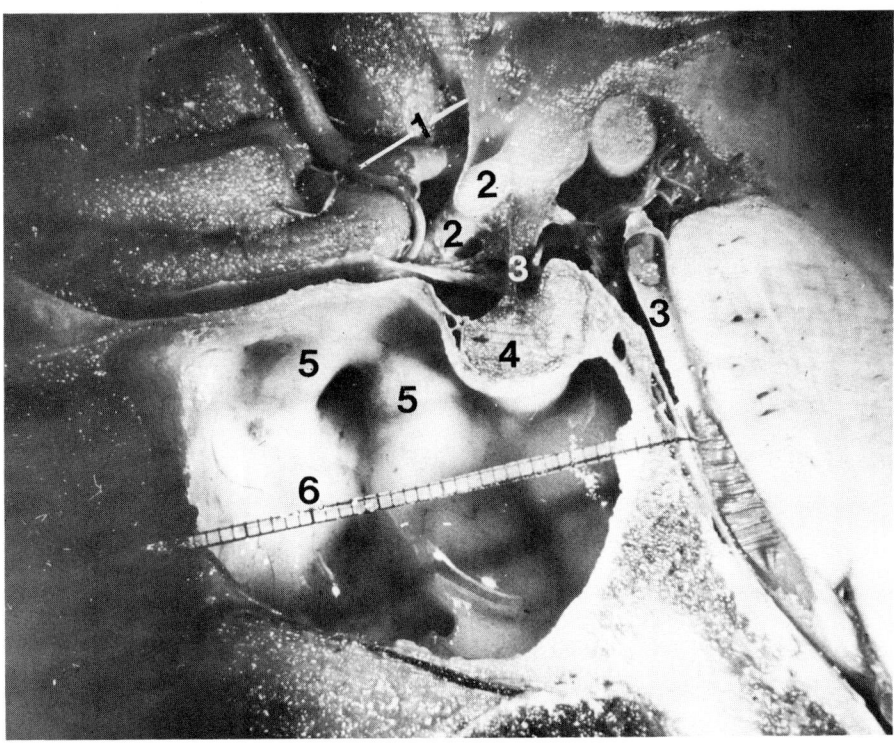

Figure 15: Large sphenoid sinus, with prominences on its lateral wall. 1. Lamina terminalis of third ventricle and anterior cerebral artery. 2. Optic chiasm and optic nerve. 3. Infundibulum and basilar artery (cut). 4. Anterior lobe of hypophysis. 5. Impressions of the optic canal and internal carotid artery. 6. Millimeter scale.

Projections within the Sphenoid Sinus Caused by Vessels and Nerves (Fig. 15)

Internal Carotid Artery: The internal carotid artery emerges from the carotid canal in the petrous portion of the temporal bone and runs posterolaterally into the cavernous sinus, leaving it anteriorly at a point medial to the anterior clinoid process. When the sphenoid sinus is well developed, its lateral wall may be indented by the internal carotid artery and the bone may occasionally have undergone resorption at this point. The internal carotid artery may produce bulges on the lateral wall of the sphenoid sinus that vary in length, prominence, and orientation, depending upon the length and breadth of the sphenoid sinus and on the course of the internal carotid artery within the cavernous sinus. As a rule, the ICA bends posteriorly in the dorsal part of the cavernous sinus. The artery then runs anteriorly and medially in the cavernous sinus at an angle of 25 to 35°.[119] The anterior curve of the ICA then extends under the anterior clinoid process, bending in a convex curve anteriorly that moves first medially and then posteriorly and superiorly (Fig. 16).

In 16 to 17% of individuals, the internal carotid artery runs in an almost straight line from the transition zone of the carotid canal to the anterior convex curve.[119] An intermediate form of the internal carotid artery has an S-shaped course (53% of our specimens). In such cases the artery ascends almost to the posterior clinoid process, then bends sharply caudally and leaves the cavernous sinus anteriorly and medially in a broad curve that is convex basally and rostrally. A straight internal carotid artery is seen most commonly in children, and its

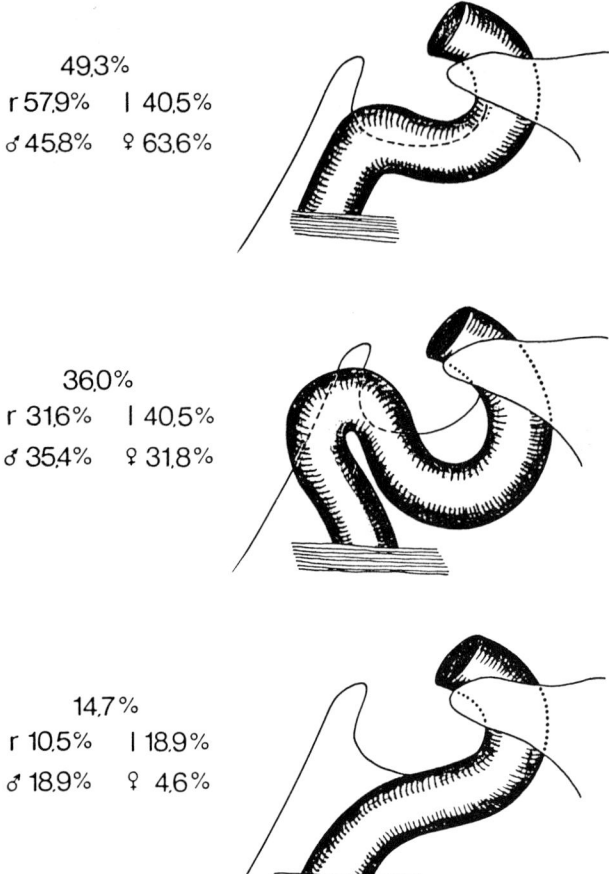

Figure 16: Course of the internal carotid artery in the cavernous sinus.

course becomes more tortuous with age.[71,98]

According to Van Alyea[4] the sphenoid sinus is deeply indented by the carotid artery in 53% of cases, and slightly indented in 12% of specimens. In 14% of skulls the entire course of the internal carotid artery along the lateral wall of the sphenoid sinus is conspicuously marked, while in 3% it is faintly marked. Seftel et al.[126] found marked paths of the internal carotid artery in 65% of the specimens studied, and in 53% of this group the path was conspicuous. In contrast, Renn and Rhoton[123] demonstrated the presence of carotid prominences in 71% of the specimens they studied, and Fujii et al.[36] state that presellar indentations are present in 98% of sinuses of the presellar type. These last investigators noted that infrasellar indentations were present in 80% of their specimens, while retrosellar indentations were visible in 78% of sphenoid sinuses of the sellar type. According to their findings, the mean length of an internal carotid artery prominence is 12.9 mm (range 8–18 mm). We found impressions of the internal carotid artery in 53% of our specimens in the anterior part.[95]

Recesses of the Sphenoid Sinus: We have described an anterior, lateral, and posterior supraoptic recess, and a recess of the dorsum sellae.[78]

When examined during surgery, the anterior lobe of the pituitary gland looks yellowish and feels relatively firm, while the posterior lobe looks gelatinous and gray. Hardy[48] states that the anterior lobe is surrounded by a potential cleft in which venous capillaries run between the pituitary gland capsule and the periosteum of the sella turcica. The posterior lobe, on the other hand, is usually firmly attached to the posterior wall of the pituitary gland fossa. In our specimens we often found the same relationships as those described by Hardy.[48]

Hardy also states that numerous colloid follicles and venous capillaries can be seen within the intermediate lobe, and that surgically they delineate the boundary between the anterior and posterior lobes. When the sphenoid sinus is of the sellar type, the periosteal layer of the dura will come into view after a thin layer of bone has been removed as dissection proceeds from the sphenoid sinus outward. The inferior cavernous sinuses are incorporated into this periosteal layer. Last comes a potential cleft and the pituitary gland capsule, the inner surface of which is attached to the pituitary gland.

Inferior Hypophyseal Artery and Capsular Artery: The inferior hypophyseal artery usually gives off small branches that run in the potential cleft between the pituitary gland capsule and the periosteal layer. Twigs from this vessel may extend in a retrograde direction to the pituitary gland, while others pierce the floor of the sphenoid bone and the mucoperiosteum of the sphenoid sinus.

Upper Nasal Cavity and Ethmoid Sinuses

The roof of the nasal cavity is very small, and is formed by the cribriform plate of the ethmoid bone. We estimated its width in our specimens to be 2 to 3 mm on each side. The length of the cribrose lamina of the ethmoid bone is larger than it appears when viewed intracranially, and in the anterior area of the roof the superior anterior nasal spine of the frontal bone may be seen. This bone supports the nasal bones, and is variable in length.

The anterior part of the sphenoid bone is situated on the posterior end of the roof, and is composed of the sphenoid concha. The aperture of the sphenoid sinus is located in this area. The olfactory nerve fiber bundles to the olfactory bulb, the anterior and posterior ethmoid nerves and vessels to the nasal cavity, and (at least in newborns) the vomeronasal nerve and the terminal nerve to the anterior cranial fossa and the area of the olfactory trigone all pass through the cribrose lamina.

Ethmoid Sinuses

In the anatomical terminology of 1977, the ethmoid labyrinth has been accepted as being composed of the ethmoid cells; the orbital lamina; the ethmoid foramina; the conchae nasalis suprema, superior, and media; the bulla ethmoidalis; the uncinate process; the infundibulum ethmoidale; and the hiatus semilunaris. The sinus ethmoidalis or cellulae ethmoidales are divided into anterior, middle, and posterior ethmoid cells, and the ethmoid bulla.[3] *Anterior ethmoid cells* have their ostia in the middle nasal meatus or its extensions (the infundibula and ducts). The ethmoid cells that develop from the superior nasal meatus are called *posterior ethmoid cells*, while cells that open into the meatus nasi supremus are called *postrem ethmoid cells*. There are many variations in the development of these cells, which are not confined to the edge of the ethmoid bone. The ethmoid labyrinth can be likened to a pyramid oriented horizontally, its base being the transition area between the ethmoid and sphenoid and its apex pointing rostrally. This pyramid is small in the area of the infundibulum (8 mm), and wide in the area of the bulla ethmoidalis, especially dorsally (15 mm) (see Figs. 17 and 18).

The anterior ethmoid cells occupy as a rule the whole width of the labyrinth, while the posterior cells are arranged in three layers. Rarely, the anterior and posterior labyrinth are each composed of a single cell.[51] However, this researcher found some labyrinths to have three cells, two of them in the anterior and one in the posterior part of the labyrinth. In a study of 100 heads, Van Alyea[3] found an average of nine (range 4 to 17) ethmoid cells. We found three ethmoid cells normally projecting from the superior nasal meatus, one directed superiorly, one superoposteriorly, and the third projecting into the

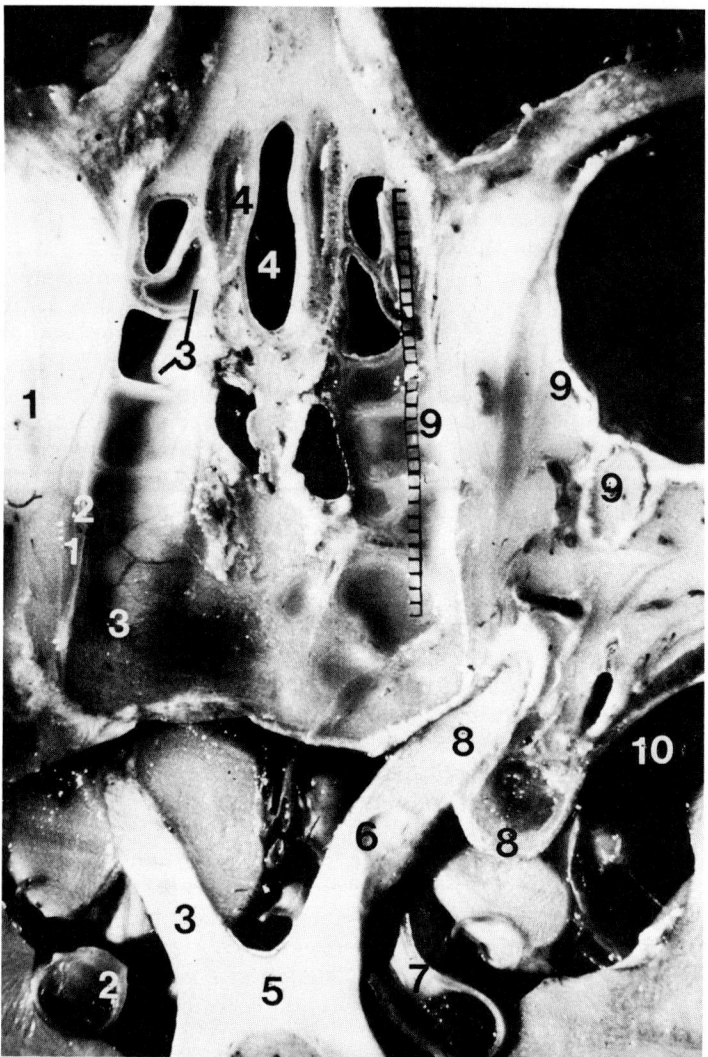

Figure 17: Roof of ethmoid labyrinth, viewed from below. 1. Medial rectus and superior oblique muscles. 2. Lamina papyracea and internal carotid artery. 3. Superior labyrinthine cells and right optic nerve. 4. Roof of nasal cavity and pneumatized crista galli. 5. Optic chiasm. 6. Left optic nerve, compressed by internal carotid artery (subdural hematoma). 7. Anterior cerebral artery (A1 segment). 8. Optic nerve, optic canal, and anterior clinoid process. 9. Millimeter scale, sclera, and optic nerve. 10. Subdural hematoma.

bulla. When a supreme nasal meatus was present (as was the case in one-third of our specimens), the cells developed dorsally and superiorly in 75% of cases.

Frontal Sinus, Ostium (Figs. 19 and 20): Hayek[51] defined the ostium frontale as the transition area between the frontal and ethmoid bones. The infundibulum enlarges to form a nasofrontal duct, which extends to the frontal ostium. The width of the infundibulum is very variable, and depends on the width of the hiatus semilunaris and neighboring ethmoid cells. A nasofrontal duct is formed when the infundibulum narrows anteriorly and superiorly to form a channel a few millimeters long between the frontal ostium and the frontal sinus. The medial wall of

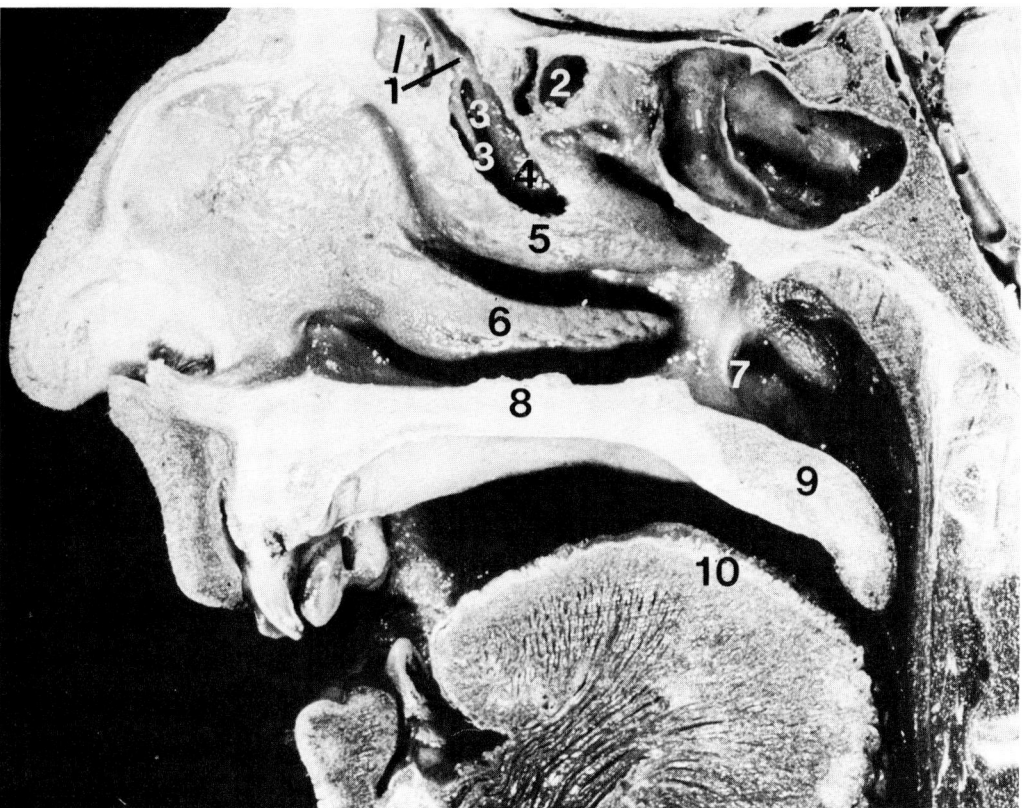

Figure 18: Nasofrontal duct and bulla frontalis (frontal cells) viewed medially. A portion of the middle concha and medial walls of the ethmoid cells have been removed. 1. Bulla frontalis (frontal cell and nasofrontal duct). 2. Superior ethmoid cell. 3. Hiatus semilunaris and uncinate process. 4. Bulla ethmoidalis. 5. Middle nasal concha. 6. Inferior nasal concha. 7. Anterior border of the pharyngeal ostium of the auditory tube. 8. Hard palate. 9. Soft palate. 10. Tongue.

the nasofrontal duct is part of the middle nasal concha, which is fixed on the agger nasi area. If ethmoid cells have developed in this area, then they border the nasofrontal duct.

When Hayek found ethmoid cells in the frontal recess, he called them cellulae recessus frontales. As a rule, he identified three to four anterior and medial recessus cells, with one contacting the frontal sinus.

Agger Cells (Fig. 21): Van Alyea[4] found one infundibular cell developed in the agger nasi in 90% of cases. When two such cells were present one of them was sometimes situated between the agger and the medial wall of the fossa lacrimalis. If one of these cells was identified in the area of the lacrimal bone it would have been called a cellula lacrimalis by earlier investigators. Ethmoid cells have been found surrounding the nasofrontal duct medially and anteriorly, and extending to the frontal process of the maxilla.

Suprainfundibular Ethmoid Cells: The upper recess of the middle nasal meatus is located superior to the transition area between the ethmoid bulla and the uncinate process. Van Alyea[3] found suprainfundibular cells with ostia in this area in 53% of the specimens he studied, and suprabullar cells in 46%.

Apex Cells: In 74% of the specimens he studied, Van Alyea[3] found only one cell, an apex cell, in the infundibulum ethmoidale. In 34% of cases agger cells also opened into this cell.

The landmarks for surgical ap-

484 • TUMORS OF THE CRANIAL BASE: DIAGNOSIS AND TREATMENT

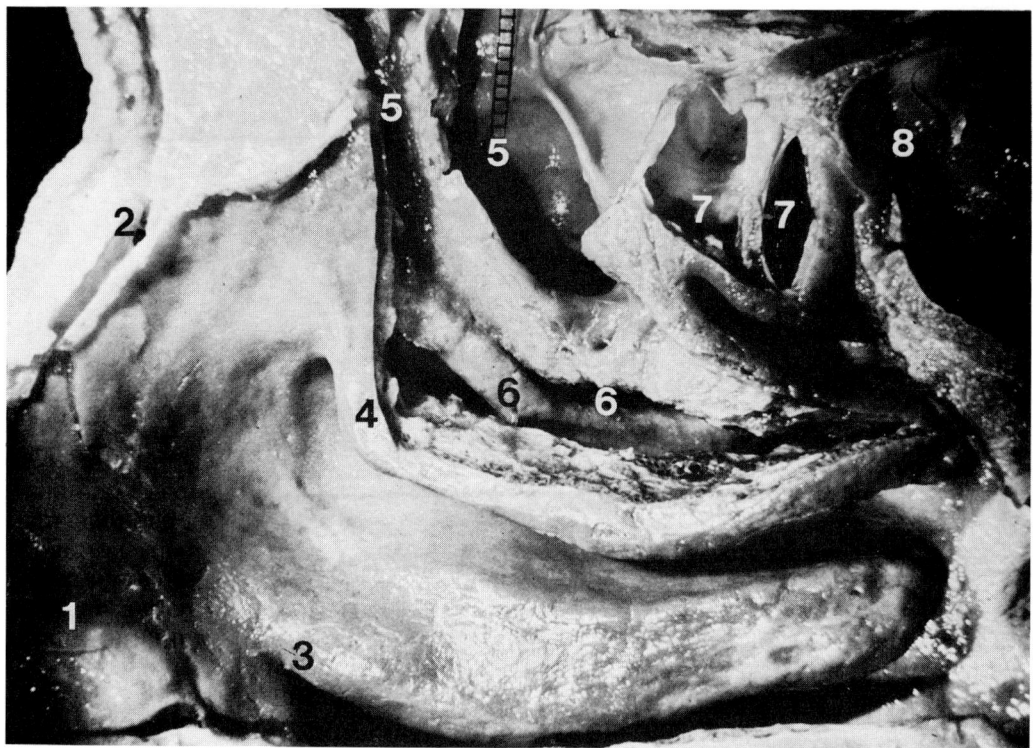

Figure 19: Large bulla ethmoidalis situated immediately posterior to the nasofrontal duct. 1. Vestibulum nasi. 2. Os nasale. 3. Inferior nasal concha. 4. Middle nasal concha (dorsal portion removed). 5. Large ethmoid bulla immediately posterior to nasofrontal duct; millimeter scale. 6. Uncinate process and hiatus semilunaris. 7. Posterior superior ethmoid cells. 8. Sphenoid sinus.

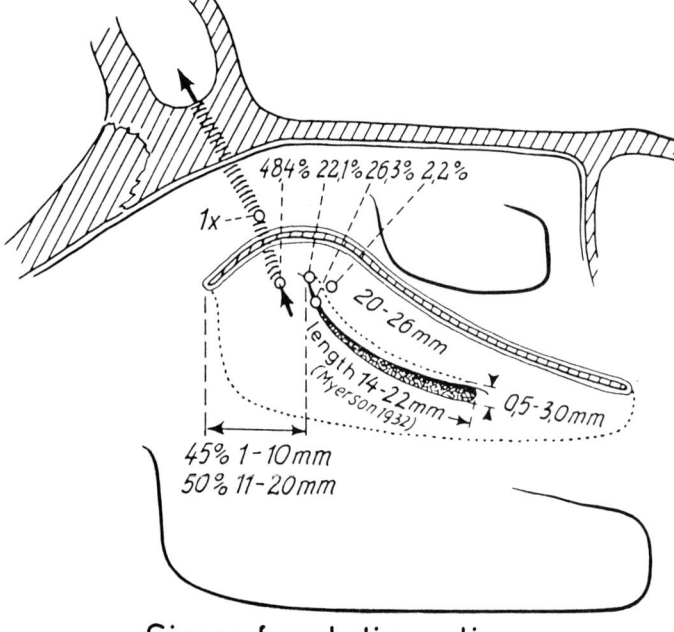

Figure 20: Frontal sinus, showing location of nasofrontal duct (infundibulum). Length and width of the hiatus semilunaris, and distances from the anterior border of the middle nasal concha are shown. In one case the ostium was above the middle concha.

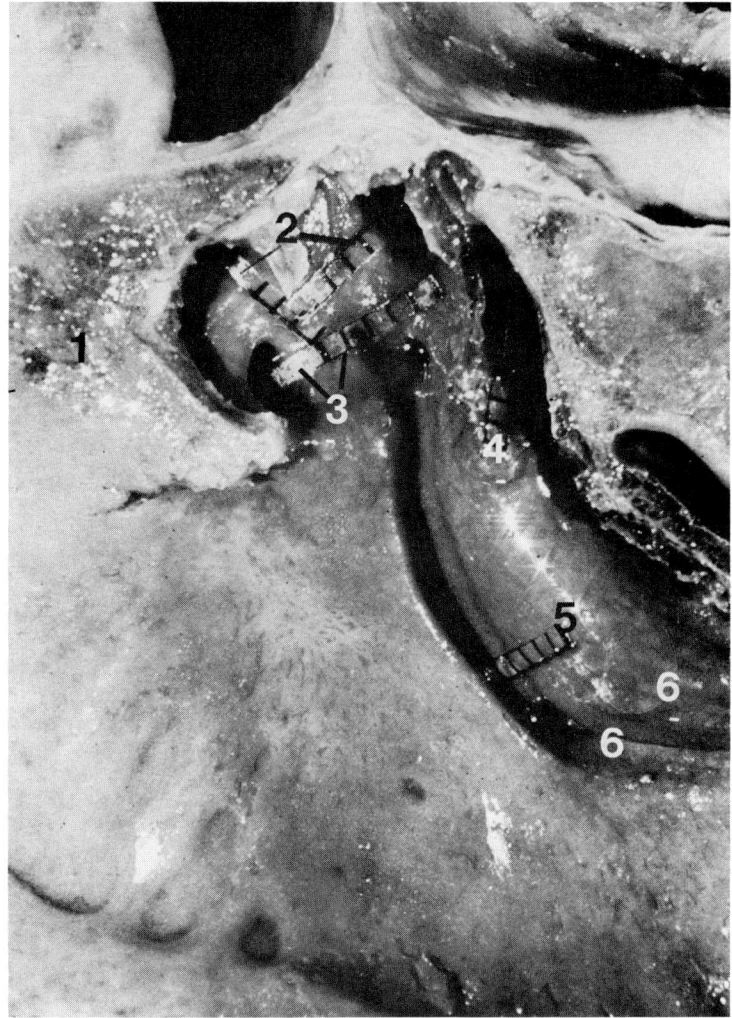

Figure 21: Ducts in the area of the hiatus semilunaris, and millimeter scale showing distance to paranasal sinuses. 1. Agger nasi on anterior border of middle concha (removed). 2. Dimensions of frontal bulla and frontal sinus. 3. Dimensions of infundibular cell. 4. Dimensions of anterior ethmoid cell. 5. Dimensions of maxillary sinus. 6. Processus uncinatus and hiatus semilunaris.

proaches to the ethmoid labyrinth are indicated in Figure 22.

Supraorbital cells were found by Van Alyea in 15% of the specimens he studied.[78]

Ethmoid cells that had developed in the area of the orbital floor were identified by Van Alyea[3] in 11% of the specimens he studied, and sometimes more than four cells had developed in this inferolateral direction. We also found the orbital plate of the vertical lamina of the palatine bone to be pneumatized, while Hayek[51] noted that this area may also be pneumatized by extension of maxillary sinus cells.

We found the maxillary sinuses to be completely divided in some cases.[87] In one specimen (from a 49-year-old woman), the posterosuperior part of this sinus was noted to open superior to the middle nasal concha, leading us to believe that it belonged to the posteroinferior ethmoid cell. In other cases the opening was behind the ethmoid bulla in the mid-

Conchae nasales, ant. borders to a vertical line on the subspinal point (in mm)

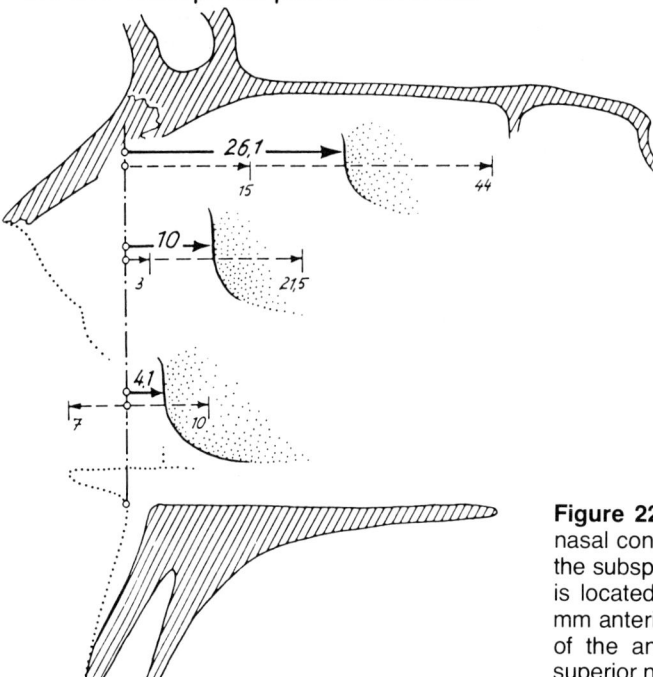

Figure 22: Distance from anterior border of nasal concha to a vertical line drawn through the subspinal point. The inferior nasal concha is located 4.1 mm behind this line (range 7 mm anterior to 10 mm posterior). Dimensions of the anterior borders of the middle and superior nasal conchae are also shown in millimeters.[90]

dle nasal meatus. In one case a hole was found in the wall between the two maxillary sinuses, perhaps the result of further pneumatization and resorption of part of the wall.

Middle Nasal Concha, Fixation (Figs. 23 and 24)

Onishi[113] stated that injury to the cranial base had occurred in 0.15% of 450,000 endonasal sinusectomies, and acute meningitis in 0.1%. Therefore, it is important for the surgeon to know how the middle nasal concha is fixed to the cranial base and the medial wall of the orbit. According to Seydel[127] and others, it is the medial ends of the lamellae of the ethmoid labyrinth that fix the nasal conchae, by reaching through the labyrinth laterally and extending superiorly to the lamina orbitalis and beyond to the lamina cribrosa of the ethmoid bone. In adults, four or five such lamellae are present.

Ground Lamellae (Turbinates): The most inferior, and an incomplete, turbinate, is formed by the uncinate process. Superior to this turbinate, the lateral extension of the bulla ethmoidalis reaches to the lamina orbitalis laterally and superiorly to the lamina cribrosa. This lamella forms the border between the nasal part (nasofrontal duct) of the frontal sinus and the ethmoid labyrinth.

The third turbinate (moving from inferior to superior) fixes the area of the middle nasal concha, and extends laterally to the lamina orbitalis of the ethmoid bone and superiorly to the lamina cribrosa. This turbinate and the turbinate of the ethmoid bulla enclose the anterior ethmoid labyrinth. The fourth turbinate extends laterally from the area of fixation of the superior nasal concha. The fifth turbinate, when present, fixes the area of the supreme nasal concha. Because the air cells between the superior and most superior conchae open into the superior nasal meatus, they are considered part of the posterior labyrinthine cells.

The *roofs of the superior ethmoid*

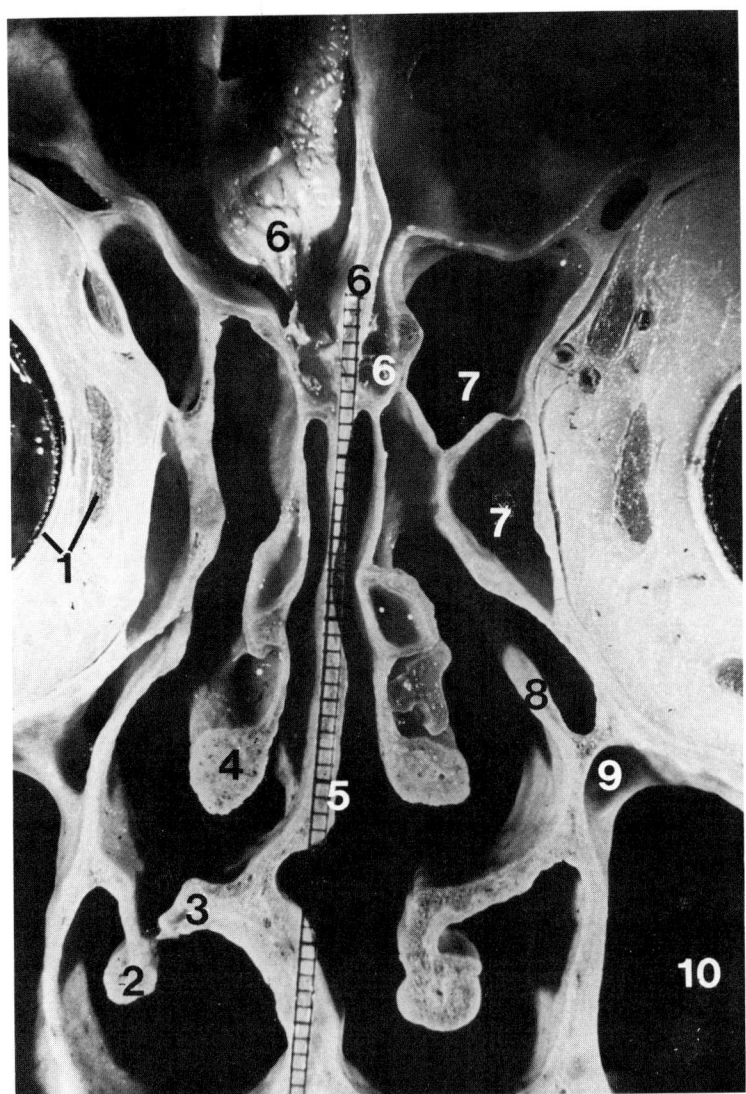

Figure 23: Coronal section through nasal cavity and surrounding structures at the level of the lamina cribrosa. 1. Sclera and medial rectus muscle. 2. Inferior nasal concha. 3. Deviation of nasal septum. 4. Middle nasal concha reaches to lateral border of the lamina cribrosa in this area. 5. Millimeter scale showing dimensions of nasal septum and crista galli. 6. Bulbus olfactorius, crista galli, and lamina cribrosa. 7. Anterior ethmoid cell and bulla ethmoidalis. 8. Processus uncinatus. 9. Infundibulum of maxillary sinus. 10. Maxillary sinus.

cells are composed in most cases of thin portions of the frontal bone, and in many cases bony dehiscences were found, and the mucoperiosteal layer of the ethmoid cells were in contact with the dura mater of the anterior cranial fossa. According to Onishi,[113] such rarefactions are identifiable in 38% of specimens, and dehiscences or defects in the bone are present in 14% of specimens in the area of the olfactory groove. If the middle nasal concha is injured or removed the olfactory fiber bundles may be avulsed and rhinorrhea may occur.

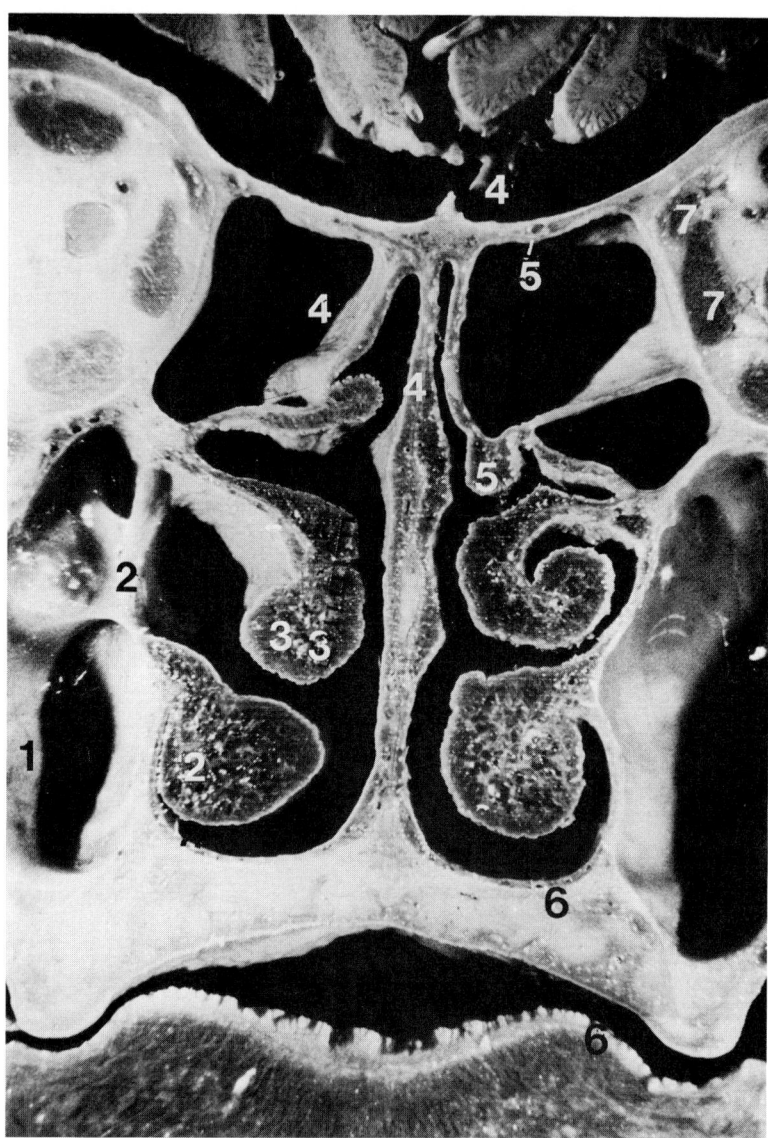

Figure 24: Coronal section through nasal cavity and surrounding structures (viewed from anteriorly) at the level of the planum sphenoidale. 1. Maxillary sinus, posterior wall. 2. Accessory aperture of maxillary sinus and inferior nasal concha. 3. Middle nasal concha dimensions (in millimeters) with continuous medial wall of orbit and planum sphenoidale. 4. Superior posterior ethmoid cell, septum nasi, and tractus olfactorius. 5. Superior nasal concha and planum sphenoidale. 6. Hard palate and tongue. 7. Superior oblique nerve and medial rectus muscle.

Superoposterior Ethmoid Cells and Sphenoid Sinus Area (Fig. 25)

The anterior wall of the sphenoid sinus is bounded by the sphenoid concha (concha sphenoidalis, ossicula Bertini), which begins to develop in the fifth month of fetal life. In addition to the ossicles of Bertin, the conchae are composed of foci of membranous bone that form in the inferior wall of the developing sphenoid sinus around the tenth month of fetal life. At birth, each concha consists of a triangular bony plate, positioned

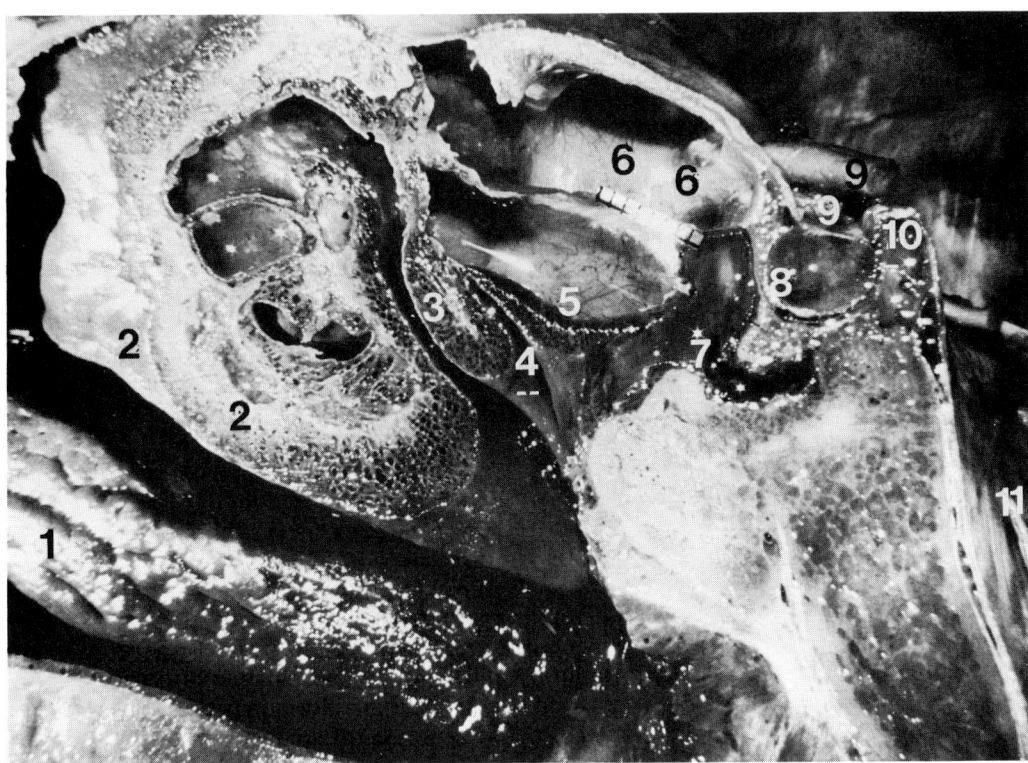

Figure 25: Posterior ethmoid cell, extending to the tuberculum sellae, viewed medially (paramedian section). 1. Inferior nasal concha. 2. Middle nasal concha, partly dissected. 3. Superior nasal concha, cut. 4. Sphenoethmoid recess. 5. Posterior inferior ethmoid cell. 6. Posterior superior ethmoid cell and medial wall of optic canal. 7. Extremely small sphenoid sinus. 8. Anterior lobe of hypophysis. 9. Optic nerve and inferior carotid artery, cut. 10. Dorsum sellae. 11. Abducens nerve.

roughly sagittally and adjacent to the primary sphenoid rostrum on each side. The inferior margins of the conchae extend to the superior margin of the vomer. During the first year of postnatal life, the conchae continue to grow, increasing chiefly in height and to a lesser extent in width.

Between the fourth and ninth years of life, the sphenoid sinus increases in width, and the conchal region covers it medially and anteriorly. During this time the bony ostium of the sphenoid sinus, the superolateral margin of which is derived from the ethmoid bone, migrates laterally. According to Toldt,[136] the sphenoid concha fuses with the body of the sphenoid between the ninth and twelfth years. If the concha remains small, the most posterior and superior ethmoid cells grow further dorsally to form the medial wall of the optic channel, or come to underlie the floor of the pituitary fossa. This was found to be the case in approximately 10% of the specimens we examined.

Chorda Dorsalis and Skull Base Development (Fig. 26)

Notochord

The development and remnants of the notochord are discussed in Chapter 25.

Foramen Magnum

The foramen magnum is discussed in detail in Chapter 25.

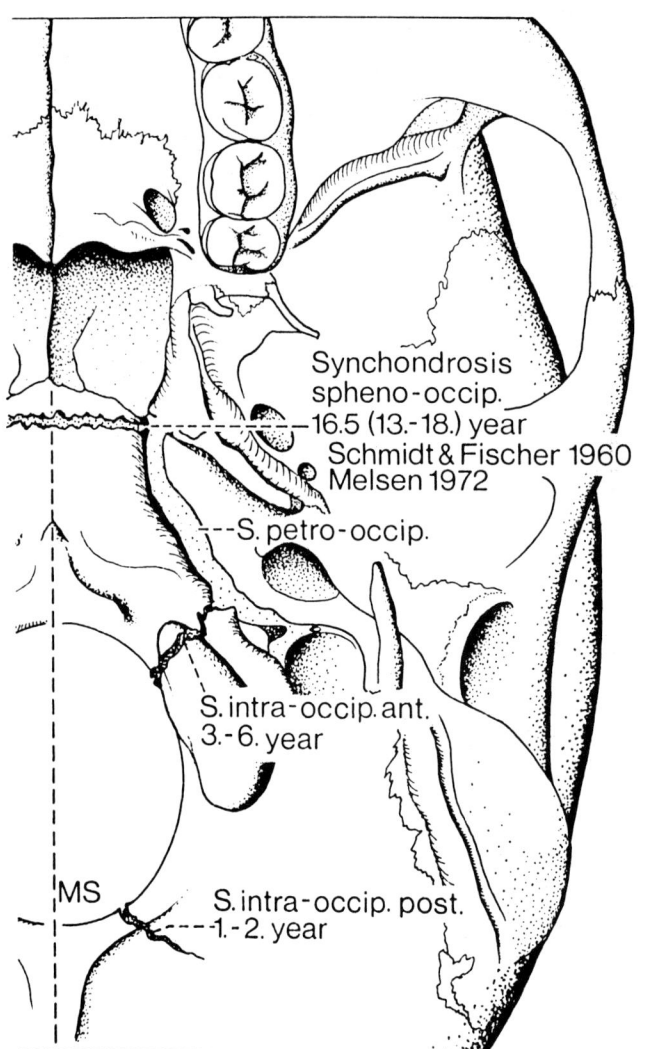

Figure 26: Skull base from below, showing most important synchondroses and time of ossification in normal individuals.

Third Condyle (Fig. 27)

Sometimes a cartilage-covered process, called a third condyle, is present near the basion.[78] This structure may result from failure of the hypochordal arch to degenerate, or perhaps it is a remnant of the proatlas. Toro and Szepe[137] found that in such cases the atlas often becomes part of the occiput. Kamieth[65,66] found that one part of the bone extended from the clivus inferiorly to articulate with the anterior arch of the atlas and apex of the dens. He also had the feeling that this was a manifestation of an occipital vertebral rudiment.

Ossicles other than the basion and the dens of the axis are known as Bergmann's ossicles, and in our specimens we found not only articulations between a third condyle and the apex of the dens axis (Bergmann's ossicles), but also particles of unattached bone below the anterior arch of the atlas.[78]

Occipitalization of the Atlas

The atlas was found to be occipitalized in 0.1 to 0.8% of cases (Figs. 28, 29). When the atlas was completely joined with the occiput, there was no atlanto-

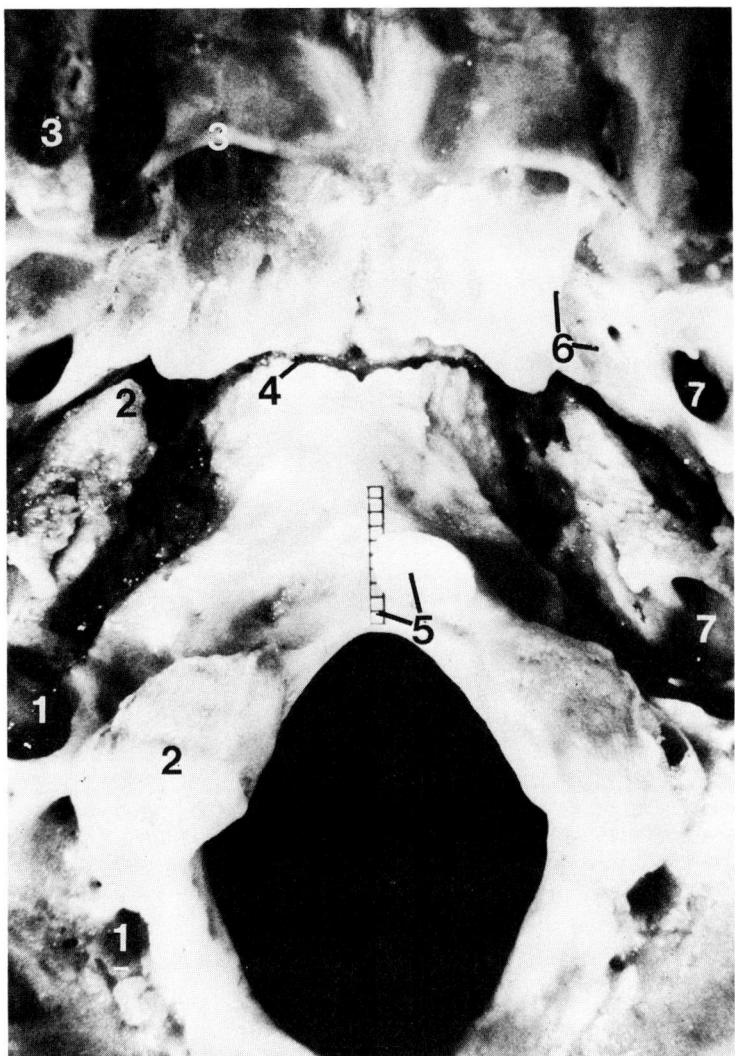

Figure 27: Third condyle, disarticulated from spheno-occipital synchondroses, from skull of an elderly individual; note variations. 1. Jugular foramen and inferior opening of condylar emissary canal. 2. Apex of petrous part and occipital condyles. 3. Alveolar process of maxilla and palatine bone. 4. Spheno-occipital synchondrosis. 5. Third condyle and millimeter scale. 6. Lamina medialis of pterygoid process and scaphoid fossa. 7. Foramen ovale and carotid canal.

occipital joint. Occipitalization was often noted to occur asymmetrically, and in such cases there was sometimes torticollis of bony origin.[78,142]

Jugular Foramen

The jugular foramen, an important point of exit from and entry to the posterior cranial fossa, most often presents in the shape of a long, sharply pointed triangle in the inner skull base. The apex of the triangle points anteriorly and medially, and the posteromedial side is formed by the pars lateralis of the occipital bone, while the anterior side is formed by the petrous part of the temporal bone. The shape of the petrous part of the bone in the jugular foramen is variable, and in some

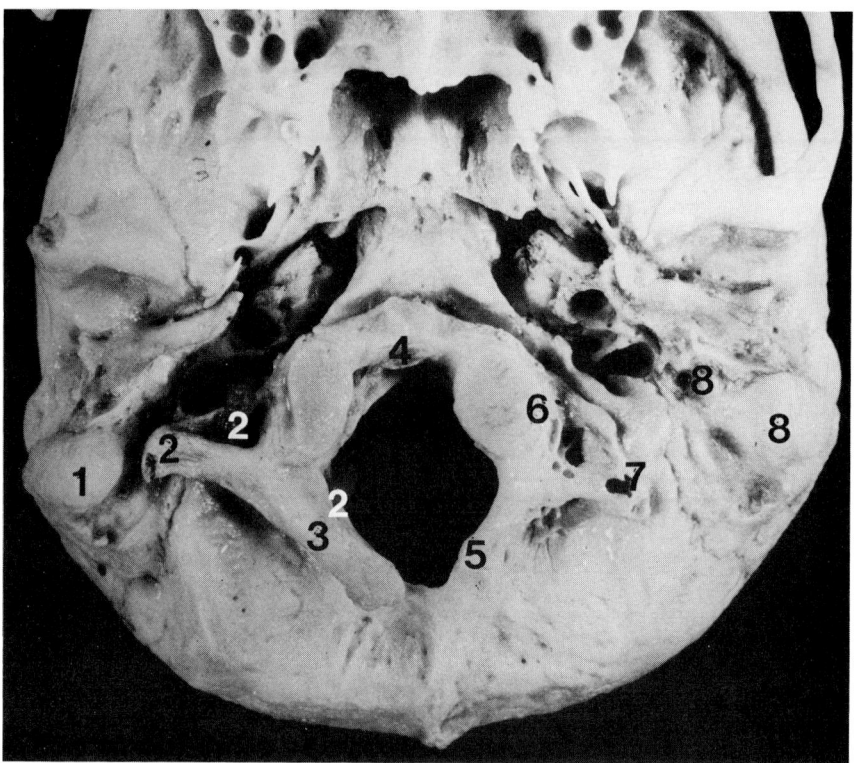

Figure 28: Assimilation of the atlas, showing asymmetry (viewed from below). 1. Mastoid process. 2. Massa lateralis atlantis and vertebral artery, course. 3. Dorsal arch of atlas with disarticulated occiput. 4. Facies articularis dentis. 5. Dorsal arch of atlas united with occipital bone. 6. Facies articularis inferior atlantis. 7. Area of massa lateralis, united with occipital bone. 8. Stylomastoid foramen and mastoid process.

specimens an intrajugular process is present; such a process is present in some bones on the occipital border as well. At the point where the sigmoid sinus enters the jugular foramen there is commonly a bony ridge, oriented from anterolateral to posteromedial, which we term the margo sigmoidea terminalis. The medial border of the jugular foramen in most specimens has a hooklike bony spur of the occipital bone located either inside or outside the skull base. Figure 4 of Chapter 25 presents our results of measuring postnatal lateral shifting of the medial border of the foramen and enlargement of the jugular foramen.[91]

Cranial nerves IX, X, and XI run in a connective tissue plate to the outer skull base. In 50% of specimens studied, this connective tissue plate contained one posterior meningeal artery, in 37.5% it contained two such branches, and in 10.5%, three smaller branches arising from the ascending pharyngeal artery were seen to travel in this tissue plate.[82]

Figure 9 shows the relative positions of the inferior petrosal sinus, cranial nerves IX, X, and XI, and the bulb of the internal jugular vein in specimens with bony spurs of the petrous portion and the occipital bone. It should be noted that the bony bridges varied, thus leading to differences in compartmentalization of the inferior petrosal sinus (ISP) and ninth cranial nerve (indicated in black on this figure).[146] In most cases (48%), the inferior petrosal sinus pierced the connective tissue/nervous tissue septum between the ninth and tenth cranial nerves, in 30% the inferior petrosal sinus extended to the

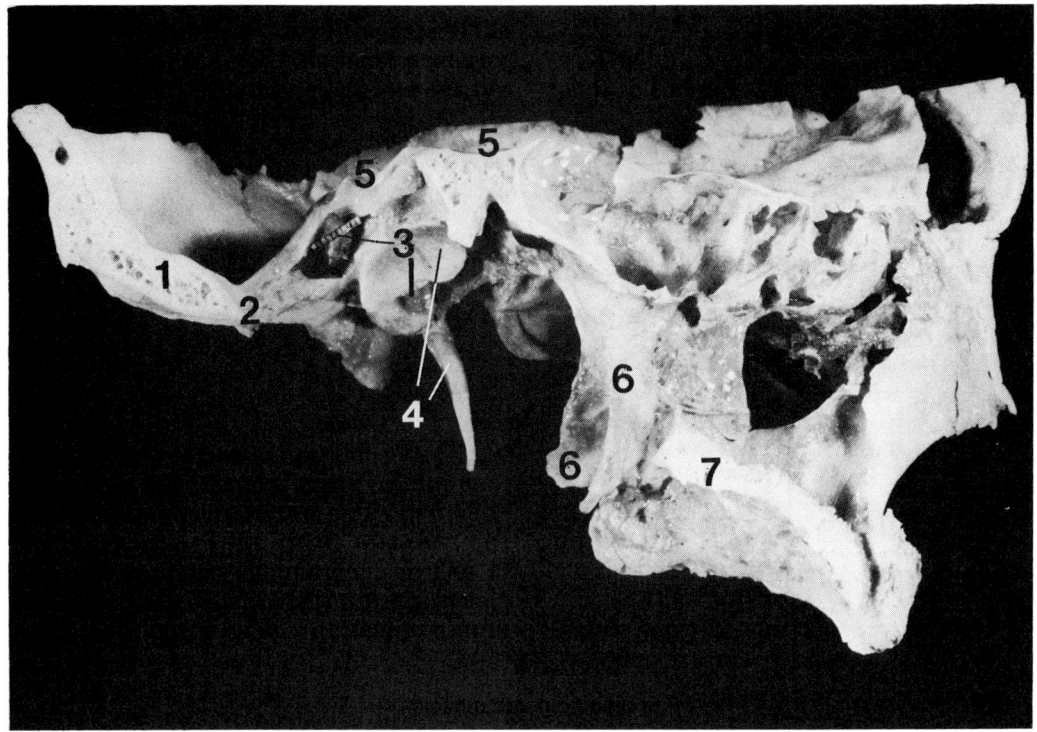

Figure 29: Basilar impression combined with atlas assimilation (left skull half, viewed from the right). 1. Internal occipital crest. 2. Opisthion. 3. Course of vertebral artery. 4. Inferior articulation of atlas and styloid process. 5. Clivus and basilar impression. 6. Pterygoid process. 7. Palatum durum.

jugular foramen anterior to the ninth cranial nerve, in 16% of specimens the sinus was posterior to the ninth cranial nerve, and in 6% the sinus was located between the tenth and eleventh cranial nerves. It is not uncommon for the sinus to have two openings within the connective tissue septum, or for the orifice to be located at the level of the jugular bulb, the level of the jugular foramen, or inferior to the skull base (for further details see Lang[78]).

We measured the foramen jugulare and the jugular fossa on the outer skull base in our specimens.[94] Figure 31 shows the results of these measurements on 178 foramina. Figure 15 shows how many of the foramina were divided or partly divided in adults and children, and Figure 16 demonstrates the most commonly seen shapes in undivided foramina. Under very rare conditions (in only one of our specimens) the foramen jugulare may be very narrow, allowing passage of only the inferior petrosal sinus.

Hypoglossal Channel (Fig. 30)

Figure 9 shows postnatal shifts in the position of the internal pore of the hypoglossal channel and its length, its intra- and extracranial widths, its volume, and its angle to the midsagittal plane. In about 39% of our specimens we found bony spurs on the superior border of the opening, which partly divided the intracranial pore. On the right side the intracranial pore was totally divided in about 15% of our specimens; this was true on the left in 27% of 142 channels examined.[125] In all cases we noted that the channels joined inside the cranium, although sometimes the channel was found divided in its middle portion.

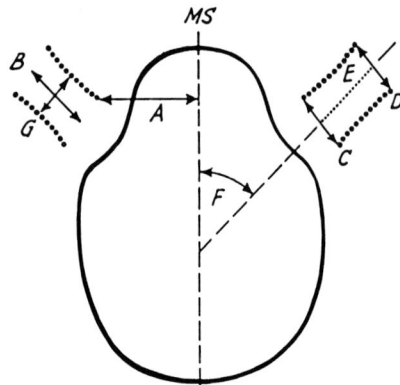

Hypoglossal canal		A Distance to MS (mm)	B Length (mm)	C Intra-cranial width (mm)	D Extra-cranial width (mm)	E Volume (mm³)	F Angle with MS (°)
Neonate	right	7.1	4.9	3.4	3.1	34.0	33.2
	left	7.0	4.9	3.6	3.1	41.3	35.0
ca 3 years	right	11.4	6.6	4.3	4.6	137.8	42.1
	left	12.0	6.6	4.4	4.7	146.4	42.4
9–11 years	right	11.8	7.6	5.0	5.4	198.0	41.6
	left	12.3	7.3	4.9	5.4	198.5	42.8
Adult	right	12.0	8.8	Width 5.7/4.1 Height (center) 5.6/4.1 (center)		216.1	45.6
	left	12.0	8.6			213.1	44.6

Figure 30: Postnatal development of the hypoglossal canal. MS = midsagittal plane.

Clivus and Related Structures

The clivus and related structures are shown in Figure 20 of Chapter 25, while Figure 27 of this chapter shows the synchondroses on the outer skull base and the time of their closure. For approaches to the clivus (and through the clivus) in the posterior fossa it is important to know the paramedian distances between different portals of the nerves and vessels in the outer skull base. Figure 6 shows measurements of distances between the two carotid channels and the jugular foramina.

Occipital Condyles

The long axis of the occipital condyles is oriented anteromedially, at a mean angle to the midsagittal plane in neonates of 35.5° and about 28° in adults.[58] The medial side of the condyle is inferior to the lateral side, and the angle of the occipital condyles to the horizontal plane has been measured to be 124° in men and 127° in women.[69] In addition, the anteroposterior length of the articular surface of the condyles is greater on the medial side than on the lateral side. The ratio between the length of each condyle and its width is about 2 to 1.

Each condyle has two convexities, along an axis directed from posteromedial to anterolateral. The anterior convexity is more pronounced, and has a radius of about 13 mm, while the shallower posterior convexity has a radius of about 21 mm.[69] In our specimens the transverse axis of rotation of the major part of the articular surfaces of the condyles was

20.53 mm (range 11.0–27.0 mm) posterior to the basion and 9.57 mm (range 6.4–13.3 mm) inferior to the Frankfort horizontal plane (Fig. 31).[35]

Many variations may be noted in the portion of bone covered by the cartilage of the *condylar surface*. Anteriorly, the articular area extends almost to the anterior margin of the hypoglossal channel, while laterally it slopes toward the condylar channel or groove. Posteriorly the articular area tapers off to the condylar fossa near the condylar channel, with individual variations being particularly pronounced in this area, where arthritic changes especially may be noted. The alar ligament of the dens attaches to the medial side of the condyle, in an area that is rough and, of course, larger in proportion to the acuity of the frontal-condylar angle.

Inferior Condylar Channel

On the inferior surface of the skull, between the opening of the hypoglossal channel and the area lateral to the occipital condyle, a bony groove is usually present. Henle[53] noted that this groove may be converted into a partially or wholly enclosed channel for a blood vessel when covered by a lamella of bone that may curve over the jugular foramen. We identified this channel in 66.5% of the 173 half heads we examined, and in 4.7% it passed directly into the exterior opening of the hypoglossal channel, while in 28.7% it ended in the immediate vicinity of this channel.

Outer Skull Base, Rare Variations

In some of our specimens we found very unusually oriented occipital condyles (see Fig. 328 in Lang[78]). Processus paracondylares may be found lateral to an occipital condyle, and posterior and medial to the stylomastoid foramen. Such prominences vary greatly in height, and may articulate with the massa lateralis atlantis.[102,105,135] A *condylus tertius* (Fig. 30) has been noted in 0.1 to 1 percent of specimens by different authors. On one of 600 skulls he examined, Hyrtl[57] found a process the size and shape of a hazelnut on the origin of the lateral rectus capitis muscle. Such a processus pneumaticus was found in one of our specimens as well.

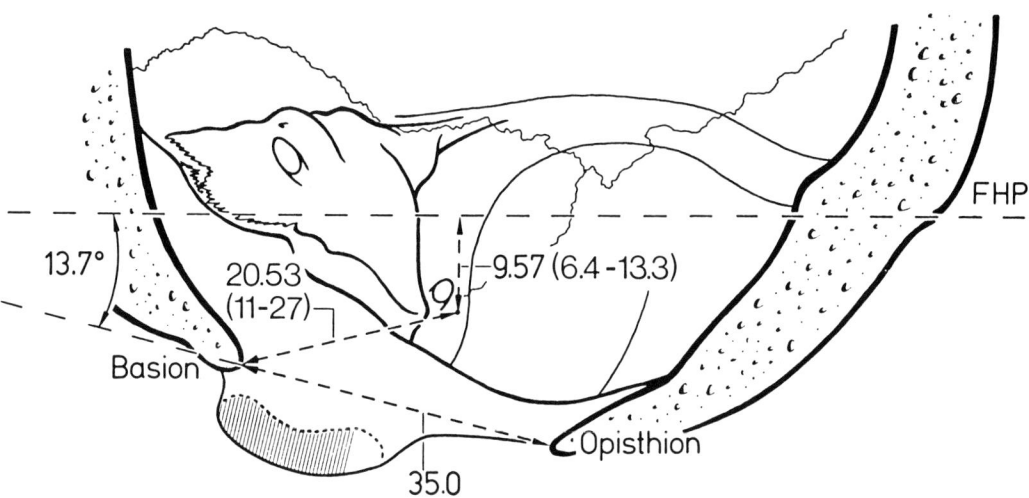

Figure 31: Rotation axis of atlanto-occipital joint. Both condylar surfaces together form a portion of an ellipse, the axis of the rotation of which was estimated to be 20.53 mm behind the basion and 9.57 mm below the Frankfort horizontal plane. Also shown are our measurements of the angle between the long axis of the foramen magnum and the Frankfort horizontal plane (13.7°) and the mean length of the foramen magnum.

A *transverse basilar fissure*, or fissure in the base of the skull at the level of the pharyngeal tubercle or slightly behind the jugular foramen, has very rarely been observed. It is thought to represent the anterior limit of the ante proatlas, and in most cases is present unilaterally.[124]

Processus Paraoccipitalis: Grunbaum[40] described a processus paraoccipitalis medial to the mastoid process (and medial to the grooves for the digastric muscle and the occipital artery). In our specimens such prominences were located in most skulls behind the lateral portion of the foramen jugulare and medial to the stylomastoid foramen. These prominences are part of the occipital bone, and vary in shape. Connective tissue may extend from these processes to the neighborhood of the outer opening of the condylar channel.

Basial Process: Small, thin, medioventrally oriented tubercles were found on the anterior portions of some occipital condyles.[13,18]

Atlas (Figs. 32, 35)

The anterior turbercle lies on the ventral aspect of the anterior arch of the atlas, while the posterior surface of the anterior arch is covered with cartilage and articulates with the dens of the axis. The larger posterior arch forms about two-fifths of the ring-shaped bone, which usually has a posterior tubercle on its dorsal surface. The anterior and posterior arches converge on the articular portions of the atlas and its lateral appendages. The fovea articularis superior is covered with cartilage, which articulates with the occipital condyle, while the long axes of the two ovoid or reniform superior articular facettes (which can be divided into anterior and posterior portions) converge an-

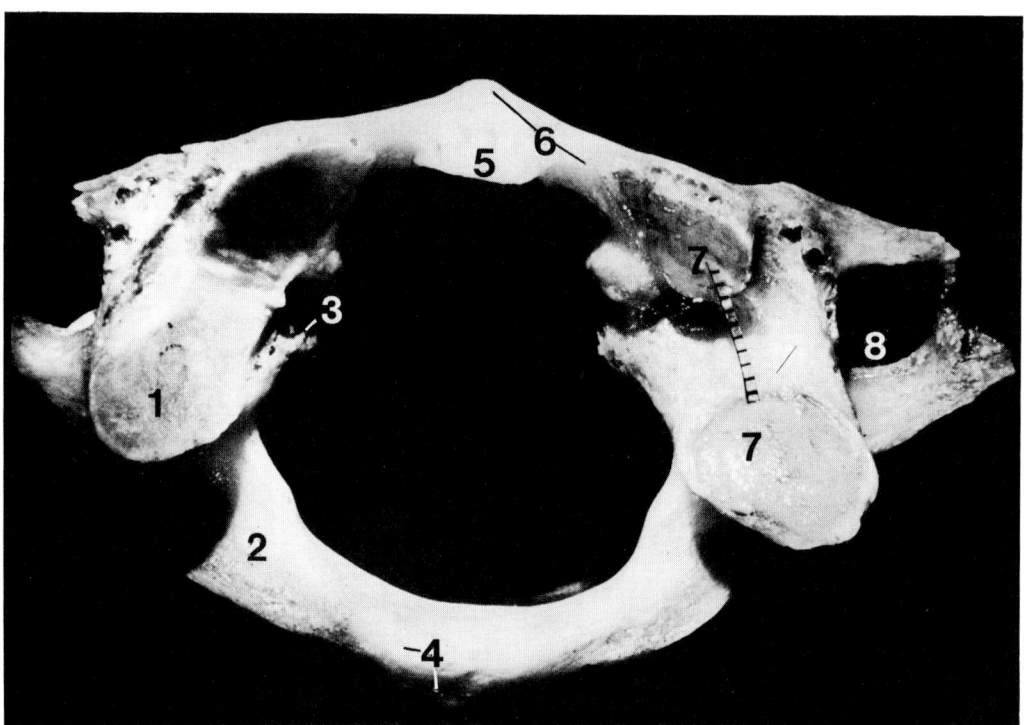

Figure 32: Atlas, viewed superior. 1. Superior articular surface, common development. 2. Sulcus for the vertebral artery. 3. Insertion of transverse ligament. 4. Posterior arch and tubercle. 5. Articulation with dens. 6. Ventral tubercle and arch. 7. Superior articular surface, divided into two parts; millimeter scale. 8. Foramen transversum.

terosuperiorly (as do the occipital condyles).

Immediately posterior to the fovea articularis superior a transverse groove for the vertebral artery may be found, along with the veins that accompany it and the first cervical nerve. This groove is usually somewhat overhung anteriorly by the lateral mass, and often there is a bony bridge over the course of the vertebral artery (in 7% of specimens bilaterally, and in 14% unilaterally). Much more frequently, however, incomplete bridges of anterior and posterior bony spurs (posterior and lateral ponticuli) are present.

Medial to the articular surface, a rough bony structure with nutrient foramina may be found, on which the transverse ligament of the atlas inserts. The greatest width of the atlas (in the area of the massae laterales atlantis) in specimens from European individuals was 83 mm (range 74-90 mm) in men and 72 mm (range 65-76 mm) in women.[29,49,139]

Between the fovea articularis superior and the massa lateralis atlantis, the foramen transversarium for the vertebral artery and its concomitant veins is located. Sometimes this foramen is open.[76,78] Most authorities state that the anterior border of the transverse foramen is a rudiment of a cervical rib and the posterior one a rudiment of the transverse process.

Atlanto-Occipital Joint (Figs. 31, 33, 34)

The principal movement at the atlanto-occipital joint is nodding, in which the head rotates transversely along an elliptical path, only parts of which are represented by actual anatomical structures, namely the cartilage-covered surfaces of the occipital condyles. Our studies show that the transverse axis of rotation (the long axis) of this articular component is located 20.93 mm (± 2.0 mm) below the Frankfort horizontal plane and 9.57 mm (± 1.6 mm) posterior to the basion.[35] Johnson et al.[60] measured the range of flexion and extension at the atlanto-occipital joint in young people and found it to be between 16.8° and 20.8°, while the range at the atlantoaxial joint was between 12.2° and 15.4°. During extension and forward flexion, the mean displacement of the anterior arch of the atlas in relation to the dens of the axis is 1.1 mm in men and 1.7 mm in women.[135] The possible range of extension exceeds that of flexion, because flexion is restricted by bony approximation of the atlas and occiput and by reflex innervation of antagonist muscles and ligaments. Forward flexion is also restricted by the ligamentum nuchae, the posterior longitudinal ligament, the tectorial membrane and the longitudinal band of the cruciform ligament of the atlas, the posterior atlanto-occipital membrane, and the dorsal muscles of the neck.

Tilting of the Atlas

Forward flexion of the neck first increases, and then in the second and third phases narrows[43] the space between the squama and the posterior arch of the atlas. The head and the atlas tilt forward on the axis during flexion, and follow exactly the reverse path during extension.

Lateral Flexion

Only slight lateral flexion is possible at the atlanto-occipital joint, and this movement is easiest during slight forward flexion. At this time the possible range is about 4° to either side, or 3° when forced rotation is performed simultaneously.

Rotation – Atlantoaxial Joint

The principal movement between the axis and the atlas (and the head) is rotation. Turning the head rotates the atlas and its transverse ligament about the dens of the axis like a wheel around its axle. The axis actually glides over the anterior and posterior articular surfaces of the dens. Movement between the lateral atlantoaxial joints occurs when the individual is looking straight ahead only when they are in their neutral positions, because these surfaces have transverse crests of

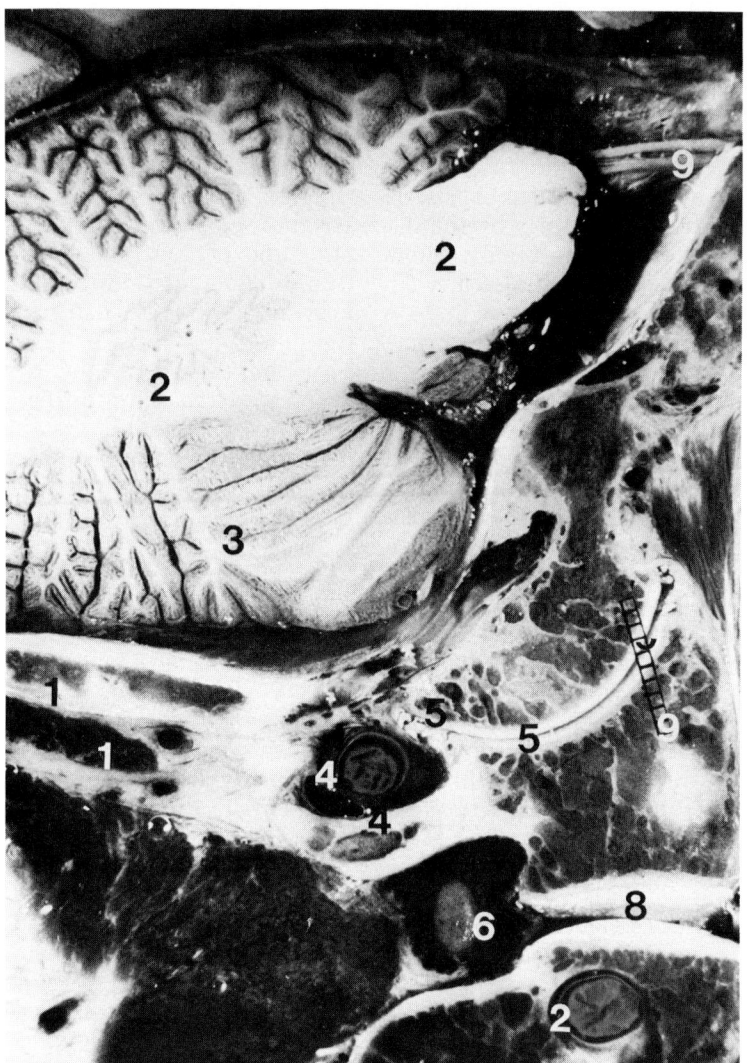

Figure 33: Craniocervical junction, seen in a nearly midsagittal section viewed medially. 1. Squama occipitalis and short muscles of the neck. 2. Nucleus dentatus and pedunculus cerebellaris medius. 3. Lobulus biventer. 4. Vertebral artery in sulcus arterius vertebralis atlantis. 5. Articulatio atlanto-occipitalis. 6. Greater occipital nerve. 7. Vertebral artery, coursing laterally and superiorly. 8. Atlanto-axial joint. 9. Trigeminal nerve and millimeter scale.

cartilage. The norm for rotation of the head from the midsagittal plane is considered to be about 35°. During this movement the head sinks approximately 2 mm downward.

Limitation of Rotation

Rotary movement of the head and atlas at the atlantoaxial articulation is limited in particular by the very strong alar ligaments that pass from the lateral surfaces of the dens to the medial sides of the occipital condyles. The origins of the ligaments lie slightly posterior to the axis of rotation, and during rotation they become taut as the distances between their origins and the attachments to the occiput increase, anteriorly on one side and posteriorly on the other. Rotation is also checked by the membrana tectoria, the posterior

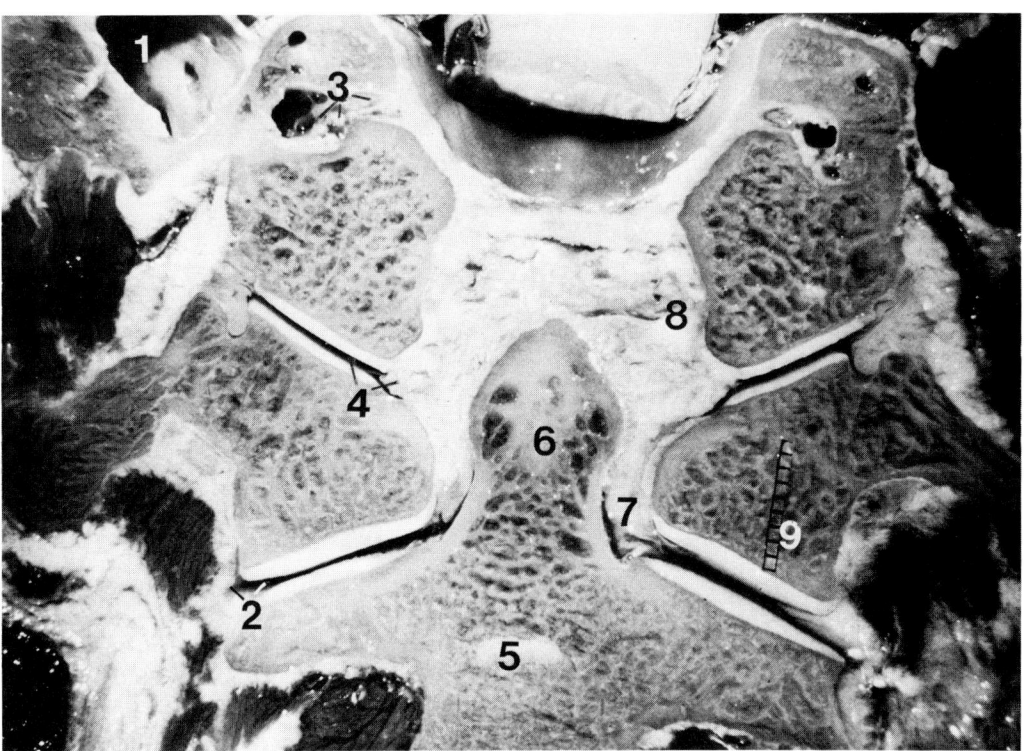

Figure 34: Coronal section through the craniocervical junction, seen from posterior. 1. Jugular foramen. 2. Articulation of atlantoaxialis lateralis; note capsule and synovial villi. 3. Hypoglossal canal and nerve. 4. Villus in atlanto-occipital joint. 5. Synchondrosis subdentalis. 6. Dens axis. 7. Transverse ligament. 8. Alar ligament. 9. Millimeter scale and atlas.

atlanto-occipital membrane, and the relatively thin articular capsules of the atlanto-occipital joints.

Flexion and Extension

The range of forward flexion and extension allowed by the atlantoaxial articulation is also small. During forward flexion, the dens of the axis moves superiorly, between the anterior arch of the atlas and the transverse ligament of the atlas. During extension it moves inferiorly between them.

Lateral Flexion of the Atlantoaxial Joints

Lateral flexion of about 5° to either side is possible at the atlantoaxial articulation, with further lateral flexion (up to 9.7°)[69] possible only in conjunction with rotation on the axis. Flexion to one side necessitates rotation toward the opposite side; thus tension on the two alar ligaments probably remains about the same during such a maneuver. The atlas is displaced posteriorly on the occipital condyle on the side toward which the head is inclined, so that the head rotates toward the opposite side and the distance between the condyles and the axis decreases. Rotation at the atlantoaxial articulation causes posterior and inferior displacement of the atlas: the skull comes nearer to the axis and the body becomes shorter. This prevents overstretching of the alar ligament on the opposite side.

Atlas, Viewed Inferiorly

Figure 35 shows our measurements of the inferior surface of the atlas, including the width of different portions of the ver-

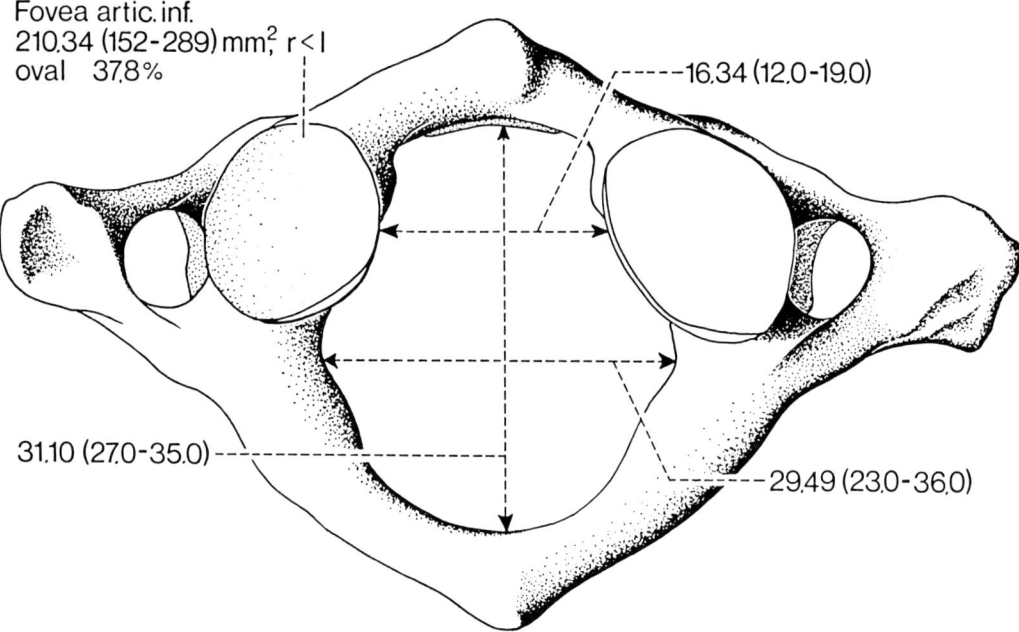

Figure 35: Atlas, seen from inferior. Dimensions of the foramen vertebrale, length of the foramen, and area of the fovea articularis inferior of the atlas are shown. In most cases, this fovea was oval. All measurements are in millimeters.

tebral channel. It is notable that in our specimens we found that the inferior articular surface of the atlas sometimes had cartilage on its medial circumference.

Axis

Our measurements of the superior surface of the axis and the diameters of the vertebral channel are shown in Figure 36, and the anterior surface of the axis is shown in Figure 37.

Helms[52] measured the angle between the axis of the dens and the lower surface of the dens roentgenographically, and found it to be between 42° and 88° (90° being straight). The dens axis is occasionally inclined laterally (scoliosis dentis); the values he obtained ranged between +10° (tilted to the right) and −6° (inclined to the left).

Ligaments of the Atlantoaxial Articulations

The posterior articulating portion of the dens is smooth, and covered with a soft layer of connective tissue about 0.5 mm thick. It articulates with the cartilage-covered anterior surface of the transverse ligament of the atlas. Several recesses of the joint cavity have been described.

Transverse Ligament of the Atlas (Figs. 36–40)

The medial surfaces of the lateral masses of the atlas usually have several tubercles, which are the sites of origin of the transverse ligament. The parallel fibers of this ligament form rounded bands near their sites of origin, but then the ligament widens out over the posterior surface of the dens. It is formed of bundles of collagenous fibers that cross one another at acute angles, allowing for slight stretching when the cervical spine and head are bent forward.[130] According to MacAlister,[102] it requires a force of 130 kg to tear this ligament.

Cruciform Ligament of the Atlas

The transverse ligament composes the major part of the cruciform ligament,

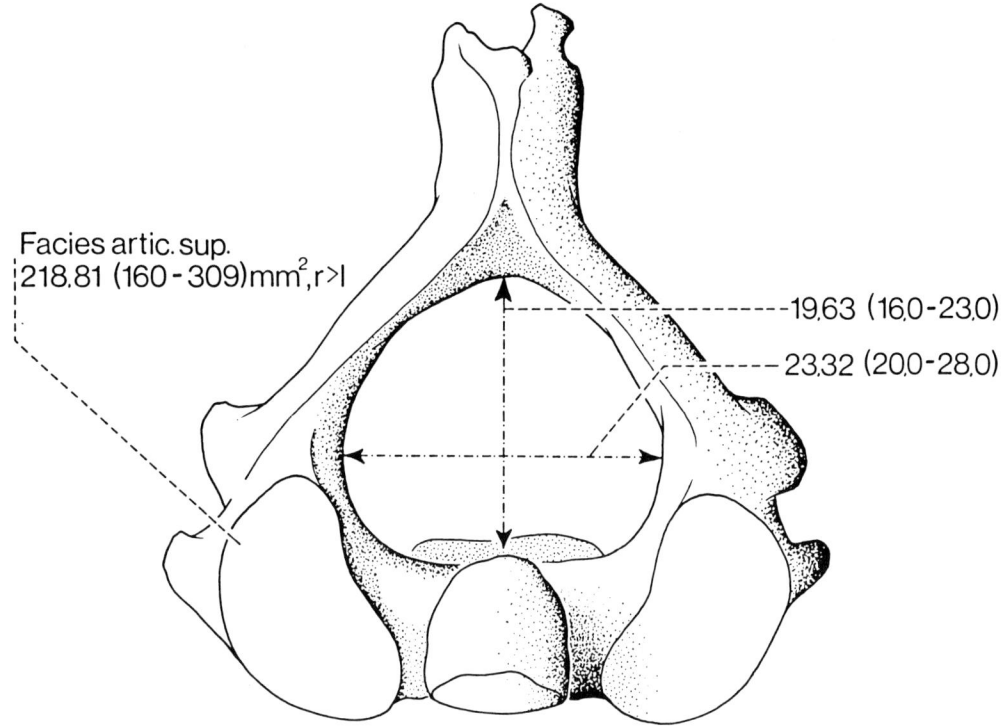

Figure 36: Axis, viewed from superior. Lengths and widths of the foramen vertebrale and facies articularis superior are given in millimeters.

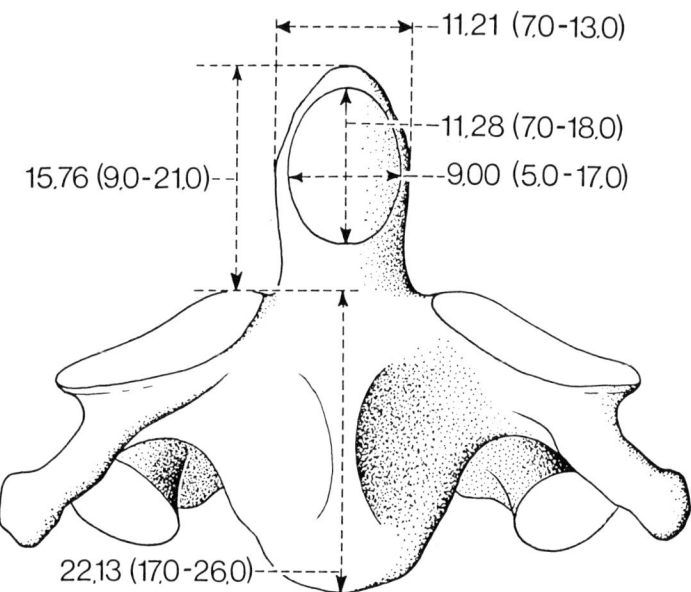

Figure 37: Axis, seen from anterior. Height of corpus and dens axis, width of dens, and dimensions of the facies articularis anterior dentis are given in millimeters (range).

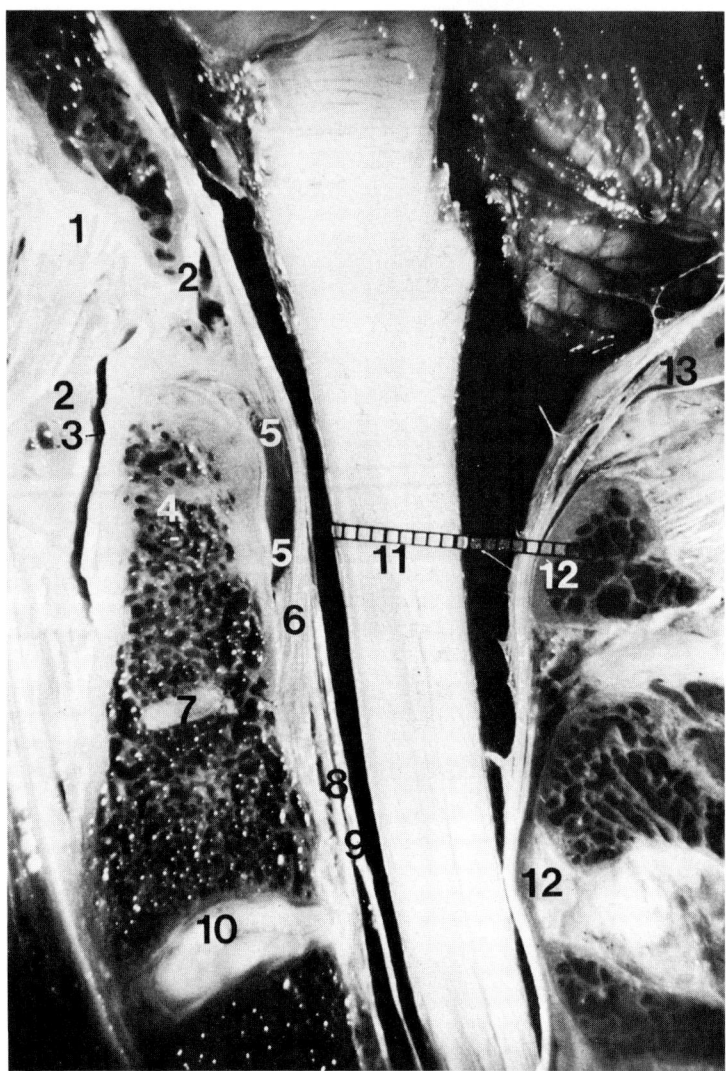

Figure 38: Craniocervical junction, seen in a midsagittal section (right side), seen from the left. 1. Membrana atlanto-occipitalis ventralis. 2. Basion and ventral arch of atlas. 3. Atlantodental joint, widened. 4. Dens axis. 5. Transverse ligament. 6. Cruciform ligament and tectorial membrane. 7. Subdental synchondroses. 8. Posterior longitudinal ligament. 9. Dura mater. 10. Discus of second/third cervical vertebrae. 11. Spinal cord; millimeter scale. 12. Posterior arch of atlas and ligamentum flavum of second/third cervical vertebrae. 13. Opisthion.

which also is made up of more dorsal bundles of fibers running longitudinally. The superior longitudinal band of the ligament is present in *all* specimens, enclosed by loose connective tissue, and merges with the anterior atlanto-occipital membrane. The inferior longitudinal band, when present, is attached to the posterior surface of the body of the axis.

Apical Ligament of the Dens

The apical ligament of the dens is of no functional significance. It is thought to be a vestige of the notochord. We found bony deposits in this ligament in several of our specimens, and have also described a process of the dens that articulates with the basion and occupies the same location as the apical ligament of the dens.[96]

Inferior Cranial Base Anatomy • 503

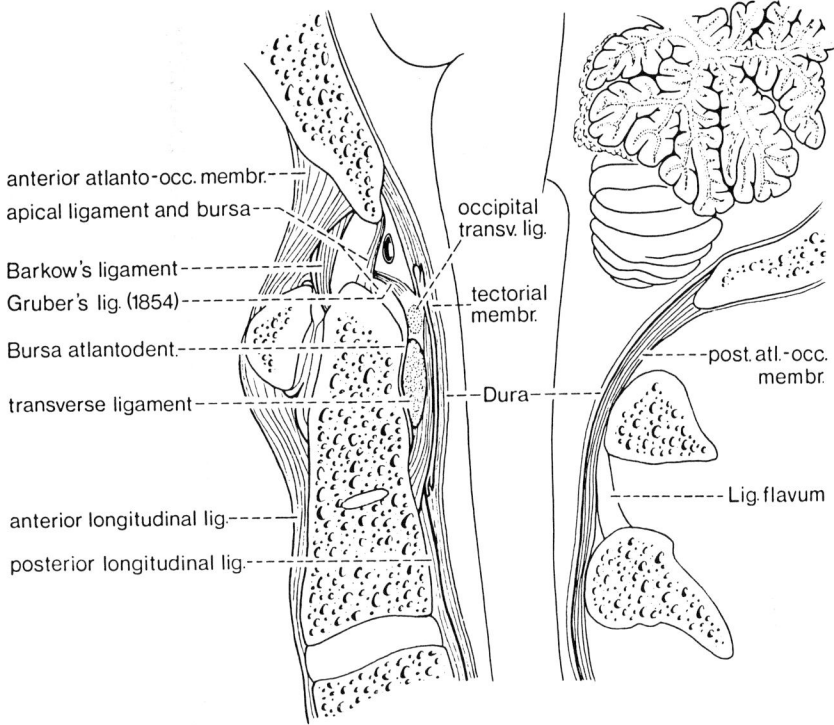

Figure 39: Ligaments of the craniocervical junction.

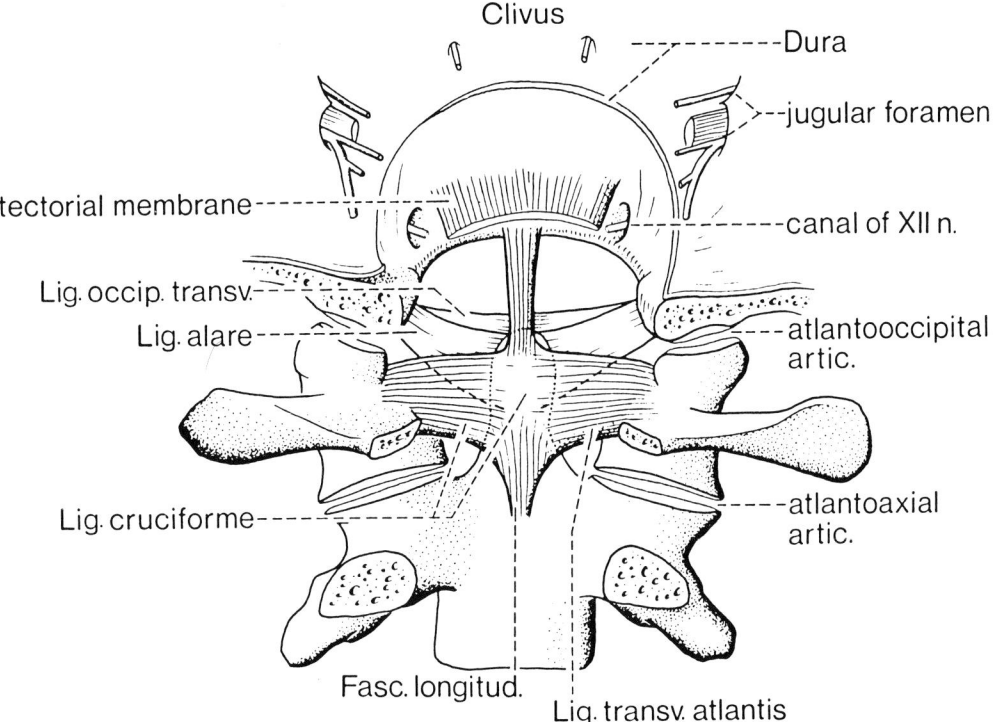

Figure 40: Craniocervical junction, showing ligaments on the posterior aspect of the dens (dura mater and tectorial membrane were resected).

Membrana Tectoria

Immediately under the anterior dura, the dens of the axis and the cruciform ligament are covered posteriorly by a broad, flat, and fairly strong ligament known as the membrana tectoria. This membrane may be regarded as a cranial continuation of the posterior longitudinal ligament of the vertebral column[143] and consists of two lamellae. The lateral portion of this ligament extends to the capsule of the atlanto-occipital joint, while the dorsal portion is continuous with the dura mater in the vicinity of the clivus, slightly superior to the foramen magnum. The inferior portion of the membrana tectoria connects superiorly to the basilar part of the occipital bone, and inferiorly to the posterior surface of the body of the axis. It also attaches close to the cruciform ligament (transverse ligament of the atlas).

Anterior and Posterior Longitudinal Ligaments of the Cervical Spine

Hayashi et al.[50] examined the vertebral columns of 62 adult and eight fetal specimens, and found that the anterior longitudinal ligament passes around the lateral surfaces of the vertebral bodies and deep to the longus colli muscle, and meets the posterior longitudinal ligament in the vicinity of the intervertebral foramina. The posterior longitudinal ligament lies against the posterior surfaces of the vertebral bodies, and is two-layered; the deep layer supplies fibers to the annulus fibrosus. The superficial layer is loosely attached to the deep layer medially, but laterally is entirely separate from it and extends outward as a connective tissue membrane to invest the dura mater, the nerve roots, and the vertebral artery. In this portion the membrane may be relatively thick, but elsewhere it may be thin or incomplete, especially posteriorly. The portions of this membrane around the nerve roots and the vertebral artery are usually clearly recognizable, however.

Alar Ligament

The alar ligaments originate on broad tuberosities, about 10 mm long and 4 mm wide, on the anterior and medial surfaces of the occipital condyles. The rounded, 8-mm wide ligaments run medially and slightly caudally to the lateral surface of the cranial two-thirds of the dens axis, with the superior fibers crossing the midline in some cases, when they are called ligamentum transversum occipitale. A deep portion of this ligament runs to the lateroposterior border of the dens axis, while a superficial portion inserts partially on the apex dentis. Other fibers of this ligament have been noted to run to the opposite side of the head. If well developed, this ligament may border on the transverse ligament of the atlas.

Inferior Cranial Base: Muscles

Lateral Pterygoid Muscle

The lateral pterygoid muscle (Figs. 41 and 42) consists of two parts, a flat superior portion called the caput infratemporale, and the lower belly, the caput pterygoideum. These two parts of the muscle are separated from each other by horizontal septa of connective tissue.[55] The proximal portions of each part of the pterygoid muscle are surrounded by fascia, and the two fasciae meet about 10 mm in front of the temporomandibular joint.

Caput Infratemporale

The origin of the infratemporal head of the lateral pterygoid muscle lies on the planum infratemporale and the infratemporal spine of the lower surface of the ala major of the sphenoid bone, medial to the infratemporal crest. The flattened pterygoid muscle is bordered laterally by the temporal muscle. It runs nearly horizontally and dorsolaterally, and it merges with the caput pterygoideum a short dis-

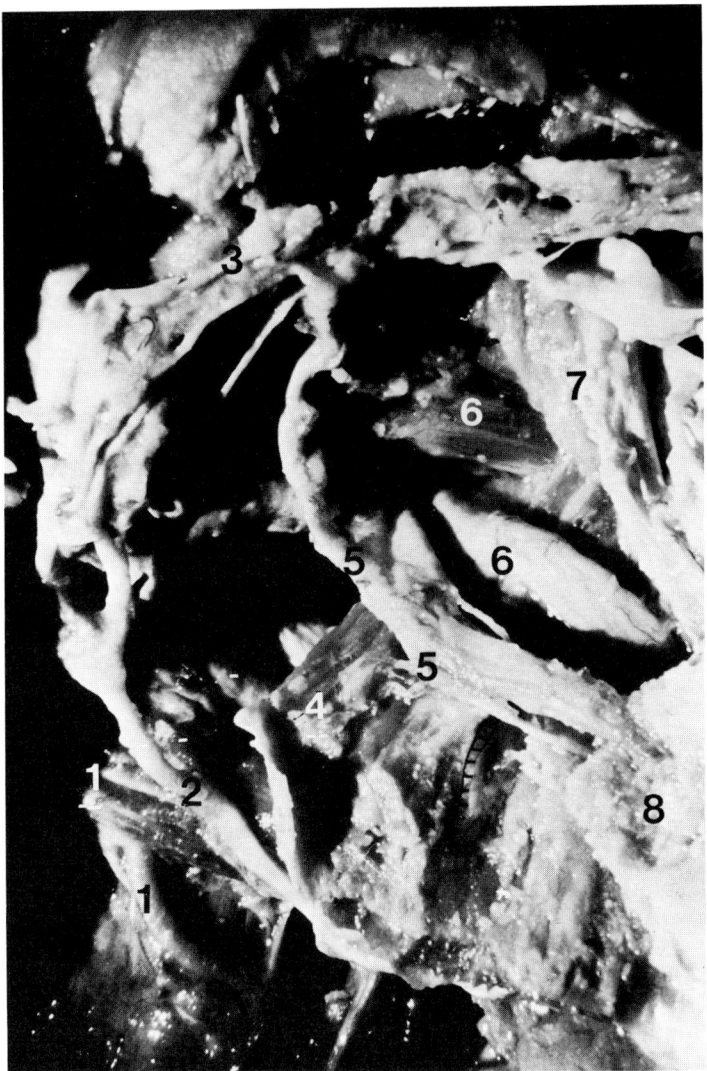

Figure 41: Masticatory space, after resection of ramus mandibulae. 1. Digastric muscle and occipital artery. 2. R. colli. 3. Branches of facial nerve, displaced superiorly. 4. Medial pterygoid muscle. 5. Inferior alveolar nerve and mylohyoideus muscle. 6. Lateral pterygoid muscle and lingual nerve. 7. Deep tendon of temporalis muscle. 8. Mandible, area of resection.

tance anterior to the temporomandibular joint. The caput infratemporale of the pterygoid muscle inserts on the medial half of the collum mandibulae, slightly superior to the insertion of the caput pterygoideum. A portion of its tendon runs in the capsule of the temporomandibular joint and its disc[55,117] and the axis of the muscle forms an angle with the zygomatic arch of about 20°.

In earlier times it was thought that the articular disc and the condyle were anterior extensions of the pterygoid muscle. Juniper[64] and others have stated that the superior head of the lateral pterygoid muscle serves to close and/or stabilize the

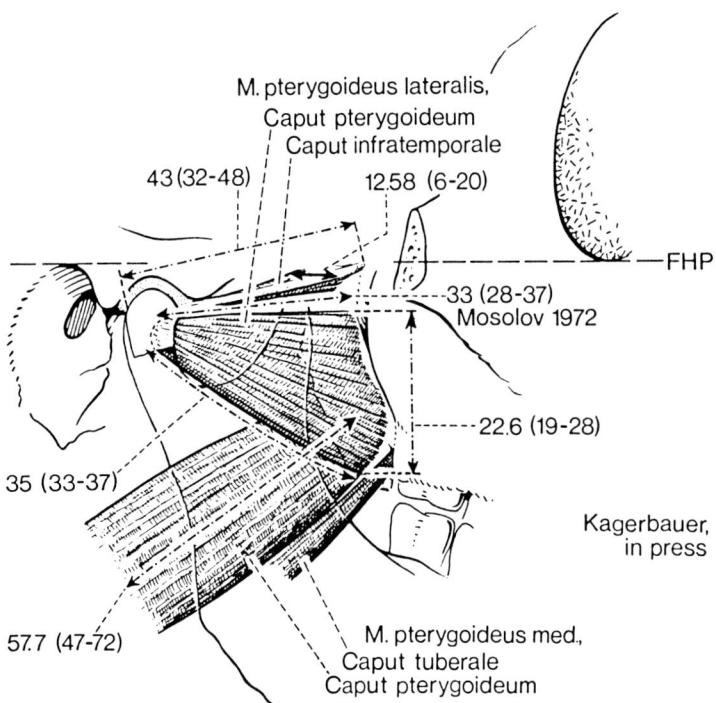

Figure 42: Measurements in the area of the lateral and medial pterygoid muscles.

temporomandibular joint, probably directing the forces of mastication to the articular eminence.

Caput Pterygoideum

The inferior head of the lateral pterygoid muscle originates in the outer surface of the lamina lateralis of the pterygoid process. The muscle fibers run dorsally and superiorly. The muscle belly contracts to effect opening of the mouth by pulling the condylar process of the mandible and the articular disc forward, while the head of the mandible rotates on the articular disc.

Musculus (M) Temporalis, Origin

Figure 43 shows the planum temporale on the lateral surface of the skull, the fossa temporalis, and the posterior border of the frontal process of the zygomatic bone. The deep portion of the temporalis muscle originates on the infratemporal spine and crest, on the sphenomaxillary surface of the sphenoid bone, or sometimes on the connective tissue of the inferior orbital fissure or the external opening of the foramen rotundum.[147]

M. Masseter, Origin

Pars Superficialis

The superficial part of the masseter muscle originates on the lower surface of the zygomatic bone, or sometimes on the zygomatic process of the maxilla. A small portion of this muscle arises on the outer surface of the zygomatic bone.

Pars Profunda

The deep part of the masseter muscle originates in the inferior and medial surface of the zygomatic arch. It extends dorsally to the capsule of the temporomandibular articulation.

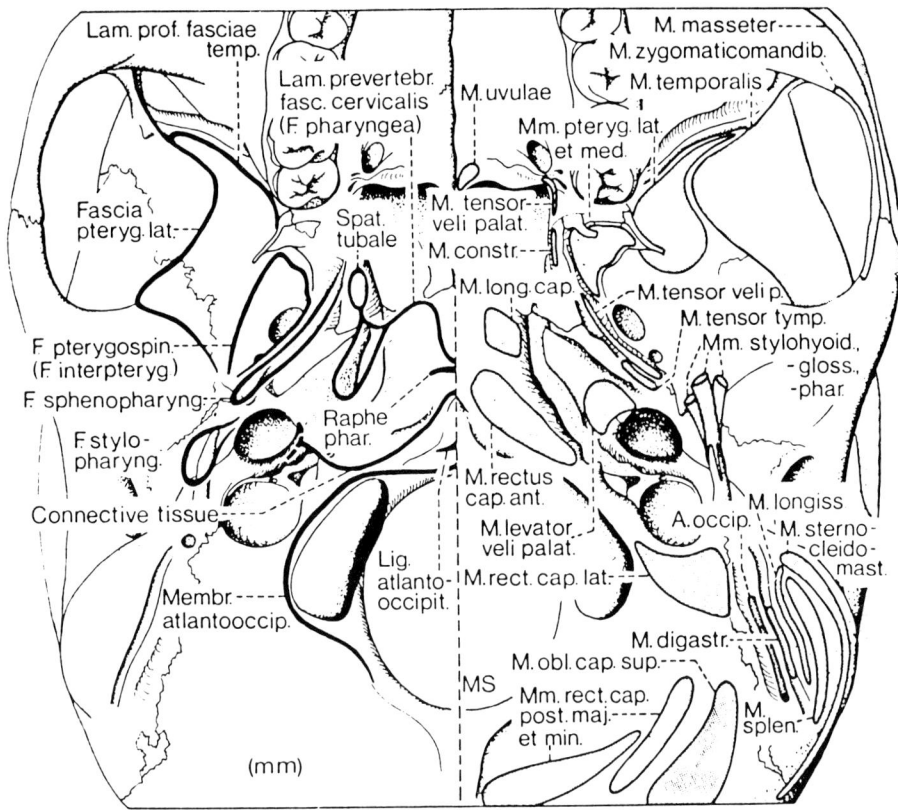

Figure 43: Left side, inferior skull. On the right, origins of muscles may be seen; on the left, insertion areas of fasciae either on the skull base or immediately inferior to it.

M. Pterygoideus Medialis, Origin

We divide this muscle into two portions. The main portion arises in the pterygoid fossa, including the pyramidal process of the palatine bone, while the smaller, accessory, portion arises from the posterior surface of the tuber maxillae.

M. Uvulae, Origin

The uvular muscle arises from the inferior surface of the horizontal lamina of the palatine bone, immediately medial to an insertion of the tensor veli palatini muscle.

M. Levator Veli Palatini, Origin

The m. levator veli palatini originates from tuberosities that lie anterior to the external aperture of the carotid channel, in an area bordered by the inferior surface of the apex of the petrous bone. Part of this area is formed by the tympanic portion of the temporal bone. Other fibers of this muscle arise on the medial lamina of the cartilaginous portion of the auditory tube.

M. Tensor Veli Palatini, Origin

Deep portions of this muscle originate in the fascia salpingopharyngea, while other fibers are loosely connected with the lower border of the lateral or anterior lamellae of the auditory tube. Fibers also arise in the semicanalis m. tensor tympani and connect with this muscle.

M. Longus Capitis

A groove for the insertion of the m. longus capitis is found lateral and posterior to the tuberculum pharyngeum in most cases, while the insertion of the m. rectus capitis anterior is located dorsal and lateral to this area. Dorsolateral to this latter muscle's origin lies the insertion of the m. rectus lateralis.

Styloid Process and Origin of Muscles

The origin of the m. stylopharyngeus is located in the superomedial styloid process, while in the lateral portion of the styloid process the origin of the m. stylohyoideus may be found. In the superior portion or along the anterior border of the styloid process the m. styloglossus arises.

Fascia of the Pharynx

The fascia of the head and neck (Figs. 44 and 45) have been topics of controversy since they were first described by Burns.[17,28,39,44,53,103,120,128,145,147] Many connective tissue layers are present between the posterior surface of the maxilla and the prevertebral muscles. These tissues limit or divert, at least temporarily, material that may be extravasated as a result of inflammatory or hemorrhagic processes, and also serve as landmarks for diagnostic and therapeutic procedures in the head and neck. In addition, some fascia support adjacent structures, and influence the direction of expansion of neoplasms or cysts.[19]

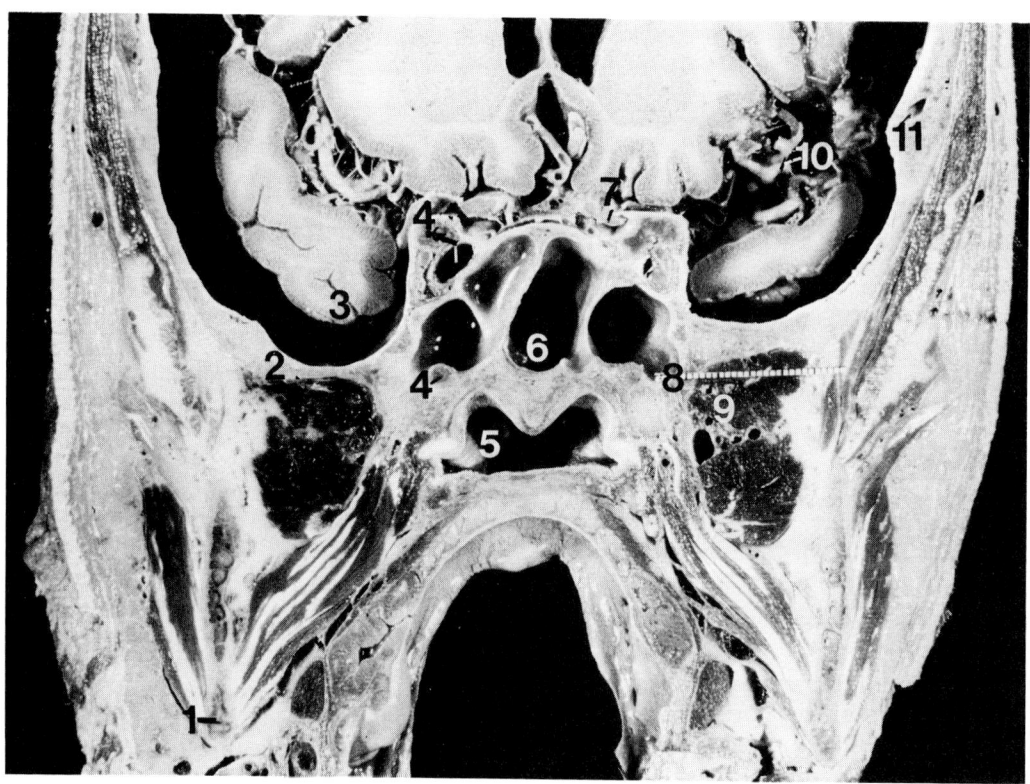

Figure 44: Coronal oblique section (seen from posterior and inferior), through the area of the masticatory muscles. 1. Angulus mandibulae. 2. Middle cranial fossa, floor. 3. Temporal lobe. 4. Anterior clinoid process, internal carotid artery, and pterygoid canal. 5. Nasopharynx. 6. Sphenoid sinus. 7. Left optic nerve. 8. Millimeter scale. 9. Infratemporal head of lateral pterygoid muscle. 10. Branches of middle cerebral artery. 11. Canal for middle meningeal artery and veins.

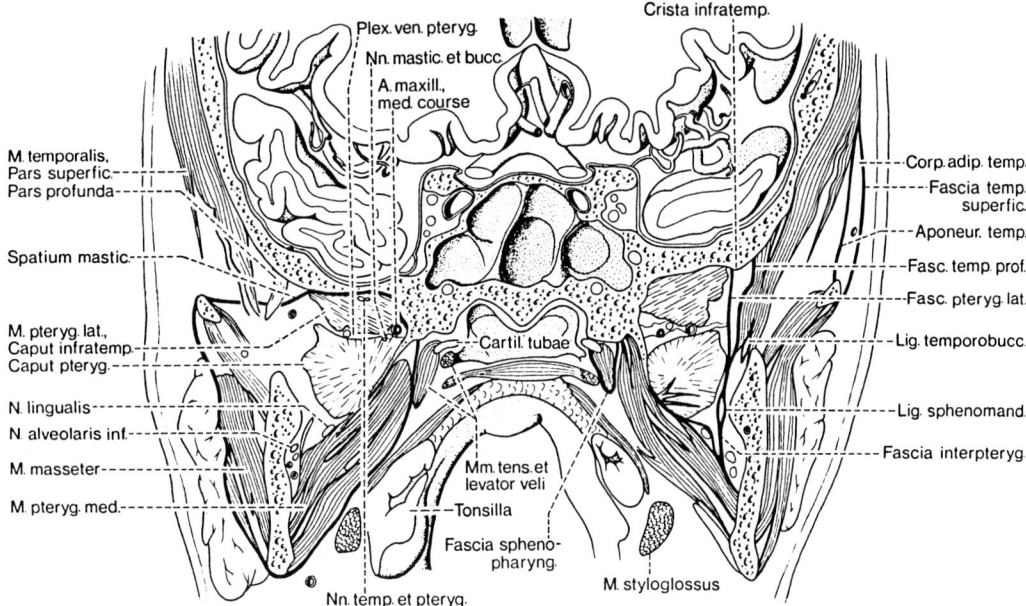

Figure 45: Schematic drawing of fasciae in the masticatory space in the same section shown in Figure 44.

The fascia facilitate movement of the mandible and neck because they permit easy displacement of the muscles, vessels, and nerves. This is partly due to the fat buds of Bichat, which fill the interstices between the muscles.

The pterygoid venous plexus can expand with additional blood, thus acting as a cushion. It may be filled from inside the skull or by veins of the foramen ovale or venosum Vesalii, by the carotid venous plexus, or by hypoglossal or condylar veins, among others. In addition, veins connect this plexus with the veins of the face, in particular with a venous network behind the temporomandibular joint that flows inferiorly to the maxillary vein.

Temporal Fascia

The temporal fascia surrounds the temporal muscle on its inner and outer surfaces: the inner layer inserts on the medial border of the zygomatic arch, while the outer layer inserts on the lateral superior rim of the zygomatic arch. The deep temporal fascia attaches to the lateral margin of the inferior temporal fissure, the inferior temporal crest, and the retromolar trigone of the mandible. The buccinator muscle fasciculi in this area are directly continuous with the most inferior 2 to 3 mm of the attachment of the deep temporal tendon,[147] while the deep temporal fascia also attaches along an oblique line following the line of the mandible to the buccinator fascia.

Lateral Pterygoid Fascia

This thin fascia extends along the lateral surface of the lateral pterygoid muscle between the sphenomaxillary crest,[53] over the infraorbital fissure, the infratemporal spine, and infratemporal crest, and dorsally to the anterior border of the capsule of the temporomandibular joint. Because portions of the venous pterygoid plexus, the maxillary artery, the temporal nerves, and branches of temporal vessels travel in this fascia, French anatomists have called it the fascia vascularis.[138]

Medial and anterior to the lateral

pterygoid fascia the so-called pterygoid process of the fat bud (Bichat) is located. The deep temporal fascia and the lateral ptyergoid fascia are separated anteriorly and unite posteriorly. On a deeper level, this fascia is fixed to the lateral lamina of the pterygoid process, to the posterior border of the sphenomaxillary fissure, and to the tuber maxillae. Anteriorly it merges with the fascia buccinatoria, and more posteriorly with the interpterygoid fascia. A small fascial pocket is present anteriorly, occupied by the pterygoid process of the masticatory fat bud. The inferior border runs obliquely to the retromolar trigone of the mandible, across the base of the coronoid process medial to the deep tendon and muscle fibers of the temporal muscle. Connections exist between this fascia and the sphenomandibular ligament.

Pterygospinose Ligament (Interpterygoid Fascia)

The interpterygoid fascia originates between the posterior border of the lateral lamina of the pterygoid process and the spina ossis sphenoidalis, the petrotympanic fissure, or the bony lamina pterygospinosa. This fascia spreads downward to the outer fascia of the medial pterygoid muscle, and carries the lingual and inferior alveolar nerves. Other insertions of this fascia include the suture between the palatine and the sphenoid bone in the pterygoid fossa, the tuber maxillae, the lingula, and the retromolar trigone of the mandible.

Temporobuccinator Band

Within the plane of fascia covering the surface of the superficial and deep tendons of the temporal muscle is a prominent regional condensation about 2 cm long and 1 cm wide, which passes inferiorly and medially. It extends from the medial surface of the superficial tendon at its attachment to the anterior edge of the coronoid process of the mandible to the buccinator fascia, slightly anterior to the pterygomandibular raphe.[37,147]

Stylopharyngeal Fascia

At the base of the spina sphenoidalis, ventrolateral to the external aperture of the carotid channel and on the vagina of the styloid process, the stylopharyngeal fascia originates. This fascia extends inferiorly in two sheets, which surround the anterior and posterior border of the m. levator veli palatini. Lateral to the stylopharyngeus and styloglossus muscles, the fascia blends into the stylomandibular ligament and the stylomandibular fascia. The outer layer of the stylopharyngeal fascia is the inner margin of the retromandibular process for the parotid gland, and another connective tissue mass is located between this fascia and the buccopharyngeal fascia.

Sphenopharyngeal (Salpingopharyngeal, Sphenopterygopharyngeal) Fascia

This fascia originates posterior to the foramina ovale and spinosum of the sphenoid bone, and unites with the stylopharyngeal fascia anterior and lateral to the external aperture of the carotid channel, the styloid process, and the medial extension of the pars tympanica. A medially oriented extension of the fascia surrounds the m. tensor veli palatini on its medial border, while a lateral extension may be seen slightly below the skull base, dorsolateral to this muscle. The two fascial sheets are connected with one another 0.5 to 1 cm posterior to the muscle.[147]

The lateral fascial layer extends into the pterygoid fossa, while the medial fascia runs along the medial side of the tensor veli palatini muscle to the lamina medialis of the pterygoid process. According to Zenker,[147] the origin of this fascia is 3 cm long and 5 mm wide, while its insertion is 1 to 2 cm long on the lateral wall of the pharynx.

Lamina Profunda Fasciae Cervicalis

The deep or pervertebral fascia is situated between the pharynx and its fascia anteriorly and the prevertebral muscles posteriorly. It is a thin connective tissue layer composed of several thin, vascularized laminae that allow movement of the pharynx medially and of the large vessels and nerves laterally. According to Hall[44] and Grodinsky and Holyoke,[39] the deepest layer of the cervical fascia consists of two main subdivisions: the alar and the prevertebral fasciae. The latter authors describe a complete layer of fascia between the visceral and prevertebral layers, which they named the alar fascia. This fascia extends across the midline, posterior to the pharynx and visceral fascia, to fuse with the prevertebral fascia at the tip of the transverse processes, to which both of these layers are attached. This alar fascia then passes anterolaterally to form the medial anterior wall of the carotid sheath.

Pharyngeal Fascia (Fascia Buccopharyngea)

The pharynx is covered by a thin connective tissue layer, in which nerves and veins are interlaced.

Spaces

Sptaium Masticatorium

The spatium masticatorium contains the masseter and pterygoid muscles, and the ramus mandibulae.[21,39] It is closed, except for the temporal muscle superiorly, and lies anterolateral to the lateral pharyngeal space and anterior to the parotid space. On the outer skull base, the masticatory space is separated into a space for the lateral pterygoid muscle, between the lateral pterygoid fascia and the pterygospinose ligament (interpterygoid fascia), and a space between the pterygospinose lamina and the sphenopharyngeal fascia where the medial pterygoid muscle originates. The sphenopharyngeal fascia surrounds the medial border of the tensor veli palatini muscle and is fixed to the membranous wall of the auditory tube.

Salpingopharyngeal Space

This space is located dorsomedial to the sphenopharyngeal fascia, and contains the auditory tube, the m. levator veli palatini, and portions of the ascending palatine artery.

Vagina Carotica

Dorsolateral to the vagina carotica the internal carotid artery, the internal jugular vein, the ascending pharyngeal artery, and cranial nerves IX to XII are located, at different levels. Anterolaterally this space is surrounded by the stylopharyngeal fascia, and dorsally it is bordered by the connective tissue of the lamina prevertebralis fasciae cervicalis.

Spatium Parapharyngeum

According to earlier authors, the parapharyngeal space is divided into an anterior compartment (spatium parapharyngeum anterius) and a posterior compartment. The anterior compartment contains lymph nodes and connective tissue, and is located between the skull base and the angle of the mandible, while the posterior compartment lies posterior to the pharynx and contains the prevertebral muscles. In the midline the connective tissues of the pharyngeal and prevertebral fasciae are fixed on the vertebral column in the cranial base. The space behind the pharynx laterally is bordered by the attachment of the pharyngeal fascia and the prevertebral fascia, and still further laterally the spatium lateropharyngeum posterius may be found, posterior to the styloid process and its muscles. The internal carotid arteries and cranial nerves IX to XII are located in this space, and the internal jugular vein and lymph nodes may also be found here. In the medial retropharyngeal space, retropharyngeal lymph nodes are found.

Prevertebral Lamina and Sympathetic Trunk

The sympathetic trunk is interwoven in the lamina prevertebralis fasciae cervicales. According to Becker and Grunt,[9] the ganglion cervicale superius is 28 mm (range 15–35 mm) long, and is located between the first and third cervical vertebrae. In 62.3% of cases (40% bilaterally and 22% unilaterally), these authors found a sympathetic ganglion anterior to the sixth cervical vertebra in most cases (although anywhere between the third and seventh cervical vertebra in the specimens they examined). This ganglion cervicale medium was a mean of 7 mm long (range 2–15 mm).

The superior cervical sympathetic ganglion is supplied mainly by twigs of the ascending pharyngeal artery,[82] and lateral to the sympathetic trunk the ventral rami of the cervical nerves pierce the lamina profunda of the cervical fascia. These rami are connected by branches to the ventral cervical branches superior and inferior to the hypoglossal nerve, and to the sympathetic trunk. It has been noted that these twigs supply other than the prevertebral muscles, and other twigs of this plexus may be found running dorsal to the nervous plexus, around the vertebral, and superiorly to the carotid arteries.

The sympathetic trunk also connects to the superior laryngeal nerve. As a rule, one or two twigs of the ganglion cervicale superius of the sympathetic trunk supply the internal carotid artery, and one twig supplies the internal jugular vein.

Between 76,000 and 1 million nerve fibers may be found in the ganglion cervicale superius, of which 5000 to 12,000 are preganglionic. Of these fibers, 1600 to 5000 are myelinated.[30] The multipolar cells of this ganglion have diameters between 20 and 60 μm, and contain one to three nuclei with diameters of about 11 μm.

Infratemporal Fossa: Masticatory Space, Vessels, and Nerves

Arteria Maxillaris, Origin

The main vessel of the infratemporal fossa is the maxillary artery, which is a branch of the external carotid artery and takes a variable course to the lateral pterygoid muscle. In our specimens this vessel originated 24.62 mm (range 17–29 mm) inferior to the head of the mandible. We estimated the lumen of this artery 5 mm distal to its origin to be 1.77 mm (range 1.1–2.7 mm). In 50% of our specimens, the maxillary artery ran parallel to the Frankfort plane or within 5° above this plane; in 35% of cases the course lay between 6° and 20° above the Frankfort plane; and in the remaining 15% of cases, the course descended at an angle of 21° to 30° to the Frankfort plane. This last was the situation in most cases in which the artery coursed lateral to the caput infratemporale of the lateral pterygoid muscle.

Maxillary Artery

The first part of the maxillary artery is the retromandibular portion, which courses behind the mandible and gives off one or two small twigs to the tympanic membrane, a twig to the a. auricularis profunda, a twig to the anterior tympanic artery, and a twig to the middle meningeal artery. The accessory middle meningeal artery branches off of this twig in most cases, but this vessel may also arise directly from the maxillary artery. The middle meningeal artery supplies part of the pterygoid muscles and the tensor veli palatini muscle.

The second part of the maxillary artery, the pars pterygoidea, extends obliquely anteromedially, and was found by different investigators to run medial or lateral to the lateral pterygoid muscle (see Fig. 46). The middle meningeal artery branches off proximal to the inferior alveolar artery in cases where this artery takes a lateral course, and vice versa when it takes a medial course.[72,73] Twigs of the pars pterygoidea of the maxillary artery run to the pterygoid muscles, the masseter muscle, and the deep temporal arteries. These last twigs course superiorly and then run in small grooves of the temporal squama.

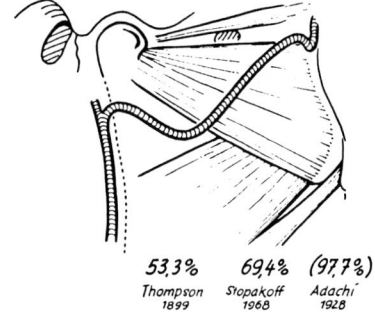

53,3% Thompson 1899   69,4% Stopakoff 1968   (97,7%) Adachi 1928

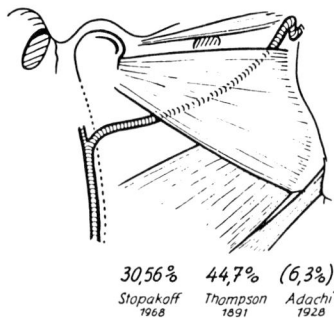

30,56% Stopakoff 1968   44,7% Thompson 1891   (6,3%) Adachi 1928

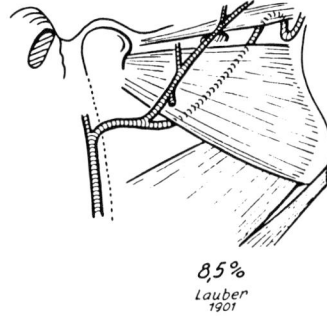

8,5% Lauber 1901

Figure 46: Course of maxillary artery to lateral pterygoid muscle (in particular, note caput pterygoideum). Adachi[2] found that the artery in most cases took a course lateral to the muscle; Lauber[93] found a branch medial to the branch lateral to the pterygoid muscle in 8.5% of cases.

The pterygopalatine part of the maxillary artery courses through the sphenopalatine fissure in the pterygopalatine fossa, and anteriorly to the pterygopalatine ganglion and veins. The twigs of this vessel are the anterior deep temporal artery, the posterior superior alveolar artery, the infraorbital artery (often the infraorbital and the superior and posterior alveolar arteries have a common trunk), the a. palatina major, and the sphenopalatine artery. Pearson et al.[116] found a sphenopalatine vein running from the sphenopalatine foramen to the inferior border of the sphenomaxillary fissure, immediately posterior to the periosteal layer of the maxillary sinus in two cases. In the other cases they examined the veins were very small.

Tumors in the infratemporal fossa cause deafness, auditory canal pain, and anesthesia of the mandibular nerve distribution, as well as asymmetry of the soft palate, trismus (when the pterygoid muscles are involved), and swelling in the area of the zygomatic arch. Aneurysms of the maxillary artery occur very rarely: only four cases had been identified up until 1966, and in all cases the diagnosis was made when the aneurysms ruptured. Rankow[121] reported on a 53-year-old woman who presented with pain in the area anterior to the left ear; during surgery, a congenital saccular aneurysm of the maxillary artery was identified in the area of the lateral pterygoid muscle.

The course of the maxillary artery to the lingual and inferior alveolar nerves is very variable (see Fig. 47).

The Mandibular Nerve

The mandibular nerve is located medial to the auditory tube and tensor veli palatini muscle, inferior to the foramen ovale, and medial to the lateral pterygoid muscle. The nerve is surrounded by the venous plexus of the foramen ovale, and close to the accessory middle meningeal artery and the meningeal branch of the mandibular nerve. The otic ganglion is

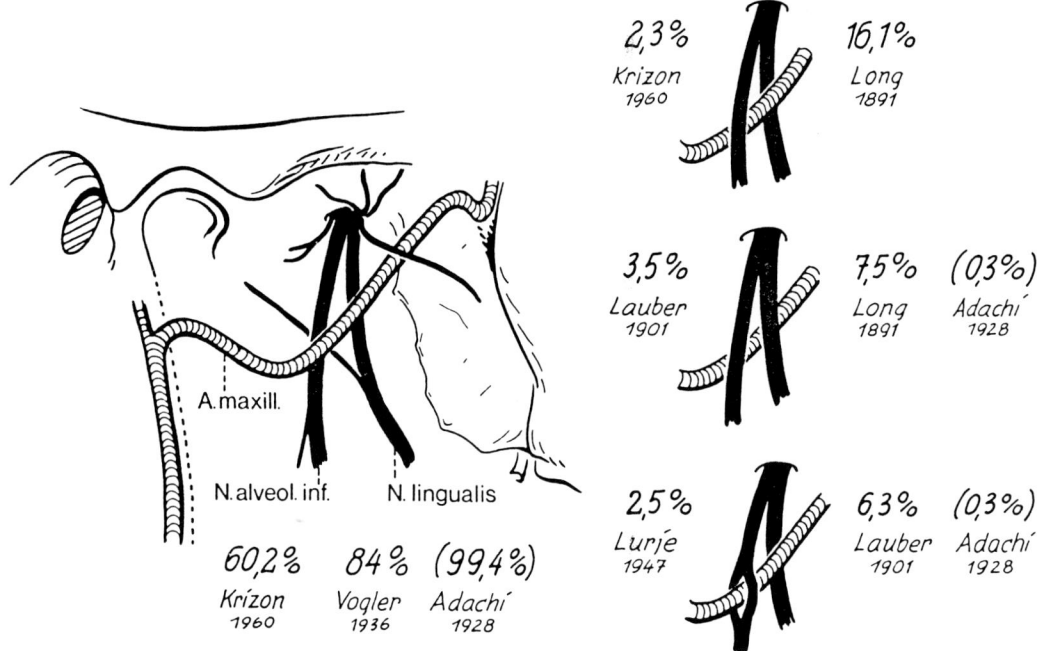

Figure 47: Maxillary artery in relation to inferior alveolar and lingual nerves.

located medial to the mandibular nerve.

The posterior branch of the mandibular nerve is the auriculotemporal nerve, which gives off two twigs that surround the middle meningeal artery and then unite later to form the nerve that extends posterior to the temporomandibular joint in the parotid region.

The chorda tympani nerve, a nerve of variable length, lies medial to the lateral pterygoid muscle. It courses between the petrotympanic fissure and the lingual nerve. Other medial and superior branches of the mandibular nerve give off twigs to the pterygoid muscle, the tensor tympani, and the tensor veli palatini muscle. The deep temporal nerves course on the superior margin of the infratemporal head of the lateral pterygoid muscle, and penetrate the temporal muscle from medial to lateral. The masseter nerve runs through the incisura mandibulae to the masseter muscle, while the buccal nerve runs between the two heads of the lateral pterygoid muscle to the outer surface of the buccinator muscle.

The lingual and inferior alveolar nerves run through the hiatus pterygoideus to the lateral border of the medial pterygoid muscle and its fascial sheath. This hiatus is bordered by the inferior limit of the caput pterygoideum of the lateral pterygoid muscle, the superior and posterior borders of the medial pterygoid muscle, and the neck of the mandible. The lingual nerve may originate as one to three roots. It may receive a branch from the inferior alveolar nerve, the sympathetic plexus, and the otic ganglion.

Parapharyngeal Space: Nerves

Glossopharyngeal Nerve

Anatomy

The glossopharyngeal nerve is illustrated in Figures 16 and 17 of Chapter 25 and in Figure 48 of this chapter. This nerve leaves the skull through the anterosuperior medial portion of the jugular foramen. Its inferior ganglion is situated on the outer skull base, in the location

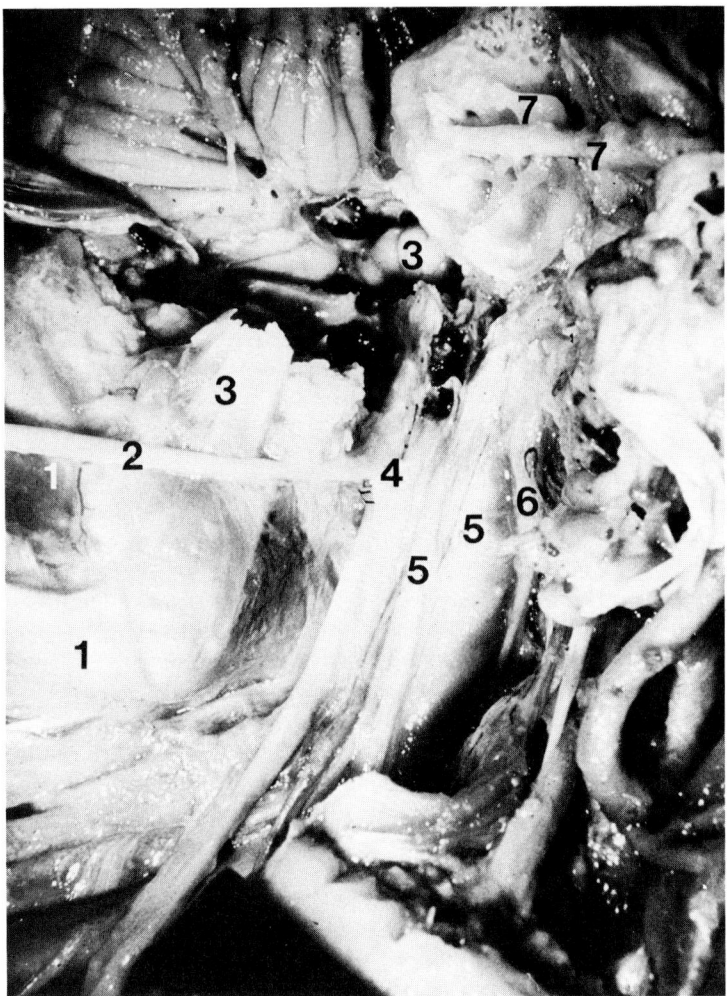

Figure 48: Upper pharyngeal space, nerve, and arteries; jugular vein has been resected from lateral to anterior. 1. Superior and inferior oblique muscles. 2. Accessory nerve, displaced dorsally, and hypoglossal nerve. 3. Lateral rectus muscle and flocculus. 4. Anastmoses between ninth and tenth cranial nerves. 5. Internal carotid nerve and internal carotid artery. 6. Glossopharyngeal nerve, displaced anteriorly. 7. Mastoid portion of facial nerve, displaced anteriorly, and short process of incus.

where a small fossa between the apertura externa of the carotid channel and the jugular fossa is sometimes seen, called the fossula petrosa.

A small twig of the ninth cranial nerve, the tympanic nerve, courses with a twig of the ascending pharyngeal artery through the canaliculus tympanicus to the middle ear cavity. Two to six glomeruli, from which chemodectomas may arise, are present in the course of this nerve.[42]

After the glossopharyngeal nerve gives off another twig to anastomose with the vagus nerve, it courses along the outer surface of the internal carotid artery and turns medial to the internal jugular vein to bury itself in the vagina carotica. The nerve then runs inferiorly and anteriorly to the internal carotid artery. The landmark for the nerve in this location is the stylopharyngeal muscle, which it also supplies; the nerve has been seen piercing this muscle in about 12% of cases.[108]

The nerve then runs in the fascia

stylopharyngea to the margin between the superior pharyngeal constrictor muscle and the middle pharyngeal constrictor muscle. Rarely, the nerve may pierce the superior constrictor muscle, but in all cases the nerve anastomoses with the auricular branch of the vagus nerve, the sympathetic trunk, and the facial nerve. In the last case, the glossopharyngeal nerve sometimes anastomoses with the extracranial portion of the facial nerve, but may anastomose with the digastric branch of this nerve. These anastomoses provide a means for the sensory fibers from the pinna to reach the ninth cranial nerve.

Inferior to the ganglion of the glossopharyngeal nerve, one or two twigs (the rr. sinus carotici), which anastomose with twigs of the tenth cranial nerve and the sympathetic trunk, run to the pressor receptive zone of the sinus caroticus and the glomus caroticum. In addition, three to four pharyngeal branches of the ninth cranial nerve run to the posterior surface of the pharynx, tonsillar branches extend to the tonsillar capsule, and lingual branches to the pharyngeal part of the tongue, the papillae vallatae, the vallecula glossoepiglottica, and the upper surface of the epiglottis.

Motor branches of the ninth cranial nerve supply the stylopharyngeal muscle and the upper constrictors of the pharynx (together with the tenth cranial nerve).

Sensory innervation of the posterior third of the tongue (taste fibers to the vallate papillae) and dorsal parts of the mouth cavity, the isthmus faucium, and the pharynx is by way of the glossopharyngeal nerve as well. Sensory areas innervated by the ninth cranial nerve include the isthmus faucium, the tonsilla palatina, the pharyngeal surface of the tongue, the posterior and lateral walls of the pharynx, the tympanic cavity, the auditory tube, and a small area posterior to the ear.

Parasympathetic secretory fibers run in the ninth cranial nerve, the tympanic nerve, and the lesser petrosal nerve to the otic ganglion and then to the parotid gland, buccal glands, molar glands, glands of the papillae vallatae, and the posterior third of the tongue.

The sensory fibers of the ninth cranial nerve run through the ventral spinocerebellar tract, in the spinal tract of the trigeminal nerve, and then caudally. One bundle of the fibers extends to the nucleus solitarius, while another runs to the nuclei cuneati medialis et lateralis and in the spinal nucleus of the trigeminal nerve.[67] The efferent fibers of the n. petrosus minor originate in the formatio reticularis pontis and the medulla oblongata,[109] while the other motor fibers of the ninth nerve are axons of the anterior portion of the nucleus ambiguus.

The neural cells of the afferent fibers are located in the inferior and superior ganglia of the ninth cranial nerve. It should be remembered that the fibers of the rami sinus carotici (Hering's nerve) may run in the ninth or twelfth cranial nerve, or in the vagus nerve to the central nervous system.[14,32,131]

Vagus Nerve (Fig. 48)

In our specimens, we counted an average of 8.65 (range 4.0–15.0) nerve fiber bundles leaving the brain stem in the retro-olivary fossa.[89] The nerve fiber bundles ran to the dural pore in the area of the jugular foramen, where the superior ganglion of the tenth cranial nerve is located. This pore is ovoid, and about 4 mm long. An average of 1.48 (range 1 to 3) anastomoses with the glossopharyngeal nerve were found in this area. The ramus internus of the accessory nerve branches off 11.34 mm (range 2–19 mm) below the margo terminalis sigmoidea of the jugular foramen. This branch is an average of 9.75 mm (range 3–24 mm) long, and intersects the vagus nerve. At more inferior levels, we found an average of 1.4 (range 1 to 3) anastomoses between the tenth and ninth cranial nerves.

The auricular branch of the vagus nerve branched off from the lower circumference of the superior ganglion of the tenth cranial nerve, and in most cases contained fibers from the glossopharyngeal nerve. This branch courses through the jugular fossa and then runs in a small channel through the petrous part of the temporal bone on the posterior or anterior circumference of the mastoid portion of the facial nerve. Anastomoses of the ninth cranial nerve with the seventh cranial nerve also occur in this area. The auricular branch of the vagus nerve then courses through the temporal bone to the tympanomastoid fissure, in rare cases in company with the facial nerve branch to the stylomastoid foramen, and provides part of the innervation of the lateral surface of the tympanic membrane and the external auditory canal. A small branch of the superior ganglion of the vagus nerve is thought to course posteriorly in the posterior fossa, in particular around the occipital sinus.

The inferior ganglion of the tenth cranial nerve is located anterior to the transverse processes of the first and second cervical vertebrae. It is 25.47 mm (range 12–38 mm) long, and its greatest diameter is 3.46 mm (range 1.83–6.1 mm). In more than 50% of our specimens, we found large veins running through the ganglion area. The vagus nerve was found to be 2.88 mm (range 1.77–5.32 mm) wide, measured 5 mm below the inferior ganglion, and 1.47 mm (range 0.36–2.44 mm) thick. In all of the cases we examined, there were anastomoses between the ganglion inferius of the vagus nerve and the ganglion cervicale superius of the sympathetic nerve, and in most cases with the superior ansa of the ventral rami of the cervical nerves as well. We did not always find anastomoses with the twelfth cranial nerve, but in 53 head halves studied, there were up to nine such anastomoses present, with an average of 2.04 (range zero to nine).

The first ramus pharyngeus branches off of the vagus nerve in the area of the inferior ganglion. In the 59 cases we studied, we found one branch in 50, two branches in seven, a triple branch in one, and one case in which this nerve could not be evaluated. The branch anastomosed with the pharyngeal branch of the ninth cranial nerve an average of 18.17 mm (range 1–46 mm) from its origin.

The superior laryngeal nerve is the next branch of the vagus nerve extracranially. This twig leaves the vagus nerve 37 mm (range 26–52 mm) inferior to the margo terminalis sigmoidea in the area of the foramen jugulare on the right side, and 35.1 mm (range 20–58 mm) on the left.

The motor fibers of the vagus nerve are axons of the nucleus ambiguus in the medulla oblongata, and supply (together with the fibers of the glossopharyngeal nerve) the constrictor muscles of the pharynx, the stylopharyngeal muscle, the levator veli palatini, and the palatoglossus and palatopharyngeal muscles.

The sensory fibers of the mucous membrane of the pharynx, the thyroid gland, and the parathyroid gland run centrally in the pharyngeal branches of the vagus nerve. It should be noted that glomerula laryngea were found on the superior laryngeal nerve by Watzka[144] and on the inferior laryngeal nerve by Kleinsasser.[68] These findings are important in understanding the origins of glomus tumors.

Accessory Nerve

In our specimens we found an average of 10.66 (range 6–16) cranial root fiber bundles of the accessory nerve anastomosing with the vagus nerve. These fibers are composed of axons of the inferior portion of the nucleus ambiguus, and run in the pharyngeal branches of the vagus nerve and in the recurrent laryngeal nerve. The spinal portion of the accessory nerve is composed of fiber bundles that leave the spinal cord between the anterior and posterior fiber bundles, sometimes as far inferior as the seventh cervical segment.

The nucleus of the accessory nerve in the spinal cord extends from the caudal third of the inferior olive to between the fourth and seventh (although usually between the fourth and sixth) cervical segments, slightly dorsal to the ventral column. The spinal roots of the accessory nerve emerge from the lateral portion of the spinal cord or, occasionally, in line with the dorsal nerve roots. The most inferior fibers may come from the sixth or the seventh cervical segment.

The roots of the accessory nerve unite to ascend between the denticulate ligament and the dorsal rootlets of the spinal nerve, and then pass through the foramen magnum posterior to the vertebral artery. We found one to three fibers from the dorsal rootlets of the first cervical nerve anastomosing with the spinal root of the accessory nerve, and occasionally with the second cervical nerve.

In the area of the anastomoses between the first cervical nerve and the spinal roots of the accessory nerve, a ganglion was visible to macroscopic inspection on the right side in 41% of specimens and on the left in 43%.[78] It is possible that sensory fibers of the first cervical nerve also go to the deeper portions of the spinal cord via the eleventh cranial nerve and its descending roots. In addition, proprioceptive fibers from the muscles supplied by the accessory nerve may enter the spinal cord via the dorsal rootlets.

In the foramen jugulare area, the accessory nerve runs immediately posterior to the vagus nerve, embedded in the nerve guide plate. The external branch of the accessory nerve is 1.28 mm (range 0.67–2.44 mm) wide, and 0.64 mm (range 0.18–1.52 mm) thick. According to Tandler,[133] this nerve then runs posterior to the internal jugular vein in 33% of cases and anterior to this vein in 66%. In 85% of our specimens the eleventh cranial nerve ran below the cranial base and in front of the jugular vein, while in the other 15% it ran behind this vein to the sternocleidomastoid muscle and anastomosed with twigs of the cervical plexus. In a few specimens, the nerve ran between deep communications of the inferior petrosal sinus with the internal jugular vein, and then coursed dorsal to the styloid process in the styloid muscles.

The sternocleidomastoid branch of the occipital artery runs a short distance with the accessory nerve. This nerve (and the cervical plexus) supply the sternocleidomastoid muscle and the trapezius muscle.

Hypoglossal Nerve

We counted the nerve fiber bundles leaving the sulcus between the pyramid and the oliva of the medulla oblongata, and found an average of 13.6 (range 7–26) root fiber bundles. The most superior fiber bundle had a length of 11.34 mm (range 7.0–24.0 mm), while the inferior bundle, in the posterior fossa, measured 11 mm (range 5.5–18.0 mm). The hypoglossal channel was noted to be divided into two channels in 12.7% of our specimens on the right, and in 25% on the left. The dural pores were duplicated in 65% of specimens, with an average distance between the pores of 4.16 mm (range 0.5–9.0 mm). In all cases the nerve fiber bundles (and their channels) united inside the hypoglossal channel.

The channel for the hypoglossal nerve was found to be 8 mm (range 6.1–14.1 mm) long, and to lie at an angle to the midsagittal plane of 44°. The nerve (and sometimes also the posterior fossa meningeal branch) was surrounded by venous plexus, a dural sheath, and an arachnoidal sheath.

On the outer skull base, the hypoglossal nerve runs on the medial surface of the internal jugular vein and on the lateral surface of the vagus nerve in 92% of cases. Then the twelfth cranial nerve curves around the occipital artery or its first branch to the sternocleidomastoid muscle to course, first to the lateral and then to the anterior surface of the external carotid artery. In about 8% of cases, the nerve curves around the external carotid artery distal to the origin zone of the occipital artery, and then takes a lateral course on the outer surface of the external carotid artery and posterior to the internal jugular vein.[101]

Distal to the hypoglossal channel, the hypoglossal nerve is 1.53 mm (range 6.8–2.44 mm) wide, and 0.9 mm (range 0.6–2.13 mm) thick. It connects with the ventral rami of C1 and C2, and the ventral ansa between these two branches. The hypoglossal nerve and ansa were estimated to be 24.72 mm (range 15–45 mm) long.

The ramus descendens n. hypoglossi leaves the main trunk of the hypoglossal nerve about 14.3 mm (range 0–34 mm) distal to the ansa. At this point the hypoglossal nerve is about 2 mm (with a spread of 3.3 mm) wide, and has a diameter of 1.16 mm (range 0.5–2 mm).[108] After the ramus descendens has split off from the hypoglossal nerve, the hypoglossal nerve is 1.79 mm (range 1.04–3.12 mm) wide and 0.4 mm (range 0–1.98 mm) thick.

In all cases, a ramus communicans cum n. lingualis was present on the outer surface of the hyoglossus muscle.[33,106] It is important to note that the fibers of the first and second cervical nerves supply the m. longus capitis, the m. rectus capitis anterior, and the infrahyoid muscles. The lingual twigs of the hypoglossal nerve supply the genioglossus, hyoglossus, styloglossus, and intrinsic muscles of the tongue, and when a lesion is present on one side of the hypoglossal nerve, the tongue (especially the genioglossus) points to the side of the lesion. When bilateral lesions of the hypoglossal nerve are present, it is impossible to move the tongue at all, and disturbances in swallowing and speech are present as well. Occasionally glossospasm and fibrillation of the tongue may be seen when such lesions are small.

Parapharyngeal Space: Vessels

Common Carotid Artery (Fig. 49)

In our specimens,[104] the length of the right common carotid artery measured 98.8 mm (range 81–125 mm), and of the left measured 121.2 mm (range 100–145 mm).

The outer diameter of the right artery is 8.9 mm (range 7–11 mm), and that of the left is 8.9 mm (range 7–11 mm). The right common carotid artery originates 19.2 mm (range 11–28 mm) from the midsagittal plane, at the level of C6 it is 30.6 mm (range 22–42 mm) from the midsagittal plane, and at the level of C4 it lies 32.9 mm (range 24–40 mm) lateral to the midsagittal plane.

The left common carotid artery originates 20.5 mm (range 15–28 mm) from the midsagittal plane, at the level of C6 it is 31.6 mm (range 25–38 mm) from the midsagittal plane, and at the level of C4 it lies 33.5 mm (range 18–43 mm) lateral to the midsagittal plane. This artery bifurcates in most cases between the second and fifth cervical vertebrae, although in about 2% of cases the bifurcation was more superior or inferior.

Sinus Caroticus

Binswanger[10] first showed that the carotid bulb was not always located on the origin of the internal carotid artery but might be found at the termination of the common carotid artery or be located so as to include both the origin of the internal and the termination of the common carotid arteries. We evaluated the carotid sinus just before the common carotid artery bifurcated into the external and internal carotid arteries. The right carotid sinus was an average of 14.8 mm (range 10–21 mm) in diameter, and the sinus on the left was 15.2 mm (range 11–20 mm) wide.

Internal Carotid Artery (Fig. 50)

The external width of the left internal carotid artery in our specimens was found to be 6.2 mm (range 4.5–8.0 mm) and on the right side to be 5.9 mm (range 4.0–7.5 mm). The artery bifurcated in most cases between the third and fourth cervical vertebrae. On the left side the bifurcation was slightly inferior to the location of bifurcation on the right. For a description of the variations possible in the origin of the common carotid artery and the twigs of the external artery, see Lang.[79,80]

The internal carotid artery ascends in the lateral parapharyngeal space to the external opening of the carotid canal in the temporal bone. According to Herrshaft,[54] the internal carotid artery may elongate, coil, or kink in 10 to 20% of cases (we found this to be true in only 10% of our specimens). Tortuosities develop in most cases only when arteriosclerosis is present, while coiling of the artery may possibly be a congenital condition, due to lack of stretching of the internal carotid arteries during descent of the carotids.[15]

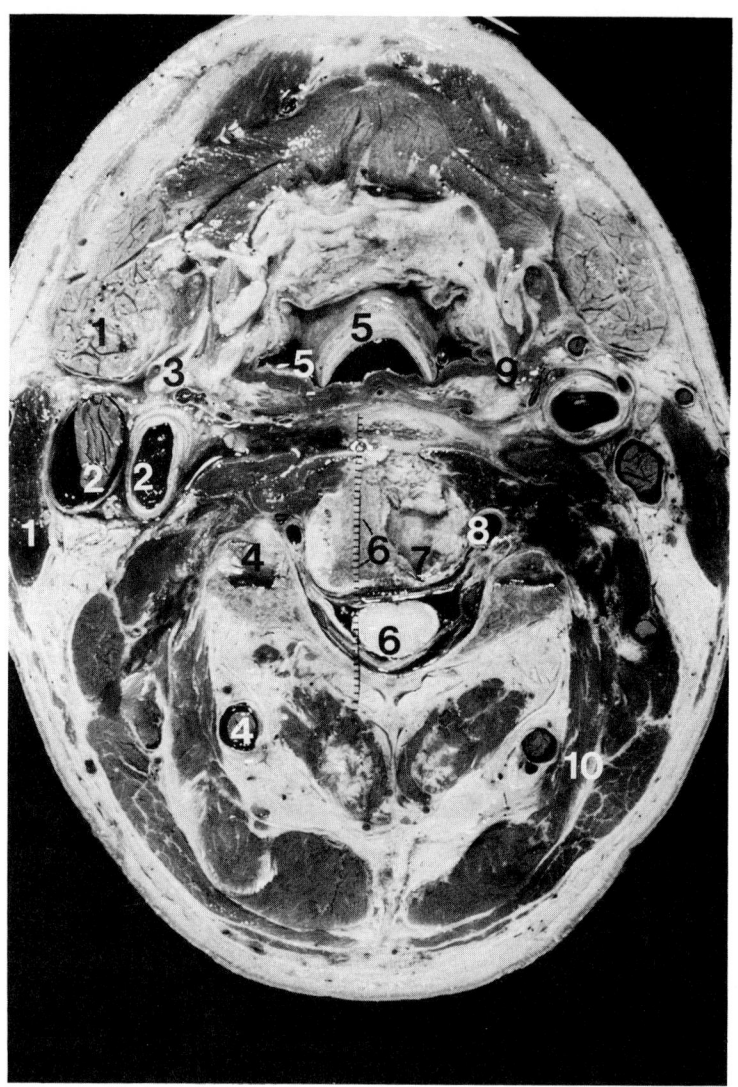

Figure 49: Transverse section through body of third cervical vertebra, viewed from superiorly. 1. Sternocleidomastoid muscle and submandibular gland. 2. Internal jugular vein and common carotid artery. 3. Hypoglossal nerve. 4. Zygapophyseal joint, exposed, and deep cervical vein. 5. Piriform recess and epiglottis. 6. Body of third cervical vertebra, millimeter scale, and spinal cord. 7. Disc between third and fourth cervical vertebrae; body of third cervical vertebra resected. 8. Vertebral artery. 9. Cornu major or hyoid bone. 10. Splenius cervicis muscle.

Kinking of this vessel is most often directed dorsally in the proximal portion and directed ventrally when it is distal. For further details, see Lang.[79,80]

Ascending Pharyngeal Artery (Fig. 51)

We studied 63 head halves, and noted that the ascending pharyngeal artery originated directly as a branch of the external carotid artery in 55.6%.[82] The origin was an average of 12.5 mm (range 6–20 mm) distal to the origin of the external carotid artery. In 11.1% of cases, the ascending pharyngeal artery was a branch of another artery that left the external carotid artery, and in 12.7% of cases the ascending pharyngeal artery originated near the bifurcation of the a. carotis com-

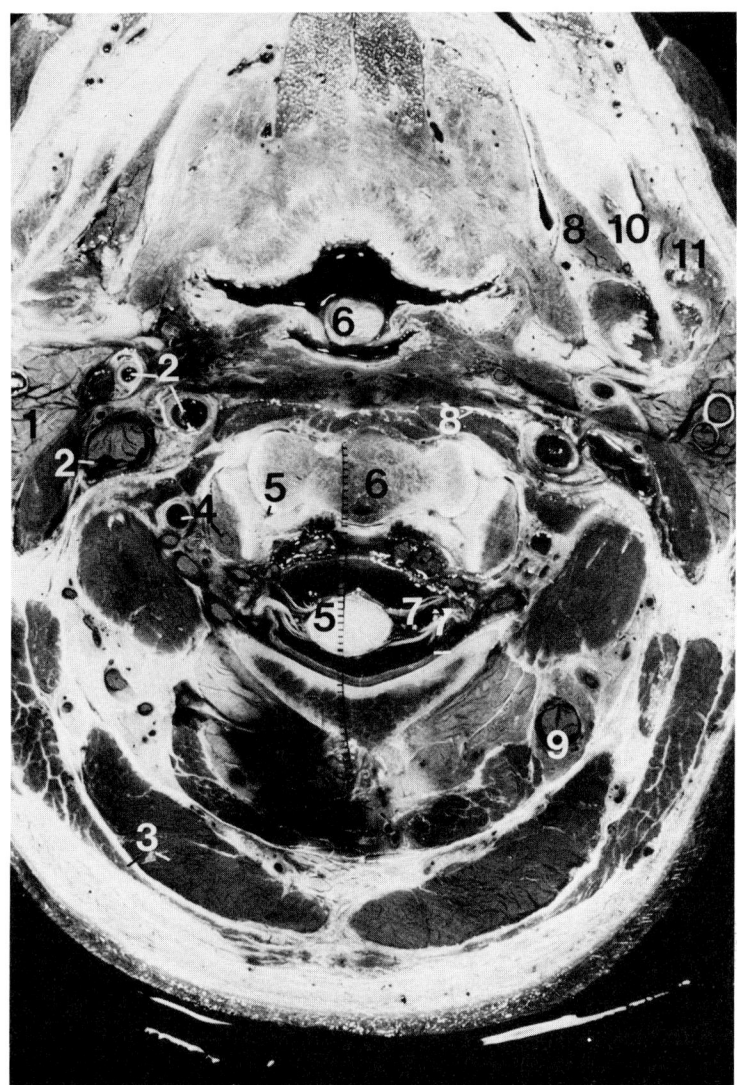

Figure 50: Transverse section through lateral atlantoaxial joint, viewed from below. 1. Parotid gland and digastric muscle. 2. Internal jugular vein and external and internal carotid arteries. 3. Transverse occipital and splenius capitis muscles. 4. Vertebral artery and atlas, cut. 5. Lateral atlantoaxial joint and spinal cord; millimeter scale. 6. Uvula and axis. 7. Ventral and dorsal root fibers of second cervical vertebra. 8. Prevertebral muscles and mylohyoid muscle. 9. Deep cervical vein. 10. Inferior alveolar nerve and artery. 11. Masseter muscle.

munis. In 8% of cases the ascending pharyngeal artery was a twig of the occipital artery, and in about 5% it was a twig of the internal carotid artery, leaving 17.7 mm (range 17–19 mm) distal to the bifurcation of the internal carotid artery. The outer diameter of the ascending pharyngeal artery was found to be 1.57 mm (range 0.9–2.3 mm). If more than one vessel had developed (accessory ascending pharyngeal arteries), one had a smaller diameter.

Ascending Pharyngeal Artery, Course

In most cases this artery runs in a straight course or with only slight deviations superior to the internal carotid artery. In 39% of cases, however, the artery

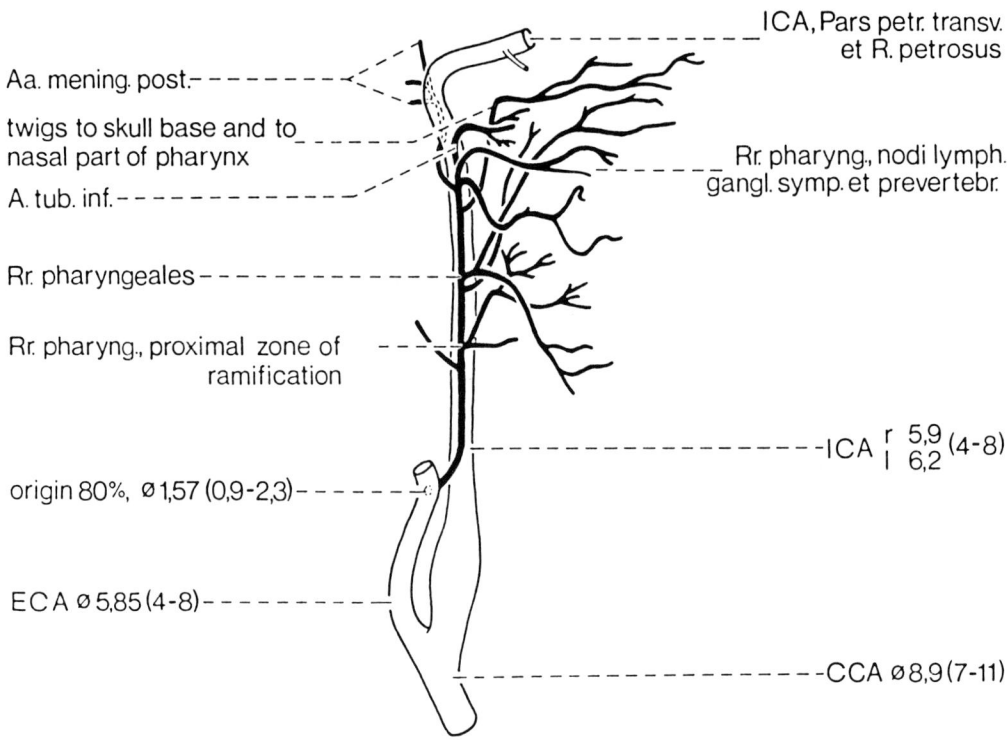

Figure 51: Origin and main twigs of ascending pharyngeal artery. Outer diameters of arteries are shown in millimeters (range).

ran medial to, and in 35%, medioanterior to, the internal carotid artery. In about 9% of our specimens, the vessel was found lateral to the internal carotid artery, and in 7.5%, it was laterorostral. In 9.25% of specimens the proximal two-thirds of the course of the ascending pharyngeal artery ran rostral to the internal carotid artery.

In approximately 80% of the cases we studied, the ascending pharyngeal artery divided 13 to 33 mm distal to its origin into twigs that ran to the muscles of the pharynx, to the tenth and twelfth cranial nerves, to the sympathetic trunk, and to lymph nodes in the para- and retropharyngeal spaces. Other twigs may extend to the pharyngeal tonsilla and to the auditory tube, to the cranial base, and to the foramina of the posterior cranial fossa. In addition, the mm. longus capitis, longus colli, and anterior rectus muscle are supplied by this vessel. Branches of the ascending pharyngeal artery may also be observed running medial to the styloglossus, stylopharyngeal, and stylohyoid muscles.

In 50% of cases we saw one branch of the ascending pharyngeal artery to the jugular foramen, two branches were present in 37.5% of cases, and three branches were seen in 10.5% of cases. These represent meningeal branches to the posterior cranial fossa (dura and bone). They were 0.63 mm (range 0.2–1.1 mm) in diameter, and most originated in the intracranial portion of the ascending pharyngeal artery, although in 30% of cases the vessels were twigs from the middle pharyngeal artery, and in 8% they derived from the proximal distribution of the ascending pharyngeal artery. In about 4% of specimens the branch to the jugular foramen was a twig of the occipital artery.

Two twigs of the ascending pharyngeal artery running to the inferior cranial base were found in about 33% of cases, three were found in 35% of cases, one was found in 19% of cases, and four branches were found in 5.4% of cases. The outer diameter of the twigs averaged 0.62 mm (range 0.3–1.1 mm).

In most cases, twigs of the ascending pharyngeal artery (distal segment) were seen running to the epipharynx, to the pharyngeal tonsilla, and to the auditory tube. In the last case, the vessel anastomosed with the ascending palatine artery, the sphenopalatine artery, and the arterial network in the tympanic cavity.

The *ascending palatine artery* was studied by Lang and Preis.[88] It originated on the facial artery in 71% of cases, and on the external carotid artery in 29% of cases. Its most important branch is the tonsillary branch, which has an outer diameter of 0.79 mm (range 0.5–1.4 mm), but the ramus palatinis branch is important for transpalatine approaches to the clivus in the upper cervical column. This branch was 1.02 mm (range 0.6–1.5 mm) wide in our specimens.

Further branches of this artery run to the medial pterygoid muscle, the fatty corpus adiposum buccae (Bichat), the pharynx, the tensor and levator veli palatini muscles, and the auditory tube. The vessel anastomoses with twigs of the ascending pharyngeal artery, the greater and lesser palatine arteries, and with contralateral vessels. For further details see Lang and Preis.[88]

Parapharyngeal Space: Veins (Fig. 52)

The most important vein in the parapharyngeal space is the internal jugular vein. The bulb of this vein is located anteriorly, at varying distances lateral to the terminal sigmoid margin of the jugular foramen. From this landmark the bulb extends superiorly 8.8 mm (range 5–14 mm) on the right and 8.2 mm (range 5–13 mm) on the left. When an extremely high jugular bulb is situated more medially, it may be found immediately lateral to the inferior area of the internal auditory meatus, and bulge into the floor of the middle ear cavity. The internal jugular vein was estimated to be 11.5 mm (range 5–18 mm) wide in the area of the jugular bulb. Variations of the entrance of the inferior petrosal sinus were discussed earlier.

In their study of 257 temporal bones, Overton and Ritter[114] found the jugular bulb to be elevated (superior to the lower perimeter of the tympanic annulus) in 6 percent. The internal jugular vein normally takes a lateral course in the parapharyngeal space, slightly posterior to the internal carotid artery.

Vertebral Artery and Veins: Prevertebral and Transverse Segments

The prevertebral segment of the vertebral artery is that segment between the artery's origin and the foramen transversarium, which is entered by this artery. This segment was first approached surgically by Crawford et al.[25] to manage lesions causing osteal stenosis.

The transverse segment of this artery is that portion between the foramen transversarium and the C2–C3 intercervical space. This segment was first approached surgically by Kuttner[74] and Oljenick,[112] while Elkin and Harris,[31] Hardin et al.,[47] and Jung[61] used this approach to treat traumatic vertebral arteriovenous aneurysms and neurovascular complications secondary to spondylosis.

Arterial Width

According to Argenson et al.,[6] the right vertebral artery has a mean diameter of 4.4 mm in Africans and 4.3 mm in Europeans, while the left artery has a mean diameter of 5.3 mm in Africans and 4.7 mm in Europeans. A dominant left vertebral artery was present in 37 and a dominant right vertebral artery in 27 of their cases.

Jung and Kehr[62] defined arterial hypoplasia as an arterial diameter of less than 2 mm, measured radiographically, and by incomplete or retarded filling with contrast material on serial x-rays. A "single" vertebral artery refers to total ab-

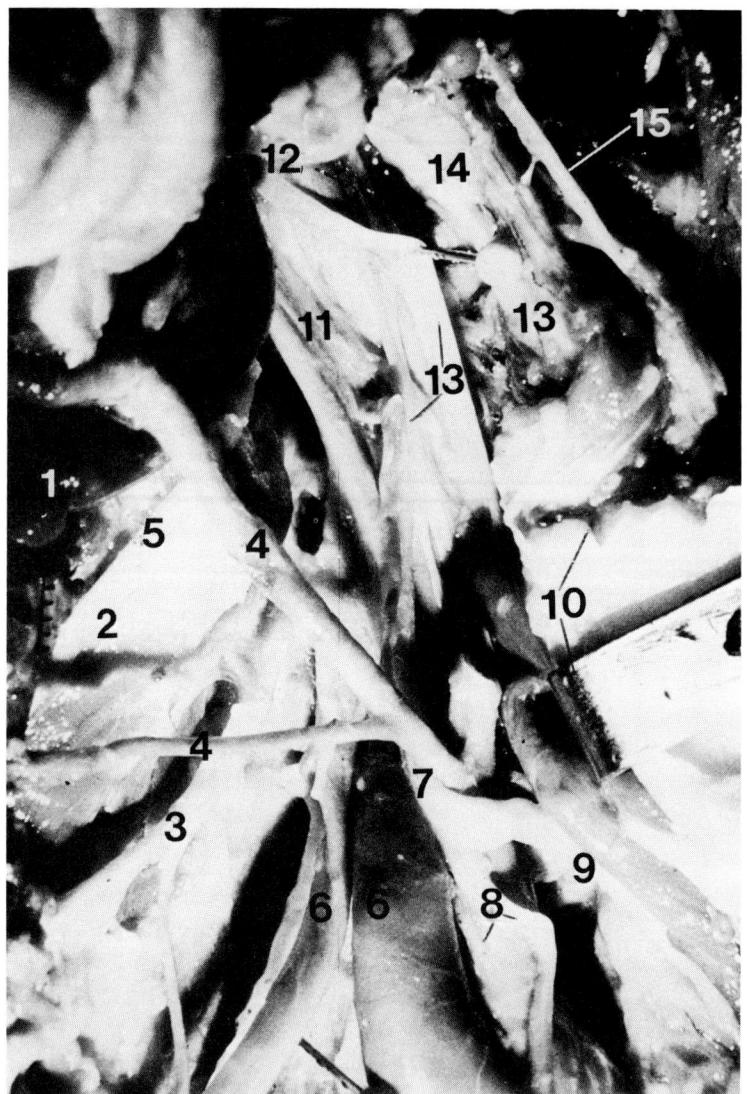

Figure 52: Parapharyngeal space, lateral view. 1. Internal jugular vein, displaced posteriorly. 2. Splenius cervicis muscle. 3. R. ventr. third cervical vertebra. 4. Occipital artery and sternocleidomastoid r. 5. Accessory nerve. 6. Inferior ganglion of the vagus nerve and internal carotid artery. 7. Hypoglossal nerve. 8. External carotid artery and descending branch of twelfth cranial nerve. 9. Thyrohyoid. 10. Mandible, severed and displaced anteriorly. 11. A. pharyngea ascendens. 12. Internal carotid artery; millimeter scale. 13. Glossopharyngeal nerve and twigs, displaced anteriorly. 14. Retroarticular cushion, displaced anteriorly. 15. Twig of inferior alveolar nerve to posterior wall of capsule of the temporomandibular joint (extremely rare variation).

sence of one artery or presence of a nonfunctional (hypoplastic) artery as identified by retarded filling with contrast material on x-ray.[6] Complete absence of the vertebral artery was found by Jung[63] in 2.5% of cases, and functional aplasia of one artery in 6%. Argenson et al.[6] noted unilateral hypoplasia of the vertebral artery in 9.3% of cases on the right and in 3.7% of cases on the left side. Jung[63] found that hypoplasia occurred three times as often on the left as on the right. Bilateral hypoplasia of the vertebral arteries was found in 3.7% of Africans.

Transverse Segment of the Vertebral Artery

Foramen Transversarium (Fig. 53)

In 60 cervical spinal columns from Europeans, the anteroposterior diameter varied only slightly between C6 and C3, from 6.5 to 5.7 mm on the left; the average transverse diameter was more constant, and close to 7 mm. It should be noted that sometimes a posterior depression continued along the transverse sulcus to form a transverse orifice. This orifice, which was studied by different methods, angled sharply from C6 to C3. The communicating rami of the vertebral nerve passed through the orifice toward cervical nerves six, five, four, and, rarely, three.

Transverse Channel: Contents (Fig. 54)

We found the average diameter of the vertebral artery lumen to be only 1 to 2 mm different from that measured by Jung.[61] The artery is surrounded by the vertebral venous system and the sympathetic elements, and lies anteromedially in the channel, in contact with the anterior root of the transverse apophysis, more or less in the region of the uncus.

Normally the artery has an undulating course from one transverse foramen to the other. As it passes between the periosteum of the uncus and the vertebral body, one or more small veins may be interposed. The largest vertebral vein ran between the artery and the periosteum of the anterior bony root of the transverse process in two cases studied.

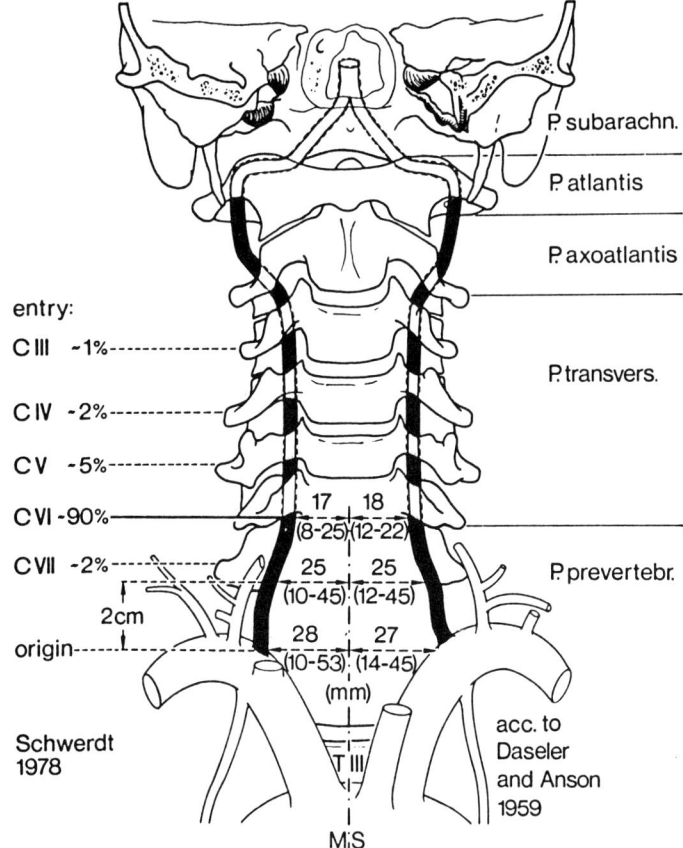

Figure 53: Vertebral artery, showing area of entrance into its canal and distances from the midsagittal plane as estimated from radiographs (the most common origin is shown).

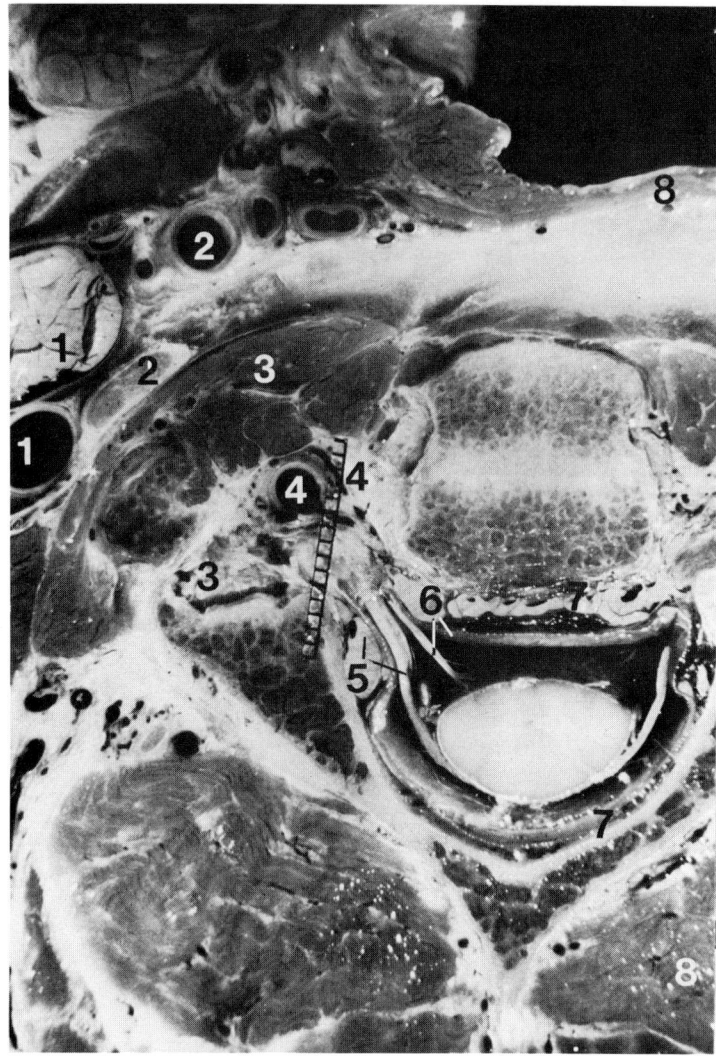

Figure 54: Transverse section through the ganglion of the third cervical vertebra, seen from above. 1. Internal jugular vein and internal carotid artery. 2. Ganglion superior trunci sympathici and external carotid artery. 3. Prevertebral muscles and articulatio zygapophysialis of second/third cervical vertebrae. 4. Vertebral artery and millimeter scale. 5. Intervertebral vein and radix dorsum of third cervical vertebra. 6. Dura and radix ventra. 7. Plexus ven. vertebr, int. ant. and dura. 8. Pharynx, displaced anteriorly, and semispinalis cervicis muscle.

In the upper cervical area, Argenson et al.[6] found a system of venules in the transverse channel. These venules come together at C5 in 30% of cases, and at C6 in 50%, to form one or two veins of variable diameter, before emerging at C7 in 40% of cases, at C6 in 50%, or at C5 in 10% of cases. In only 20% of the cases did the veins continue, one to the last centimeter of the intratransverse course.

Collaterals at Each Intertransverse Space

Posteromedially, the vertebral veins receive the veins of the intervertebral foramina, which spread around the spinal nerve and radicular arteries to form a venous channel that may attain a diameter of 10 mm and forms an anastomosis between the anterior longitudinal intraspinal plexus and the vertebrotransverse sinus.

Posterolaterally, the sinus anastomoses with a knot of transverse venules that may run posteriorly toward the posterior jugular vein (v. jugularis posterior).

Anteromedially, in the superior portion of the intertransverse space, the venous sinus may give off transverse branches anterior to the vertebral bodies. The longitudinal rami of these branches have been seen to form a descending cervical vein along the vertebral bodies, which often ended in the terminal segment of the vertebral vein.

The vertebral nerve in the specimens studied by Argenson et al.[6] was almost always located on the posterior or posteromedial surface of the artery, against the adventitia, to which it adheres. Therefore, it lies in direct contact with the disc or uncus. The transverse diameter of the nerve was measured to be 1 to 2 mm, and its posterior diameter to be 0.8 mm. In one case these researchers found a swelling resembling a ganglion in the region of the fifth cervical segment. The nerve diameter decreased rapidly at the level of C5, quite rarely at C3, to become lost to view. According to other researchers, the filaments in this area form at least one nerve plexus around the artery, and at each level the vertebral nerve sends out filaments to the nerve plexus of the artery.

The communicating rami to the spinal roots may be seen to arise in the intertransverse spaces, to ascend the anterior surface of the posterior articular complex, and then to traverse the transverse foramen lying superiorly, to finally come in contact with its posterior edge. They then join the corresponding cervical spine nerve. Often the rami produce a notch in the transverse groove, which on occasion gives rise to an accessory foramen by ossification of the fibroperiosteal covering on its anterior surface. Normally the communicating ramus is accompanied by a venule.[122]

Superior Vertebral Nerves of Guerrier[41]

The superior vertebral nerves of Guerrier contain twigs of the middle cervical ganglion, the superior cervical ganglion, or the interganglionic rami. They run transversely medially, crossing the anterior surface of the anterior intertransverse channel along the external surface of the uncovertebral apophysis. In most cases these nerves are twigs of the middle cervical ganglion or branch off directly from the inferiorly or superiorly adjacent sympathetic root; they rejoin the transverse channel at C4/C5 or C5/C6. Sometimes sympathetic ganglia were found in the transverse canal.[6,27,41]

Uncoarterioradicular Junction

The uncus, artery, and radicle meet at the exit zone of the intervertebral foramen. Anglo-Saxon authors call the sulbus nervi spinalis the "bony gargoyle."

The root of the transverse process of the vertebral body is usually found between C2/C3 and C5/C6. Superiorly, the inferior surface of the transverse process and the anterior wall are formed by the posterior interapophyseals. The anterior medial wall of the passage is composed of a succession of uncovertebral joints, and when a degenerative disc lesion is present they may form a disco-osteophytic nodule that impinges on the spinal roots and causes brachialgia. Anterolaterally, the junction bulges toward the transverse channel, flattening or even causing a depression on the medial surface of the vertebral artery, thereby greatly reducing the functional diameter of the lumen, by up to four-fifths in some cases examined by Argenson et al.[6] These investigators noted that the artery was attached to the uncus, adhering to its periosteum, and thus subject to osteophytic compression because it was separated from the bone by only an average distance of less than 1 mm, and not protected by a venous system medially.

Atlantoaxial Part

The atlantoaxial portion of the vertebral artery courses slightly laterally, between the third and second transverse processes of the cervical vertebrae. It winds in a variable path between the second and the first vertebrae. In our specimens, we found, between the axis and the atlas, anteriorly curving arteries that were indented by the ventral branch of the second cervical nerve. The ventral artery in this segment has extra length, permitting head and atlas rotations. However, it seems possible that excessive length of this segment of the artery may cause a deficit in the blood supply to several brain structures, especially the vestibular nuclei.

Atlantic Part

After passing the transverse foramen of the first cervical vertebra, the vertebral artery courses dorsomedially in the sulcus a. vertebralis of the atlas, surrounded by the venous plexus. Then the vessel usually curves sharply ventrally to pierce the atlanto-occipital membrane, the dura mater, and the arachnoid membrane.

In about 10% of specimens, a ponticulus of the atlas is present, which overlaps the vertebral artery and the vertebral vein. There are posterior and lateral ponticuli, defined by their positions (for further details see Lang[77,78,80]). It should be remembered that the walls of the internal carotid artery and the vertebral artery become significantly thinner between their extracranial and intracranial courses. In addition to this thinning of the wall in the tunica media, relatively more muscle tissue and less elastic and collagen material were found intracranially than extracranially.[75]

Variations

Persistent Hypoglossal Artery

Until 1966, persistence of the hypoglossal artery had been demonstrated in only four pathological specimens.[8,107,110,132] In the case described by Morris and Moffat,[107] the persistent hypoglossal artery originated on the internal carotid artery, 13 mm inferior to the massa lateralis atlantis. The diameter of this vessel was 4.5 mm, and the diameter of the internal carotid artery 4.3 mm. The persistent hypoglossal artery extended to the hypoglossal channel, through this channel, and intracranially, to run first caudally, then dorsomedially, and finally rostrally. From this vessel, a small branch was seen to run extracranially to the suboccipital region, and intracranial branches included the anterior spinal artery and all of the arteries that in other cases arise from the posterior inferior cerebellar artery, except the labyrinthine artery. The final branches of the vessel were the posterior cerebral arteries. The left vertebral artery had a diameter of 1.4 mm in the specimens studied, and branched from the aortic arch between the origins of the a. carotis communis and the left subclavian artery. The right vertebral artery had a diameter of 1.2 mm, and gave off the posterior spinal artery and the posterior inferior cerebellar artery. More distally, the vessel united with the persistent hypoglossal artery.

During embryonic development, the hypoglossal artery connects a portion of the dorsal aorta to the developing basilar artery (longitudinal neural artery) and the primitive lateral basilovertebral anastomoses in the region of the hypoglossal nerve rootlets. The hypoglossal artery normally regresses at the 8-mm stage, when the embryological basilar artery receives its main blood supply from the proatlantal artery, or embryological fourth intersegmental artery. This artery then becomes correspondingly larger. The vertebral artery develops during the 7- to 9-mm stage by fusion of the cervical intersegmental arteries, and is completed by fusion with the proatlantal artery rostrally and with the seventh cervical intersegmental artery caudally, which becomes the subclavian artery later in development.[22,26,115]

Blain and Logothetis[11] described a 46-year-old white woman who seized when moving her head and eyes to the left; she also evidenced chewing movements and had a positive Babinski's sign. An anomalous hypoglossal artery was found: it lay lateral and dorsal to the hypoglossal nerve rootlets, in contrast to the embryological stage when it lies medial and ventral to the nerve rootlets.

Several researchers have demonstrated persistent hypoglossal arteries angiographically since 1961: Bruetman and Fields,[16] Jackson,[59] Gerlach et al.,[38] and others. Springer et al.[129] demonstrated an aneurysm at the origin of the superior cerebellar artery in a patient with a primitive hypoglossal artery, and Udvarhelyi and Lai[140] recorded a subarachnoid hemorrhage due to rupture of an aneurysm on a persistent left hypoglossal artery.

According to Springer et al.,[129] persistence of the hypoglossal artery has been reported in 24 cases, and may be seen on 0.1 to 0.2% of angiograms. According to Lie,[100] the anatomy and angiographic presentation of the primitive hypoglossal artery may take one of four forms:

1. the artery arises from the internal carotid artery at C1–C3;
2. the artery enters the skull via the hypoglossal channel (anterior condyloid foramen);
3. the basilar artery is filled only beyond the point where the hypoglossal artery enters it; or
4. the posterior communicating artery is absent. Usually the vertebral artery is either absent on the ipsilateral side and hypoplastic on the opposite side, or hypoplastic on both sides.

Proatlantal Intersegmental Artery with Absence of Bilateral Vertebral Arteries

The proatlantal intersegmental artery originates from the internal carotid artery, curves dorsally, and courses between the atlas and occiput to join the stem of the basilar artery.[50] Normally this and the other anastomotic channels between the carotid and basilar circulatory systems involute by 35 to 40 days of gestation,[115] but persisting proatlantal arteries were demonstrated by Abe and Suzuki,[1] Anderson and Sondheimer,[5] and Hutchinson and Miller.[52]

According to Anderson and Sondheimer,[5] the proatlantal artery curves sharply dorsally to rest upon the superior aspect of the transverse process of the atlas. Its suboccipital horizontal course is identical to that of the vertebral artery, except that it does not pass through the foramen transversarium of any vertebra. The proatlantal artery originates from the external carotid artery or the internal carotid artery, and enters the skull through the foramen magnum. The vertebral arteries may be absent or hypoplastic.

References

1. Abe K, Suzuki T: Persistence of embryonic carotid vertebrobasilar anastomoses. *Folia Psychiatr Neurol Jpn* 18:257-276, 1964.
2. Adachi B: Das Arteriensystem der Japaner, I. and II. Verlag der Kaiserlich-Japanischen Universitat, 1928.
3. Alyea OE, Van: Ethmoid labyrinth. *Arch Otolaryngol* 29:881-902, 1939.
4. Alyea OE, Van: Sphenoid sinus anatomic study with consideration of the clinical significance of the structural characteristics of the sphenoid sinus. *Arch Otolaryngol* 34:225-253, 1941.
5. Anderson RA, Sondheimer FK: Rare carotid-vertebrobasilar anastomoses with notes on the differentiation between proatlantal and hypoglossal arteries. *Neuroradiology* 11:113-118, 1976.
6. Argenson C, Francke J, Sylla S, et al: The vertebral arteries (segments V_1 and V_2). *Anat Clin* 2:29-41, 1980.
7. Bartels P: Uber Geschlechtsunterschiede am Schadel. Inaug. Diss. Berlin, 1897.
8. Batujeff N: Eine seltene Arterienanomalie (Ursprung der A. basilaris aus der A. carotis interna), 1889.
9. Becker RF, Grunt JA: The cervical sympathetic ganglia. *Anat Rec* 127:1-14, 1957.
10. Binswanger: Anatomische Untersuchungen uber die Ursprungsstelle und den Anfangsteil der Carotis interna. *Arch Psychiatr* 9:351, 1879.
11. Blain JG, Logothetis J: The persistent hypoglossal artery. *J Neurol Neurosurg Psychiatr* 29:346-349, 1966.
12. Blumenbach JF: Geschichte und Beschreibung der Knochen des menschlichen Korpers. Gottingen, Dietrich, 1786.

13. Bolk L: Die verschiedenen Formen des Condylus tertius und ihre Entstehungsursachen. *Anat Anz* 54:335-347, 1921.
14. Brauecker W: Neue Untersuchungsergebnisse uber das pressorezeptorische Nervensystem und seine praktische Bedeutung in der Chirurgie. *Zentralbl Chir* 15:854-857, 1933.
15. Brosig HJ, Vollmar J: Chirurgische Korrektur der Knickstenosen der A. carotis interna. *Munch Med Wochenschr* 116/19, 1974.
16. Bruetman ME, Fields WS: Persistent hypoglossal artery. *Arch Neurol* 8:369-372, 1963.
17. Burns A: Observations on the surgical anatomy of the head and neck, Edinburg, 1811, In Merkel, F: Uber die Halsfascie. *Anat Hefte* 1:77-111, 1892.
18. Bystrow AP: Assimilation des Atlas und Manifestaton des Proatlas. *Z Anat Entwicklungsgesch* 95:210-242, 1931.
19. Casberg MA: The clinical significance of the cervical fascial planes. *Surg Clin North Am* 30:1415-1434, 1950.
20. Chorobsky J, Penfield W: Cerebral vasodilator nerves and their pathway from the medulla oblongata: With observations on the pial and intracerebral vascular plexus. *Arch Neurol Psychiatr* 28:1257-1289, 1932.
21. Coller FA, Yglesias L: Infections of the lip and face. *Surg Gyn Obstet* 60:277-290, 1935.
22. Congdon ED: Transformation of the aortic arch system during the development of the human embryo. *Contrib Embryol Carnegie Inst* 14:47-110, 1922.
23. Cope VZ: The internal structure of the sphenoid sinus. *J Anat* 51:127-136, 1917.
24. Corner EM: The processes of the occipital and mastoid regions of the skull. *J Anat Physiol* 30:386-388, 1896.
25. Crawford E, de Baker M, Fields W: Roentgenographic diagnosis and surgical treatment of basilar artery insufficiency. *JAMA* 168:509-514, 1958.
26. Dandy WE: *Intracranial Arterial Aneurysms*, New York, Comstock Publishing Co, 1944.
27. Dechaume J, Antonietti C, Bouvier A, et al: Sympathique et arthrose cervicales. *Doc Anat J Med* (Lyon) 42:493-530, 1961.
28. Dittel L: Die Topographie der Halsfascien, Wien, 1857, In Grodinsky M, Holyoke EA: The fasciae and fascial space of the head, neck and adjacent regions. *Am J Anat* 63:367-408, 1938.
29. Dubreuil-Chambardel: Variationes sexuelles de l'atlas. *Bull Soc Anthropol* (Paris) 5 and 8, 1907.
30. Ebbesson SOE: Quantitative studies of superior cervical sympathetic ganglia in a variety of primates including man. I. The ratio of preganglionic fibers to ganglionic neurons. *Gegenbaurs Morphol Jahrb* 124:117-131, 1968.
31. Elkin DC, Harris MH: Arteriovenous aneurysm of the vertebral vessels: Report of 10 cases. *Ann Surg* 124:934-951, 1946.
32. Ferris EB, Capps RB, Weiss S: Relation of the carotid sinus to the autonomic nervous system and the neuroses. *Arch Neurol Psychiatr* 37:365-384, 1937.
33. Fitzgerald MJT, Law ME: The peripheral connections between the lingual and hypoglossal nerves. *J Anat* 92:178-188, 1958.
34. Frommer J: Anatomic variations in the stylohyoid chain and their possible clinical significance. *Oral Surg* 38/5:659-667, 1974.
35. Fuchs E: Untersuchung uber die Gelenkflachen der Articulatio atlantooccipitalis. Inaug Diss Wurzburg, 1980.
36. Fujii K, Lenkey C, Rhoton AL: Microsurgical anatomy of the choroidal arteries, fourth ventricle and cerebellopontine angles. *J Neurosurg* 52:504-524, 1980.
37. Gaughran GRL: Fasciae of the masticator space. *Anat Rec* 129:383-400, 1957.
38. Gerlach J, Jensen HP, Spuler H, et al: Traumatic caroticocavernous fistula combined with persisting primitive hypoglossal artery. *J Neurosurg* 20:885-887, 1963.
39. Grodinsky M, Holyoke EA: The fasciae and fascial space of the head, neck and adjacent regions. *Am J Anat* 63:367-408, 1938.
40. Grunbaum AS: Some points in the anatomy of the suboccipital region. *J Anat Physiol* 25:428-432, 1891.
41. Guerrier Y: Le sympathique cervical. These Medecine, Montpellier, 1944.
42. Guild SR: A hitherto unrecognized structure, the glomus jugularis in man. *Anat Rec* 79:29, 1941.
43. Gutmann G: *Die Halswirbelsaule. Die funktionsanalytische Rontgendiagnostic*, Stuttgart, Fischer, 1981.
44. Hall C: The parapharyngeal space: An anatomical and clinical study. *Ann Otol Rhinol Laryngol* 43:793-812, 1934.
45. Hamberger CA, Hammer G, Norlen G, et al: Surgical treatment of acromegaly. *Acta Otolaryngol* (Stockh) (Suppl) 158:168-172, 1960.

46. Hammer G, Radberg C: The sphenoidal sinus. *Acta Radiol* 56:401-422, 1961.
47. Hardin C, Williamson W, Steegmann A: Vertebral artery insufficiency produced by cervical osteoarthritic spurs. *Neurology* 10:855-858, 1960.
48. Hardy J: Transsphenoidal microsurgery of the normal and pathological pituitary. *Clin Neurosurg* 16:185-217, 1969.
49. Hasebe K: Die Wirbelsaule der Japaner. *A Morphol Anthropol* 15, 1913.
50. Hayashi K, Yabuki T, Kurokawa T, et al: The anterior and the posterior ligaments of the lower cervical spine. *J Anat* 124:633-636, 1977.
51. Hayek M: Pathologie und Therapie der entzundlishen Erkrankungen der Nebenhohle der Nase. Leipzig, Wien, Deutige, 1909.
52. Helms J: Uber den Winkel zwischen Dens und Epistropheus. Inaug Diss Munchen, 1963.
53. Henle J: *Handbuch der Systematischen Anatomie des Menschen*, Vol 3, Part II, Vieweg Braunschweig, 1871.
54. Herrschaft H: Cerebral Durchblutungsstorungen bei extremer Schlingenbildung der A. carotis interna. *Munch Med Wschr* 46:2694-2702, 1968.
55. Honee GLJM: The anatomy of the lateral pterygoid muscle. *Acta Morphol Neerl Scand* 10:331-340, 1972.
56. Hutchinson NA, Miller DR: Persistent proatlantal artery. *J Neurol Psychiatr* 33:524-527, 1970.
57. Hyrtl J: Wahre und Falsche Schaltknochen in der Pars orbitaria des Stirnbeines. *Sitzb Akad Wissensch* 42:213, 1860.
58. Ingelmark BE: Uber das craniovertebrale Grenzgebiet beim Menschen. *Acta Anat (Suppl)* 6:1-116, 1947.
59. Jackson FE: Syncope associated with persistent hypoglossal artery: Case report. *J Neurosurg* 21:139-141, 1964.
60. Johnson RM, Hart DL, Simmons EF, et al: Cervical orthoses: a study comparing their effectiveness in restricting cervical motion in normal subjects. *J Bone Joint Surg* 59/3:332-339, 1977.
61. Jung A: Resection de l'articulation uncovertebrale et ouverture de trou de conjugaison par boie anterieure dans le traitment de la neuralgie cervicobrachiale. Technique operatoire. *Mem Acad Chir* 89:361-367, 1963.
62. Jung A, Kehr P: *Pathologie de l'Artere Vertebrale et des Racines Nerveuses dans les Arthrose et les Traumatismes du Rachis Cervical*, Paris, Masson, 1972.
63. Jung FM: Les traumatismes du rachis cervical avec lesions de l'artere vertebral. These Medecine, Trasbourg, 1974.
64. Juniper RP: The superior pterygoid muscle. *Br J Oral Surg* 19:121-128, 1981.
65. Kamieth H: Ein nicht sicher einzuordnender Knochenkeil am Unterrand des Clivus. *Rofo* 91:334-339, 1959.
66. Kamieth H: Ventrales Okzipitalwirbelrudiment, verbunden mit einer Assimilisation eines Ossibulum terminale mit dem verderen Atlasbogen. *Rofo* 119:632-633, 1973.
67. Kerr FWL: Facial, vagal, and glossopharyngeal nerves in the cat. *Arch Neurol (NY)* 6:264-281, 1962.
68. Kleinsasser O: Das Glomus laryngicum inferior. Ein bisher unbekanntes nicht chromaffines Paraganglion vom Bau der sog. Carotisdruse im Menschlichen Kehlkopf. *Arch Ohr Nas Kehlk Heilk* 184:214-224, 1964.
69. Knese KH: Kopfgelenk, Kopfhaltung und Kopfbewegung des Menschen. *Z Anat Entwicklungsgesch* 114:67-107, 1949/50.
70. Krauss J: Wissenschaftliche Arbeit am Anatomischen Institut Wurzburg, 1985.
71. Krayenbuhl H, Yasargil MG: *Die Zerebrale Angiographie*. Stuttgart, Georg Thieme Verlag, 1965.
72. Krizan A: Beitrage zur deskriptiven und topographischen Anatomie der A. maxillaris. *Acta Anat* 41:319-333, 1960a.
73. Krizan A: Uber die fraglichen Korrelationen und uber die Entwicklung einiger Typen der A. maxillaris. *Acta Anat* 42:71-87, 1960b.
74. Kuttner E: Die Verletzungen und traumatischen Aneurysmen der Vertebralgefasse am Halse und ihre operative Behandlung. *Beit Klin Chir* 108:1-160, 1917.
75. Lang J: Feinstruktur der Arterienwand. *Verh Dtsch Kreislaufforschg* 40:1-14, 1974.
76. Lang J (ed): *Praktische Anatomie*, New York, Berlin, Springer Verlag, 1979.
77. Lang J: *Klinische Anatomie des Kopfes: Neurokranium, Orbita, kraniozervikaler Ubergang*, Berlin, Heidelberg, Springer Verlag, 1981.
78. Lang J: *Clinical Anatomy of the Head: Neurocranium, Orbit, Craniocervical Regions*, Wilson RR, Winstanley DP (trans), New York, Springer Verlag, 1983.
79. Lang J: Zur Anatomie und Topographie der A. vertebralis. In Gutmann G von (ed): *Arteria Vertebralis: Traumatologie und Funktionelle Pathologie*, Berlin, Heidelberg, New York, Tokyo, Springer

Verlag, 1985, pp 3-63.
80. Lang J: *Craniocervical Region, Osteology and Articulations*, Vienna, Springer Verlag, 1985.
81. Lang J, Baldauf R: Beitrag zur Gefassversorgung des Ruckenmarks. *Gegenbaurs Morphol Jahrb* 129:57-95, 1983.
82. Lang J, Heilek E: Anatomische-klinische Befunde zur A. pharyngea ascendens. *Anat Anz* 156:177-207, 1984.
83. Lang J, Hetterich A: Beitrag zur postnatalen Entwincklung des Processus pterygoideus. *Anat Anz* 154:1-32, 1983.
84. Lang J, Keller H: Uber die hintere Pfortenregion der Fossa pterygopalatina und die Lage des Ganglion pterygopalatinum. *Gegenbaurs Morphol Jahrb* 124:207-214, 1978.
85. Lang J, Niederfeilner J: About the face of the cleft of the articulus mandibulae. *Anat Anz* 141:398-400, 1977.
86. Lang J, Oder M: Uber die Biomorphose der Mandibula. *Gegenbaurs Morphol Jahrb* 130:185-234, 1984.
87. Lang J, Papke J: Uber die klinische Anatomie des Paries inferior orbitae und dessen Nachbarstrukturen. *Gegenbaurs Morphol Jahrb* 130:1-47, 1984.
88. Lang J, Preis KH: A. palatina ascendes, Ursprung, Verlauf und Zweige. *HNO* 29:391-396, 1981.
89. Lang J, Reiter U: Uber die intrazisternale Lange der Hirnnerven VII-XII. *Neurochirurgia* 28:153-157, 1985.
90. Lang J, Sakals E: Uber den Recessus sphenoethmoidalis, die Apertura nasalis des Ductus nasolacrimalis und den Hiatus semilunaris. *Anat Anz* 152:393-412, 1982.
91. Lang J, Schafhauser O, Hofmann S: Uber die postnatale Entwicklung der transbasalen Schadelpforten: Canalis caroticus, Foramen jugulare, Canalis hypoglossalis, Canalis condylaris und Foramen magnum. *Anat Anz* 153:315-357, 1983.
92. Lang J, Schiller A: Caput mandibulae: Anteversio, Flachenwert und Scheitelkrummungsradius. *Verh Anat Ges* 70:605-612, 1976.
93. Lang J, Schlehahn FA: Uber die postnatale Entwicklung der Fissurae orbitales. *Gegenbaurs Morphol Jahrb* 127:849-859, 1981.
94. Lang J, Schreiber T: Uber Form and Lage des Foramen jugulare (Fossa jugularis), des Canalis caroticus und des Foramen stylomastoideum sowie deren postnatale Lageveranderungen. *HNO* 31:80-87, 1983.
95. Lang J, Tisch-Rottensteiner KF: Uber Form und Formvarianten der Sella turcica. *Verh Anat Ges* 71:1279-1282, 1977.
96. Lanz T, Wachsmuth W: In Lang J (ed): *Praktische Anatomie: Ein Lehr- und Hilfsbuch der Anatomischen Grundlagen Arztlichen Handelns*, Vol. 1, Part IB, Berlin, Heidelberg, New York, Springer Verlag, 1979.
97. Lauber H: Ein Fall von teilweiser persistenz der hinteren Cardinal-venen beim Menschen. *Anat Anz* 19:590-594, 1901.
98. Lazorthes G: *Vascularisation et Circulation Cerebrales*, Paris, Masson, 1961.
99. Lesoine W: Das Stylo-Kerato-Hyoidale Syndrom. *D A* 38:2381, 1976.
100. Lie TA: Congenital anomalies of the carotid arteries including the carotid-vertebral anastomoses; an angiographic study and review of the literature. Amsterdam, Excerpta Medica, 1968.
101. Lowy R: Uber das topographische Verhalten des Nervus hypoglossus zur Vena jugularis interna. *Anat Anz* 37:10-12, 1910.
102. MacAlister A: Notes on the development and variations of the atlas. *J Anat Physiol* (Lond) 27:518-542, 1893.
103. Merkel F: Uber die Halsfascie. *Anat Hefte* 1:77-111, 1892.
104. Meuer HW: Anatomische Befunde zu den Aa. thyreoideae. Inaug. Diss. Wurzburg, 1983.
105. Misch M: *Beitrage zur Kenntnis der Gelenkfortsatze des Menschlichen Hinterhauptes und der Varietaten in Ihrem Bereich*, Berlin, Gunther, 1905.
106. Mizuno N, Akimoto C, Mochizuki K, et al: Experimental studies of afferent fibers in the hypoglossal nerve in the cat: A scanning electron microscopic observation on the lingual mucosa following transection of the nerve, and a degeneration study with silver impregnation methods. *Arch Histol Jap* 35:99-113, 1973.
107. Morris ED, Moffat DB: Abnormal origin of the basilar artery from the cervical part of the internal carotid and its embryological significance. *Anat Rec* 125:701-711, 1956.
108. Muller T: Uber die Verbreitung des N. glossopharyngeus im Bereich des Gaumens und die Anastomosen des N. hypoglossus im Spatium parapharyngeum. Inaug. Diss. Wurzburg, 1985.
109. Nomura S, Mizuno N: Central distribution of afferent and efferent components of the glossopharyngeal nerve: An HRP

study in the cat. *Brain Res* 236:1-13, 1982.
110. Oertel P: Uber die Persistenz embryonaler Verbindungen zwischen der A. carotis interna und der A. vertebralis cerebralis. *Verh Anat Ges* 31:281-295, 1922.
111. Oliveira Y, de: Le processus retroarticulaire ou tubercule retromandibulaire du squelette cranien chez l'homme. *Acta Anat* 104:211-219, 1979.
112. Oljenick I: Uber die Unterbindung der arteria vertebralis. *Zentralbl Chir* 44:1067-1069, 1917.
113. Onishi T: Bony defects and dehiscences of the roof of the ethmoid cells. *Rhinology* 19:195-202, 1981.
114. Overton SB, Ritter FN: A high-placed jugular bulb in the middle ear. A clinical and temporal bone study. *Laryngoscope* 83:1986-1991, 1973.
115. Padget DH: The development of the cranial arteries in the human embryo. *Contr Embryol Carnegie Inst* 212/32:205-261, 1948.
116. Pearson BW, MacKenzie RG, Goodman WS: The anatomical basis of transantral ligation of the maxillary artery in severe epistaxis. *Laryngoscope* 79/1:969-984, 1969.
117. Peterson H: Braus' Lehrbuch der Anatomie. *Roux Arch Entwicklungsmech* 106:26-32, 1925.
118. Platzer W: Zur Anatomie der 'Sellabrucke' und ihrer Beziehung zur A. carotis interna. *Rofo* 87:613-616, 1957.
119. Platzer W: Die Variabilitat der Arteria carotis internal im Sinus cavernosus in Beziehung zur Variabilitat der Schadelbasis. *Gegenbaurs Morphol Jahrb* 98:220-243, 1957.
120. Pousen K: Uber die Fascien und die interfascialen Raume des Halses. *Z Chir* 23:223-272, 1886.
121. Rankow RM: Congential aneurysm of the maxillary artery. *Plast Reconstr Surg* 37:291-294, 1966.
122. Remy I: Anatomie du canal transversaire. These Medecine, Lille, 1971.
123. Renn WH, Rhoton AL: Microsurgical anatomy of the sellar region. *J Neurosurg* 43:288-298, 1975.
124. Sauser G: Intrakraniale Manifestation des letzten Occipital-Wirbels. *Z Anat Entwicklungsgesch* 104:159-168, 1935.
125. Schmidt T: Der Canalis hypoglossi, Topographie, Form, Lange, Durchmesser und Volumen. Inaug. Diss. Wurzburg, 1975.
126. Seftel DM, Kolson H, Gordon BS: Ruptured intracranial carotid artery aneurysm with fatal epistaxis. *Arch Otolaryngol* 70:52-60, 1959.
127. Seydel O: Uber die Nasenhohle der hoheren Saugethiere und des Menschen. *Gegenbaurs Morphol Jahrb* 17:44-99, 1891.
128. Singer E: *Fasciae of the Human Body and their Relation to the Organs They Envelop*, Baltimore, Williams & Wilkins Company, 1935.
129. Springer TD, Fishbone G, Shapiro R: Persistent hypoglossal artery associated with superior cerebellar artery aneurysm. *J Neurosurg* 40:397-399, 1974.
130. Stofft E: Das Ligamentum transversum atlantis als funktionell-strukturierter Dens-Halteapparat. *Anat Anz* 123:157-168, 1968.
131. Sunder-Plassmann P: Untersuchungen uber den Bulbus carotidis bei Mensch und Tier im Hinblick auf die 'Sinusreflexe' nach HE Hering; ein Vergleich mit anderen Gefassstrecken; die Histopathologie des Bulbus carotidis; das Glomus caroticum. *Z Anat Entwicklungsgesch* 93:567-622, 1930.
132. Sutton D: Anomalous carotid-basilar Anastomosis. *Br J Radiol* 23:617-619, 1950.
133. Tandler J: Die Entwicklung der Lagebeziehung zwischen N. accessorius und V. jugularis interna beim Menschen. *Anat Anz* 31:473-480, 1907.
134. Terracol J, Corone A, Guerrier Y: *La Trompe d'Eustache*, Paris, Masson, 1949.
135. Tischendorf F: Zur Frage der Manifestation des Occipitalwirbels beim Menschen. *Anat Anz* 102:217-223, 1955/56.
136. Toldt C: Osteologische Mitteilung. 1. Entstehung und Ausbildung der Conchae und des Sinus sphenoidalis etc. *Lotus Jahrb Naturwiss* Parts 3,4 61:1-20, 1882.
137. Toro I, Szepe L: Untersuchungen uber die Frage der Assimilation und Manifestation des Atlas. *Z Anat Entwicklungsgesch* 111:186-200, 1942.
138. Truffert P: Les espaces peripharynges. Les voies d'acces les suppurations qui s y developpent. *Press Med* 55:580-581, 1924.
139. Tsusaki T: Uber den Atlas und Epistropheus bei den Eingeborenen Formosanern. *Folia Anat Jap* 2:221-246, 1924.
140. Udvarhelyi GB, Lai M: Subarachnoid haemorrhage due to rupture of an

aneurysm on a persistent left hypoglossal artery. *Br J Radiol* 36:843-847, 1963.
141. Velpeau A: *A Treatise on Surgical Anatomy of the Anatomy of the Regions*, Vol 1, New York, Wood and Sons, 1830.
142. Wackenheim A: *Roentgendiagnosis of the Craniovertebral Region*, New York, Berlin, Heidelberg, Springer Verlag, 1974.
143. Warwick R, Williams PL: *Gray's Anatomy*, 35th edition, London, Longman Group, 1973.
144. Watzka M: Uber Paraganglien in der Plica ventricularis des menschlichen Kehlkopfes. *Deutsch Med Forsch* 1:19-20, 1963.
145. Weber-Liel FE: *Uber das Wesen und die Heilbarkeit der Haufigsten Form Progressiver Schwerhorigkeit*, Berlin, Hirschwald, 1873.
146. Weigel-Kunzel M: Uber die Topographie von Nerven und Gefassen am Foramen jugulare. Inaug Diss Wurzburg, 1982.
147. Zenker W: Das 'Spatium buccotemporale' und die anderen Fascienraume der tiefen seitlichen Gesichtsregion. *Z Anat Entwicklungsgesch* 118:371-390, 1955.
148. Zolotarewa T, Strynck E: Characteristics of the surgical anatomy and information of the human pterygopalatine ganglion. *Tr Charkovsk Gosud Med Inst* 93:32-36, 1971.

27

Clinical Syndromes of the Posterior Fossa

Benjamin H. Eidelman, M.D.

Introduction

The posterior fossa which is enclosed by bone and dura contains the brain stem, cerebellum, and cranial nerves in addition to vascular structures, cartilage, and chordal remnants. Pathological processes arising from any of these elements may produce intriguing syndromes which are the most challenging in clinical neurology. The proximity of the posterior fossa to the nasopharynx and the middle ear provides an added dimension as infiltrating lesions from these adjacent sites may invade the posterior fossa, giving rise to symptoms while the primary process still remains occult.

The syndromes of the posterior fossa are, for the most part, related to the site of origin of the pathological process. The anatomy of the region has been well described elsewhere in this volume. However, for the purpose of this discussion, it is important to review certain anatomical details. The posterior fossa is a bowl-shaped structure which houses the cerebellum and brain stem. It is bounded ventrally by the clivus which extends from dorsum sella, rostrally to the anterior lip of the foramen magnum caudally. The basilar artery and ventral brain stem are important related structures. The petrous portion of the temporal bones lie on either side of the clivus forming a slight concavity then rising rapidly to form the petrous ridge. The petrous ridges are posteriorly related to occipital bone which forms the major concavity, housing the cerebellum. The foramen magnum which is oval in shape lies within the depth of the occipital concavity bounded anteriorly by the clivus and is encircled posterolaterally by the occipital bone (Fig. 1).

The present discussion will be limited to pathological processes arising extrinsic to the brain stem, from basally situated structures in the posterior fossa. There are three major regions of clinical importance. First, there is the clivus itself with the closely related basilar artery which lies in the prepeduncular region of the posterior fossa. The second area is the bony space bounded by the lateral border of the clivus medially and its petrous ridges laterally (Fig. 1). This triangular region, which extends caudally to the occipital fossa, contains the cerebellopontine (CP) recess and also encompasses the

From: Sekhar LN, Schramm VL Jr, eds: *Tumors of the Cranial Base: Diagnosis and Treatment*. Mount Kisco, New York, Futura Publishing Co, Inc, © 1987.

536 • TUMORS OF THE CRANIAL BASE: DIAGNOSIS AND TREATMENT

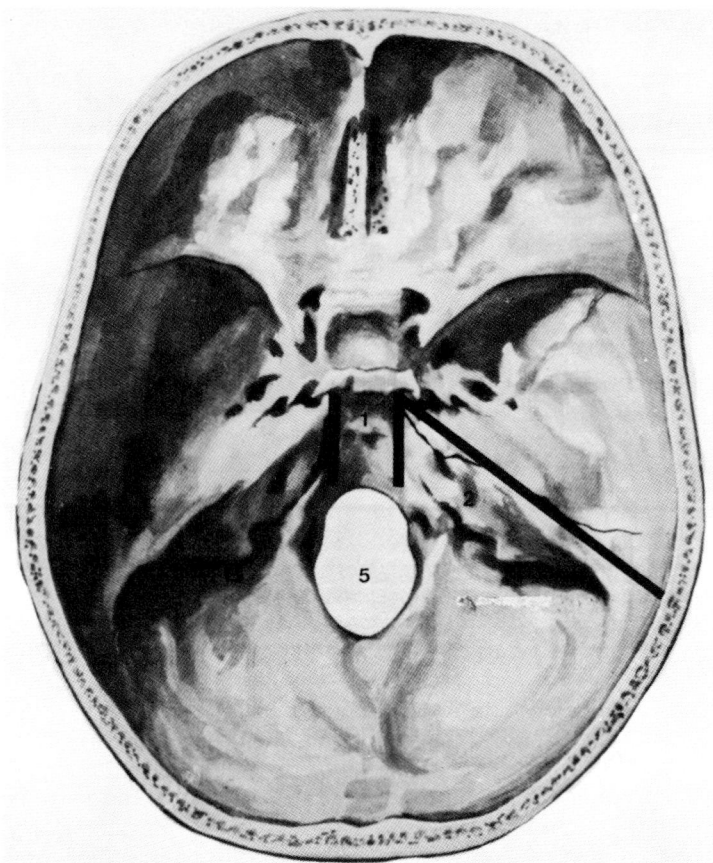

Figure 1: This view of the skull base outlines important bony landmarks of the posterior fossa. The clivus (1) lies ventrally and is bordered laterally by the petrous ridges (2) which together with the anterior lip of the occipital fossa (6) demarcate a triangular area. The cerebello pontine recess is situated in the middle of this triangular region and the jugular foramen (4) and hypoglossal canal (3) are situated at the inferomedial aspect of the triangle. (5) Foramen magnum.

jugular canal. The foramen magnum and its adjacent neural structures constitutes the third region.

Clinical Syndromes of the Posterior Fossa

Syndromes of the posterior fossa may be considered on the basis of the anatomical regions described above. These may be divided into the following: (1) syndromes of the clivus and prepeduncular region of the posterior fossa, (2) the CP recess syndromes, (3) syndromes of the jugular foramen, and (4) syndromes of the foramen magnum.

Syndrome of the Clivus and Prepeduncular Region of the Posterior Base

In considering the clinical manifestations of pathological processes which arise in this area, it is important to appreciate certain clinical principles. The descending motor tracts lie ventrally in the brain stem, and all of the cranial nerves except the 4th emerge from the ventral aspect of the brain stem and then generally take a lateral course as they run towards their point of exit from the cranial cavity. Thus, lesions which arise extra-axially in the region first involve the cranial nerves and the early symptoms are referrable to a disturbance of cranial nerve function. The abnormality is initially unilateral but as the pathological process becomes more extensive, bilateral signs may be evident. The 6th cranial nerves, however, arise close to the midline and both nerves may be involved simultaneously by an infiltrating process developing in the vicinity of the emergent nerves and bilateral 6th nerve signs may be present at an early stage.

The prepeduncular area is relatively narrow and an expanding tumor tends to encroach upon the ventral brain stem, compressing the descending motor tracts producing motor signs at a relatively early stage. The involvement is typically bilateral and is usually symmetrical. The combination of bilateral motor tract signs together with single or multiple cranial nerve lesions which in turn may be unilateral or bilateral is highly suggestive of a pathological process situated in the prepeduncular region of the posterior base.

As the lesion expands, the brain stem will be compressed further and structures within the tegmentum may be compromised producing additional signs such as sensory disturbance, paralysis of conjugate gaze, choreo-athetotic movements, and cerebellar ataxia but these tend to occur as late manifestations.

Occasionally diagnostic difficulty may arise with ventrally situated intrinsic brain stem lesions which have a tendency to interrupt the motor tracts in the early stages of their development. It should be noted that the tracts in the basis pedunculi are somatotopically organized with the fibers destined for the face ventral, and the leg fibers lie dorsally with the arm fibers in between. Thus, with small intrinsic, infiltrating lesions, only one group of fibers may be predominantly involved producing paresis in the contralateral limb. Also, an intrinsic process will involve the descending motor tract and the emergent cranial nerves on the same side, and as the motor tracts decussate distally, the clinical syndrome is one of a contralateral hemiplegia and ipsilateral cranial nerve dysfunction; this combination is the hallmark of an intrinsic brain stem lesion. In contrast, the extrinsic process will usually manifest initially with cranial nerve dysfunction followed later by evidence of disturbed motor function which is often bilateral from the outset.

There are further points of difference between extrinsic and intrinsic lesions. In an extrinsic process, signs of nerve irritation are much more obvious and phenomena such as hemifacial spasm, trigeminal neuralgia, glossopharyngeal neuralgia, and tinnitus are prominent features. Lesions arising from within the brain stem are much less frequently associated with such manifestations although facial myokymia, which presents as a gentle, undulating involuntary facial movement, is sometimes seen and may be mistaken for hemifacial spasm.

The two most important pathological entities which occur in this region are: chordomas of the clivus and ectasia of the basilar artery.

Chordomas of the Clivus

Chordomas are tumors originating in remnants of the notochord which is the primitive skeleton of the fetus and extends from the buccopharyngeal membrane to the terminal coccygeal segment.[26] With the development of the axial skeleton, the notochord becomes incorporated for most of its length into the vertebral column, contributing to the formation of the nucleus pulposus of the intervertebral disc. Nodular remnants of notochordal cord tissue may occur throughout the neural axis but tend to be most common in the clivus and at the coccygeal region.[13] The development of chordomas in adult life correlates well with the location of these nodular remnants and the majority occur in the clivus and sacrococcygeal region but may develop at other sites along the course of the spinal column.[15,26]

Incidence

Chordomas are uncommon and account for 0.1–0.2% of intracranial tumors.[43] Symptoms may develop in early life[26] but the majority present in the third or fourth decade.[31] The tumors tend to be more common in men than in women.[31]

Clinical Features

Lying at the base of the skull, the tumor develops very slowly and, while not malignant in the sense of metastasizing or killing rapidly, it grows in a persistent, insidious manner, deeply indenting the ventral surface of the brain, distorting and compressing the cranial nerves, and sometimes may infiltrate the pituitary, orbit, and other nerve structures. The nasopharynx may be entered destroying the turbinates and even involving the maxillary antrum.[26]

Symptoms and signs can be divided into those relating to invasion of bone and extracranial structures and into those arising from invasion of the nervous system.

Nasopharyngeal Manifestations

The nasopharyngeal structures are involved as the tumor invades forward from the clivus into the nasopharynx and adjacent paranasal sinus. Symptoms of nasal stuffiness, pain, and purulent, bloody nasal discharge occur. Large tumor masses may cause mechanical obstruction and produce dysphagia. Nasopharyngeal symptoms may antedate neurological disturbances and patients may seek advice regarding these before disturbances of neurological function develop.

Neurological Symptoms and Signs

Headache is a common symptom and occurs in a majority of cases. The pain is usually dull and aching in character and, while often generalized, may be referred to the front or back of the head.[26] It may be present for many years prior to the diagnosis of the tumor and has no specific characteristic features and may thus be dismissed as a muscle contraction headache. The pain is probably related to the slow, gradual erosion of bone.

The most characteristic feature of the chordoma relates to its propensity to infiltrate the cranial nerves as they course intracranially from their origin in the brain stem to the various exit foramina in the skull base. Cranial neuropathies, which are frequently multiple, are thus the hallmark of the condition. One or more cranial nerves may be affected but the 6th nerve is the most commonly involved.[24] Cranial nerve involvement may be bilateral[29] but is usually unilateral particularly if the tumor extends into the middle or anterior fossa. Cranial nerves 3 to 12 may be involved with resulting combination of diplopia, facial numbness, facial weakness, hearing loss, tinnitus, dysphagia, dysphonia, and dysarthria. Dorsal extension of the tumor may result in indentation of the brain stem with the development of cortico-spinal and sensory symptoms,[26] although such manifestations generally occur late. Supratentoral extension of the tumor results in symptoms referrable to the optic nerves and chiasm with resultant visual loss and optic atrophy.[24] Involvement of the pituitary gland may produce hypopituitarism.[15] In some instances, the tumor may progress anteriorly and erode through the posterior wall of the orbit producing proptosis. Anosmia may rarely occur if the tumor invades the olfactory nerve.[15] Hydrocephalus develops as a late manifestation of the chordoma and may be produced by aqueductal, or fourth ventricular outflow obstruction.[36] Subarachnoid hemorrhage occurs as a rare complication and results from hemorrhage into the tumor and subsequent extravasation into the subarachnoid space.[46]

Differential Diagnosis of Chordomas of the Clivus

The most characteristic feature of a chordoma arises out of its propensity to infiltrate the cranial nerves and the condition shows itself initially through involvement of multiple cranial nerves. Progression is usually slow, developing over several years and in some patients nasopharyngeal symptoms are present. There are a number of pathological conditions which give rise to a similar combination of signs and symptoms and these are considered individually.

Nasopharyngeal Carcinoma: Nasopharyngeal carcinomas are common in men and have a mean age of onset in the late 40's.[7] These tumors often develop deep within the region of the nasopharynx and may remain latent for a long period of time. Nasopharyngeal manifestations such as blockage of a nasal passage and epistaxis may be the first manifestations but neurological symptoms develop initially in 25% of cases[41] with signs of the local disease appearing later. Symptoms of 5th nerve involvement are the most common primary manifestations with persistent, unilateral facial pain, usually in the distribution of the second division being an early manifestation. There may be accompanying stabbing pain but other symptoms such as paresthesia and numbness tend to develop later. The 6th nerve is involved next in numerical order followed by paralysis of the 9th, 10th, 11th, and 12th cranial nerves, occurring independently or together. The third and fourth nerves may also be involved and visual failure from optic nerve infiltration may also occur. The 7th and 8th cranial nerves may also be compromised, usually from invasion of the petrous bone.[39]

Although the clivus chordoma and nasopharyngeal carcinoma may both involve cranial nerves and manifest nasopharyngeal symptoms, there are important differences in their presentation. The clivus chordoma tends to present with 6th nerve paresis as the initial sign while the nasopharyngeal carcinoma signals itself through infiltration of the 5th nerve, producing pain in the cheek. The chordoma tends to progress more slowly, developing over years while the nasopharyngeal carcinoma spreads rapidly with signs and symptoms evolving over several months although there are rare exceptions. In addition, the chordoma usually presents with unilateral multiple cranial nerve involvement while bilateral signs are more common with the nasopharyngeal carcinoma.

Radiological studies are helpful in differentiating the two conditions. The clivus chordoma tends to show selective erosion of bone within the region of the clivus while the nasopharyngeal carcinoma, except early in the course, causes massive destruction of the skull base. The ultimate differentiation, however, rests on biopsy of the lesion. When nasopharyngeal symptoms are evident, clinical examination of the nasopharynx and nasal space by a surgical expert is mandatory and, if negative, should be repeated at frequent intervals combined with nasopharyngeal biopsies or currettage if a nasopharyngeal carcinoma is strongly suspected.[7]

Carcinomatous Meningitis: Systemic neoplasms, especially adenocarcinomas, may spread to the meninges of the subarachnoid space producing carcinomatous meningitis. Symptoms and signs arising from meningeal invasion may be the first indication of malignant disease and, in some instances, the presentation may be primarily that of a meningeal syndrome with headache, nausea, vomiting, neck stiffness, and alteration in consciousness. Cranial nerve involvement, however, may be the first symptom and among the manifestations of this mode of presentation, visual symptoms are common and result from infiltration of the optic nerve or chiasma, producing rapid visual loss.[4] Other visual complaints include diplopia due to paralysis of the 3rd or 6th nerves.[34] Seventh nerve palsy occurs relatively frequently and the 5th and 8th nerves may also be involved, the latter sometimes being the first manifestation of carcinomatous meningitis.[2] Dysarthria and dysphagia from 9th and 10th cranial nerve infiltration tend to be late manifestations and the 12th cranial nerve is occasionally involved. Symptoms referrable to the cranial nerves are often the only manifestation of the disorder and this can lead to diagnostic confusion as initial attention is drawn to the possibility of a primary process arising in the vicinity of the ventral brain stem. The propensity to involve the optic nerves and rather rapid progression of symptoms help differentiate the condition from the chordoma where symptoms evolve more slowly and tend to be confined initially to the oculomotor nerves.

Glomus Jugulare Tumors: Tumors of the glomus jugulare tend to infiltrate cranial nerves and thus require consideration in the differential diagnosis of patients presenting with multiple cranial neuropathy. These tumors arise from clusters of chemoreceptor cells situated in the vicinity of the bulb of the jugular vein and have the structure of chemodectomas. They are locally invasive and infiltrate the jugular vein, involving the 9th, 10th, and 11th nerves in and around the jugular foramen then often spreading medially towards the hypoglossal canal involving the 12th cranial nerve.[45] It is rare for the tumor to involve other cranial nerves except for the 6th, although totally unilateral involvement of cranial nerves from the 3rd and 12th has been described.[22] These tumors, which are more common in the female, tend to occur in the 5th and 6th decades of life and progression is extremely slow. Aural symptoms from the middle ear invasion invariably precede cranial nerve involvement and a deafness and pulsatile tinnitus are frequent initial symptoms. Pain and discharge from the ear are also important features indicative of the diagnosis. Symptoms and signs referable to the brain stem are exceedingly uncommon but may develop when the tumor mass is large enough to compress the brain stem.

Non-Neoplastic Conditions: Non-neoplastic conditions, particularly chronic meningitis, may present primarily with disturbances of cranial nerve function. Conditions such as tuberculosis, sarcoidosis, syphilis, fungal infections, and parasitic disease may all produce a chronic leptomeningeal infiltration manifesting with cranial nerve dysfunction. In addition, cranial neuropathy may be a complication of the diabetes which largely tends to involve the 3rd, 4th, and 6th cranial nerves but other cranial nerves may also be affected and this condition should always be considered in the differential diagnosis. Collagen vascular diseases complicated by arteritis and ischemic neuropathy may produce multiple cranial nerve lesions. These entities require consideration in the differential diagnosis of a pathological process in the prepeduncular region, and should there be a high index of clinical suspicion for one of these disorders, appropriate tests should be done to identify the pathology.

Ectasia of the Basilar Artery

The basilar artery lies ventral and in close proximity to the brain stem. The vessel may become tortuous and ectatic with advancing age.[33] The enlarged, sinuous basilar artery may protrude dorsally beyond its normal confines compressing the brain stem and redundant loops extending laterally may impinge upon the cranial nerves as they run from the brain stem laterally toward their points of exit from the cranial cavity. The condition, although uncommon, has been well documented pathologically and is usually seen in individuals above the age of 50 years.[33] In the majority of patients, onset is insidious, although in some reported instances, symptoms may come on suddenly.[33] In the latter, however, the acute presentation may relate to a coincidental ischemic event rather than from a direct pressure effect of the ectatic basilar artery. The most prominent symptoms are related to cranial nerve dysfunction, and of these, hemifacial spasm with or without additional symptoms referable to other cranial nerves or the brain stem, is most common. The initial presentation, however, may relate to the development of brain stem disturbances and the patient may notice weakness of an arm and leg, experience sensory symptoms, or have difficulty with coordination due to cerebellar dysfunction.

As would be expected, the most prominent physical signs are referable to the cranial nerves. The 7th nerve is most commonly involved and may take the form of a hemifacial spasm or a peripheral-type facial palsy. The 8th cranial nerve is the next most frequently affected while the 5th is involved in order of frequency.[33] The latter may present in the form of facial numbness but trigeminal neuralgia-like symptoms may also be prominent.[27] The lower four cranial nerves can also be involved and oculomotor findings occur although they are less common. Brain stem findings usually take the form of cerebellar ataxia or hemiparesis with hyperflexia and an extensor plantar response. The close proximity of the basilar artery to the ventrally situated motor tracts in the brain stem probably accounts for the frequency of involvement of the latter. Dementia is relatively rare but is a well-described complication[20] and may be evidenced by apathy, impaired memory, decreased initiative, inappropriate affect, and lack of insight. Patients with dementia may occasionally exhibit gait apraxia in addition to signs of pyramidal tract dysfunction.[20]

Differential Diagnosis of Ectasia of the Basilar Artery

The typical presentation of a patient with ectasia of the basilar artery is an elderly, hypertensive individual showing signs of multiple cranial nerve involvement with irritative phenomenon such as hemifacial spasm or trigeminal neuralgia often dominating the clinical picture. In addition, signs of brain stem dysfunction may be present. The cranial nerve signs tend to evolve slowly over several years. Many conditions may produce a similar clinical picture and while these have been discussed in the preceding section, it is important to emphasize that neoplastic and inflammatory conditions tend to evolve at a much more rapid rate and, for the most part, do not produce the irritative symptoms so characteristic of vascular compressive lesions. Chordomas may evolve slowly and have been well described in late middle age, and as such, may be similar in presentation. The presence of signs of nasal passage involvement, however, usually clarifies the diagnosis. A meningioma arising ventral to the brain stem and slowly growing over many years may produce an identical clinical picture but is readily differentiated by CT scanning of the head.

The Cerebellopontine Recess Syndromes

Anatomical Considerations

The bony landmarks that define this triangular region are the lateral margin of the clivus medially, the petrous ridge laterally, and the cerebellar fossa of the occipital bone inferiorly (see Fig. 1). The neural structures contained in this bony region include the brain stem medially, the middle cerebellar peduncle and cerebellum posteriorly, and the 9th, 10th, and 11th cranial nerves caudally. The 5th, 7th, and 8th cranial nerves pass through the midregion. Specifically, the space bounded by the brain stem medially, the middle cerebellar peduncle and the cerebellum posteriorly, the petrous temporal bone anteriorly, the 9th, 10th, and 11th cranial nerves inferiorly and by the tentorium cerebelli superiorly, is known as the CP angle or recess, the latter being a more accurate term for this three-dimensional space and will be used henceforth. The CP recess, in addition to being traversed by the 5th, 7th, and 8th cranial nerves, also contains a number of vessels including the loops of the posterior inferior cerebellar artery, anterior inferior cerebellar artery, and its internal auditory branch. Pathological processes may arise from neural elements, vessels, bone, cartilage, and embryonal remnants. Also, the area may be infiltrated by metastatic tumors arising from contiguous as well as distant sites.

Lesions of the CP recess usually produce characteristic signs and symptoms which may be grouped according to the structures involved.[16] The CP recess syndrome is typically produced by a tumor, particularly the acoustic neurilemmoma. The signs of such a lesion relate primarily to the anatomical structures involved, although exceptions may occur if the syndrome evolves through the following stages: (1) findings confined to the 8th cranial nerve; (2) involvement of the 8th nerve with signs referrable to either the 5th or 7th, or both cranial nerves in addition to cerebellar dysfunction; (3) involvement of the 5th, 7th, and 8th cranial nerves, the cerebellum and brain stem; (4) any or all of the above manifestations plus signs of raised intracranial pressure.

Clinical Features: Stage 1

The tumor typically produces gradual deafness, and for many months or years no other symptoms may occur. The deafness is unilateral and progressive, particularly affecting high frequency sounds early in the course of the disorder. It has all the characteristics of sensorineural deafness, and voice perception is particularly poor. Tinnitus may occur in the affected ear as an initial symptom but usually follows the deafness. Tinnitus, which occurs in somewhat less than 50% of cases, is usually high-pitched, irritating, and often intermittently intensifying.

True vertigo with a sense of rotation may also occur and may be spontaneous or induced by changes in position. The most common symptom referrable to this, however, is a feeling of insecurity of balance or unsteadiness when walking. Clinical evidence of vestibular dysfunction may be found in the form of horizontal or rotatory nystagmus with the slow component towards the affected side as well as a tendency to sway towards the affected side.

The symptoms at this stage are relatively mild and diagnosis is often delayed because little concern is paid to this seemingly innocuous, mild hearing loss in one ear. At this stage, a history of localized pain in the occipital region, ipsilateral to the tumor, occasioned by straining at stool may often be obtained. Examination, in addition to revealing signs of 8th nerve involvement, may also demonstrate a subtle ipsilateral loss of the corneal reflex which is an early and most important sign.

Clinical Features: Stage 2

This stage is characterized by additional involvement of cranial nerves. However, with slowly growing tumors, displacement occurs gradually and functional loss is minimal. The nerves most frequently involved in the early stages are the 5th and 7th. Symptoms referrable to the former are fleeting attacks of unilateral numbness of the face on the side of the deafness, which clearly follow the distribution of the 5th nerve. These symptoms are often so dramatic that a lesion of the trigeminal nerve cannot be doubted even though the sensory examination may be normal.

With involvement of the 7th nerve early in the curse, there is a slight facial asymmetry, the nasolabial fold will be less developed on the side of the lesion, and when smiling, the facial movements will be more pronounced on the opposite side. There is less complete closure of the eyelid on the affected side. The latter observation is very important for it indicates a peripheral rather than a central origin of the facial palsy. Cerebellar dysfunction may appear early and the patient or observer will note an unsteadiness of gait which at this stage may be intermittent. There may be a deviation to one side when walking or skilled movements of the hand on the affected side may be less effectively executed.

This is usually the stage at which most patients seek medical advice. Signs of raised intracranial pressure have not developed and the clinical diagnosis rests on careful observation to determine the presence of abnormalities in the involved cranial nerves together with a disturbance of cerebellar function.

Clinical Features: Stage 3

Signs of 5th and 7th nerve involvement become more overt and, in addition, growth of the tumor in a caudal direction may produce involvement of 9th, 10th, and 11th nerves with asymmetry of the palate, dysarthria and dysphagia. The 6th nerve may also be involved, albeit rarely with resulting diplopia. Compression of the brain stem gives rise to hemiplegia and/or hemianesthesia, both usually contralateral to the tumor, as well as exaggeration of the tendon reflexes with an extensor plantor response. Signs of cerebellar dysfunction become more obvious with marked staggering of gait with deviation to the side of the lesion, and a tendency to fall to one side during the Romberg test.

Clinical Features: Stage 4

Signs of raised intracranial pressure become obvious as a result of obstruction of the aqueduct and the development of hydrocephalus. Papilledema becomes apparent and headaches are a major complaint. The headache is usually bilateral, situated both frontally and suboccipitally

Unusual Findings in Cerebellopontine Tumors

Occasionally hearing and vestibular function are intact while other cranial nerves are severely involved and in some instances hemifacial spasm may be the dominant feature.[14]

Differential Diagnosis

The most common CP recess lesion is the acoustic neurilemmoma.[37] These tend to be slow-growing and evolve through the stages outlined above over several years. Meningiomas of this region may present in an identical manner.[35] Cholesteatomas or epidermoid tumors which occur in adult life and progress slowly may present with similar signs and symptoms but more frequently show hemifacial spasm.[9] Gliomas arising from the cerebellum or brain stem and projecting laterally into the recess may initially compress cranial nerves and may mimic a CP recess tumor.[8] These tumors tend to occur in younger individuals and progress more rapidly with signs of brain stem involvement occurring earlier. Ependymomas may grow laterally, extending through the foramen of Luschka and presenting as a CP recess syndrome. These tumors tend to grow rather rapidly and other signs of brain stem involvement rapidly intervene.[38] Vascular causes of the CP syndrome include cirsoid aneurysms of the basilar artery,[23] arteriovenous malformation, and tortuosity of the vertebral and basilar arteries.[27] Arachnoiditis of the posterior fossa,[1] local infections close to the facial nerve, and cross-compression by aberrant loops of the posterior inferior cerebellar artery may also produce the syndrome.[19] Metastatic tumors may develop in the course producing signs of a mass lesion;[8] however, the course of evolution is usually rapid.

and is a manifestation of the raised intracranial pressure rather than a direct effect of the tumor.

The progressive deafness seen in the early course of the syndrome combined with episodic vertigo may mimic Meniere's syndrome. Symptoms may be entirely aural in the early phase and the two conditions may be very difficult to separate, requiring the use of additional diagnostic aids.

Separation of the various conditions requires specialty testing including audiological evaluation, EMG, brain stem evoked responses, radiological studies including angiography, contrast cisternography, and magnetic resonance imaging (MRI).

Syndromes of the Jugular Foramen

Lying at the inferomedial aspect of the triangular region bounded by the brain stem, petrous ridge, and lower three cranial nerves, the jugular foramen is situated in a well-defined anatomical area, and recognition of the neurological syndromes that develop from pathology at this site is of great importance. The jugular foramen (foramen lacerum posterius) is actually a canal that crosses in an antero-infero-lateral direction from its intracranial origin to an extracranial exit. The foramen is divided by a fibrous or bony septum into a pars-nervosa and pars-vascularis. The jugular canal is traversed by three cranial nerves, the 9th, 10th, and 11th. Non-neural structures that traverse the canal include the inferior petrosal sinus, the posterior meningeal artery, and jugular vein. The jugular canal is in close proximity to the hypoglossal canal through which passes the 12th cranial nerve. The intracranial orifice of the latter lies within 8 mm of the posteromedial border of the jugular foramen which is of clinical significance as a relatively localized pathological process at the jugular foramen may involve the 12th nerve as well. The hypoglossal canal is separated extracranially from the jugular foramen by only a thin ridge of bone, usually a few millimeters thick; consequently, an extracranial mass (encroaching upon the jugular foramen) or a mass that has infiltrated through the foramen itself will very often involve the 12th nerve as it emerges from the hypoglossal canal. Also, the cervical sympathetic chain lies close to the lower four cranial nerves as they exit at the base of the skull. Appreciation of these anatomical details is essential to the understanding of clinical syndromes which may involve this region.

Clinical Syndromes

The pure jugular foramen syndrome also called Vernet's syndrome, consists of unilateral loss of taste over the posterior third of the tongue due to involvement of the 9th cranial nerve, paralysis of the trapezius and sternocleidomastoid muscles resulting from 11th nerve involvement, and paralysis of the vocal cord and palate which relates to a disturbance of 10th nerve function. Several other syndromes have been described with involvement of various combinations of the lower cranial nerves, and of the sympathetic chain, with or without brain stem signs. Of practical importance is Villaret's syndrome, which includes involvement of cranial nerves 9, 10, 11, and 12 in addition to signs of cervical sympathetic dysfunction. The posterior lacero-condylar Collet-Sicard syndrome is characterized by the isolated involvement of the cranial nerves 9, 10, 11, and 12, differing from the former by an absence of sympathetic dysfunction.

Pathological Considerations

Pathological conditions which may produce the jugular foramen and allied syndromes include: thrombosis of the jugular vein at the jugular foramen; primary or metastatic tumors at the base of the skull; chronic meningitis; neurilemmomas of any of the lower four cranial nerves or adjacent nerves in the cerebellopontine recess; features of the base of the skull; and extension of pathology from neighboring pharyngeal and retropharyngeal areas, usually malignant. But suppurative conditions such as a retropharyngeal abscess of tuberculous adenitis may also involve these nerves.

Neurilemmomas

Neurilemmomas of the four lowest cranial nerves are uncommon causes of the jugular foramen syndrome. Columella, Delzanno, and Nicola,[12] in their review of the subject, found that no more than seven cases of neurilemmomas of the 12th and 9th cranial nerves had been reported in the literature and the same number had been described involving the 10th and 11th cranial nerves. Similar findings were reported by Williams and Fox.[48] Neurilemmomas of the 8th cranial nerve are much more common and may eventually involve the lowest four cranial nerves but evidence of involvement of these occurs late and they are preceded by clinical manifestations of the 8th nerve involvement.[12] Intracranial tumors that may produce the syndrome include meningiomas arising near the foramen magnum[40] as well as dermoids.[30]

The most common extracranial primary tumor producing this syndrome is the glomus jugulare tumor. These tumors arise from chemoreceptor tissue in the region of the jugular bulb and frequently involve the nerves passing through the jugular foramen, albeit only at a late stage. In reviewing 33 cases, Siekert[45] found that the 9th, 10th, 11th, and 12th nerves were involved in about one-third of the cases, but the clinical manifestations were not limited to these nerves. Usually, auditory symptoms are the first manifestations with tinnitus, distortion of hearing, and pain in the ear predominating. Paralysis of the 7th nerve follows with the lower four cranial nerves being involved subsequently.

Metastatic infiltration from a variety of sources is a common cause of the jugular foramen syndrome. Malignancy may extend from adjacent lymph nodes or from a primary source within the nasopharynx but may also arise from distant sites such as the breast, lung, and prostate.[25]

Vascular lesions may also give rise to the syndrome and both aneurysms of the vein of Galen and arteriovenous malformation have been described as causes.[18] Thrombophlebitis of the jugular vein, as well as other infectious conditions including arachnoiditis and osteitis of the skull base, and fractures of the skull base and trauma due to missile wounds[3] are additional causes.

Diagnostic Principles

Clinical examination yielding evidence of lesions of cranial nerves 9 through 12 provides initial information that leads to anatomical localization of the lesion within the confines or general region of the jugular foramen. Further neurological evaluation is required to determine whether additional features are present and thus the presence of long tract signs is of vital importance. The latter manifestations may indicate a primary process intrinsic to the brain stem but a mass lying outside the brain stem may also produce such signs through secondary compression of the brain stem although these occur late. The presence of brain stem signs directs attention to the intracranial cavity and appropriate investigations including skull x-rays, CT head scan, and MRI would be in order. If the clinical features indicate involvement of the cranial nerves without other signs, the mode of onset of symptoms may provide important diagnostic clues. The slow development of abnormalities over many years would indicate a benign process such as a neurilemmoma or a glomus jugulare tumor which is notoriously insidious in evolution as symptoms may develop over many years. The rapid development of symptoms with or without signs of a more generalized process suggests a malignancy of an inflammatory disorder. Further information may be obtained from the general examination and, in this respect, attention must be directed to the cervical region which may reveal the presence of local masses. Inspection of the ears is of vital importance as this may yield evidence of a glomus tumor or local infection. The nasopharynx deserves careful evaluation to determine whether a nasopharyngeal tumor or perhaps a retropharyngeal mass is present. The presence of a mass lesion at any of these sites dictates the need for biopsy which may usually provide the diagnosis. In those patients where local examination proves negative, further diagnostic studies are indicated including x-rays of the skull base, tomograms of the jugular foramen, CT scanning, contrast cisternography, and MRI. All patients deserve careful general examination with the appropriate clinical testing to exclude neoplastic conditions arising from distant sites and systemic diseases such as tuberculosis, sarcoidosis, diabetes, collagen-vascular disease and, although uncommon in modern medicine, syphillis is also a diagnostic consideration.

Syndromes of the Foramen Magnum

The foramen magnum demarcates the craniocervical boundary and may be involved by pathological processes originating within the basal part of the cranium which may then extend into the upper cervical canal. In some instances a tumor may originate within the cervical canal and extend superiorly into the cranial cavity. Both entities produce a wide range of clinical syndromes arising out of involvement of related structures including the brain stem, emergent cranial nerves, and bony structures of the cranial base and upper cervical cord. In addition, distal effects such as hydrocephalus, hydromyelia, and syringomyelia may further complicate the picture. Two major pathological entities in this region require consideration, namely (1) the Arnold-Chiari malformation, and (2) tumors arising at the craniocervical junction.

The Arnold-Chiari Malformation

This congenital malformation was elegantly described by Chiari.[10,11] Arnold[6] described a single example, and the two authors' names were subsequently linked to encompass the various varieties of malformation that occur in this region.

In essence, the abnormalities that constitute the Arnold-Chiari malformation relate to downward displacement of the cerebellum and brain stem into the spinal cord and encompass two major components: (1) a tongue of cerebellar tissue which extends posterior to the medullary spinal cord for several centimeters into the cervical canal, and (2) displacement of the medulla oblongata into the cervical canal together with the inferior part of the fourth ventricle. Displacement of these structures is variable and it is customary to divide the Arnold-Chiari malformation into types 1 and 2, depending on the extent of displacement.

Type I Arnold-Chiari Malformation

This consists of displacement of the medulla oblongata through the foramen magnum into the cervical spinal canal. There is accompanying herniation of the cerebellum which presents on the dorsal surface of the medulla as two elongated masses of tissue. The latter may extend from the level of C2 to C7 and often enshroud the medulla. The mass of displaced tissue usually wedges tightly into the foramen magnum and the intracranial portion of the cerebellum which is often small may also be displaced, obliterating the cisterna magnum. The lower cranial nerves tend to be displaced and often run an ascending course from their points of emergence from the brain stem to their exit foramina. In addition, the arachnoid around the brain stem and herniated cerebellar tongue is thickened and fibrotic. Additional components include hydromyelia and syringomyelia of the cervical cord.

Type II Arnold-Chiari Malformation

This type, as in type I, includes displacement of the cerebellum and fourth ventricles into the cervical canal. In addition, the entire medulla oblongata and lower pons lie below the foramen magnum and usually the dorsal surface of the spinal cord is kinked by the bulbous expansion of the caudal extension of the fourth ventricle. A meningomyelocele is a frequent associated anomaly. The central canal of the spinal cord may be dilated and there is also thickening of the arachnoid membrane in the vicinity of the displaced tissue. The lower cranial nerves also are displaced and run an ascending course from the brain stem. A number of additional components have been described including: abnormalities of the cerebrum, displacement of the lower spinal cord, atrophy of the displaced cerebellar tissue, flattening of the superior vermis by the occipital lobes which may herniate through the enlarged incisura, elongation and attenuation of the medulla and pons, the foramena of Luschka, and Magendie opening into the cervical canal and part of the inferior vermis lying within the fourth ventricle. Also, the tectal plate at the level of the inferior colliculus may have a posterior beaked appearance. The internal nuclei of the medulla may also be displaced.

Bony abnormalities are also present in the form of a small posterior fossa and enlargement of the foramen magnum which may be moved posteriorly. The cervical canal is often widened and the cranial bones may be thinned with incomplete development of the falx cerebri. The base of the skull may be flattened and basilar impression with displacement of the odontoid process may be apparent. Hydrocephalus may be a prominent associated finding in both type I and type II malformations.

Clinical Manifestations

In patients with type I Arnold-Chiari malformation, there are no external signs of dysraphism, and while the condition frequently presents in childhood, it may remain silent for many years, manifesting ony in middle age or beyond. The diagnosis rests on clinical features indicating disorders of structures centered around the medulla oblongata, cerebellum, and upper cervical cord. In addition, symptoms may arise from raised intracranial pressure secondary to the hydrocephalus. Several neurological syndromes may occur:

Symptoms Arising from Increased Intracranial Pressure

Headache and vomiting may be the first features and may be present for months or years and thus may be attributed to tension headache, migraine, or degenerative arthritis of the cervical spine. The pain is usually localized to the occiput but may include frontal and other regions. The headache may be increased by cough, exertion, and other maneuvers which raise intracranial pressure but these features may often be absent which further reinforces the contention of "benign headaches." The neurological examination may be unrevealing with the development of additional signs appearing only as the condition progresses.

Progressive Cerebellar Ataxia

In some instances, signs of raised intracranial pressure may be absent and the primary disturbance is related to an abnormality of cerebellar function. This may be progressive in nature with a course extending over many years but in some instances, signs and symptoms may be episodic, giving rise to the suspicion of multiple sclerosis.

Posterior Base Upper Cervical Syndrome

Various combinations of disturbed neurological function may occur with disorders of cranial nerves, cerebellum, medulla, and spinal cord developing without an associated headache. The signs and symptoms are often complex and apparently multifocal which once again may give rise to the diagnosis of multiple sclerosis. Of the cranial nerves, the lowest tend to be most affected, and when the 10th nerve is involved, the vocal cords may be weakened producing dysphonia, although laryngeal stridor is a prominent sign of this in the young child.[28] Twelfth nerve dysfunction may produce weakness or atrophy of the tongue and, if the 11th nerve is involved, one of the sternomastoid muscles may be atrophic. Signs and symptoms of auditory and vestibular dysfunction, relating to involvement of the 8th cranial nerve have also been described[42] and reports also indicate that the 3rd, 6th, and 7th nerves may also be involved.[35] Facial numbness due to involvement of the 5th cranial nerve have also been described.[42]

There may be accompanying cerebellar ataxia which may be asymmetrical affecting an arm and leg on one side more than the other, although it is often bilateral with an altered gait. Signs of descending motor symptom dysfunction may be evident with spastic weakness affecting one limb, following a hemiplegic distribution or involving all four limbs. There may be accompanying small muscle wasting of the hands, and a cape-like segmental sensory loss over the shoulders and arms may be present.

Signs referrable to the brain stem include faintness on neck flexion, sudden loss of postural control on neck extension, down-beat nystagmus, hiccups, and palatal myoclonus.

Syringomyelia

A number of cases of Arnold-Chiari malformation develop syringomyelia even without dysrhaphism of the spinal cord. Features suggestive of this are: loss of sensitivity to thermal stimulation producing painless injury, atrophic weakness of the arm, and unexplained pain in the neck, arm, or thorax with segmental sensory loss.

Diagnosis of the Arnold-Chiari Malformation

Arnold-Chiari Type I

This may pose considerable diagnostic difficulty as signs of dysrhaphism are absent. The condition should always be considered in patients who present with signs and symptoms referrable to the brain stem, lower cranial neres, and spinal cord. The course is generally progressive but episodic symptoms may occur and the latter should not dissuade one from the diagnosis. The following features provide a hint of the condition: low hairline, large skull circumference due to arrested hydrocephalus, down-beat nystagmus, sensory loss in the C2–C3 area, dissociated sensory loss in the upper limbs, and small muscle wasting for the hands.

Radiological studies may be of use and x-rays of the cervical spine and base of the skull occasionally reveal abnormalities such as: widening of the cervical canal, fusion of vertebral bodies, unfused posterior arch of C1, and occipitovertebral fusion.[5]

Further radiological studies are required to confirm the diagnosis and, until recently, metrizamide CT study was the investigation of choice; however, the recent advent of MRI has altered established concepts and recent studies indicate that MRI may be the most valuable method of demonstrating the condition.[17]

Arnold-Chiari Type II

The majority of such patients exhibit signs of spinal dysrhaphism with a meningo-myelocele of the lumbosacral region being the most prominent presenting feature. Signs of hydrocephalus are initially absent. Suspicion of an associated Arnold-Chiari malformation may be suspected in a newborn who becomes less alert, exhibiting rapid enlargement of the head which demonstrates unusually wide and tense fontanelles. At this stage, the problem is essentially one of hydrocephalus and all the symptoms can be attributed to the effect of enlarging ventricles and compression of neural structures. In some instances, the condition may manifest as a result of abnormalities of the cranial nerves and, in this respect, laryngeal stridor due to weakness and/or paralysis of the vocal cords is a striking and important feature.[28,32] Multiple cranial nerve deficits have been described,[44] and these may result in weakness and fasciculation of the tongue, dysphagia, head lag due to sternomastoid weakness, facial weakness, disturbed ocular motility secondary to third and sixth nerve involvement, as well as deafness due to involvement of the 8th nerve. If the child survives, other neurological abnormalities described in the type I Arnold-Chiari malformation may become evident at any stage of adolescent or adult life.

Tumors in the Vicinity of the Craniocervical Junction

Tumors of this region whether they are primarily of intracranial origin with secondary extension into the spinal cord, or primarily extracranial with secondary involvement of intracranial structures have characteristics that may mimic the Arnold-Chiari malformation. The signs and symptoms reflect traction and compression of neighboring nerve structures[47] which include the cervical cord and emergent nerves, lower cranial nerves, brain stem, and cerebellum. Distal effects due to raised intracranial pressure secondary to hydrocephalus may also occur.

Tumors in this region are, for the most part, exra-axial and include meningiomas, neurilemmomas, and dermoids.[47] Aneurysms or ectasia of the vertebral artery may occasionally mimic a tumor in this region.[47] Tumors of this region are not easily recognized because the initial symptoms are sensory and signs of objective neurological dysfunction may be absent or at best subtle and variable. There are a number of important features that draw attention to a lesion in this region.

Sensory Symptoms

One of the most common initial complaints relates to craniocervical pain, which is usually referred to the second cervical dermatomal distribution on one or both sides but lower cervical segments may be involved as well.[21] The pain is usually felt in the neck and occipital region, is often aching in nature and is increased on movement of the head. As a result, the head is held in a stiff, fixed position. Pain may antedate other symptoms by several years and, in the absence of additional clinical findings, gives rise to the mistaken diagnosis of tension headache or degenerative disease of the cervical spine. Later, additional sensory symptoms develop including numbness and tingling which may be referred to the ipsilateral arm, forearm, and hand. Tingling may be confined to isolated fingers or, in some instances, may be referred to the whole hand. These symptoms tend to progress increasing in severity as the lesion expands. Unusual symptoms such as "a feeling of a tight band" around the neck region and episodic paraesthesia have also been described. Other characteristic sensory symptoms relate to the feeling of intense coldness experienced in one or more limbs.[21] It occurs most often in the contralateral lower extremity although the upper limb may also be affected. This tends to be most severe at night and may awaken the patient from sleep. Little relief is obtained by warmth applied to the affected region.

Sensory Signs

Frequently, sensory examination reveals the presence of a contralateral dissociated sensory loss with tactile sensibility preserved in the presence of a marked disturbance of pain and temperature sensation. The latter may take the form of a hemisensory loss extending from the second cervical segment downward to involve the one side of the body. In some instances, however, loss of pain and temperature may be minimal and largely confined to the second and third cervical segments. Joint position sense is less frequently involved and will often be confined to the upper limbs, another characteristic of lesions in this area. Vibration sense may be lost together with disturbances of joint position sensibility. In some instances there may be a dissociation between these modalities of sensation with vibration sense preserved while the joint position sense is lost and the reverse may also hold true.[21]

Motor System

Spastic weakness of the extremities is a prominent feature of tumors in this region. Weakness begins in the ipsilateral upper limb, then progresses to the lower limb of the same side followed by weakness of the contralateral lower limb and finally, weakness becomes apparent in the contralateral upper limb. This distinct progression of motor symptoms is an important characteristic.[47] Localized muscular wasting of the intrinsic muscles of the hands, which develops ipsilateral to the lesion, is a further important feature. In some instances, the wasting may extend to involve the forearms.[21] Tendon reflexes tend to be abnormally brisk with absence of abdominal reflexes and extensor plantar responses on the same side. The cervical sympathetic may occasionally be involved with an ipsilateral Horner's syndrome present. Sphincter control is not disturbed except as a late feature when spinal cord compression is extreme. Signs of cerebellar dysfunction are usually absent unless the intracranial extent of the tumor is very large. Local abnormalities of the neck region are usually absent, although in some instances, focal tenderness may be apparent when pressure is applied over the vertebrae adjacent to the site of the tumor.

Differential Diagnosis of an Abnormality in the Craniocervical Region

There are a number of prominent features which indicate the presence of an abnormality in the craniocervical region and these include: occipital headaches with fixed head posture; presence of signs of lower cranial nerve dysfunction in combination with motor and sensory features suggesting spinal cord localization; prominent sensory symptoms, particularly the feeling of intense coldness in the lower extremities; loss of sensation in the second and third dermatomes with sensory disturbances over the opposite half of the body; dissociated sensory loss; and, finally, intrinsic muscle wasting of the hands which may be asymmetrical.

The type I Arnold-Chiari malformation and tumors of this region are similar in clinical presentation. The type II Arnold-Chiari malformation usually signals its presence through additional dysrhaphic abnormalities and poses less of a diagnostic challenge.

If a lesion of this region is suspected, careful scrutiny may reveal the presence of a low hairline, short neck, or large head, strongly in favor of the diagnosis of an Arnold-Chiari malformation. The combination of brain stem, cerebellar, and spinal cord signs may suggest a spinocerebellar degeneration and there the presence of skeletal abnormalities such as kyphoscoliosis and pes cavus deformity are important collateral findings. A positive family history of similar skeletal abnormalities with or without neurological disturbances would support this diagnosis. Multiple sclerosis, which may present with brain stem, cerebellar, and spinal cord signs, is an additional diagnostic consideration, particularly as fluctuating symptoms are common to both conditions. Intrinsic tumors of the lower brain stem and upper cervical cord, aneurysms of the vertebral artery, and granulomas are additional pathological entities that may give rise to a similar clinical presentation.

The differentiation of the various conditions that may develop in the craniocervical region relies on diagnostic testing using a variety of methods. Plain x-rays of the neck and skull bone may be useful in demonstrating bony abnormalities. CT myelography with metrizamide is extremely helpful in delineating pathology in the region, and MRI gives promise of being the choice of investigation for detecting abnormalities in this area. The latter technique has a further advantage in that it is noninvasive and does not require the use of iodine contrast agents.

Conclusion

Lesions of the posterior base, arising extrinsic from the brain stem, usually signal their presence at an early stage by involving cranial nerves. Subsequent compression of the brain stem by an enlarging mass may produce long tract and other signs related to disturbances of brain stem function but these generally occur as a second readvent. The localization of the lesion is to a large extent dependent on a combination of cranial nerve and brain stem signs. The presence of multiple cranial nerve abnormalities with or without signs suggests a ventrally placed lesion in the vicinity of the clivus or prepeduncular region of the posterior fossa. The CP recess mass is characterized by a combination of 5th, 7th, and 8th cranial nerve abnormalities together with signs of cerebellar dysfunction. Involvement of the 9th and 12th cranial nerves suggests a process in the area of the jugular canal. The presence of lower cranial nerve abnormalities, cerebellar dysfunction, and signs referrable to the upper cervical cord is indicative of a pathological process in the vicinity of the craniocervical junction. Thus, careful correlation of anatomical principles and clinical abnormalities can provide important information about both the site and pathological nature of the lesion, and such information is vital to the planning of an appropriate plan of investigation.

References

1. Adeloye A, Ogan O, Olumide AA: Arachnoiditis presenting as a cerebello pontine angle tumor. *J Laryngol Otol* 92:911-3, 1978.
2. Alberts MC, Terrence CF: Hearing loss in carcinomatous meningitis. *J Laryngol Otol* 92:233-241, 1978.
3. Aldrich EM, Baker GS: Injuries of the hypoglossal nerve: report of ten cases. *Mil Surgeon* 103:20-25, 1948.
4. Altrocchi PA, Eckman PB: Meningeal carcinomatous and blindness. *J Neurol Neurosurg Psychiatr* 36:206-210, 1973.
5. Appleby A, Foster J, Hankinson J, et al: The diagnosis and management of the Chiari anomalies in adult life. *Brain* 91:131-140, 1968.
6. Arnold J: Myelocyste, transposition von gewebskeimen und sympodie. *Beitr Path Anat* 16:1-28, 1894.

7. Batsakis JG: *Tumours of the Head and Neck: Clinical and Pathological Considerations*, 2nd Edition, Baltimore, Williams and Wilkins, 1979.
8. Brackman DE, Bartels LJ: Rare tumors of the cerebellopontine angle. Otolaryngol Head Neck Surg 88:555-9, 1980.
9. Cawthorne T, Griffith A: Primary cholesteatomata of the temporal bone. Arch Otolaryngol 73:252-61, 1961.
10. Chiari H: Ueber Veranderungen des Kleinhirns infolge von hydrocephalie des grosshirns. Deutsch Med Wschr 17:1172-1175, 1891.
11. Chiari H: Ueber Veranderungen des Kleinhirns des Pons der Medulla oblongata in Folge von congenit haler Hydrocephalie des grosshirns. Danschr Akad Wiss Wien 63:71-116, 1896.
12. Columella F, Delzanno GB, Nicola GC: Les neurinomes des quatre demiers nerfs craniens. Neuro-chirurgie 5:280-295, 1959.
13. Congdon CC: Benign and malignant chordomas. Am J Pathol 28:793-821, 1952.
14. Cushing HW: *Tumors of the Nervus Acusticus and the Syndrome of the Cerebellopontine Angle*, Philadelphia, WB Saunders, 1917.
15. Dahlin DC, MacCarty CS: Chordomas Cancer 5:1170-1178, 1952.
16. Dandy WE: *The Brain*, Hagerstown, W.F. Prior, 521, 1966.
17. Dela Pas RL, Brady TJ, Buonanno FS, et al: Nuclear magnetic resonance (NMR) imaging of Arnold Chiari Type I malformation with hydromyelia. J Comput Assist Tomogr 7:126-129, 1983.
18. DiChiro G, Fisher R, Nelson K: The jugular foramen. J Neurosurg 21:447-60, 1964.
19. Eidelman BH, Nielsen VK, Moller M, Jannetta PJ: Vascular compression, hemifacial spasm and multiple cranial neuropathy. Neurology (Cleveland) 35:712-716, 1985.
20. Ekbom K, Greitz T, Kugelberg E: 20 Hydrocephalus due to ectasia of the basilar artery. J Neurol Sci 8:465-477, 1969.
21. Elsberg CA, Strauss I: Tumors of the spinal cord which project into the posterior cranial fossa. Arch Neuro Psych 28:261-273, 1928.
22. Figi FA, Weisman PA: Cancer and chemodectoma in middle ear and mastoid. JAMA 156:1157-1162, 1954.
23. Gardner WT, Sawa GA: Hemifacial spasm: A reversible pathophysiologic state. J Neurosurg 19:240-7, 1962.
24. Givner I: Ophthalmologic features of intracranial chordoma and allied tumors of the clivus. Arch Ophthalmol 33:397-403, 1945.
25. Greenberg HS, Deck MD, Vikram B, et al: Metastasis to the base of the skull: Clinical findings in 43 patients. Neurology 31:530-537, 1981.
26. Hass GM: Chordomas of the cranium and cervical spine. Arch Neurol Psych 32:300-327, 1934.
27. Kerber CW, Margolis MT, et al: Tortuous vertebrobasilar system: A cause of cranial nerve signs. Neuroradiology 4:74-7, 1972.
28. Kirsch WM, Duncan BR, Black FO, et al: Laryngeal palsy in association with myelomeningocele, hydrocephalus and the Arnold-Chiari malformation. J Neurosurg 28:207-214, 1968.
29. Kline LB, Glaser JS: Bilateral abducens nerve palsies from clivus chordomas. Ann Ophthalmol 13:705-707, 1981.
30. Love JG: Jugular foramen syndrome (Jackson's syndrome) due to intracranial epidermal tumor: Successful surgical treatment. Proc Mayo Clin 26:252-1951.
31. Meaney TF, Greenwald CM, Phalen GS: Chordoma. Clin Orthop 7:103-112, 1956.
32. Morley AR: Laryngeal stridor, Arnold-Chiari malformation and medullary haemorrhages. Develop Med Child Neurol 11:471-574, 1969.
33. Moseley IF, Holland IM: Ectasia of the basilar artery: the breadth of the clinical spectrum and the diagnostic value of computed tomography. Neuroradiology 18:83-91, 1979.
34. Olson ME, Chemick NL, Posner JB: Infiltration of the leptomeninges by systemic cancer. Arch Neurol 30:122-137, 1974.
35. Penfield W, Coburn DF: Arnold-Chiari malformations and its operative treatment. Arch Neurol Psych (Chic) 40:328-336, 1938.
36. Plaut HF, Blatt ES: Chordomas of the clivus. Am J Roentgenol 100:639-649, 1967.
37. Revilla AG: Neurinomas of the cerebellopontine recess: A clinical study of one hundred and sixty cases including operative mortality and end results. Bull John Hopkins Hosp 80:254-96, 1947.
38. Revilla AG: Differential diagnosis of tumors at the cerebello pontine recess. Bull John Hopkins Hosp 83:187-212, 1948.
39. Riggs HE, Rupp C, Ray H. Yaskin JC: Cranial nerve syndromes associated with nasopharyngeal malignancy. Arch Neurol Psych (Chicago) 77:473-482, 1957.
40. Rivers MH, Svien HJ, Baker HL: Diagnostic principles in the jugular foramen syndrome. Surg Clin N Am 43:1129-1133, 1963.
41. Rosenbaum HE, Seaman WB: Neurological

manifestations of nasopharyngeal tumors. *Neurology* 5:868-874, 1955.
42. Rydell RE, Pulec JL: Arnold-Chiari malformation. *Arch Otolaryngol* 94:8-12, 1971.
43. Schisamo G, Tovi D: Clivus chordoma. *Neurochirurgia* (Stuttg) 5:99-120, 1962.
44. Sieben RL, Hamida MB, Shulman K: Multiple cranial nerve deficits associated with the Arnold-Chiari malformation. *Neurology* 21:673-681, 1971.
45. Siekert RG: Neurologic manifestations of tumors of the glomus jugulare: chemodectoma, nonchromaffin paraganglioma or carotid body-like tumor. *A Ma Arch Neurol with Psychiat* 76:113, 1956.
46. Simonsen J: Fatal subarachnoid haemorrhage originating in an intracranial chordoma. *Acta Pathol Microbiol Scand* 59:13-20, 1963.
47. Symonds CP, Meadows SP: Compression of the spinal cord in the neighborhood of the foramen magnum. *Brain* 60:52-84, 1937.
48. Williams JM, Fox JL: Neurinoma of the intracranial portion of the hypoglossal nerve: review and case report. *J Neurosurg* 19:248-250, 1962.

28

Otoneurological Evaluation of Patients with Posterior Fossa Tumors

Margareta B. Møller, M.D.

Introduction

Because tumors in the posterior fossa give early signs of involvement of the 8th nerve, audiological and vestibular tests are useful in the diagnosis of such tumors. The symptoms that patients with tumors in the posterior fossa often present with include tinnitus, unilateral hearing loss, and dysequilibrium, but rarely true vertigo. To assess involvement of the cochlear portion of the 8th cranial nerve, pure tone audiometry, speech audiometry, and recordings of the acoustic middle ear reflex (AR), and of the brain stem auditory evoked potentials (BAEP) are of value. Involvement of the vestibular portion of the 8th cranial nerve can be assessed by recording nystagmus, either spontaneous nystagmus or that induced by caloric or rotational stimulation. State-of-the-art testing gives quantitative measurements of these values.

The tests just delineated make it possible to differentiate between a lesion of the sensory organ (inner ear) and the 8th cranial nerve. This is important because, while such tumors primarily affect the nerve, they can also affect the inner ear by impairing its blood supply. When posterior fossa tumors also compress adjacent cranial nerves, the results are specific neurological symptoms such as numbness of the face, facial weakness, otalgia, and occasional paroxysmal pain in the distribution of the trigeminal nerve. Large tumors often cause symptoms such as headache, nausea and vomiting, diplopia, and gait ataxia.

Tinnitus is present in 70% of patients with posterior fossa tumors, and in patients with acoustic tumors, it may be the only symptom for many years. The tinnitus is usually of moderate intensity and is described as a ringing or hissing sound, or occasionally as a severe roaring. As the tumor grows in size and causes either occlusion of the internal auditory artery or compression of the neural structures of the brain stem, the tinnitus may change in character, becoming very intense and disabling to the patient.

From: Sekhar LN, Schramm VL Jr, eds: *Tumors of the Cranial Base: Diagnosis and Treatment*. Mount Kisco, New York, Futura Publishing Co, Inc, © 1987.

Audiometry

The audiological results most often seen in patients with posterior fossa tumors are a gradually sloping, unilateral high frequency hearing loss resembling that seen in advanced presbyacusis, ototoxic lesions, and severe acoustic traumas, but speech discrimination scores on the affected side are much lower than could be expected from such an audiogram.[9,13,14] Because cerebellopontine angle (CPA) tumors cause unilateral hearing loss with poor speech discrimination scores, they are easily distinguishable from other causes of high frequency hearing loss just discussed. In some other cases, however, patients with posterior fossa tumors may have a low frequency hearing loss, a notched audiogram, or a flat sensorineural hearing loss.

In a recent study of 27 patients with surgically confirmed CPA tumors,[21] 16 were found to have a high frequency hearing loss as revealed by their pure tone audiograms, while only two patients had a low frequency hearing loss similar to that found in Meniere's disease. Eight patients showed a "notch" audiogram with maximum hearing loss in the mid-frequency range. This audiometric configuration is pathognomonic for an auditory nerve lesion.

Patients are often deaf on the affected side at the time of their initial examination. Palva et al.[25] found that 39% of their patients with acoustic tumors had a deaf ear at the time of the first evaluation, while Johnson[10] reported that 18% of such patients had a deaf ear. In our study, however, only one patient had a deaf ear, an incidence of 3%.[21] The difference in the incidence of deaf ears at the initial examination may reflect many things: among others, the availability of otologic or neurologic evaluation and the availability of radiological evaluation for the time period when each patient was studied (the 1960s versus the 1980s).

When speech discrimination tests are used in the diagnosis of auditory nerve lesions, the pure tone threshold must be considered since a sensorineural hearing loss in itself can impair speech discrimination.[13] This was confirmed in one study of 27 patients with CPA tumors,[21] in which eight patients with pure tone thresholds better than 25 dB had discrimination scores ranging from 52 to 100%, and seven patients with hearing losses in the range 26 to 40 dB had discrimination scores between 8 and 96%; on the other hand, those patients with a pure tone hearing loss greater than 40 dB usually had severely reduced speech discrimination scores, and in some cases no discrimination at all.[21]

Brain Stem Auditory Evoked Potentials

The most sensitive way to detect auditory nerve and brain stem lesions is to record brain stem auditory evoked potentials (BAEP). BAEP are the farfield potentials that are generated by the auditory nerve, and nuclei and fiber tracts of the ascending auditory pathway in response to transient sound stimulation. Clinically, BAEP are usually recorded from electrodes placed at the vertex, or forehead, and mastoid when one ear at a time is stimulated with repetitive clicks or short tonebursts. The responses are small in amplitude and, therefore, as many as 2,000 to 4,000 responses must be averaged in order to obtain an interpretable recording. Several advantages of this test are that it does not require any cooperation from the patient, it is not measurably affected by the patient's state of alertness, and it is not affected by most self-administered drugs and medications.

Because peak V of the BAEP is the largest and the most robust of the evoked potentials in man,[21,27] it has been the most studied. The results of previous studies show that when a patient has a confirmed 8th cranial nerve tumor or a brain stem lesion, wave V of the BAEP, when recorded from the ipsilateral ear, has a prolonged latency or abnormal morphology, or later waves are reduced or absent.[3,4,11,26,27] An interaural latency difference (ILD) for wave V of 0.3 msec or longer is considered to be abnormal and indicative of a lesion involving the auditory nerve.[21,27]

A hearing loss, either sensorineural or conductive, can alter the latency of wave I on the affected ear, thus also the latency of wave V. In order to minimize this effect of hearing loss, the interpeak latency interval (IPL) from wave I to wave V is used, as representing a more accurate measure of the "central conduction time" than the absolute values of the latencies of various waves.

Recordings made directly from the auditory nerve in man during microvascular decompression (MVD) operations have shown that the auditory nerve is the main generator of both waves I and II, and that the cochlear nucleus is the main generator of wave III (see Fig. 1).[16-18,20] Wave IV most likely represents activ-

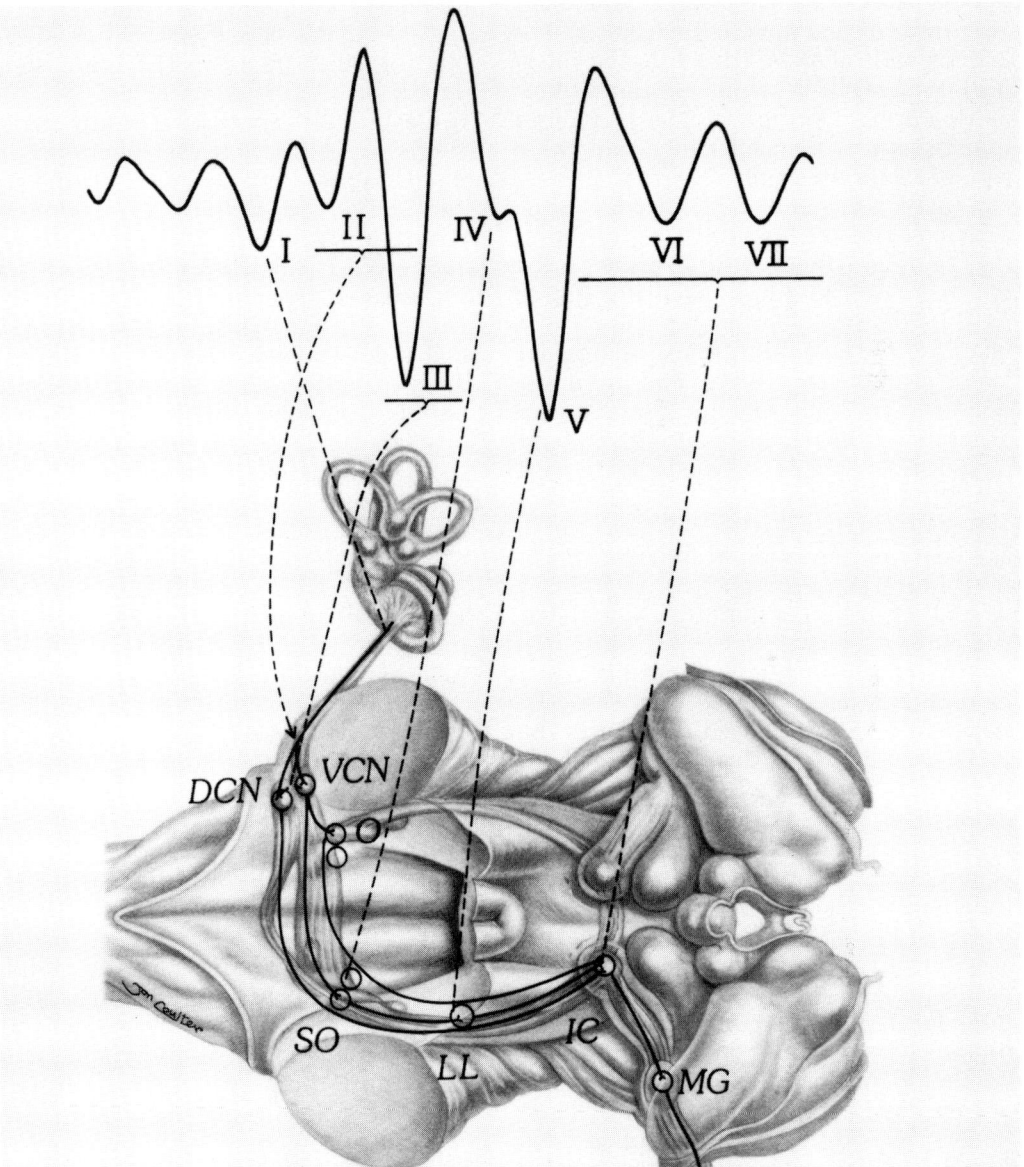

Figure 1: Schematic outline of the main neural generators of the human brain stem auditory evoked potentials (BAEP). (From Moller AR and Jannetta PJ: Neural generators of the brain stem auditory evoked potentials (BAEP). In: *The Auditory Brain Stem Response*, JT Jacobson (ed), San Diego, California, College Hill Press, 1984.) DCN = dorsal cochlear nucleus; VCN = ventral cochlear nucleus; SO = superior olive; LL = lateral lemniscus; IC = inferior colliculus; MG = medial geniculate.

ity from the superior olivary complex, while wave V has a more complex origin: the sharp tip originates in the fiber tracts of the lateral lemniscus, while the slow vertex negativity that follows it originates in the inferior colliculus.[19,22] In view of these findings, a tumor affecting the auditory nerve may be expected to cause a prolonged latency of wave II and/or a reduced amplitude of this wave with a subsequent latency shift of wave III, while the interpeak interval III-V can be expected to remain normal, except in cases of large tumors causing displacement or compression of the brain stem.

In our study of 27 patients with surgically confirmed CPA tumors,[21] we found that 24 of 26 patients with hearing on the affected side had a prolonged IPL I-III or an ILD for wave III prolonged by ≥ 0.3 msec. Only two patients had normal latencies of the early waves and prolongation of wave V only. Figures 2 and 3 give examples of the results of audiometry and recording of BAEPs in two patients with acoustic neuromas.

Large tumors in the posterior fossa can cause prolongation of the latencies of the later waves in the BAEP obtained when the ear on the nontumor (contralateral) side is stimulated.[12,24,28] Also, abnormal amplitudes and abnormal wave morphology have been seen in the contralateral BAEP. Increased IPL I-III in the BAEP recorded from the contralateral ear in patients with large tumors in the posterior fossa may be caused by a displacement of the cerebellum and, subsequently, of the flocculus on the side that is contralateral to the tumor. Since the later waves of the BAEP (IV and V) are generated mainly by the crossed auditory pathways and, consequently, by structures located on the contralateral side, a prolongation of these waves in the contralateral BAEP is a natural consequence of compression of the brain stem by large tumors (see Fig. 4). Some studies have found that large tumors cause greater changes in BAEP than small tumors,[3,4,6,27] but other studies have not found any correlation at all between tumor size and BAEP changes, and in fact BAEP responses can be absent in small intracanalicular tumors.[26]

Intrinsic brain stem tumors usually cause the same changes in BAEP as do large extrinsic tumors, namely, abnormal later waves (III to V). However, these tumors usually cause early and rapidly progressive symptoms of involvement of adjacent cranial nerves, as well as of descending fiber tracts in the brain stem (Fig. 5).

Despite the fact that recording BAEP is the most sensitive test presently available to diagnose lesions involving the auditory nerve, it is not always possible to obtain interpretable BAEPs. Further, BAEP give "false-positive" results in 0 to 33% of cases, depending upon the criteria used.[3,4,21,27,29] A "positive" response is usually determined to be false when the results of radiographic tests, particularly computerized tomography, are negative. However, small tumors may not be detected even with high-resolution scanners. We have also found[7] that the BAEP and results of other audiological tests in patients with vascular compression of cranial nerves VII and VIII can show abnormalities similar to those found in patients with confirmed tumors of the posterior fossa: of 30 patients seen consecutively who underwent MVD for disabling vertigo, 27 had BAEP changes similar but not as pronounced as those found in patients with 8th nerve tumors.[23]

The Acoustic Middle Ear Reflex Response

The threshold of the acoustic middle ear reflex, usually called the stapedial or acoustic reflex (AR), is elevated when a lesion is affecting the auditory and facial nerves and their brain stem connections,[1,5,8,9,14] but the threshold is usually not elevated in patients with hearing loss of cochlear origin. This makes the acoustic middle ear reflex a valuable test in the diagnosis of posterior fossa tumors. The acoustic middle ear reflex involves the

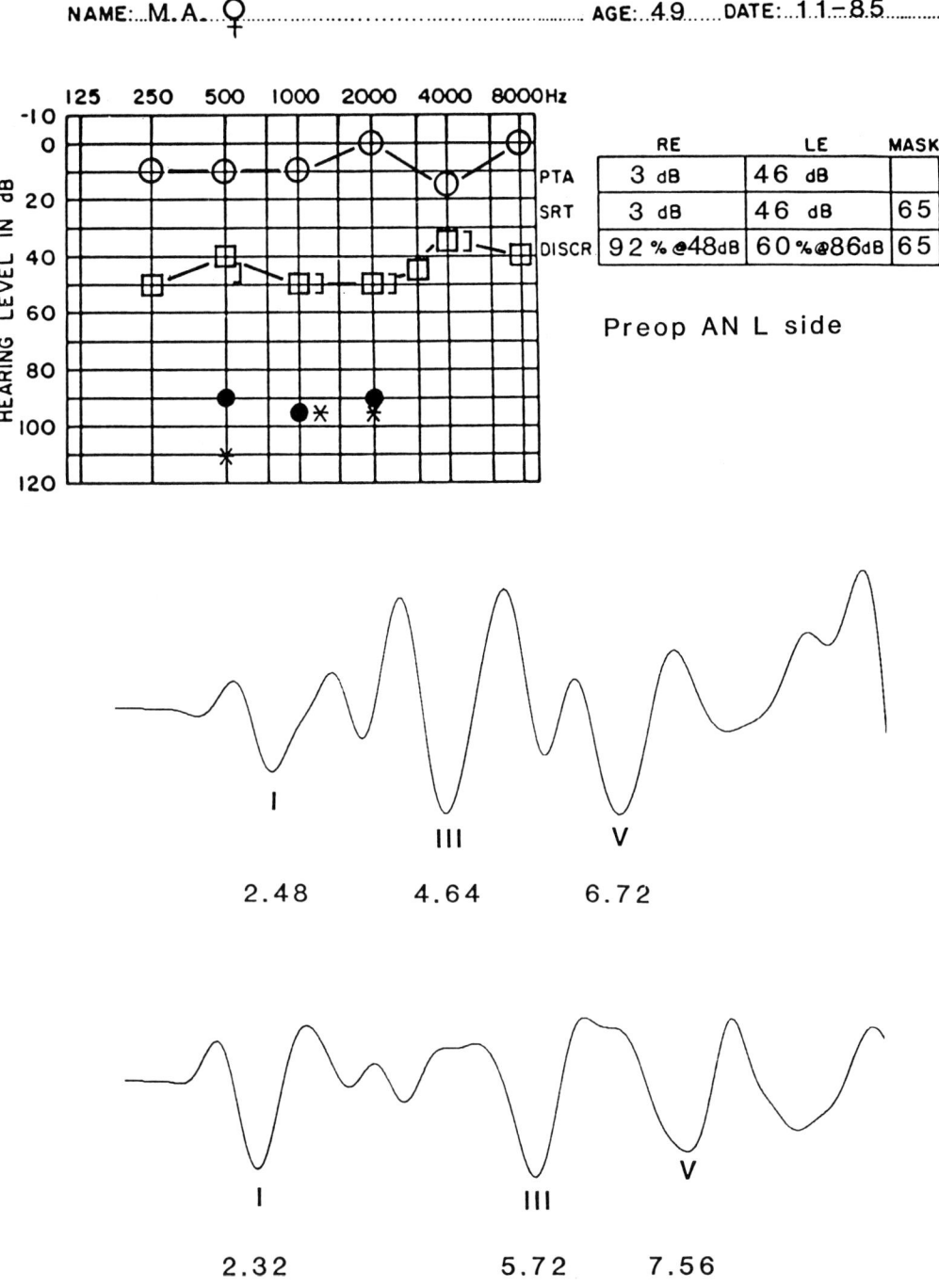

Figure 2: Results from audiometry and BAEP in a patient with a large acoustic neuroma on the left side. Upper tracing of BAEP is from the unaffected side and the lower tracing from the tumor side. IPL for waves I to III is prolonged on the affected side, while IPL III to V is normal (stimulus, 2,000-Hz tonebursts of 1 msec duration, 10 stimulations/sec).

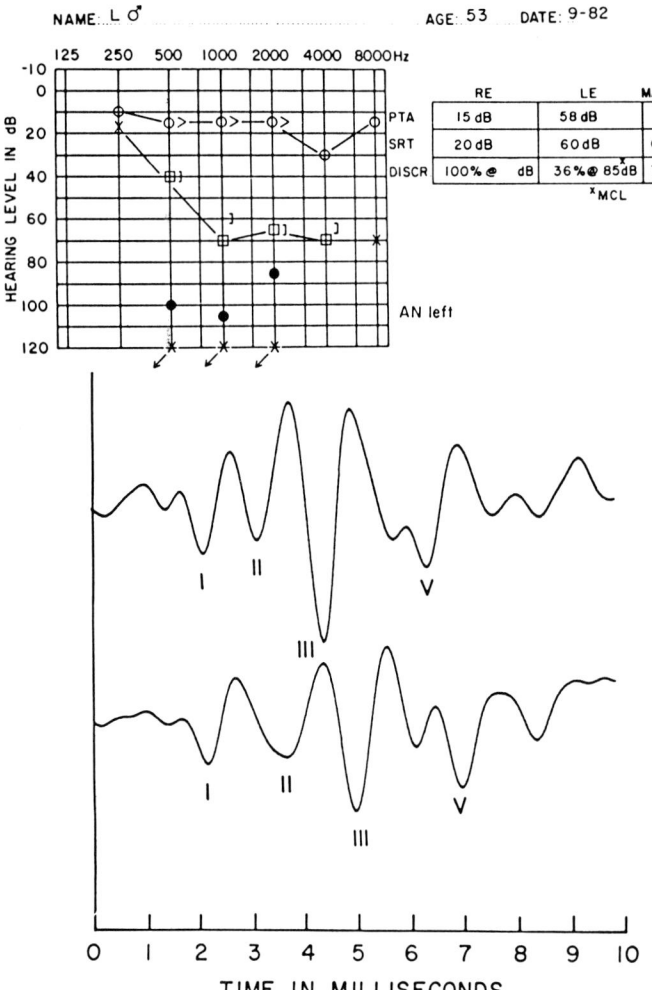

Figure 3: Results from audiometry and BAEP in a patient with a medium-sized acoustic neuroma on the left side. Upper tracing of BAEP is from the unaffected side and lower tracing from the tumor side. The latency of wave I is the same for both ears, despite a 60-dB hearing loss on the affected side. (Stimulus, 2,000-Hz tonebursts of 1 msec duration, 10 stimulations/sec.) IPL for waves I to III is prolonged on the affected side, while IPL III to V is normal.

stapedial muscles (innervated by cranial nerve VII), and it can be elicited by a loud sound, such as a pure tone or white noise. When such sound stimulus is applied to only one ear, bilateral contraction of the stapedius muscle occurs. This contraction can be recorded noninvasively, using an electroacoustic device placed in the ear canal, because the contraction of the stapedius muscle changes the acoustic impedance of the middle ear.

When tested clinically, the stapedial reflex response is usually recorded from the ear opposite to the stimulation (crossed acoustic reflex response), and the stimulus is usually pure tones of the frequencies 500, 1,000, and 2,000 Hz. The amplitude of the reflex response is slightly lower on the contralateral side and the reflex threshold is higher,[15] but recording the response on the same side from which it is elicited leads to many technical difficulties.

In a normal ear, the threshold for the acoustic middle ear reflex is 85 to 95 dB above hearing threshold.[1,13] In patients with a sensorineural hearing loss due to a cochlear lesion, the reflex threshold is unchanged, but when a lesion involves the 8th cranial nerve, the reflex threshold is elevated (>95 dB), often above the level of maximum stimulus intensity (120 dB).

In our study of 27 patients with CPA tumors, the acoustic reflex threshold was found to be abnormal (elevated or absent at the maximum level of stimulation) in

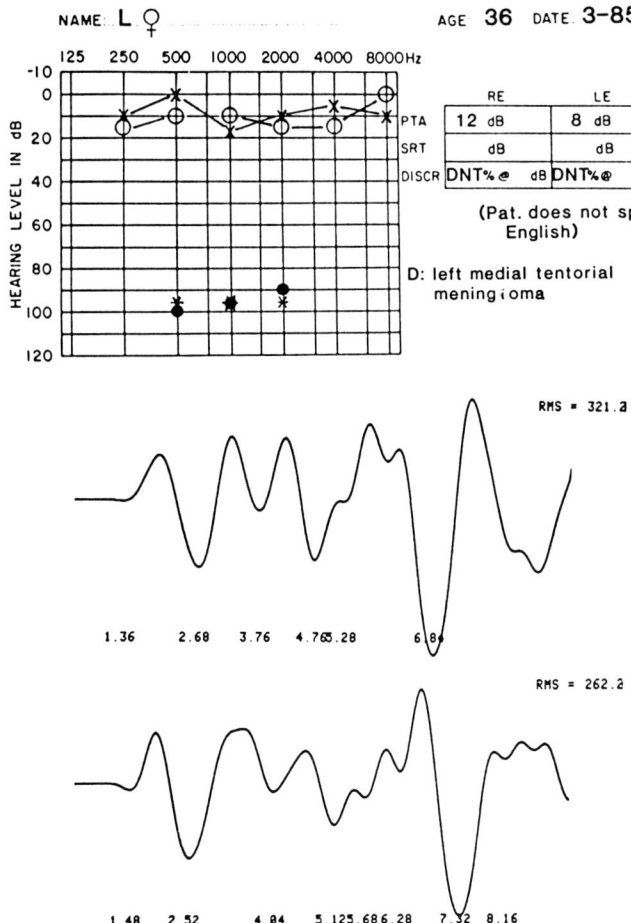

Figure 4: Results of audiometry and BAEP in a patient with a large meningioma in the posterior fossa, left side. Upper tracing of BAEP from the unaffected side and lower tracing from the tumor side. The latencies of waves I and II are normal while wave III is broad and split, and, subsequently, a delay of later waves (IV and V). (Stimulus, 2,000-Hz tonebursts of 1 msec duration, 10 stimulations/sec.)

92%, and in 8% the reflex threshold was abnormal at one of the three frequencies tested.[21] When elicited from the normal ear and recorded on the tumor side, the reflex was abnormal in 44% of the patients, indicating facial nerve involvement on the side with the tumor.

Usually, it is the threshold of the acoustic middle ear reflex that is used in diagnosis. However, the way in which the response grows with increasing stimulus intensity above threshold is of great diagnostic value. Thus, some patients have a relatively normal threshold but poor growth of the reflex response above threshold. Such poor growth of the reflex response is commonly seen in patients with 8th nerve lesions.

A lesion of the facial nerve on the side where the reflex response is recorded will naturally impair the reflex response or cause it to become absent. Recording of the acoustic reflex response is therefore valuable in assessing the location of a lesion of the facial nerve, since when a lesion is peripheral to the stapedial branch of the facial nerve, the reflex response will be normal even when facial paralysis is present.

Vestibular Tests

Acoustic nerve tumors almost always arise from the vestibular nerve and they cause a slowly progressive loss of function on the affected side. Usually, patients with a small or medium-sized tumor have few symptoms of vestibular involvement such as vertigo because the vestibular sys-

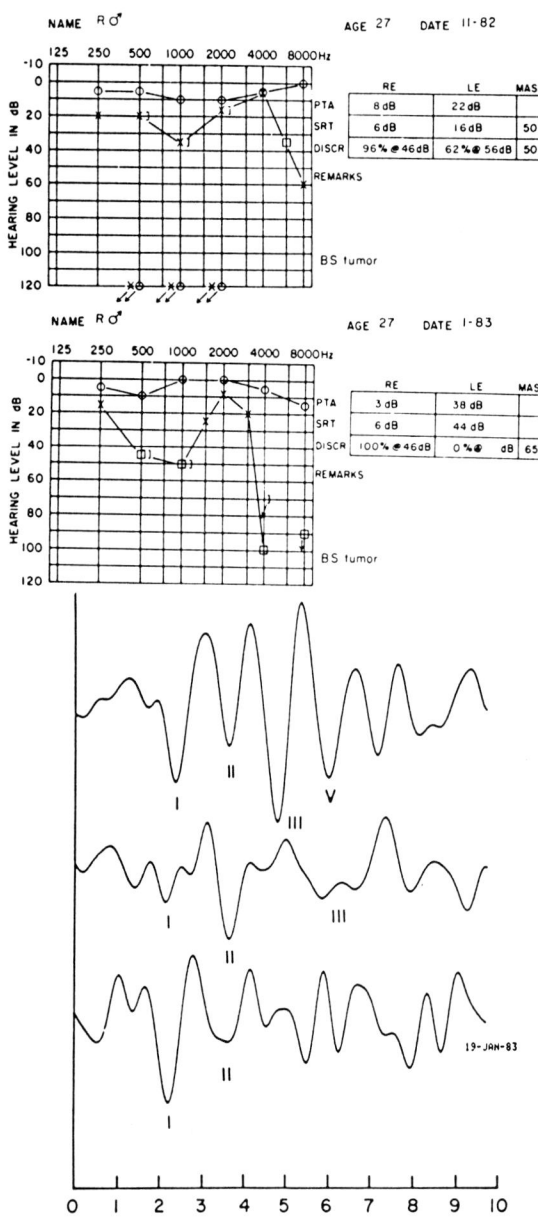

Figure 5: Results of audiometry and BAEP in a patient with a brain stem astrocytoma involving the left pontine and brain stem area. The patient's hearing deteriorated between testings done in November 1982 and January 1983. Upper tracing of BAEP obtained from the right ear shows normal latencies of waves I to V. Lower two tracings of BAEP were obtained from the side of the tumor in November 1982 and January 1983. Only waves I and II are discernible, while later waves are missing. There is a marked deterioration of the BAEP results from the left side over a 2-month period.

tem adapts to a gradual loss of function. Thus it is reported that vertigo occurs in less than 20% of patients with acoustic neuromas, while more nonspecific symptoms such as loss of balance and dysequilibrium occur in 50%. Occasionally, a patient with a posterior fossa tumor can experience a sudden onset of severe vertigo, usually associated with a sudden decrease in hearing on the affected side. These sudden symptoms most likely represent sudden expansion of the tumor due to intracapsular bleeding.

When a tumor increases in size and compresses the brain stem, the patient will notice increasing ataxia, gait disturbance, and a feeling of being off-balance. These symptoms are frequently related to other signs such as headaches and facial numbness or weakness. A classical finding in patients with large posterior fossa tumors is Brun's nystagmus, characterized by a coarse, irregular nystagmus in gaze toward the side of the tumor and a fine, rapid nystagmus in gaze toward the unaffected side. The presence of Brun's nystagmus is almost pathognomonic for a brain stem and/or cerebellar compression.

A more detailed examination of the vestibular system can be made by electronystagmography (ENG). ENG recordings utilize the differences in electrical potentials between the cornea (which is positive) and the retina (which is negative) to measure eye movements. Thus, as the eyes move from side to side, small changes in the potentials can be recorded differentially from electrodes placed on each side of the eye. To record vertical eye movements electrodes are also placed below and above each eye.

Nystagmus is an involuntary movement of the eyes with a fast and a slow component. By definition, the direction of the nystagmus is in the direction of the fast component. However, it is the slow component that is the physiological movement of the eyes. Nystagmus can be induced by rotation, stimulation of one or both ears with cold or warm water or air (30° and 44° Celsius), or by visual tracking (optokinetic nystagmus). Pathological nystagmus includes spontaneous nystagmus, nystagmus recorded with the head and/or body in different positions (positional nystagmus), and nystagmus evoked by gaze. Spontaneous nystagmus is a sign of a vestibular disturbance which may be due to a lesion involving the labyrinth, the vestibular nerve, or its central connections. When spontaneous nystagmus is due to a peripheral lesion, it may be inhibited by visual fixation, but when it is caused by a central lesion the opposite is true: visual fixation does not alter the nystagmus. A unilateral peripheral lesion (loss of function) will cause a nystagmus directed toward the healthy side, while an irritation of the labyrinth and vestibular nerve causes nystagmus, the fast component of which beats toward the involved side. A direction-fixed positional nystagmus indicates that a disturbance is affecting both the peripheral and the central vestibular system, while a direction-changing nystagmus in different positions indicates that the disturbance is mainly of central origin, including the proximal portion of the 8th nerve. Gaze-evoked nystagmus is commonly caused by drugs (valium, barbiturates, alcohol, etc.), or it may be a sign of cerebellar/brain stem involvement (Brun's nystagmus). Stimulation of one or both ears (alternate or simultaneous bithermal testing) with air or water at 30° and 44° Celsius causes a physiological nystagmus. As a general rule, a reduced vestibular response to bithermal caloric stimulation indicates a peripheral lesion, while a directional preponderance can indicate both a peripheral and a central lesion. Rotatory testing can give additional information about the function of the vestibular system but is not particularly useful in identifying unilateral vestibular lesions.[2] On the other hand, rotatory testing is most useful in evaluating patients with bilateral peripheral vestibular lesions.

In general, vestibular tests have relatively low specificity in diagnosis of posterior fossa tumors and any given test result can be caused by a variety of disorders. Also, the fact that the patient needs to be highly alert during testing in order to obtain accurate results adds uncertainty to vestibular testings.

In summary, the state-of-the-art of auditory and vestibular tests allows us to diagnose involvement of the 8th cranial nerve and its central connection in the brain stem from tumors in the posterior fossa. The auditory tests today have a higher specificity in revealing 8th cranial nerve pathology than did the vestibular tests.

References

1. Anderson H, Barr B, Wedenberg E: Early diagnosis of VIIIth nerve tumors by acoustic reflex tests. *Acta Otolaryngol* (Stockh) (Suppl) 263:232-237, 1970.
2. Baloh RW: Dizziness, hearing loss and tinnitus. *The Essentials of Neurotology*, Philadelphia, F.A. Davis Co., 1984.
3. Clemis JD, McGee T: Brainstem electric re-

sponse audiometry in the differential diagnosis of acoustic tumors. *Laryngoscope* 89:31-42, 1979.
4. Eggermont JJ, Don M, Brackmann DE: Electrocochleography and auditory brainstem electric responses in patients with pontine angle tumors. *Ann Otol Rhinol Laryngol* 89:1-19, 1980.
5. Hirsch A, Anderson H: Audiological test results in 96 patients with tumours affecting the eighth nerve. *Acta Otolaryngol (Stockh) (Suppl)* 369, 1980.
6. Hyde ML, Blair RL: The auditory brainstem response in neurology: Perspectives and problems. *J Otolaryngol* 10:117-125, 1981.
7. Jannetta PJ, Møller MB, Møller AR: Disabling positional vertigo. *New Engl J Med* 310:1700-1705, 1984.
8. Jerger J, Hartford E, Clemis J, et al: The acoustic reflex in eighth nerve disorders. *Arch Otolaryngol* 99:409-413, 1974.
9. Johnson EW: Auditory test results in 500 cases of acoustic neuroma. *Arch Otolaryngol* 103:152-158, 1977.
10. Johnson EW: Results of auditory tests in acoustic tumor patients. In House WF, Luetje CM (eds): *Acoustic Tumors*, Baltimore, University Park Press, 1979, Vol. 1, pp 209-224.
11. Josey AF, Jackson CG, Glasscock ME: Brainstem evoked response audiometry in confirmed eighth nerve tumors. *Am J Otolaryngol* 1:285-290, 1980.
12. Kinney SE, Nodar RH: Brainstem auditory evoked potentials for detection of retrocochlear pathology. *Ann Otol Rhinol Laryngol* 89:291-295, 1980.
13. Liden G.: Speech audiometry. *Acta Otolaryngol (Stockh) (Suppl)* 114, 1954.
14. Liden G, Korsan-Bengsten M (aka Møller MB): Audiometric manifestations of retrocochlear lesions. *Scand Audiol (Stockh)* 2:29-40, 1973.
15. Møller AR: The acoustic reflex in man Special issue in honor of Professor Georg von Bekesy. *J Acoust Soc Am* 34:1524-1534, 1962.
16. Møller AR, Jannetta PJ, Bennett M, Møller MB: Intracranially recorded responses from the human auditory nerve: New insights into the origin of brainstem evoked potentials (BSEPs). *Electroencephalogr Clin Neurophysiol* 52:18-27, 1981a.
17. Møller AR, Jannetta PJ, Møller MB: Neural generators of brainstem evoked potentials. Results from human intracranial recordings. *Ann Otol Rhinol Laryngol* 90:591-596, 1981b.
18. Møller AR, Jannetta PJ: Auditory evoked potentials recorded intracranially from the brainstem in man. *J Exp Neurol* 78:144-157, 1982a.
19. Møller AR, Jannetta PJ: Evoked potentials from the inferior colliculus in man. *Electroencephalogr Clin Neurophysiol* 53:612620, 1982b.
20. Møller AR, Jannetta PJ, Møller MB: Intracranially recorded auditory nerve response in man: New interpretations of BSER. *Arch Otolaryngol* 108:77-82, 1982.
21. Møller MB, Møller AR: Brainstem auditory evoked potentials in patients with cerebellopontine angle tumors. *Ann Otol Rhinol Laryngol* 92:645-650, 1983.
22. Møller AR, Jannetta PJ: Neural generators of the auditory brainstem response. In Jacobson JT (ed): *The Auditory Brainstem Response*, San Diego, California, College Hill Press, 1984, pp 13-31.
23. Møller MB, Møller AR, Jannetta PJ, Sekhar L: Diagnosis and surgical treatment of disabling positional vertigo. *J Neurosurg* 1985, in press.
24. Nodar RH, Kinney SE: The contralateral effect of large tumors on the brain stem auditory evoked potentials. *Laryngoscope* 90:1762-1768, 1980.
25. Palva T, Jauhiainen T, Sjoblom CJ, et al: Diagnosis and surgery of acoustic tumors. *Acta Otolaryngol (Stockh)* 86:233240, 1978.
26. Rosenhall U: Brain stem electrical response in cerebellopontine angle tumors. *J Laryngol Otol* 95:931-940, 1981.
27. Selters WA, Brackmann DE: Acoustic tumor detection with brain stem response audiometry. *Arch Otolaryngol* 103:181-187, 1977.
28. Shanon E, Gold S, Himelfarb MZ: Auditory brain stem responses in cerebellopontine angle tumors. *Laryngoscope* 91:254-259, 1981.
29. Thompson J, Terkildsen K, Osterhammel P: Auditory brainstem responses in patients with acoustic neuromas. *Scand Audiol (Stockh)* 7:179-184, 1978.

29

Acoustic Neurinomas: Neurosurgical Approaches and Results

Peter J. Jannetta, M.D.

Introduction

Despite the major technological advances that have been applied to acoustic neurinomas over the last 20 years, major difficulties persist in some lesions. These include, to a significant degree, lesions at either end of the spectrum. In the huge lesions, problems of total excision, brain stem dysfunction, and facial nerve preservation persist. In the larger lesions, facial nerve preservation remains an area of significant difficulty. In small lesions, where threat to life and facial nerve loss are not areas of such major concern, the question of hearing preservation remains an area of difficulty. In this chapter we will update our experience with staging of huge tumors, review our technique for intermediate-sized tumors and discuss the technique of hearing preservation in smaller lesions, elaborate upon electrophysiologic monitoring of auditory and facial nerve function, and review our series of tumors.

I. The Two-Stage Excision of Huge Tumors

We define huge acoustic neurinomas as those causing marked distortion and indentation of the brain stem and cerebellum, as well as malfunction of multiple cranial nerves. These tumors measure 4 cm or greater in diameter and usually extend to or across the midline.[55]

Dissection of the tumor from the brain stem with preservation of its arterial supply and root entry zones of the involved cranial nerves is the most important and meticulous portion of the procedure. Unfortunately, in huge tumors, this part of the procedure frequently takes place near the end of a long operation when the surgical team is fatigued. This is especially true when the tumor is dense and fibrous in nature, and the integrity of the facial nerve has been preserved. The velocity of decompression of the distorted brain stem as the tumor moves away from the pons is another serious factor in morbidity and

---

From: Sekhar LN, Schramm VL Jr, eds: *Tumors of the Cranial Base: Diagnosis and Treatment*. Mount Kisco, New York, Futura Publishing Co, Inc, © 1987.

mortality. In our first patient in this series, the operation was terminated because of marked changes in the vital signs (asystole) while the medial portion of the tumor was being removed from the brain stem. As a result, a significant amount of tumor was left attached to the brain stem. Reoperation was performed one week later, and the residual tumor was found to have extruded into the vacant space in the cerebellopontine angle left by the initial removal of lateral tumor (Fig. 1). The brain stem was no longer distorted. The cleft between the arachnoid layers of the brain stem and the tumor was easily identified as it was virgin territory that had not been entered at the prior procedure. Removal of the remaining tumor was quite easy, and the patient suffered no abnormalities of the vital signs when the residual neurinoma was removed from the brain stem. This prompted our use of the two-stage procedure in similar cases of huge acoustic neurinomas.

Clinical Materials and Methods

Patient Population

This series consists of 27 patients ranging in age from 10 to 68 years, with a mean age of 36.9 years. There were 19 females and 8 males. All the patients had extensive neuro-otological and neuroradiological evaluations, as well as clinical and radiographic evidence of huge acoustic neurinomas. All had preoperative CT scans and most had vertebral angiography. Varying combinations of multiple cranial-nerve deficits associated with brain stem and/or cerebellar dysfunction were present in all. Five patients had papilledema and obstructive hydrocephalus severe enough to necessitate the insertion of preoperative ventriculoperitoneal shunts.

Operative Technique

Our earlier procedures were carried out with the patient in the semi-sitting position. We now use the lateral position in all patients:[24] the skull secured with a three-point head holder and a soft roll under the axilla to protect the brachial plexus. A standardized anesthetic technique is used, consisting of narcotic, nitrous oxide, and controlled hyperventilation. All patients are monitored with electrocardiography and direct arterial and venous pressure lines and intermittent blood gas analysis. Expiratory CO_2 levels and urinary output are monitored. The pulse rate is monitored via a Doppler ultrasonic detector. Brain stem auditory evoked potentials (BAEP) are monitored from the opposite ear primarily to

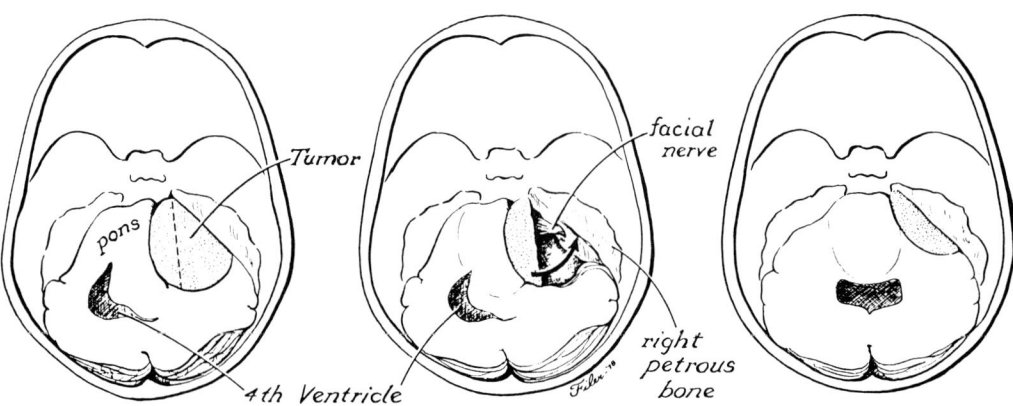

Figure 1: Schematic views of removal of a huge acoustic neurinoma. Left: Preoperative view. Center: View after multiple tumor removal in stage-one procedure. Right: Before stage-two procedure, showing the decompression of the brain stem and extraction of remaining tumor laterally.

evaluate wave V, which is a brain stem wave on the operative side.[18,31,32] Facial nerve electromyography is utilized for facial nerve identification and preservation.[33] In our experience, air embolism has not been a problem in the lateral position and we use a central venous line but do not place it in or near the right atrium. Osmotic agents and adrenal cortical steroids are utilized.

A 6 or 7 cm linear incision is made over the occipital bone two fingerbreadths behind the mastoid eminence parallel to and behind the hairline. A unilateral retromastoid craniectomy is then carried out, with the bone removed to the posterior border of the sigmoid sinus. We have followed the basic neurosurgical technique of the suboccipital transmeatal approach as outlined by Rand and Kurze[45-48] and modified by Yasargil[66,67] and ourselves.[24,25,55] The dural arterial feeders to the tumor on the posterior lip of the meatus are coagulated and divided as early as possible. After the facial nerve is identified and separated from the tumor in the internal auditory canal, the bulk of the tumor is decompressed. Initial internal decompression may be necessary to find the internal auditory meatus. The layers of arachnoid over the tumor are opened. Beginning laterally, resection proceeds from the posterior direction down to the pons, and care is taken to identify the 9th, 10th and 11th nerves. In addition, branches of the anterior inferior cerebellar artery are also identified and spared. Tumor from above is then resected down to the pons, and the 5th nerve is identified and spared. Any tumor within the incisura is brought down and removed. The tumor is also dissected clear of the facial nerve anteriorly, and the facial nerve is marked with heavy suture or a Silastic sling for ease of identification at the second stage. About this time, a decision is made of whether to proceed with complete tumor removal in one stage. If the procedure has been long or difficult, considerable time has been spent dissecting a stretched, thinned-out facial nerve, the operation is usually terminated. It is not unusual to have been operating for 3 to 5 hours up to this point.

In recent years, serial computerized tomography (CT) scans have been performed postoperatively, and compared to the preoperative scans (Figs. 2A and 2B). The tumor gradually decompresses out of the pons, swiveling laterally like a gate with the anterior edge of tumor acting as a fulcrum (the hinges of the gate) so that the transected tumor surface comes to lie flush against the petrous bone. Approximately 7 to 14 days after the first stage, depending on the rate of decompression and the status of the patient, the second stage is performed. For various reasons the interval between the first and second procedure has been stretched to 3 to 4 weeks on several occasions, and one patient early in the series underwent the second stage 3 months after her first operation.

Using the same anesthetic and monitoring techniques as before, the wound is reopened and the major reference points are re-identified using constant gentle irrigation to flush away the material in the operative site. The previously marked facial nerve is identified using a previously placed sling and the electromyographic probe. In addition, the other major structures are identified. The now-smaller tumor lies in the cerebellopontine angle with a more normal relationship to its surrounding neural and vascular structures. The tumor fills up the void previously left at the termination of the first procedure and has moved away from the pons. The lateral pontine region is virgin territory which was not entered during the first stage. The proximal facial nerve and anterior inferior cerebellar arteries are usually identified and preserved with relative ease. The second-stage basically involves removal of the remaining tumor from the brain stem and adjacent zones of the involved cranial nerves. Great care is taken to preserve the anterior inferior cerebellar artery and its perforating branches. We have found that it is easy to identify the arachnoid plane between the brain stem and the tumor, and have not had any problems with changes in vital signs occurring when we removed the remaining portion of the tumor from the brain stem. Once the facial nerve had been identified and saved during the first stage

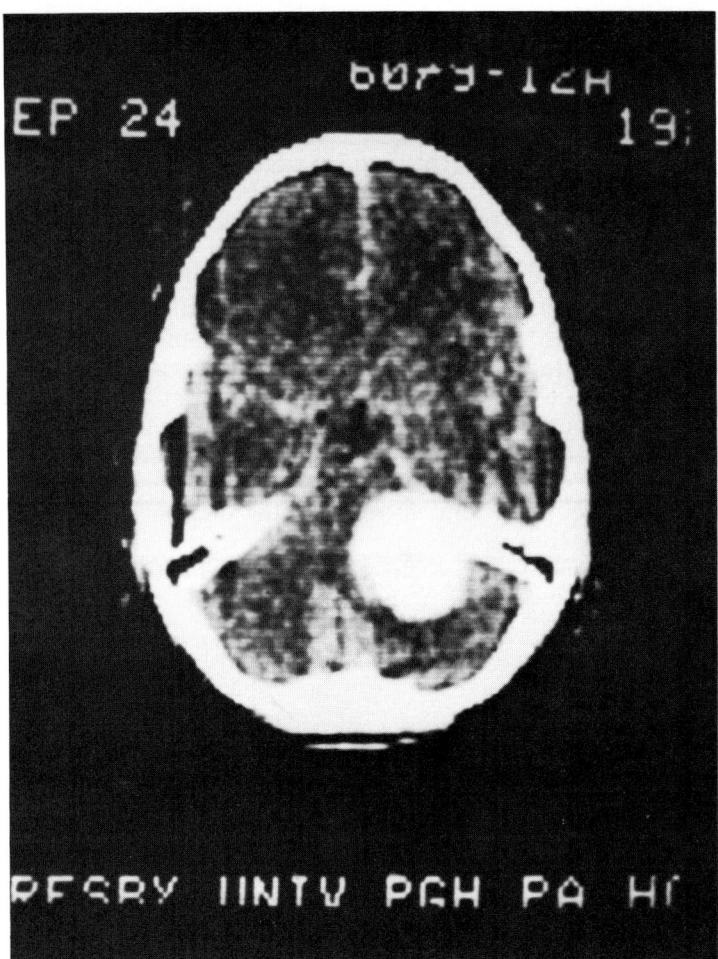

Figure 2: Preoperative CT scan (A), and after first stage excision (B). Note that the tumor has shifted laterally with its cut surface now against the petrous bone.

of the procedure, it was always possible to save it in the second stage. The operating time for the second stage of the procedure is approximately 2 to 4 hours.

On four occasions early in the series it was necessary to resect a portion of the lateral cerebellar hemisphere when it became apparent that prolonged retraction had contused the cerebellar tissue.

Operative Results

All patients in this series had two separate, staged procedures with successful total excision of their acoustic tumors. Five of these patients had preoperative ventriculoperitoneal shunts inserted for the control of obstructive hydrocephalus and papilledema. There was no operative mortality and no deaths have occurred in a follow-up period ranging from 1 to 11 years. Good results have been obtained in 24 (89%) of our patients, who have returned to normal activities or full-time employment. Three patients (11%) have residual preoperative neurological deficits causing a reduced level of activity. Of these, only one is unable to care for himself. Of the five patients who had shunts placed preoperatively, four have resumed routine activity, while the fifth remains under custodial care because of a persistent residual preoperative mental dysfunction and ataxia. None of our patients was made significantly worse by the operative procedures (Table I).

The only significant intraoperative morbidity that occurred was that of a pa-

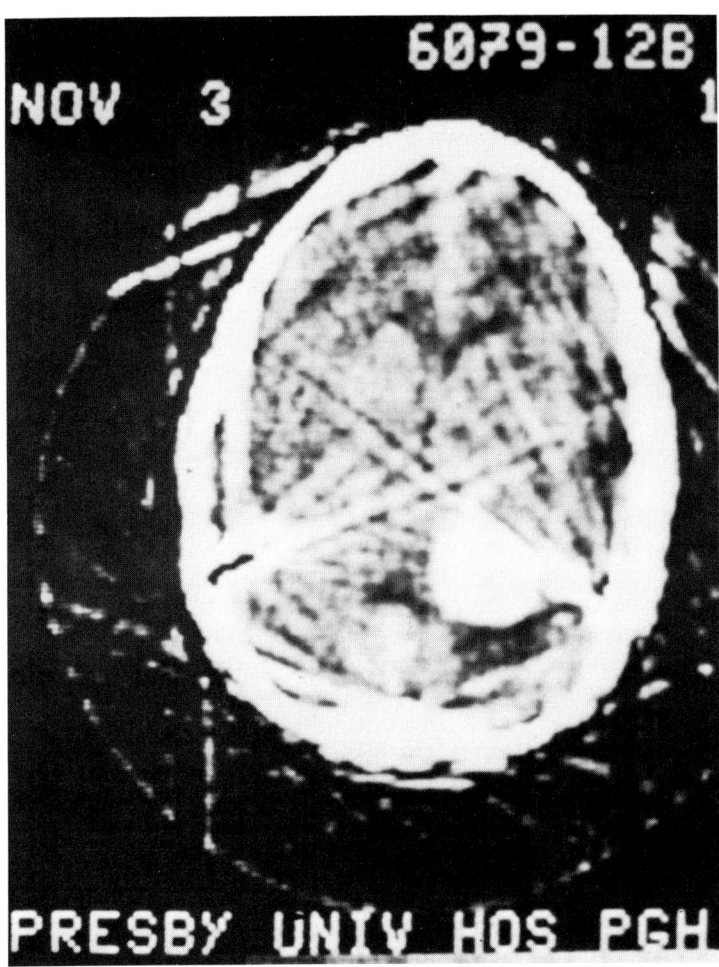

tient who had the first stage of her procedure terminated when she developed massive air embolism with resultant serious cardiac arrhythmia and hypotension. The patient subsequently had an uneventful second-stage procedure performed 3 weeks later.

Table I
Quality of Patient's Life:
Staged Excision of Huge Acoustic Neurilemmomas

Quality of Life	Cases No.	(%)
Fulltime activity or employment	24	89
No improvement over preop status	3	11
Worse after surgery	0	0
Total	27	100

Postoperative morbidity (Table II) included 10 patients (38%) who demon-

Table II
Operative Results:
Staged Excision of Huge Acoustic Neurilemmomas

Operative Results	Cases No.	(%)
Mortality	0	0
Total excision	26	96.3
Recurrence	1	3.7
Morbidity		
CSF circulation	10	38
V_1 hypesthesia	5	19
meiosis, ipsilateral	1	3.7
transient nerve VI paresis	1	3.7
IX neuralgia	1	3.7
massive air embolism	1	3.7

strated cerebrospinal fluid (CSF) circulation problems. Nine patients developed evidence of pseudomeningocele formation with some signs of increased intracranial pressure. The tenth developed a CSF leak at the surgical site. Eight patients with pseudomeningocele formation were successfully treated by lumbar spinal subarachnoid drainage as described by McCallum et al.[30] One of the patients required insertion of a postoperative ventriculoperitoneal shunt. The patient with the CSF leak underwent wound revision. Five patients with postoperative facial paresis and fifth-nerve deficit needed temporary tarsorrhaphies for control of potential keratitis. One man developed a transient 6th nerve paresis postoperatively, and one woman developed postoperative intractable glossopharyngeal neuralgia on the operated side approximately 3 months after her second-stage surgical procedure. This was successfully treated by microvascular decompression of the 9th and 10th nerves.

Anatomic continuity of the facial nerve was preserved in 21 patients (78%). In the remaining six patients, the facial nerve was so frayed that primary intracranial anastomosis was not feasible. Five of these six patients have had a subsequent facial-hypoglossal anastomosis performed. Of the 21 patients with preserved facial nerves, 18 have recovered facial function. Fourteen of these have exhibited full recovery, and four demonstrate partial cosmetically acceptable function. All of our patients with intact facial function had either total or partial facial weakness at the conclusion of their second-stage procedure. Recovery of facial movement took place over a period of 2 to 14 months.

Discussion

Staging of brain-tumor surgery is not a new concept. Such procedures have been carried out for many years, especially with certain supratentorial gliomas, meningiomas, and arteriovenous malformations. Deliberate planned staging of acoustic neurinoma surgery was reported by us in 1979.[55]

Recent reports by many authors[10-13, 22,26,27,29,34,37,44,50,55,58,61,64,66,67] have shown a marked reduction in the operative mortality from acoustic neurinoma surgery. However, if one analyzes the results of these series carefully, it becomes apparent that large acoustic tumors are still a problem, for almost all of the mortality in these reports occurred in patients with large tumors. In addition, incomplete tumor removal with subsequent recurrence remains a serious consideration. In MacCarty's series,[27] 15 of 132 patients had subtotal excisions, and of these, five needed reoperation for recurrence. In the series of Ojemann et al.,[35-37] 19 patients were reported as having large tumors, greater than 2 cm in diameter. Of these tumors, only 10 were totally removed; at the time of that report, three patients had recurrence within 15 to 24 months after their initial operative procedure. DiTullio et al.[10] were able to obtain complete removal in 89% of their 45 patients with large tumors. They gave no indication as to whether any procedure for recurrence was carried out. Yasargil[67] and Fox[66] are the only authors to report a series in which all patients had total excision of acoustic neurinomas in one stage. In their series, 44 tumors (33.6%) were described as being very large. There was a 6.8% mortality in this group of patients with very large lesions.

Satisfactory postoperative facial function in large tumors in the 65% to 80% range is presently acceptable. The rate of return of facial function in our patients corresponds to reports of others.[42,49]

We suggest that a two-stage procedure may be the operation of choice for huge acoustic neurinomas. There is no doubt that some of these huge lesions can be removed effectively in one stage with low mortality and morbidity and with preservation of the facial nerve. However, there is also no doubt that in many instances large tumors are incompletely removed because of problems that occur not only with the dissection and the vital signs of the patient, but also because of fatigue of the surgical team, especially during the dissection of tumor from the brain stem. As a result, such procedures are terminated and the patients are allowed to leave the hospital with residual tumor still in place. Re-exploration is carried out only when evidence of recurrence becomes apparent.[49] We consider that patients with incomplete tumor removal can be safely operated on for the residual tumor within a short period of time, thus negating the consequences of tumor recurrence. This result can best be accomplished by a two-stage procedure.

This operative approach has changed our attitude toward these huge acoustic neurinomas. We believe that converting a long, tedious, and potentially hazardous procedure into two shorter operations may be easier for the patient as well as for the surgeon. We suggest that an elective two-stage procedure may offer a better chance for complete tumor removal, lessened mortality and morbidity, and good quality of survival for the patient. With modern neuro-anesthetic techniques, the two-stage procedure offers no unusual problems and gives us an alternative in a very difficult situation.

II. Large to Medium Tumors

These lesions measuring >2.5 cm to <4.0 cm in diameter include the majority of acoustic neurinomas upon which we operate. The technique for their removal is generally the same as for the huge tumors except that it is one continuous procedure.[55] We have occasionally planned a two-stage procedure, only to find that the lesion, although large, was soft, not especially vascular, and gradually decompressed from the pons as we dissected laterally so we have been able to remove it in toto in one stage.

We generally drill away the posterior wall of the porus acusticus and identify the facial nerve in the canal first, but follow the surgical dictum which states that one does what he is doing while it is going on and then stops, before an impasse is reached, to do something else. The specific areas of dissection are as follows.

Operative Technique

Drilling the Porus and Identifying the Facial Nerve in the Canal

The electromyographic probe is extremely helpful in facial nerve identification. Drilling to the point where the transverse crest can be identified with a small nerve hook will help to ensure that the facial nerve is in the rostral and anterior part of the canal beyond the tumor. Once the facial nerve is identified (the vestibular nerves, having been sectioned beyond the tumor), the lesion is swept back toward the lip of the porus using sharp dissection.

Debulking of the Tumor

It appears to this author that the blood supply to an acoustic neurinoma is segmental. The blood supply to lateral and rostral-lateral portions of the tumor comes from the small dural arteries along the lip of the porus. These should be coagulated before opening into the tumor. The rostral-medial and medial tumor is supplied by the anterior inferior cerebellar artery (AICA). There are usually three branches of AICA to the tumor, each of which must be coagulated and divided. The caudal and caudal-anterior tumor is fed by the posterior inferior cerebellar artery (PICA) (inconstant). If possible, coagulation and division of as many feeding vessels as possible should be performed early in the procedure so as to reduce bleeding.

Initial debulking is performed through a small posterior opening in the capsule, incised after coagulation and after scanning the posterior capsule with the EMG probe to be sure that the facial nerve is not posterior. We use the Cavitron after a biopsy specimen is taken, first working in the lateral half of the lesion, using the CT as a guide so as not to plunge through the tumor, and then working medially. With a small slit-like opening which just fits the Cavitron probe, bleeding is controllable during aspiration of the tumor. Any excessive tumor bleeding after removal of the probe is usually controlled with Surgicel® and small cotton balls placed inside the cavity. Occasionally Avetine® is necessary.

After the initial debulking, the EMG probe is passed over the entire exposed capsule. If the facial nerve is not in this area, a large circular segment of capsule is coagulated along its periphery and excised. Large chunks of posterior tumor are removed in this way. The Cavitron, laser, or bipolar forceps may then be used for further removal of tumor inside the capsule.

Rostral Tumor Resection

The rostral tumor capsule is grasped with a Rush forceps or rotated slightly with a double-ended ganglion knife, and the EMG probe used to locate the facial nerve which frequently runs rostrally into the region of the trigeminal nerve at the brain stem. Presuming that nerve VII is not found, debulking of the rostral tumor is carried out, and the capsule shrunken down with coagulation and excised piecemeal, always preserving a lip of capsule as a handle. A soft friable capsule can be "toughened up" to be a better handle by running the bipolar coagulation forceps across the full thickness of the capsular edge. The trigeminal nerve is identified much more easily than nerve VII. The superior petrosal venous complex is in the region. It is better to take it than to tear it.

Caudal Tumor Resection

This is similar to the rostral dissection except that there is more potential trouble—with PICA, AICA, injury to the glossopharyngeal and vagus nerves, and injury to the labyrinthine artery or arteries in the region. Once nerves IX and X are decompressed, one should be very cautious in the region anterior to these nerves. It is better to leave more tumor here than you want while you clarify the AICA and PICA relationships. If you are lucky, by gently elevating the tumor, you will see a broad expanse of tumor (check again for nerve VII) and the arteries with branches to tumor which may be coagulated and divided. The labyrinthine artery, which may be multiple, may be seen here. We feel that this artery must be preserved to avoid temporary facial palsy (sometimes delayed) and incomplete return of function.

Medial Dissection

Throughout the capsular dissection, the surgeon must stay in the right plane, just adjacent to the capsule and deep to the arachnoid layers. This is especially true on the medial side of the tumor if one is to avoid brain stem arteries and veins and pontine injury. As careful debulking is performed, the posterior lip of capsule is reflected anteriorly and laterally. The tumor becomes tougher as the area from which it arises in the proximal nerve VIII is reached. PICA is in the area against the brain stem. Nerve VIII at the brain stem is just rostral to IX and X and the choroid plexus of the lateral recess of the fourth ventricle is between them although it may be displaced posteriorly. The facial nerve is just anterior to VIII at the brain stem, but rather than running laterally it is pushed away, anteriorly against the pons and usually rostrally, just beyond the brain stem. The lateral pontomedullary venous complex (sometimes multiple) may be posterior to VIII, anterior to VII, or between VII and VIII. It is too inconstant to be useful in identifying VII and is deep to the arachnoid. It may be coagulated and divided safely if violated. The EMG is most useful in finding VII against the pons in this region.

Facial Nerve Preservation

Once the nerve is identified both at the brain stem and inside the internal auditory canal, large pieces of tumor can be removed easily, to the point where the remaining tumor is attached to the facial nerve just medial to the porus acusticus. The facial nerve may be of good conformation or may be splayed out. Dissection of the area just medial to the lip of the porus is critical because not only may the nerve be splayed out, but the tumor and nerve are intimately attached here adjacent to the point where the nerve makes a 90° turn. Sharp dissection is necessary to separate the tumor from nerve VII at this point. The dissection should take place alternately, laterally, and medially. The audio on the EMG will reflect injury to and stimulation of the nerve as it is manipulated primarily or secondarily and while this *sharp* dissection is performed. In general, the nerve can look terrible and function beautifully if the blood supply via the labyrinthine artery is intact. Unfortunately, the reverse is also true: the nerve can look perfect and function poorly if the blood supply is taken.

After Tumor Removal

The area of bone removal in the porus should be treated with bone wax and a pledget of Gelfoam® placed in the porus (held in place with wax) to prevent cerebrospinal fluid leak. Multiple Valsalva maneuvers are performed with multiple gentle irrigation to stress both the venous and arterial systems to decrease the chance of postoperative hemorrhage. The dura mater is closed in a watertight fashion. The bone chips from the craniectomy, except those which include mastoid air cells, are replaced as a layer over a piece of Gelfoam on the dura to fill the upper part of the bony opening. The remaining closure is routine.

Patients are usually kept in the intensive care unit for 24 to 48 hours and then returned to their rooms. They are given intravenous fluids at the rate of 100 ml per hour and allowed to eat and drink ad lib. They usually are allowed to the bathroom on the first postoperative day and allowed to ambulate fully on the second or third day.

Mortality and Morbidity

We have had no operative deaths in this group consisting of over 200 patients. We have been able to preserve the facial nerve anatomically in every patient since we began using intraoperative electromyography. Facial nerve function has been good to excellent in all but one patient since we started using this technique (50 patients), compared to approximately 70% good to excellent function in the prior 150 (no recent follow-up).

III. Technique of Hearing Preservation in Small Acoustic Neuromas

Advances in diagnostic testing over recent years have enabled surgeons to see a higher proportion of patients with small acoustic tumors, some of whom have preserved hearing. Similarly, the application of advanced technology to operations for acoustic neurinomas have allowed surgeons progressively to decrease operative mortality, to save facial nerve function in a higher proportion of patients, and, more recently, to preserve useful hearing in selected patients. A number of investigators have now presented series of patients in whom attempts were made to preserve hearing.[10,13,15-17,19-23,25-29,34,37-41,44,45,48,50,52,56-61,63,65] Some patients have had useful hearing function preserved and documented and, in a rare patient, function has improved over the preoperative status. Buried in several of these published papers are technical details that may be useful in preservation of hearing function,[2,29,32,33,51,53,54,56-60] but no one has described a detailed technique until we did so recently.[25] The details of this technique of acoustic tumor removal are now described.

Anesthetic Techniques, Monitoring, and Patient Position

The patient with his head at the foot of the operating table (to allow knee room for the surgeon) is anesthetized and intubated. Inhalation anesthesia is used. Arterial and central venous pressure (CVP) lines and a Foley catheter are utilized. It is not necessary that the CVP line be near the right atrium. Monitoring of brain stem auditory evoked responses (BAER)[31,36,38,42,46] and direct auditory compound action potentials[32] during the operation are utilized as an aid in hearing preservation. We use a facial electromyographic technique[33] similar to the one described by Delgado et al.[9] for recording the contraction of facial muscles. While Delgado et al. used surface electrodes, we find needle electrodes more convenient. These electromyographic electrodes are placed in the musculi (m.) orbitalis oris and m. orb. oculi. Needles are placed at the vertex (Cz) and just above the ipsilateral pinna for recording of BAER. A ground electrode is placed on the forehead. Sound is delivered by an insert earphone placed in the ipsilateral ear using standard earmolds.[31,32] After placement of a three-point fixation headholder, the patient is turned into the contralateral lateral decubitus position with an axillary roll in place to protect the brachial plexus, and the headholder connected with the neck slightly stretched, flexed, and rotated a few degrees to the ipsilateral side. The ipsilateral shoulder is taped caudally and anteriorly out of the way. The purpose of these details of position is to expose the ipsilateral occipital boss. A retromastoid craniectomy is performed extending to the lateral and sigmoid sinuses and to the floor of the occipital bone.

The bone chips are preserved. If mastoid air cells are entered during the craniectomy (common in dolichocephalic patients), they are heavily waxed along with the bony edge of the craniectomy. The dura mater is opened in curvilinear fashion, incised into the corners, and the rostral, lateral, and caudal flaps are sewn back out of the way. The usual craniectomy is about 3.0 to 3.5 cm in diameter in these small tumors.

Intracranial Techniques

The surgical binocular microscope with a straight eyepiece and 250 mm focal length lens is used throughout the intradural part of the procedure. The cerebellum is elevated over the occipital floor with a narrow (0.5 cm wide) retractor blade (Fig. 3). Cranial nerves (CN) IX and X are identified. The cerebellum is protected by a piece of rubber dam (rubber does not adhere to tissue) cut from an old rubber glove and slightly larger than a 0.5 × 2 inch cottonoid strip which is placed between the rubber dam and the retractor blade or by Biocol®. The subarachnoid cistern over CN IX and X is opened. Any bridging veins coursing from cerebellum through IX and X that may be torn with retraction (seen in about 30% of patients) are coagulated and divided. The cerebellum is elevated over the glossopharyngeal-vagal complex. Lateral-to-medial retraction of the cerebellum is avoided as much as possible at this time as this is deleterious to hearing function. This initial exposure is similar to that used in microvascular decompression for hemifacial spasm.[24] The recording electrode for direct auditory compound action potentials is placed on the 8th nerve.[32] Once this electrode is in place, medial retraction of the cerebellum can be performed safely.

The tumor and its relationships to CN VII and VIII are evaluated (Fig. 4). The two arachnoidal layers over the tumor are opened, the medial side of the tumor and its relationship are clarified, and the posterior rim of the internal auditory meatus is identified and palpated using a 45° microhook. The facial nerve is usually seen supramedially, stretched away from CN VIII by the tumor mass (Fig. 4). The cochlear portion of CN VIII is not clearly seen at this point because the proximal superior vestibular nerve, from which the tumor commonly arises, lies posterior to it and, therefore, between the surgeon and the nerve. With the microscope on high magnification (15×, 25×), a cleft between superior and inferior vestibular nerves can be seen, usually just medial to the medial aspect of the tumor bulge (Fig. 4).

The facial nerve is definitively identified using monopolar electrical stimulation. The active electrode consists of a thin Teflon-insulated silver wire placed on a handle. The tip is freed of insulation. The stimulus is delivered by a Grass SD9 type nerve stimulator with a built-in stimulus isolation unit. The stimulus parameters used are of 150 sec duration at

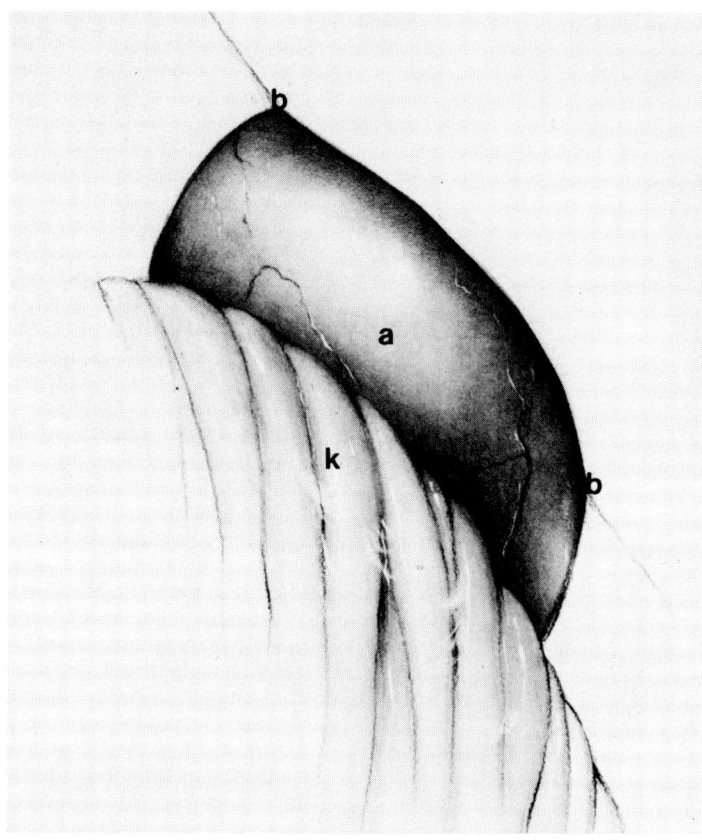

Figure 3: Drawing of right acoustic neurinoma. Patient in left lateral decubitus position. Exposure via retromastoid craniectomy. Initial view of tumor (a) extending into cerebellopontine angle from a dilated internal auditory canal (b). Flocculus of cerebellum (k).

10 pulses/sec and 0.5 to 0.7 V. The response from the facial muscles is amplified using a Grass P511K differential amplifier. The output of the amplifier is displaced on an oscilloscope that is triggered by the stimulation. It is also connected to an audio-amplifier via a gate that is closed during the stimulation. The stimulus artifacts are totally eliminated in this way and only the muscle potentials are audible.[33] This auditory feedback is valuable because it gives a clear impression of how close the stimulating electrode is to the nerve. Using this method, the nerve can quickly be identified by moving the stimulating electrode over the tumor and nerves in progressively smaller sweeps. No assistance from anesthetists, etc., is needed because the surgeon can hear the response without having to move from the microscope. A gradual increase occurs as the electrode tip comes close to the 8th nerve. This response is a result of using monopolar stimulation. The stimulus parameters we use produce less current through the nerve, minimizing the risk of damaging the nerve from the electrical stimulation.

Recordings of the BAER are made during the entire procedure. The potentials are amplified using a Grass P511K amplifier and averaged using a signal averager. The bandpass of the amplifier is usually set at 3 to 3000 Hz but, occasionally, the lower cut-off is set at 30 or 100 Hz. The sound consists of bursts of 2000 Hz pure tones of a 1 msec duration. This is the same stimulus as used in the preoperative testing, which enables easy comparison of results. The tonebursts have an equivalent intensity of about 100 dB and they are presented at an interstimulus interval of 100 msec (or occasionally 70 msec). In addition to recording BAER from scalp electrodes, we also record compound action potentials from the au-

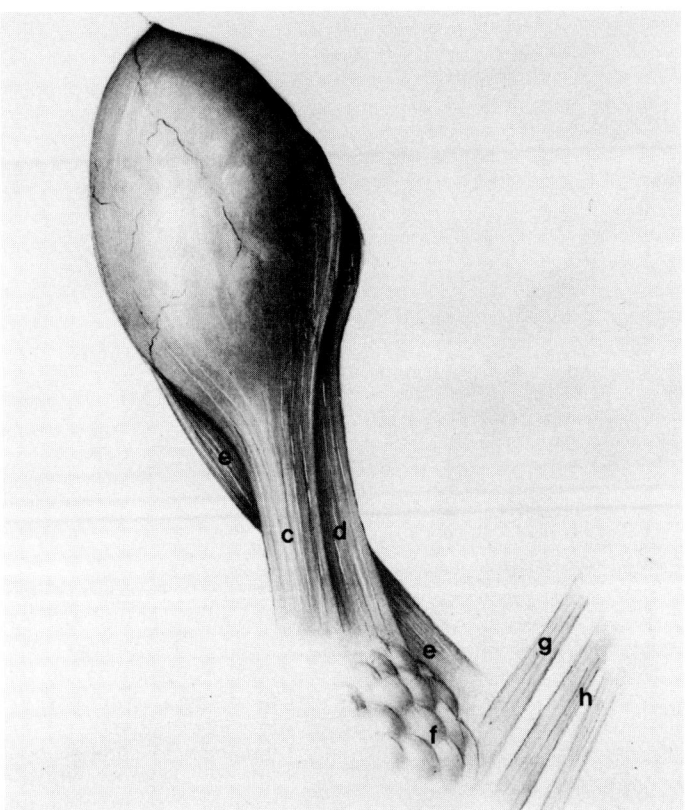

Figure 4: Same exposure as Figure 3. Cerebellum not shown in this and subsequent figures. Tumor is growing from superior vestibular nerve (c). Tumor and nerve are separable from inferior vestibular nerve (d). Facial nerve (e) arises anterior to auditory nerve and is stretched away from it by tumor mass. Choroid plexus of lateral recess of fourth ventricle (f), glossopharyngeal (g) and vagus (h) nerves shown.

ditory nerve by placing an electrode directly on the 8th nerve as soon as it becomes accessible. The technique is the same as previously described for monitoring of auditory function during microvascular decompression of the 7th and 5th cranial nerves.[31,32] The electrode used consists of a fine malleable Teflon-insulated silver wire. The insulation is removed from the tip, which is bent over, and a small cotton wick is sutured to the tip. A needle electrode is placed through the skin to serve as a reference electrode. The potentials are amplified using a Grass P511K amplifier set at 3 Hz (or 100 Hz) to 3 kHz and the potentials are displayed on an oscilloscope. Usually, the amplitude is so large that no averaging is necessary. The same ground electrode as was used for the BAER recorded from the scalp is used. The intracranial potentials are simultaneously recorded with the potentials from scalp electrodes, and the same sound stimulation is used for both recordings.

Direct recording of the response from the auditory nerve is of some value in identifying the 8th nerve, but it most importantly provides instantaneous monitoring of auditory function, making it possible to reverse the effect of direct compression or neural distraction from retraction before it has reached the level at which permanent damage to the nerve occurs. If possible, the labyrinthine artery (single or multiple) is identified early on. This artery *must* be preserved if hearing function is to be preserved.

The posterior wall of the internal auditory canal is cleared of overlying dura mater, drilled away for a distance of 1 cm, and the transverse crest is identified by palpation (Fig. 5). It is important that the internal ear not be injured by drilling too far. Before this drilling is begun and the dura cleared away, the dural arteries over the posterior lip of the porus to the tumor are coagulated, making sure to use relatively high volumes of irrigation with the suction irrigation to prevent heat-spread

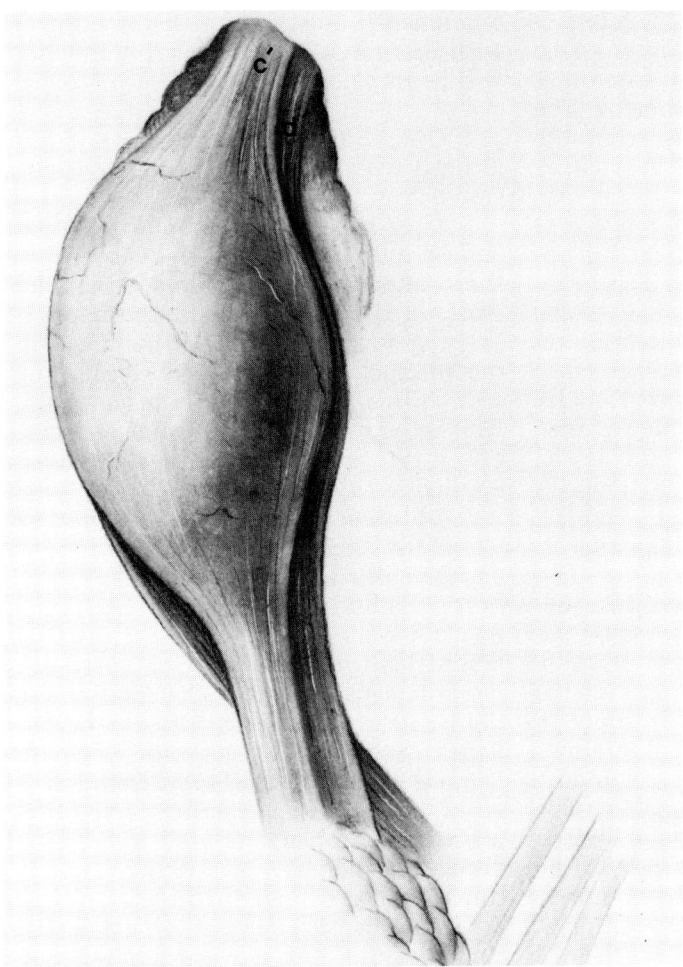

Figure 5: Posterior wall of internal auditory canal has been drilled away for a distance of 1 cm. Distal superior vesticular nerve (c) and distal inferior vestibular nerve (d) shown.

to CN VII and VIII. High volume, low velocity irrigation is important during drilling, again to prevent injury by transmitted heat. We have seen improvement in auditory nerve function as measured by the evoked potentials as the canal is opened and the intracanalicular nerve decompressed.

The facial nerve stimulating electrode is passed over the tumor to ensure that the facial nerve does not lie within it although this relationship is probably rare in small tumors. Ultrasonic aspiration or laser removal is acceptable after a satisfactory biopsy has been taken. Capsular bleeding is controlled with bipolar coagulation and intratumoral bleeding is controlled with Surgicel® packing, if necessary. It is not necessary to remove much tumor at this point but it is critical that the tumor mass not be moved about during debulking.

Specific Technical Considerations

1. Sharp dissection is necessary in separating tumor from neural tissue. Blunt dissection, even using small microinstruments to sweep tumor away from CN VII or VIII, may cause immediate and permanent hearing loss.

2. Gentle rostral-to-caudal and caudal-to-rostal retraction of CN VIII will not usually interfere with neural function.

3. However, lateral-to-medial retraction of the cerebellum, even if apparently minimal, can be particularly injurious to function of CN VIII and even of CN VII,

often irreversibly and totally. Such retraction of cerebellum should therefore be performed in conjunction with careful attention to direct CN VIII monitoring. The pia-arachnoidal connections from the nerves to cerebellum should be sharply transected to avoid traction on the nerves.

4. The superior vestibular nerve is usually connected to the hearing apparatus in the temporal bone. The nerve must be sectioned sharply, distal to the tumor, being careful to avoid traction on the nerve, if hearing is to be preserved.

5. The usually tortuous, occasionally multiple labyrinthine artery may course right through the tumor. If such is the case, hearing is lost when the tumor is removed. In this situation, which Ojemann has described,[38] BAERs and direct auditory recording disappear immediately as the artery is taken. This occurred in our case #5.

6. Usually, however, the labyrinthine artery courses on the caudal side of the tumor and gives off a branch to tumor in the region of the mesial internal auditory canal. This branch must be coagulated and divided sharply as the tumor mass is elevated, making sure not to tear it off at its origin. If this occurs, hearing will be lost in achieving hemostasis by compression of neural tissue and/or coagulation of the labyrinthine artery.

7. Sharp dissection, as noted above, is the only technique of separation of tumor from cranial nerves compatible with consistent preservation of hearing. This technique implies that tumor is gently elevated off the nerves without distracting the nerves during the dissection.

8. The cochlear nerve is almost always splayed out by the tumor. Any further distraction or compression of this nerve can cause immediate and total hearing loss.

9. The facial nerve is intimately attached to the tumor at and just medial to the internal auditory meatus. It is important that the sharp dissection at this point not inadvertently enter the nerve. The audio feedback on the EMG is helpful for avoiding such injury.

10. The facial nerve is adherent to the cochlear nerve just inside the canal. This relationship must not be disturbed even with sharp dissection as hearing function will be impaired or lost.

The above technical details are utilized wherever pertinent to the discussion below.

After the tumor is moderately debulked and the porus acusticus drilled, the sequence may continue either medially or in the canal. It is not important that the surgeon start in either area, but the surgical principle of continuing dissection in an area where things are going well and moving to another area of dissection if things have reached a stalemate is applied to this operation.

Attention is turned to the medial extent of the tumor and adjacent superior (or occasionally inferior) vestibular nerves from which tumor is growing. Starting at this point on the nerve, and using high magnification, the superior vestibular nerve is separated from the inferior vestibular nerve for a short distance using a Rosen dissector. The superior vestibular nerve is gently elevated away from the inferior nerve at the superior nerve-tumor junction with a 45° angled micronerve hook. The superior vestibular nerve is transected proximal to the tumor with scissors. The distal end of the nerve adjacent to tumor can now be grasped with forceps and held away from cochlear and inferior vestibular nerves. Further tumor is debulked if necessary. The cochlear nerve electrode may need to be repositioned at this point. The tumor is elevated and separated from adjacent nerves in a medial-to-lateral dissection using the Rosen dissector and scissors. The technique is repeated serially: debulking, elevating, and separating are repeated sequentially. It is important that the cochlear nerve not be manipulated or moved in any direction throughout the dissection (Fig. 6).

As dissection continues around the equator of the tumor and nears the internal auditory meatus, the facial nerve-tumor junction becomes more intimate. EMG monitoring of the facial muscles using the audiomonitor provides useful feedback to the surgeon since mechanical

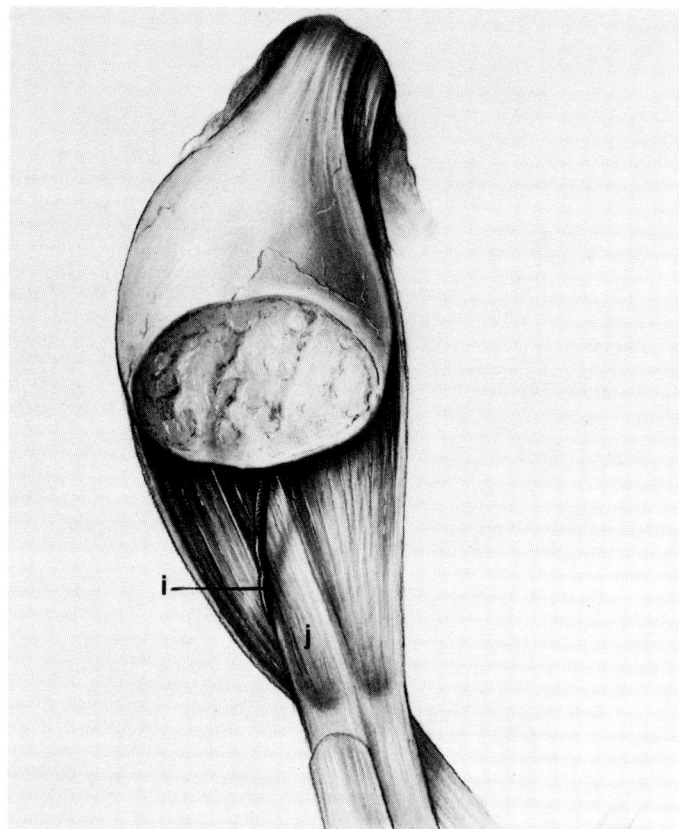

Figure 6: Proximal superior vestibular nerve has been divided sharply and medial tumor resected. A labyrinthine artery (i) and cochlear nerve (j) are now visualized.

manipulation of the nerve causes stimulation of the nerve.[9,33] The resulting EMG of the facial muscles is made audible using the above-described facial nerve monitor. If CN VII is injured, even minimally, there will be a spontaneous activity that can last for several minutes.

At or just inside the internal auditory meatus, the arterial branch to tumor, mentioned above, will be seen, but only if the tumor is elevated from the cranial nerves (Fig. 7). This branch should be coagulated and divided. Because the tissue planes may become unclear in this area, the dissection may be stopped and the procedure in the internal auditory meatus instituted.

In the lateral portion of the dissection, the facial and cochlear nerves are identified just beyond the tumor. The superior vestibular nerve is gently elevated with a 45° hook and transected with scissors, being certain that no traction is placed on the distal nerve (see above). The tumor may then be elevated and dissected medially, but not for any great distance if the tumor-arterial branch has not been previously found and transected medially because of the tumor-vascular supply arrangement as noted. Attention is then turned to the proximal side, again with debulking, if necessary, and sharp dissection extended laterally until the tumor is out (Fig. 8). The bony canal dissection area is waxed to avoid cerebrospinal fluid leak. The one or more labyrinthine arterial branches should be intact.

Closure

After multiple Valsalva maneuvers, the retractor, rubber dam and cottonoids or Biocol® are removed and the dura mater is closed in a watertight fashion. The caudal deeper fascial and muscle layers are approximated. A piece of Gel-

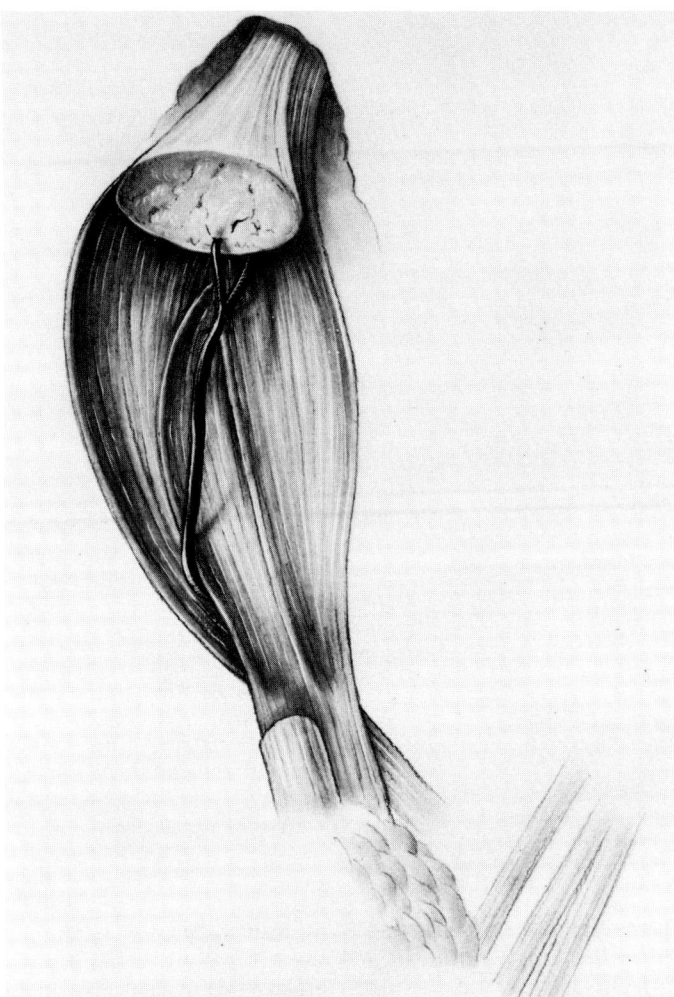

Figure 7: More tumor has been removed. Branch of labyrinthine artery to tumor is visualized. The area where the facial and cochlear nerves are conjoined is not disturbed.

foam, cut to fit the craniectomy site, is put into place over the dura mater, and the bone chips are placed in a layer on the Gelfoam.

The bone chips will be partly absorbed in time and will not look at all substantial roentgenographically, and yet they form a satisfactory fibrous fusion. Therefore, there is no depression in the skull or "soft spot." The remainder of the wound closure is completed, and a small wound dressing is applied.

Patients are kept in the intensive care unit overnight. Fluids are not restricted after surgery. The arterial and central venous lines are removed in the morning of the first postoperative day. The patient may resume a normal diet as desired, may ambulate on the first postoperative day, and can usually be discharged on the seventh postoperative day.

Patient Material

We have divided our patient population into two groups. The first consists of three women operated upon in 1975 and 1976, each of whom had some hearing before surgery and in whom we attempted to save hearing. The tumors were located on the right in all three and were 1.0, 1.5, and 1.5 cm in diameter, respectively. We did not use intraoperative auditory monitor-

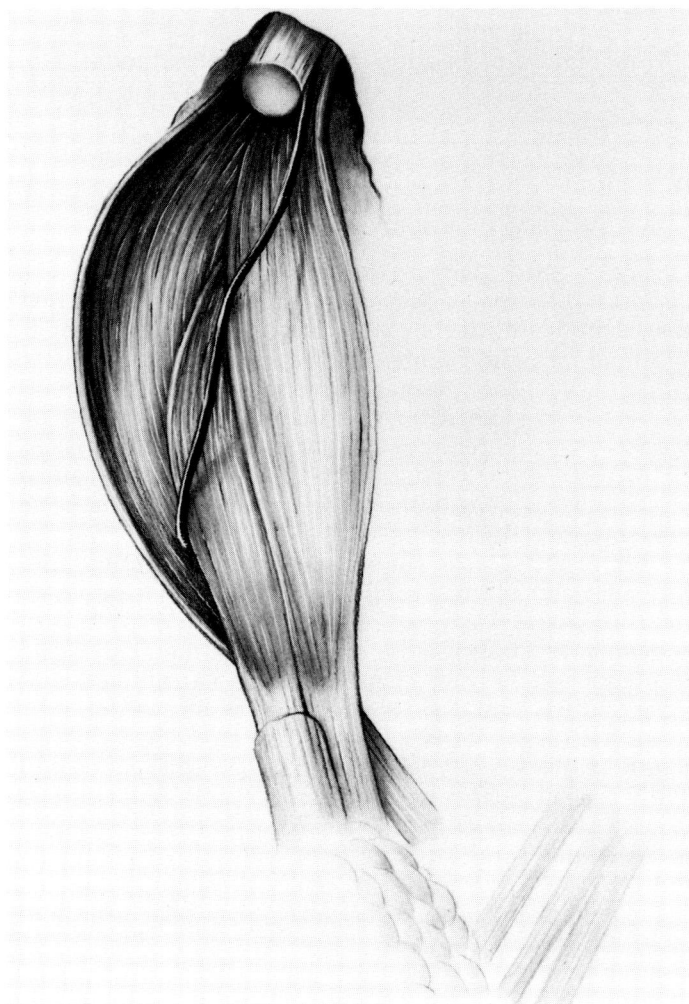

Figure 8: Distal superior vestibular nerve has been transected using sharp dissection. Tumor has been removed.

ing. We were unable to preserve useful hearing (Table III). Review of each operative videotape demonstrated errors of technique. With the information gained from this experience, we developed the current technique.

The patient population in whom we have used this technique consists of three men and three women aged 29 to 53 years. The tumor was located on the left in three and on the right in the other three. One tumor was intracanalicular. The remainder were 1.3, 1.5, 1.5, 1.7, and 2.5 cm in diameter, respectively. In three patients (nos. 1, 3, 4), it was possible to preserve useful hearing after tumor removal, while in an additional two patients (nos. 2, 5),

there was measurable postoperative response on pure tone audiometry but no useful hearing for speech. In one patient (no. 1), the discrimination score for the tumor-ear improved 18% after surgery (at 1 year), while in two patients, the speech discrimination scores decreased from 100% to 70% and 72%, respectively (Table IV).

Patient no. 2 was at the same level of hearing immediately after operation as he had had preoperatively, but within 4 months hearing deteriorated and repeated hearing tests revealed a flat sensorineural hearing loss with 28% discrimination (at 4 years). The threshold for the middle ear acoustic reflexes were obtained at normal

Table III
Prior Series: Attempted Preservation of Hearing in Acoustic Neurinoma

Patient #	Age (Years)	Sex	Year	Side	Size (cm)	Preoperative Hearing	Postoperative Hearing
1 (EP)	58	F	1975	R	1.0	A2	F5
2 (SF)	57	F	1976	R	2.0	A4	F5
3 (RS)	63	F	1976	R	1.5	C3	D5

levels, indicating a cochlear lesion with complete recruitment. Computerized tomography shows no evidence of tumor recurrence.

Special Situations

1. The tumor arises from the inferior vestibular nerve. Although this lesion is supposed to cause early severe loss of hearing by compression of the cochlear nerve in the internal auditory canal, we have seen one such patient with preoperative preservation of useful hearing. In this case, the cochlear nerve was badly stretched and attenuated by the main tumor mass, which had apparently arisen in the cerbellopontine angle rather than in the canal and had somehow dislocated the cochlear nerve rostrally along with the facial nerve. Both nerves were preserved anatomically but the single labyrinthine artery was engulfed by the tumor with no separate tumor branch, and hearing function was lost as the artery was transected. The patient also awoke with severe facial paresis, which gradually returned to normal except for modest synkinesis over a 5 month period.

2. The tumor is located totally in the cerebellopontine angle. Such tumors in the past were commonly not diagnosed until they were large, apparently because the cochlear nerve is not compressed in the internal auditory canal by the tumor. The internal auditory meatus may be flared, but if normal nerve can be visualized distal to the tumor, the nerve can be sharply transected with little or no bone drilling.

3. The tumor extends laterally into the temporal bone and beyond the crista transversalis and cannot be removed totally via the cerebellopontine angle. This has not occurred in the current series of small lesions but only in large tumors.

4. We have noted an invasive tumor in one patient with neurofibromatosis in whom we sacrificed CN VIII. She also had an adjacent facial nerve neurinoma and had severe facial paresis, which improved. She recently died of generalized neoplasm related to her neurofibromatosis.

Discussion

Forty-two contributions that described preservation of hearing in acoustic neurinomas were published prior to our 1984 paper were reviewed.[1-8,10,13,15-17,19-23,26-29,34-37,39,41,44,45,48-52,56-65] Before the

Table IV
Current Series: Attempted Preservation of Hearing in Acoustic Neurinoma

Patient	Age (Years)	Sex	Year	Side	Size (cm)	Preoperative Hearing	Postoperative Hearing
1 (BF)	37	M	1977	L	1.7	B3	A2
2 (GR)	35	M	1978	L	1.5	C3	C3 E4
3 (MS)	38	F	1980	R	2.5	A1	B2
4 (SE)	32	F	1980	R	1C	A1	B2
5 (NC)	29	F	1983	R	1.3	A3	D2
6 (JL)	53	M	1983	L	1.5	B2	D5

application of microsurgical techniques to acoustic neurinomas, with two exceptions,[5,13] hearing was preserved only in some of those patients who had internal debulking of the tumor. Of these 42 papers, 15 were updates of series by several authors or were specific reports of certain groups of patients in such series. It was difficult to be certain that all such duplications were noted in analyzing these data. With the caveat that there were difficulties in avoiding such duplications, it appears that by 1984, 30 authors or groups of authors published case reports or series of patients in whom it was stated that hearing was preserved in the nerve compromised by the acoustic tumor. The testing criteria for preservation of hearing vary naturally with the era in which the operations were performed. Some surgeons clarified the presence of useful hearing by use of hearing testing. Others did not clearly do so. Some claims were made for preservation of hearing that were not substantiated by the published auditory function data. Other papers were purely anecdotal with no data. Several of these were in sequential papers where the "hard" data were published in another paper of the series. Interpretation of findings and results were frequently difficult. The following summary is as accurate as was possible:

Over 201 patients were reported who had preservation of hearing before surgery and in whom hearing preservation was attempted. This number is probably much higher (over 500), as a number of studies did not discuss this number. One hundred and seventy-six of these over 201 patients had "preservation" of hearing reported, i.e., the operation was successful in preserving hearing according to the text. Further analysis of the data showed that 49 patients clearly had documented preservation of useful hearing and that another 12 possibly had preservation of useful hearing. Several patients who had hearing preserved had only partial removal of their tumors and are not included as successful procedures. One or more papers confused anatomic preservation of the cochlear nerve with hearing preservation. One in particular stated that hearing was preserved and showed a totally deaf ear on testing. This paper is quoted frequently in the above literature as showing hearing preservation. What it demonstrated was that the cochlear nerve could be anatomically preserved. In a number of papers, there is some dichotomy between the announced degree of preservation and the primary data. Other reports have not validated the presence of useful hearing. Authors who had convincingly demonstrated preservation of useful hearing function (pure tone and discrimination) by the time of publication of our 1984 paper[25] include House,[22] Hitselberger et al.,[21] Smith et al.,[56-58] Harker and McCabe,[20] Cohen[6] and Cohen and Ransohoff,[7] Palva et al.,[39] Sterkers,[59,60] Ojemann,[36] Ojemann and Crowell,[35] Wigand et al.,[65] Samii and Ohlemutz,[52] Portman and Sterkers,[43] and Tarlov.[62] More recent well documented cases include those by Ojemann et al.,[38] Palva et al.,[40] and Tator and Nedzelski.[63]

It appears that the rate of hearing preservation has been significantly improved with increased experience. Such is the case in our patients as we learned which maneuvers were injurious to CN VIII function. Videotape reviews of our first series of three patients were most meaningful as a learning experience. Case #1 was instructive in showing us that manipulation of the badly distorted cochlear nerve was incompatible with hearing preservation. Case #2 taught us about the vascular relationships of the inner ear and tumor. From case #3, we learned about the need for sharp transection of the distal superior vestibular nerve because of its physical attachment to the hearing apparatus in the temporal bone. With the application of BAER monitoring, we learned that lateral-to-medial cerebellar retraction could be deleterious to hearing. But BAERs, although extremely useful, have limitations, specifically delayed feedback, and falsely unchanged potentials due to gradual changes in delay of impulses.

By the time we did case #1 in the current series, we had the principles of the technique described in this chapter reasonably well developed. Despite this, we still have cases of small tumors in which hearing has not been preserved. In case #5, the labyrinthine arterial supply coursed into and through the tumor, an arrangement that is, for us, incompatible with preservation of hearing. Further, a recent patient with a larger (2.5 cm diameter) tumor (case #6), in whom all the technical suggestions described in this paper were utilized and in whom no deterioration of BAERs or of direct auditory nerve potentials was noted during surgery, has some preservation of hearing but no useful function. Therefore, although application of these technical points are helpful in preservation of hearing, they certainly do not guarantee preservation of function.

Some important technical and anatomic observations regarding preservation of hearing are found in the literature, factors that we were frequently unaware of as we developed our own techniques. These important technical points include Smith and Clancey and Lang's 1973 statement regarding preservation of the labyrinthine arteries,[56] and Rhoton's description in 1974 of the arterial supply to the labyrinth.[51] Smith's 1982 paper[57] is significant in two ways. First, he mentioned the deleterious effects of lateral-to-medial cerebellar retraction on CN VIII function as measured by BAERs. Second, he stated that the facial and cochlear nerves are fused in the area of the porus acusticus and should not be separated or hearing will be lost. The use of bipolar stimulation of the facial nerve in conjunction with electromyographic evaluation of facial nerve function as described by Delgado et al. in 1979[9] is an outstanding advance in regard to preservation of the facial nerve, especially in larger tumors. This technique has been modified by Sugita and Kobayashi,[61] who used accelerometers, and by Møller and Jannetta[33] in the application of monopolar constant voltage facial nerve stimulation. The monopolar set-up is helpful even in small tumors because of the intimate association of tumor and facial nerve at the porus acusticus and the clear delineation of facial and cochlear nerves. Minimal trauma or movement of facial stimulation of the nerve is audible on the loudspeaker from mechanical stimulation of the nerve.

The application of these techniques, most of which pertain to gentle treatment of CN VIII in smaller tumors may increase the chances that hearing function will be preserved by other surgeons. Two specific techniques of tumor removal have not been discussed here. First is the ultrasonic dissector (Cavitron, CUSA). If the CUSA is used in small acoustic tumors, the surgeon must be especially careful that the vacuum is set low as the tumor and CN VIII can move, indeed flutter, with the use of this instrument causing immediate, permanent, and total loss of function. The laser is useful because the CN VIII is not disturbed *in situ*. However, heat transmission is a problem and the laser beam can easily destroy tissue one is trying to preserve. For these reasons, we do not recommend a specific technique or instrument for tumor debulking or final removal. Certainly, grasping tumor with pituitary forceps and pulling fragments out piecemeal is more traumatic than either of the above. Bipolar coagulation with high volume suction irrigation and sharp dissection with scissors for piecemeal removal is effective and can be performed without trauma. Many of these small tumors (1.5 cm diameter) can be removed *in toto* using the latter technique and larger ones by the same technique after first debulking. The surgeon can do what he does best in this regard, and if he performs the necessary technical maneuvers while monitoring BAERs, direct auditory potentials, and facial EMG, he will find which technique is least injurious to neural function in his hands. Samii and Ohlemutz[52] have preserved useful hearing in some large tumors in patients who had good preservation before surgery. We agree with Samii that the surgeon should try to save hearing in all patients who have preserved before surgery, despite size of tumor.

Since this section of the chapter deals with preservation, our criteria for evaluation of hearing preservation are necessarily stringent and include objective evidence of such preservation. We may be penalizing certain investigators in interpreting these contributions in such a manner, but we feel that such a perspective is important if we are to set up valid criteria for determining hearing preservation.

The following is a recently published set of rules for analysis of hearing preservation followed by a set of criteria for preservation of hearing in acoustic neurinoma removal.[25]

Rules for Evaluation of Hearing

1. Preoperatively, the patient must have full evaluation of hearing including pure tone and speech discrimination. It is conceivable that a rare patient in whom hearing will be preserved may have no measurable hearing before surgery, but the data should be collected.
2. All patients in whom hearing preservation is attempted are included in the series.
3. Total excision of the tumor is performed.
4. After surgery, the patient must have the same evaluation of hearing as was done before surgery. This should be done in the immediate postoperative period (i.e., postoperative day 6 or 7), and at 3 months, 6 months, and yearly.

Criteria for Preservation of Hearing

Criteria for hearing functions are based on two measurements: (1) pure tone average for 500, 1000, and 2000 Hz, and (2) discrimination score, using recorded one-syllable words and presented under earphones at 40 dB above Pure Tone Average or at the most comfortable listening level. Our criteria are described in Tables V and VI. These criteria are based on both common guidelines regarding compensation as well as clinical experience with patients with hearing loss and the benefit from amplification.

We find that in our hands the retromastoid approach is a safe and efficient way to preserve function of the auditory and facial nerves, even in patients with small intracanalicular tumors. We cannot agree that the middle fossa method offers any advantages that would make that method a choice over the retromastoid one[17] and are somewhat concerned about the unnecessary risks of postoperative hemorrhage and epilepsy with the middle fossa approach. With the use of current operative and monitoring techniques, hearing preservation is possible in more patients with acoustic tumors. With the use of strict rules for patient evaluation and a set of criteria to determine hearing function and its preservation, the state of function can be objectively evaluated.

Table V
Classification with Regard to Pure Tone Audiograms

Pure Tone Score Average (dB)	Hearing Status	Grade
0–26	Normal	A
26–40	Mild loss	B
41–55	Moderate loss	C
56–70	Moderate severe loss	D
71–90	Severe loss	E
90+	Profound	F

Table VI
Classification with Regard to Speech Discrimination

Discrimination Score (%)	Hearing Status	Grade
92–100	Normal	1
72–88	Mild deficit	2
48–68	Moderate deficit	3
20–44	Severe deficit	4
20	Non-useful hearing	5

References

1. Belal A, Linthicum FH, House WF: Acoustic tumor surgery with preservation of hearing: A histopathologic report. Am J Otolaryngol 4:9-16, 1982.
2. Brackmann DE: Middle cranial fossa approach. In House WF, Luetje CM (eds): Acoustic Nerve Tumors. Baltimore, University Park Press, 1979, pp 15-42.

3. Bremond G: Le probleme de la conservation de l'audition aux cours de l'excese des tumeurs de l'angle ponto-cerebelleux. *Rev Laryngol Otol Rhinol* 100:111-114.
4. Buchheit WA: Comment on Ref. #12. *Neurosurgery* 7:159, 1980.
5. Chai W: Preservation of facial and acoustic nerves in the total removal of large and small acoustic tumors. Report of two cases. *J Neurosurg* 54:268-272, 1981.
6. Cohen NL: Acoustic neuroma surgery with emphasis on preservation of hearing. *Laryngoscope* 89:886-896, 1979.
7. Cohen NL, Ransohoff J: Preservation of hearing in acoustic neurinoma surgery. In Samii M, Jannetta PJ, (eds): *The Cranial Nerves*. New York, Springer-Verlag, 1981, pp 561-568.
8. Daspit CP, Raudzens P, Shetter A: Monitoring of intraoperative auditory brain stem responses. *Otolaryngol Head Neck Surg* 90:108-116, 1982.
9. Delgado TE, Buchheit WA, Rosenholtz HR, et al: Intraoperative monitoring of facial muscle evoked responses obtained by intracranial stimulation of the facial nerve: a more accurate technique for facial nerve dissection. *Neurosurgery* 4:418-421, 1979.
10. DiTullio MV, Malkasian D, Rand RW: A critical comparison of neurosurgical and otolaryngological approaches to acoustic neuromas. *J Neurosurg* 48:1-12, 1978.
11. Drake CG: Surgical treatment of acoustic neuroma with preservation or reconstitution of the facial nerve. *J Neurosurg* 26:459-464, 1967.
12. Drake CG: Total removal of large acoustic neuromas: A modification of the McKenzie operation with special emphasis on saving the facial nerve. *J Neurosurg* 26:554-561, 1967.
13. Elliott FA, McKissock W: Acoustic neuroma early diagnosis. *Lancet* 267:1189-1191, 1954.
14. Erikson DL, Ausman JI, Chou SN: Prognosis of seventh nerve palsy following removal of large acoustic tumors. *J Neurosurg* 47:31-34, 1977.
15. Fischer G, Costantini JL, Mercier P: Improvement of hearing after microsurgical removal of acoustic neurinoma. *Neurosurgery* 7:154-159, 1980.
16. Glasscock ME, Hays JW, Jackson CG, et al: A one-stage combined approach for the management of large cerebellopontine angle tumors. *Laryngoscope* 88:1563-1576, 1978.
17. Glasscock ME, Hays JW, Joseph AF, et al: Middle fossa approach for acoustic tumor removal and preservation of hearing. In Brackmann DE (ed): *Neurological Surgery of the Ear and Skull Base*. New York, Raven Press, 1982, 223-226.
18. Grundy BL, Jannetta PJ, Procopio PT, et al: Intraoperative monitoring of brain stem auditory evoked potentials. *J Neurosurg* 57:674-681, 1982.
19. Hardy RW, Kinney SE, Lueders H, et al: Preservation of cochlear nerve function with the aid of brain stem auditory evoked potentials. *Neurosurgery* 11:16-19, 1982.
20. Harker LA, McCabe BF: Iowa results of acoustic neuroma operations. *Laryngoscope* 88:1904-1911, 1978.
21. Hitselberger WE, Hughes RL: Bilateral acoustic tumors and neurofibromatosis. *Acta Otolaryngol* 88-700-711, 1968.
22. House WF. Case summaries. *Arch Otolaryngol* 88:586-591, 1968.
23. Hullay J, Tomits GH. Experiences with total removal of tumors of the acoustic nerve. *J Neurosurg* 22:127-135, 1965.
24. Jannetta PJ, Abbasy M, Maroon JC, et al: Etiology and definitive microsurgical treatment of hemifacial spasm: Operative techniques and results in forty-seven patients. *J Neurosurg* 47:321-328, 1977.
25. Jannetta PJ, Møller AR, Møller MB: Technique of hearing preservation in small acoustic neuromas. *Ann Surg* 200:513-523, 1984.
26. King TT, Morrison AW: Translabyrinthine and transtentorial removal of acoustic nerve tumors: Results in 150 cases. *J Neurosurg* 52:210-216, 1980.
27. MacCarty CS: Acoustic neuroma and the suboccipital approach (1967-1972). *Mayo Clin Proc* 50:15-16, 1975.
28. Mackey IS, King IJ: Pre- and post-operative brain stem responses in a case of acoustic neuroma, sparing the VIII nerve. *Clin Otolaryngol* 2:233-238, 1977.
29. Malis LI: Microsurgical treatment of acoustic neurinomas. In Handa H, (ed): *Microneurosurgery*. Baltimore, University Park Press, 1975, pp 105-120.
30. McCallum J, Maroon JC, Jannetta PJ: Treatment of postoperative cerebrospinal fluid fistulas by subarachnoid drainage. *J Neurosurg* 42:434-437, 1975.
31. Møller AR, Jannetta PJ, Bennett M, et al: Intracranially recorded responses from the human auditory nerve: New insights into the origin of brain stem evoked potentials (BSEPs). *Electroencephalog Clin Neurophysiol* 52:18-27, 1981.
32. Moller AR, Jannetta PJ: Monitoring auditory functions during cranial nerve microvascular decompression operations by

direct recording from the eighth nerve. *J Neurosurg* 59:493-499, 1984.
33. Møller AR, Jannetta PJ: Preservation of facial function during removal of acoustic neuromas: use of monopolar constant voltage stimulation and EMG. *J Neurosurgery* 61:757-760, 1984.
34. Nedzelski JM, Tator CH: Surgical management of cerebellopontine angle tumors. *J Otolaryngol* 9:105-112, 1980.
35. Ojemann RG, Crowell RC. Acoustic neuromas treated by microsurgical suboccipital operations. *Progr Neurologic Surg* 9:337-373, 1978.
36. Ojemann RG: Microsurgical suboccipital approach to cerebellopontine angle tumors. *Clin Neurosurg* 25:461-479, 1978.
37. Ojemann RG, Montgomery WW, Weiss AD: Evaluation and surgical treatment of acoustic neuroma. *N Engl J Med* 287:895-899, 1972.
38. Ojemann RG, Levine RA, Montgomery WM, et al: Use of intraoperative auditory evoked potentials to preserve hearing in unilateral acoustic neuroma removal. *J Neurosurgery* 61:938-948, 1984.
39. Palva T, Troupp H, Jauhiainen T: Team surgery for acoustic neurinomas and the preservation of hearing. *Acta Otolaryngol* 91:37-45, 1981.
40. Palva T, Troupp H, Jauhiainen T: Hearing preservation in acoustic neurinoma surgery. *Acta Otolaryngol (Stockh)* 99:1-7, 1985.
41. Pertuiset B, Maspetiol R, Semette D, et al: La conservation des fonctions auditive et faciale au cours de l'acoustique par voie sous occipitale. *La Presse Medicale* 74:2327-2330, 1966.
42. Poole JL, Pava AA, Greenfield EC: *Acoustic Nerve Tumors: Early Diagnosis and Treatment*, ed 2. Springfield, Ill, Charles C. Thomas, 1970.
43. Portmann M, Sterkers JM: The internal auditory meatus. In Portmann M, Sterkers JM, Charachon R, et al, (eds): *Tumors of the Internal Auditory Meatus and Surrounding Structures*. New York, Churchill Livingstone, 1975, pp 193-426.
44. Pulec JL, House WF, Britton BH, et al: A system of management of acoustic neuroma based on 364 cases. *Trans Am Acad Ophthal Otol* 75:48-55, 1971.
45. Rand RW, Kurze T: Case reports and technical notes. Preservation of vestibular, cochlear, and facial nerves during microsurgical removal of acoustic tumors: Report of two cases. *J Neurosurg* 28:158-161, 1968.
46. Rand RW, Kurze T: Facial nerve preservation by posterior fossa transmeatal microdissection and total removal of acoustic tumors. *J Neurol Neurosurg Psychiatry* 28:311-316, 1965.
47. Rand RW, Kurze T: Micro-neurosurgical resection of acoustic tumors by a transmeatal posterior fossa approach. *Bull Los Angeles Neurol Soc* 30:17-20, 1965.
48. Rand RW: Postoperative edema and preservation of hearing in acoustic tumor surgery. In Brackmann DE, (ed): *Neurological Surgery of the Ear and Skull Base*. New York, Raven Press, 1982, pp 247-255.
49. Ransohoff J, Potanos J, Boschenstein F, et al: Total removal of recurrent acoustic tumors. *J Neurosurg* 18:804-810, 1961.
50. Rhoton AL: Microsurgical removal of acoustic neuromas. *Surg Neurol* 6:211-219, 1976.
51. Rhoton AL: Microsurgery of the internal acoustic meatus. *Surg Neurol* 2:311-318, 1974.
52. Samii M, Ohlemutz A: Preservation of eighth cranial nerve in cerebellopontine angle tumors. In Samii M, Jannetta PJ (eds): *Cranial Nerve*. New York, Springer-Verlag, 1981, pp 586-590.
53. Sekiya T, Møller AR: Cochlear nerve injuries caused by cerebellopontine angle manipulations: An electrophysiological and morphological study in dogs. *J Neurosurg* (Accepted for publication 1987.)
54. Sekiya T, Iwabuchi T, Andoh A, et al: Changes of the auditory system after cerebellopontine angle manipulations. *Neurosurgery* 12:80-85, 1983.
55. Sheptak PE, Jannetta PJ: The two-stage excision of huge acoustic neurinomas. *J Neurosurg* 51:37-41, 1979.
56. Smith MFW, Clancy TP, Lang JS: Conservation of hearing in acoustic neurilemmoma excision. *Trans Am Acad Ophthal Otol* 84:704-709, 1977.
57. Smith MFW: Hearing conservation and the CO_2 laser in acoustic neurilemmoma excision. In Brackmann DE (ed): *Neurological Surgery of the Ear and Skull Base*. New York, Raven Press, 1982, pp 243-245.
58. Smith MFW, Miller RN, Cox DJ: Suboccipital microsurgical removal of acoustic neurinomas of all sizes. *Trans Am Otol Soc* 61:119-126, 1973.
59. Sterkers JM: Retro-sigmoid approach for preservation of hearing in early acoustic neuroma surgery. In Samii M, Jannetta PJ (eds): *The Cranial Nerves*. New York, Springer-Verlag, 1981, pp 579-585.

60. Sterkers JM: Removal of bilateral and unilateral acoustic tumors with preservation of hearing: a comparison of the retrosigmoid and translabyrinthine approach. In Silverstein H, Norell H (eds): *Neurological Surgery of the Ear*, Vol 2. Aesculapius, Birmingham, 1979.
61. Sugita K, Kobayashi S: Technical and instrumental improvements in the surgical treatment of acoustic neurinomas. *J Neurosurg* 57:747-752, 1982.
62. Tarlov E: Total one-stage suboccipital microsurgical removal of acoustic neuromas of all sizes with emphasis on arachnoid planes and on saving the facial nerve. *Surg Clin North Am* 60:565-591, 1980.
63. Tator CH, Nedzelski JM: Preservation of hearing in patients undergoing excision of acoustic neuromas and other cerebellopontine angle tumors. *J Neurosurg* 63:168-174, 1985.
64. Thomsen J: Suboccipital removal of acoustic neuromas: Results of 125 operations. *Acta Otolaryngol* 81:406-414, 1976.
65. Wigand ME, Haid T, Berg M, et al: Early diagnosis and transtemporal removal of small nerve VII and VIII tumors. In Samii M, Jannetta PJ (eds): *The Cranial Nerves*. New York, Springer-Verlag, 1981, pp 569-574.
66. Yasargil MG, Fox JL: The microsurgical approach to acoustic neurinomas. *Surg. Neurol* 2:393-398, 1974.
67. Yasargil MG, Smith RD, Gaser JC: Microsurgical approach to acoustic neurinomas. In Krayer H (ed): *Advances and Technical Standards in Neurosurgery*. New York, Springer-Verlag, 1973, pp 93-128.
68. Zappulla RA, Greenblatt, E, Karmel BZ: The effects of acoustic neuromas on ipsilateral and contralateral brain stem auditory evoked responses during stimulation of the unaffected ear. *Otolaryngology* 4:118-122, 1982.

30

Acoustic Neuromas: Otologic Approaches and Results

Peter S. Roland, M.D.
Michael E. Glasscock, III, M.D.
Dennis I. Bojrab, M.D.

Introduction

Tumors arising from the vestibulocochlear nerve were first described in the early 19th century in autopsy specimens. In 1917, a clinical picture of hearing loss associated with facial anesthesia, facial paralysis, cerebellar ataxia, and death was developed by Cushing. Pre-morbid diagnosis of acoustic neuroma was made with increasing frequency during the first half of the 20th century.[5] Cushing developed a suboccipital approach to acoustic neuromas and performed intracapsular (incomplete) tumor removals. Facial paralysis and deafness were regular postoperative sequelae in those patients, and many of the patients died subsequently due to tumor regrowth. Walter Dandy subsequently showed that total tumor excision could be performed even when the tumors were very large, with a reduction in mortality. In the late 1950s, Dr. William House refined the translabyrinthine approach to acoustic tumor originally developed by Panse. In the 1960s, House developed the middle fossa approach for hearing conservation in small tumors. The suboccipital approach was progressively refined by adding microsurgical and laser technology to the standard approaches of Cushing and Dandy. In the future, we will see increased utilization of all approaches as more tumors are diagnosed at earlier stages. We look forward to further decreases in surgical mortality and ever-increasing conservation of both facial movement and hearing.

Pathology

Acoustic neuromas are more accurately termed *schwannomas* since the tumors arise from the schwann cells inversing the axon. The pathology of these lesions has been described in detail elsewhere in this book, and in other publications.[1] The neoplasms arise most commonly from the inferior vestibular nerve, and rarely from the cochlear nerve.

From: Sekhar LN, Schramm VL Jr, eds: *Tumors of the Cranial Base: Diagnosis and Treatment*. Mount Kisco, New York, Futura Publishing Co, Inc, © 1987.

The site of origin of the tumor is usually within the porus acusticus, although it may originate along the intracranial course of the 8th cranial nerve. Reports of tumor cells found within the cochlear nerve and labyrinth, even in tumors arising from the vestibular nerves, have raised concern about operative techniques designed to preserve hearing. Histological differences may be found in acoustic tumors of patients with von Recklinghausen's disease.

Recent Developments in the Management of Acoustic Neuromas

During the last 20 years, the use of the operative microscope, a progressive refinement in microsurgical technique, and improvement in postoperative care have greatly reduced the mortality and morbidity associated with the excision of acoustic schwannomas. Preservation of the facial nerve has become commonplace, and preservation of hearing, while still unusual, is now a reasonable goal in selected patients with smaller tumors.

We believe that the neurotologist-neurosurgeon team provides the most comprehensive and flexible approach to the patient with acoustic neuroma. The combined expertise of the team will provide the best results for some of these difficult operations. The use of the microscope and microsurgical technique are absolutely essential.

Increased awareness and understanding of corneal exposure has led to effective techniques for preventive care. Use of protective eye "bubbles" and the prophylactic use of artificial tears and ointment greatly lessens ophthalmologic complications in those with temporary facial nerve paralysis. Early consultation with an ophthalmologist familiar with facial nerve paralysis and the liberal use of temporary lateral tarsorrhaphy minimizes the long-term problems in those patients for whom the usual preventive measures are not adequate. Chemical meningitis and brief periods of communicating hydrocephalus in the immediate postoperative period are now well managed by lumbar puncture and steroid therapy.

Significant strides have been made in rehabilitation of the paralyzed face. Patients in whom sacrifice of the facial nerve is mandated in order to achieve complete tumor removal are now most commonly treated either by primary reanastomosis of the nerve, or by cable graft reconstruction. Usually this is accomplished at the time of the primary procedure, speeding up the recovery of function as well as avoiding a second operative procedure. Patients who are not candidates for immediate facial nerve repair are offered a facial-hypoglossal anastomosis during the initial hospitalization. Only 2 to 3 days are added to the hospital stay and satisfactory results are the rule. For those patients who are not candidates for nerve reconstruction procedures and/or those few in whom such procedures fail, very satisfactory rehabilitative techniques have developed for both static and dynamic repair. Muscle transfers, fascial sling procedures, tarsal springs, and lid weights are all examples of the techniques available.

Evaluation of the Patient

A high index of suspicion is mandatory if acoustic neuromas are to be diagnosed early.[2] Morbidity and mortality are proportional to tumor size. Small tumors most often present with minimal and often nonspecific signs and symptoms. Acoustic neuromas may grow to substantial size before even the most subtle symptoms occur. Careful review of the clinical history of many patients with large tumors reveals that changes in hearing, onset of tinnitus, or dysequilibrium occurred only weeks or a few months prior to diagnosis when the tumor was already large. Therefore, *the otologist must definitively exclude acoustic neuroma in every patient with unilateral otologic symptoms.*

Any unilateral hearing loss, however minor, requires investigation. In no case should it be assumed to be of viral or "idiopathic" etiology. The literature is replete with patients with acoustic neuroma who had normal or near normal hearing at presentation. Sudden hearing loss is a relatively frequent presenting symptom in our experience. Patients with all the manifestations of Meniere's disease are occasionally found to have tumors.

The audiometric hallmark of the acoustic neuroma is markedly decreased speech discrimination, often out of proportion to the pure tone loss. Five percent of patients with acoustic neuroma will have normal hearing. High frequency loss is most common but other patterns of hearing loss occur in about one-third of patients. About 75% will have word discrimination scores below 60%. Moreover, many patients will have significant "rollover."[2] Generally, the ability to understand words increases if the word is presented to the listener at higher loudness levels. In retrocochlear lesions, the *opposite* often occurs: understanding *diminishes* even though the words are presented at higher loudness levels. The combination of a unilateral, high frequency hearing loss with poor word discrimination scores and positive "rollover" is suspicious for an acoustic neuroma.

Tinnitus *alone* is the presenting complaint in about 10% of patients with an acoustic neuroma. Unfortunately no characteristic type of tinnitus is found. It may be high pitched, low pitched, or with changing pitch. It may be described as roaring, whistling, or like machinery. It need not be constant but may come and go.

Vestibular ablation is so slow that balance disturbances are rarely apparent to the patient and, if present, are often subtle. Typically, patients report balance disturbance only when directly questioned about it. Even then, they often admit only to a mild sense of dysequilibrium or "clumsiness." True rotatory vertigo is quite uncommon except as a very brief accompaniment to rapid position changes. Occasionally, more sustained episodes of true vertigo associated with nausea and vomiting (mimicking Meniere's disease) are encountered.

Neurological symptoms are generally late. Paresthesia or hypesthesia within the distribution of the 5th cranial nerve occurs in large tumors, especially those with anteriorly directed growth. The motor division of the 5th nerve seems more resistant to pressure effects and is only very rarely involved. Hypesthesia of the floor of the external auditory canal is the most common, earliest 5th nerve change (Hitselberger's sign). Despite the profound distortion of the facial nerve seen intraoperatively, facial nerve weakness is quite uncommon. Occasionally tumors with inferiorly directed growth patterns will produce impairment of cranial nerves IX and X—usually dysphonia or dysphagia.

Large tumors will eventually exert pressure on the cerebellum and brain stem and cause a brain stem shift toward the contralateral side. Typical symptoms of cerebellar dysfunction that may be found include ataxia, wide-based gait, dysdiadochokinesia, and slurred speech. Obstructive hydrocephalus from brain stem compression will produce headache, visual loss from papilledema and, if allowed to advance, will eventually result in death from brain stem herniation and respiratory failure.

Signs

Otologic signs are limited to positive findings on the neurotologic examination. Neurosensory hearing loss may be of any pattern and will usually be asymmetric compared with the contralateral side. Complete hearing loss usually occurs in large tumors as a late finding but occasionally lesions originating in the lateral portion of the internal auditory canal will invade the cochlea. Those rare instances in which the tumor originates from the cochlear nerve may also have complete hearing loss even though the tumor is small.

Special audiometric testing has changed dramatically within the last 10 years. The older "retrocochlear" test battery which included SISI, ABLB, tone decay, and Bekesy audiometry has been replaced by stapedius reflex studies and auditory brain stem response (ABR). In addition to being more sensitive and specific, these newer tests are not dependent on the amount of attention or effort given the task by the patient.

The acoustic reflex provides a good, inexpensive screening test for retrocochlear pathology. The test measures contraction of the stapedius muscle which occurs when a high intensity sound is presented to the ear. This is apparently a protective reflex. The reflex contraction of the stapedius muscle is normally maintained as long as the test tone is presented. The patient with a retrocochlear lesion will demonstrate "decay" of the contractile response manifested as a rapid return to baseline. The use of this test is limited to patients without conductive hearing losses and without profound neurosensory hearing loss. It will be positive in 90% or more of patients wtih acoustic neuroma, and false positives are uncommon.

The auditory brain stem response (ABR) is the most useful and reliable audiometric test in the work-up of acoustic neuroma.[8] This test measures the electrical response in the cochlea, 8th nerve, and brian stem to auditory stimulation by summating several hundred responses. The brain stem responses have been classified into five identifiable "waves," each thought to originate from a specific area in the brain stem. The fifth wave is thought to arise from the inferior colliculus. Patients with acoustic neuromas will have a "delay" of one to several milliseconds in appearance of the fifth wave. This is termed an "increased latency" of the fifth wave response. The test will be positive (i.e., there will be an increased latency) in many varieties of retrocochlear pathology but it is reliably negative in cases of cochlear pathology. Thus, more than 95% of patients with acoustic neuroma will have a positive test. The ABR is limited to those patients with some residual hearing. As hearing loss increases, there will be an increase in wave V latency attributable to the hearing loss itself. However, the progressive increase in latency is predictable. This is, in effect, a repeatable "strength-duration" curve and sophisticated interpreters of the ABR are still able to determine latency increases greater than that attributable to hearing loss alone that are indicative of retrocochlear pathology. The test cannot be performed on patients with more than 60 dB to 70 dB of neurosensory hearing loss. It has become an important part of the standard evaluation of patients with nonconductive hearing losses (Fig. 1).

Electronystagmography will be abnormal in over 80% of patients with an acoustic neuroma. Reduced or absent caloric responses ipsilateral to the tumor is the usual finding. Various degrees of spontaneous or positional nystagmus are less common but may still be seen in greater than 50% of patients. "Directional preponderance," a measure of differential sensitivity to either warm or cold stimuli, has not been a useful measurement.

Medical Imaging

Plain transorbital roentgenographs of the petrous apex are the most basic and readily accessible of radiographic examinations. They can be performed with simple equipment, are inexpensive, and are available in many physicians' offices. They demonstrate the internal auditory canals clearly and should be carefully examined for asymmetry. A difference between the two sides of 2 mm in height or 3 mm in length is significant and mandates further assessment. Marked flaring of one porus acusticus or globular deformity of the midportion of one side is significant. Fifty percent of patients with acoustic neuromas will have positive plain films. Polytomography will increase the yield to 80% but has been supplanted by computerized tomographic (CT) examination.

CT examination is, at present, the single most useful radiographic technique.[4] Contrast enhancement is absolutely essential as even large tumors may not be detected on unenhanced studies. Care must be taken to assure that contrast is administered in adequate doses and that sufficient time has elapsed for the contrast media to diffuse into the tumor. Cuts of 1.5 mm through the internal auditory canals and cerebellopontine angle should be obtained. If a mass is present,

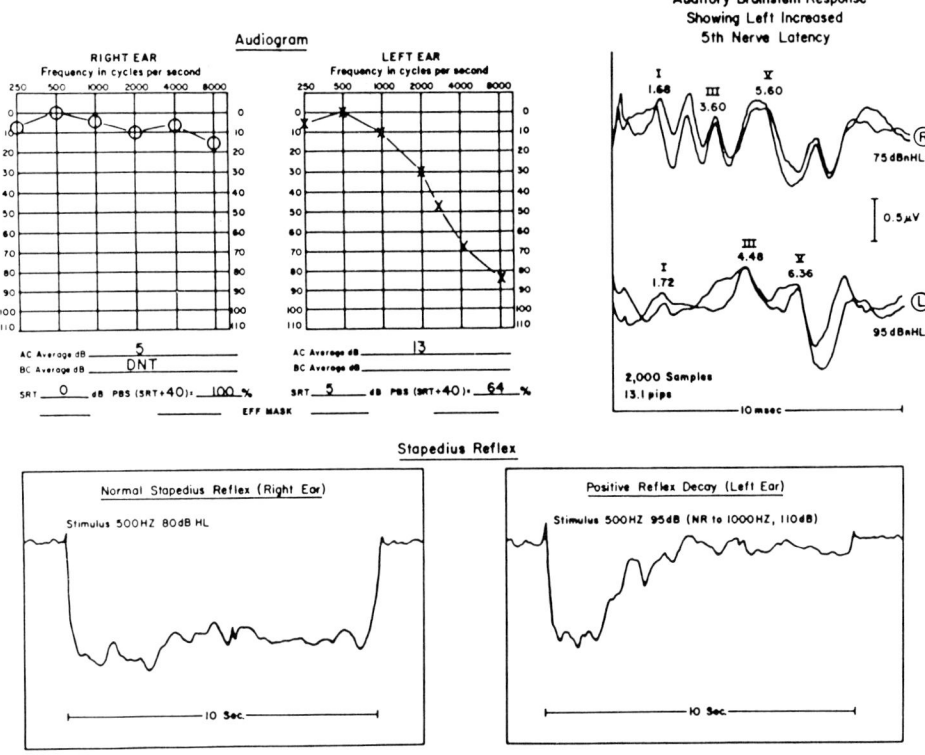

Figure 1: Typical audiometric findings for patients with acoustic neuroma. This patient had a left high frequency neurosensory hearing loss with reduced word discrimination. The ABR was abnormal with prolonged I-V latency. Marked "decay" of the stapedius reflex is shown on the left.

the study should be carefully scrutinized to determine if the internal auditory canal on the involved side is enlarged or if the porus acusticus is flared. A normal canal or eccentric placement of the mass with respect to the porus acusticus should raise suspicions of meningioma. Anterior extension should be determined and the relationship of the tumor to the vertebral and basilar artery noted. The superior and inferior limits of the tumor should be ascertained and thought given to possible displacement of cranial nerves IV through XII. Brain stem "shift" and secondary hydrocephalus may be seen in larger tumors. The relative size of the sigmoid sinus should be assessed to determine whether or not it is the dominant or, rarely, the only sinus. The position of the sigmoid sinus and its relationship to the bony labyrinth should be noted especially when planning a translabyrinthine approach. The contralateral cerebellopontine angle needs to be very carefully examined for bilateral acoustic tumors which are not uncommon. The presence of a second, contralateral acoustic tumor may significantly alter the patient's management.

Patients who have negative CT scans and either complete hearing loss or audiometric indications of retrocochlear pathology need contrast cisternography. Pantopaque posterior fossa myelography has been the standard study until recently. It is extremely accurate, rapidly performed, and requires only standard x-ray equipment. Computerized tomographic air contrast cisternography has recently replaced the posterior fossa myelogram. It does not require the introduction of a foreign substance and there is a much lower incidence of postspinal headache. It can be performed as an outpatient procedure. Some distressing "false positive" examinations have been reported but experienced examiners are able to distinguish between the actual presence of a mass lesion within the internal auditory canal and simple failure of the canal to fill. The 7th and 8th cranial nerves are usually well demonstrated and a negative study insures the absence of even very small tumors.

The role of magnetic resonance imaging (MRI) in the diagnosis of acoustic neuroma is still emerging. The study is very sensitive to the presence of a very small mass, is noninvasive, and involves no exposure to ionizing radiation. The possibility, still in the future, of making firm determinations of tissue type from this study alone is intriguing. It suffers the disadvantages of eliminating all bony detail and thus makes assessment of the relationship of the tumor to temporal bone landmarks difficult. It is especially attractive in special situations such as during pregnancy, or for frequent assessment of tumor growth in patients with unresected tumors or with bilateral tumors.

Differential Diagnosis

Ten to fifteen percent of the mass lesions identified within the cerebellopontine angle will be lesions other than acoustic neuroma. They will have a clinical presentation indistinguishable from typical acoustic neuromas. CT scanning has helped enormously in differential diagnosis.[9]

Meningiomas are the most common lesions of the cerebellopontine angle other than acoustic neuromas. Preoperative identification of this lesion is still difficult. Suspicion should be raised in cases where the cerebellopontine angle mass is eccentrically placed with respect to the internal auditory canal or if the internal auditory canal is neither widened nor shortened. Occasionally, calcification within the mass will suggest meningioma. They have an identical appearance on CT scan and no sure method of differentiation has evolved. MRI may, in the future, solve this problem.

Cholesteatomas arising from the petrous apex frequently extend into the cerebellopontine angle. They account for about 5% of "angle" lesions. They grow slowly and are somewhat more likely to produce facial nerve symptoms. The 5th nerve is commonly involved. The very low density of these lesions on CT has made preoperative diagnosis routine rather than exceptional.

A variety of other lesions occur uncommonly and include gliomas, osteomas, lipomas, and vascular neoplasms. Non-neoplastic lesions such as arachnoid cysts, cholesterol granulomas, and aneurysms are rarely encountered.

Classification

The classification of acoustic tumors has historically been by size measurement in the tumor's greatest diameter. Small tumors are less than 1.5 cm, medium tumors are from 1.5 cm up to 2.9 cm, and large tumors are 3.0 cm or larger. Some surgeons size these tumors at surgery while others make this determination by preoperative radiographic studies. Today, with high resolution CT scanning, one can quite accurately determine the size of acoustic tumors preoperatively. Recently there has been a suggestion of volume averaging these tumors which is accomplished by taking various cross-sectional measurements of the tumor during CT scanning. This technique has promise in the determination of growth characteristics of particular tumors. This may become extremely important in determining the role of nonoperative management in elderly patients.

It is necessary to assess accurately the size of these lesions in order to counsel patients. Morbidity and mortality, as well as facial nerve and hearing preservation, are usually determined by the size of the lesion. Specific results with various classifications will be discussed later in this chapter.

Management

Once the diagnosis of a cerebellopontine angle tumor has been made, an organized and unified team approach to the problem is begun. The various specialists involved are the neurotologist, the neurosurgeon, the internist, the ophthalmologist, and the nursing staff. Elderly patients, patients with medical problems, or patients with large tumors are seen preoperatively by an internist who will follow the patient postoperatively until a stable course is obtained.

Postoperatively, the patient is observed overnight in the intensive care unit or recovery room. Patients are monitored with an arterial line, Foley catheter, and hourly neurological examinations. Most patients are transferred to a neurosurgical ward the first postoperative day. Patients are encouraged to ambulate with assistance the first day. From that point, progressive ambulation is individualized. Those patients with facial nerve trauma during surgery are monitored for ocular complications. All patients with facial paralysis are managed with an eye bubble moisture chamber, artificial hypoallergenic tears throughout the day on an hourly basis, and an ophthalmologic ointment at night. These patients are at great risk for ophthalmologic complications. This is due to exposure of the cornea resulting from closure problems of the eyelid and decreasing tear production secondary to trauma to the greater superficial petrosal nerve parasympathetic fibers. The ophthalmologist may elect to perform a lateral tarsorrhaphy to prevent a keratitis. Many patients will have a progression of a headache by the second to fourth day. This is usually due to a chemical meningitis from blood breakdown products and may be dramatically relieved in the majority of the cases by lumbar puncture. Spinal fluid is sent to the laboratory for routine spinal fluid analyses including culture. The large mastoid-type dressing is removed on the sixth day. The skin staples are removed by the seventh day. The average postoperative stay is from 7 to 12 days. Once discharged from the hospital, straining and lifting are discouraged for 3 to 6 months, depending on the type of procedure employed. Otherwise patients resume routine daily activities or jobs within 4 to 6 weeks of surgery.

Surgical Approaches to Tumor Removal

Middle Cranial Fossa Approach (Figs. 2 and 3)

This approach is selected for patients with reasonable hearing and for tumors that are either intracanalicular or extend out of the internal auditory canal not more than 1.5 cm.[3] Reasonable hearing is considered hearing with pure tone averages within 30 dB and speech discrimination of at least 76%.[7] The advantages of this approach are extradural dissection, direct examination of the lateral-most part of the internal auditory canal, and direct visualization of the facial nerve throughout the dissection. This lowers morbidity and allows total removal of the tumor with the preservation of the facial nerve. The disadvantage of this approach is that one must work under the facial nerve for tumor removal and one has limited access to the posterior fossa.

Technique of Middle Fossa Tumor Removal

Incision

The surgeon operates from the head of the table. A generous head shave is required because of the length of the incision. The area is then draped off with self-adhering plastic and a 10-minute Betadine scrub is completed. The ear is draped in the usual fashion and a craniotomy sheet with a collection bag is placed at the top of the table. Intravenous steroids and mannitol are begun at the time of the incision.

The incision is begun at the level of the root of the zygoma and extends superiorly for approximately 10 cm. Bleeding is controlled with cautery. The temporalis muscle is incised, beginning at the root of the zygoma and ending as the temporalis fascia inserts into the pericranium. The base of the temporalis muscle is then cut in a "T" fashion over the root of the zygoma for approximately 2 cm

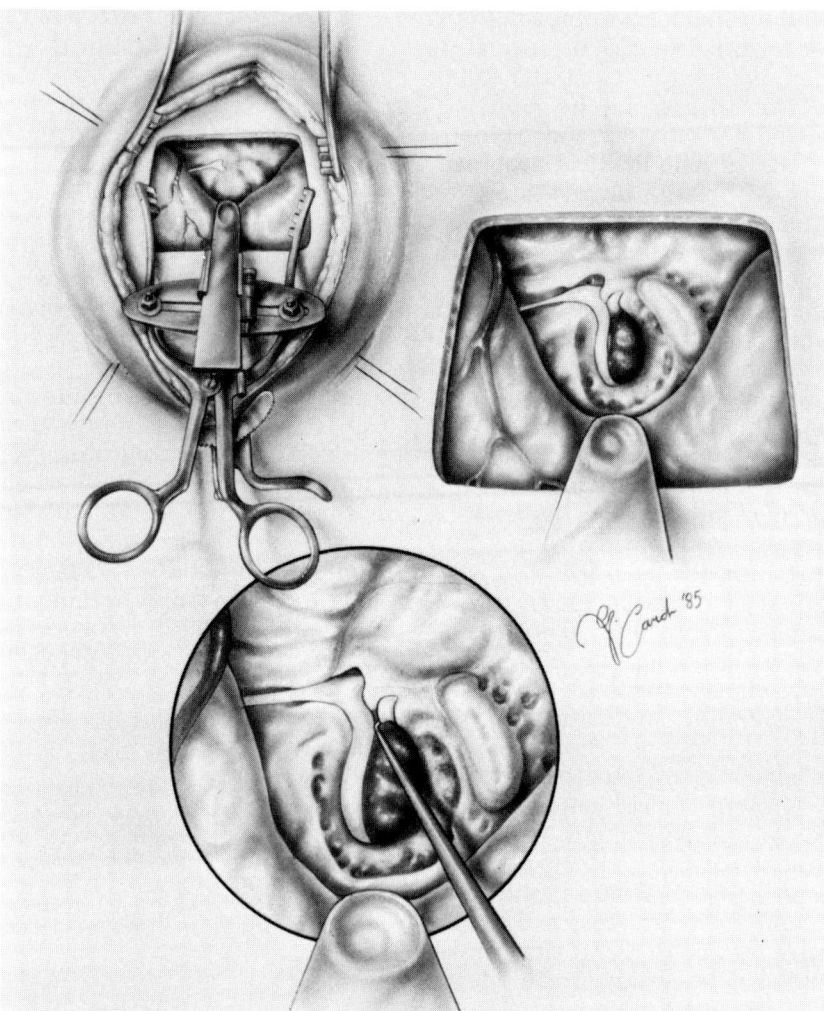

Figure 2: Middle fossa removal of acoustic neuroma. *Upper left:* Through a 4×4 cm craniotomy in the inferior temporal squamosa, the dura mater over the superior petrous portion of the temporal bone is elevated. The House-Urban retractor has been inserted and the temporal lobe elevated superiorly. The greater superficial petrosal nerve and its take-off from the geniculate ganglion is seen because the overlying bone is dehiscent. *Upper right:* The internal auditory canal has been widely opened from above, exposing an acoustic tumor arising from the superior vestibular nerve. The superior semicircular canal has been "blue-lined" so that the posterolateral portion of the IAC can be safely opened. *Lower left:* A small right-angle hook is used to avulse the superior vestibular nerve in the lateral IAC. Great care must be exercised in removing the tumor in order to avoid disruption of the cochlear blood supply.

to allow for a maximal view of the base of the temporal bone. Muscle is harvested at this time and placed into a sterile saline basin for closure of the internal auditory canal at the completion of the procedure. During the initial incision, a branch of the superficial temporal artery may be encountered and this artery should be ligated with a nonabsorbable suture to prevent postoperative bleeding and hematoma formation. The periosteum is elevated from the squamous portion of the temporal bone and a self-retaining retractor is placed.

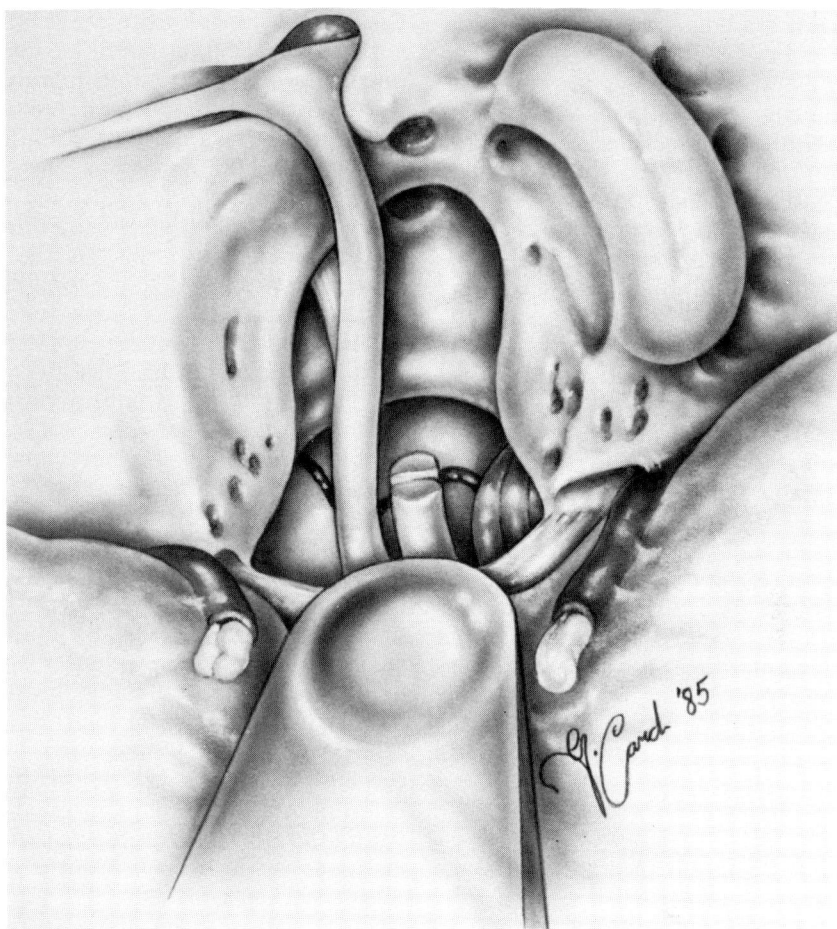

Figure 3: Middle fossa removal of acoustic neuroma, continued. Tumor removal is complete. The cut ends of the superior and inferior vestibular nerves are seen. The facial nerve is intact as is the cochlear nerve beneath it. The superior petrosal sinus has been divided and packed with Surgicel in order to provide access to the posterior fossa.

Elevation of Bone Flap

A craniotomy is made in the squamous portion of the temporal bone. The opening is a total of 3 cm square with 2 cm placed anterior to the root of the zygoma and 1 cm placed posterior to the root of the zygoma. It is important to make the inferior limit of the bone flap near the root of the zygoma and zygomatic arch so as to enter at the floor of the middle cranial fossa. Retraction by an assistant will help with this inferior exposure.

A cutting burr and continuous suction irrigation are used. The bone is drilled away until the dura is visualized through a thin plate of bone. A diamond burr is then used for the final bone plate removal. The bone flap is elevated from the dura using a freer elevator and placed in sterile saline. This is used later for closure of the defect and is sutured in place at that time.

Elevation of Dura

The dura is elevated gently from the floor of the middle fossa and hemostasis is secured with bipolar cautery. The dura must remain intact. In approximately 8%

of the cases, the bone over the geniculate ganglion of the facial nerve will be dehiscent. Blind and abrupt elevation might result in damage to the facial nerve. The posterior limit of dissection will be at the arcuate eminence. At times this may be an indistinct landmark. A positive point of identification is the greater superficial petrosal nerve which passes parallel to the petrous ridge and is anterior to the geniculate ganglion and goes toward the geniculate ganglion via the facial hiatus. This nerve lies medial and usually posterior to the anterior limit of dissection which is the middle meningeal artery. Troublesome bleeding from the venous plexus around the foramen spinosum or from various diplopic veins encountered in the dissection may be controlled by microfibrillar collagen hemostat (Avitene). At this point, the House-Urban retractor blade is firmly set into place, medial to the geniculate ganglion, as near as possible to the superior petrosal sinus for maximum exposure of the floor of the middle fossa.

Exposure of the Internal Auditory Canal

A small diamond burr is used since the ampullary end of the superior semicircular canal lies only a fraction of a millimeter posterior to the facial nerve at this point and the cochlea lies anterior to the facial nerve. The labyrinthine portion of the facial nerve lies almost parallel to the plane of the superior semicircular canal. There may be a layer of cystic bone overlying the otic capsule beneath the arcuate eminence. After removal of this layer, the hard white bone of the otic capsule becomes apparent. The superior semicircular canal is seen as a thin line in the matrix of the otic capsule and exposure is from the superior petrosal sinus laterally to the ampulla and vestibule. This delineates the posterior limit of dissection. The internal auditory canal makes an angle 45° to 60° with the superior semicircular canal. After exposing the dura of the internal canal, attention is turned toward identification of the triangular piece of bone at the lateral extent of the canal, Bill's bar. This separates the facial nerve anteriorly from the superior vestibular nerve posteriorly. It marks the actual junction of the labyrinthine portion of the facial nerve canal and the canal for the superior vestibular nerve. Once these landmarks have been identified, bone removal is continued medially until the entire surface of the internal auditory canal is exposed. As the surgeon proceeds medially, it is possible to enlarge the exposure because the superior semicircular canal courses posteriorly and the dissection is medial to the cochlea.

Bone removal is continued medially up to the porus acusticus. Care is taken to remove the bone without entering the dura because the facial nerve lies directly beneath the dura at this point. It is best to leave an eggshell thickness of bone over the entire surface of the internal auditory canal until total exposure of the canal is completed. Bone removal should be extensive at the porus acusticus to allow exposure of approximately three-quarters of the circumference of the internal auditory canal. One may now remove this thin eggshell of bone overlying the dura of the internal auditory canal and open the dura lining the internal auditory canal. The incision is made from the porus acusticus over the posterior aspect of the internal auditory canal to its lateral extent. This allows the dissection to be over the tumor and away from the area of the facial nerve.

Removal of Tumor

Having reflected the dura, the superior vestibular nerve is identified at the ampulla of the superior semicircular canal and the nerve is followed medially until the surface of the tumor is identified. The plane between the facial nerve and tumor can then be developed because identification of the freed nerve fibers at the lateral extent of the canal has been established prior to the actual dissection of the tumor. The vestibulo-facial anastomotic fibers are cut, and the superior vestibular nerve is avulsed out of the end of the internal auditory canal.

Separation of the tumor from the facial nerve is now begun. The tumor will be delivered from under the facial nerve posteriorly. As the inferior pole of the tumor is freed, the cochlear nerve will be seen. The internal auditory artery runs in the plane between the cochlear nerve and facial nerve. The artery may lie between the tumor and cochlear nerve itself. Care must be taken to stay as close to the tumor as possible for preservation of this vessel. It is important not to retract medially on the cochlea nerve avulsing the nerve as it enters the cochlear cribosa area. Hearing preservation is a function of not only an intact cochlear nerve, but also of an intact arterial supply. Direct 8th nerve action potentials and/or brain stem evoked responses are monitored throughout this dissection to alert the surgeon to possible cochlear nerve damage.

After the tumor has been dissected free in the internal auditory canal, any medial extension into the posterior fossa should be removed. One must remember the varied anatomic position of the anterior inferior cerebellar artery. Occasionally, this artery or a lateral branch may contact the surface of the tumor and in some instances extend into the internal auditory canal. Sometimes it is necessary to remove part of the intracapsular component of the tumor to allow for removal of the entire tumor without trauma to the facial nerve or anterior inferior cerebellar artery.

When removing larger tumors by the middle cranial fossa approach, it may be necessary to ligate the superior petrosal sinus in order to extend exposure in the posterior fossa.

Closure

After total removal of the tumor, the area is irrigated profusely and the anesthesiologist is asked to Valsalva the patient to check for hemostasis. Most bleeding subsides with profuse irrigation. At times, larger vessels will require bipolar cautery. The dural opening of the internal auditory canal is closed using a free muscle graft obtained from the temporalis muscle to prevent spinal fluid leakage. The House-Urban retractor is removed and the middle fossa dura is allowed to expand. The rectangular temporal bone flap is sutured back into place. The temporalis muscle is reapproximated with interrupted sutures. The skin and subcutaneous tissue are closed in separate layers using interrupted absorbable sutures. A drain is not generally used. A dry, sterile dressing is applied and the patient is observed overnight in the intensive care unit.

Translabyrinthine Approach (Figs. 4 and 5)

The translabyrinthine approach is the most direct route to the cerebellopontine angle. It is the preferred method by The Otology Group (Nashville, TN) for acoustic neuromas up to approximately 3 cm in diameter. We routinely use this approach for small acoustic neuromas with poor hearing or larger tumors where hearing preservation is not possible. Dissection of the lateral end of the internal auditory canal insures complete tumor removal from that area and also allows identification of the facial nerve throughout the dissection. Another advantage of this approach is that if the facial nerve is transected during acoustic tumor removal, the translabyrinthine approach offers the best opportunity for immediate repair by either direct end-to-end anastomosis or by interposition of a nerve graft. The most important advantage to this procedure is that it carries a very low morbidity and mortality.

Technique of the Translabyrinthine Approach

The patient is placed in the supine position with the head turned toward the opposite side. The postauricular area is shaved just prior to surgery by the circulating nurse in the holding area. The postauricular skin and ear are prepped with a Betadine solution for 10 minutes in the operating suite. Prophylactic antibiotics are not used in acoustic neuroma removal. Ten milligrams of dexamethasone

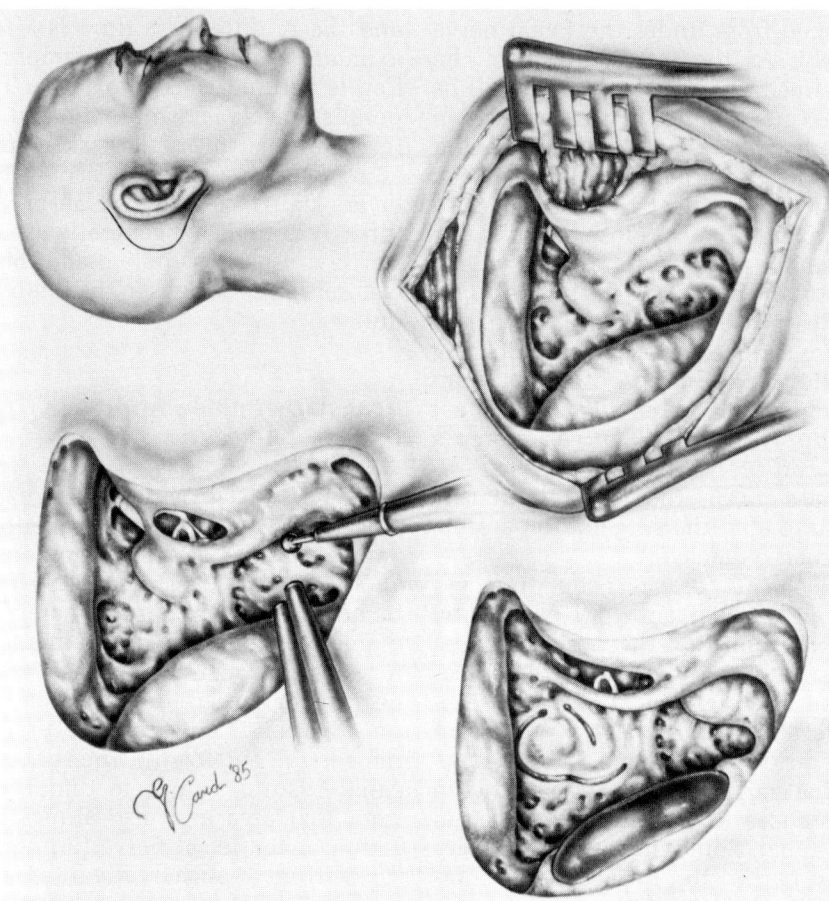

Figure 4: Translabyrinthine removal of acoustic neuroma. *Upper left:* A postauricular flap 2–3 cm posterior to the postauricular fold is elevated. *Upper right:* Simple mastoidectomy is completed. *Lower left:* The bony labyrinth is outlined and the facial recess opened. *Lower right:* The incus has been removed and the eustachian tube packed with sterilized Proplast. The labyrinth has been opened to begin labyrinthectomy. Bone has been completely removed from sigmoid sinus.

are given intravenously at the time of the skin incision. Mannitol is given during the labyrinthectomy part of this procedure. The usual incision is made approximately 2 cm to 4 cm behind the postauricular fold. The incision is carried through the subcutaneous tissue to the areolar tissue over the temporalis fascia. Next, an incision is made in a similar shape into the temporalis muscle and lateral mastoid periosteum leaving this area attached to the subcutaneous tissue of the postauricular flap. The Lempert periosteal elevator is used to free the postauricular tissues from the underlying cortex, posterior to the sinodural angle and forward until the spine of Henle and the external auditory canal are identified. The skin of the external auditory canal should be left intact in order to prevent postoperative infection and CSF leakage.

Cortical Mastoidectomy

After adequate exposure of the cortex has been obtained, bone removal is carried out in the usual fashion with a large cutting burr and suction irrigation. The entire dissection is accomplished with the aid of the operating microscope. Dissection is continued until only a thin plate of

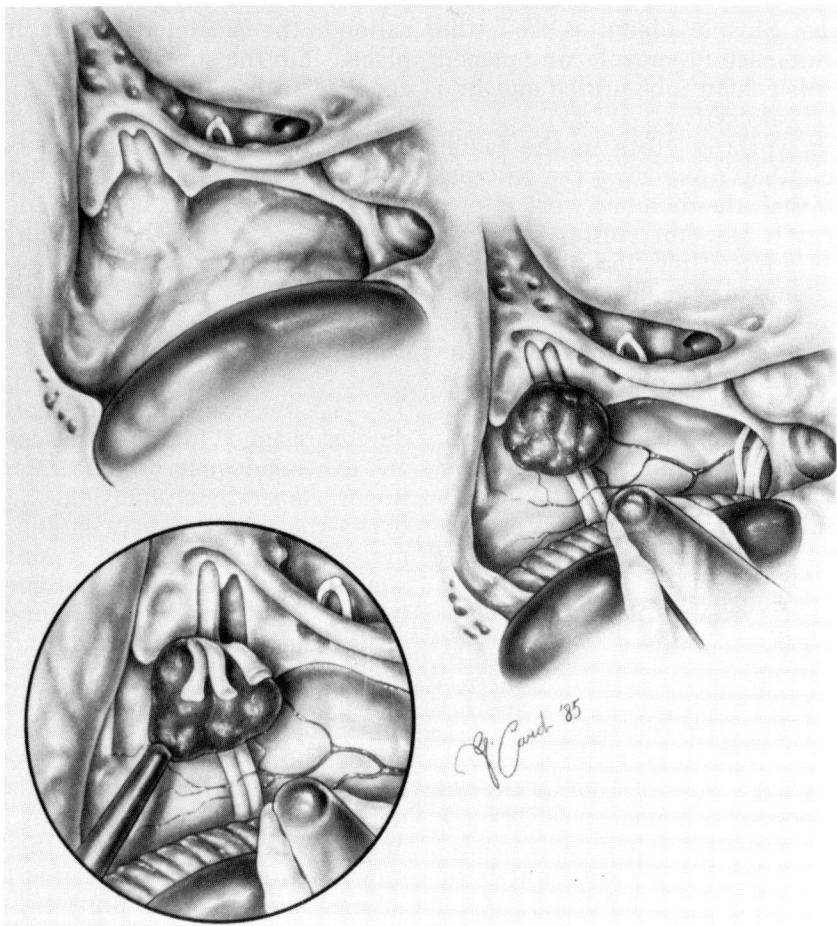

Figure 5: Translabyrinthine removal of acoustic neuroma continued. *Upper left:* Labyrinthectomy has been completed. Bone has been completely removed from the sigmoid sinus, posterior fossa dura, middle fossa dura, and the internal auditory canal. Tumor can be seen bulging in the lateral IAC and CP angle. *Middle right:* The dura mater has been opened. The small tumor can be seen extending into the CP angle but free from the brain stem. *Lower left:* The cut ends of the superior vestibular, inferior vestibular, and cochlear nerves are seen. The facial nerve remains intact.

bone is left overlying the dura. Bone removal is continued, outlining the external auditory canal. The simple cortical mastoidectomy is completed by defining the tegmen, sinodural angle, and sigmoid sinus. Often an emissary vein is found running perpendicularly from the sigmoid sinus, posteriorly. Care is taken not to injure this.

A complete, simple mastoidectomy is then performed down at the level of the horizontal semicircular canal. It is important that the antrum be opened and the horizontal canal be identified as it is the basic landmark for location of the facial nerve. The semicircular canals are clearly identified and air cells surrounding the otic capsule are removed. Next, a medium-sized diamond burr is utilized to skeletonize the facial nerve from the area of the second genu to the stylomastoid foramen.

The facial recess approach is used to enter the middle ear. The incudostapedial joint is separated and the incus is removed and placed into a bone bank. The head of the malleus is amputated. Sterilized Proplast is packed into the eustachian tube. Muscle pledglets from the sternocleidomastoid muscle are placed over the eustachian tube orifice and into the middle ear cavity.

When working close to the facial nerve and finally exposing the internal auditory canal, the diamond burr is preferred. First, the horizontal canal is opened. It is traced inferiorly to the posterior sermicircular canal. The posterior canal is followed inferiorly and anteriorly until the crus commune is identified. The superior canal is then followed anteriorly and superiorly until the ampulla is located. At the ampullary end of the superior canal, a very important landmark is identified. The landmark is the macula cribosis superiorus. It marks the lateral extent of the internal auditory canal where the superior vestibular nerve perforates the ampullary end of the superior semicircular canal.

Internal Auditory Canal Dissection

The bone is removed from the area of the superior petrosal sinus, posterior fossa dura plate, and jugular bulb. The dissection is continued anteriorly until the cochlear aqueduct is apparent. It is essential that the internal auditory canal be exposed a full 180° or there will be insufficient exposure for controlled tumor removal. Having outlined the internal auditory canal, attention is next directed to the area of the facial nerve and the lateral extent of the canal.

Final Identification of the Facial Nerve

Attention is now directed to the superior vestibular nerve. This is done by first finding the nerves innervating the ampulla of the horizontal and superior semicircular canals. Once these are identified, the diamond burr is used to remove the bone overlying the nerve endings and the superior vestibular nerve is identified. The next step is to identify Bill's bar which corresponds to the vertical bar of bone that separates the facial and vestibular nerves. This will identify the exact location of the facial nerve. A small hook is placed into the superior vestibular nerve canal. The hook follows Bill's bar medially until it drops anteriorly into the facial canal. The hook is placed back into the superior vestibular canal and rotated 90% inferiorly. The hook is then lifted posteriorly avulsing the superior vestibular nerve from its canal.

Dural Incision

The incision into the posterior fossa dura is designed to protect the cerebellum and to give adequate room to approach the tumor. Generally an incision midway between the porus acousticus and the sigmoid sinus is adequate. A small right angle hook is placed into the dura which is elevated laterally and a number 11 blade is utilized to make the initial incision into the dura. Microscissors are used to extend the incision. The incision is continued inferiorly toward the area of the jugular bulb and then superiorly to the area of the superior petrosal sinus. Lateral traction of the dura prevents any injury to deeper venous structures or the cerebellum. Next the dura is incised at the most inferior and posterior limit of the bony internal auditory canal. By staying close to the posterior-inferior limit of the internal auditory canal, the facial nerve will not be injured. This incision is continued from a lateral to a medial fashion going down to the area of the previous dural incision posteriorly. Also the dura of the most superior part of the internal auditory canal is incised from a lateral to an anterior approach connecting the previously incised dura. Many times this rectangular piece of dura outlined between the initial incision of the dura and the porus acusticus is actually removed. In some large tumors, the dura up to the sigmoid sinus must be removed.

Isolating the Tumor

The junction of the cerebellum and the capsule of the tumor is identified. A large moistened telfa strip is placed at this junctional point and medial retraction of the cerebellum is undertaken. Usually the lateral cerebellar cistern is encountered around the posterior aspect of the tumor. This is opened with an arachnoid knife and cerebrospinal fluid is allowed to escape. This will allow shrinkage of the cerebellum and medialward retraction. Often a large vein will be encountered at this point, corresponding to one of the petrosal veins which originate in the cerebellum and drain into the superior petrosal sinus near the level of the internal auditory canal. Care is taken not to injure this vein.

The tumor is now isolated by surrounding the field with cottonoids. The cottonoids are used to completely surround the tumor in various planes. Medially, tumor separation from the brain stem in larger tumors is also accomplished in this fashion. The microsurgical technique of acoustic tumor removal has greatly improved the resection of these tumors and preservation of important vascular structures. Individual, small bleeding vessels are initially cauterized with bipolar cautery and then cut with fine microscissors.

Inferiorly, an attempt is made to localize cranial nerves IX, X, and XI. In large tumors, these nerves may be stretched over the surface of the tumor. The plane is carefully developed and isolated using cottonoids.

Next, the superior aspect of the tumor capsule is developed. The petrosal vein will be encountered and in this location must be separated from the tumor. The 5th cranial nerve is identified at the medial superior aspect of the tumor, and these structures are gently separated from the capsule and packed away with cottonoids.

Identification of the Facial Nerve

After locating Bill's bar, a hook is used to remove the inferior vestibular nerve and dura of the internal auditory canal. Gentle facial nerve dissection is continued medially in the internal auditory canal into the posterior fossa. Once in the posterior fossa, the facial nerve becomes quite thinned and spread over the anterior or superior surface of the tumor. The separation of the nerve in this region is tedious and difficult but if a persistent effort is made, the tumor can normally be delivered without excessive trauma to the facial nerve.

Removal of the Tumor

The approach to tumor removal is mandated by the type of tumor and its growth characteristics. In most tumors, the facial nerve is splayed at the porus acusticus area and persistent removal of the tumor from the nerve is quite dangerous. Because of this, the dissection is turned medially toward the area of the brain stem. If the tumor is not in direct continuity with the brain stem, the root entry zone of the 7th cranial nerve can be identified and dissection can then be continued from the inferior limit of the tumor laterally sparing the facial nerve throughout its course and utilizing the facial nerve as an important landmark. In moderate-sized tumors, removal of tumor from the brain stem and other structures may be quite dangerous due to the proximity of the blood vessels arising from the vertebral and basilar arteries. In larger tumors, we have found it expedient to utilize the CO_2 laser. The laser is used to incise the posterior aspect of the tumor capsule and the tumor is removed by initially removing the bulk of the tumor intracapsularly. Only those vessels that actually enter the tumor capsule or matrix are coagulated. Peripheral vessels are carefully freed from the tumor capsule. The remainder of the tumor removal is accomplished going from a medial to a lateral direction, identifying clearly the root entry zone of the facial nerve. The root entry zone of the 8th nerve is identified and this is sectioned prior to the lateral removal.

Hemostasis and Closure

After total tumor removal, the wound is profusely irrigated to remove any blood clots. Cottonoids are then removed and all bleeding points are controlled with bipolar cautery. Absolute hemostasis must be obtained and this may require considerable time and effort. The anesthesiologist is asked to Valsalva the patient to assure hemostasis.

The dural opening and mastoidectomy cavity are obliterated with strips of fat taken from abdomen. These strips measure approximately 1 cm by 3 cm. One-half centimeter of the fat strip is placed intradurally and the remainder of the strip is placed into the mastoid defect. Multiple strips are placed so as to tightly seal the dural defect. Subcutaneous soft tissues and subcuticular layers are closed in layers and with interrupted absorbable sutures. Skin closure is accomplished with metallic clips. A tight mastoid dressing is then placed at the completion of the procedure.

One-Stage Combined Translabyrinthine-Suboccipital Approach (Figs. 6 and 7)

This procedure is used for tumors over 4 cm.[6] A large postauricular flap is created in order to expose the mastoid and occipital bones. This flap is created in order to expose the mastoid and occipital bones. This flap is retracted forward and held in place with dural hooks. A complete translabyrinthine dissection, as previously described, is carried out. Bone is removed from behind the sigmoid sinus for approximately 3 to 4 cm. The dura

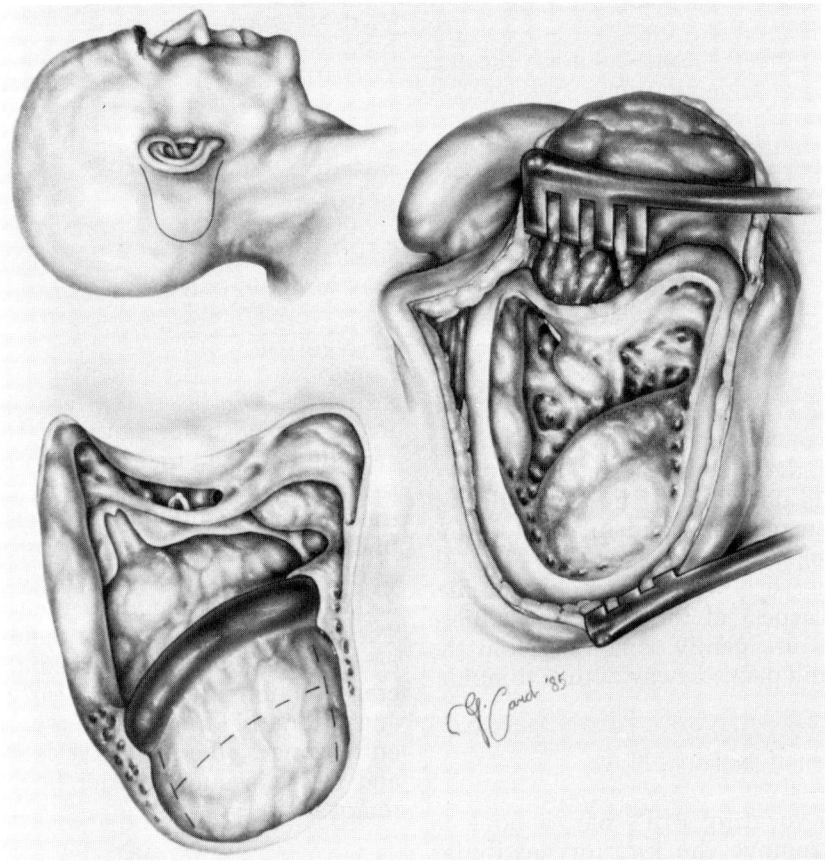

Figure 6: Combined suboccipital-translabyrinthine removal of acoustic neuroma. *Upper left:* A large flap extending 4–6 cm posterior to the postauricular fold is created. *Middle right:* The mastoidectomy is completed. Bone removal is carried 2–3 cm posterior to the sigmoid sinus. *Lower left:* Bone has been completely removed from the posterior fossa dura both anterior and posterior to the sigmoid sinus.

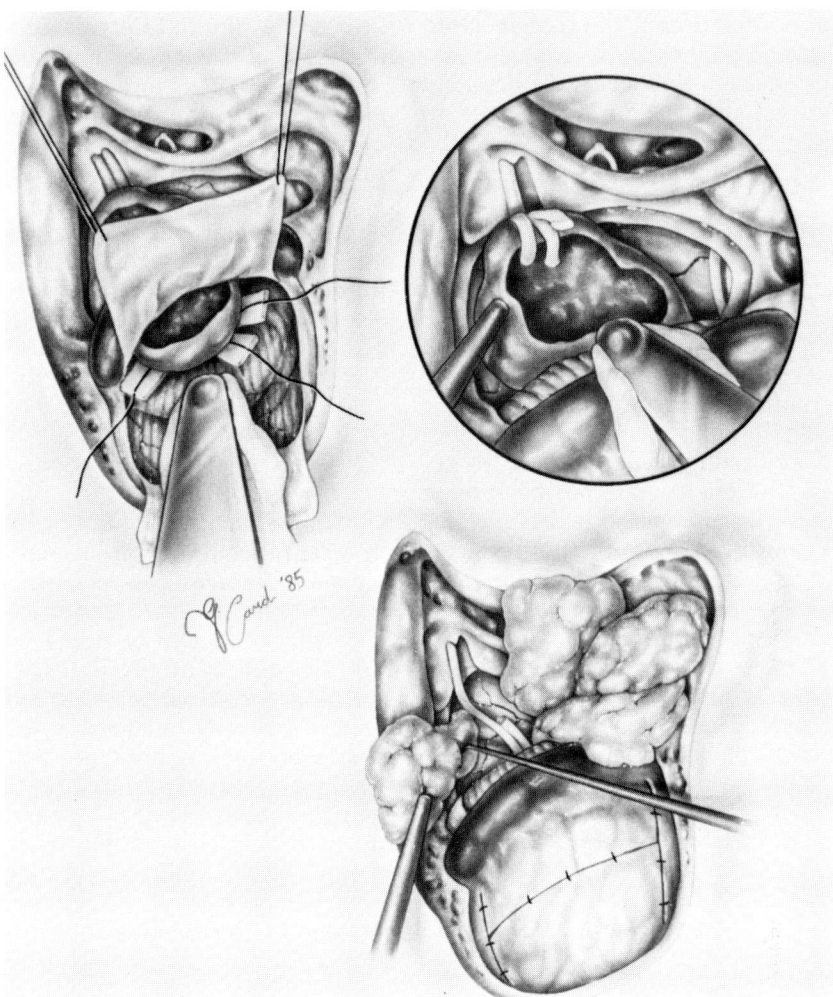

Figure 7: Combined suboccipital-translabyrinthine removal of acoustic neuroma continued. *Upper left:* The posterior fossa behind the sigmoid sinus has been opened, exposing a large acoustic neuroma indenting the brain stem and cerebellum. Cottonoid pledgelets are used to isolate the tumor from underlying brain. The tumor is then "debulked" using the CO_2 laser until it can be reflected anteriorly under the sigmoid sinus. *Upper right:* Debulking is continued anterior to the sigmoid sinus until it is possible to mobilize the entire tumor capsule. Prior to mobilization, the lateral IAC is opened so that the facial nerve can be identified where its position is undistorted by tumor growth. *Lower right:* 4-0 silk sutures are used to achieve water tight closure of the retrosigmoid dura mater. The bony defect anterior to the sigmoid is carefully filled with strips of fat obtained from the abdomen.

over the cerebellum is retracted laterally with a right angle hook and the dura is incised with a number 11 blade. Stay sutures of 4-0 silk are then placed and lateral retraction of the dura is accomplished. Double strips are then placed over the cerebellum and a Jannetta posterior fossa retractor is inserted to retract the cerebellum. Once this has been accomplished, the tumor is isolated with cottonoids, the capsule is incised, and the mass is gutted. The tumor is reduced to a size of approximately 2 to 3 cm. The remainder of the surgery is performed through the translabyrinthine route.

At the completion of tumor removal, the posterior fossa incision behind the sigmoid sinus is closed with 4-0 silk sutures. Fat obliteration of the transmastoid defect is accomplished in the routine fashion. Once again, a tight mastoid dressing is placed and the patient is observed in the recovery room overnight.

Suboccipital Approach

The unilateral suboccipital approach to the cerebellopontine angle is discussed elsewhere in this book. Highlights of the technique will be mentioned.[10]

The unilateral suboccipital approach to the cerebellopontine angle has been the standard neurosurgical approach. In recent years, the microscope has been used on a routine basis and the technique improved upon by removal of the posterior lip of the internal auditory canal for identification and preservation of the facial nerve and occasionally the cochlear nerve.

The major disadvantages of this approach are that the surgeon does not have the benefit of the bony landmarks of Bill's bar, the dissection is quite deep, requiring extra long instruments, and dissection of the lateral portion of the internal auditory canal is done blindly.

Special Problems in Acoustic Neuroma Surgery

Observation

Life expectancy in America is continuing to increase. Acoustic neuroma growth is slow but progressive. There have been isolated case reports of very rapid growth. In elderly patients (over the age of 65) or surgically high risk patients, observation may be the most appropriate management. The senior author has operated on an 81-year-old with an aggressive acoustic neuroma who had an uneventful postoperative course.

With new techniques of high resolution CT scanning, the volume of an acoustic tumor can be determined. It is recommended that a repeat CT scan be performed at 6-month intervals and a growth rate for the particular tumor calculated. The surgeon needs to weigh the risk of an operative procedure against the risk of neurological complications from continued tumor growth.

Radiation of these tumors is not recommended. One must consider the possibility of malignant transformation of these tumors secondary to the radiotherapy. Stereotactic gamma knife radiation in lieu of surgery deserves further study.

Bilateral Tumors

Bilateral acoustic tumors, often felt to represent a central form of von Recklinghausen's disease, pose a particular challenge to the acoustic neuroma surgeon. Early diagnosis can be achieved by clinical awareness of the disease, through radiologic evaluation and appropriate family screening. Bilateral tumor removal should be total, if possible, with hearing preserved on at least one side. Early diagnosis is mandatory if postoperative hearing is to be preserved, and rehabilitation in high risk patients should be planned early before hearing is jeopardized. Associated hydrocephalus and additional intracranial tumors may complicate the overall clinical picture. Hearing preservation with total tumor removal through either a suboccipital or middle fossa approach is probable if the lesion is not larger than 1 cm in size. Hearing preservation with total tumor removal is doubtful if the tumor is larger than 2 cm in size.

These tumors appear to have a different type of growth pattern than the usual acoustic neuroma in that often the cochlear nerve is surrounded by the tumor mass in a lobulated form. This makes the actual dissection and total tumor removal with hearing preservation much more difficult. The Otology Group uses a middle fossa approach to preserve hearing and totally remove the tumor. If hearing preservation is accomplished and maintained for at least 1 to 2 years, the other side is observed until intracranial complications occur.

Large Tumors

Large tumor removal has already been described via the translabyrinthine-suboccipital, one-stage approach.[6] Tumors that present in a patient with other central nervous system signs are individualized in their management.

Most patients presenting with marked hydrocephalus will have papilledema. Usually these patients are medically stable enough to be thoroughly evaluated preoperatively and surgical management can be planned in an organized fashion. At the time of surgery, these patients are taken to the operating room with a half-head shave and abdominal prep. Through a superior burr hole, the ventricular system is tapped and relieved of the excess cerebrospinal fluid and the tumor is removed. The patient is then taken to the recovery room or intensive care unit where close monitoring is undertaken. A permanent ventriculo-peritoneal shunt is not placed at the time of surgery. The patient is closely observed for neurologic signs and symptoms and repeat CT scans are obtained 24 hours and 72 hours postoperatively. The necessity for a permanent peritoneal shunt is decided upon during the postoperative period.

Results

The results are based on over 600 acoustic neuromas personally removed by the senior author. The mean age is 47 years with an age range from 4 years to 81 years.

Tumor size is evaluated by preoperative CT scanning. In the past, the size was measured by either posterior fossa myelogram or measurements taken at the time of surgery. Small tumors, those that measure up to 1.5 cm, have amounted to approximately 17% of this series. Medium tumors, which are considered those from 1.5 cm to 2.9 cm, constitute approximately 53% of the tumors in this series. Large tumors, those that are greater than 3 cm, account for approximately 30% in this series.

Sixty-nine percent of the procedures were translabyrinthine approaches. The combined translabyrinthine-suboccipital approach was used in approximately 21% of the cases. The middle fossa surgical approach was used only in hearing preservation attempts and this amounted to approximately 9% of this series. The suboccipital approach was employed in approximately 2% of the surgical patients. Depending on the tumor characteristics, a combination of approaches was used and there were a combined middle fossa and suboccipital, combined middle fossa and translabyrinthine, and combined translabyrinthine and transcochlear approach. Total tumor removal was 98.5%. Two patients had planned subtotal removals due to age and general health.

Facial nerve preservation is a major advantage to the translabyrinthine approach. Facial nerve preservation was accomplished in 82% of the patients. In small tumors, the facial nerve was preserved in 99% and in medium tumors, the facial nerve was preserved in approximately 91%. In larger tumors, the facial nerve was preserved in 57%.

Cerebrospinal fluid leak was detected either through the middle ear or eustachian tube, and eventually in the nasopharynx, or out of the incision site. Treatment for cerebrospinal fluid leak is dependent on the site of escape. Those patients who had leakage through the nasopharynx all required a second operative procedure at which time the eustachian tube was obliterated with muscle or Proplast. If a direct site of leakage was found at the dural defect, it was treated with an additional adipose tissue graft. Patients who presented with spinal fluid leak through the incision site were usually managed conservatively. Additional cutaneous sutures, bedrest, and daily spinal taps were performed until the leakage stopped. The technique currently employed has dramatically decreased the incidence of spinal fluid leak. The insertion of Proplast into the eustachian tube, obliteration of the middle ear with muscle, adipose strip grafts layered in the dural defect, postoperative pressure dressing that remains for 6 days, and a third-day lumbar puncture has drastically reduced the incidence of spinal fluid leak. The incidence of postoperative meningitis was approximately 5%. This generally occurred in those patients who developed some type of cerebrospinal fluid leak. Currently there have been four postoperative deaths attributed to acoustic neuroma surgery in this series (0.67%). There has been one recurrence.

Conclusions

The goal of acoustic tumor surgery is total tumor removal without neurologic deficit. We prefer the translabyrinthine approach in the majority of our patients so that the facial nerve is viewed throughout the surgical extirpation of the tumor. In small tumors, where hearing preservation is important, the middle fossa approach is selected. The suboccipital approach is reserved for those patients with serviceable hearing and tumors greater than 1.5 cm.

References

1. Batsakis JG: *Tumor of the Head and Neck: Clinical and Pathologic Consideration.* Baltimore, Williams and Wilkins, 1979, p 573.
2. Brackmann DE: A review of acoustic tumors. *Am J Otology* 5:233-244, 1984.
3. Clemis JD: Hearing conservation in acoustic tumor surgery: Pro's and con's. *Otolaryngol Head Neck Surg* 92:156-161, 1984.
4. Creed L, Seeger JF: Radiologic evaluation of the acoustic neuroma. *Ariz Med* 41:739-743, 1984.
5. Cushing H: *Tumors of the Nervous Acousticus and the Syndrome of the Cerebellopontine Angle,* Edition 2. New York, Haefner Publishing Co., 1963.
6. Glasscock ME, Hays JW, Jackson CG, et al.: A one-stage combined approach for the management of large cerebellopontine angle tumors. *Laryngoscope* 88:1563-1576, 1978.
7. Glasscock ME, Hays JW, Miller GW, et al.: Preservation of hearing in tumors of the internal auditory canal and cerebellopontine angle. *Laryngoscope* 88:43-55, 1978.
8. Hart RG, Davenport J: Diagnosis of acoustic neuroma. *Neurosurgery* 9:450-63, 1981.
9. Morrison AW, King TT: Space-occupying lesions of the internal auditory meatus and cerebellopontine angle. *Adv Otolaryngol* 34:121, 1984.
10. Smith MF, Miller RH, Cox DS: Suboccipital microsurgical removal of acoustic neuromas of all sizes. *Ann Otol Rhinol Laryngol* 81:409, 1983.
11. Thomsen J, Terkildson K, Tos M: Acoustic neuromas: Progression of hearing impairment and function of the eighth cranial nerve. *Am J Otology* 5:20-33, 1983.

31

Management of Cranial Chordomas

Patrick J. Derome, M.D.
Andre Visot, M.D.
J.P. Monteil, M.D.
J.L. Maestro, M.D.

Surgical Management: Principles and Complications

The surgical management of clivus chordomas is certainly one of the most difficult problems encountered by the neurosurgeon. This is due to several factors: (1) tumors are usually located deep and medially, at the center of the skull base; (2) it is difficult to remove the lesion completely, and yet this must be attempted; and (3) many surgical approaches are possible, and each has advantages and limitations.

Chordomas are embryonal tumors originating from the remnants of the notochord, which is the first axial skeleton of vertebrates. The preferential sites of development of these tumors are the extremities of the notochord in the cranial and caudal areas. When the mesodermal tissue that will become the base of the skull envelops the primary notochord between the hypophyseal fossa and the vertebral column, some remnants of the notochord may remain free and superficial; they are found in the sellar or parasellar areas, posterior to the clivus and extending backward to the posterior fossa, or anterior to the clivus and extending toward the pharyngeal epithelium. Because cranial chordomas originate from remnant cells of the axial notochord or its extensions, the tumors that develop are variable, and the surgical approach chosen depends upon the extent and location of bone destruction, and on the main direction and extension of the tumor at the base of the skull.

The surgical difficulties of chordoma removal also vary with the macroscopic morphology of the tumor. Many chordomas have a smooth, semigelatinous consistency; this explains why quite large lesions may be removed through a relatively narrow surgical approach. However, other chordomas have a firmer consistency, which makes the surgical removal more difficult and less complete than may be expected; in our experience this type of tumor appears more frequently at the occipitovertebral junction. Chordomas may sometimes appear to be encapsulated, but this is deceptive, and

From: Sekhar LN, Schramm VL Jr, eds: *Tumors of the Cranial Base: Diagnosis and Treatment*. Mount Kisco, New York, Futura Publishing Co, Inc, © 1987.

bone will be found to be widely infiltrated. Total removal of such chordomas is therefore difficult.

The relationship of the tumor to the dura is also important. Chordomas are primarily extradural lesions, and they may usually be removed by an extradural approach. However, as the tumor increases in size, it will infiltrate and destroy the basal dura to become both an intradural and extradural lesion. When this occurs, some surgical approaches become difficult or impossible, and this must be taken into consideration when choosing the best approach. Predicting dural involvement before surgery is very difficult; however, some clival chordomas remain totally extradural despite their invasive nature, instead extending far toward the posterior fossa, as visualizable on computed tomography or magnetic resonance imaging. In contrast, retrosellar and retroclival chordomas that do not destroy the clivus are frequently totally intradural tumors. Dural invasion decreases the possibility of wide removal, and is one factor indicating a poor prognosis.

Because they are located at the base of the skull, are of variable consistency, and invade locally, these tumors are usually not able to be removed completely. However, the goal of surgery is total (or subtotal) removal, since radiotherapy for such lesions is of questionable value.[15,18,25] Radiotherapy is usually administered postoperatively,[12,14,20,21,24,26] but it is very difficult to assess its results. We believe that the prognosis for patient survival is dependent on the extent of operative resection, and if postoperative radiation therapy has any effect, it will be enhanced if the residual tumor volume is as small as possible.

Microsurgical techniques have allowed neurosurgeons to become more aggressive in the management of cranial chordomas. Because maximally complete removal is presently the main determinant of long-term survival (or possibly cure), this attitude seems valid. The principles governing treatment of cranial chordomas are: (1) to choose the approach that will allow the widest tumor removal; this will depend on the main direction in which the tumor has extended; (2) to improve the extent of removal by combining several approaches in one or several stages; and (3) to reoperate on tumor recurrences, without hesitating to vary the approaches used according to the site of recurrence (recurrences develop frequently from remnants of the primary lesion that had not been removed initially).

Surgical Approaches

Many different approaches may be used to reach a tumor of the skull base. The surgical approach must be chosen according to whether the tumor is located in the midline or has extended laterally, according to the relationship of the tumor to the dura, and according to the degree to which tumor has destroyed the bone at the base of the skull. A final consideration in choosing the surgical approach is resolution of neurological symptoms. Intradural and the extradural approaches will be discussed in detail.

Intradural Approaches

The main indication for an intradural approach is a chordoma that has involved and destroyed the dura to extend intracranially, coming in close proximity to neural structures and basal vessels. Most extradural approaches are too risky in such cases because of the dangers of cerebrospinal fluid (CSF) leakage and secondary infection; this results from the difficulty in restoring complete dural integrity following wide destruction of the dura. The cavernous sinus is frequently involved as well in patients with intradural chordomas, and this often limits the surgical removal of the lesion.

Parasellar location of a cranial chordoma is another indication for an intradural approach to its removal. Figure 1 summarizes the different approaches that may be used, depending upon the site of the lesion.

Pterional Approach

A pterional approach to a cranial chordoma allows the surgeon to reach the

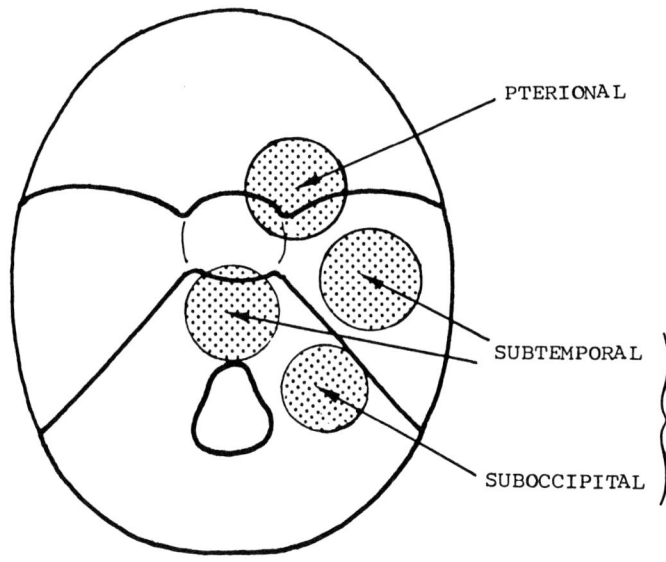

Figure 1: Intradural approaches to cranial chordomas; the approach chosen will depend on the location of the lesion. Subtemporal and suboccipital approaches may be combined.

tumor located in the suprasellar area (Fig. 2), and to relieve any intradural compression of the optic apparatus. This operative approach, in which the Sylvian fissure is opened, is well known.

We have also used this approach to reach three totally extradural tumors that had invaded the cavernous sinus, producing visual disturbances (two of these three patients were already blind in one eye and had begun to lose their vision in the opposite eye). The protrusion of the cavernous sinus facilitates exposure between the frontal and temporal lobes in such cases, while blood vessels and cranial nerves, particularly the internal carotid artery and the oculomotor nerve, are usually displaced by the underlying tumor (Fig. 3). The dura is incised medial or lateral to the oculomotor nerve, according to where the main protrusion of the chordoma lies; such transdural removal is necessarily incomplete, but may improve neurological symptoms when chordomas have invaded the cavernous sinuses. We then repair the dura of the skull base to prevent subdural hematoma in the postoperative period.

Subtemporal Approach

A subtemporal approach to a cranial chordoma is indicated when the lesion has involved the middle cerebral fossa between the greater sphenoid wing anteriorly and the petrous bone posteriorly, growing into the paracavernous area as would a trigeminal schwannoma. The extradural tumor is reached through the basal dura; in these cases, the intradural approach is the best route, even though the lesion is extradural.

However, such cases occur rarely. Thus, the main indication for a subtemporal approach is location of the chordoma in the upper half of the clivus, even when it is in the midline (Fig. 4). A subtemporal approach is absolutely essential when the clival bone has not been destroyed, and when there is no extension of the tumor into the sphenoid; when the dorsum sellae, the adjacent clivus, and the sphenoid sinuses are involved, the transsphenoidal route may be considered.

The side of the subtemporal approach is chosen according to the main lateralization of the tumor (ipsilateral to cranial nerve palsies, contralateral to displacement of the basilar artery); if the tumor is strictly in the midline, the lesion should be approached from the side of the patient's nondominant hemisphere. Particular care must be taken not to injure veins draining the temporal lobe to avoid postoperative complications related to venous infarction and edema. Division of the ten-

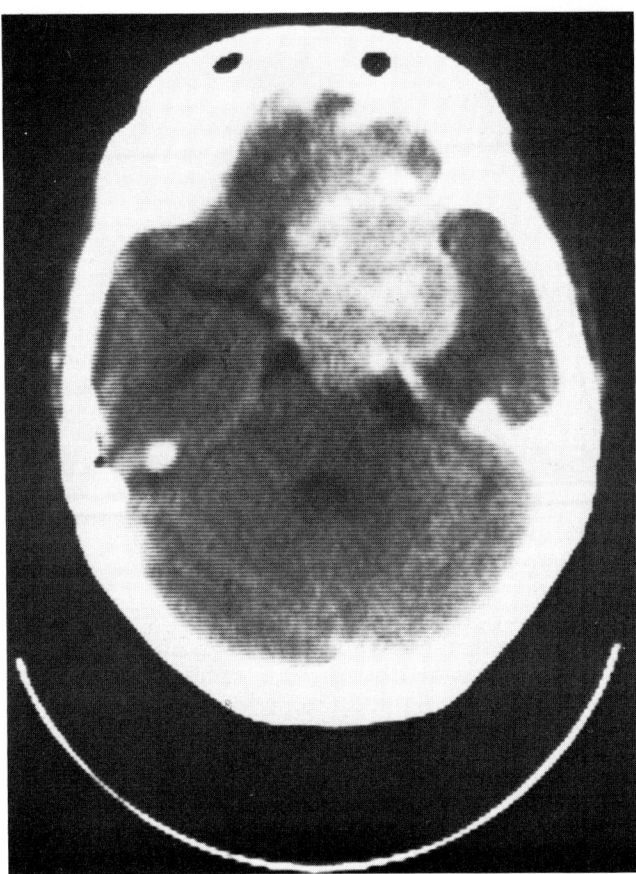

Figure 2: Supra- and parasellar chordoma; indication for a pterional approach.

torium provides wide exposure between the 3rd and 5th cranial nerves; the tumor increases the space available so that the larger the lesion, the better will be the possibility of reaching the lower part of the clivus. However, even if the tumor is large, the exposure obtained by such subtemporal and transtentorial exploration is limited, and it is difficult to expose the lower third of the clivus sufficiently to reach tumor extending to the foramen magnum. Reaching the lateral part of the posterior fossa and the cerebellopontine angle is also difficult if the tumor extends toward the 7th and 8th cranial nerves. Such extension requires other surgical approaches.

Suboccipital Approach

A suboccipital approach is recommended to reach tumor extending laterally in the posterior fossa, particularly when it extends to the cerebellopontine angle. As with subtemporal approaches, extradural tumor involving the petrous bone or the adjacent occipital bone must be removed through the basal dura, which is repaired at the end of the procedure whenever possible. Wide opening of the foramen magnum, and a laminectomy of the first and second cervical vertebrae, will be necessary when the tumor extends toward the upper cervical spine. In such cases, the suboccipital approach is made more difficult and limited by the proximity of the brain stem, the lattice of the lower cranial nerves, and the cerebellar and vertebral arteries.

Combination Suboccipital/Subtemporal Approach

It may be extremely useful to combine a suboccipital aproach and a subtemporal

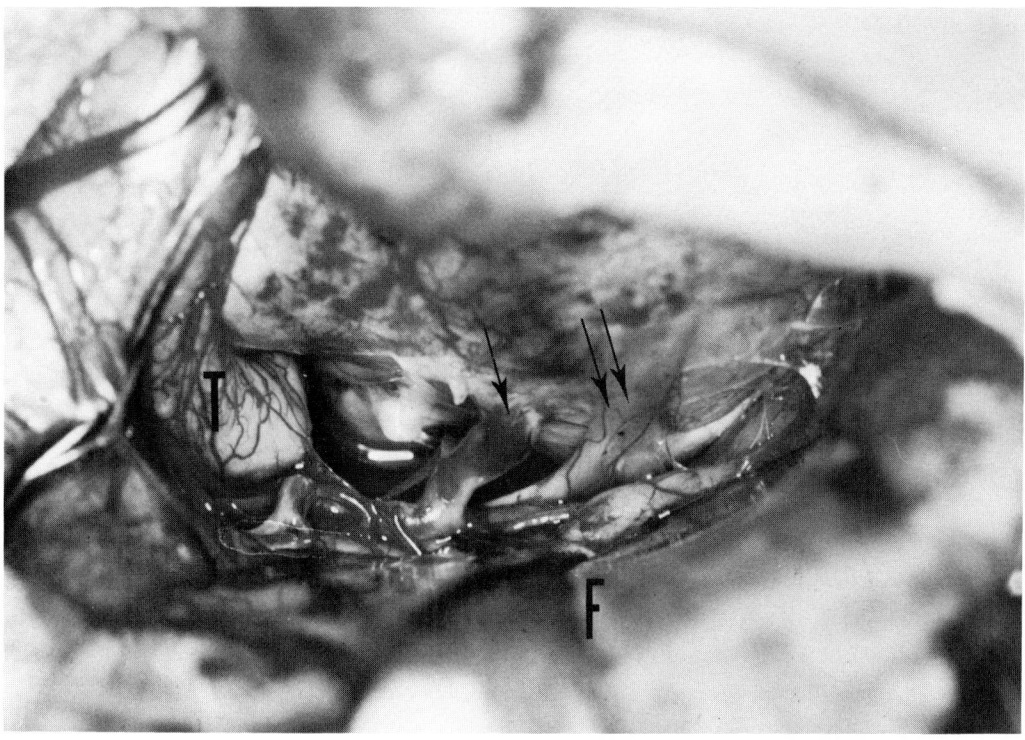

Figure 3: Pterional approach. Bulging of an extradural chordoma involving the left cavernous sinus is visible between the frontal lobe (F) and the retracted temporal lobe (T). Single arrow, left internal carotid artery; double arrows, optic chiasm tract.

approach in the same surgical procedure to reach large tumors extending from the upper part to the lower part of the clivus, or when portions of the tumor are located at the limits of these two approaches.

In such cases, the transverse sinus is dissected free and severed just anterior to the opening of the vein of Labbè; then the tentorium is divided. This provides wide exposure below the temporal lobe and between the clivus and the petrous bone anteriorly, and the brain stem and cerebellum posteriorly, permitting, in the same procedure, removal of a chordoma extending from the interpeduncular cistern down to the foramen magnum or the jugular foramen. However, the indications for this combined approach are relatively rare, as most such large tumors destroy the clivus and extend anteriorly toward the cavum; because of extensive bony involvement, their removal is easier through a transoral approach.

Anterior Extradural Approaches

An anterior extradural approach is particularly useful when a chordoma is in the midline and purely extradural extension is suspected. Such extradural development is sometimes obvious from bulging of the pharyngeal mucosa with minimal destruction of the bone of the clivus, odontoid, and body of the first and second cervical vertebrae; in addition, a tumor may extend posteriorly into the posterior fossa, with clival destruction and bone involvement, and still not invade the dura. A regularly shaped tumor border in the posterior fossa is in favor of an extradural location. On the other hand, tumors located in front of the brain stem, without destruction of the bone, are probably intradural. The risk of CSF leakage postoperatively must be considered in choosing some of these anterior approaches.

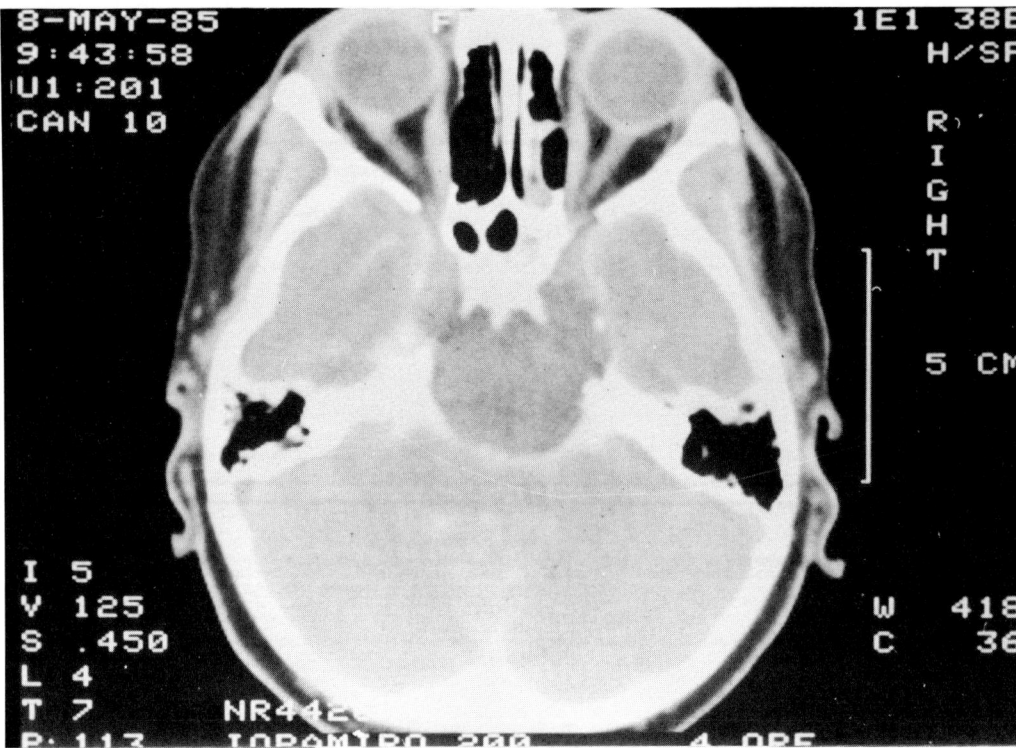

Figure 4: Chordoma of the upper half of the clivus, without destruction of bone, is an indication for a subtemporal approach.

The approach chosen also depends upon the level of the chordoma along the base of the skull and clivus. The difficulties associated with the anatomical limits of each extradural approach will be discussed below. When a chordoma is located between the cervical and sphenoid areas, one may use a transcervical, transoral, transsphenoid, or transbasal approach (Fig. 5).

Transcervical, Transclival Approach

Stevenson et al.[23] described this approach, which permits exposure of the lower third or lower half of the clivus. In the case they describe, a chordoma of the foramen magnum and adjacent clivus was reached by resection of the odontoid and the anterior arch of the atlas. They succeeded in excavating a 4.5 cm square area of clivus to extirpate the tumor radically. The approach in this case was between the neck vessels and the trachea, similar to the approach to the cervical spine. Many measures were undertaken to prevent postoperative complications in their case, including postoperative immobilization with Crutchfield tongs, muscle grafts in the clival window, and continuous spinal drainage to avoid postoperative CSF leakage.

We consider this approach to be of most value in cases of intentional or accidental dural opening, because it can preclude CSF leakage and infection since the paranasal sinuses and nasopharynx are not opened. In addition, closure of any dural defect through this approach is more likely to be effective. The disadvantages of using this approach are the depth of the operative field (even though an operating microscope is used), the relatively limited lateral extent of the operative field, and the partly lateral approach to the midline, in contrast to the transoral or transsphenoid approach.

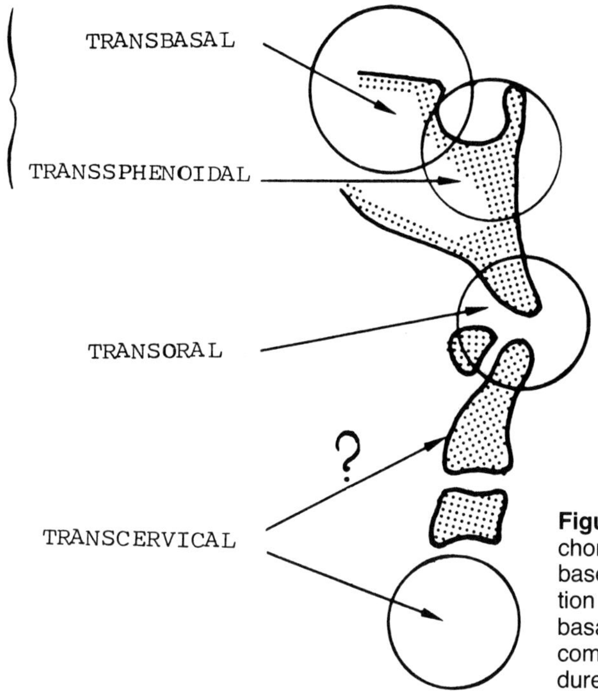

Figure 5: Anterior extradural approaches to chordomas. The specific approach is chosen based on the level of the chordoma with relation to the spheno-occipital area. The transbasal and transsphenoid approaches may be combined during the same surgical procedure.

In our opinion, the transcervical, transclival approach is most useful in cases of inferior and lateral extensions of chordomas in the cervical region, below the level of the second cervical vertebra.

Transoral Approach

We believe that the transoral approach is technically easy to perform: the lower half of the clivus is reached without deviating from the midline, and tumor extensions down to the second and third cervical vertebrae may be removed readily through the same approach.[1,4,6,17,19] The most obvious indication for using this approach is a tumor extending anteriorly to bulge significantly into the pharyngeal muscosa, causing swallowing difficulties and sometimes respiratory problems (Fig. 6). However, chordomas that have destroyed the lower half of the clivus and involved the posterior fossa may also be easily removed by this approach, after first resecting the anterior arch of the atlas, the odontoid, and even the body of the second cervical vertebra if it is involved.

For this approach, the patient is placed in a semi-sitting position (similar to that used for transsphenoidal pituitary surgery) to permit intraoperative fluoroscopy to visualize the extent of bone removal and the positions of the instruments (Fig. 7). Tracheostomy is performed only when respiratory obstruction or major swallowing difficulty is present. The soft palate is incised vertically, from the hard palate to the uvula, and retracted laterally. The anterior aspects of the bodies of the first two (or three, if necessary) cervical vertebrae are exposed through a midline, vertical incision through the pharyngeal mucosa.

This incision should be extended as far laterally as possible. Wide exposure in the area of the foramen magnum and of the first two cervical vertebrae may be obtained in this way, but the operative field narrows progressively superiorly because of the triangular field afforded by vertical incision of the soft palate; it is impossible to obtain surgical exposure above the lower half of the clivus, and repair of the upper part of the pharyngeal incision is often difficult because the clival area at

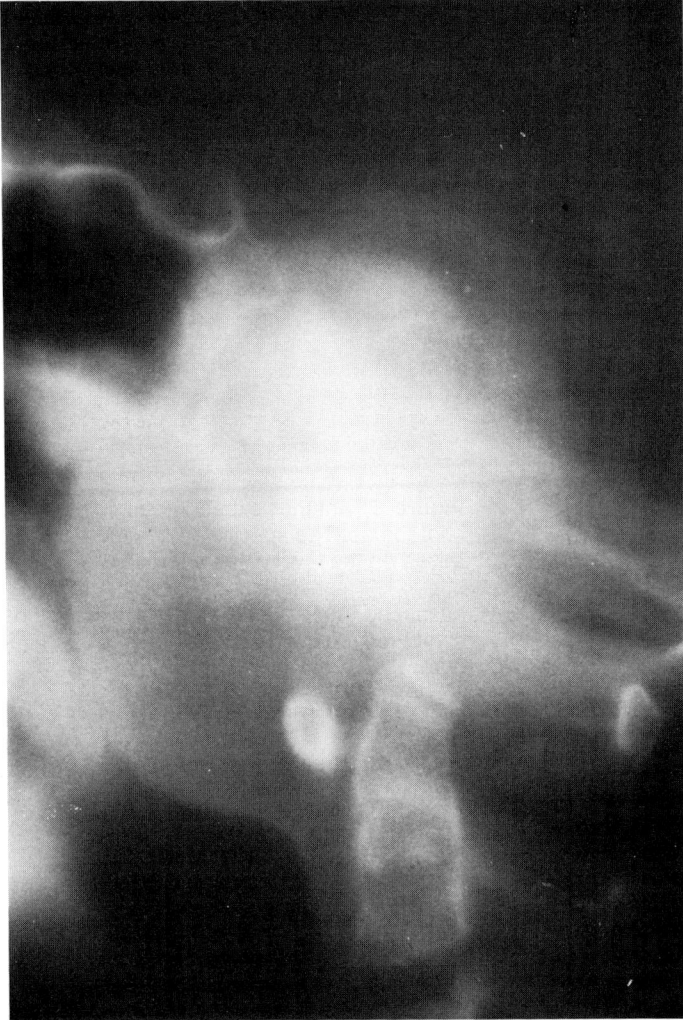

Figure 6: Extremely large chordoma bulging into the pharyngeal spaces and posterior fossa is an indication for a transoral approach.

the boundary between the upper limit of the transoral approach and the lower limit of the transsphenoid approach is a "blind spot."

Exposure may be improved by making an additional incision, from the midline incision of the soft palate to the mucosa of the hard palate (Fig. 8). This incision creates two mucosal flaps turned laterally around the hook of the pterygoid processes, and vascularized by the pterygopalatine arteries. Thus, instead of providing a narrow triangular exposure at the upper limit of the transoral approach, this transpalatal approach provides a broad quadrangular exposure when the posterior edge of the hard palate has been removed. With this combined approach, it is possible to remove, under direct visualization, a chordoma extending more superiorly on the clivus up to the level of the sella. This additional incision also makes suturing of the pharyngeal incision easier, and permits watertight closure of the dura in two planes, which is essential if it is suspected that any CSF leakage might have occurred with tumor removal.

Leakage of CSF remains the major complication of the transoral and transpalatal approach when the clival dura has been involved by tumor or destroyed. Very often the dura is uninvolved, and the transoral route is totally safe. When the dura is partially involved, we have merely

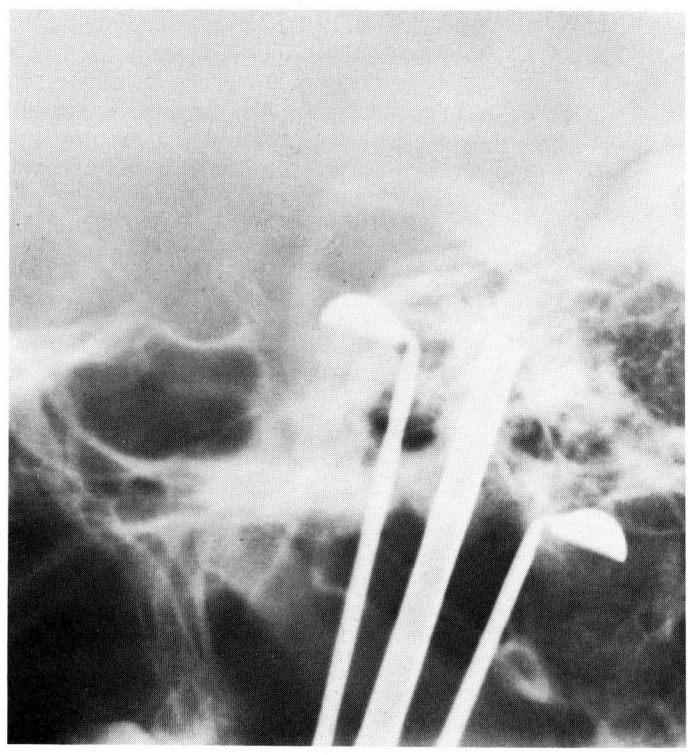

Figure 7: Same patient as in Figure 6, showing control of instruments for removal of a chordoma through a transoral approach.

coagulated the affected area. However, when the dura has been extensively invaded and destroyed, as happened in two of our patients, it is necessary to take steps to prevent CSF leakage. In such cases we pack muscle into the operative cavity, without removing the intradural portion of the chordoma. This tumor is left to plug the dura, rather than creating a fistula through which CSF would leak. After careful closure and total cicatrization of the extradural planes, the posterior part of the tumor is removed through an intradural approach.

Others have suggested different ways to provide watertight closure of the dura,[1,11,16,27] but in most of these cases the dural defect was the result of an incision made during management of a basilar or vertebrobasilar aneurysm, rather than a large meningeal defect such as may result from wide invasion of a chordoma. Nevertheless, the enlargement of this approach in the future may facilitate watertight closure of the pharyngeal incision and obviate an additional surgical procedure.

In our experience, it was not necessary to stabilize the patient's head after resection of the anterior arch of the first cervical vertebra, odontoid, and part of the body of the second cervical vertebra, or clivus, except in these situations: (1) lateral extension of the chordoma at the occipitocervical junction with destruction of the lateral portion of the occiput and first cervical vertebra or (2) after performing a complementary posterior approach to the cervical spine, particularly in a young patient.

A final consideration in resection of chordomas is use of a nasogastric tube. A nasogastric tube should be inserted when

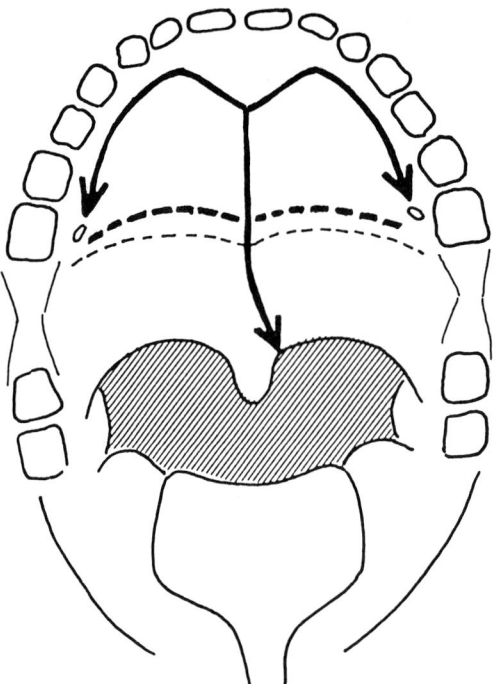

Figure 8: Transoral approach, showing incision of the palatal fibromucosa and soft palate (arrows), and separation of the two muscosal flaps from the posterior edge of the hard palate (dotted lines).

the tumor caused swallowing difficulties, and it should be placed after the pharyngeal mucosa has been sutured, but before the soft palate has been sutured; the tube should be attached carefully to the nasal septum. The tube should never be introduced blindly after completion of the surgical procedure, as this may result in secondary reopening of the pharyngeal suture line with resultant leakage of CSF, as occurred in one of our cases.

It should be emphasized that the transoral approach is no more difficult to use than the transsphenoidal approach currently being used to resect pituitary adenomas. Further, it is unnecessary to divide the tongue and the mandible with this approach, as some others have proposed. Septic complications occur rarely after removal of chordomas, and the transoral approach remains the best for removal of tumors located around the foramen magnum or the occipitocervical junction.

Transsphenoidal Approach

The sellar area, sphenoid sinuses, and upper half of the clivus can be reached by the transsphenoidal approach. In many cases this approach is used for tumor biopsy, but it may also be used for extensive subtotal (or possibly total) removal of a chordoma, despite the relative narrowness of the operative field.[6,8,22,26] Tumors of soft consistency that invade the sphenoid sinuses and destroy the bone are more readily removed by this route.

When a chordoma extends intradurally, and a CSF leak occurs intraoperatively, the leak is more easily controlled in this area when a transsphenoidal approach is used than when a transoral approach has been used. In this case, the sphenoid sinus is packed with muscle (or fat), and lumbar punctures or a lumbar drain are used to remove excess CSF, as for pituitary surgery. Extradural chordomas are particularly accessible by the transsphenoidal approach, even when they extend behind the sella and the dorsum sellae.

The major limitation of the transsphenoidal approach is the narrow operative field. This is bounded by the cavernous sinuses laterally, and extends inferiorly to below the level of the choanae and soft palate and superiorly to the bulge of the sellar dura, if the sella has not been invaded. This field may be extended by using fluoroscopy intraoperatively to complete removal and permit precise placement of instruments. Because this approach permits direct visualization of the clival dura, it may be combined with the transbasal approach during the same surgical procedure.

Transbasal Approach

The transbasal approach has been described for tumors involving the ethmoid and sphenoid in the anterior and/or middle cranial fossa; for chordomas this approach was used in a few cases to reach clival tumors bulging anteriorly. However, although we have photographic documentation of impressive exposure obtained through this approach, and it may be of benefit for dissection and preservation of the pharyngeal mucosa should an unexpected CSF leak occur,[5,6] we have given up this approach for removal of chordomas for two reasons. First, the surgical field is limited laterally by the optic canals and extradural portion of the optic nerves, and posteriorly by the bulge of the sellar dura. Second, reaching the anterior arch of the first and second cervical vertebrae is feasible, but it is impossible to enlarge the area of tumor removal at this depth.

Nevertheless, the transbasal approach is definitely indicated whenever a chordoma has invaded the anterior fossa on the midline in the sphenoethmoid area, when the tumor has caused extradural compression of the optic nerves in the optic canals, or when it extends laterally, toward the pterygoid fossa, around the orbit, destroying and/or invading the lesser and greater sphenoid wings (Fig. 9). In such cases, a bifrontal extradural approach becomes necessary for tumor removal and basal reconstruction. However, chordomas that extend superiorly and anteriorly to the anterior fossa usually also grow posteriorly into the upper half of the clivus, below the sella; in such cases the transbasal approach is not sufficient for tumor removal and must be combined with the transsphenoid approach.

Combined Approaches

It may be necessary to combine two approaches to enlarge exposure to permit the widest resection possible; this is particularly true when a chordoma overlaps one or more boundaries of a single approach. The advantages of a combined subtemporal-suboccipital approach were addressed in the section on intradural approaches. When an extradural approach is planned, it is particularly useful to combine transbasal and transsphenoid approaches during the same surgical procedure[5,6] when a chordoma has invaded the sphenoethmoid area and the anterior

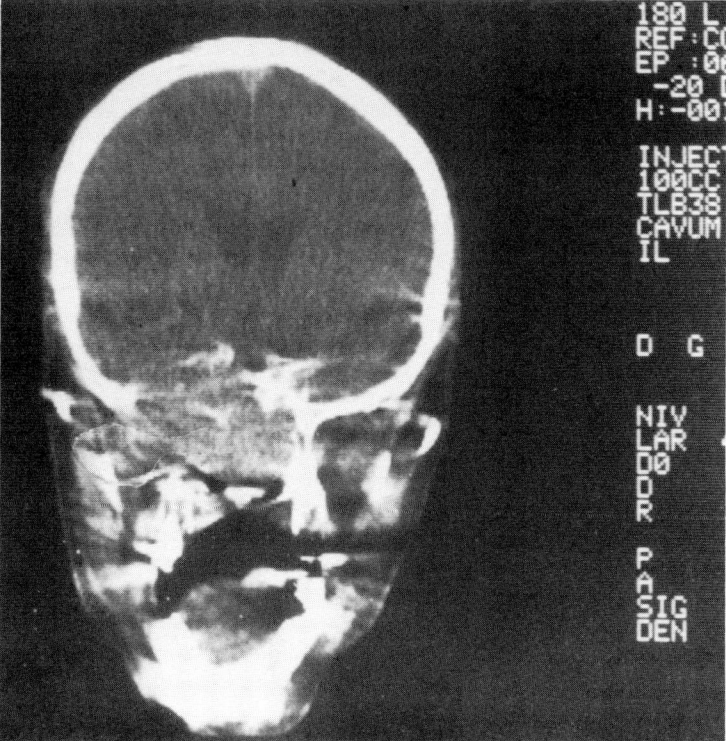

Figure 9: Lateral and medial involvement of the anterior skull base by a chordoma. A bifrontal extradural and transbasal approach was indicated for removal of the lesion.

fossa, and extended posteriorly below the sella, behind the dorsum sellae, and into the clival area. The bifrontal approach is used to remove tumor invading the nasal fossae, the ethmoid, and the sphenoid body through exposure between the optic nerves (Fig. 10). The transbasal approach permits enlargement of the lateral and posterior fields, and removal through a rhinoseptal approach of tumor bulging posteriorly below the sellar dura. Such a combined approach has permitted very extensive removal of particularly invasive chordomas (Fig. 11): two of the three patients in whom this combined approach was used have survived 14 and 11 years after surgery, and the third survived 1 year.

It is very difficult to combine an extradural and an intradural approach in one surgical procedure. However, it may be considered for removal of a chordoma that has grown into the sphenoid sinus or pharyngeal space but has also destroyed dura and invaded the posterior fossa. When the choice of surgical approach is not obvious, it seems advisable to do the extradural resection first, and then, in a second stage, to complete intradural resection followed by careful, complete dural closure and total cicatrization. This reduces the risk of CSF leakage and sub-

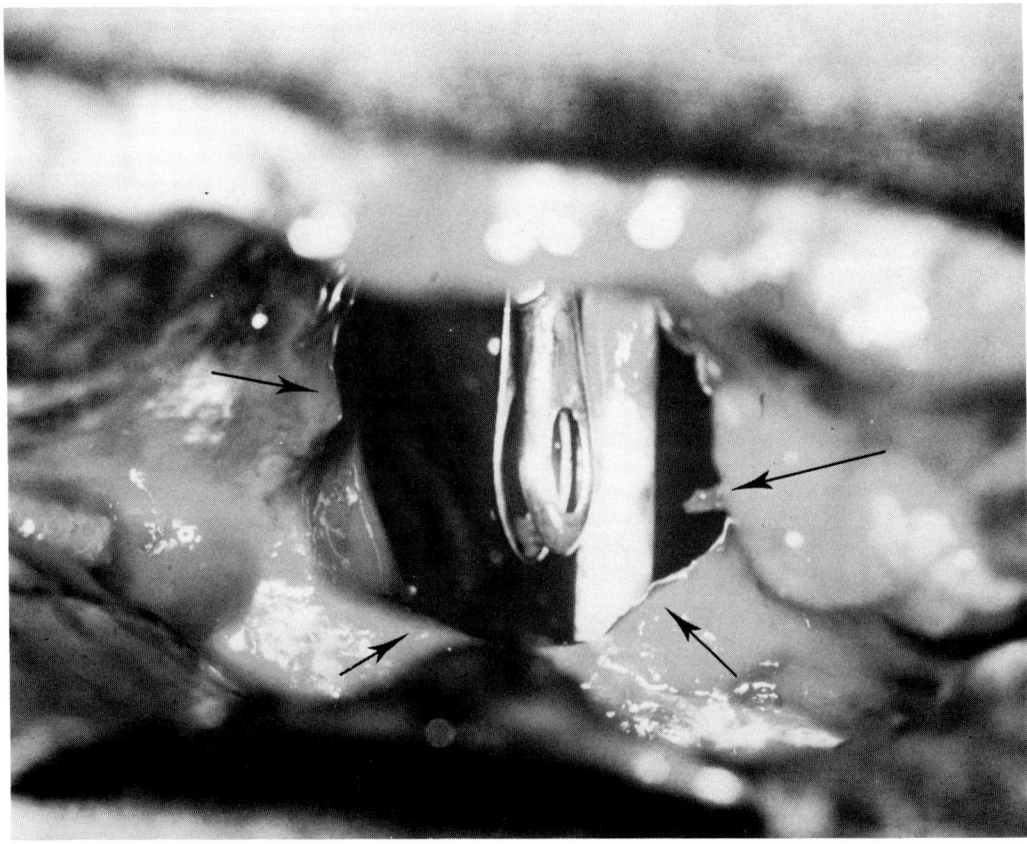

Figure 10: Same patient as in Figure 9, showing combined transbasal and transsphenoid approaches. The medial ethmoidsphenoid portion of the chordoma was removed between the periorbitum and optic nerves (arrows). The instruments introduced through the nasal septum for removal of the subsellar and retrosellar portions of the tumor are visible through the medial defect in the anterior fossa.

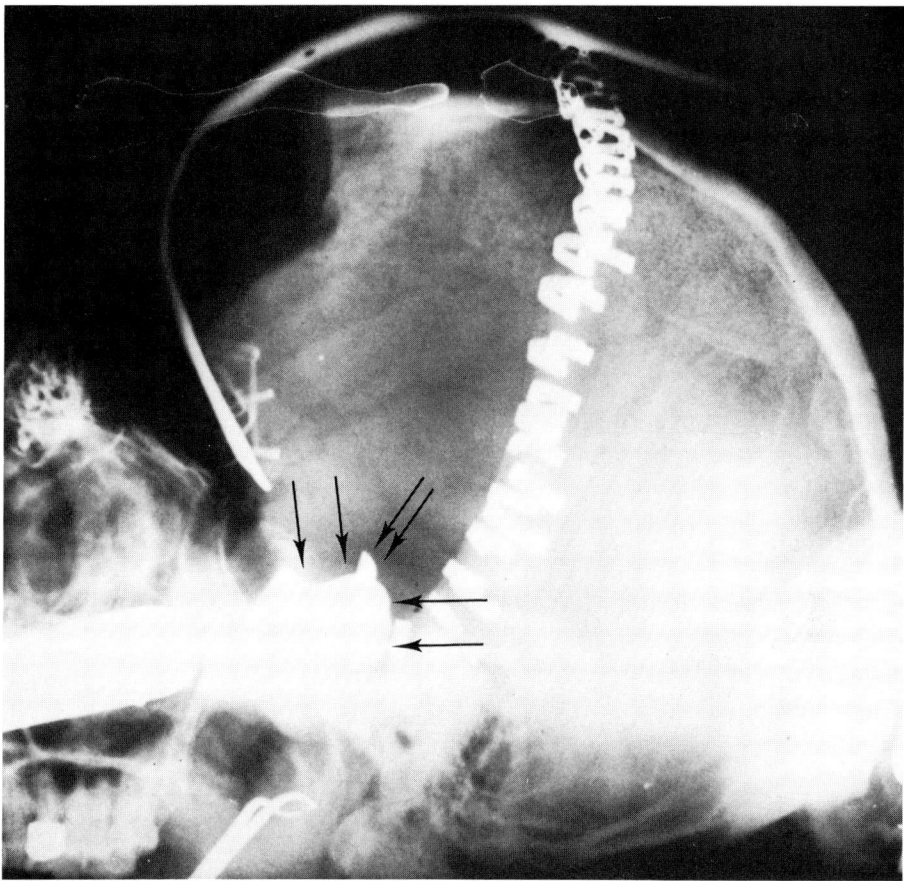

Figure 11: Combined transbasal and transsphenoid approaches. The operative defect was filled with Pantopaque after removal of the sphenoid chordoma. Arrows indicate the sellar dura and the clival dura (double arrows indicate removal of the tumor behind the dorsum sellae).

sequent infection that may occur following extensive procedures in the nasopharyngeal cavities when wide destruction of tissue and a dural defect are present.

Other Approaches

Other otorhinolaryngological approaches have been described in the literature. However, they are less often used than the approaches described in this chapter, and may have been chosen because of the particular skills of the neurosurgeon or the availability of specialists in maxillofacial or otorhinolaryngological surgery. In addition, it is difficult to determine whether these approaches actually improve the extent of tumor removal. When a tumor lies in the midline, a specialized approach may be used to augment extradural exposure; such specialized approaches may include transnasal, transpalatal, lateral rhinotomy, translabiomandibular, or translabioglossomandibular approaches.[2,3,9,10,17] The infratemporal approach,[7,13] used for the removal of glomus tumors or jugular foramen tumors, may also be considered, but we do not believe that this approach significantly improves the extensiveness of chordoma removal, and it carries additional risks of destruction of the conductive hearing apparatus, and of facial paralysis.

General Management

The management of a cranial chordoma begins with surgical resection of as much of the tumor as possible, whenever operative removal is performed. Tables I and II summarize the different approaches used to reach 45 chordomas treated at Hopital Foch between 1955 and 1985: 35 patients underwent one operation, and 10 patients had combined operations (in one or multiple stages) to improve the extent of tumor removal or for recurrences. The frequency of transsphenoidal approaches before 1970 was related to the frequency of biopsies; in 1970 we became more aggressive in our management of cranial chordomas, notably by developing other extradural anterior approaches.

The role of radiotherapy in treatment of cranial chordomas is not clear, as no one knows if this type of embryonal tumor is susceptible to radiation, although the survival rate following postoperative radiotherapy for sacrococcygeal chordomas seems improved.[18] Nevertheless, because most of the patients with cranial chordomas reported on in the literature have undergone radiotherapy,[12,14,15,18,21,26] it is difficult to estimate what percentage would have survived had this therapy not been used. Radiation therapy was used postoperatively for all patients in our series whose tumors were known to be incompletely resected.

The optimal amount of radiation to be administered postoperatively is also controversial. Many authors recommend using high dosages;[12,14,20] our patients usually received between 50 and 60 grays.

For the last 2 years, as a result of advances in surgical techniques and the ease of following patients with CT scanning or MRI, we have modified our protocol slightly: radiation therapy is combined with surgery when the removal of the tumor is obviously incomplete and the extent of resection cannot be improved by any additional surgical approach, but when "total" or near-total resection has been achieved, we do not administer radiation therapy. Should the tumor recur, however, we reoperate and administer radiation therapy after this second procedure.

When more is known about the biological behavior of chordomas, it may be possible to predict the effects of radiation therapy more accurately. However, their biological behavior does not depend upon the pathological findings, although some authors have speculated that the prognosis might be better for "chondroid" chordomas than for classic chordomas.[21,26] We hesitate to adopt this hypothesis, for chordomas in children in particular, because even though such tumors may appear to be, and often are, benign, they may also be very aggressive and thus carry a poor prognosis.

Some authors have recently proposed other types of adjunctive treatment, including heavy-particle beam therapy or chemotherapy.[18,24,28] It will be necessary

Table I
Single Approaches Used to Remove 35 Chordomas

Approach	No. of Patients	
Intradural approaches:		
Subfrontal—pterional	4	
Subtemporal	5	
Suboccipital	3	
		12
Extradural approaches:		
Transsphenoid	15	
Transbasal	3	
Transoral	5	
		23
Total		35

Table II
Combined Approaches Used in Removing 10 Chordomas

Approach	No. of Patients
Transbasal + transsphenoid	3
Transbasal + transoral	1
transsphenoid + transoral	1
transsphenoid + subtemporal	1
transoral + subtemporal	1
Transsphenoid + subtemporal	3
Transoral + subtemporal	1

to review the long-term follow-up results of a large group of patients treated with such radiation before these results can be evaluated fully.

In the Hopital Foch series, 9 of our 45 patients were lost to follow-up. Of the 36 patients followed for 6 months to 15 years, 56% are alive at this time. However, only 30% of these 36 patients have survived for 6 or more years postoperatively, although we have been impressed with the quality of life most of them enjoy, despite the fact that we know many of them are probably not cured.

Quality of life remains one of the most difficult problems in the management of tumors invading the cranial base, particularly chordomas, which continue to grow despite surgical excision and postoperative radiation therapy. Is it reasonable to continue to perform ever more complex operations to remove residual tumor, when often each additional procedure adds new neurological deficits to those already present? Each neurosurgeon must know his or her capabilities in this regard, and base recommendations to the patient and family on this knowledge and on evaluation of the possible results of each proposed procedure. When managing cranial chordomas, deciding when to cease further surgical attempts to remove recurrent tumor is most difficult. Unfortunately, this decision must be made by the physicians involved in each case; no rules can be given.

References

1. Crockard HA, Bradford R: Transoral transclival removal of a schwannoma anterior to the craniocervical junction: Case report. J Neurosurg 62:293-295, 1985.
2. Decker RE, Malis LI: Surgical approaches to midline lesions at the base of the skull. Mt Sinai J Med 37:84-102, 1970.
3. Delgado TE, Garrido E, Harwick RD: Labiomandibular transoral approach to chordomas in the clivus and upper cervical spine. Neurosurgery 8:675-679, 1981.
4. Derome PJ: La voie transbuccopharyngee et al pathologie tumorale du clivus. Neurochir (Paris) 23:298-306, 1977.
5. Derome PJ: The transbasal approach to tumors invading the base of the skull. In Schmidek HH, Sweet WH (ed): Current Techniques in Operative Neurosurgery. New York, Grune & Stratton, 1977, pp 223-245.
6. Derome PJ, Guiot G: Surgical approaches to the sphenoidal and clival areas. Adv Tech Stand Neurosurg 6:101-136, 1979.
7. Fisch U: Infratemporal fossa approach for glomus tumors of the temporal bone. Ann Otorhinolaryngol 91:474-479, 1982.
8. Guiot G, Rougerie J, Bouche J: The rhinoseptal route for removal of clivus chordomas. Johns Hopkins Med J 122:329-335, 1968.
9. Guthkelch AN, Williams RG: Recurrent chordoma of the clivus. Acta Neurol Scand 46:622-630, 1970.
10. Guthkelch AN, Williams RG: Anterior approach to recurrent chordomas of the clivus: Technical note. J Neurosurg 36:670-672, 1972.
11. Hayakawa T, Kamikawa K, Ohnishi T, et al: Prevention of post-operative complications after a transoral transclival approach to basilar aneurysms: Technical note. J Neurosurg 54:699-703, 1981.
12. Higginbotham NL, Phillips RF, Farr HW, et al: Chordoma: Thirty-five year study at Memorial Hospital. Cancer 20:1841-1850, 1967.
13. Jenkins HA, Fisch U: Glomus tumors of the temporal region. Arch Otolaryngol 107:209-214, 1981.
14. Kamrin BP, Potonos JL, Pool JL: An evaluation of the diagnosis and treatment of chordoma. J Neurol Neurosurg Psychiatr 27:157-165, 1964.
15. Krayenbuhl H, Yasargil MG: Cranial chordomas. Prog Neurol Surg 6:380-434, 1975.
16. Litvak J, Summers TC, Barron JL, et al: A successful approach to vertebrobasilar aneurysms: Technical note. J Neurosurg 55:491-494, 1981.
17. Mullan S, Naunton R, Hekmat-Panah J, et al: The use of an anterior approach to ventrally placed tumors in the foramen. J Neurosurg 24:536-543, 1966.
18. O'Neill P, Bell BA, Miller JD, et al: Fifty years experience with chordomas in south-east Scotland. Neurosurgery 16:166-170, 1985.
19. Pasztor E, Vajda J, Piffko P, et al: Transoral surgery for craniocervical space-occupying processes. J Neurosurg 60:276-281, 1984.
20. Pearlman AW, Friedman M: Radical radiation therapy of chordoma. Am J Radiol 108:333-341, 1970.

21. Raffel C, Wright DC, Gutin PH, et al: Cranial chordomas. Clinical presentation and results of operative and radiation therapy in twenty-six patients. Neurosurgery 17:703-710, 1985.
22. Rougerie T, Guiot G, Bouche J, et al: Les voies d'abord des chordomes du clivus. Neurochir (Paris) 13:559-570, 1967.
23. Stevenson GC, Stoney RJ, Perkins RK, et al: A transcervical transclival approach to the ventral surface of the brain stem for removal of a clivus chordoma. J Neurosurg 24:544-551, 1966.
24. Suit HD, Goiten M, Munzenrider J, et al: Definitive radiotherapy for chordoma and chondrosarcoma of base of skull and cervical spine. J Neurosurg 56:377-385, 1982.
25. Trotoux J, Vilde F, Astier P, et al: Chordome de la base du crane. Ann Otolaryngol (Paris) 96:565-582, 1979.
26. Wold LE, Laws ER Jr: Cranial chordomas in children and young adults. J Neurosurg 59:1043-1047, 1983.
27. Yamaura A, Makino H, Isobe K et al: Repair of cerebrospinal fluid fistula following transoral transclival approach to a basilar aneurysm: Technical note. J Neurosurg 50:834-836, 1979.
28. Zoltan L, Fenyes I: Stereotactic diagnosis and radioactive treatment in a case of spheno-occipital chordoma. J Neurosurg 17:888-900, 1960.

32

Petroclival and Medial Tentorial Meningiomas

Laligam N. Sekhar, M.D.
Peter J. Jannetta, M.D.

Introduction

The operative management of petroclival and medial tentorial meningiomas continues to be a difficult problem for neurosurgeons. The total removal of these tumors is often difficult and hazardous because of the critical location in front of the brain stem, their involvement of the cranial nerves, displacement or encasement of the vertebral-basilar arteries and their branches, and the extension of the tumors into multiple anatomical sites, making it difficult to remove them by a single operative approach. Until recently, the surgical excision of these lesions was often accompanied by high operative mortality and morbidity. Several advances have been made in their management, but many problems remain to be solved. The material presented in this chapter is based on the experience gained at the University of Pittsburgh during the removal of 30 petroclival and 15 medial tentorial meningiomas. The majority of the operations were performed by either of the authors between 1973 and 1985.

Clusters of meningothelial cells are found in normal individuals around the venous sinuses of the cranial base, and around the exit sites of the cranial nerves. Even though basal meningiomas may originate primarily in one site, they soon spread to involve adjacent areas. Thus a lesion originating in the petrous ridge may soon extend into the clival region, the tentorial notch, the Meckel's cave, and the cavernous sinus. Classifications are, therefore, artificial and may be spurious. However, they do help the surgeon in planning the operative approaches and in comparing the results of different series. The majority of petroclival and medial tentorial meningiomas have reached a large (2.5–5 cm) or a giant (more than 5 cm) size before becoming symptomatic. This remains true despite the fact that the availability of the CT scanner is facilitating early diagnosis. Presumably, the slow growth of these lesions provides time for the cranial nerves and the brain stem to adapt to the distortions created by the tumor, and symptoms do not appear until adaptation mechanisms are exhausted.

From: Sekhar LN, Schramm VL Jr, eds: *Tumors of the Cranial Base: Diagnosis and Treatment*. Mount Kisco, New York, Futura Publishing Co, Inc, © 1987.

Clinical Signs and Symptoms

The clinical signs and symptoms of the patients in both groups are summarized in Table I. Cerebellar signs and symptoms are equally common in both groups. Cranial nerve signs and symptoms are somewhat more frequent in the petroclival group. Dementia, hemiparesis, and hemisensory loss are more frequent in the medial tentorial meningioma group. In addition, psychomotor seizures and intermittent or persistent coma are also observed occasionally in some of the patients with medial tentorial tumors. Seizures are presumably due to medial temporal lobe compression, and coma presumably results from severe compression of the midbrain or from obstructive hydrocephalus.

Preoperative Studies

Cranial CT scans in the axial and coronal planes are the most useful preoperative studies (Table II). The coronal scans reveal the relationship of the tumor to the tentorium and this is useful in planning operative approaches. In general, in unenhanced CT scans, the tumors are hyperdense in comparison with the brain, and following contrast infusion, the tumors enhance significantly in a homogenous fashion. When the lesion is located in the petroclival area, the following features are useful to distinguish it from acoustic neurinomas: meningiomas have a broader base and may be more oval in shape in contrast to acoustic neurinomas which have a smaller base and are more circular; the porus acusticus is usually flared with acoustic neurinomas and usually not widened with meningiomas; meningiomas enhance uniformly following contrast infusion whereas acoustic neurinomas have varying patterns of contrast enhancement and may also have areas of low density within the lesion indicating cyst formation or necrosis; meningiomas may extend into the tentorial notch, middle fossa, and the cavernous sinus area in a sheet-like

Table I
Symptoms and Signs of Patients with Petroclival and Medial Tentorial Meningiomas

	Petroclival (n = 30)	Tentorial (n = 15)
Dementia	4	5
Psychomotor Seizure	—	5
Coma: Intermittent or Persistent	—	4
Cranial Nerve Problems		
II Visual Loss (Postpapilledemic)	1	1
III Paresis	—	3
IV Paresis	—	3
V Trigeminal Neuralgia	11	3
Numbness	16	7
VI Paresis or Palsy	3	2
VII Hemifacial Spasm	4	1
Paresis or Palsy	10	4
VIII Vertigo, Dysequilibrium	4	3
Tinnitus	8	—
Hearing Loss	18	1
X Paresis	3	1
XII Paresis	2	3
Hemiparesis	3	5
Hemisensory Loss	1	1
Cerebellar Deficit		
Gait Ataxia	17	12
Extremity Ataxia	7	8

Table II
Petroclival Meningiomas:
Computed Tomographic Findings

Size of Lesion	
Small <1 cm	1
Medium 1 to 2.5 cm	2
Large >2.5 cm	27*
Tumor Extension	
Tentorial Notch	9
Clivus	11
Foramen Magnum	1
Relationship to Internal Auditory Canal (IAC)	
Anterior	23
Posterior	7
Bony Changes	
Erosion of Petrous Apex	2
Hyperostosis of Petrous Bone	7
Widening of IAC	1
No Change	21

*Majority of tumors >5 cm in size.

fashion, and this does not occur with acoustic neurinomas.

Cerebral angiography is essential. It demonstrates the relationships of the tumor to the arteries and branches of the vertebrobasilar circulation and to the internal carotid artery when the medial tentorial area is involved. The vascular supply of most of these tumors is derived from the meningohypophyseal branch of the internal carotid artery, and less commonly from the middle meningeal, the occipital, the ascending pharyngeal, and the vertebral-meningeal arteries. The tumors may also receive some blood supply from branches of the vertebrobasilar circulation and the internal carotid circulation. In the evaluation of medial tentorial meningiomas which encase the internal carotid artery in the petrous apex region and extend into the cavernous sinus, when radical removal is planned, we feel that it is essential to perform a balloon occlusion test of the internal carotid artery along with cerebral blood flow measurement during the test occlusion.

Magnetic resonance imaging (MRI) scans have been found to be very useful in demonstrating the relationship of the tumor to the brain as well as to the blood vessels. The flowing blood within arteries creates a black image in the scans and this can help the surgeon to clarify preoperatively whether the arteries are encased or merely displaced by the lesion, and their precise location.

Neurophysiological studies such as audiography, brain stem evoked responses, and electromyographic examinations are performed preoperatively. Such tests are useful when intraoperative monitoring is planned, and for postoperative follow-up.

Preoperative embolization of vascular basal meningiomas has been suggested but has not been used by us for petroclival and medial tentorial meningiomas. Such embolization may be considered if the predominant blood supply of the tumor is from the external carotid circulation, rather than from the internal carotid artery or from the vertebral-meningeal artery.

Anesthesia and Monitoring

A neuroanesthesiologist well versed in the anesthetic management of basal cranial tumors is an essential member of the operative team. Because of the requirements for monitoring of EMG activity from the facial or extraocular muscles during the operation, an inhalational rather than a balanced anesthetic technique is preferred. Short-acting muscle relaxants may be used on induction. Hyperventilation is employed during the operation, and either mannitol or furosemide may be used to achieve further cerebral relaxation. Cerebrospinal fluid drainage is always accomplished by the opening of subarachnoid cisterns during the operation, or by means of a lumbar subarachnoid catheter. Hypotensive anesthesia is avoided, since the combination of hypotension and brain retraction can increase injury to the retracted brain.

Monitoring of the functions of the brain and of the functions of the cranial nerves has been found to very useful to avoid injury to these structures. The brain stem evoked responses (BSER) are generally monitored by placing click electrodes in the opposite ear, since wave V is an indicator of the activity of the contralateral brain stem. Somatosensory evoked responses and central conduction time may also be monitored and combined with the monitoring of BSER. When the eighth cranial nerve is exposed in the operative field and preservation of hearing function is important, it would be helpful to monitor the BSER from the ipsilateral ear and, if possible, also to monitor action potentials recorded by an electrode placed directly on the nerve. Facial nerve activity is monitored by EMG electrodes placed in the facial muscles, with intermittent monopolar stimulation of the nerve. The activity of the third, fourth, and sixth cranial nerves is monitored by electrodes placed adjacent to extraocular muscles, with monopolar stimulation of these nerves when feasible. Monitoring of brain retraction pressure, and of the evoked somatosensory potential from the retracted brain have not become popular due to technical problems.

Operation

General Principles

The surgeon should be familiar with a variety of operative approaches to the tentorial notch, petrous ridge, and the clivus area, and select the best approach, or the best combination of approaches for that particular patient. Often, a portion of the tumor that is difficult to expose by one approach may be easily exposed by another, and such combination of procedures may make the total removal of the tumor an easy matter. After the initial exposure of the tumor with minimal brain retraction, the surface of the tumor is carefully inspected and, if appropriate, monopolar stimulation is performed to identify cranial nerves. Any arteries lying on the surface of the tumor may be dissected at this stage and moved away from the region to be debulked. Then, using either the bipolar cautery and suction-irrigation, or the carbon dioxide laser, the core of the tumor is removed. For vascular meningiomas, we usually use the defocused beam of the CO_2 laser at about 50–60 watts power in the continuous mode. The laser should not be used near cranial nerves or major arteries. The surgeon can usually locate the edge of the dural attachment of the tumor relatively early especially in tentorial lesions, and this can help in understanding the relationships to the cranial nerves and also in getting to the tumor base so as to devascularize the rest of the tumor.

After initial debulking, the tumor is dissected away from cranial nerves, the cerebellum, and the brain stem. This process is continued progressively until the entire lesion is removed. When there is doubt about the thickness of the remaining tumor and the proximity to the cranial nerves or major blood vessels, it is better to avoid the use of the laser and rely on the bipolar cautery. The dural attachments of these tumors may be dealt with by removal of the dura, burning with the bipolar cautery, or with the laser. If there is a bony exostosis, it should be drilled away using a cutting or a diamond drill. After the drilling, the defect in the dura may be covered with a piece of fascia, pericranium, or lyophilised dura. When there is a considerable extradural extension of the tumor, this often has to be removed as a separate operation.

Retromastoid Approach

The retromastoid paracerebellar approach is very good for removing tumor from the petrous ridge region, the intradural jugular foramen area, the foramen magnum region, and the middle and lower clivus area below the trigeminal root. It may be inadequate for the resection of the tumor from the tentorial notch area. In addition, when the brain stem has been deeply indented by the tumor, dissection of the tumor from the midbrain and pons may be difficult from this approach.

Following a vertical retroauricular incision, a craniectomy is performed up to the transverse sinus superiorly, and laterally just beyond the sigmoid sinus, carefully unroofing it. Inferiorly, the craniectomy usually extends to the level of the floor of the posterior fossa. If there is extension through the foramen magnum, the lip of the foramen magnum and the arch of C_1 may have to be removed, taking care not to injure the extradural portion of the vertebral artery in this region. The dura may be opened in a cruciate fashion and sutures placed on the lateral edge to rotate the sigmoid sinus out of the way, to provide a more direct approach to the tumor. After dural opening, the lateral cerebello-medullary cistern is opened to drain the CSF and to relax the cerebellum. The cerebellum should never be retracted more than 2 cm from the lateral wall of the posterior fossa. The remainder of the operation proceeds as detailed above.

The relationship of the seventh and eighth cranial nerves to the tumor during this exposure depends upon whether the lesion arises posterior or anterior to the internal auditory canal, and this can be often determined preoperatively. The ninth and tenth cranial nerves have a variable relationship and may even be invaded by tumor. The trigeminal nerve may be displaced superiorly, posteriorly, anteriorly, or inferiorly, depending upon the location of the tumor. The fourth cranial nerve is almost always dorsolateral to the tumor and may have to be sacrificed if the tumor invades the tentorial edge attaching to the cavernous sinus (Table III). The oculomotor nerve is generally pushed medially and upwards by these tumors but this relationship is more easily apparent through one of the other approaches.

Posterior Subtemporal Approach

The incision for this approach can either be preauricular, extending from the zygomatic arch to the frontal scalp or postauricular as an upward continuation of the incision used for the retromastoid paracerebellar approach. The craniotomy is centered on the base of the mastoid eminence and is performed down to the floor of the middle fossa, with the transverse sinus barely exposed. When the

Table III
Petroclival Meningiomas: Cranial Nerve Relationships

Cranial Nerve	Relation to Tumor	Number
IV	Superior, Lateral	25
	Superior, Anterior	5
V	Superior, Anterior	18
	Anterior	9
	Inferior	1
	Posterior	1
	Invaded	1
VI	Anterior, Inferior	30
VII, VIII	Posterior	20
	Inferior	3
	Superior	1
	Anterior	7
IX, X	Inferior	18
	Anterior	2
	Posterior	2
	Surrounded	1
	Not Closely Related	7

dura is opened, care must be taken not to injure the vein of Labbè. Spinal fluid drainage from a lumbar catheter is often necessary to relax the temporal lobe adequately. After identifying the structures in the region of the medial tentorial notch, the tentorium is divided posterior to the superior petrosal sinus and posterior to the insertion of the trochlear nerve. The trochlear nerve is the only cranial nerve superficial to the tumor by this approach.

In a modification of this approach, it may be combined with the retromastoid approach at the same sitting. When this is done, one may elect to divide the transverse sinus at its junction with the sigmoid sinus, anterior to the drainage of the vein of Labbè. If this is to be considered, a preoperative angiogram is essential to ensure that there is good flow through the opposite transverse sinus and that there is good communication between the two sinuses at the Torcula. The preoperative angiogram will also show the drainage site of the vein of Labbè.

The posterior subtemporal approach provides optimal exposure of the tentorial notch area. However, the morbidity of retracting the posterior temporal lobe is high. The authors generally do not use this approach where it can be avoided.

Anterior Subtemporal Approach

The incision for this approach is similar to that of a pterional craniotomy for anterior circulation aneurysms but extends somewhat posteriorly. When necessary, the incision may be continued downwards over the root of the zygoma and the zygomatic arch may be temporarily divided to provide a more basal approach. After removal of the bone flap and dural opening, the tip of the temporal lobe may be elevated from the floor of the middle fossa if it has been already displaced considerably by the middle fossa extension of the tumor. When this has not occurred, the anterior 4 cm of the inferior temporal gyrus and a portion of the middle temporal gyrus are removed. The medial temporal lobe structures (the uncus and the hippocampus) are carefully preserved. This provides the surgeon with excellent exposure of the tentorial notch and the cavernous sinus area without any need for temporal lobe retraction and without any of the postoperative problems associated with it. The authors prefer this approach to the posterior subtemporal because of the low morbidity associated with it. Dissection of the tumor from the midbrain, pons, and the major arteries in the upper and middle clival region is easier with this approach. It may also be combined with the infratemporal fossa approach detailed below.

Trans-Sylvian Approach

The craniotomy for this approach is similar to that of the anterior subtemporal approach. The pterion and the lateral wall of the orbit are removed to the lateral edge of the superior orbital fissure. The Sylvian fissure is then opened widely from a lateral to a medial direction. The internal carotid, anterior cerebral, and the middle cerebral arteries are coated thoroughly with papaverine to relax any spasm. After coagulating and dividing the bridging veins of the medial temporal lobe, the medial temporal lobe is retracted laterally. The surgeon approaches the tumor inferolateral to the internal carotid and medial to the temporal lobe. Although the exposure of the upper clivus area and the anterior tentorial notch region is adequate with this approach, the space available to work within is very small. In addition, there is also a greater risk of injuring the internal carotid artery or the middle cerebral artery when the surgeon is concentrating on tumor resection at a depth and these vessels are out of the focal plane of the surgical microscope.

Infratemporal Fossa Approach

The details of the preauricular infratemporal fossa approach are discussed in another chapter. This approach is used primarily for extradural clival lesions. However, it may also be used on occasion for the removal of the intradural clival lesions. The exposure of the petrous internal carotid artery may be important when it is encased by tumor. Following a preauricular incision, and the displacement or resection of the mandibular condyle, the petrous internal carotid artery is unroofed in the carotid canal, and is mobilized forward after displacing it out of the carotid canal or after dissecting it free of tumor. The region of the petrous apex and the lateral clivus is then drilled away using a high-speed drill with a cutting or diamond bit, being careful not to injure the cochlea and the facial nerve which lie posterosuperior and slightly lateral to the genu of the petrous carotid artery. Once the dura has been exposed, the superior petrosal sinus is found running horizontally in the middle of the field to enter the cavernous sinus and is divided. However, this sinus may have been already occluded by tumor invasion. After opening the dura, tumor can thus be removed from the region of the tentorial notch and from the clivus below the trigeminal nerve. The sixth cranial nerve and the midbasilar artery along with its branches and the pons are readily exposed by this approach. At the conclusion of the tumor resection, the defect in the dura is covered by a fascial graft and a portion of the temporalis muscle may be rotated to cover the defect. Alternatively, a free rectus abdominis flap may be placed to fill the dead space and to prevent the possibility of CSF leakage through the sphenoid sinus or through the wound. If such a leak occurs, it is easily managed by placing a lumbar subarachnoid drain for a few days.

Illustrative Cases

Patient #1: Medial Tentorial Meningioma

This 66-year-old man presented with progressive ataxia and dementia for 6 months. Axial and coronal CT scans revealed a very large medial tentorial meningioma extending into the region of the petrous ridge and the cavernous sinus (Figs. 1A–C and 2A, B). Cerebral angiography showed that the tumor was fed predominantly by the meningohypophyseal branch of the internal carotid artery and that it was displacing the posterior cerebral, the superior cerebellar, and the basilar arteries. The operation combined the posterior subtemporal and retromastoid approaches (Figs. 3 and 4). The tumor was completely resected, except for the portion within the cavernous sinus. the cavernous sinus was not entered because he had no extraocular muscle palsies. The trochlear nerve coursed through the tumor and was resected. The superior cerebellar artery entered the tumor and had to be dissected a fair amount in order to preserve it. The trigeminal nerve was displaced downwards below the level of the seventh and eighth cranial nerves. The seventh and eighth nerves were displaced posteriorly and inferiorly. Postoperatively, the patient exhibited transient right facial palsy and left hemiparesis, both of which resolved subsequently. In follow-up 2 years later, he was ambulatory and his dementia had improved.

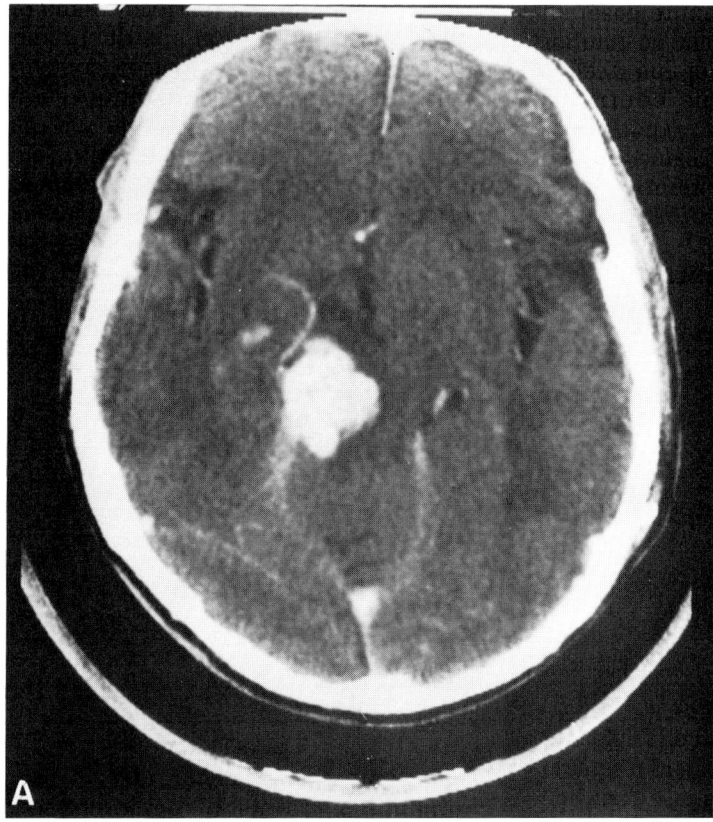

Figure 1 A-C: Axial CT scans on patient no. 1 illustrating tumor high up in the tentorial notch area with extension to the petroclival region with significant compression of the midbrain and pons, and with slight extension into the cavernous sinus.

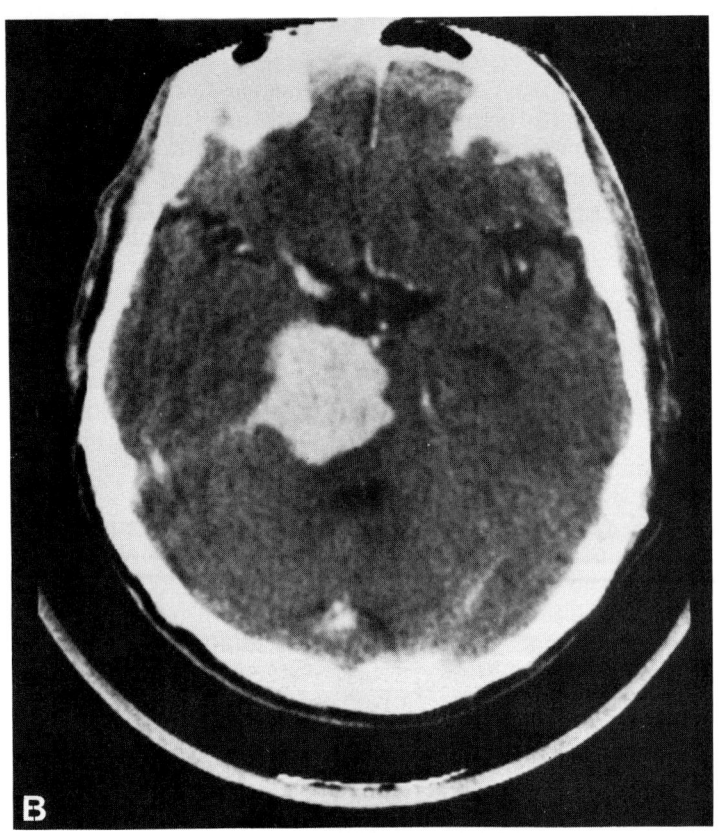

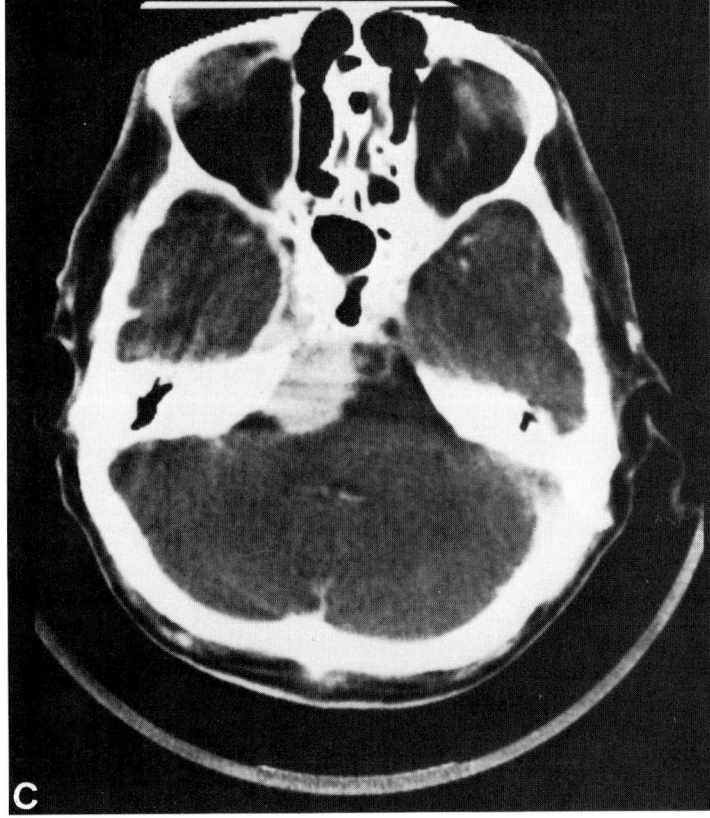

Figure 1C.

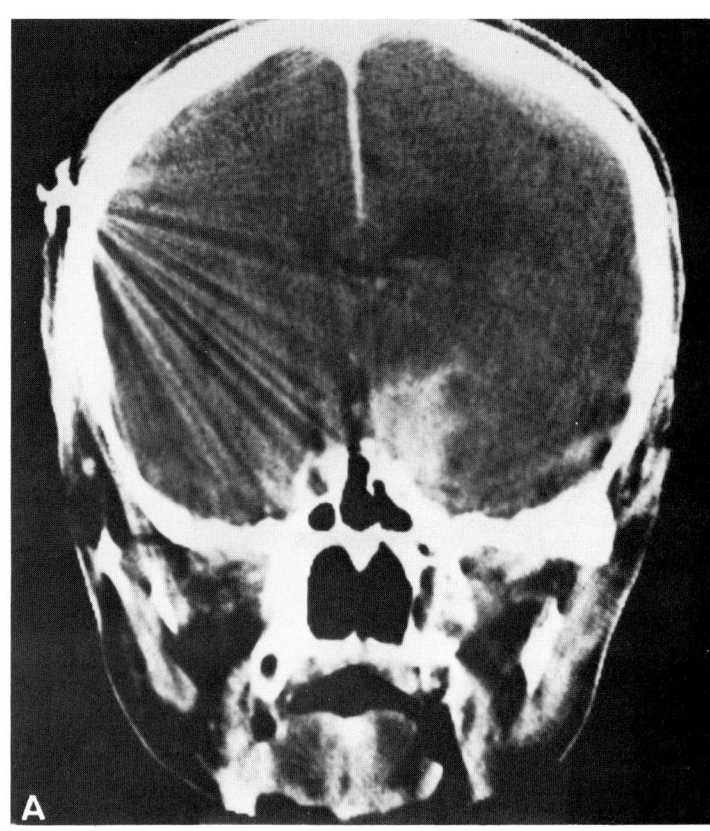

Figure 2A, B: Coronal CAT scans on patient no. 1 illustrate the extension of the tumor both above and below the tentorium.

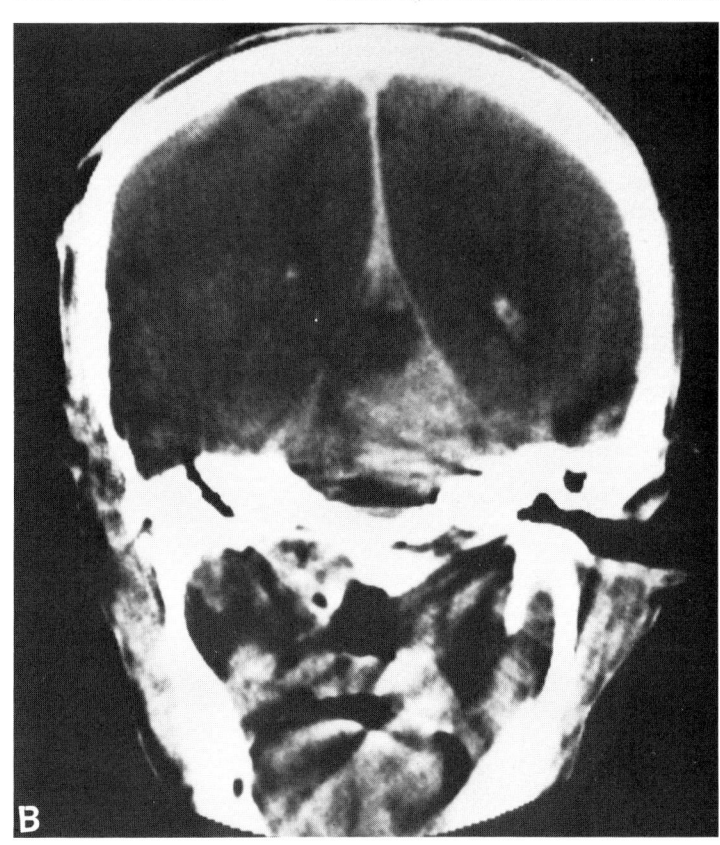

Figure 2B.

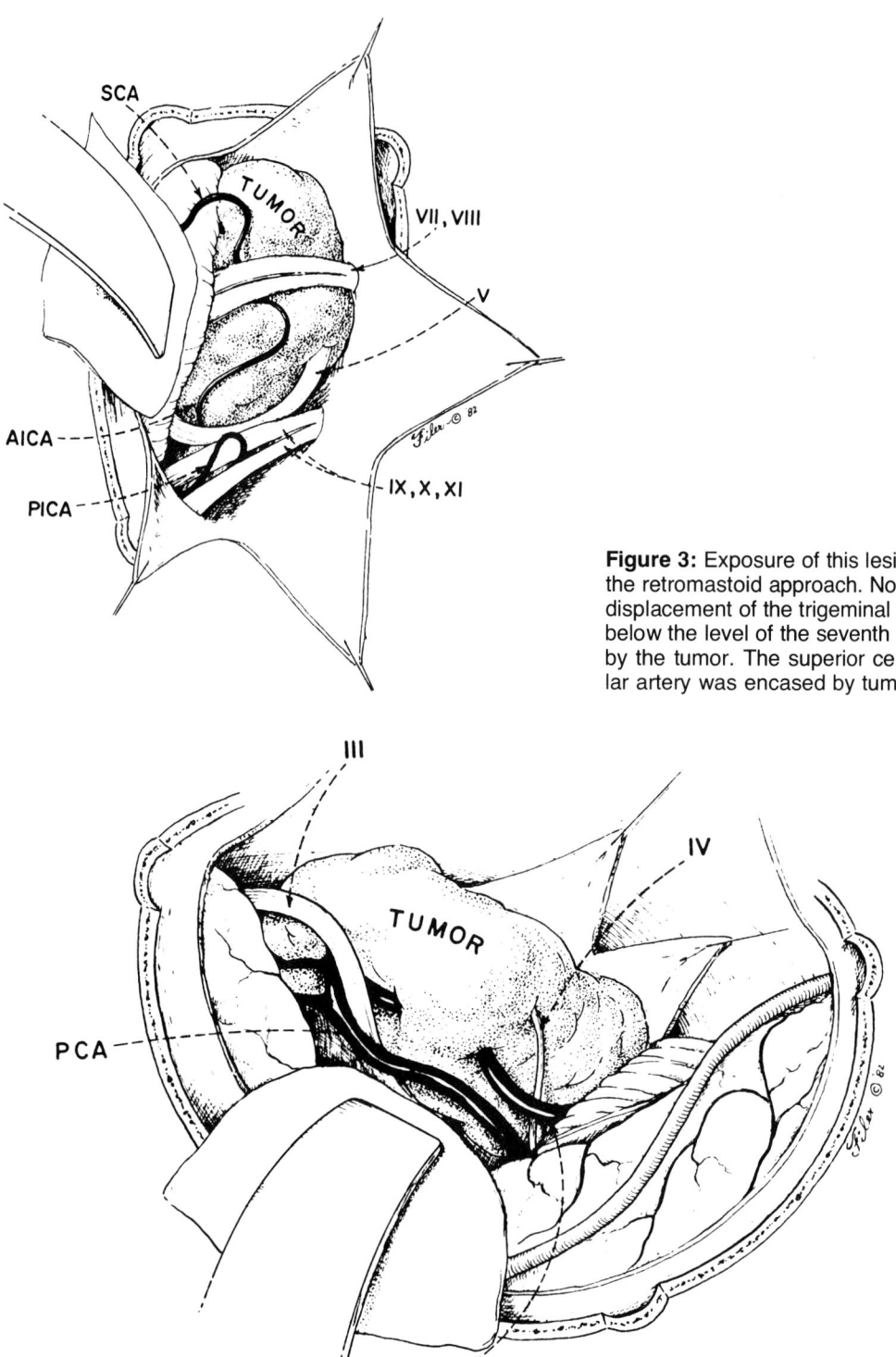

Figure 3: Exposure of this lesion by the retromastoid approach. Note the displacement of the trigeminal nerve below the level of the seventh nerve by the tumor. The superior cerebellar artery was encased by tumor.

Figure 4: Exposure of the same tumor by a simultaneous posterior subtemporal approach. The fourth nerve was running into the tumor and was sacrificed. The superior cerebellar artery is encased by tumor. All of the tumor with the exception of the portion within the cavernous sinus was resected.

Patient #2: Petroclival Meningioma Anterior to Internal Auditory Canal

This 36-year-old woman presented with a pseudobulbar syndrome and a mild right hemiparesis which had become progressively worse during the past 2 years. Preoperatively, she had good seventh and eighth cranial nerve function. CT scans revealed a large petroclival and medial tentorial meningioma about 5 cm in maximal diameter (Fig. 5). The lesion was exposed by a retromastoid paracerebellar approach. It lay in front of the seventh and eighth nerves, and the trigeminal nerve was displaced below the level of the seventh nerve by the tumor (Figs. 6 and 7). After considerable debulking and dissection, the third cranial nerve was identified high up in the tentorial notch, superior and medial to the tumor (Fig. 8). Monitoring the electromyographic activity of the extraocular muscles innervated by the third nerve and direct monitoring of cochlear nerve action potentials were very useful to prevent injury to these nerves during the tumor resection. The tumor was thought to be totally removed and postoperative scans have not shown any residual tumor 1 year after the operation. She is neurologically normal on follow-up examination.

Patient #3: Petrous Ridge, Tentorial Notch, and Foramen Magnum Meningioma

This 48-year-old man had undergone partial resection of a posterior fossa

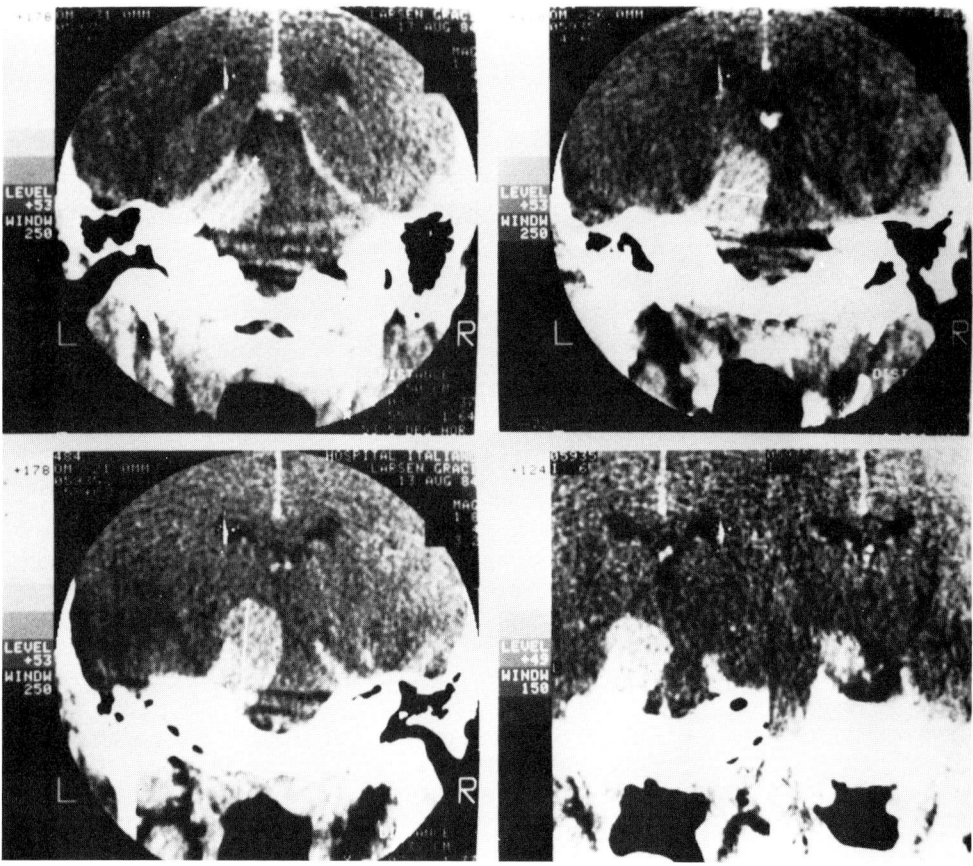

Figure 5: Coronal CAT scans of patient no. 2 illustrating the location of a petroclival meningioma predominantly below the tentorium but with also an extension into the tentorial notch area.

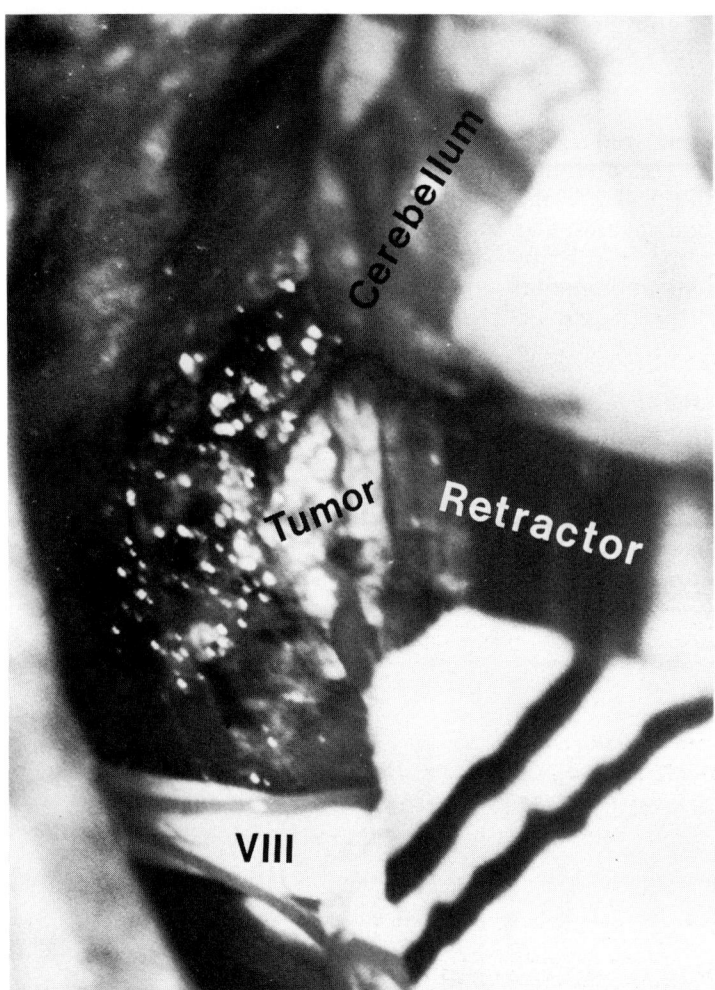

Figure 6: Patient No. 2 Initial exposure by the retromastoid approach. Note the eighth and the seventh nerve superficial and slightly caudal to the tumor and the tumor itself.

meningioma elsewhere 2 years ago and was referred to us because of recurrence from residual tumor. His only symptom was intractable headache, and he had no neurological deficits. Preoperative studies revealed that the tumor involved the left sigmoid sinus and extended through the foramen magnum (Figs. 9, 10A, B, and 11). The lesion was completely removed in two stages. During the first stage, the main bulk of the tumor was removed from the posterior fossa by a retromastoid approach. The posterior inferior cerebellar artery was surrounded by tumor and was dissected entirely free of it. The fascicles of the ninth nerve were encased by tumor and were resected. The seventh and eighth nerves were markedly stretched anterior to the tumor as was the trigeminal nerve, and these were carefully preserved. During the second stage, the sigmoid sinus and the jugular bulb were exposed by drilling away the temporal bone. Tumor was removed from within the sigmoid sinus and the jugular bulb after opening them. The dural origin of the neoplasm was also totally resected. The postoperative course was uneventful. In view of the rapid regrowth following the prior operation, the patient was given

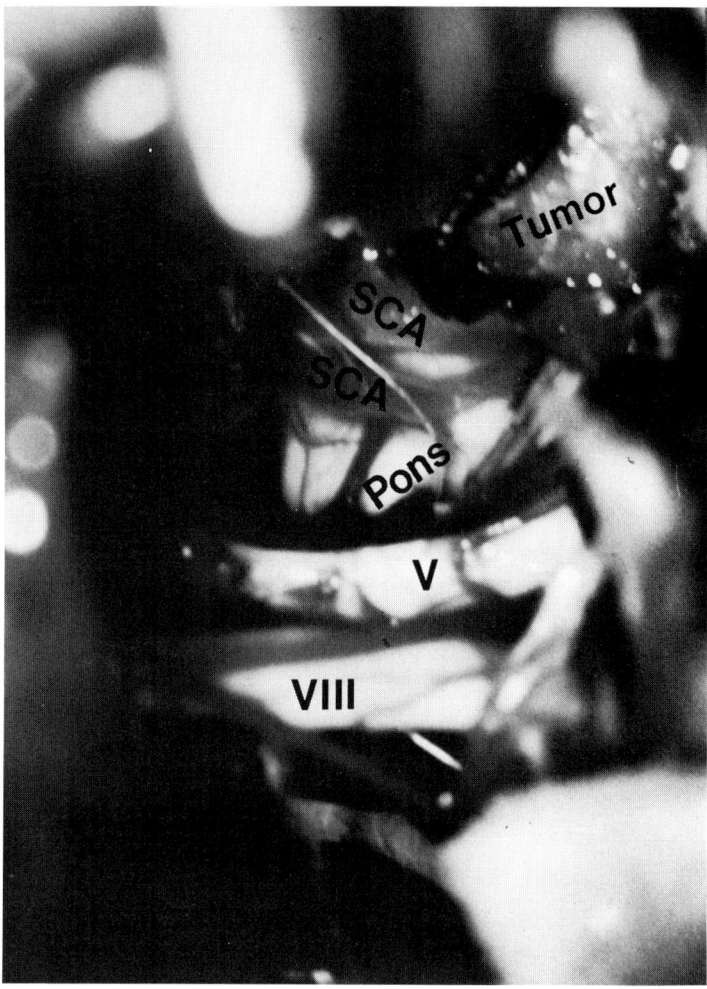

Figure 7: Patient No. 2 After considerable debulking and dissection of the tumor, the trigeminal nerve was seen which had been pushed down below the level of the seventh and eighth nerves by the tumor. The pons and two branches of the superior cerebellar artery lying on it are also seen.

radiation therapy even though the tumor was histologically benign. Two years postoperatively, he remains free of tumor recurrence and is asymptomatic.

Patient #4: Petrous Ridge Meningioma from the Internal Auditory Canal

This 70-year-old woman presented with a one year history of facial paralysis and hearing loss. She was thought to have an acoustic neuroma on the basis of her preoperative studies (Figs. 12A, B). At operation, however, the lesion proved to be a petrous ridge meningioma arising from within the internal auditory canal, invading the seventh and eighth nerves in the internal auditory canal. The tumor was removed completely. The facial nerve was divided just proximal to the area of tumor invasion. A sural nerve graft was

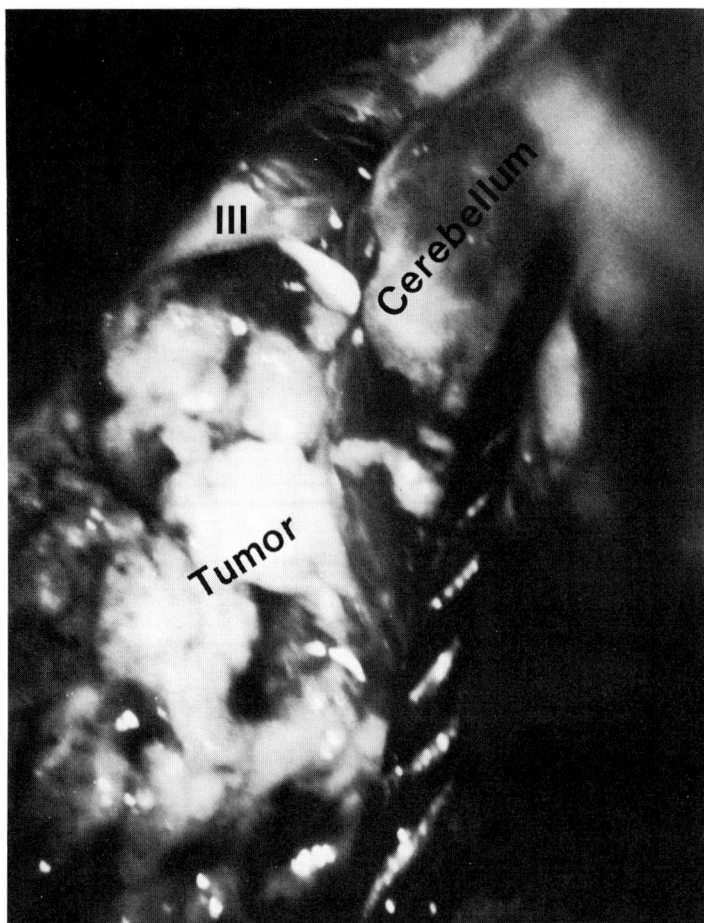

Figure 8: Delivery of the tumor from the tentorial notch area. Note the tumor and the oculomotor nerve displaced way up cranially and medially by the tumor.

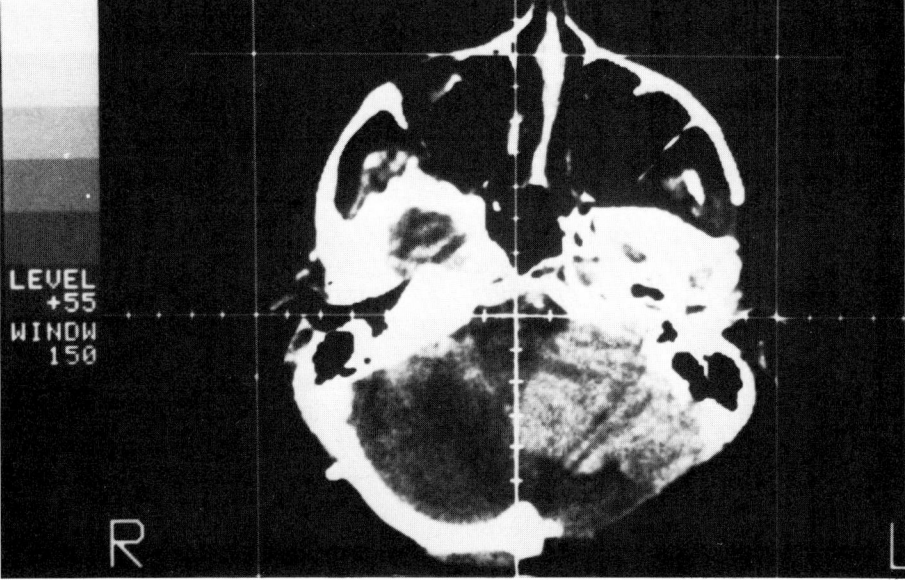

Figure 9: A large meningioma arising from the dura of the petrous bone is illustrated in the axial CT scan of patient no. 3.

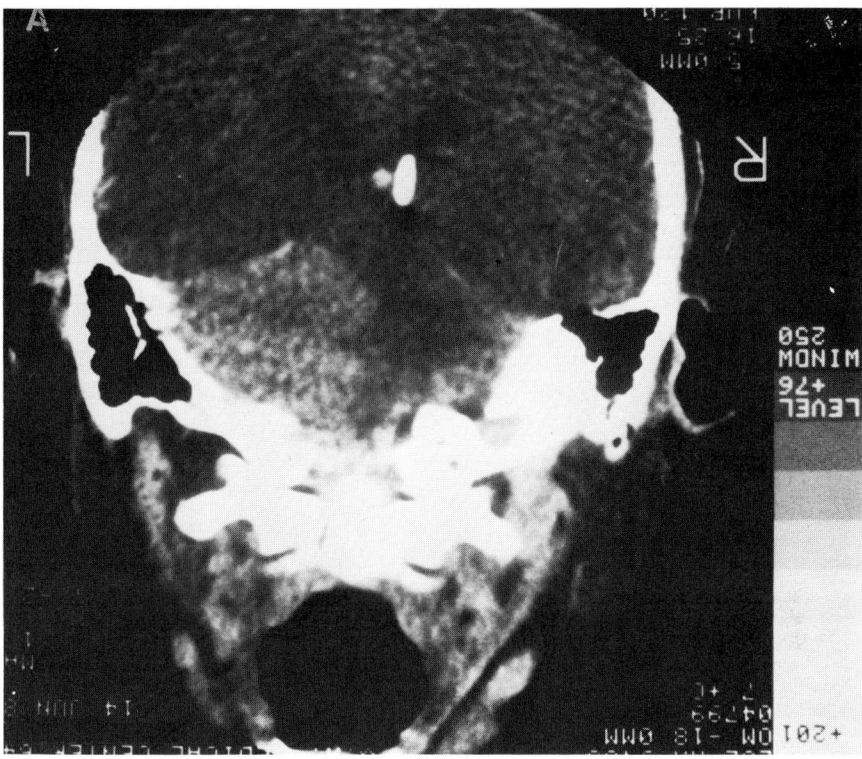

Figure 10A, B: These figures illustrate the extension of the tumor to the tentorium cranially, to the midline medially, and through the foramen magnum area caudally.

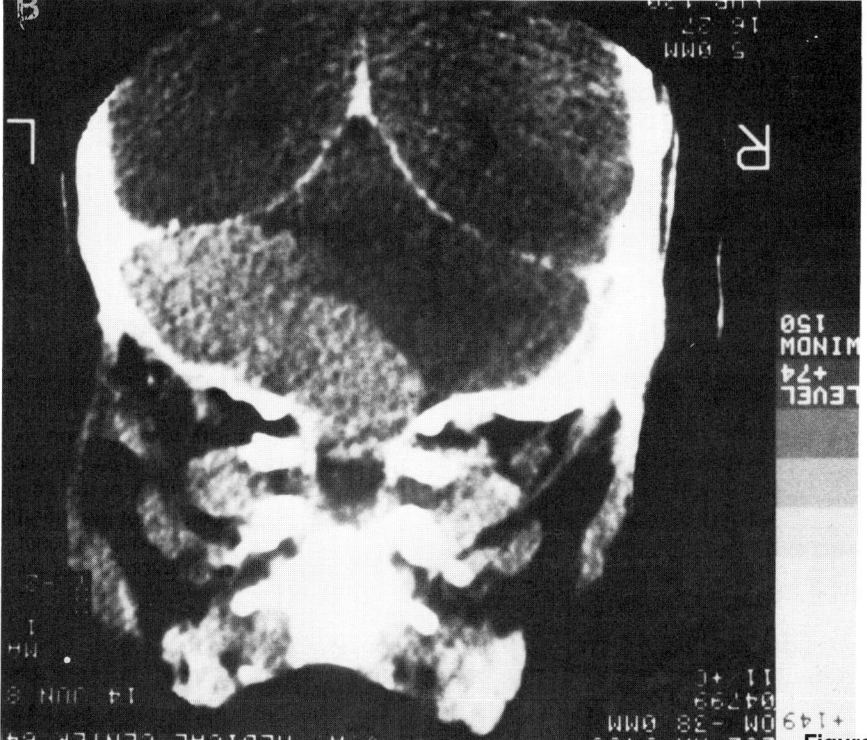

Figure 10B.

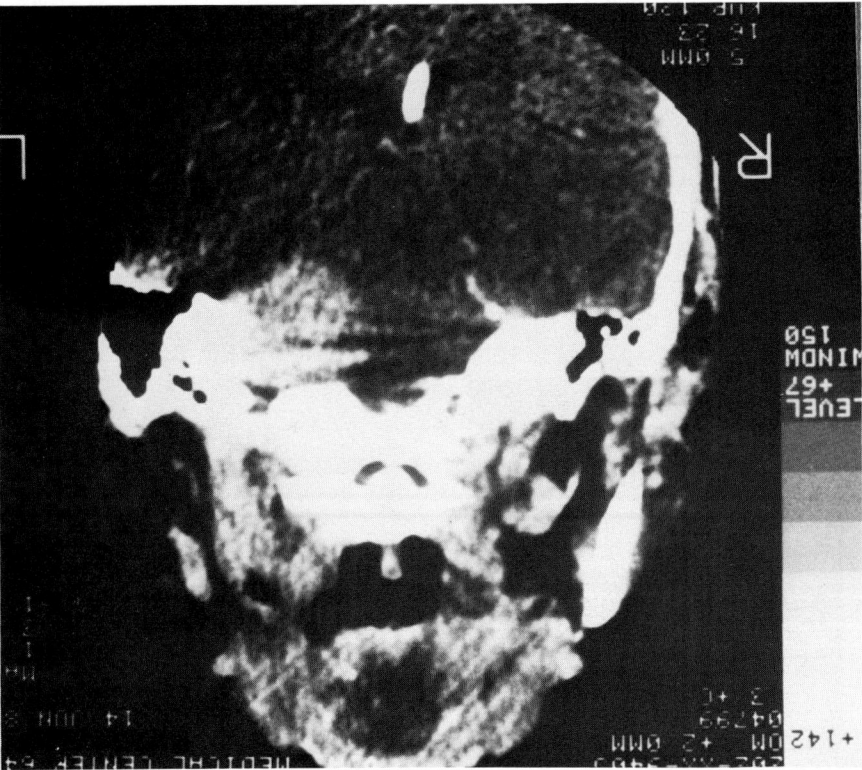

Figure 11: This coronal CAT scan illustrates the extension of the tumor into the temporal bone in the jugular bulb area.

placed from the proximal facial nerve stump to the distal aspect of the facial nerve at the stylomastoid foramen. The postoperative course was uneventful. She remains tumor-free 6 months postoperatively. It is too early to comment about recovery of facial function.

Operative Results

The results of the operative excision of 30 petroclival and 15 medial tentorial meningiomas at the University of Pittsburgh are summarized in Tables IV and V. There was no operative mortality in either group. With increasing experience, it has become progressively easier to remove the tumors completely with minimal or no morbidity.

Problems to be Solved

The invasion of the cavernous sinus by these tumors, involvement of the temporal bone, and of the petrous carotid artery were limitations for radical tumor resection in the past. However, with improvements in surgical techniques, these problems are being resolved.[4,5] Preservation and/or reconstruction of cranial nerves, and the avoidance of occasional major morbidity or mortality remains a continuing challenge. When the patient is elderly, or when there is encasement by tumor of the basilar artery, the surgeon may choose to leave some residual tumor behind. In these cases, a decision must be made regarding postoperative radiation therapy. Several reports suggest that such radiation therapy may be of value in preventing further regrowth of residual tumor.[1,6]

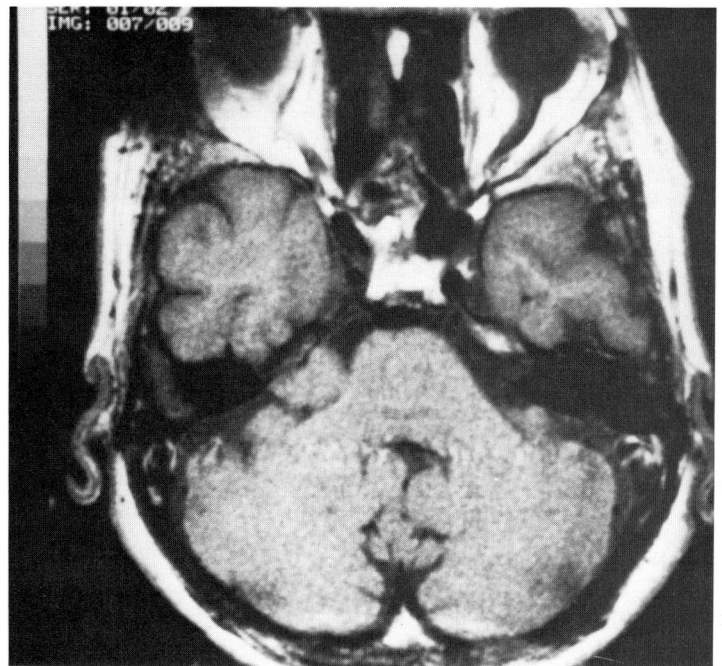

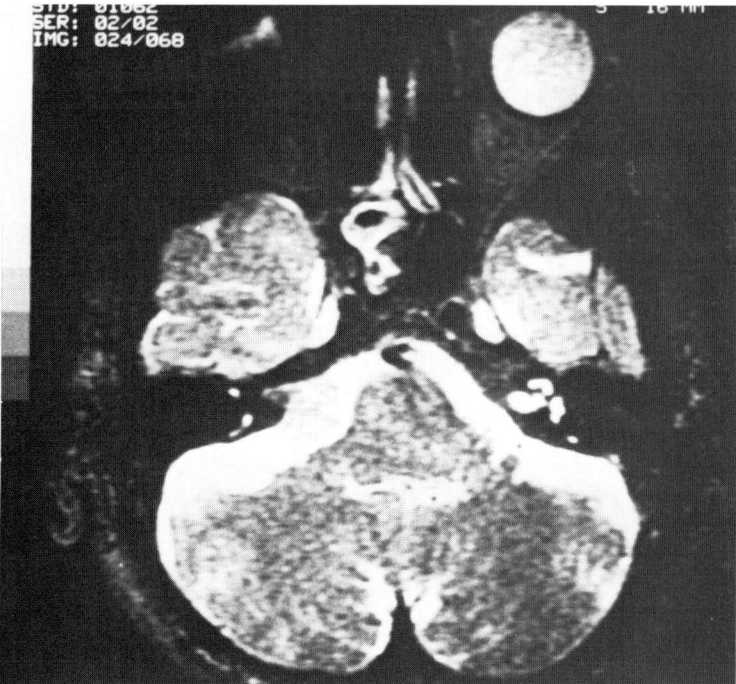

Figure 12 A, B: T_1 weighted (A) and T_2 weighted (B) magnetic resonance images of patient no. 4. The appearance is typical of an acoustic neurinoma with the widening of the porus acusticus, and the globular shaped lesion. At operation, the tumor was found to be a meningioma which had arisen within the porus acusticus and had invaded the seventh and eighth cranial nerves.

Table IV
Petroclival Meningiomas:
Operative Results and Complications

Postoperative Results Operative Approach	Total Cases	Outcome			
		Good	Fair	Poor	Dead
Retromastoid Paracerebellar					
Total Removal	19	18	1	0	0
Subtotal Removal	8	5	3	0	0
Posterior Subtemporal					
Total Removal	2	1	1	0	0
Subtotal Removal	1	0	1	0	0
Complications					
Death	None				
Pneumonia	1				
CSF Leakage	1				
Cranial Nerve Deficits					
IV Permanent	1				
V Permanent	1				
Temporary	7				
VII Permanent	2				
Temporary	4				
VIII Permanent	2				
IX,X Temporary	2				
Follow Up and Recurrence Rates					
Factor	Complete Excision		Subtotal Excision		
Follow-Up (years)					
Mean	5		5		
Range	1–11		1–8		
Recurrence or Regrowth	1 (small)		1		
Reoperation	0		1		

Table V
Medial Tentorial Meningiomas:
Operative Results and Complications
(n = 15)

Operations	Number
Cerebrospinal Shunt Only	2
Retromastoid Approach	
Total Excision	1
Subtotal Excision	3
Retromastoid-Subtemporal	
(Posterior)	2
Subtemporal	
Total Excision	5
Subtotal Excision	—
Frontotemporal Sylvian	1
Infratemporal Fossa	
(With Subtemporal)	1
Complications	
Death	None
Permanent Hemiparesis	2
Cranial Nerve Deficits	5

References

1. Petty AM, Kun LE, Meyer GA: Radiation therapy for incompletely resected meningiomas. *J Neurosurg* 62:502-507, 1985.
2. Sekhar LN, Jannetta PJ: Cerebellopontine angle meningiomas: Microsurgical excision and follow up results. *J Neurosurg* 60:500-505, 1984.
3. Sekhar LN, Jannetta PJ, Maroon JC: Tentorial meningiomas: Surgical management and results. *Neurosurgery* 14:268-275, 1984.
4. Sekhar LN, Moller A: Operative management of tumors involving the cavernous sinus. *J Neurosurg* 64:879-889, 1986.
5. Sekhar LN, Schramm VL, Jones NF: Combined excision of large lateral and posterior cranial base neoplasms. In Sekhar LN, Schramm VL (eds): *Tumors of the Cranial Base: Diagnosis and Treatment*, Mount Kisco, NY, Futura Publishing Co., 1987.
6. Wara WM, Sheline GE, Newman H, et al: Radiation therapy of meningiomas. *AJR* 123:453-458, 1975.

33

Paragangliomas ("Glomus Tumors") of the Temporal Bone

Donald B. Kamerer, M.D.
Barry E. Hirsch, M.D.

History

Identification of paragangliomas was reported in the German literature over 200 years ago. The carotid body received most of the attention until 1941, when Guild first described the "glomus jugularis."[13] Four years later, Rosenwasser[24] removed a middle ear tumor that histologically resembled the carotid body, but was considered to be a glomus jugularis. These paraganglionic formations were anatomically defined by Guild in 1953.[12] In 88 temporal bones obtained from asymptomatic patients, he identified 248 formations. Most were located in the adventitia of the dome of the jugular bulb. Others were found in the submucosa of the cochlear promontory within the tympanic plexus. The afferent (sensory) nerves innervating these areas are branches of Jacobson's nerve (glossopharyngeal) and Arnold's nerve (vagus). These structures are histologically similar to the carotid body, a receptor organ responsive to changes in pH, PO_2, temperature, and certain drugs such as cyanides, sulfides, and nicotine.[28] They were therefore termed chemodectomas. However, chemoreceptor activity of these formations has yet to be verified.

Terminology

Paragangliomas, carotid body tumors, and pheochromocytomas have similar features on light and electron microscopy. However, when prepared with dichromate salts, pheochromocytomas routinely and readily pick up this stain, whereas paragangliomas and carotid body tumors are usually weakly reactive, thus, the name nonchromaffin paraganglioma. This term was ascribed by Watzka in 1943.[33]

Subsequent to the identification of glomus jugulare tumors, the nomenclature was further confused when additional authors coined terms based upon the histologic appearance and presumed functional activity. Phrases such as chemodectoma, glomus jugularis tumors,[34] nonchromaffin paragangliomas,[19] receptoma,[9] glomerocytoma,[35] tympanic

From: Sekhar LN, Schramm VL Jr, eds: *Tumors of the Cranial Base: Diagnosis and Treatment.* Mount Kisco, New York, Futura Publishing Co, Inc © 1987.

body tumors,[20] and chemoreceptoma[22] have all been popularized in the literature.

Clarification and classification of lesions arising from the paraganglionic nervous system was provided by Glenner and Grimley in 1974.[11] These formations are minute macroscopic collections of cells that are distributed along the para-axial region of the trunk in close association with the ganglia of the autonomic nervous system. Paraganglions in the head and neck approximate the arterial vasculature and cranial nerves of the branchial arches. Formations found in this area are termed branchiomeric paraganglions. Included in this category are the jugulo-tympanic, intercarotid, subclavian, laryngeal, coronary, aortico-pulmonary, and pulmonary. Orbital and sinonasal locations would also be included with these areas. As intravagal paragangliomas are not associated with a specific branchial arterial vessel, they are considered a separate group. However, branchiomeric and intravagal formations cannot be distinguished microscopically or cytochemically. The remaining groups of the paraganglionic system are the aortico-sympathetic, visceral autonomic and the adrenal gland itself.

Like the adrenal gland, paraganglia have their embryologic origin from the neural crest, i.e., neuroectoderm. Histologic examination of these formations shows a central compact nest of epitheloid cells called the Zellballen pattern (Fig. 1). These are comprised of type I or chief cells, which contain dense cored granules that store catecholamines, particularly norepinephrine. The stromal tissue and rich blood supply has its origin from the mesoderm. The supporting framework is provided by type II cells, or sustentacular satellite cells. These cells compartmentalize the tumor cells into Zellballen. The vascularity is extensive both surrounding and infiltrating the cellular matrix.

Methods other than dichromate stain-

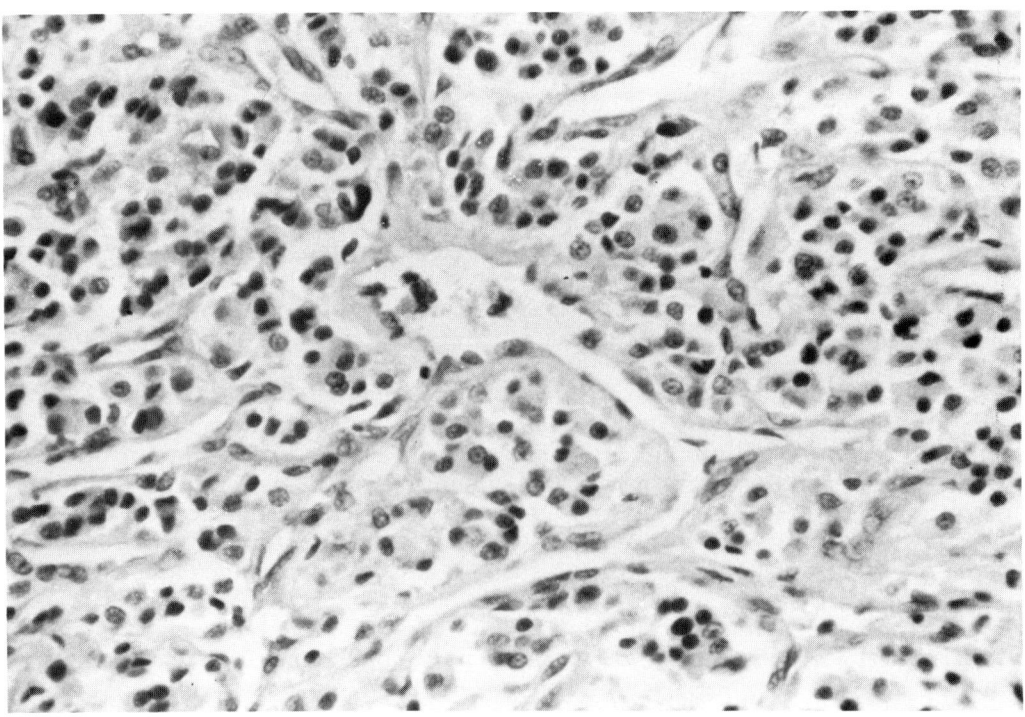

Figure 1: Typical appearance of paraganglioma demonstrating nests of epithelioid cells and "Zellballen" pattern.

ing are available for more accurate catecholamine assays. Fixation of paraganglioma specimens with hot formaldehyde vapors can emit a blue-green fluorescence using ultraviolet excitation. A more recent technique using neuron-specific enolase (NSE), a glycolytic enzyme, has demonstrated the presence of other neuropeptide hormones in most, if not all, of these tumors.[32]

Proper anatomic and histologic classification should incorporate the term paraganglioma. A glomus body is actually a normal structure located at end arterioles, comprised of endomyoepithelial cells and is responsible for regulating local capillary blood flow. In fact, a true glomus tumor is an arteriovenous malformation that is a benign hamartoma or hyperplasia of the normal structure.[14] However, the term glomus tumor has persisted in the literature and is often used interchangeably with paragangliomas.

Signs and Symptoms

Patients with paraganglioma of the temporal region and skull base can present with a myriad of otologic and neurologic signs and symptoms depending on the size and extent of the lesion. Isolated tympanic paragangliomas are limited to the middle ear and sinus tympani, originating from the cochlear promontory and hypotympanum. Patients usually complain of pulsatile tinnitus and hearing loss. Microscopic examination of the intact tympanic membrane would reveal a reddish-blue pulsatile mass within the middle ear (Fig. 2). Pneumatic otoscopy with compression of the lesion produces a diminution of pulsation and blanching of the erythematous mass (Brown's sign). Tuning fork and audiologic evaluation may reveal a conductive hearing loss. As the lesion expands, the mastoid and facial nerve become in-

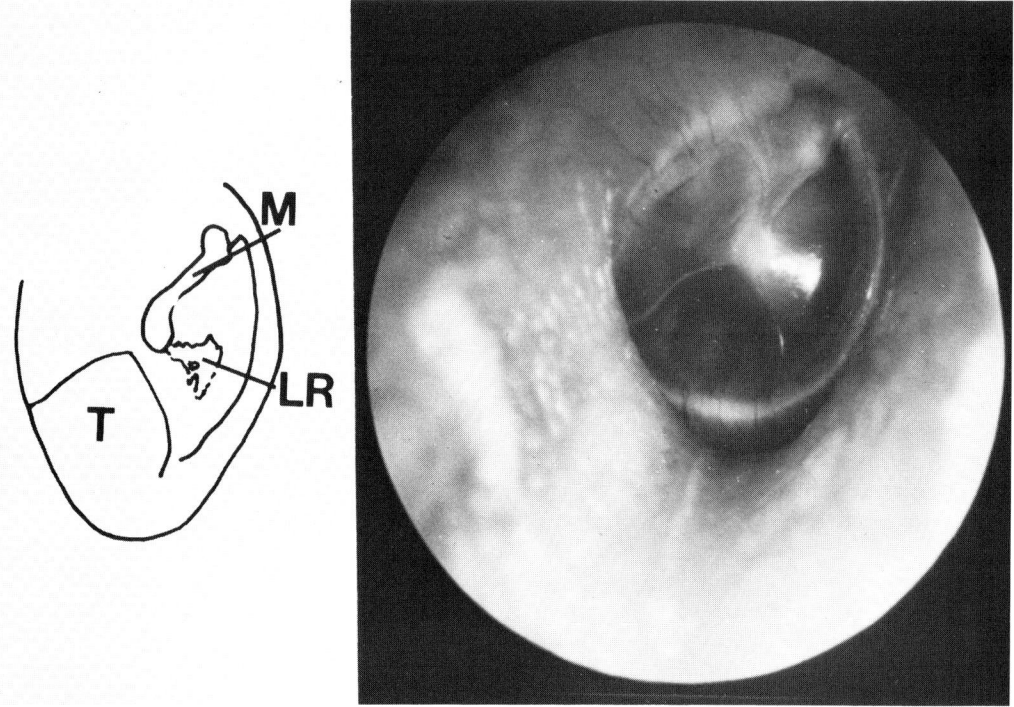

Figure 2: Otoscopic view of tympanic membrane revealing intratympanic paraganglioma. M = malleus handle, LR = light reflex, T = tumor.

volved with a subsequent facial paresis or paralysis. Infiltration in and through the tympanic membrane would give rise to an aural polyp and a sanguinous discharge, especially if manipulated.

Tumor expansion with erosion of the hypotympanum encroaches on the jugular fossa and dome of the jugular bulb. When lesions approach this extent and location, differentiation of a tympanic from a jugular paraganglioma becomes difficult. The clinical relevance of this distinction is minimal because management depends on the location of the lesion and the patient's status rather than the tumor's origin.

Numerous studies have shown the higher incidence of jugular paraganglioma in women. In a review of 231 cases, Brown found that these lesions were six times more common in women than in men.[2] The usual patient presents in the sixth decade of life. Jackson reported that 87% of patients with tympanic, jugular, and vagal paragangliomas were females, with ages ranging from 13 to 76 years.[16] In a recent series of our patients with paraganglioma, 82% were female, typically in the sixth decade of life.

Lesions of the temporal region and skull base place numerous vital structures at risk. Cranial nerve involvement of the jugular fossa entails compromise of the glossopharyngeal, vagus, and spinal accessory nerves (IX, X, XI). Symptoms of dysphagia, hoarseness, aspiration, and coughing would typify skull base destruction in this area. Tumor expansion medially and anteriorly encroaches upon the carotid artery, hypoglossal nerve (XII), and sympathetic chain. When paretic, the facial nerve (VII) is typically infiltrated in the vertical mastoid segment of the fallopian canal, but can also be involved in the soft tissue of the stylomastoid foramen. Further growth medially into the infratemporal fossa and parapharyngeal space would compromise swallowing and nasal breathing by its mass effect. Erosion of the temporal bone and otic capsule causes progressive sensorineural hearing loss. Acute vertigo would result from rapid destruction of the otic capsule. Trigeminal nerve involvement from extensive skull base destruction presents with facial hypesthesia, trismus, or problems with mastication. Regardless of the extent of the tumor, the most common symptoms are tinnitus and hearing loss with associated ear pain and fullness.

An initial report by Glenner indicated that vasoactive pressor substances were secreted by paragangliomas.[10] Signs and symptoms would be similar to those seen in the patients with pheochromocytomas. Paroxysmal labile hypertension, headaches, tachycardia, palpitations, profuse sweating, flushing, weight loss, and syncope are hallmarks that a metabolically active tumor is likely to be present. The incidence of secreting and functioning paragangliomas is apparently quite low but may reach 3%.[25] However, if the above signs or symptoms are present, the physician should pursue further diagnostic studies.

Norepinephrine is the most common catecholamine secreted by these tumors, but epinephrine and dopamine are seen rarely. Norepinephrine has alpha activity while epinephrine causes beta receptor stimulation. The end metabolic product of all of these substances is vanillylmandelic acid (VMA) and 24 hour urine levels of greater than 7.0 mgm should alert one to the possibility of secretory activity. When elevated urine VMA levels are present (particularly when accompanied by clinical symptoms), selective venous catheterization for serum levels of VMA, metanephrines, and catecholamines should be done. Certain food and drugs must be accounted for when determining urine VMA levels. These include coffee and tea (caffeine), vanilla, bananas, citrus fruit, vasopressors, tetracycline, and MAO inhibitors. Failure to identify secretory activity and initiate preoperative alpha and/or beta blockade may result in catastrophic intraoperative or postoperative hypertensive or arrhythmic crises. Recognition of catecholamine secretion will also allow the anesthesiologist to avoid halothane which sensitizes the myocardium.

Diagnostic Studies

A patient presenting with pulsatile tinnitus, dysphagia, and shoulder weakness with a red-blue pulsatile mass in the middle ear, a conductive hearing loss, unilateral pharyngeal hypesthesia, vocal cord paralysis, and paresis of the sternocleidomastoid and trapezius muscles would not pose significant difficulty towards establishing an appropriate diagnosis. On the other hand, finding a vascular lesion in the middle ear without cranial nerve deficits would require further investigation and evaluation.

In addition to paragangliomas, the differential diagnosis of an isolated reddish-blue mass in the middle ear includes a congenital dehiscence of the jugular bulb, an aneurysm of or aberrance of the internal carotid artery, a persistent stapedial artery, metastatic disease, cholesterol granuloma, and encephalocele. In most cases, accurate assessment can be achieved with radiographic tests. If a pathologic process other than vessel aberrance is suspected in an isolated middle ear lesion, an exploratory tympanotomy may be necessary to establish the histologic diagnosis.

A thorough history and complete neurotologic examination is mandatory initially. Should auditory signs or symptoms be identified, audiometric testing is obtained to determine if the hearing loss is purely conductive, sensorineural, or mixed. A tympanogram may reflect the pulsatile nature of the middle ear mass.

Previously, evaluation of these lesions included polydirectional tomography, arteriography, and retrograde venography. The fifth generation high resolution CT scan has increased the diagnostic and staging capabilities necessary for accurate tumor assessment. The features available which greatly facilitate precise imaging are 1.5 mm cuts, contrast enhancement, and windowing with bone algorithm software. If an enhancing middle ear lesion is identified and the scan determines that the bony walls separating the carotid artery and the jugular bulb from each other and the middle ear are intact, then a tympanic paraganglioma is most likely present. If a pathologic process other than vessel aberrancy is suspected in an isolated middle ear lesion, an exploratory tympanotomy may be necessary to establish the histologic diagnosis.

In this situation, arteriography would not be required if the tumor was shown to be confined to the middle ear.

The high resolution CT scan is most valuable in assessing larger lesions. With this modality, the presence of intracranial intradural disease, medial extension, the relationship of the tumor to the carotid artery and facial nerve, and the inferior extent of the lesion can be determined.[4] The most characteristic high resolution CT signs of paraganglioma include jugular fossa expansion, soft tissue mass in the hypotympanum and sinus tympani, invasion of the cochlear promontory, dural compression by mass effect, anterior displacement of parapharyngeal fat planes, and extension into the eustachian tube orifice.[3]

The diagnosis of enlarged or atypical enhancing lesions present in the skull base or parapharyngeal space is facilitated with selective arteriography. Paragangliomas are typified by the characteristic radiographic blush due to their marked vascularity. This finding often obviates the need for operative biopsy. Four-vessel angiography provides additional information that is important and necessary for comprehensive tumor assessment and management. Angiography not only identifies the tumor by its blush, but defines the tumor's blood supply, extent, and carotid involvement. The four-vessel study can also determine the adequacy of the cerebral circulation and identify multiple tumors in other areas of the head and neck. In addition, the venous "run-off" phase of the arteriogram often outlines the jugular drainage system making retrograde venography unnecessary.[6] Magnetic resonance imaging has recently provided better information beneath the skull base due to the flow void in large vessels, but CT scanning with bone algorithms continue to provide superior information within the temporal bone.

Natural History

Management of skull base paragangliomas demands a thorough understanding of the tumor's natural history. In addition to identifying the location and extent of these vascular lesions, the potential problems of multicentricity, malignancy, and familial tendencies must all be considered.

Most patients with clinical paragangliomas do not have a positive family history of these vascular lesions. In approximately 8% of reported cases, a family history is positive. The inheritance pattern of familial paraganglioma is considered to be autosomal dominant, carried by a single gene. Penetrance would therefore be expected to be 50% in subsequent generations. However, the degree of penetrance was noted to be 85% in the second generation and 24% in the third generation in a genetic survey done by vanBaars.[30] Identification of the familial form of the disease has numerous implications. Given the significant degree of penetrance, evaluation of other family members would be indicated. In addition, patients with familial paragangliomas have a much higher incidence of multicentric lesions (Fig. 3). Bilateral tumors are present in 33% to 50% of the familial cases.[7,30] This is in contrast with multicentricity in nonfamilial cases. Multiple tumors can present synchronously or metachronously in as many as 10% of patients with nonfamilial paragangliomas.[29] A noninvasive means for evaluating asymptomatic family members or screening for multicentric lesions utilizes technetium 99m methylene diphosphonate. Routinely used for bone scanning perfusion scintigraphy, it is capable of identifying tumors of 2 cm or greater.[31]

Paragangliomas of the head and neck usually are slow-growing tumors. Although progressive morbidity from tumor invasion and expansion is inevitable, the mortality of nonmalignant lesions is very low. In two series of 148 patients, deaths

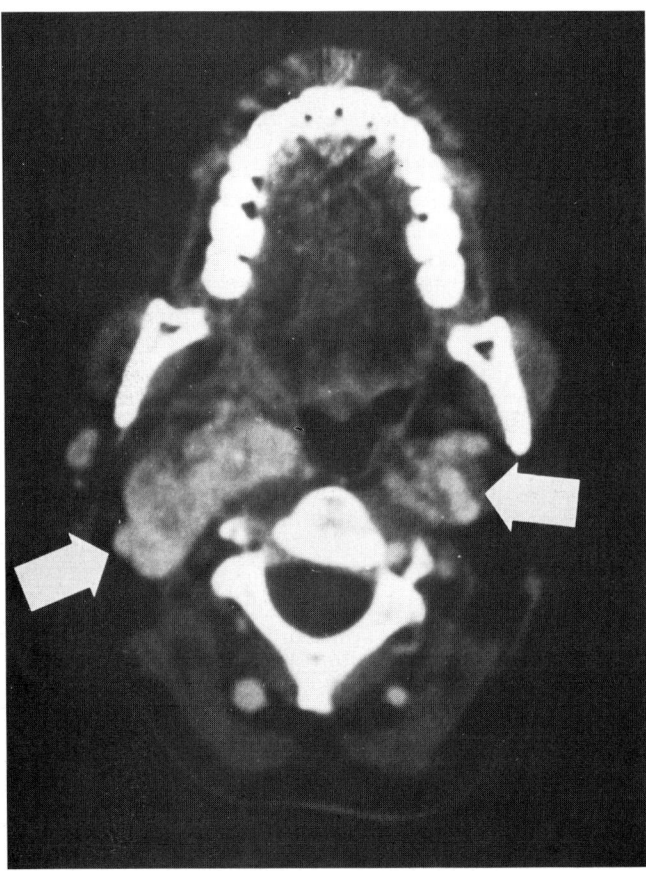

Figure 3: CT scan of skull base, showing bilateral and multiple paragangliomas of jugular, carotid, and vagal origin.

were reported only in those tumors exhibiting metastatic disease.[15,21]

Malignancy

Paragangliomas of the head and neck are usually slow-growing tumors that are locally invasive and destructive. Those occurring in the base of the skull (jugulotympanic and vagal paragangliomas) often involve cranial nerves VII through XII and typically exhibit a protracted course prior to presentation. Carotid body paragangliomas, by comparison, are usually identified earlier and undergo more rapid growth. When these tumors are locally aggressive, malignant degeneration is often questioned. Histologic sections of these lesions are considered benign with a low index of mitotic cells. The diagnosis of malignant disease, therefore, is defined by identifying metastatic foci in lymph nodes, bone marrow, the liver, pancreas, or epicardium. The method of spread is by vascular tumor embolization.

Despite the relatively low occurrence of malignancy in most paragangliomas, tumors of vagal origin are reported to have the highest incidence of metastatic disease. In a series of 37 patients, Druck reported 19% of patients had evidence of distant metastasis.[5] Next in frequency would be carotid body paragangliomas. Metastatic tumor identification may occur in as many as 9% of these patients. The time course for presentation is also quite variable. Distant disease has been verified in patients 16 years following management of primary carotid paraganglioma.[18]

Jugulotympanic paragangliomas not only are slower growing but also have a lower incidence of metastatic disease. Alford and Guilford compiled a series of 316 cases with jugular paragangliomas. They reported a rate of 1%, demonstrating four patients with distant spread.[1]

Autopsy microscopic findings of incidental asymptomatic pulmonary paragangliomas have been observed and are of no clinical significance.[26] However, those lesions that are identified in the parenchyma of the lung with routine radiographic techniques do represent probable metastatic disease. It must be realized that identification of lesions exhibiting a vascular blush does not necessarily mean metastatic disease. Multifocal presentation of paragangliomas must also be considered.

Classification

Many classifications for paragangliomas have been proposed, but that devised by Fisch[8] is most succinct and successful in addressing the surgeon's need for anatomic landmarks. His classification is shown in Table I. A survey of cases

Table I
Fisch's Classification of Paragangliomas

Class A:	Tumors limited to the middle ear cleft.
Class B:	Tumors limited to the tympanomastoid area without destruction of bone in the infralabyrinthine compartment.
Class C:	Tumors extending into and destroying bone of the infralabyrinthine and apical compartments of temporal bone.
C_1:	Tumors destroying the bone of the jugular foramen and jugular bulb with limited involvement of the vertical portion of the carotid canal.
C_2:	Tumors destroying the infralabyrinthine compartment of the temporal bone and invading the vertical portion of the carotid canal.
C_3:	Tumors involving the infralabyrinthine and apical compartments of the temporal bone with invasion of the horizontal portion of the carotid canal.
Class D:	Tumors with intracranial intradural extension.
D_1:	Tumors with an intracranial intradural extension up to 2 cm in diameter.
D_2:	Tumors with an intracranial intradural extension greater than 2 cm in diameter that require a combined two-stage otologic and neurosurgical removal.
D_3:	Tumors with inoperable intracranial intradural extension.

treated at the Pittsburgh Eye and Ear Hospital during a recent 5 year period is shown in Table II. The greatest number of cases were types B and C, and only one malignant lesion was identified. The use of modern radiographic imaging has greatly contributed to the accuracy of classification. This preoperative evaluation provides the necessary information for the skull base surgeons to determine the presence and degree of carotid, intracranial, and intradural extension. Classification is, quite simply, a method of determining tumor size and location preoperatively, and for planning the proper approach.

Treatment

At the present time, surgery is considered the preferred method of treatment in nearly all cases. It is estimated that between 80% and 90% of tumors are completely resectable and a high percentage of cure should be obtained. Despite the low incidence of malignancy, local recurrence is marked by progressive cranial nerve involvement, pain, and generalized disability. For this reason, a complete resection should be planned and achieved in a high percentage of cases.

Radiation therapy has been advocated by some, but is not utilized by the authors as primary treatment, with few exceptions. Elderly or poor risk patients are candidates for radiation without fear of long-term radiation risk. Although fibrosis has been shown to occur following radiation to paragangliomas, there is little evidence to suggest significant sensitivity of the tumor cells per se. For these reasons, radiation is probably best viewed as palliative. Chemotherapy has not been widely used, which is again appropriate in view of the benign characteristics of most of these lesions.

Surgical Approaches

The histologically benign nature of most paragangliomas allows for utilization of classic temporal bone surgical approaches without need of en bloc resection. The removal of extensive areas of bone is often necessary and is accomplished with cutting and diamond-stone burrs in order to isolate the lesion from its surrounding osseous perimeters. These techniques also allow for preservation and/or rerouting of essential neural and vascular structures.

Type A tumors (Fig. 4) can often be extirpated via the external auditory canal. Superior reflection of the tympanic membrane and removal of inferior canal bone will expose the hypotympanum and allow for removal of most intratympanic lesions, as popularized by Shambaugh[8] (Fig. 5). Using this approach, one is usually able to preserve hearing and normal tympanic architecture. When superior extension into the epitympanum or posterior extension into the mastoid are encountered (Fig. 6), a postauricular mastoidectomy is necessary to expose these areas. Preservation of the posterior canal wall and tympanic membrane may be possible with smaller type B tumors; certainly, this is not to be encouraged in larger type B or C tumors. Extension of paraganglioma into the petrous apex and infralabyrinthine structures will necessitate open cavity procedures when viable hearing remains. This is feasible as long as major vascular and neural structures are covered and will allow for amplification devices to be worn easily as well as providing easy access for viewing in follow-up of the patient. When hearing has been lost and complete tumor removal is assured, it is helpful to ablate the surgical defect with local muscle flaps and external meatal closure. Incomplete

Table II
Recent 5 Year Experience at Pittsburgh Eye and Ear Hospital

Tumor Type	Number
A	7
B	27
C	13 (1 metastatic)
D_1	5
D_2	4
Total	56

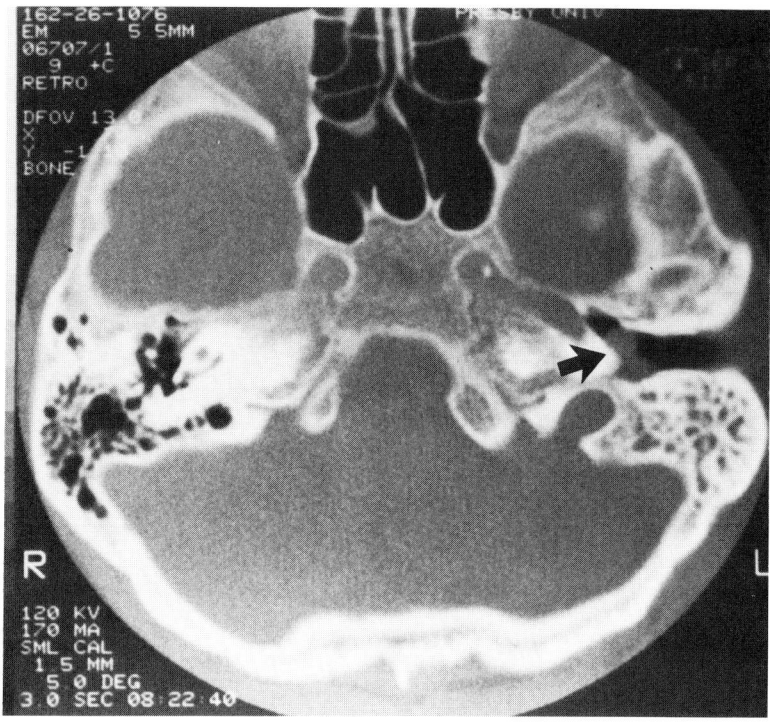

Figure 4: Axial CT scan demonstrating class A tumor entirely limited to the middle ear.

removal, of course, should dictate an open cavity procedure.

As might be expected, the facial nerve is commonly involved in its horizontal, vertical, or extratemporal portions. Complete eradication of tumor will, therefore, often require mobilization of the nerve from its bony canal for varying distances (Fig. 7). This technique will permit access to virtually all portions of the temporal bone between the carotid artery and sigmoid sinus. Transcochlear or translabyrinthine exposure of the medial extent of tumor may be achieved easily when hearing is poor, and is rarely necessary in the event of good hearing.

Intracranial extension of tumor may be extra- or intradural and will usually involve the posterior rather than middle fossa (Figs. 8 and 9). Invasion of the cranial cavity occurs through three major routes; along blood vessels (intra- or extraluminal), through cranial nerve foramina, and via the hypotympanic air cell tracts (Fig. 10). Collaboration between the otologist and neurosurgeon is obviously necessary for success with these larger lesions. In addition, ablation with local or distant flaps is most often required due to the large surgical defects that result following removal.

Finally, paragangliomas may extend anteromedially into the infratemporal fossa. This approach will not be discussed here since it is considered elsewhere in this book.

In all tumors, with the exception of type A and smaller type B tumors, it is advisable to initially seek and ligate the feeding vessels which have been identified during arteriography (Fig. 11). The occipital and ascending pharyngeal arteries are most often involved. Bleeding is often brisk throughout the tumor removal, but easily controlled with packing. In larger tumors, blood replacement should always be anticipated.

A word is in order about the effects of

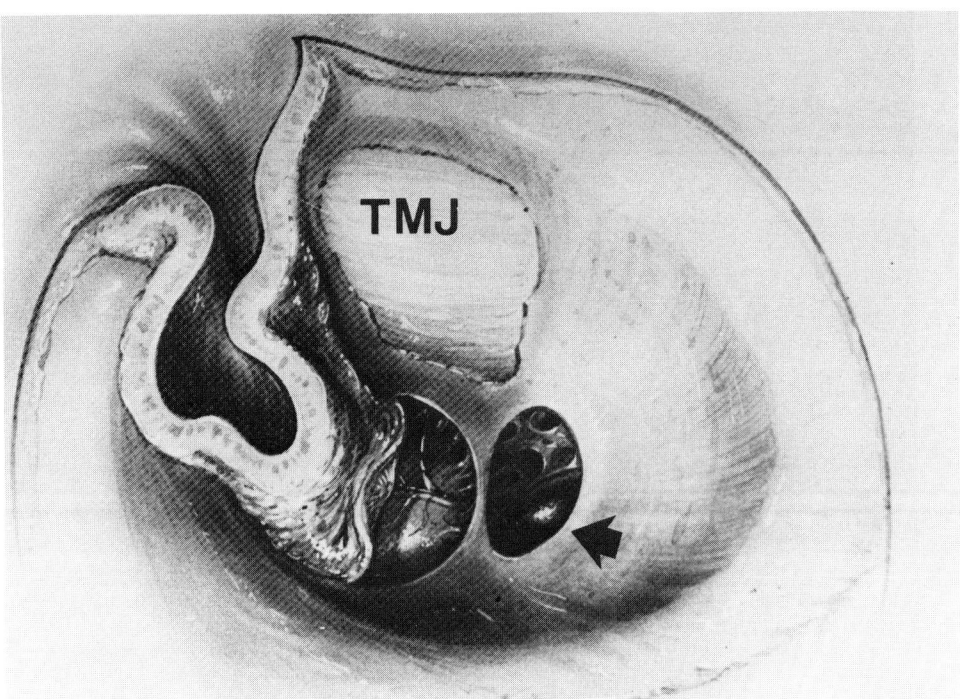

Figure 5: Surgeon's view of a right ear with transcanal, hypotympanotomy approach. Canal skin and tympanic membrane are reflected superiorly. Arrow = jugular bulb, TMJ = temporomandibular joint. (HH Naumann (ed): *Head and Neck Surgery.* Stuttgart, Georg Thieme Verlag, Vol. 3, Fig. 9.25, p 438, 1982.)

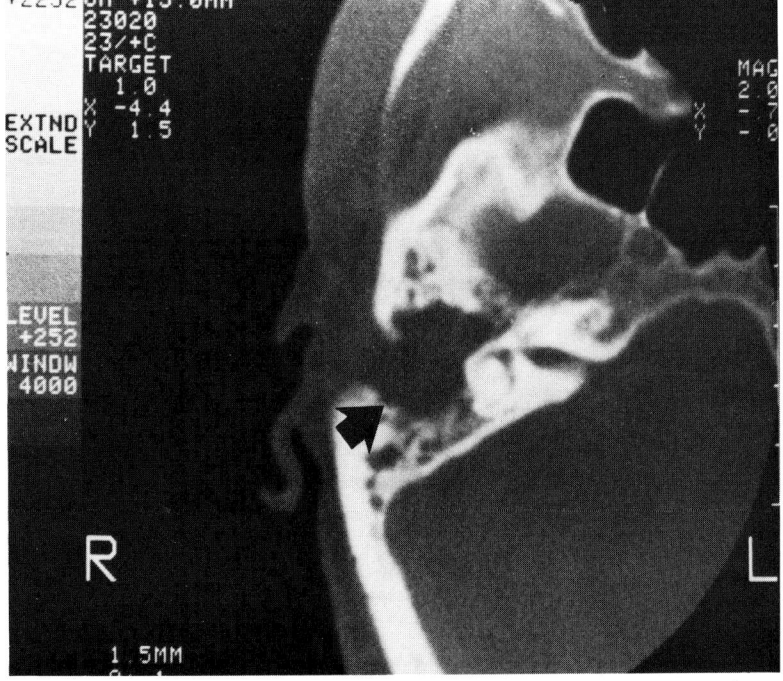

Figure 6: Axial CT scan showing a class C tumor with destruction of mastoid and apical portions of temporal bone.

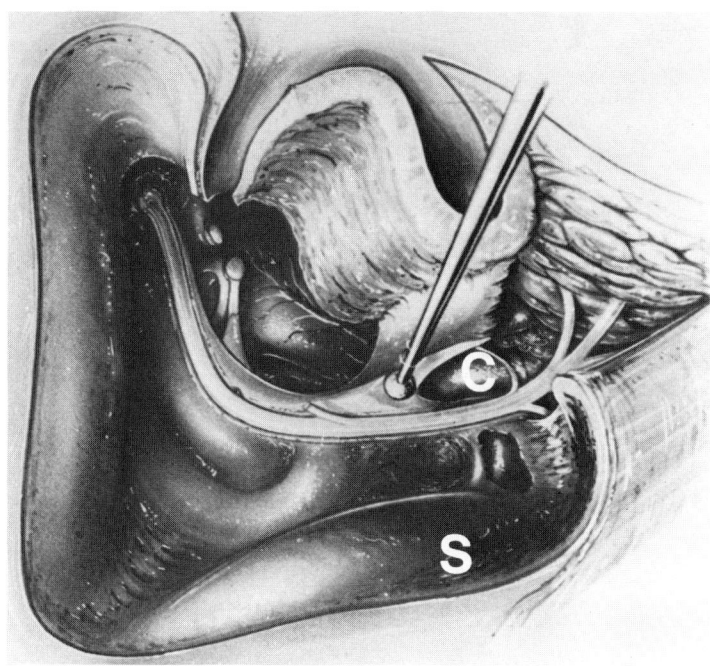

Figure 7: Surgeon's view of a right temporal bone with posterior canal wall removed and facial nerve skeletonized to allow anterior mobilization of the nerve. C = Internal carotid artery, S = sigmoid sinus. (HH Naumann (ed): *Head and Neck Surgery.* Stuttgart, Georg Thieme Verlag, Vol. 3, Fig. 9.30, p 440, 1982.)

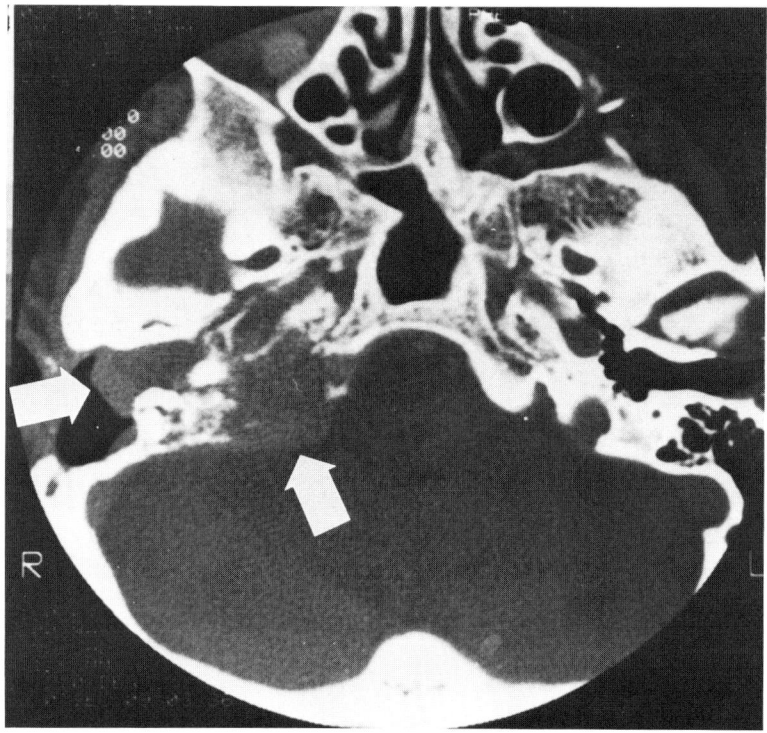

Figure 8: Axial CT scan of a large class D_2 tumor with posterior fossa extension.

652 • TUMORS OF THE CRANIAL BASE: DIAGNOSIS AND TREATMENT

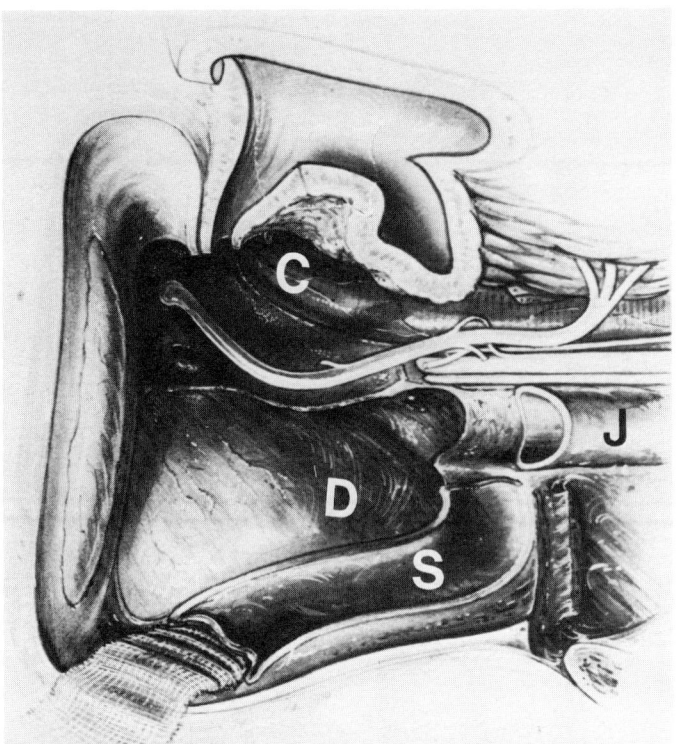

Figure 9: Surgical view of exposure necessary for extirpation of class D tumor. Facial nerve is reflected anteriorly. C = carotid artery, D = posterior fossa dura, S = opened sigmoid sinus, J = internal jugular vein. (HH Naumann (ed): *Head and Neck Surgery.* Stuttgart, Georg Thieme Verlag, Vol. 3, Fig. 9.36, p 446, 1982.)

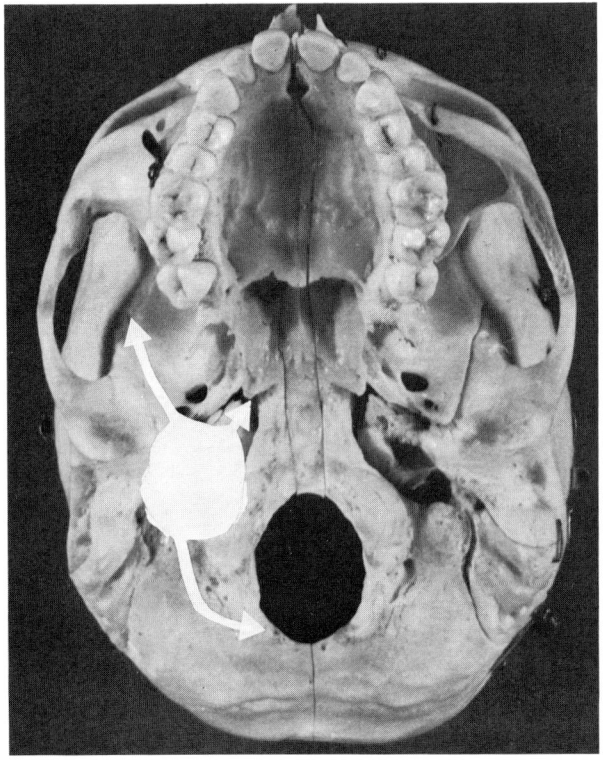

Figure 10: Paragangliomas of skull base origin extend via three chief pathways. As illustrated by the arrows, these are: (1) along blood vessels, (2) through cranial nerve foramina, (3) along mastoid air cell tracts into the petrous apex.

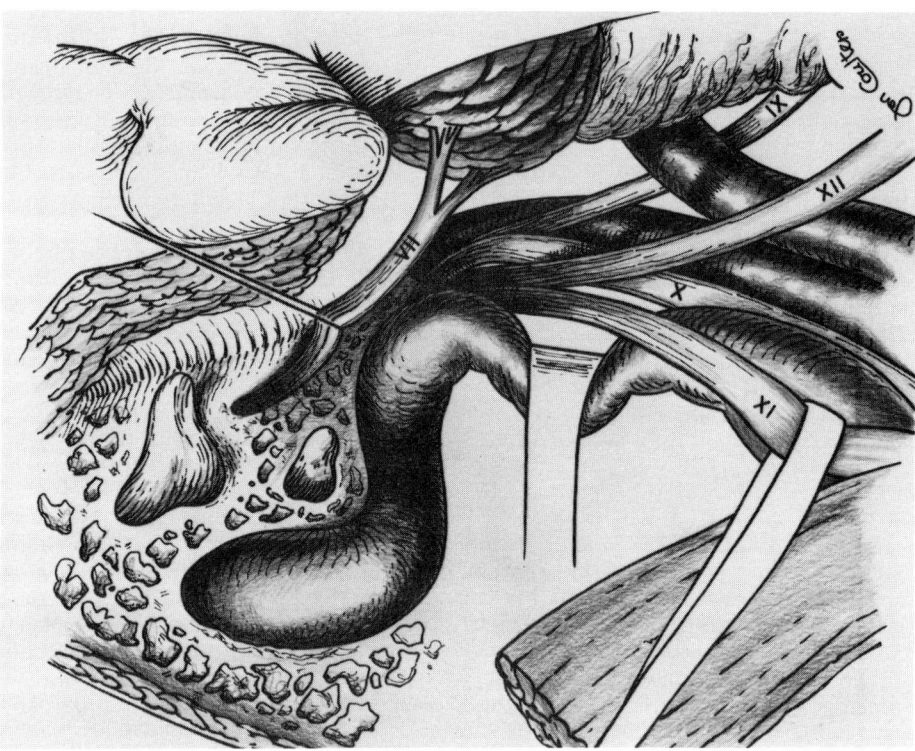

Figure 11: Surgical exposure of skull base with cranial nerve and large vessel identification with larger tumors. Initial neck dissection will allow for ligation of feeder vessels and control of the internal carotid artery and jugular vein.

vascular embolization on surgical removal. Early efforts, using absorbable gelatin sponge were largely ineffectual from the surgeon's standpoint. Recent techniques using polyvinyl alcohol and histoacrylic polymers have shown much greater promise in reducing blood loss at the time of surgery. Whenever possible, preoperative arteriography and embolization should be done concurrently with an appropriate planned interval prior to surgery.

Complications of paraganglioma surgery are similar to those of any major head and neck extirpative procedure and include cranial nerve loss, cerebrospinal fluid leakage, and infection.

Summary

Paragangliomas of the temporal bone are invasive, slow-growing, and most often benign. It is not unusual for patients to forego treatment until tumor size is surprisingly large. The location of these unusual lesions at the skull base requires not only excellent preoperative assessment, but the utmost in skill from those who surgically manage them.

References

1. Alford BR, Guilford FR: A comprehensive study of tumors of the glomus jugulare. *Laryngoscope* 72:765-787, 1962.
2. Brown JS: Glomus jugulare tumors revisited: A ten year statistical follow-up of 231 cases. *Laryngoscope* 95:284-288, 1985.
3. Chakeres D, LaMasters D: Paragangliomas of the temporal bone; high resolution CT studies. *Radiology* 150:749-753, 1984.
4. Curtin HC: Radiologic approach to paraganglioma of the temporal bone. *Radiology* 150:837-881, 1984.
5. Druck NS, Spector GJ, Gralsky RH, et al: Malignant glomus vagale: Report of a case

and review of the literature. *Arch Otolaryngol* 102:634-636, 1976.
6. Errin D, Osgothorpe JD: Multicentric paragangliomas. *Ann Otol Rhinol Laryngol* 93:96-71, 1984.
7. Farr WH: Carotid body tumors: A 40 year study. *CA (Cancer J for Clinicians)* 30:260-265, 1980.
8. Fisch U, Fagan P, Valavanis A: The infratemporal fossa approach for the lateral skull base. *Otolaryngol Clin North Am* 17(3):524, 1984.
9. Gaffney JC: Carotid-body-like tumors of the jugular bulb and middle ear. *J Pathol Bacteriol* 66:157-170, 1953.
10. Glenner GG, Crout JR, Roberts WC: A functional carotid-body-like tumor secreting levarterenol. *Arch Pathol* 73:230-240, 1962.
11. Glenner GG, Grimley PM: Tumors of the extra adrenal paraganglion system (including chemoreceptors). *Atlas of Tumor Pathology*, Second series, fascicle 9, AFIP, Washington, DC, 1974.
12. Guild SR: Glomus jugulare, a nonchromaffin paraganglion in man. *Ann Otol Rhinol Laryngol* 62:1045-1071, 1953.
13. Guild SR: Hitherto unrecognized structure, glomus jugularis in man. *Anat Rec* 79(Suppl):28, 1941.
14. Hirsch BE, Johnson JT, Black FO, et al: Paragangliomas of vagal origin. *Otolaryngol Head Neck Surg* 90:708-714, 1982.
15. Irons GB, Weiland LH, Brown WL: Paragangliomas of the neck: clinical and pathologic analysis of 116 cases. *Surg Clin North Am* 57:575-583, 1977.
16. Jackson CG, et al: Glomus tumor surgery, the approaches, results and problems. *Otolaryngol Clin North Am* 15(4):897-916, 1982.
17. Koegel L, Levine H, Waldman S: Paraganglioma of the sphenoid sinus appearing as labile hypertension. *Otolaryngol Head Neck Surg* 90:704-707, 1982.
18. Lack CE, Cubilla AL, Woodruff JM, et al: Paragangliomas of the head and neck region. *Cancer* 39:397-409, 1977.
19. Lattes R, Waltner JG: Nonchromaffin paraganglioma of the middle ear. *Cancer* 2:447-468, 1949.
20. Lundgren N: Tympanic body tumors in the middle ear; tumors of carotid body type. *Acta Otolaryngol* 37:367-379, 1949.
21. McCable BF, Fletcher M: Selection of therapy of glomus jugulare tumors. *Arch Otolaryngol* 89:183-185, 1969.
22. Mulligan RN: Chemodectoma in the dog. *Am J Pathol* 28:680-681, 1950.
23. Persson A, Frusha J, Dial P, et al: Vagal body tumor: Paraganglioma of the head and neck. *CA (Cancer J for Clinicians)* 35:232-237, 1985.
24. Rosenwasser H: Carotid body tumor of the middle ear and mastoid. *Arch Otolaryngol* 41:64-67, 1945.
25. Schwaber M, et al: Diagnosis and management of catecholamine secreting glomus tumors. *Laryngoscope* 94:1008-1015, 1984.
26. Schwartz ML, Israel HL: Severe anemia as a manifestation of metastatic jugular paraganglioma. *Arch Otolaryngol* 109:269-272, 1983.
27. Shambaugh G: Surgical approach for so-called glomus tumors of the middle ear. *Laryngoscope* 65:185-198, 1955.
28. Shamblin WR, ReMine W, Sheps SG, et al: Carotid body tumor (chemodectoma). *Am J Surg* 122:732-739, 1971.
29. Spector GJ: Multiple glomus tumors in head and neck. *Laryngoscope* 85:1066-1075, 1975.
30. vanBaars F, Cremers C, vandenBrock P, et al: Genetic aspects of nonchromaffin paragangliomas. *Hum Genet Co* 60:305-309, 1982.
31. Veldman JE, et al: Early detection of asymptomatic hereditary chemodectoma with radionuclide scintiangiography. *Arch Otolaryngol* 106:547-552, 1980.
32. Warren WH, et al: Neuroendocrine markers in paragangliomas of the head and neck. *Ann Otol Rhinol Laryngol* 94:555-559, 1985.
33. Watzka J: Die paraganglien handb. *Mikro Anat Menschen* 6:262-308, 1943.
34. Winship T, Klopp CT, Jenkin NH: Glomus-jugularis tumors. *Cancer* 1:441-448, 1948.
35. Zettergren L, Lindstrom J: Glomus tympanicum, its occurrence in man and its relation to middle ear tumors of carotid body type. *Acta Pathol Microbiol Scand* 28:157-164, 1951.

34

Operative Management of Large Neoplasms of the Lateral and Posterior Cranial Base

Laligam N. Sekhar, M.D.
Victor L. Schramm, Jr., M.D.
Neil F. Jones, M.D.

Introduction

The collaborative efforts of neurosurgeons, otolaryngologists, and plastic surgeon have made it possible to remove many large intra- and extracranial skull base neoplasms, some of which were previously considered inoperable. The proper selection of operative approaches, the exposure and the management of the petrous and cavernous segments of the internal carotid artery (ICA), and a careful reconstruction of the cranial base enables the removal of such neoplasms with minimal morbidity. In this chapter, we will describe our experience with the management of 32 patients with such neoplasms involving the middle and posterior cranial base. Four patients who underwent temporal bone resection for carcinoma are excluded since they are discussed in another chapter.

Patient Material

Between July 1983 and August 1986, 32 patients with large neoplasms involving the lateral and posterior cranial base were operated on (Tables I and II). Many of these tumors involved the intradural compartment, the cranium, and the extracranial spaces. All of these patients initially underwent a careful physical, neurological, and otolaryngological examination. Computed tomographic (CT) scanning was performed in the axial and coronal planes, using both soft tissue and bone algorithms. Magnetic resonance imaging (MRI) was performed in all of the recent patients and was especially useful to delineate the relationship of the arteries to the neoplasms, and to identify the presence of residual neoplasm on follow-up examination.

All the patients underwent cerebral

From: Sekhar LN, Schramm VL Jr, eds: *Tumors of the Cranial Base: Diagnosis and Treatment*. Mount Kisco, New York, Futura Publishing Co, Inc, © 1987.

Table I
Large Lateral and Posterior Cranial Base Neoplasms Operated During 1983–1986

		Group A Subtemporal and Preauricular Infratemporal Fossa Approach	Group B Postauricular Transtemporal and Infratemporal Fossa Approach
I.	Benign Neoplasms		
	Angiofibroma, juvenile*	1	—
	Epidermoid cyst	2	—
	Glomus jugulare tumor†	—	3
	Glomus vagale tumor	1	—
	Meningioma†	5	1
	Neurilemmoma IX†	1	—
	Neurilemmoma X†	—	2
	Teratoma, benign	—	1
II.	Malignant Cartilaginous Neoplasms		
	Chordoma*†	2	—
	Chondrosarcoma*†	1	—
III.	Other Malignant Neoplasms		
	Adenoid cystic carcinoma†	2	1
	Basal cell carcinoma	1	—
	Parotid adenocarcinoma	—	1
	Rhabdomyosarcoma	—	1
	Squamous cell carcinoma†	3	—
	Undifferentiated carcinoma (recurrent)	3	—
	TOTAL	22	10

*An anterior extradural approach, either transbasal or transethmoidal was also used simultaneously or in a different stage for tumor removal.

†An intradural approach, either retromastoid or frontotemporal was used in the same or different stage for tumor removal.

and cervical angiography. A balloon occlusion test of the appropriate ICA was performed in the majority of the patients, with the monitoring of the patients' clinical status, postocclusion stump pressure, and cerebral blood flow (CBF), before and after test occlusion. This test was used to estimate the risk of temporary or permanent occlusion of the ICA during the operation. Neurophysiological tests such as audiogram, brain stem evoked response, blink reflex, and visual evoked response were performed preoperatively when appropriate.

Operative Management

Two intradural and two extradural approaches were used for tumor resection. The intradural approaches were the retromastoid paracerebellar and the frontotemporal. The extradural approaches were the postauricular transtemporal and infratemporal fossa approach ("infratemporal approach" of Fisch), and the subtemporal-preauricular infratemporal fossa approach. Although we attempted to remove all of the tumor in a single operation, staging of tumor removal was necessary in 10 patients for the following reasons: (1) The tumor was very large in both the intra- and extradural compartments, and a single stage removal was impractical even with a team approach. (2) The tumor removal exposed the nasopharynx or the air sinuses, and occlusion of these was considered an important first step prior to removal of intradural tumor. (3) The presence of residual tumor was dis-

Table II
Location of Tumors

	Group A	Group B
Intracranial		
Middle cranial fossa	3	—
Cavernous sinus	11	2
Posterior fossa-cerebellopontine angle	6	8
clivus	5	—
foramen magnum	1	1
Cranial (Bone Involvement)		
Clivus (excluding body of sphenoid)	12	8
Sphenoid bone	11	1
Petrous bone, medial region	17	8
Petrous bone, lateral region	0	10
Extracranial		
Orbit	6	—
Ethmoid sinus	4	—
Sphenoid sinus	10	—
Maxillary sinus	6	—
Middle ear	—	7
External ear canal	—	1
Infratemporal fossa	18	5
Retropharyngeal space	9	2
Parapharyngeal space	7	7
Upper cervical area	1	5
Nasopharynx	5	2

covered on follow-up scans. All patients with malignant neoplasms were given radiation therapy postoperatively, and three patients underwent chemotherapy as well. One patient with a meningioma (patient PK) also underwent radiation therapy postoperatively.

Operative Technique

The selection of the operative approaches is based on the location of the tumor. When the neoplasm involves the cerebellopontine angle, the retromastoid approach is used; when the intradural middle cranial fossa, cavernous sinus, the tentorial notch, or the upper clivus region (intradural) are involved, the frontotemporal approach is utilized. A postauricular transtemporal and infratemporal fossa approach is used when the jugular foramen, hypotympanic area, and the facial recess region were invaded by neoplasm. When the petrous apex, the clivus, and the infratemporal fossa are involved, the subtemporal and preauricular infratemporal fossa approach is utilized. Both approaches provide a good exposure of the clivus extradurally, but we prefer the latter whenever possible.

Anesthetic Management

For the extradural operations, a lumbar subarachnoid drain is placed whenever possible. During intradural operations, cerebrospinal fluid (CSF) drainage is accomplished by cisternal drainage. Intravenous furosemide or mannitol are used for brain relaxation only when such drainage is not feasible. For most of the operations, patients receive only short-acting muscle relaxants during the anesthetic induction to permit neurophysiological monitoring of muscles supplied by the cranial nerves. Hypotension is avoided during the operation to minimize potential damage from brain retraction or from vascular occlusion. Induced hypertension of about 20 torr above the normal mean arterial pressure is used whenever major arteries (vertebral or carotid) are temporarily occluded. A very close dialogue is maintained during the operation between the surgeon and the anesthesiologist to maintain homeostasis. Following our experience with two wound hematomas, both in patients with impaired coagulation postoperatively, we electively transfuse one unit of fresh frozen plasma for every four units of packed red blood cells replaced. In addition, the platelet count is checked during and after the operation, and platelets are transfused whenever the count is lower than 100,000/cc. Prophylactic antibiotics are used during all operations. When an operation is contaminated (exposure of nasopharynx), or when a foreign body is left in the wound (drains or Doppler monitors), the antibiotics are continued for 4 days or until the foreign body is removed.

Retromastoid Paracerebellar Approach

The technical details of this approach are well known and have been emphasized in other chapters. The patients are generally in the lateral position, or in the supine position with the head turned away from the surgeon and with a roll under the shoulder to minimize stretch of the cervical veins. A craniectomy is performed in the retromastoid area measuring 4 × 4 cm, exposing the margin of the transverse sinus superiorly, the sigmoid sinus laterally, and the floor of the posterior fossa inferiorly. Following dural incision, the cerebellum is elevated under magnification provided by the operation microscope. The lateral cerebellomedullary cistern is opened to drain CSF and to relax the cerebellum. Then, using minimal cerebellar retraction, cranial nerves V through XII are exposed, and the neoplasm is removed piecemeal. The core of the tumor is initially gutted with bipolar cautery or with the CO_2 laser. The remainder of the neoplasm is dissected away from cranial nerves, basal blood vessels, and the brain stem using bipolar cautery, suction irrigation, and sharp microinstruments.

This approach is especially good for the removal of the tumors in the cerebellopontine angle and in the foramen magnum area. When the tumor occupies the tentorial notch, the clivus area without extension into the cerebellopontine angle, or is deeply indenting the brain stem, the exposure achieved may be suboptimal.

Frontotemporal Approach

The frontotemporal approach is used when the neoplasm involves the sphenoid ridge, the middle fossa, the cavernous sinus, the tentorial notch, or the upper clivus region. The craniotomy extends from just above the root of the zygoma to just above the junction of the middle and lateral thirds of the eyebrow. When greater subfrontal exposure is desired, as with neoplasms involving the tuberculum sella region, or as in cases where the superior approach to the cavernous sinus is utilized, the craniotomy extends medially to the supraorbital notch. Following dural opening, CSF is drained from the chiasmatic and the carotid cisterns to relax the brain. If the neoplasm involves the medial sphenoid ridge region, the sylvian fissure is split initially to drain CSF, and to expose the middle cerebral artery (MCA). The MCA is then traced towards the cranial base, dissecting tumor away from the arteries. Such a technique can prevent injury to the internal carotid artery when it is encased by tumor. When the cavernous sinus is invaded, the tumor is removed by a lateral, superior, or inferior approach to the cavernous sinus as detailed in a previous chapter. For tumors involving the tentorial notch or the upper clivus area, a limited resection of the temporal lobe is performed to minimize postoperative problems due to temporal lobe retraction. The anterior 4 cm of the temporal pole is resected starting in the lower portion of the middle temporal gyrus, and sparing the uncus and hippocampus. Such resection is not necessary when the temporal lobe has already been displaced by a large neoplasm in the middle fossa. The tentorium is then divided, and the removal of the neoplasm proceeds as described elsewhere. We do not use a posterior subtemporal approach at the moment because of the danger of injuring the vein of Labbè, and the problems of temporal lobe edema and hemorrhagic infarction which often follow such injury.

Postauricular Transtemporal and Infratemporal Fossa Approach

This is similar to the "infratemporal approach" of Fisch and is utilized when the lesion involves the jugular bulb, facial recess, or the hypotympanic area. Conductive hearing is permanently lost. A facial paralysis always results, with a 6 to 10 month recovery period, and some cases with incomplete recovery and/or synkinesis. Typical lesions that are removed by this approach are glomus jugulare tumors. This approach is easily combined with the retromastoid intradural approach.

The skin incision extends from the temporal area behind the ear into the neck (Fig. 1). The external ear canal is divided and reflected forward with the skin and subcutaneous tissues (Fig. 2). A mastoidectomy is then performed, unroofing the bony labyrinth, the sigmoid sinus, and the facial nerve in the fallopian canal. The facial nerve is exposed from the geniculate ganglion to the stylomastoid foramen by drilling away the bone, and then to its bifurcation in the parotid gland. The bone of the external ear canal is drilled away, after removing the remaining skin of the canal and the tympanic membrane. The malleus and incus are removed. The facial nerve is displaced anterosuperiorly. The condyle of the mandible is dislocated anteroinferiorly if it is necessary to expose the vertical segment of the petrous ICA. The sigmoid sinus and the internal jugular vein are ligated if necessary. The neoplasm can then be removed from the jugular bulb and the hypotympanic area. Working behind the ICA, the lesion can be removed from the lower clivus region as well (Figs. 3 and 4). During the closure of the wound, the external ear canal is sutured shut. Further reconstruction is discussed below (Figs. 5 and 6).

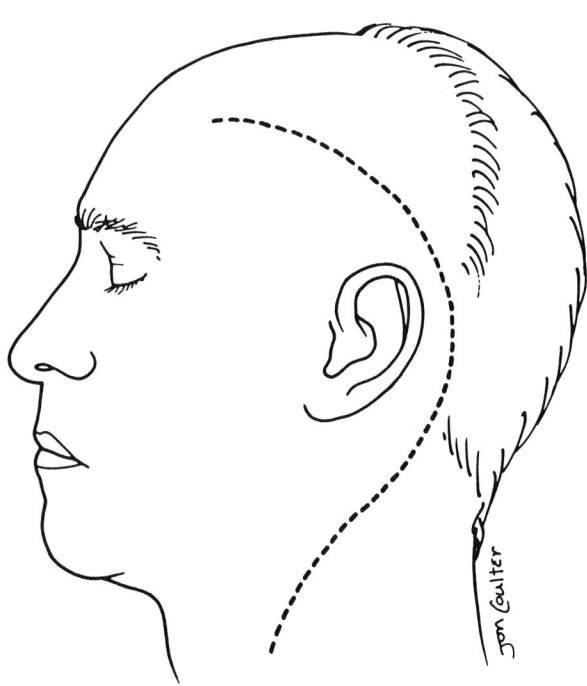

Figure 1: Skin incision for the transtemporal approach.

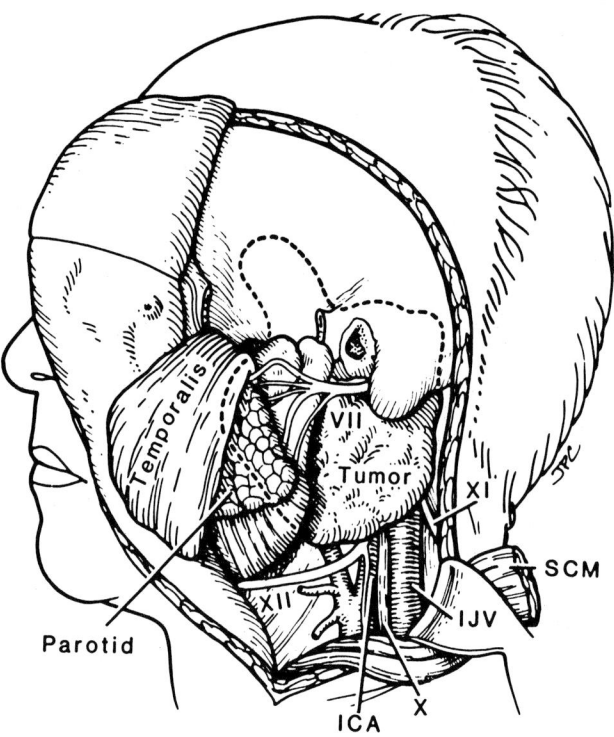

Figure 2: The skin and subcutaneous tissue flap has been turned forward. The facial nerve has been dissected and mobilized from the stylomastoid foramen through the parotid gland. After division of the zygomatic arch, the temporalis muscle has been reflected downward and forward. The major vessels and cranial nerves have been exposed in the neck. Tumor is exposed in the neck and the extent of the tumor within the temporal bone, middle fossa, and the cavernous sinus and nasopharynx is indicated by dotted lines. ICA = internal carotid artery; IJV = internal jugular vein; SCM = sternocleido mastoid muscle; VII, X, XI, XII = cranial nerves.

Subtemporal and Preauricular Infratemporal Fossa Approach

This approach is different from the "infratemporal approach" of Fisch in that the facial nerve is not displaced from the temporal bone reducing the incidence and duration of postoperative paralysis, and in that the hearing conduction mechanism is preserved. The exposure achieved is also more extensive and the reconstruction is different for some patients.

The incision is started in the temporal area, curves in front of and below the ear, and extends anteriorly on the neck along a skin crease. The main trunk of facial nerve and its upper branches are dissected from the stylomastoid foramen through the parotid gland. The skin and subcutaneous tissues are then reflected forwards. The temporalis muscle is reflected downwards and forwards after dividing the zygomatic arch. The lateral and superior walls of the orbital rim may also be resected temporarily to improve the exposure. The superficial temporal artery is ligated. The mandibular condyle and the capsule of the temporomandibular joint are dislocated downwards after the division of the lateral pterygoid muscle and the stylomandibular and sphenomandibular ligaments. Alternatively, if more space is needed, the neck and head of the mandibular condyle are resected. Dissection is performed in the neck to expose the ICA, internal jugular vein, and cranial nerves X, XI, and XII. The digastric muscle is divided, and the styloid process is resected either at this stage or later, after division of muscles and ligaments attached to its tip (Fig. 7).

A small temporal craniotomy is then performed to include the root of the zygoma. CSF is removed through the spinal drain to relax the temporal lobe. The dura of the middle fossa is then dissected under magnification to expose the arcuate eminence, greater superficial petrosal nerve (GSPN), the middle meningeal ar-

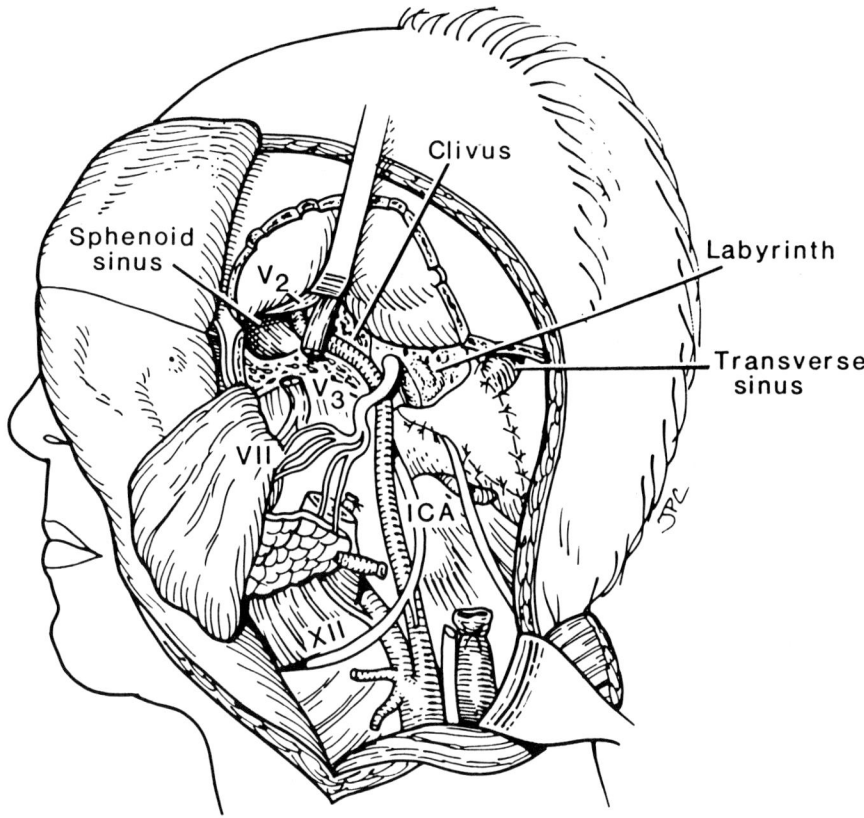

Figure 3: The tumor has been entirely resected. The facial nerve has been mobilized up to the geniculate ganglion and displaced upward and forward. The lower portion of the petrous temporal bone and the lower clivus have been drilled away as part of the tumor resection, and the labyrinth and cochlea have been spared. The defect in the posterior fossa dura after excision of the tumor has been repaired with a graft. The mandibular nerve has been divided because of tumor invasion. The sphenoid sinus is exposed after the tumor removal. The mandibular condyle and neck have been resected. The exposed nasopharynx is not shown. V_2, V_3 = maxillary and mandibular division of the trigeminal nerve.

tery, and the mandibular nerve (V_3). The middle meningeal artery is divided, and the greater wing of the sphenoid bone is rongeured to unroof the foramen ovale laterally and anteriorly. After placing a self-retaining retractor to protect the temporal dura, drilling is started deep to the temporomandibular joint to expose the eustachian tube and the tensor tympani muscle which are divided. The genu of the petrous ICA is exposed immediately deep to the eustachian tube. Using the drill and fine bone punches, it is followed downwards to expose the vertical segment of the petrous ICA. The upper cervical ICA (above the level of the facial nerve) is then dissected free after dividing the dense fibrocartilaginous ring at the entrance to the cranial base. The horizontal segment of the petrous ICA is unroofed after the division of the GSPN, and with temporary retraction of V_3. V_3 may have to be divided for better exposure of the upper clival area, or for the exposure of the basal cavernous sinus. Care must be taken not to remove the bone postero-

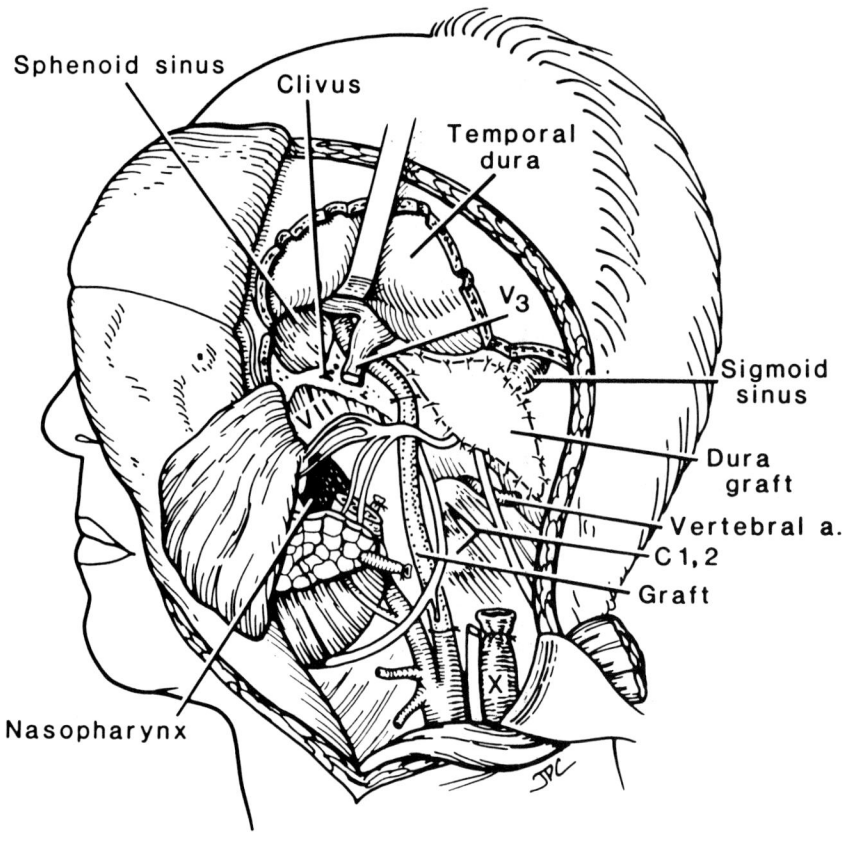

Figure 4: A slight modification of the previous operation, similar to what was done with patient MM. The entire temporal bone has been resected including the tumor contained within and the facial nerve. Tumor has been resected from the intradural clivus area as well as the cavernous sinus area. V_3, which was involved by tumor, has been resected. The facial nerve has been reconstructed by a greater auricular nerve graft from its proximal stump to its distal stump in the parotid gland. The upper cervical and petrous carotid artery have been resected in part and reconstructed by a vein graft (not performed in patient MM). Notice the exposed vertebral artery above the transverse process of C_1.

superior to the genu of the ICA, to avoid injury to the facial nerve and the cochlea. The entire petrous ICA along with its surrounding periosteal sheath is dissected from the carotid canal, and after the upper cervical ICA is mobilized, the vessels are displaced forward.

The petrous bone lying immediately deep to the carotid canal, the petrous apex region superomedial to the horizontal segment of the petrous ICA, and varying amounts of the clival bone are drilled away. This provides excellent exposure of the extradural clival region and dura from the level of the trigeminal nerve to the foramen magnum craniocaudally, and from about the level of the internal auditory canal laterally to the opposite petrous apex medially (Fig. 8). The foramen rotundum can be unroofed exposing the maxillary nerve (V_2) from the middle fossa through the pterygopalatine fossa. The superior orbital fissure can also be unroofed by removing the greater and lesser sphenoid wings. Removal of the sphenoid bone at the root of the pterygoid processes and medial to the foramen rotundum exposes the sphenoid sinus. From this loca-

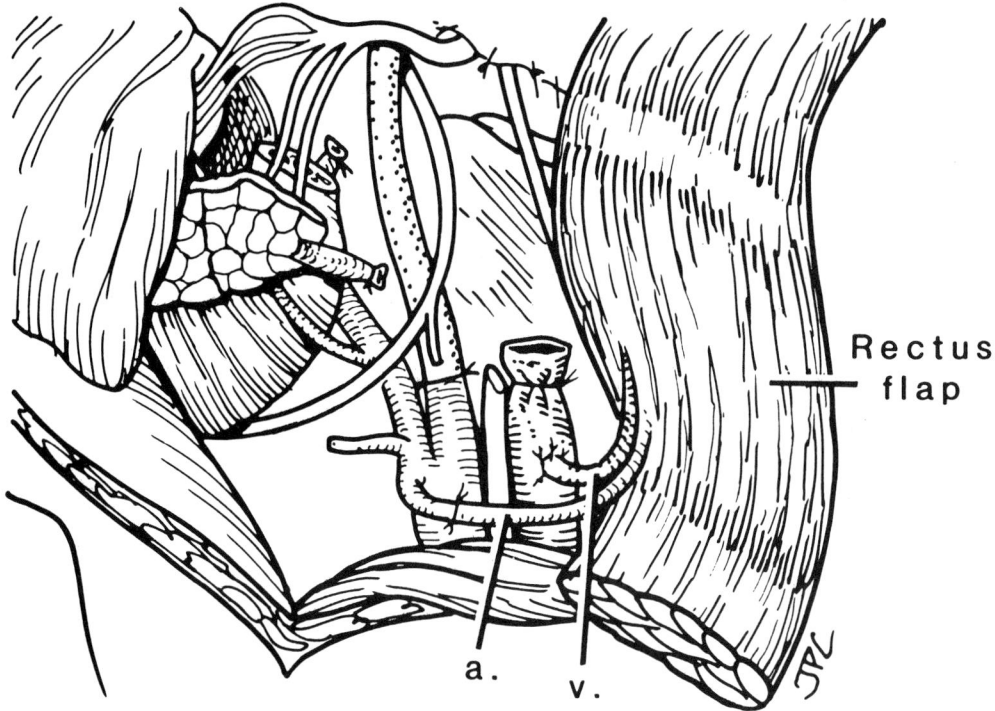

Figure 5: Reconstruction with rectus abdominis flap. The rectus abdominis flap has been harvested from the abdomen along with the inferior hypogastric artery (a) and vein (v), both of which have been attached to a branch of the external carotid artery and the internal jugular vein.

tion, one can also enter the cavernous sinus between the leaves of dura, following V_2, between V_2 and V_3, or between V_1 and V_2.

This approach is ideally suited to the resection of neoplasms involving the infratemporal fossa, the parapharyngeal area, and nasopharynx, the petrous apex region, the clivus, the sphenoid sinus, and the basal cavernous sinus. When the neoplasm involves the facial recess, the hypotympanic area, and the jugular bulb, a postauricular transtemporal and infratemporal fossa approach ("infratemporal approach" of Fisch) is more appropriate.

Management of the Petrous and Upper Cervical ICA

The exposure and management of the petrous and upper cervical ICA are detailed in a previous chapter (see Chapter 12). The intraoperative arterial management depends on the nature of the neoplasm, the results of the preoperative balloon occlusion test, and the intraoperative findings. There are four management options: (1) Exposure and decompression of the artery, dissection away from tumor, with temporary clipping and suture if the vessel is torn during dissection. (2) Intraoperative or preoperative arterial occlusion. This is preferred, especially for malignant neoplasms which encase the artery, if the patient tolerated the balloon occlusion test with minor or no changes of CBF. Such occlusion should be performed as close as possible to the ophthalmic artery to prevent a stroke due to emboli originating in the stump. (3) Excision of the encased or invaded arterial segment and vein graft reconstruction. This is recommended in all patients with benign neoplasms, and in patients with malig-

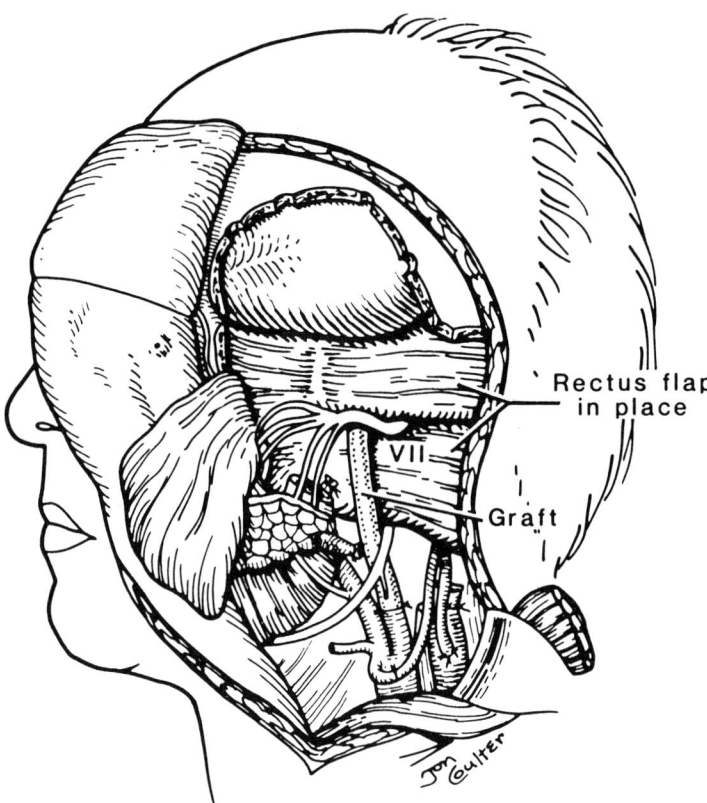

Figure 6: The rectus flap has been used to isolate the nasopharynx and the sphenoid sinus from the remainder of the wound. A tongue of the flap is covering the petrous carotid artery on both sides and the vein graft is isolated from the nasopharynx by the remainder of the graft.

nant neoplasms that tolerated the balloon occlusion test clinically, but with a reduction of the CBF to between 15 and 30 ml/100 gm/min. (4) External carotid to middle cerebral artery saphenous vein graft. If the patient was unable to tolerate the balloon occlusion test clinically, and the artery is encased or invaded by neoplasm, a microvascular bypass capable of carrying a large volume of blood acutely is recommended prior to ICA occlusion and excision. A technically more difficult alternative would be to perform direct vein graft reconstruction after placing an intraluminal shunt.

Reconstruction

Reconstruction is extremely important to prevent meningitis and to avoid infection of the wound ascending from an exposed nasopharynx, paranasal sinus, or from the skin surface. When the ICA or a vein graft is exposed, such an infection may result in carotid ulceration followed by stroke or death. A good cosmetic result is a less important reason for reconstruction.

When there is a dural defect, it is repaired using a graft of pericranium or of cadaver dura. With adequate bone removal, the dura can always be sutured, but watertight closure may not be possible. The dural repair has to be covered with another layer of vascularized tissue. The temporalis muscle or a portion of it will suffice for small defects. However, larger defects and the presence of an open nasopharynx require a more extensive reconstruction. For such cases, we have preferred to use a vascularized rectus abdominis free flap and found it to be very satisfactory (see Chapter 14 for details). Others have advocated the use of a pectoralis major myocutaneous flap, a

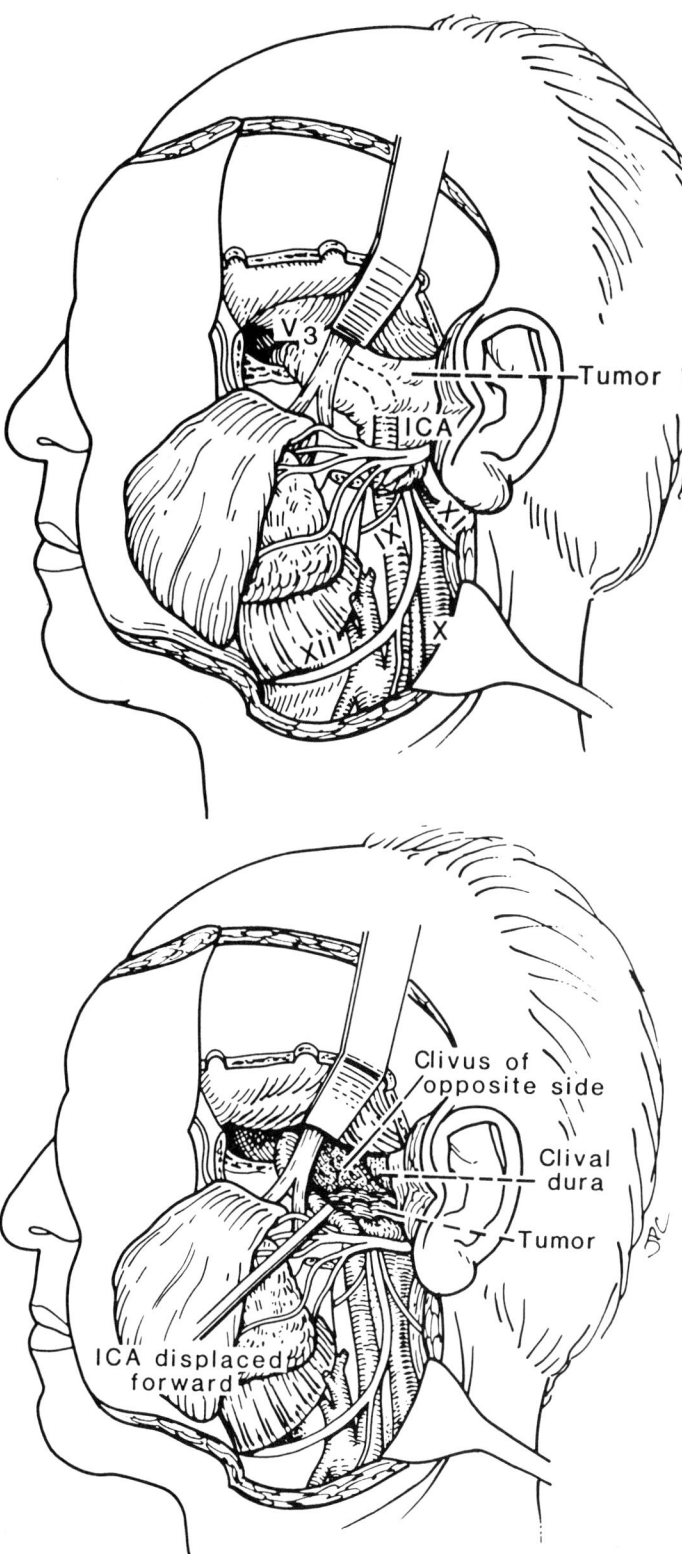

Figure 7: Preauricular infratemporal fossa approach to lesions involving the petrous apex, clivus, infratemporal fossa, and nasopharynx. The incision is preauricular. The facial nerve has been mobilized from the stylomastoid foramen through the parotid gland. The condyle and neck of the mandible are resected. V_3 has not been divided here, but may be divided temporarily if needed. The tumor is seen to be surrounding the petrous portion of the internal carotid artery extending into the cavernous sinus.

Figure 8: The petrous carotid artery has been exposed and completely dissected free of tumor all the way into the cavernous sinus. It has been displaced temporarily forward after mobilization of the upper cervical ICA. Tumor has been removed from the region of the middle and lower clivus down to the foramen magnum area. The exposed dura of the clivus on the ipsilateral side and the remaining clivus of the opposite side are seen. Reconstruction is similar to the transtemporal approach as in Figures 5 and 6.

trapezius rotation flap, or a rotated scalp flap.

A large length of rectus abdominis muscle is removed from the patient along with the deep inferior hypogastric artery and vein (Fig. 5). The artery and vein are sutured to a branch of or the main trunk of the external carotid artery and the internal jugular vein. The muscle flap is then sutured to the defect in the wall of the nasopharynx as much as possible, used to occlude the sphenoid sinus and to separate the exposed dura and the ICA from the nasopharynx. The muscle may be split into two parts to cover the ICA on both sides (Fig. 6).

Complications (Table III)

Two patients suffered strokes postoperatively, one of whom also died subsequently. One patient (WL) was a 3-year-old boy with an extensive clivus chordoma. Following an initial subfrontal and transnasal operation and a subsequent right infratemporal fossa operation, the tumor was thought to be totally excised. Follow-up CT scans revealed an intradural invasion by tumor with the displacement of the brain stem. Another operation was undertaken through a left subtemporal intradural approach to debulk the tumor 3 weeks later. He awoke well from the operation, but sustained an acute hemiplegia several hours later. Subsequent CT and MRI scans and transcranial Doppler studies have revealed an embolic occlusion of the right middle cerebral artery presumably secondary to occlusion of the ICA. The ICA occlusion may have been caused by unrecognized ICA injury during the previous operation, kinking caused by extreme head rotation, or perioperative hypercoagulability. He has recovered a significant degree of motor function and has undergone radiation therapy. He had no evidence of local tumor and was attending school when a pulmonary tumor metastasis was discovered. Another patient (MC) suffered a bilateral ICA rupture, right hemispheric stroke, and an infection of the infratemporal fossa because of inadequate exclusion of the nasopharynx by a temporalis muscle flap. She died as a consequence of the infection. This complication may have

Table III
Postoperative Complications

Death (bilateral carotid rupture, infection)		1
Cerebral Infarction		1
Carotid pseudoaneurysm (occluded without event)		1
Cerebrospinal fluid leak (one reexploration)		4
Wound hematoma		2
Wound infection		2
Temporomandibular dysfunction		2
Temporary		10
Permanent		None
Cranial nerve paralysis or weakness		
Nerve	Temporary	Permanent
II	—	1
III	3	0
IV	1	0
VI	3	2
VII	10	1 (reconstructed)
VIII Conductive	2	5
Sensorineural	—	—
IX, X	3	6
XI	1	—
XII	1	—

been avoided by the early use of a rectus abdominis muscle flap. Patient JKV suffered a postoperative wound infection and ICA pseudoaneurysm, requiring balloon occlusion of the ICA, removal of the bone flap, and intravenous antibiotics. He recovered uneventfully. Patient JMC also suffered a postoperative wound infection, but recovered after removal of the bone flap, debridement, and the placement of a vascularized rectus abdominis flap. The infection in patients MC and JMC is thought to be due to the inadequate exclusion of the nasopharynx with poorly vascularized temporalis muscle. In patient JKV, a vascularized rectus abdominis flap was used, but the sphenoid sinus was not occluded, resulting in spread of infection.

Failure to occlude the sphenoid sinus adequately resulted in CSF rhinorrhea in four other patients, necessitating reexploration with packing of the sphenoid sinus in one and dural repair in the other. Two patients with extensive intraoperative blood loss developed postoperative wound hematomas, due to abnormal coagulation studies. Both patients had an uneventful outcome after wound reexploration, and correction of the coagulation status.

The cranial nerve complications can be seen in Table III. The paralysis of cranial nerves II, III, IV, or VI were related to operations within the cavernous sinus. Facial nerve paralysis was temporary in all but one patient. When the facial nerve was displaced from the fallopian canal as part of the transtemporal approach, the paralysis took a longer time to recover (6 to 10 months) with incomplete recovery in one patient and failure to recover in another. The last patient has undergone graft reconstruction of the facial nerve. Permanent conductive hearing loss followed the transtemporal approach to remove tumor in the hypotympanic and tympanic area, whereas temporary loss was related to hemotympanum or to serous effusion after the excision of the eustachian tube. Permanent loss of glossopharyngeal and vagal function was due to tumor invasion, and required Teflon injection of the vocal cord.

Follow-Up, Results, and Outcome

The patients may be considered under three categories: benign neoplasms, malignant cartilaginous neoplasms, and other malignant neoplasms. Follow-up of all patients has ranged from 3 months to 3 years postoperatively. Among the 14 benign neoplasms, 12 were resected totally, and two subtotally. None has evidence of recurrence or regrowth to date, and all patients have a good quality of life. Among the cartilaginous malignant neoplasms, two were thought to be totally resected, and were radiated. Both are doing well without evidence of tumor recurrence. The other patient underwent subtotal resection in three stages followed by radiation therapy. He has no evidence of local disease but has a lung metastasis (WL). Among the 13 other malignant neoplasms, 10 were thought to be resected totally, and three subtotally. In the total resection group, a patient treated for recurrent rhabdomyosarcoma has local tumor regrowth despite chemotherapy (SP), and a patient with parotid acinar cell carcinoma has no local disease but a spine metastasis (MM). In the subtotal resection group, a patient with recurrent adenoid cystic carcinoma had a local regrowth and died (WS), and a patient with squamous cell carcinoma died postoperatively (MC). Nine patients surviving without evidence of disease in this group of patients are either in good (returned to previous occupation) or in fair (independent but not working) condition, but one patient is in poor condition (dependent for daily living) because of preoperative deficits.

Illustrative Cases

Patient GS: Vagus Schwannoma

This 34-year-old man presented with an 8 year history of tongue paralysis and a 2 month history of hoarseness of voice, dysphagia, and occipital headache. On examination, he had a total paralysis of the right cranial nerves VIII and XII, a partial paralysis of the cranial nerves IX, X, and XI, a mild left arm weakness, and a gait ataxia. CT scans revealed a large tumor occupying the posterior fossa, the petroclival bone, and extending into the parapharyngeal region (Figs. 9A–D). The first operation was by a retromastoid approach to excise the intradural portion of the tumor which was invading the cranial nerves IX and X. The second operation was through a transtemporal approach with the displacement of the facial nerve, and with the exposure and displacement of the vertical segment of the petrous ICA. The neoplasm was found to be arising from the vagus nerve and was totally excised. The dead space remaining after tumor removal was filled with a portion of the temporalis muscle. Postoperative problems included a temporary facial paralysis (recovered after 6 months, mild synkinesis), worsened weakness of nerve XI (recovered), worsened hoarseness, and swallowing (recovered without Teflon injection), and temporary temporomandibular joint dysfunction. There is no residual tumor apparent on CAT scans 1 year postoperatively, and he has returned to his former occupation (Figs. 9E and F).

Patient MB: Clivus Chordoma

This 40-year-old woman presented with a 1½ year history of severe occipital-nuchal headaches, a recent onset of right hypoglossal nerve palsy, paresis of the vagus, and right-sided tinnitus.

CT scan revealed a large neoplasm of the clivus extending craniocaudally from the midclivus to the first cervical vertebra, anteroposteriorly from the retropharyngeal area to the pons, and laterally displacing the right ICA (Figs. 10A–D). Because of the close relationship to the ICA, a preauricular infratemporal fossa approach was used to resect the tumor totally. Postoperatively, she had a temporary facial paralysis (complete recovery within 3 months) and temporary dysphagia and dysphonia. She has undergone proton beam radiation therapy subsequently, and is entirely asymptomatic 8 months postoperatively with no evidence of recurrent tumor.

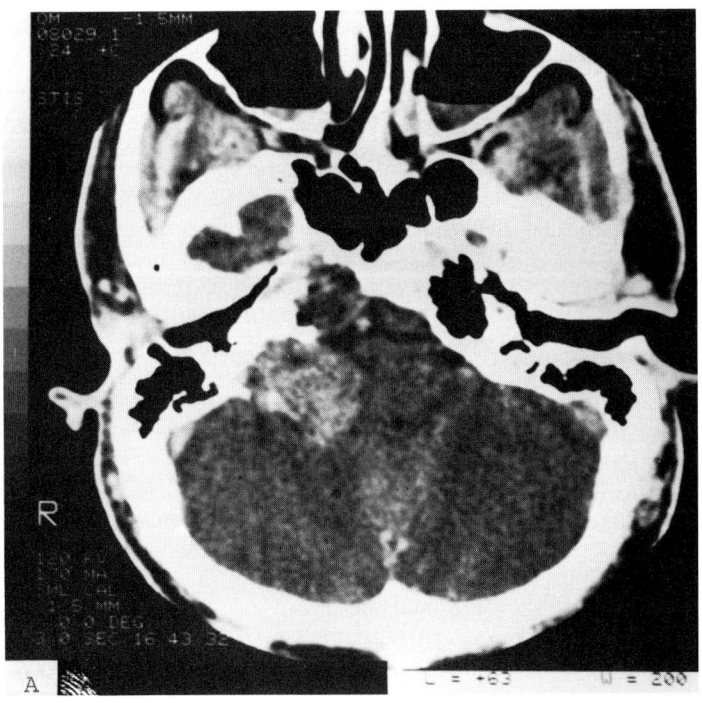

Figure 9A: CT scan of patient GS showing the extent of the tumor within the posterior fossa.

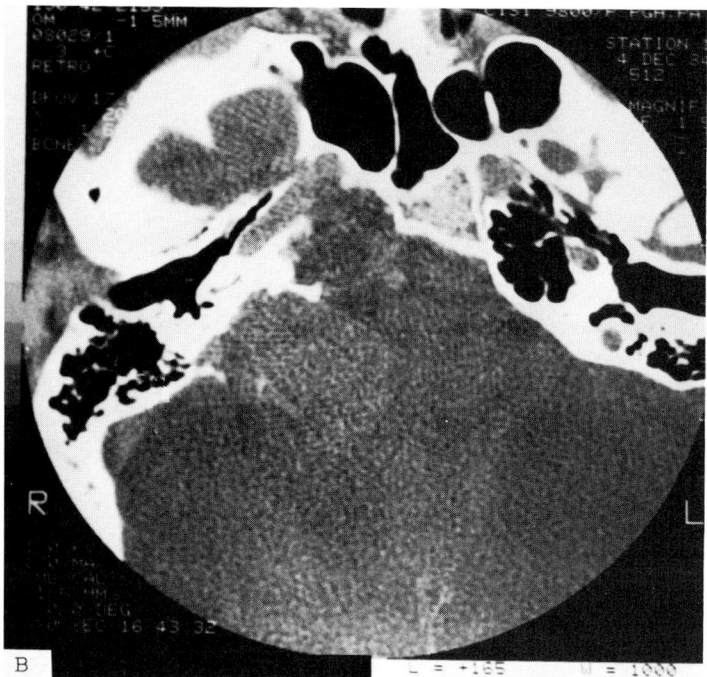

Figure 9B: Tumor involving the right half of the clivus extending just behind the horizontal segment of the petrous carotid artery.

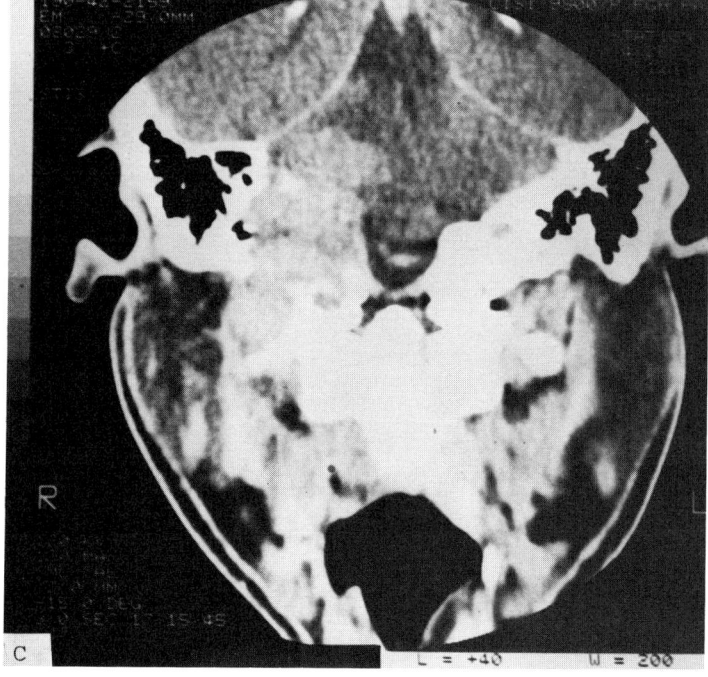

Figure 9C: Coronal CT scan showing the intra and extracranial extension of the tumor through the jugular foramen.

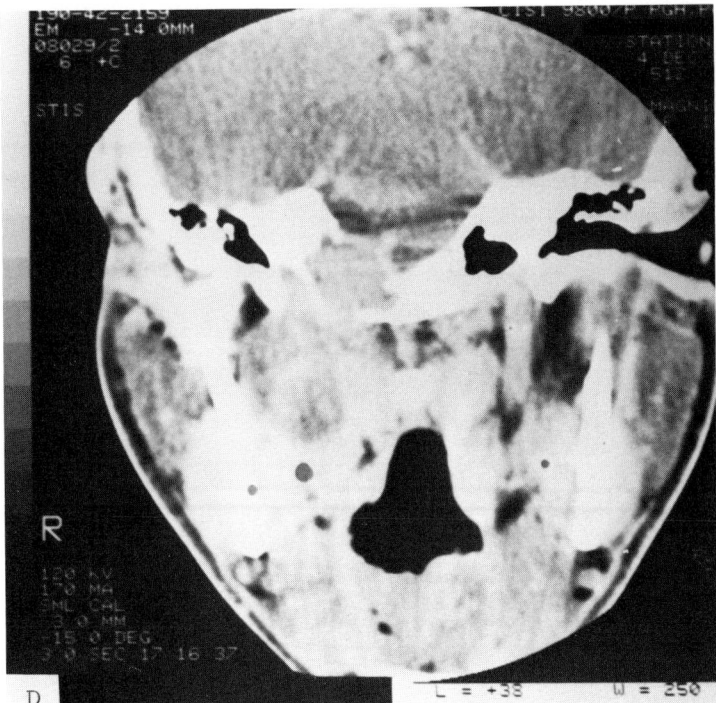

Figure 9D: The large tumor at the outer extent of the jugular foramen is clearly seen.

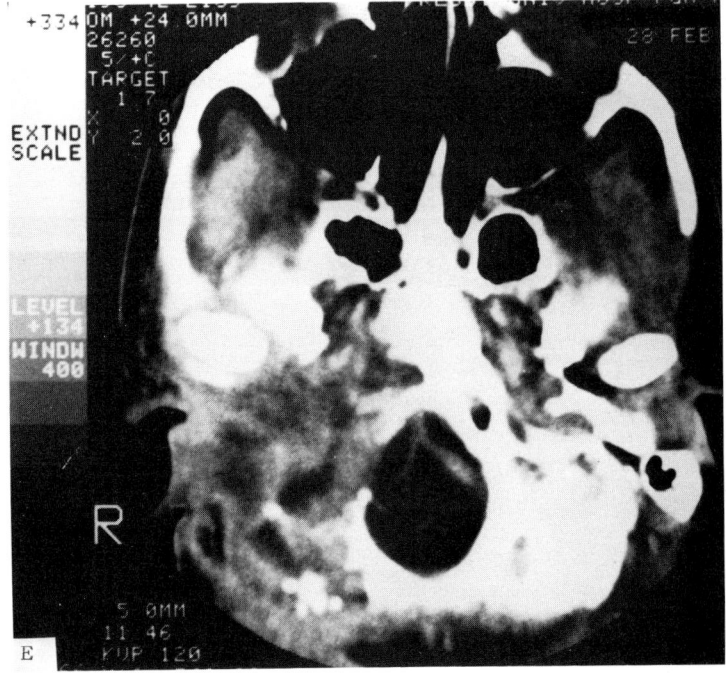

Figure 9E and F: After resection of the tumor and reconstruction with temporalis muscle.

Operative Management: Lateral and Posterior Cranial Base • 671

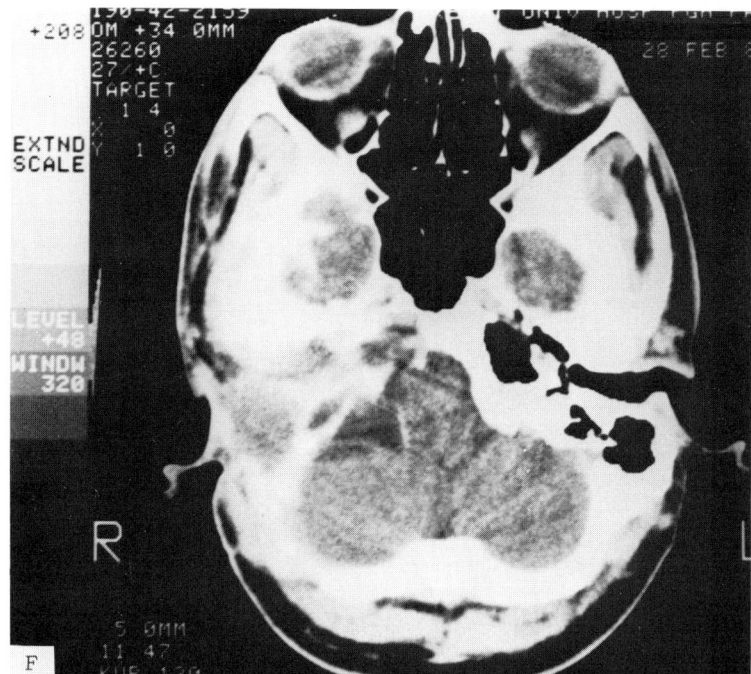

Figure 9F.

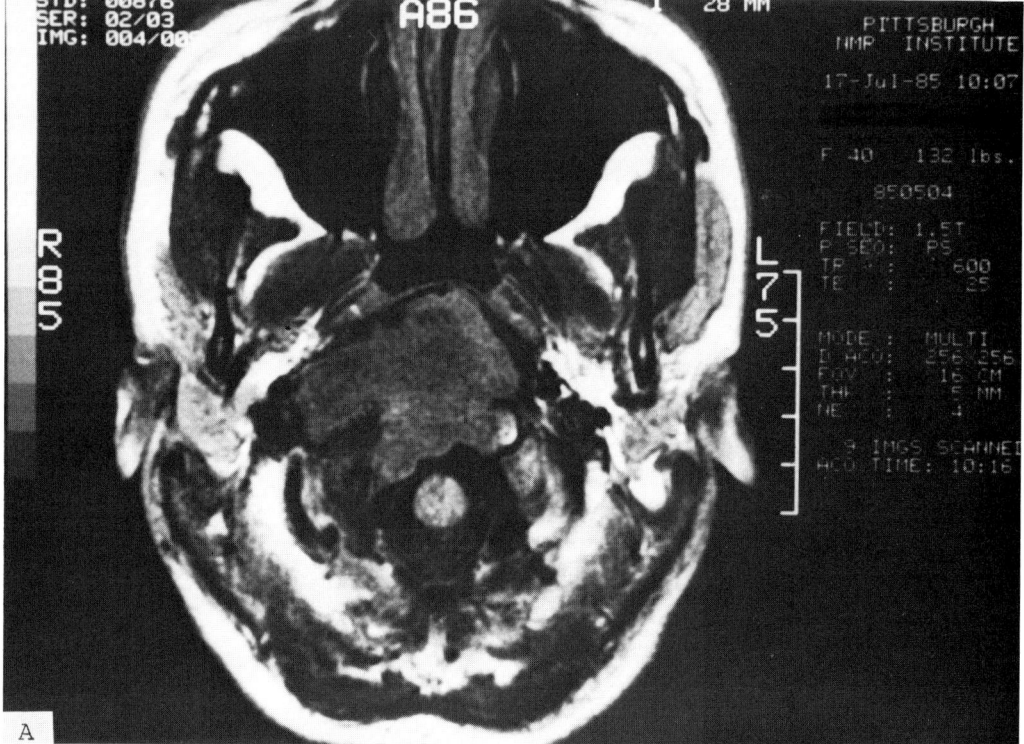

Figure 10A: MRI scan of patient MB revealing the extensive destruction of the clivus, with tumor extending anteriorly to the nasopharynx, laterally to the right ICA (arrow) and posteriorly to the spinomedullary junction.

672 • TUMORS OF THE CRANIAL BASE: DIAGNOSIS AND TREATMENT

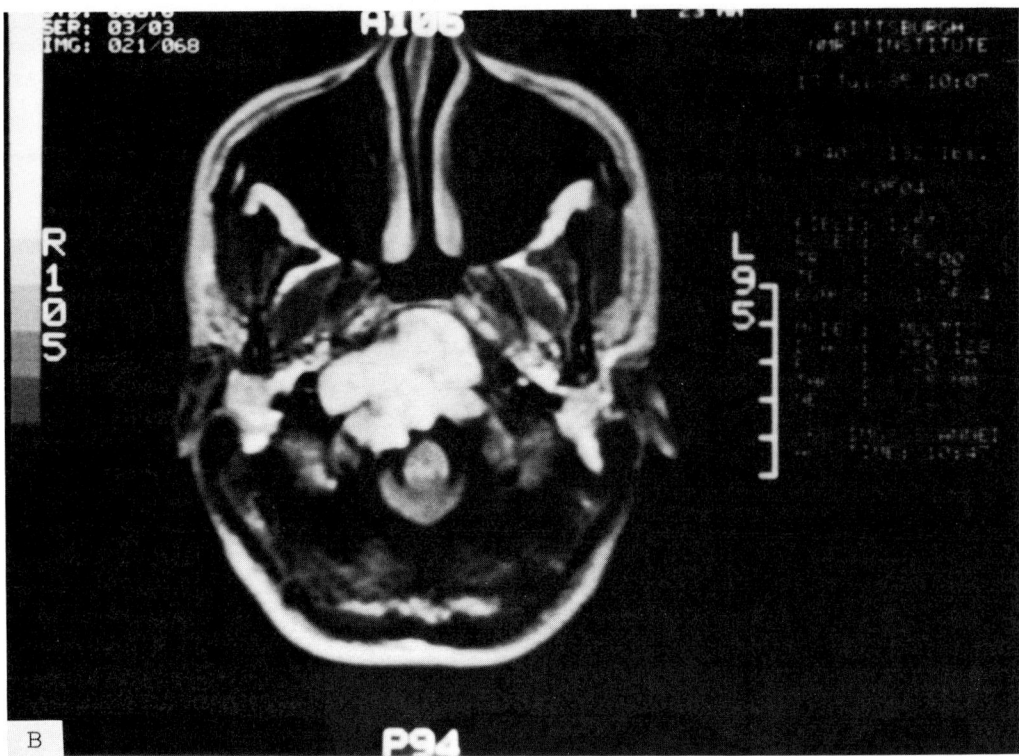

Figure 10B: A T$_2$ weighted image showing the tumor very clearly.

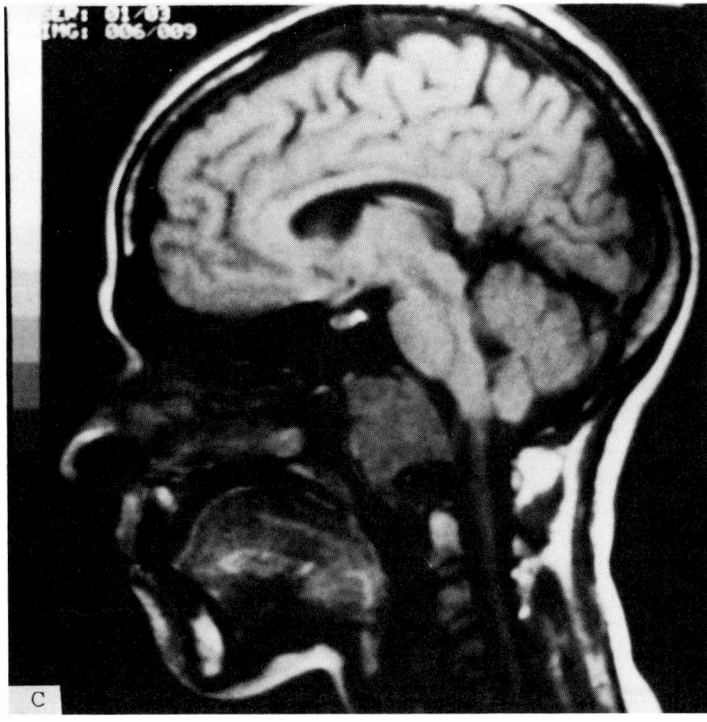

Figures 10C and D: Sagittal MRI images showing the cranial caudal extent of the tumor.

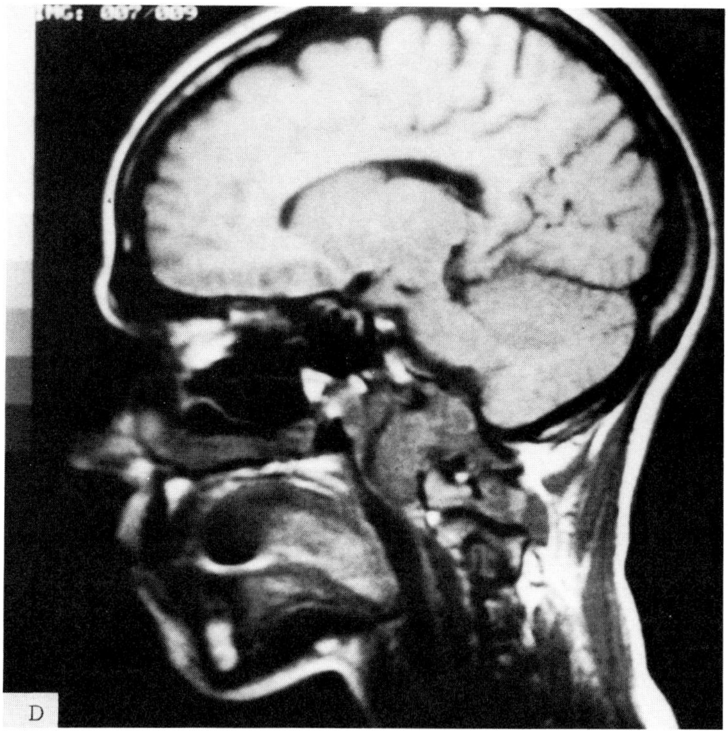

Figure 10D.

Patient MM: Parotid Acinar Cell Carcinoma

This 40-year-old man presented with a 3 year history of left facial paralysis, facial numbness, and hearing loss, and the recent onset of hoarseness and dysphagia. Five months prior to admission, a diagnosis of parotid acinar cell carcinoma infiltrating the skull base was made by computed tomography and biopsy. A course of chemotherapy was given and no response was noted. At the time of his referral, the patient had numbness in the distribution of the trigeminal nerve, and a complete paralysis of cranial nerves VI, VII, VIII, IX, and X on the left side. CT scans revealed a tumor involving the left parotid gland, parapharyngeal space, posterior fossa, clivus, left cavernous sinus, and the mandibular nerve extending into the mandible (Figs. 11A–E).

Following a tracheostomy, a radical neck dissection was first performed. The incision was then extended into the retroauricular area, and into the temporal scalp. The left parotid gland including the facial nerve, the majority of the left mandible, the temporalis muscle, and the zygomatic arch were excised. A temporal and posterior fossa craniotomy were performed. After exposing the petrous ICA, the tumor invaded mandibular and maxillary divisions of the trigeminal nerve were removed from the lateral wall of the cavernous sinus. The neoplasm was also removed from the cerebellopontine angle by a retromastoid approach. Cranial nerves VII through X were noted to be invaded but not the cerebellum or the brain stem. A total resection of the left temporal bone and one-half of the clivus were then performed. The remainder of the neoplasm occupying the intradural clival region was removed, dissecting it away from the abducens nerve. The dural defect was reconstructed with a pericranial graft, and a vascularized rectus abdominis free flap was used to fill the dead space and cover the exposed ICA. Unfortunately, the

674 • TUMORS OF THE CRANIAL BASE: DIAGNOSIS AND TREATMENT

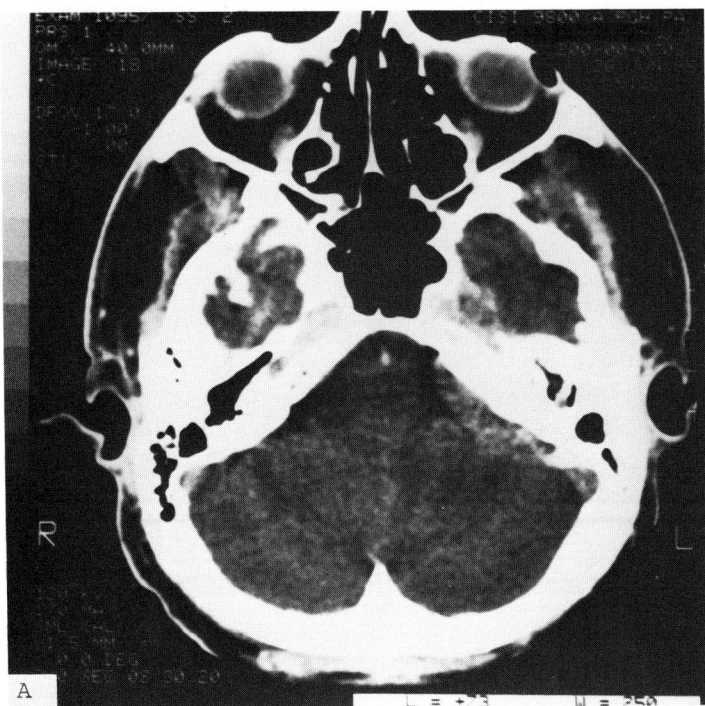

Figure 11A: Axial CT scan of patient MM showing the tumor in the cerebellopontine angle and the cavernous sinus area.

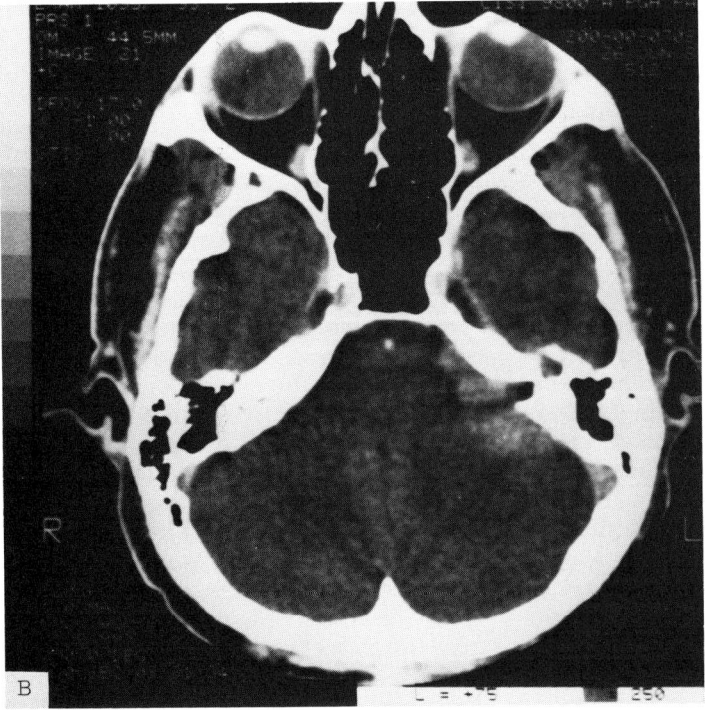

Figure 11B: Tumor extension into the internal auditory canal is seen and the appearance is suggestive of a petroclival meningioma.

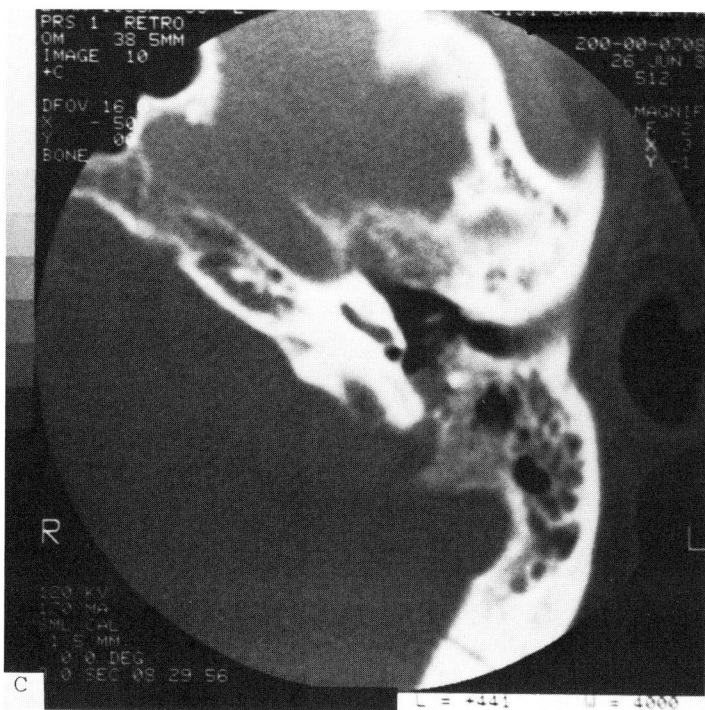

Figure 11C: Destruction of the temporal bone by neoplasm is seen with extension around the horizontal segment of the petrous carotid artery.

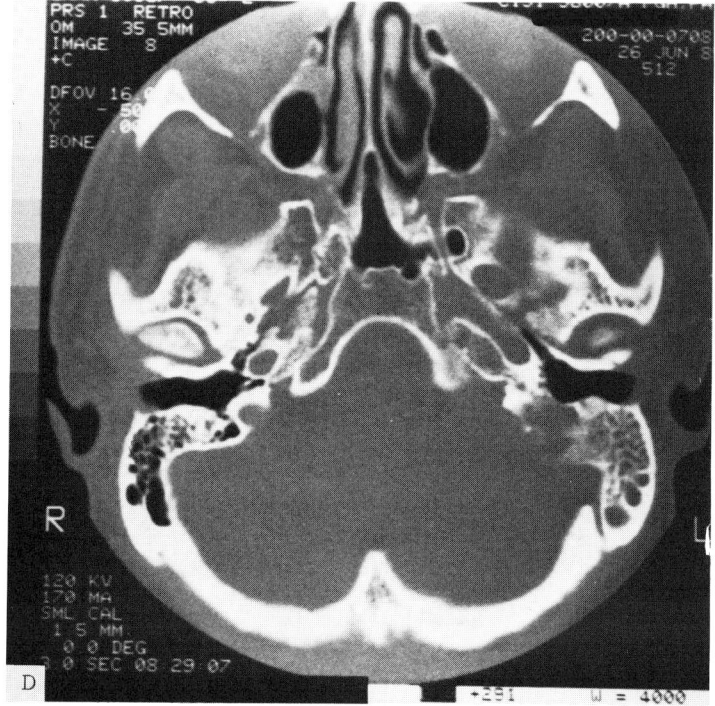

Figures 11D and E: The enlargement of the right V_3 due to invasion by tumor is seen at the cranial base (11D and in the mandible 11E).

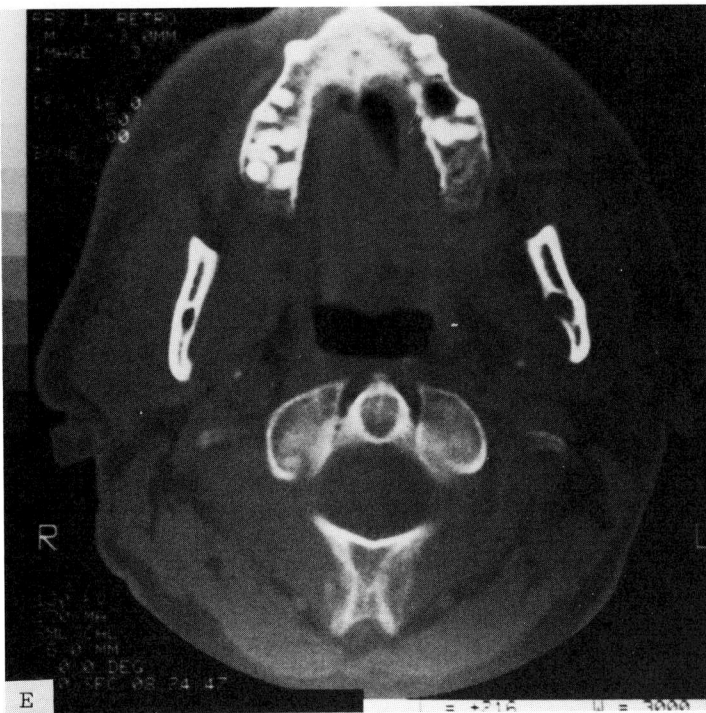

Figure 11E.

exposed sphenoid sinus was not adequately covered.

Postoperatively, the patient developed CSF rhinorrhea, necessitating reexploration, and packing of the sphenoid sinus with abdominal fat. Subsequent recovery was uneventful and radiation therapy was administered. On follow-up exam 7 months later, the abducens paresis had improved. There was no evidence of tumor local regrowth in the CT scans obtained 1½ years postoperatively, but the patient was noted to have a spine metastasis recently, and he is rapidly going downhill.

Patient TE: Chondrosarcoma

This 24-year-old man was discovered to have a very large clivus, sphenoidal, and ethmoidal chondrosarcoma extending into the suprasellar area and both cavernous sinuses, after a minor head injury (Figs. 12A and B). Except for a longstanding amblyopia involving the right eye, he was free of neurological deficits. An operation was performed by a combined lateral (subtemporal-preauricular infratemporal fossa approach) and anterior (transethmoidal) approach to remove this extensive neoplasm. Tears of the clivus dura resulting from a previous biopsy could not be repaired. A rectus abdominis muscle flap was brought in through the infratemporal fossa and laid on the clival-sphenoidal-subfrontal dura for reconstruction. Cerebrospinal fluid rhinorrhea occurred postoperatively and persisted. Upon reexploration by a subfrontal approach, this was discovered to be through the dural opening in the foramen cecum area. Dural repair and galeopericranial flap reconstruction resulted in resolution of this problem. Follow-up MRI scans revealed tumor remaining in the suprasellar region and the left cavernous sinus. This remaining tumor was then removed by a frontotemporal intradural approach. This patient has received supplementary radiation therapy and is doing quite well.

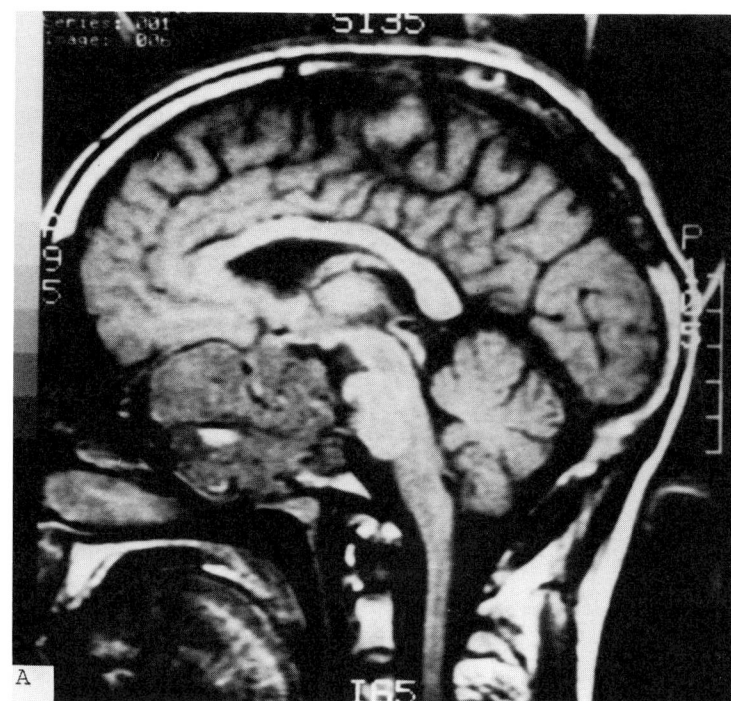

Figures 12A and B: Sagittal (A) and coronal (B) MR images of patient TE demonstrating a massive neoplasm involving the upper and midclivus, the sphenoid and ethmoid sinuses, the suprasellar region, and both cavernous sinuses. Both the petrous and cavernous carotid arteries are displaced laterally, and partially encased by neoplasm.

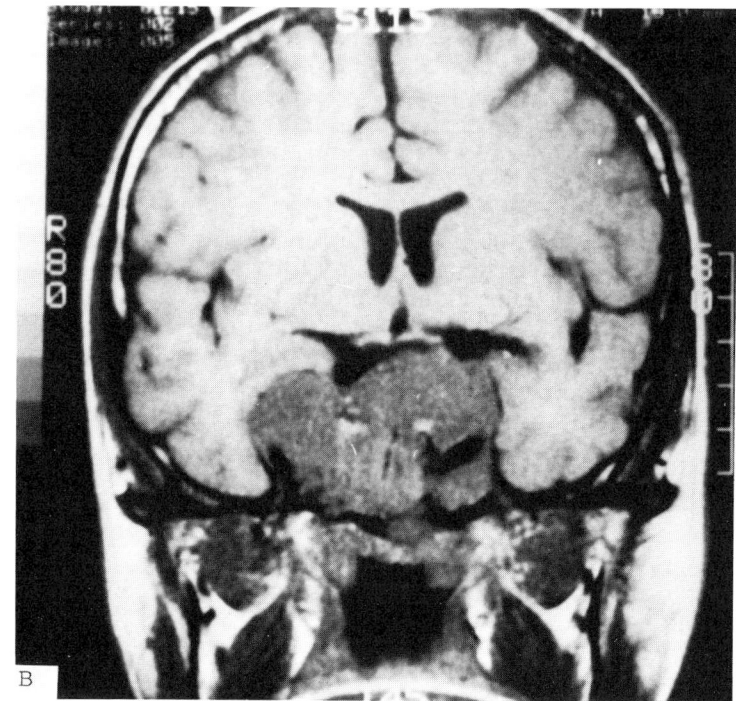

Figure 12B.

Discussion

In order to justify extensive operative procedures to remove cranial base neoplasms, one must show that such procedures can be safely performed, and that the outcome is better than with alternative treatment methods, namely radiation or chemotherapy. We have established the safety of these procedures in this small series, but are making efforts to further reduce the morbidity. Whether the outcome is better than existing treatment modalities will be known only after longer follow-up of a larger number of patients. A discussion of the current treatment outlook for the different neoplasms involving the cranial base follows. We will also discuss other available operative techniques.

Schwannomas

The majority of intra- and extracranial schwannomas are those arising from the jugular foramen, although facial nerve schwannomas and trigeminal schwannomas may also present in this fashion. Jugular foramen schwannomas may arise from cranial nerves IX, X, or XI, and the exact nerve of origin is often difficult to determine. These tumors may be primarily intra- or extracranial or both intra- and extracranial. Operative resection is the preferred treatment because these lesions are benign and relatively radio-resistant. There are two recent series presenting good results with combined otological-neurosurgical approaches to these lesions.[7,30]

Meningiomas

The majority of meningiomas that occur extracranially are extensions of intracranial basal meningiomas, although rarely meningiomas may primarily arise in the middle ear.[5,35] It has been well documented that incomplete resection of intracranial meningiomas is associated with a significant regrowth rate, and the involvement of the bone of cranial base and of the extracranial spaces may be an important reason for recurrence.[39] Pompili et al. have shown the value of radical operative resection of extensive sphenoid wing meningiomas involving the cranial base, but the invasion of the cavernous sinus, the carotid artery, the body of the sphenoid bone, and the temporal bone were limitations to radical excision.[42] The complications of the operations were due to carotid thrombosis, or to infection.[41,42] Maniglia described nine meningiomas which involved the temporal bone. Only two were removed totally, and two patients died of pulmonary infection.[35] Goin and House et al. have described the excision of petroclival meningiomas by a middle fossa or transcochlear approach.[21,26] The value of radiation therapy for histologically benign meningiomas is controversial but recent reports suggest some benefit.[39] Since most meningiomas are slow-growing, treatment should be individualized with respect to the age and physiological condition of the patient. Radical operative resection using techniques described should be considered especially in younger individuals.

Glomus Tumor

Glomus tumors arising in the middle ear (glomus tympanicum) or around the jugular bulb (glomus jugulare) are histologically benign, but often are extremely invasive locally. Large lesions may involve the jugular bulb and hypotympanic area, the petrous apex, clivus, upper cervical area, extend into the posterior fossa intradurally, and extend retrograde along the sigmoid sinus up to the torcula and antegrade along the internal jugular vein as low as the clavicle. Several authors have reported the successful surgical resection of extensive glomus tumors (type C or D tumors of Fisch or type III or IV tumors of Glassock-Jackson) using otological, neurosurgical, or combined approaches.[4,13,15,17,18,27,28,31,38,40,46,47] Long-term control of growth has also been reported in a number of patients with external beam radiation therapy, although the cure rate is only about 30%.[3,6,8,34,46] Reported complication rates for surgical therapy and radiation therapy are similar, but the cure rate is much higher with operative excision.[46,47] When tumor removal is known to be incomplete, and for very extensive lesions that are thought to be totally excised, postoperative radiation therapy is advisable. Using the operative techniques described earlier, all patients with localized glomus tumor would be considered operable, and previously described limitations do not apply.[47] The use of vascular and cranial base reconstruction techniques described by us should decrease the incidence of postoperative complications due to cerebrospinal fluid leakage or due to vascular occlusion.

Chordomas

Chordomas are tumors arising from remnants of the notochord. About 35% of the tumors involve the cranial base arising either in the upper clival-parasellar area, in the midclival area, or the lower clival-foramen magnum area. Histologically these tumors appear benign, and approximately 30% of the lesions are classified as the chondroid variety, on the basis of intercellular matrix. The treatment of chordomas has been very difficult until recently. Their location at the cranial base has generally precluded radical surgical removal. They have also been resistant to conventional doses of radiation therapy. The older literature suggests that patients with chondroid chordomas may survive many years, even after partial operative resection.

Recently, Wold et al. reported that in children and in young adults, a good long-term outcome may be possible with subtotal resection and conventional radiation.[53] The delivery of a much higher dose of radiation (equivalent of 60 to 80 Gy of cobalt-60) to the tumor is now feasible by using the Bragg-Peak effect of proton beams or helium ions.[44,48] This may considerably improve the outcome for these patients although follow-up is short. It is our feeling that the combination of total or subtotal operative resection and proton beam or helium ion radiation offers these patients the best chance of long-term survival.[9,11,43,44,48,53]

Nasopharyngeal Carcinoma

Nasopharyngeal carcinomas may be classified as anaplastic, lymphoepitheliomatous, transitional cell, or squamous cell varieties. Invasion of the skull base by these lesions occurs in about 20% of the cases.[49] When the skull base is involved, the lesion is staged as T4 or stage IV by the American Joint Committee on Cancer.[51] When such cancers are treated by radiation therapy, prognosis depends upon the tumor type and extent. For all stages of cancer treated with external beam radiation therapy, 5 year survival was 65% and 63% for lymphoepithelioma and anaplastic carcinoma, but only 40% for transitional cell carcinoma, and 31% for squamous cell carcinoma.[16] For all types of carcinoma, invasion of the skull base reduces the 5 year survival to about 19%.[2,16,49] When the lesion is well differentiated, and the cranial base is involved (T4), the 5 year survival with radiation therapy is close to 0%.[2] Recurrent disease can be reirradiated, with a 5 year survival of 16%.[37] An increase of the radiation dose from 6000 to 7000 rads may improve 5 year survival considerably.[51] An alternative approach is to use 125-iodine implants as an adjuvant to external beam radiation therapy.[36] A gross total resection of nasopharyngeal carcinomas invading the cranial base is possible using the techniques described by us, but en bloc resection is not feasible. Extensive operative resection in combination with radiation therapy must be tried for such lesions since the prognosis is grim with current treatment methods.

Temporal Bone Carcinoma

Temporal bone resection for carcinomas involving the temporal bone is discussed in Chapter 35. Radical temporal bone resection was first described by Parsons and Lewis, and modifications have been described by Hilding and Selker, and Graham et al.[24,33] Ariyan et al. described the use of the pectoralis myocutaneous flap to reduce postoperative problems of local and meningeal infection.[1] For patients with deep temporal bone involvement by carcinoma (squamous cell, basal cell, or salivary gland carcinoma) treated by operation and radiation therapy, the 5 year survival rate was 27% to 29%. The major reason for failure was incomplete resection of disease. Postoperative radiation was of no benefit when the cancer could not be completely excised. When compared with surgery alone, radiation therapy improved local control in patients with completely excised lesions, but did not demonstrate a corresponding increase in 5 year survival.[22] A more complete resection of neoplasms extending beyond the temporal bones may improve the outlook for this group of patients.

Operative Approaches

The surgical team responsible for the management of cranial base neoplasms must be aware of many operative approaches, one of which may be more applicable to the individual case.[19,20] Of the lateral approaches, the transcochlear approach described by House and Hitselberger is worth mentioning. In this extension of the translabyrinthine approach, the facial nerve is completely mobilized from the internal auditory canal to the stylomastoid foramen and displaced backward. The cochlea and the rest of the temporal bone are removed to the petrous ICA which becomes the anterior limit of the exposure. Lesions of the cerebellopontine angle and the clivus can be removed this way.[26] We have used this approach to clip an aneurysm of the basilar artery.[45] At the moment, we do not prefer this approach because of the extensive drilling needed and the consistent postoperative facial paralysis with slow recovery. Fisch has popularized the "infratemporal approach" for all lesions of the middle and posterior skull base. Our transtemporal approach is similar to his type A approach. The preauricular infratemporal fossa approach is different from his type C approach in that the incision is preauricular, the external ear canal is not divided, and the entire petrous and upper ICA is mobilized and moved forward. It also incorporates elements of the middle fossa and petrous apex approaches to the posterior fossa.[29,50] Modifications of the Fisch approach have been described which include mobilization of only a portion of the facial nerve in the fallopian canal[13] or only skeletonization and no displacement of the facial nerve.[10]

The anterior approaches to be considered are the transsphenoidal,[25] the transbasal approach of Derome, and the transoral. The anterior approaches provide a more direct view of the midline structures, but are limited craniocaudally, and also limited laterally by the petrous ICAs. In the event of intraoperative injury to the ICA, control of the hemorrhage is very difficult and reconstruction impossible. The reconstruction of dural defects is also very difficult. In practice, such approaches may have to be combined with lateral approaches for complete tumor removal (see Chapter 31 by P.J. Derome).

Conclusion

The radical resection of tumors of the posterior and the lateral cranial base, including those that are intra- and extracranial, can be safely performed. Such operations will definitely improve the outlook for patients with benign lesions. Whether such improvement will occur for those with malignant lesions will require further study. Prevention of infection spreading from the nasopharynx remains a problem, and is probably best solved by the use of a vascularized rectus abdominis flap to reconstruct defects of the nasopharynx. The management of bilateral ICA encasement by malignant neoplasms also remains an unsolved problem.

References

1. Ariyan S, Sasaki CT, Spencer D: Radical en bloc resection of temporal bone. Am J Surg 142:443-447, 1981.
2. Banfi A, Milani F, Zucali R: Risultah della radioterapie nei tumori della rinofaringe. Radiologica Medica 65:71-78, 1979.
3. Bataini JP, Kasdorf P, Brugere J, et al:

Radiotherapy des tumeurs du glomus jugulaire. *Ann Otolaryngol* (Paris) 98:239-242, 1981.
4. Black FO, Myers EN, Parnes SM: Surgical management of vagal chemodectomas. *Laryngoscope* 87:1259-1269, 1977.
5. Chen KTK, Dehner LP: Primary tumors of the external and middle ear. II. A clinicopathologic study of 14 paragangliomas and three meningiomas. *Arch Otolaryngol* 104:253-259, 1978.
6. Cole JM: Panel discussion: Glomus jugulare tumors of the temporal bone. Radiation of glomus tumors of the temporal bone. *Laryngoscope* 89:1623-1627, 1979.
7. Crumley RL, Wilson CB: Schwannomas of the jugular foramen. *Laryngoscope* 94:772-778, 1984.
8. Cummings BJ, Beale FA, Garrett PG, et al: The treatment of glomus tumors in the temporal bone by megavoltage radiation. *Cancer* 53:2635-2640, 1984.
9. Dahlin DC, MacCarty CS: Chordoma. A study of fifty-nine cases. *Cancer* 5:1170-1178, 1952.
10. Donald PJ, Chole RA: Transcervical transmastoid approach to lesions of the jugular bulb. *Arch Otolaryngol* 110:309-314, 1984.
11. Falconer MA, Bailey JC, Duchen LW: Surgical treatment of chordoma and chondroma of the skull base. *J Neurosurg* 29:261-275, 1968.
12. Farrior JB: Anterior hypotympanic approach for glomus tumor of the infratemporal fossa. *Laryngoscope* 94:1016-1024, 1984.
13. Farrior JB: Infratemporal approach to skull base for glomus tumors: Anatomic considerations. *Ann Otol Rhinol Laryngol* 93:616-622, 1984.
14. Fisch U: Infratemporal fossa approach for lesions in the temporal bone and base of skull. *Adv Otol Rhinol Laryngol* 34:254-266, 1984.
15. Fisch U, Kumar A: Infratemporal surgery of the skull base. In RW Rand (ed): *Microneurosurgery*, 3rd Ed. St. Louis, MO, CV Mosby, 1985, p 832.
16. Frommhold H, Leipner N, Herberhold C: Zur straahlentherapie des nasopharynakarzinoms-behandlungsergebnisse und optimierungsteriterian. *Strahlentherapie* 155:441-450, 1979.
17. Gardener G, Cocke EW, Robertson JT, et al: Glomus jugulare tumors-combined treatment. Part I. *J Laryngol Otol* 95:437-454, 1981.
18. Glasscock III, ME, Jackson GC, Dickens JRE: Panel discussion: glomus jugulare tumors of the temporal bone. The surgical management of glomus tumors. *Laryngoscope* 89:1640-1654, 1979.
19. Glasscock III, ME, Miller GW, Drake FD, et al: Surgery of the skull base. *Laryngoscope* 88:905-923, 1978.
20. Glasscock III, ME, Pensak ML, Gulya J: Surgery of the skull base. In RW Rand (ed): *Microneurosurgery*, 4th ed, St. Louis, MO, CV Mosby, 1985, p 832.
21. Goin PW: Surgical management of petrous apex meningioma. *Laryngoscope* 89:204-213, 1979.
22. Goodwin WJ: Malignant neoplasms of the external auditory canal and temporal bone. *Arch Otolaryngol* 106:675-679, 1980.
23. Gracek RR, Goodman M: Management of malignancy of the temporal bone. *Laryngoscope* 87:1622-1634, 1977.
24. Graham MD, Sataloff RT, Wolf GT: Total en bloc resection of the temporal bone and carotid artery for malignant tumors of the ear and temporal bone. *Laryngoscope* 94:528-533, 1984.
25. Hardy J, Vezina JL: Transsphenoidal neurosurgery for intracranial neoplasm. *Adv Neurol* 15:261-274, 1976.
26. House W, Hitselberger W: The transcochlear approach to the skull base. *Arch Otolaryngol* 102:334-342, 1976.
27. Jackson CG, Glasscock III ME, Harris PF: Glomus tumors. Diagnosis, classification, and management of large lesions. *Arch Otolaryngol* 108:401-406, 1982.
28. Jackson CG, Glasscock III ME, Nissen AJ, et al: Glomus tumor surgery: the approach, results, and problems. *Otolaryngologie Clin North Am* 15(4):897-917, 1982.
29. Kawase T, Toya S, Shiobara R, et al: Transpetrosal approach for aneurysms of the lower basilar artery. *J Neurosurg* 63:857-861, 1985.
30. Kaye AH, Hahn JF, Sinney SE, et al: Jugular foramen schwannomas. *J Neurosurg* 60:1045-1053, 1984.
31. Kempe LG, VanderArk GD, Smith DR: The neurosurgical treatment of glomus jugulare tumors. *J Neurosurg* 35:59-64, 1971.
32. Kinney SE: Glomus jugulare tumors with intracranial extension. *Am J Otol* 1:67-71, 1979.
33. Lewis JS: Temporal bone resection. Review of 100 cases. *Arch Otolaryngol* 101:23-25, 1975.
34. Lybert MLM, Van Andel JG, Eykenboom WMH, De Jong PC, et al: Radiotherapy of paragangliomas. *Clin Otolaryngol* 9:105-109, 1984.

35. Maniglia AJ: Intra and extracranial meningiomas involving the temporal bone. Laryngoscope 88 (Suppl 12):1-58, 1978.
36. Martinez A, Goffinet DR, Fee W, et al: 125-Iodine implants as an adjuvant to surgery and external beam radiotherapy in the management of locally enhanced head and neck cancer. Cancer 51:973-979, 1983.
37. McNeese M, Fletcher GH: Retreatment of recurrent nasopharyngeal carcinoma. Radiology 138:191-193, 1981.
38. Menzel J: Glomus jugulare tumoren. Diagnostik and operation. Neurochirurgische therapie extensiver glomus-jugulare tumoren. Laryngol Rhinol 57:281-286, 1978.
39. Mirimanoff RO, Dosoretz DE, Linggood RM, et al: Meningioma: analysis of recurrence and progression following neurosurgical resection. J Neurosurg 62:18-24, 1985.
40. Oldring D, Fisch U: Glomus tumors of the temporal region: surgical therapy. Am J Otol 1:7-18, 1979.
41. Pellerin P, Lesoin F, Dhellemes P, et al: Usefulness of orbitofrontomalar approach associated with bone reconstruction for frontotemporosphenoid meningiomas. Neurosurgery 15:715-718, 1984.
42. Pompili A, Derome PJ, Visot A, et al: Hyperostosing meningiomas of the sphenoid ridge-clinical features, surgical therapy, and long-term observations: review of 49 cases. Surg Neurol 17:411-416, 1982.
43. Raffel C, Wright DC, Gutin PH, Wilson CB: Cranial chordomas: Clinical presentation and results of operative and radiation therapy in twenty-six patients. Neurosurgery 17:703-710, 1985.
44. Saunders WM, Chen GTY, Austin-Seymour M, et al: Precision high dose radiotherapy. II. Helium ion treatment of tumors adjacent to critical central nervous system structures. Int J Radiation Oncol Biol Phys 11:1339-1347, 1985.
45. Sekhar LN, Estonillo R: Transtemporal approach to the skull base. Neurosurgery (in press).
46. Spector GJ, Fierstein J, Ogura JH: A comparison of therapeutic modalities of glomus tumors in the temporal bone. Laryngoscope 86:690-6, 1976.
47. Spector GJ, Sobol S: Surgery for glomus tumors at the skull base. Otolaryngol Head Neck Surg 88:524-530, 1980.
48. Suit HD, Goitein M, Munzenrider J, et al: Definitive radiation therapy for chordoma and chondrosarcoma of the base of skull and cervical spine. J Neurosurg 56:377-385, 1982.
49. Van Andel JG: Carcinoma of the nasopharynx treated in the RRTI. Radiol Clin 46:50-69, 1977.
50. Vaneecloo FM, Jomin M, Camuzet JP, et al: Suprapetrosal approach to the anterosuperior surface of the petrosa for the treatment of rare lesions of the sphenoid bone, trigeminal nerve, and internal carotid artery. Ann Otolaryngol (Paris) 101:95-101, 1984.
51. Vikram B, Strong EW, Manolatos S, et al: Improved survival in carcinoma of the nasopharynx. Head Neck Surg 7:123-128, 1984.
52. Wang CC: Radiation therapy in the management of carcinoma of the external auditory canal, middle ear, or mastoid. Radiology 116:713-715, 1975.
53. Wold LE, Laws JR, ER: Cranial chordomas in children and young adults. J Neurosurg 59:1043-1047, 1983.

35

Temporal Bone Resection

Victor L. Schramm, Jr., M.D.

Introduction

Surgical treatment of benign or malignant disease involving the temporal bone is technically the most difficult of skull base procedures and philosophically the most challenging. This is easily understood when one views the anatomy of the region. From a surgical perspective, the temporal bone is surrounded by the carotid artery and venous channels, traversed by multiple cranial nerves, and backed by a fluid-filled sac containing the brain. Published reports of surgical treatment of tumors in this area, especially the extensive experience of Lewis,[1,2] document cure rates in the 25% range, operative mortality of 5% to 10%, and high morbidity from bleeding, postoperative cerebrospinal fluid leakage, and meningitis. Attempts to improve cure rates by increasing the extent of resection have increased the morbidity from postoperative cerebrovascular complication, pulmonary embolism, and chronic aspiration.[3] Kinney[4] suggests that formal temporal bone resection might be supplanted by total tumor removal followed by radiation therapy.

Radiation therapy as an alternative course of management may produce fewer complications but also provides an even lower cure rate and often little relief of pain. Goodwin[5] has reported that radiation therapy alone is infrequently curative, especially if bone invasion is present and is of little benefit as adjunctive therapy if total tumor excision has not been achieved. Poor survival with primary radiation therapy is also reported by Wagenfeld[6] with death resulting in 18 months for patients deemed "unresectable" and less than 10% survival without salvage surgery in patients who would have been "operable" primarily. Equally disturbing is the 25% survival with salvage surgery in previously "operable" patients.

The evolution of surgical techniques for the treatment of temporal bone tumors has provided currently useful procedures when properly applied. However, the technique which includes placing a chisel cut medial to the arcuate eminence and posterior to the carotid and then removing the temporal bone with a "careful rocking motion," hoping the ensuing blood loss would not be fatal is a chapter for history. The management of temporal bone tumors described in this chapter will undoubtedly be only another plateau in the evolution of therapy but utilizing current tech-

---

From: Sekhar LN, Schramm VL Jr, eds: *Tumors of the Cranial Base: Diagnosis and Treatment.* Mount Kisco, New York, Futura Publishing Co, Inc, © 1987.

nology, survival has been improved while morbidity has been minimized and fatality from therapy eliminated.

Biological Behavior and Routes of Tumor Spread

Tumors of varying histology may involve the temporal bone. In order of frequency, squamous cell carcinoma, basal cell carcinoma, adenocarcinoma, rhabdomyosarcoma, and miscellaneous tumors such as chondrosarcoma have been treated. These tumors vary in their ability to extend locally to dura, perineurally and along the carotid artery and eustachian tube. Regional metastases are infrequent but may occur in the peritubal area, parapharyngeal, or neck regions. Distant metastases are unusual but should be considered for rhabdomyosarcoma and adenocarcinoma.

Evaluation

All patients should undergo imaging of the temporal bone and surrounding region as well as the neck and lung with computerized tomography and magnetic resonance scans. Angiography with balloon occlusion and quantitative xenon cerebral blood flow studies are also essential. Fortunately, by utilizing these techniques, it is possible to judge the proximity of the tumor to dura, cranial nerves, and the petrous carotid artery, as well as to document the cerebral cross-circulation and the patient's ability to withstand carotid occlusion.

Sequela of Surgery

When viewed with the perspective that nonsurgical treatment of temporal bone malignancy rarely eliminates ensuing pain and death, the sequela of surgical management of temporal bone tumors is of relatively less importance. Untreated patients with temporal bone malignancy usually die of local tumor or commit suicide within 6 to 12 months. Alternative therapy with radiation therapy and chemotherapy usually results in death within 18 months. However, if sequela of surgical therapy are considered before the operative procedure is initiated, many of the consequences may be eliminated or circumvented.

Cranial nerve deficits are to be expected. Resection of the facial nerve is frequently mandatory but nerve grafting at the time of surgery or temporal muscle transfer and subsequent eyelid reanimation with an eyelid weight or spring can minimize disability. Injury or resection of cranial nerves VIII, IX, XI, and XII produces alteration in physiology which cannot be corrected and these structures should be preserved if possible. However, compensation for vagal nerve injury and vocal dysfunction can be obtained by early postoperative vocal cord injection with either Gelfoam or Teflon paste. Tumor dissection adjacent to the cavernous sinus may result in sixth nerve paralysis, but if the nerve is preserved, function frequently will return.

Manipulation of the carotid artery is often necessary but cerebrovascular complications may be eliminated by proper preoperative evaluation and intraoperative management. Bleeding at the time of surgery in an amount greater than four units is common and clotting factor replacement is frequently necessary. Older patients should be monitored with a Swan-Ganz catheter and care taken to avoid cardiopulmonary overload with excessive crystalloid transfusion. Masticatory function is interfered with to some degree and muscle exercises and stretching are necessary to regain satisfactory mouth opening. Preoperative patient counseling regarding the loss of facial function as well as preparation for cosmetically filling surgical defects with muscle flaps or external prostheses is necessary. Rotation of a hair-bearing scalp flap to resurface the defect produced by external ear resection should be avoided.

Complications of Surgery

Previously observed complications involve the central nervous system as well as the cardiopulmonary system. Cerebrospinal fluid leakage should not occur if adequate dural grafting and repair as well as viable muscle flap reinforcement are accomplished. Meningitis, particularly with *Pseudomonas aeruginosa*, must be considered and perioperative third generation cephalosporin intravenous antibiotic prophylaxis is recommended. Vascular complications most frequently result from embolism or propagation of a clot from the stump of a ligated carotid. When absolutely necessary, ligation of the carotid artery should be done at the level of the cavernous sinus proximal to the ophthalmic artery, but whenever possible, a saphenous vein interposition graft should be performed. The consequences of cerebellar and brain stem retraction and compression can be minimized by lumbar subarachnoid spinal fluid drainage, intraoperative hyperventilation, and the occasional use of diuretic therapy.

The majority of patients requiring temporal bone resection are in the older age group and the possibility of intraoperative fluid overload must be considered and monitored by a Swan-Ganz catheter. Postoperative prolonged aspiration may be initially managed by tracheostomy and nasogastric feedings and subsequently by vocal cord injection. Pneumonia is a frequent problem and early mobilization of the patient as well as vigorous respiratory therapy is suggested. Though pulmonary embolism is reportedly a frequent complication, we have not had this experience, presumably because of a shorter operation time and the use of mild fluid expansion intraoperatively.

Contraindications to Surgery

The "limits" of surgical resection are currently more the limitations of the surgeon's experience and ability. Relative contraindications include direct brain invasion by malignant disease, extensive regional or distant metastasis, and a patient's unsatisfactory psychological or physiological status. Palliative resection may be considered and the pain relief and hygiene from exophytic tumor removal are often greatly appreciated by both the patient and the family.

Indication for Surgical Technique

A lateral temporal bone resection is appropriate for ear canal malignancy and as an aid to obtain a margin for parotid malignancy. A subtotal temporal bone resection is advised for tumors with limited middle ear involvement and no extension anteriorly into the eustachian tube or the area of the petrous carotid artery. An extended total temporal bone resection is recommended for management of patients with anterior tumor involvement including radiographic evidence of carotid artery or infratemporal fossa involvement.

Lateral Temporal Bone Resection Technique

The patient is placed on the operating table in a supine position with the head rotated 45° to the contralateral side. Oral endotracheal anesthesia is usually adequate. The surgical incision begins in the temporal area at the temporal line and extends 3 to 4 cm behind the postauricular crease and then into an upper cervical skin crease. A complete mastoidectomy and posterior tympanotomy are first accomplished. The incudo-stapedial joint is disarticulated and then bone removal is continued over the head of the malleus to the glenoid fossa. The ear canal is totally transected medial to the tympanic membrane. The mandibular condyle is removed if necessary and a lateral or total parotidectomy is done as required. Reconstruction can usually be accomplished satisfactorily by lining the resulting cavity with a split-thickness skin graft held in place with a surgical bolus.

Subtotal Temporal Bone Resection

Following a preliminary tracheostomy, the patient is positioned with the ipsilateral shoulder elevated and the head rotated 45° to the contralateral side. Surgical preparation includes the head, face, neck, and entire chest. The surgical incision begins above the anterior portion of the temporal line and continues in the postauricular area 4 cm behind the ear, into the upper cervical region, and continues anteriorly to the submental area. Modifications of the incision may be required, depending on the extent of external ear and facial skin resection if necessary. The cervicofacial flap is elevated as for infratemporal fossa dissection with the flap elevated at the level of the temporalis fascia superiorly and preserving an envelope of soft tissue around the upper division of the facial nerve. The dissection is carried anteriorly to the orbit and the anterior border of the masseter muscle. A lower McFee incision is done for purposes of neck dissection. Initially a standard or modified neck dissection with preservation of the facial artery and submandibular gland is completed. The greater auricular nerve or the fourth cervical cutaneous nerve is retained for later use as a free graft for the facial nerve.

The zygomatic arch is then divided above the glenoid fossa and at the posterior orbit and the temporalis muscle is elevated to the level of the foramen ovale and the zygomatic arch reflected along with it inferiorly. The mandibular condyle and surrounding joint capsule are dissected from the glenoid fossa and the neck of the mandible is transected and the condyle removed. The parotidectomy is completed as indicated by the disease with transection of the facial nerve. The internal carotid artery is dissected in the cervical region to the styloid process and the styloid process is removed to expose the carotid inferior to the carotid canal. Initial carotid exposure in the depths of the glenoid fossa may then be done with a drill and cutting burr (Fig. 1).

Prior to doing a low temporal craniotomy, cerebrospinal fluid is removed from the lumbar drain and hyperventilation is employed to lower the pCO_2. The temporal craniotomy is performed beginning above the foramen ovale and extending posteriorly to the level of the sigmoid sinus, including the zygomatic root and lateral portion of the glenoid fossa. This provides the upper margin of the temporal bone resection. Exposure of the petrous carotid artery is then continued by unroofing it with a drill and bone punches after mobilizing the third division of the trigeminal nerve. The carotid artery may be transposed from its canal to ensure its protection (Fig. 2). Dural elevation is then continued in the middle fossa past the arcuate eminence, greater and lesser superficial petrosal nerves with coagulation and division of the middle meningeal artery. If tumor involves dura, the dura should be dissected free from the tumor with bipolar cautery and dural resection completed after the temporal bone specimen is removed. Bone excision across the bony eustachian tube and tensor tympani muscle is then done with a drill. The posterior exposure begins by elevating dura from the posterior aspect of the temporal craniotomy inferiorly and removing the occipital bone with a drill and rongeur posterior to the sigmoid sinus to a level posterior to the mastoid tip. The craniotomy is then enlarged over the sigmoid sinus for subsequent sigmoid sinus ligation. Bleeding from the mastoid emissary vein may be controlled with bone wax. The dissection of the undersurface of the temporal bone is begun by transecting and removing the posterior belly of the digastric from its most posterior attachments and removing muscle from the undersurface of the occipital bone, avoiding or dissecting out the vertebral artery.

The sigmoid sinus is ligated superiorly by passing intradural ligatures after making a dural incision posterior and anterior to it. The distal stump of the jugular vein is then dissected toward the jugular foramen and jugular bulb, identifying and preserving cranial nerves IX through XII if possible. The petrous bone is transected through the otic capsule, between the arcuate eminence and the internal auditory canal with a drill dissection from above downward and from the

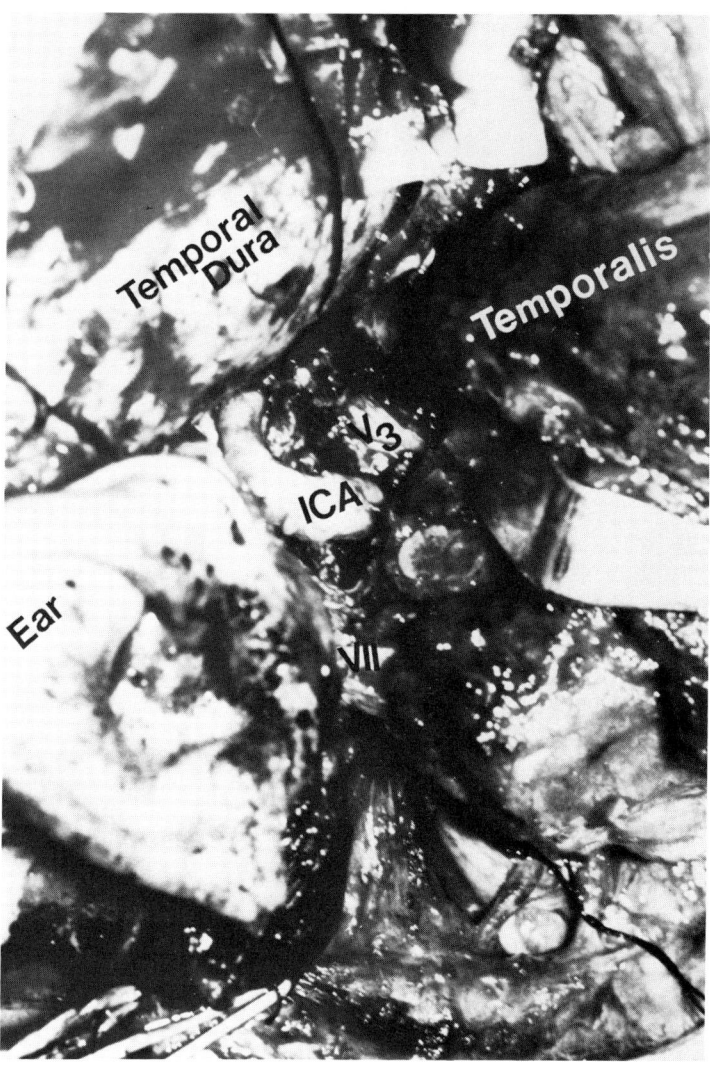

Figure 1: Exposure and partial decompression of petrous carotid artery (ICA). Mandibular condyle resected but facial nerve (VII) still intact at stylomastoid foramen. Low temporal craniotomy completed.

infratemporal fossa along the carotid from anterior to posterior. The nerves of the internal auditory canal should be sharply transected and the area packed to obtain temporary hemostasis rather than to cauterize the facial nerve.

The posterior margin of the sigmoid sinus should then be opened and a plug of muscle placed in the inferior petrosal sinus. Elevation or resection of dura over the posterior fossa plate then allows removal of the specimen.

Dural repair and grafting with pericranium or temporalis fascia is completed and a cable graft from the proximal facial nerve to the distal branches of the facial nerve is then done (Figs. 3 and 4). Consideration may be given at this point to immediate temporalis muscle transfer for reanimation of the perioral area. A pectoralis myocutaneous flap is utilized to fill the temporal bone defect (Fig. 5). If the skin defect necessitated by resection is too high for the pectoralis myocutaneous flap to reach, a lattisimus myocutaneous free flap or rectus muscle free flap with split-

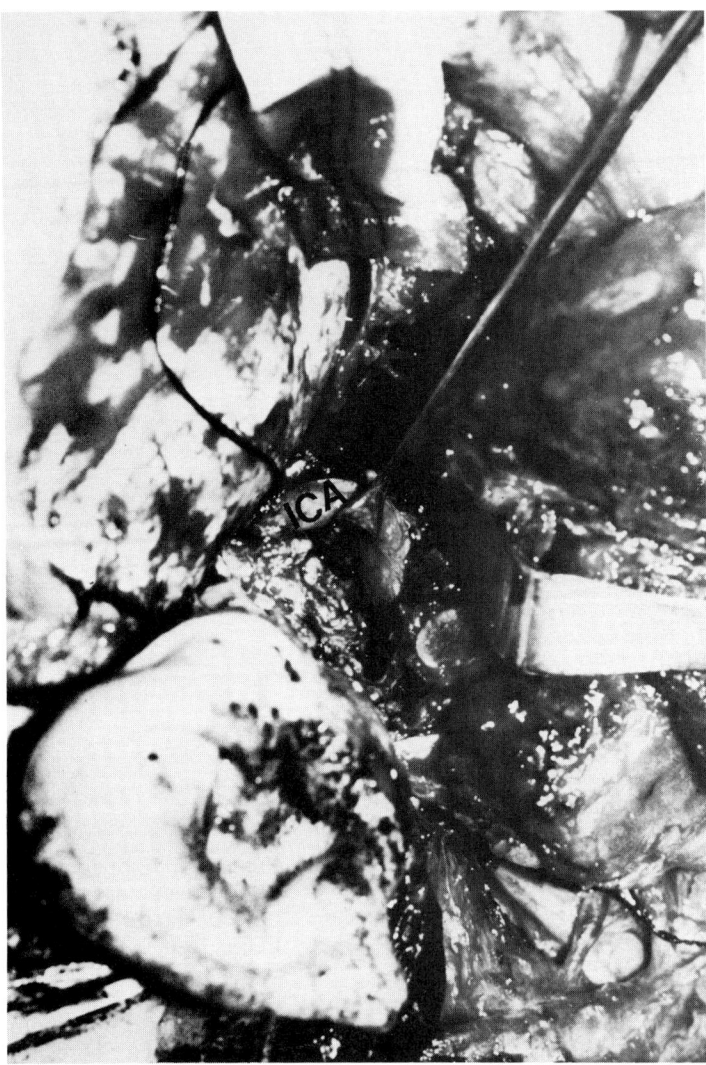

Figure 2: Carotid artery (ICA) transposed out of canal exposing area of petrous apex.

thickness skin graft are alternative reconstructive techniques. The zygomatic arch is secured anteriorly with 0 monofilament nylon or with titanium wire.

Extended Total Temporal Bone Resection

Following initial tracheostomy, the patient is positioned again with the ipsilateral shoulder slightly elevated and surgical preparation is completed from the vertex of the skull including the face, neck, upper chest, entire abdomen, groin, and leg. The extension from the subtotal temporal bone resection includes removal of the entire eustachian tube and parapharyngeal soft tissue with total transposition or resection and grafting of the petrous carotid artery.

Modification of the neck dissection is necessary to preserve the lower portion of the jugular vein and superior thyroid vein for subsequent microvascular anastomosis. The parotid is reflected over the

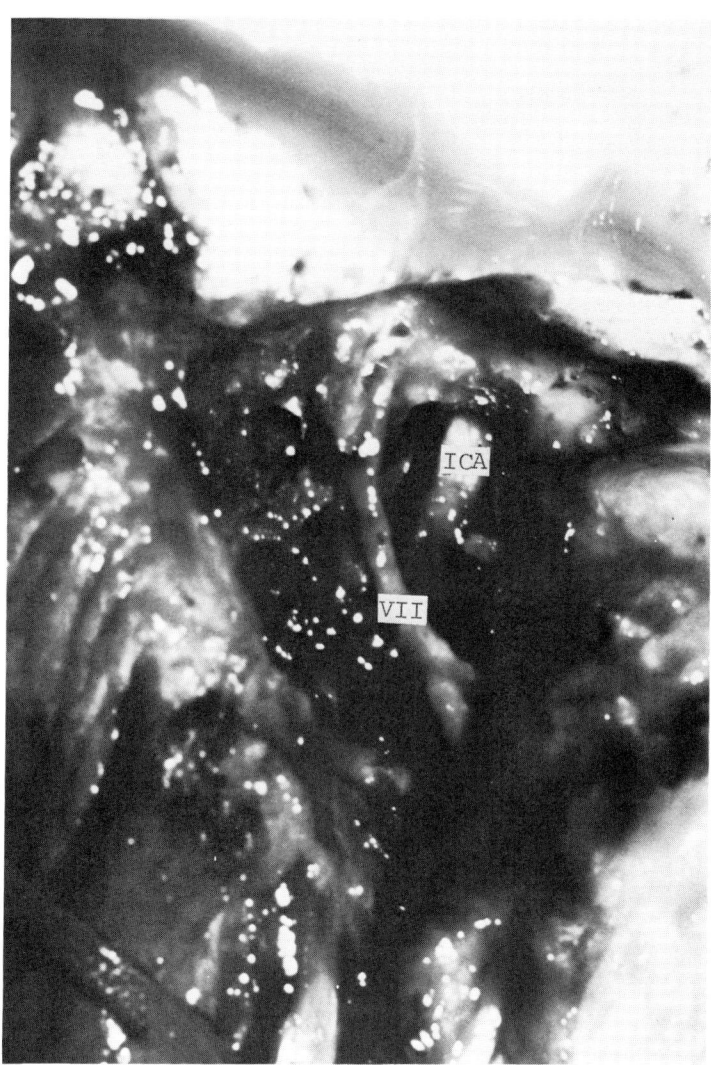

Figure 3: Facial nerve graft (VII) posterior to dissected petrous carotid following subtotal temporal bone resection.

posterior mandible and the masseter muscle is divided or elevated from the mandibular notch to the angle of the mandible. The temporal artery and vein should be dissected and preserved to the level of the midparotid for microvascular anastomosis at the time of reconstruction. The mandible is divided from the anterior portion of the notch to the angle and removed. The temporal craniotomy is extended anteriorly to the pterion and the petrous carotid artery dissection is continued anteriorly to the cavernous sinus after dividing V_3 intracranially. The petrous carotid artery may then be mobilized and transposed or resected, depending on requirements for tumor removal. Bone in the area posterior to the carotid is removed across the petrous apex with coagulation of the superior petrosal sinus and extending the bone dissection beneath the internal auditory canal to the clivus and then along the petroclival synostosis. Bone is then removed between the anterior petrous carotid and the inferior orbital fissure and the pterygoid

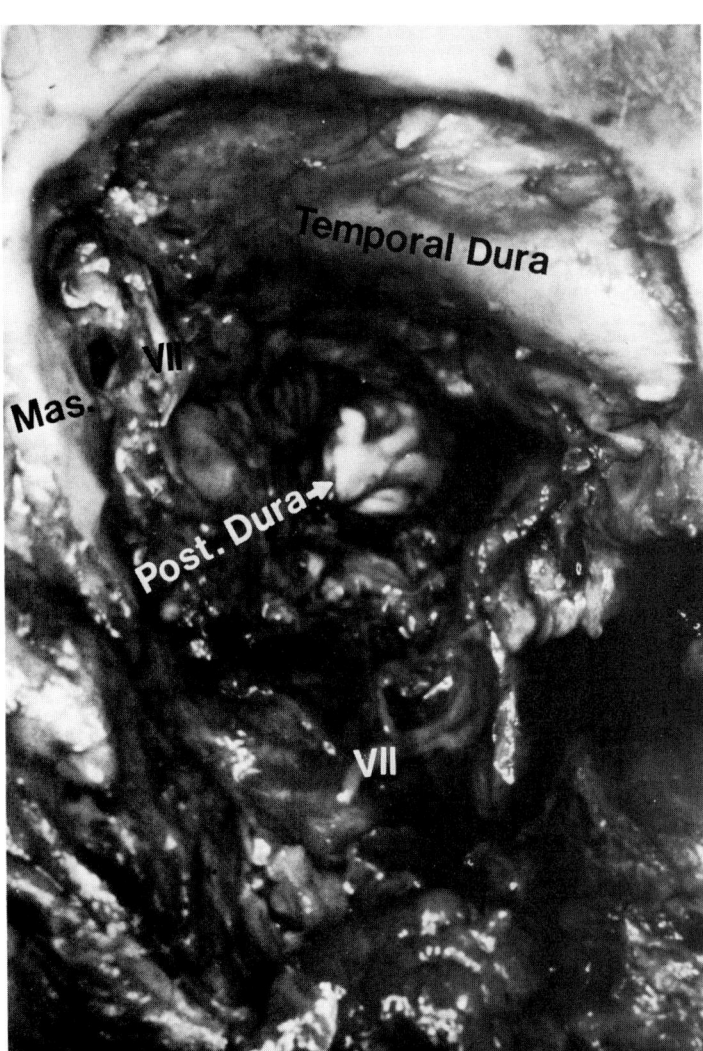

Figure 4: Temporal bone defect following subtotal resection (laboratory demonstration). Moderate area of resected dura (post dura) exposing cerebellum and brain stem. Carotid preserved. Safe reconstruction requires pectoralis myocutaneous (PCM) flap or free muscle flap. Facial nerve grafting should be done and temporalis transfer for mouth reanimation possible. Mas = mastoid.

musculature is mobilized off of the lateral pterygoid plate. The lateral pterygoid plate is removed and the medial pterygoid muscle is resected to expose the medial pterygoid plate. The nasopharynx is entered, by removing the medial pterygoid plate above and anterior to the torus tubarus. Subsequent dissection is carried posterior and medial to the carotid on the preclival fascia to the midline and the nasopharyngeal mucosa and superior constrictor muscle are divided at the midline to the level of the soft palate so that specimen removal includes the entire infratemporal fossa as well as the parapharyngeal space contents and eustachian tube. The surgical resection and some of the problems involved are further illustrated by the patient demonstrated in Figures 6 through 12.

Reconstruction is performed most commonly with a vascularized free flap transfer, either of rectus muscle or latissimus muscle. The muscle is sutured to the nasopharyngeal mucosa and secured along the infraorbital fissure, temporal

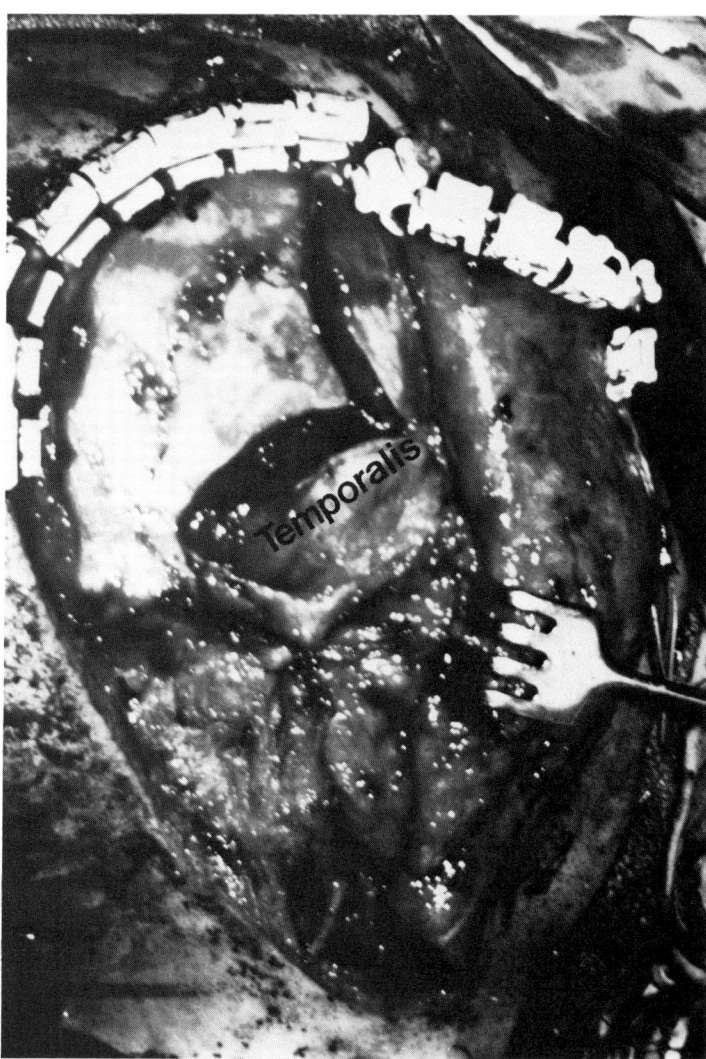

Figure 5: Division and rotation of posterior half of temporalis muscle to fill small temporal defect and surround facial nerve graft. Temporalis muscle inadequate for larger defects, for coverage of dural grafts or if infratemporal vascular supply has been compromised.

dura, and upper neck, extending posteriorly to fill the temporal bone defect and to provide coverage for any cutaneous defect created by the resection. Hemovac drains are placed away from the nasopharyngeal and dural closure as well as any microvascular anastomosis.

Postoperative Care

Patients undergoing total temporal bone resection require constant intensive nursing care and intensive monitoring. The patient should be nursed with the head elevated but should be helped from bed as early as possible to minimize pulmonary and venous thrombosis complications. The lumbar subarachnoid drain is left in place for 1 to 3 days, depending on the extent and security of the dural repair. Perioperative antibiotic therapy is limited to 24 or 48 hours. Nasogastric feeding and airway maintenance and suctioning via tracheostomy are frequently necessary for several days.

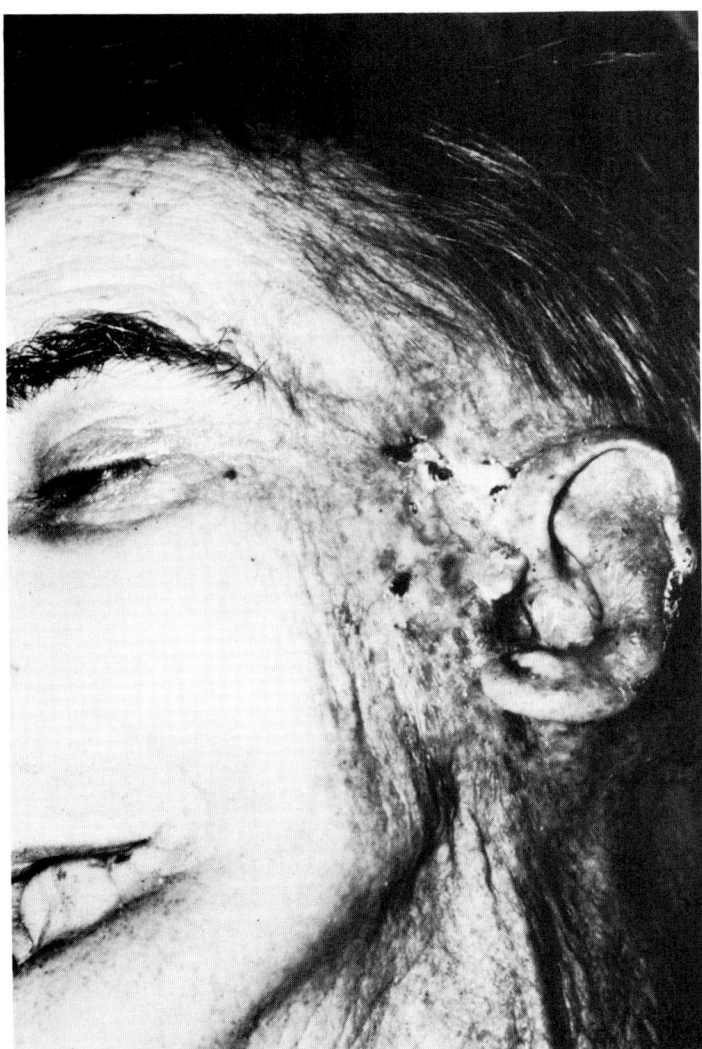

Figure 6: Elderly male with squamous cell carcinoma of skin and temporal bone with eustachian tube extension 40 years following radiation for nasopharyngeal carcinoma.

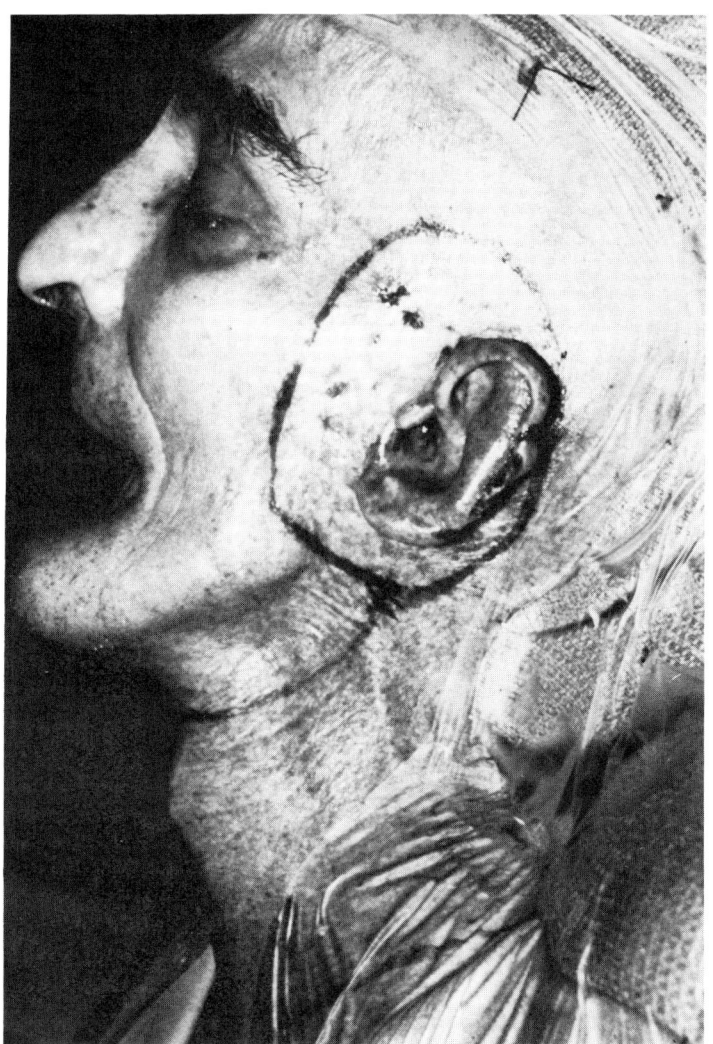

Figure 7: Resection includes external ear, surrounding skin, neck dissection, lateral parotidectomy, and extending total temporal bone resection. Plan includes pectoralis major myocutaneous flap reconstruction but defect extends superior to limits of PCM flap and free flap considered.

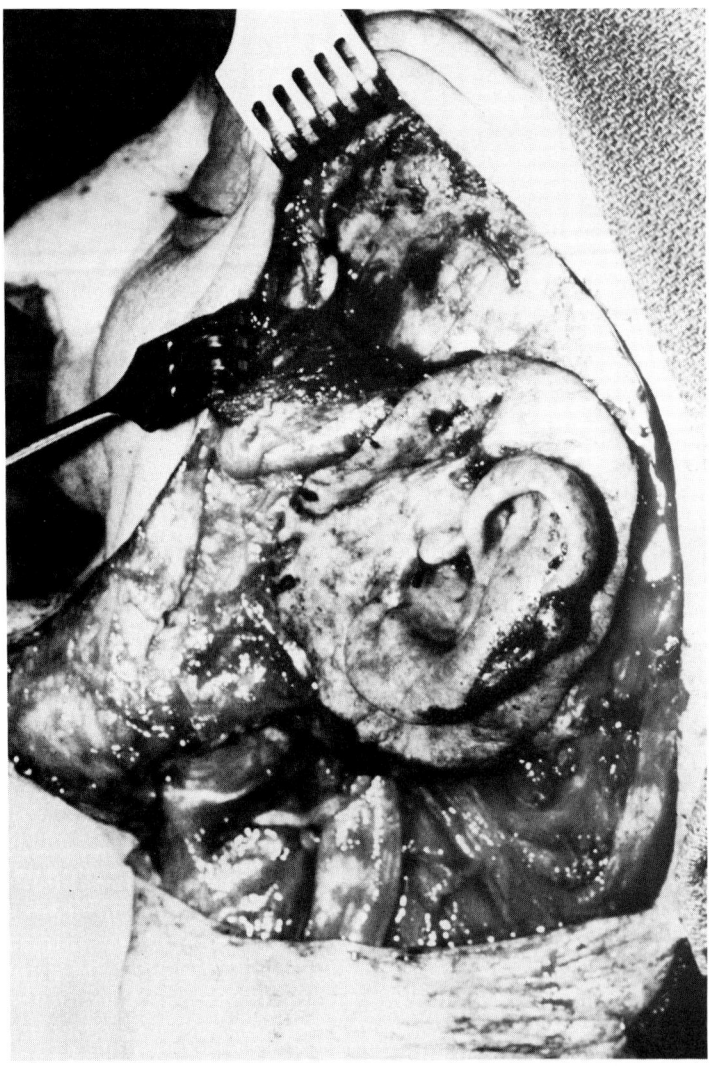

Figure 8: Intraoperative exposure of infratemporal fossa following neck dissection and parotidectomy. Temporalis muscle transposed inferiorly for temporal craniotomy.

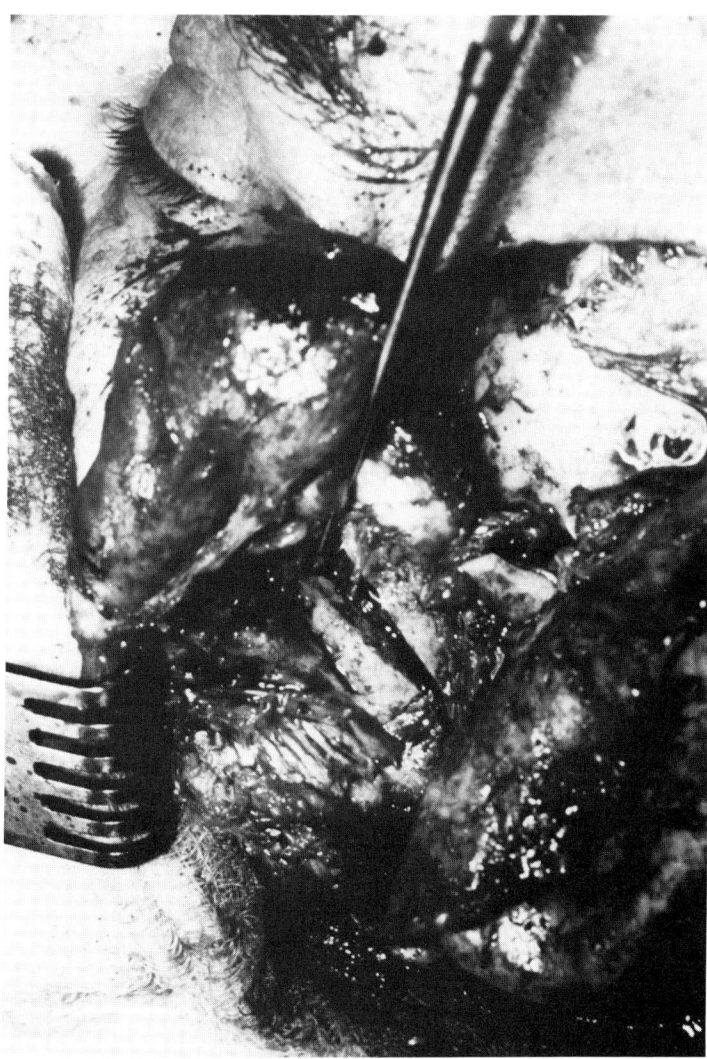

Figure 9: Mandible divided between notch and angle for anterior infratemporal fossa resection. Zygomatic root included with temporal bone resection.

696 • TUMORS OF THE CRANIAL BASE: DIAGNOSIS AND TREATMENT

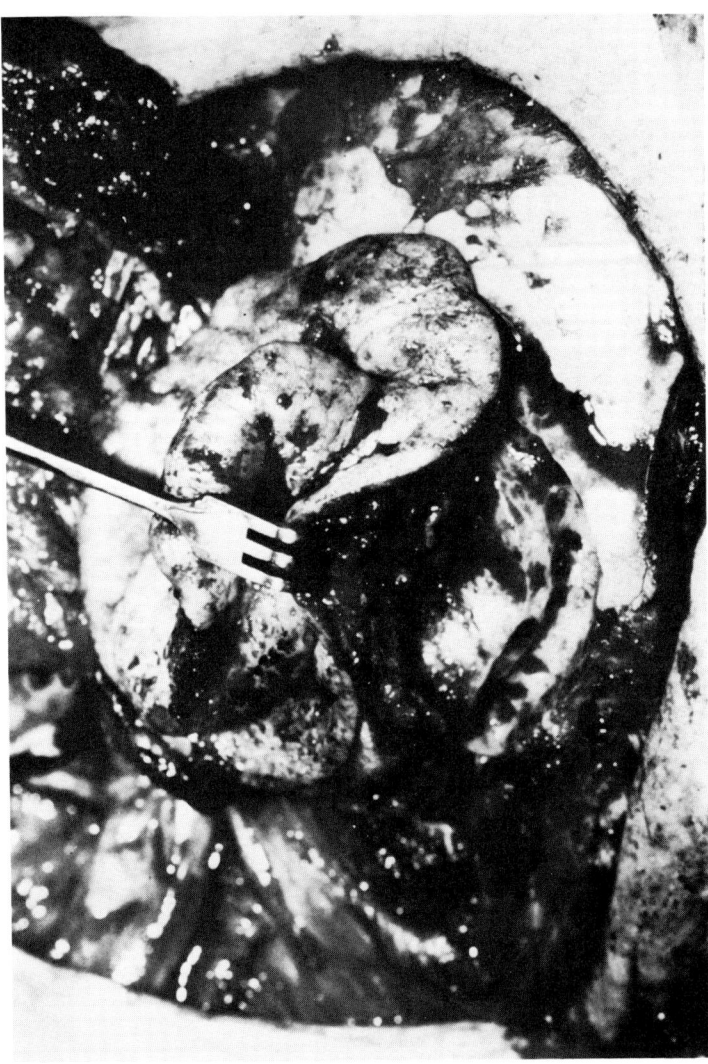

Figure 10: Posterior exposure of sigmoid sinus begun with drill. Bone removal continues inferiorly through occipital bone posterior to mastoid tip.

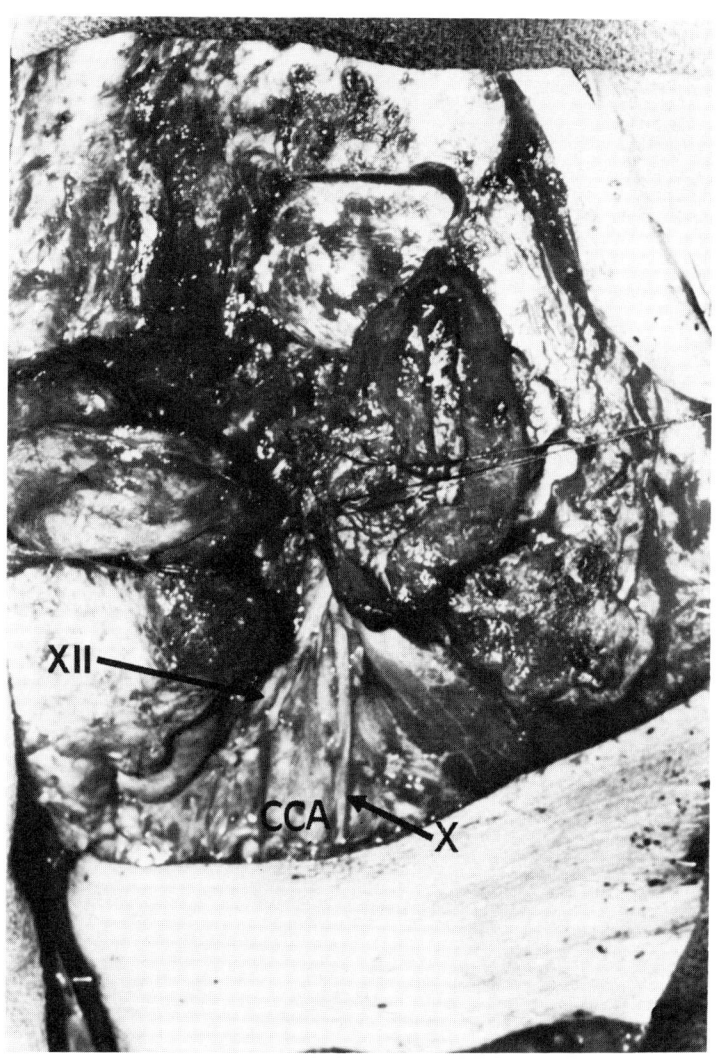

Figure 11: Exposure of petrous apex and infratemporal fossa prior to final medial temporal bone transection. Cranial nerves IX–XII dissected through skull base. Despite preservation of nerves, patient had prolonged postoperative aspiration requiring tracheostomy, vocal cord injection, and gastrostomy. X, XII = cranial nerves; CCA = common carotid artery.

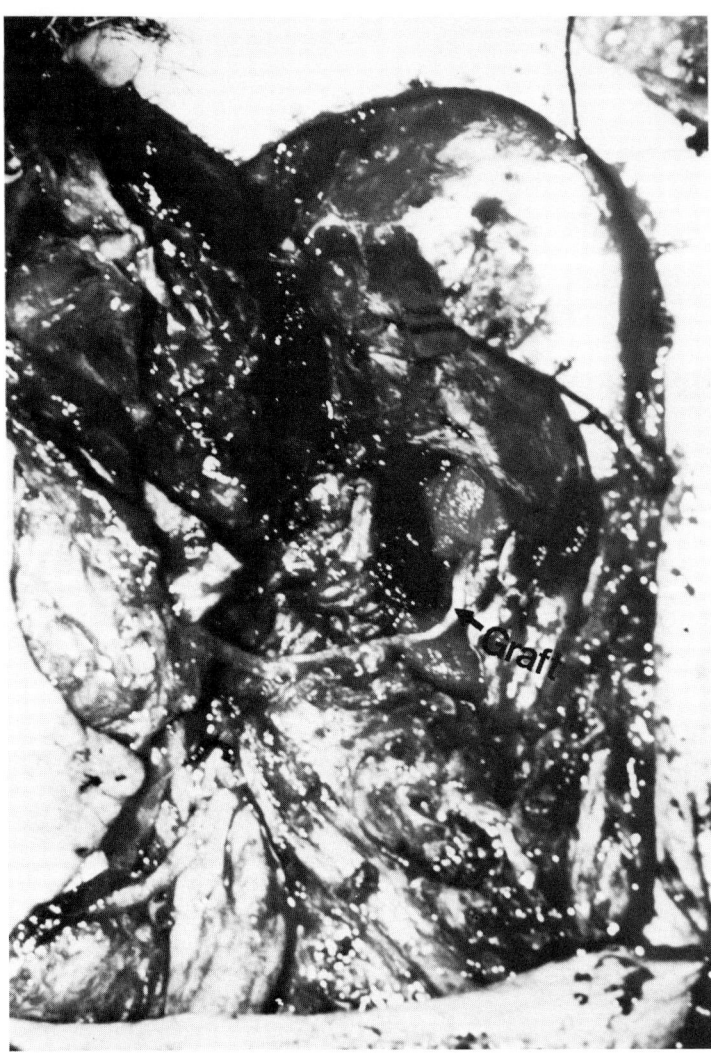

Figure 12: Facial nerve graft from brain stem to parotid and dural repair prior to transposition of PCM flap.

References

1. Lewis JS: Temporal bone resection. Arch Otolaryngol 101:23-25, 1975.
2. Lewis JS, Page R: Radical surgery for malignancy of the ear. Arch Otolaryngol 83:114-119, 1966.
3. Graham MD, Sataloff RT, Kemink JL, et al: Total en bloc resection of the temporal bone and the carotid artery for malignant tumors of the ear and temporal bone. Laryngoscope 94:528-533, 1984.
4. Kinney SE, Wood BG: Surgical treatment of skull-base malignancy. Otolaryngology—H/H Surg 92:94-99, 1984.
5. Goodwin WJ, Jesse RH: Malignant neoplasms of the external auditory canal and temporal bone. Arch Otolaryngol 106:675-679, 1980.
6. Wagenfeld DJH, Keane T, Van Nostrand AWP, et al: Primary carcinoma involving the temporal bone: Analysis of twenty-five cases. Laryngoscope 90:912-919, 1980.

Index

A

Abducens nerve. *See* Cranial nerves
Accessory nerve. *See* Cranial nerves
Acoustic meatus, internal, 449–455
Acoustic neurinoma. *See* Neurinoma, acoustic
Acoustic neuroma. *See* Neuroma, acoustic
Acoustic reflex, 556–559
Adenoidcystic carcinoma. *See* Carcinoma
Adenomas, pituitary. *See* Pituitary
Anesthesia
  cerebral blood flow, 107–108
  complications, 115–117
  effects, 109–112
  during electrophysiological monitoring of cranial nerves, 126, 129
  inhalation anesthetics, 109–110
  intracranial pressure, 108
  intravenous anesthetics, 111–112
  isoflurane, 110–111
  management of, 112–114
Aneurysms, 15–17, 61
Angiofibroma. *See* Juvenile nasopharyngeal angiofibroma
Angiography, cerebral, 48–50
Anterior cranial base
  anatomy, 247–263
  blood vessels, 253–254
  bones of, 249–252
  bony lesions, 295–309
  craniofacial resection, 265–278
  dura mater, 252–253
  meningiomas, 279–292
  orbit and optic canal, 255–261
  paranasal sinuses, 255
  reconstructive surgery, 234–238

Arachnoid cysts, 14
Arnold-Chiari malformation, 545–548
Arteries
  basilar, 540–541
  maxillary, 512–513
  vertebral, 523–529
  See also Cerebral arteries; Occlusion
Articular eminence, 463
Articular tubercle, 463
Atlas, 490–491, 496, 497–504
Audiometry, 544
Auditory canal, tumors of, 66–73, 77–81, 176–178
Axis, 500–504

B

Basilar artery. *See* Arteries
Biopsy, 151–154
Bony lesions
  of anterior and middle cranial fossa, 295–309
  fibrous dysplasia, 304–307
  meningiomas, 302–304
  surgery, 295–302
Brachytherapy, interstitial, 156
Brain stem, 447–448
Brain stem auditory evoked potentials, 554–556

C

Carcinoma, 20–21
  adenoidcystic, 200
  mucoepidermoid, 200
  nasopharyngeal, 25–28, 182, 195–196, 679
  parotid acinar cell, 673–676
  squamous cell, 200
  temporal bone, 679–680

Carotid arteries. *See* Cerebral arteries
Carotid sinus. *See* Sinuses
Cavernous sinus. *See* Sinuses
Cerebellopontine angle, 77–81, 449–455
Cerebellopontine recess, 541–543
Cerebral angiography. *See* Angiography, cerebral
Cerebral arteries
  in anterior cranial base, 253–254
  canals for, 470, 471, 495
  carotid, 116, 217–223, 519–523
  exposure, preservation, and reconstruction, 213–225
  hypophyseal, 327–328
  See also Occlusion
Cerebral veins, 217
  in anterior cranial base, 254
  bleeding in cavernous sinus, 402
  internal jugular, 523
  See also Occlusion
Cerebrospinal fluid, 402
Chemoembolization, 99
Chemotherapy
  for cranial base tumors, 191–201
  for esthesioneuroblastoma, 199–200
  for juvenile nasopharyngeal angiofibroma, 191–192
  for lymphomas, 198–199
  for meningiomas, 195
  for mid-line reticulosis, polymorphic reticulosis, and lymphomatoid granulamatosis, 193–194
  for mucoepidermoid and adenoidcystic carcinomas, 200
  for mucosal malignant melanoma, 194–195
  for nasopharyngeal carcinoma, 195–196
  for plasmacytomas, 196–198
  for rhabdomyosarcomas, 192–193
  for squamous cell carcinoma, 200
Chondrosarcoma, 32–33, 62, 63, 676–677
Chordomas, 679
  biology of, 29–30
  of cavernous sinus, 406–408
  clivus, 143, 537–540, 668–672
  cranial, 607–621
  pathology of, 14–15
  radiation treatment of, 167–170
  of the sphenoid, 62
Circulatory system. *See* Arteries; Cerebral arteries; Cerebral veins; Occlusion
Clivus, 63, 143, 455–458, 494, 536–540, 668–672
Colloid cysts, 15
Computed tomography of sphenoid bone, 39–42, 52
Condyles
  occipital, 494–495, 497
  third, 490
Congenital tumors. *See* Tumors, congenital, embryonic, and malformative
Cranial base tumors
  anesthesia for surgery, 107–117
  balloon occlusion techniques, 102–104
  biology of, 25–33
  chemotherapy, 191–201
  classification of, 3–5
  congenital, embryonic, and malformative tumors, 14–19
  cranial nerve monitoring during surgery, 123–132
  ectodermal tumors, 11–14
  embolization techniques, 95–102
  empty sella syndrome, 21
  inflammatory lesions, 19–20
  laser resection of, 135–148
  mesodermal neoplasms, 7–11
  metastatic tumors, 20–21
  neuroepithelial neoplasms, 5–7
  neurotological approaches to, 139–140
  pathology of, 3–21
  radiation therapy, 163–186
  radiological diagnosis, 39–92
  reconstruction after resection, 213–241
  stereotactic surgery, 151–161
  See also Anterior cranial base; Inferior cranial base; Middle cranial base; Posterior cranial base
Cranial nerves
  abducens, 229
  accessory, 231, 517–518
  canals for, 471, 472
  in cavernous sinus surgery, 401–402
  deficits, 116–117
  electrophysiological monitoring of during surgery, 123–132
  facial, 229–230
  glossopharyngeal, 230–231, 514–516
  hypoglossal, 231, 518–519
  oculomotor, 228–229
  olfactory, 228
  optic, 228, 381
  of posterior cranial base, 447–448
  preservation and reconstruction of, 227–232
  stimulation, 115
  trigeminal, 229
  trochlear, 229
  vagus, 230–231, 516–517
  vestibulocochlear, 230
Craniocervical junction, 548–550
Craniopharyngiomas
  diagnosis, 350–353
  pathology, 11–12, 349
  radiation treatment, 170–172, 357–359
  radiology, 59
  surgery, 160, 353–357
Craniotomy, 353–355
Cribiform plate, 55–57, 142
Cysts, 14–15, 18–19

D

Dermoid cysts, 14
Dura mater, 252–253, 298–299, 322, 381, 445–446
Dysplasia, fibrous, 304–307

E

Ear. *See* Auditory canal; Otoneurological evaluation
Ectasia, 540–541
Ectodermal tumors
  craniopharyngiomas, 11–12
  myoblastoma, 13–14
  pituitary adenomas, 12–13
Electrophysiological monitoring
  amplifiers and display, 125–126, 128
  anesthesia during, 126, 129
  of cranial nerve II, 130–131
  of cranial nerves III, IV, VI and VII, 123–126
  of cranial nerve VIII, 126–130
  electrical safety, 131–132
  electrode placement, 124–125, 127–128, 131
  interpretation, 129–130
  stimulation, 126, 128
Embolism, air, 115–116
Embolization
  complications, 104
  effects of, 95–98
  material used, 102
  technical strategies and indications, 99–102
Embryonic tumors. *See* Tumors, congenital, embryonic, and malformative
Empty sella syndrome, 21
Encephalocele, 57, 62
Epidermoid cyst, 14
Esthesioneuroblastoma, 28–29, 57, 199–200
Ethmoid sinuses. *See* Sinuses
Eustachian tube, 469–470
Eye. *See* Optic canal; Orbit

F

Facial nerve. *See* Cranial nerves
Fascia of pharynx, 509–511
Fibrous dysplasia, 304–307
Fissures
  inferior orbital, 461
  petrotympanic, 465
  sphenomaxillary, 462
Foramina
  foramen lacerum, 473
  foramen magnum, 63, 143–145, 540–550
  foramen ovale, 318–319
  foramen rotundum, 317, 319
  foramen spinosum, 319
  foramen venosum of Vesalius, 319–320
  jugular foramen, 443–445, 470–471, 491–493, 543–544

Fossae
  mandibular, 463–464
  posterior cranial, 441–443, 445–446, 535–550, 553–561
  pterygopalatine, 88–92, 462
  See also Infratemporal fossa
Fungal lesions, 20

G

Gamma knife, 159
Germ cell tumors, intracranial, 17–18
Germinomas, 17–18
Gliomas, 5–6
Glomus tumors, 678–679
  biology of, 30–31
  laser resection of, 145
  radiation therapy of, 178–180
  temporal bone, 641–653
Glossopharyngeal nerve. *See* Cranial nerves
Granulamatosis, lymphomatoid, 193–194
Granulomas, 19–20

H

Hamartoma, hypothalamic, 18
Hematopoietic tumors, 63
Hypoglossal channel, 493
Hypoglossal nerve. *See* Cranial nerves
Hypophyseal arteries. *See* Cerebral arteries
Hypothalamic hamartoma, 18

I

Inferior cranial base
  arteries, 512–513, 523–529
  fascia of pharynx, 509–511
  muscles, 504–508
  nerves, 513–518
  nerves and vessels, openings for, 468–504
  osteology, 461–468
  spaces, 511–512
Inflammatory lesions. *See* Lesions, inflammatory
Infratemporal fossa, 461
  postauricular technique, 430–433
  preauricular technique, 424–430
  radiology, 81–84
  reconstruction, 433–435
  surgery, 421–437
Infundibuloma, 18
Infusion, 98–99
Internal acoustic meatus, 449–455
Internal carotid artery. *See* Cerebral arteries
Internal jugular vein. *See* Cerebral veins
Intrasellar masses, 57–59
Irradiation, intracavitary, 154–156

J

Jugular bulb, 66–73

Jugular foramen. See Foramina
Jugular vein, internal. See Cerebral veins
Juvenile nasopharyngeal angiofibroma, 182–183, 191–192

L

Laser
    case histories, 141–147
    heat and evoked potentials, 137–138
    systems and function, 135–137
Lateral cranial base. See Middle cranial base
Lesions, cranial. See Cranial base tumors
Lesions, inflammatory
    fungal, 20
    granulomas, 19–20
    parasitic, 20
Lymphomas, 183, 198–199
Lymphomatoid granulamatosis, 193–194

M

Magnetic resonance imaging, 42–48, 52–55
Malformative tumors. See Tumors, congenital, embryonic, and malformative
Malignancy. See Carcinoma; specific tumor type
Mandibular fossa. See Fossae
Mandibular nerve, 513–514
Mastoid process, 467–468
Mastoid tumors, 176–178
Melanoma, mucosal malignant, 194–195
Meningiomas, 678
    of anterior cranial base, 279–292
    biology, 31–32
    bony lesions, 302–304
    in cavernous sinus, 402–405, 410–413
    chemotherapy, 195
    laser resection, 141–142, 143–145
    olfactory groove, 281–285
    orbital roof, 292
    pathology, 7–11
    petroclival and medial tentorial, 623–640
    radiation therapy, 166–167, 388–390
    radiological diagnosis, 55, 59–61, 63, 376
    of sphenoid wings, 373–390
    suprasellar, 285–292
    surgery, 378–388
Metastatic tumors, 20–21, 62, 63, 184–186
Middle cranial base
    anatomy, 313–333
    bony lesions, 295–309
    cavernous sinus tumors, 393–419
    craniopharyngiomas, 347–360
    dura mater, 322
    fossa orifices, 315–322
    infratemporal fossa surgery, 421–437
    neoplasms, 655–680
    pituitary region, 322–333, 335–343
    reconstructive surgery, 238–240
    sphenoid wing meningiomas, 373–390

Mucocele of sphenoid sinus, 17, 62
Mucoepidermoid carcinoma. See Carcinoma
Mucosal malignant melanoma, 194–195
Muscles, inferior cranial base, 504–508

N

Nasal cavity, 84–88, 180–182, 473–477, 481–487
Nasopharyngeal angiofibroma, juvenile. See Juvenile nasopharyngeal angiofibroma
Nasopharyngeal carcinoma. See Carcinoma
Nasopharyngeal carcinoma. See Carcinoma
Neoplasms
    of lateral and posterior cranial base, 655–680
    malignant, 20–21
    mesodermal, 7–11
    neuroepithelial, 5–7
Nerve, mandibular. See Mandibular nerve
Nerves, cranial. See Cranial nerves
Nerve sheath tumors, 6–7
Neurilemmoma, 6–7, 544–545
Neurinoma, acoustic
    hearing evaluation and preservation, 583
    surgery, 563–583
Neuroblastomas, 6
Neuroepithelial neoplasms. See Neoplasms
Neuroma, acoustic, 145–147
    hearing preservation, 571
    imaging, 590–592
    otology, 587–606
    surgery, 583–606
Neurotological approaches, 139–140
Nose. See Nasal cavity; Olfactory groove

O

Occlusion, 213–215
    balloon, 102–104
    carotid artery, 116
    test, 50
Oculomotor nerve. See Cranial nerves
Olfactory groove, 55–57, 281–285
Olfactory nerve. See Cranial nerves
Optic canal, 261–263
Optic nerve. See Cranial nerves
Orbit, 255–261, 292, 315–317, 461
Osteochondroma, 62
Otoneurological evaluation
    acoustic reflex, 556–559
    audiometry, 554
    brain stem auditory evoked potentials, 554–556
    vestibular tests, 559–561

P

Paragangliomas. See Glomus tumors
Paranasal sinuses. See Sinuses
Parapharyngeal space, 81–84
Parasellar masses, 59–62, 143

Parasitic lesions, 20
Parotid acinar cell carcinoma. See Carcinoma
Parstympanica, 465
Perineural extension, 88–92
Petrotympanic fissure. See Fissures
Petrous apex, 73–77
Pharynx, fascia of, 509–511
Pituitary
  adenomas, 12–13, 142, 159, 409–410
  hypophyseal arteries, 327–328
  intrasellar/suprasellar masses, 57–59
  large tumors, 335–344
  osteology of region, 323–327
  parasellar masses, 61–62
  radiation therapy, 173–176
Planum sphenoidale, 55–57
Plasmacytomas, 196–198
Pneumocephalus, 117
Posterior cranial base
  anatomy, 441–458
  brain stem and cranial nerves, 447–448
  cerebellopontine angle and internal acoustic meatus, 449–455
  cerebellopontine recess, 541–543
  clivus region, 455–458, 536–540
  craniocervical junction, 548–550
  dura mater, 445–446
  foramen magnum, 545–550
  fossa, 441–443, 445–446, 535–550, 553–561
  jugular foramen, 443–445, 543–544
  neoplasms, 655–680
  reconstructive surgery, 240–241
Pterygoid process, 461
Pterygopalatine fossa. See Fossae

R

Radiology
  cerebral angiography, 48–50
  computed tomography, 39–42, 52
  diagnostic, 39–92, 376
  magnetic resonance imaging, 42–48, 52–55
  radiation therapy, 163–186, 357–359, 388–390
  sphenoid bone, 39–63
  stereotactic radiosurgery, 158–159
  temporal bone, 66–81
Rathke cleft cyst, 18–19
Reconstruction. See Surgery
Resection. See Surgery
Reticulosis, 193–194
Rhabdomyosarcomas, 183–184, 192–193

S

Schwannoma, 6–7, 61, 667–668, 678
Sinuses, 84–88, 180–182, 255
  carotid, 519
  cavernous, 329–333, 393–417
  ethmoid, 481–486, 488
  paranasal, 180–182, 255
  radiology of, 84–88
  sphenoid, 17, 62–63, 373–390, 477–481, 488
Skull, tumors. See Cranial base tumors
Sphenoid body, 62–63
Sphenoid bone
  bone destruction, 51
  calcification, 52
  cerebral angiography, 48–50
  computed tomography of, 39–42, 52
  diagnosis by area, 55–63
  films, 40
  magnetic resonance imaging, 42–48, 52–55
  meningiomas of, 373–390
  radiology of, 39–63
  soft tissue mass, 51
Sphenoid sinus. See Sinuses
Sphenomaxillary fissure. See Fissures
Squamous cell carcinoma. See Carcinoma
Stereotaxy
  biopsy, 151–154
  clinical applications, 159–161
  for diagnosis and treatment of skull base lesions, 151–161
  interstitial brachytherapy, 156
  intracavitary irradiation, 154–156
  radiosurgery, 158–159
  technique, 156–157
Styloid process, 465–467
Suprasellar masses, 57–59, 141–142, 285–292
Surgery
  on acoustic neurinomas, 563–583
  on acoustic neuroma, 583–606
  anesthesia, 107–117, 126, 129
  anterior craniofacial resection, 265–278
  on bony lesions, 295–298, 301–302
  on cavernous sinus, 393–417
  on cranial chordomas, 607–621
  electrophysiological monitoring of cranial nerves during, 123–132
  infratemporal fossa, 421–437
  laser resection, 135–148
  of meningiomas of sphenoid wings, 378–388
  on neoplasms of lateral and posterior cranial base, 655–680
  on petroclival and medial tentorial meningiomas, 623–640
  reconstructive, 213–241, 299–301, 433–435
  stereotactic, 151–161
  temporal bone resection, 683–697

T

Temporal bone
  auditory canal, 66–73, 77–81
  carcinoma, 679–680
  cerebellopontine angle, 77–81
  jugular bulb, 66–73
  paragangliomas of, 641–653
  petrous, 73–77, 320–322

Temporal bone (cont.)
  radiology of, 66–81
  resection, 683–697
Tension pneumocephalus, 117
Teratomas, 14
Transfusion, 116
Trigeminal nerve. See Cranial nerves
Trochlear nerve. See Cranial nerves
Tuberculum sellae, 55–57
Tumors, congenital, embryonic, and malformative
  aneurysms, 15–17
  chordomas, 14–15
  cysts, 14–15, 18–19
  germinomas and intracranial germ cell tumors, 17–18
  hypothalamic hamartoma or infundibuloma, 18
  mucocele of sphenoid sinus, 17
  teratomas, 14
Tumors, cranial base. See Cranial base tumors
Tumors, ectodermal. See Ectodermal tumors
Tumors, glomus. See Glomus tumors
Tumors, mastoid. See Mastoid tumors
Tumors, metastatic. See Metastatic tumors
Tumors, nerve sheath. See Nerve sheath tumors
Tumors, skull. See Cranial base tumors

V

Vagus nerve. See Cranial nerves
Vascular system. See Arteries; Cerebral arteries; Cerebral veins; Occlusion
Veins. See Cerebral veins; Occlusion
Vertebral artery. See Arteries
Vestibular tests, 559–561
Vestibulocochlear nerve. See Cranial nerves